NEW, REVISED, AND RETIRED NURSING DIAGNOSES FOR 2009–2011

ineffective Activity Pattern
risk for Bleeding
readiness for enhanced Childbearing Process
impaired Comfort
risk for Electrolyte Imbalance
neonatal Jaundice
risk for disturbed Maternal/Fetal Dyad
dysfunctional gastrointestinal Motility
risk for dysfunctional gastrointestinal Motility
self Neglect
ineffective peripheral tissue Perfusion
risk for decreased cardiac tissue Perfusion
risk for impaired renal Perfusion
risk for ineffective cerebral tissue Perfusion
risk for ineffective gastrointestinal Perfusion
readiness for enhanced Relationship
impaired individual Resilience
readiness for enhanced Resilience
risk for compromised Resilience
risk for Shock
risk for vascular Trauma

REVISED NURSING DIAGNOSES, 2009–2011
risk-prone health Behavior
defensive Coping
risk for imbalanced Fluid Volume
ineffective self Health Management (previously titled ineffective Therapeutic Regimen Management)
readiness for enhanced self Health Management (previously titled readiness for enhanced Therapeutic Regimen Management)
disturbed personal Identity
risk for impaired Liver Function
chronic low Self-Esteem
disturbed Sleep Pattern

RETIRED NURSING DIAGNOSES, 2009 [RETAINED IN THIS EDITION]
Rape-Trauma Syndrome: compound reaction
Rape-Trauma Syndrome: silent reaction
effective Therapeutic Regimen Management
ineffective community Therapeutic Regimen Management
disturbed Thought Processes
total Urinary Incontinence

Nursing Diagnosis Manual

**Planning, Individualizing,
and Documenting
Client Care**

Nursing Diagnosis Manual

Planning, Individualizing, and Documenting Client Care

Marilynn E. Doenges, APN, BC—Retired
Clinical Specialist—Adult Psychiatric/Mental Health Nursing, Retired
   Adjunct Faculty
Beth-El College of Nursing and Health Sciences, CU–Springs
Colorado Springs, Colorado

Mary Frances Moorhouse, RN, MSN, CRRN, LNC
Nurse Consultant, TNT-RN Enterprises
Adjunct Nursing Faculty, Pikes Peak Community College
Colorado Springs, Colorado

Alice C. Murr, BSN, RN—Retired
Collins, Mississippi

EDITION 3

 F. A. DAVIS COMPANY • Philadelphia

F. A. Davis Company
1915 Arch Street
Philadelphia, PA 19103
www.fadavis.com

Printed in the United States of America

Last digit indicates print number: 10 9 8 7 6 5 4 3 2

Publisher, Nursing: Joanne Patzek DaCunha, RN, MSN
Director of Content Development: Darlene D. Pedersen
Project Editors: Kim DePaul, Tyler Baber
Design and Illustrations Manager: Carolyn O'Brien

As new scientific information becomes available through basic and clinical research, recommended treatments and drug therapies undergo changes. The author(s) and publisher have done everything possible to make this book accurate, up to date, and in accord with accepted standards at the time of publication. The author(s), editors, and publisher are not responsible for errors or omissions or for consequences from application of the book, and make no warranty, expressed or implied, in regard to the contents of the book. Any practice described in this book should be applied by the reader in accordance with professional standards of care used in regard to the unique circumstances that may apply in each situation. The reader is advised always to check product information (package inserts) for changes and new information regarding dose and contraindications before administering any drug. Caution is especially urged when using new or infrequently ordered drugs.

Library of Congress Cataloging-in-Publication Data

Doenges, Marilynn E., 1922–
    Nursing diagnosis manual : planning, individualizing, and documenting client care / Marilynn E. Doenges, Mary Frances Moorhouse, Alice C. Murr.—3rd ed.
        p. ; cm.
    Includes bibliographical references and index.
    ISBN-13: 978-0-8036-2221-0
    ISBN-10: 0-8036-2221-X
1. Nursing diagnosis—Handbooks, manuals, etc. 2. Nursing assessment—Handbooks, manuals, etc. 3. Nursing—Planning—Handbooks, manuals, etc. I. Moorhouse, Mary Frances, 1947– II. Murr, Alice C., 1946– III. Title.
    [DNLM: 1. Nursing Diagnosis. 2. Nursing Records. 3. Patient Care Planning. WY 100.4 D649n 2010]
    RT48.6.D643 2010
    616.07′5—dc22

2007050302

To our spouses, children, parents, and friends, who much of the time have had to manage without us while we work and dream, as well as cope with our struggles and frustrations.

The Doenges families: the late Dean, Jim; Barbara and Bob Lanza; David, Monita, Matthew, and Tyler; John, Holly, Nicole, and Kelsey; and the Daigle families: Nancy, Jim; Jennifer, Brandon, Annabelle, Will, and Henry Smith-Daigle; and Jonathan, Kim, and Mandalyn JoAn.

The Moorhouse family: Jan; Paul; Jason, Thenderlyn, Alexa, and Mary Isabella.

To my children: Kevin and Tammy Carroll, Darin and Ck Carroll and the best grandchildren ever: Chelsea-Jane, Matthew, Joseph, Nathan, and Ben. You are my rock. Mom/Grammy Murr.

To our FAD family, especially Joanne DaCunha and Kimberly DePaul, and our production who assisted us in meeting deadlines and completing this new edition, and Robert Allen for teaching old nurses new technology.

To the nurses we are writing for, who daily face the challenge of meeting the needs of clients in varied settings and are looking for a practical way to organize and document this care. We believe that nursing diagnosis and these guides will help.

And to NANDA-I and the international nurses who are facilitating the development and dissemination of nursing diagnoses—we continue to champion your efforts and the work of promoting standardized languages.

The American Nurses Association (ANA) *Social Policy Statement* of 1980 was the first to define nursing as the diagnosis and treatment of human responses to actual and potential health problems. This definition, when combined with the ANA *Standards of Practice*, has provided impetus and support for the use of nursing diagnosis. Defining *nursing* and its effect on client care supports the growing awareness that nursing care is a key factor in client survival and in the maintenance, rehabilitative, and preventive aspects of healthcare. Changes and new developments in healthcare delivery in the past decade have given rise to the need for a common framework of communication to ensure continuity of care for the client moving between multiple healthcare settings and providers.

This book is designed to aid the student nurse and the practitioner in identifying interventions commonly associated with specific nursing diagnoses as proposed by NANDA International. These interventions are the activities needed to implement and document care provided to the individual client and can be used in varied settings from acute to community/home care.

Chapter 1 presents a brief discussion of the nursing process and introduces the concept of evidence-based practice. Standardized nursing languages (SNLs) are discussed in Chapter 2 with a focus on NANDA-I (nursing diagnoses), NIC (interventions), and NOC (outcomes). NANDA-I has 206 diagnosis labels with definitions, defining characteristics, and related or risk factors used to define a client need or problem. NIC is a comprehensive standardized language providing 542 direct and indirect intervention labels with definitions and a list of activities a nurse might choose to carry out each intervention. NOC language provides 385 outcome labels with definitions, a set of indicators describing specific client, caregiver, family, or community states related to the outcome, and a 5-point Likert-type measurement scale that can demonstrate client progress even when outcomes are not fully met. Chapter 3 addresses the assessment process using a nursing framework for data collection such as the Diagnostic Divisions Assessment Tool.

A creative approach for developing and documenting the planning of care is demonstrated in Chapter 4. Mind or Concept Mapping is a new technique or learning tool provided to assist you in achieving a holistic view of your client, enhance your critical thinking skills, and facilitate the creative process of planning client care. For more in-depth information and inclusive plans of care related to specific medical/psychiatric conditions (with rationale and the application of the diagnoses), refer to the larger work also published by the F. A. Davis Company: *Nursing Care Plans: Guidelines for Individualizing Client Care Across the Lifespan*, ed. 8 (Doenges, Moorhouse, & Murr, 2010) which includes psychiatric/mental health and maternal/newborn plans of care on the CD-ROM accompanying the text.

Chapter 6 contains 850 disorders and health conditions reflecting all specialty areas with associated nursing diagnoses written as client problem/need statements to aid you in validating the assessment and diagnosis steps of the nursing process.

In Chapter 5, the heart of the book, all the nursing diagnoses are listed alphabetically for ease of reference and include the diagnoses accepted for use by NANDA-I 2009–2011. The alphabetization of diagnoses follows NANDA-I's own sequencing, whereby diagnoses are alphabetized first by their key term, which is capitalized. Subordinate terminology or descriptors of the diagnosis are presented in lowercase words and are alphabetized secondarily to the key term (for example, chronic Pain is alphabetized under P, following acute Pain). Each approved diagnosis includes its definition and information divided into the NANDA-I categories of Related or Risk Factors and Defining Characteristics. Related/Risk Factors information reflects causative or contributing factors that can be useful for determining whether the diagnosis is applicable to a particular client. Defining Characteristics (signs and symptoms or cues) are listed as subjective and/or objective and are used to confirm actual diagnoses, aid in formulating outcomes, and provide additional data for choosing appropriate interventions. We have not deleted or altered NANDA-I's listings; however, on occasion, we have added to their definitions and suggested additional criteria to provide clarification and direction. These additions are denoted with brackets [ ].

NANDA-I nursing diagnosis labels are designed to be multiaxial with seven axes or descriptors. An *axis* is defined as a dimension of the human response that is considered in the diagnostic process (see Appendix). Sometimes an axis may be included in the diagnostic concept, such as ineffective community Coping in which the unit of care (i.e., community) is named. Some are implicit, such as Activity Intolerance in which the individual is the unit of care. At times, an axis may not be pertinent to a particular diagnosis and will not be a part of the nursing diagnosis label. For example, the time frame (e.g., acute, intermittent) or body part (e.g., cerebral, oral, skin) may not be relevant to each diagnostic situation.

Desired Outcomes/Evaluation Criteria are identified to assist you in formulating individual client outcomes and to support the evaluation process. Suggested NOC linkages to the nursing diagnosis are provided.

Nursing priorities are used to group the suggested interventions, which are primarily directed to adult care, although interventions designated as across the lifespan do include pediatric and geriatric considerations and are designated by an icon. In general, the interventions can be used in multiple settings—acute care, rehabilitation, community clinics, home care, or private practice. Most interventions are independent or nursing originated; however, some interventions are collaborative orders (e.g., medical, psychiatric), and you will need to determine when this is necessary and take the appropriate action. Icons are also used to differentiate collaborative interventions, diagnostic studies, and medications, as well as transcultural considerations. All of these "specialized" interventions are presented with icons, rather than being broken out under separate headings, to maintain their sequence within the prioritization of all nursing interventions for the diagnosis. Additionally, in support of evidence-based practice, rationales are provided for the interventions and references for these rationales are cited.

The inclusion of Documentation Focus suggestions is to remind you of the importance and necessity of recording the steps of the nursing process.

As noted, with few exceptions, we have presented NANDA-I's recommendations as formulated. We support the belief that practicing nurses and researchers need to study, use, and evaluate the diagnoses as presented. Nurses can be creative as they use the standardized language, redefining and sharing information as the diagnoses are used with individual clients. As new nursing diagnoses are developed, it is important that the data they encompass are added to assessment tools and current data bases. As part of the process by clinicians, educators, and researchers across practice specialties and academic settings to define, test, and refine nursing diagnosis, nurses are encouraged to share insights and ideas with NANDA-I at the following address: NANDA International, 100 North 20th Street, 4th Floor, Philadelphia, PA 19103; e-mail: info@nanda.org.

Marilynn E. Doenges
Mary Frances Moorhouse
Alice C. Murr

CONTRIBUTORS

Diane Bligh, RN, MS, CNS
Associate Professor, Nursing
Front Range Community College
Westminster, Colorado

Mary F. Johnston, RN, MSN
Retired Program Director, Nursing
Front Range Community College
Westminster, Colorado

Sheila Marquez, RN, BSN, PNP—Retired
Former Executive Director, Vice President/Chief
   Operating Officer
The Colorado SIDS Program, Inc.
Denver, Colorado

Susan Moberly, RNC, BSN, ICCE (Deceased)
Childbirth Educator
Obstetric Nursing and Lactation Consultant
Colorado Springs, Colorado

Alma Mueller, RN, MEd
Retired Chair and Professor of Nursing
Front Range Community College
Westminster, Colorado

CONTENTS

CHAPTER 1

The Nursing Process: The Foundation of Quality Client Care

Defining the Profession

In the world of healthcare, nursing has long struggled to establish itself as a profession. Dictionary terms describe nursing as "a calling requiring specialized knowledge and often long and intensive academic preparation; a principal calling, vocation, or employment; the whole body of persons engaged in a calling."[1] Throughout the history of nursing, unfavorable stereotypes (based on the view of nursing as subservient and dependent on the medical profession) have negatively affected the view of nursing as an independent entity. In its early developmental years, nursing did not seek or have the means to control its own practice. Florence Nightingale, in discussing the nature of nursing in 1859, observed that "nursing has been limited to signify little more than the administration of medicines and the application of poultices."[2] Although this attitude may persist to some degree, the nursing profession has defined what makes nursing unique and has identified a body of professional knowledge. As early as 1896, nurses in America banded together to seek standardization of educational programs and laws governing their practice. The task of nursing since that time has been to create descriptive terminology reflecting specific nursing functions and levels of competency.[3] Erickson, Tomlin, and Swain stated the belief that "nursing will thrive as a unique and valued profession when nurses present a theory and rationalistic model for their practice, correct misleading stereotypes, locate control with clients, and actively participate in processes for change."[4]

In the past several decades, more than a dozen prominent nursing scholars (e.g., Rogers, Parse, Henderson) have developed conceptualizations to define the nature of nursing. Because much of nursing is nonphenomenological or nonobservable, the nature of nursing cannot be explained using the usual parameters of scientific investigation. Kikuchi proposes that conceptualizations about nursing are philosophic in nature and as such are still testable.[5] As nursing research continues the work of establishing the profession as independent in its own right, the value of nursing goals is understood and the difference between nursing and other professions is being delineated. Nursing is now recognized as both a science and an art concerned with the physical, psychological, sociological, cultural, and spiritual concerns of the individual. The science of nursing is based on a broad theoretical framework; its art depends on the caring skills and abilities of the individual nurse. The importance of the nurse within the healthcare system is noted in many positive ways, and the profession of nursing is acknowledging the need for its practitioners to act professionally and be accountable for the care they provide.

Barely a century after Miss Nightingale noted that "the very elements of nursing are all but unknown," the American Nurses Association (ANA) developed its first Social Policy Statement in 1980, defining nursing as "the diagnosis and treatment of *human responses* to actual or potential health problems."[6] Human responses (defined as people's experiences with and responses to health, illness, and life events) are nursing's phenomena of concern. In 1995, this statement was revisited, updated, and titled "Nursing's Social Policy Statement." This policy statement acknowledged that since the release of the original statement, "nursing has been influenced by many social and professional changes, as well as by the science of caring."[7]

The statement delineated four essential features of today's contemporary nursing practice:

1. Attention to the full range of human experiences and responses to health and illness without restriction to a problem-focused orientation
2. Integration of objective data with knowledge gained from an understanding of the client's or group's subjective experience
3. Application of scientific knowledge to the processes of diagnosis and treatment
4. Provision of a caring relationship that facilitates health and healing[7]

Thus, nursing's role includes promotion of health as well as performance of activities that contribute to recovery from or adjustment to illness. This is reflected in ANA's 2003 Nursing's Social Policy Statement, which recognized nursing's full scope of care by defining nursing as "the protection, promotion, and optimization of health and abilities, prevention of illness and injury, alleviation of suffering through the diagnosis and treatment of human response, and advocacy in the care of individuals, families, communities, and populations."[8] Also, nurses support the right of clients to define their own health-related goals and to engage in care that reflects their personal values. Emphasis is placed on the mind-body-spirit connection with a holistic view of the individual as nurses facilitate the client's efforts in striving for growth and development.

In your readings, you will likely encounter other definitions of nursing. As your knowledge and experience develops, your definition of nursing may change to reflect your personal nursing philosophy, your focus on a particular care setting or population, or your specific role. For example, although the definition of nursing developed by Erickson, Tomlin, and Swain is more than 25 years old, it remains viable and timely because it incorporates the concepts noted previously with today's holistic approach to care. Their definition includes what nursing is, how it is accomplished, and the goals of nursing: "Nursing is the holistic helping of persons with their self-care activities in relation to their health. This is an interactive, interpersonal process that nurtures strengths to enable development, release, and channeling of resources for coping with one's circumstances and environment. The goal is to achieve a state of perceived optimum health and contentment."[4]

An understanding of human nature is certainly important in the development of a philosophy of nursing. Understanding that "needs motivate behavior" helps the nurse to determine the client's needs at a particular moment in time. Maslow's hierarchy of needs[9] provides a basis for understanding that unmet needs can interfere with an individual's holistic growth and may even result in physical or mental distress and illness. Other theorists have also studied how people are similar, providing the nurse with more information to help understand the client. For example, Erik Erikson's observations on the stages of psychological development suggest that the individual is a "work in progress" accomplishing age-specific maturational tasks throughout the life span. Piaget's cognitive stages address how thinking develops and how individuals adapt to and organize their environment intellectually.[4] However, in the end, the individual is the primary source of information about himself/herself. The nurse needs to listen with an open mind and empathic, unconditional acceptance to what the client is relating. Knowing how people are alike provides a basis to understanding human nature. However, each person is unique, and the nurse needs to look for the client's model of the world and how it relates to the client's own situation.

The nursing profession is further defined by fundamental philosophical beliefs that have been identified over time as essential to the practice of nursing. These values and assumptions offer guidance to the nurse and need to be kept in mind to enhance the quality of nursing care provided:

- The client is a human being who has worth and dignity.
- Humans manifest an essential unity of mind/body/spirit.[7]
- There are basic human needs that must be met (Maslow's Hierarchy of Needs).
- When these needs are not met, problems arise that may require intervention by another person until the individuals can resume responsibility for themselves.
- Human experience is contextually and culturally defined.[7]
- Health and illness are human experiences.[7]
- Clients have a right to quality health and nursing care delivered with interest, compassion, and competence with a focus on wellness and prevention.
- The presence of illness does not preclude health, nor does optimal health preclude illness.[7]
- The therapeutic nurse-client relationship is important in the nursing process and provision of individualized care.

Finally, the Code of Ethics for Nurses[10] addresses the need for nurses to respect human dignity, acknowledge the uniqueness of each client, and honor the client's right to privacy. The Code also calls on nurses to assume responsibility for individual nursing judgments and actions and for the delegation of nursing activities to others. Nurses are encouraged to maintain competence in nursing, contribute to the ongoing development of the profession, and participate in implementation and improvement of standards. This last goal can be accomplished by using the results of nursing research to engage in evidence-based nursing practice.

The roots of evidence-based practice lie in the efforts of many in the past. Hippocrates described the symptoms and course of illnesses and related them to the seasons, geographical area, and types of people associated with each. These hypotheses founded the rational approach to the understanding of disease. As knowledge grew and the germ theory of disease was accepted, epidemiology began to count disease events, leading to the establishment of a central government agency to collect and record data. This led to the posing of questions in the form of testable hypotheses, the collection of data to support or refute hypotheses, and the development of statistical tools to summarize numerical data.[11] The work of Pasteur and Koch expanded the understanding of causal relationships between bacterial causes of many diseases, leading to reducing illness and mortality.

Florence Nightingale used statistics to measure health, identify causes of mortality, evaluate health services, and reform institutions. After the Crimean War, she began organizing committees, assembling data, and preparing reports and hearings on how administrative inadequacies affected clients' health. Her work resulted in British Army Hospital and government reform in the interest of preventing death and disease. She became an honorary member of the American Statistical Association in 1874, and her papers were read at a National Social Science Congress in 1863 and at the nurses' congress of the Chicago World's Fair in 1893. The efforts of these pioneers laid the groundwork for the development of evidence-based practice.

Barnsteiner and Provost note that "the current definition [of evidence-based practice] is the integration of best research evidence with clinical expertise and patient values"[12]—that is, both research and nonresearch components are combined to create evidence-based practice. Quantitative research is invaluable in measuring the effectiveness of nursing interventions, while qualitative studies capture the preferences, attitudes, and values of healthcare consumers. However, the nurses' clinical judgment and individual client needs and perspectives must also be included. As nurses work to provide cost-effective care in the best setting for the client, "the most important [and challenging] requirement for practicing nurses in the 21st century will be to utilize [appropriate] evidence available to improve practice."[13]

Nursing leaders have identified a process that "combines the most desirable elements of the art of nursing with the most relevant elements of systems theory, using the scientific method."[14] This *nursing process* incorporates an interactive and interpersonal approach with a problem-solving and decision-making process that serves as a framework for the delivery of nursing care.[15–17]

The concept of nursing process was first introduced in the 1950s as a three-step process of assessment, planning, and evaluation based on the scientific method of observing, measuring, gathering data, and analyzing the findings. Years of study, use, and refinement have led nurses to expand the nursing process to five distinct steps that provide an efficient method of organizing thought processes for clinical decision making, problem-solving, and delivery of higher-quality, individualized client care. The nursing process now consists of the following:

- *assessment* or the systematic collection of data relating to clients;
- *diagnosis or need identification* involving the analysis of collected data to identify the client's needs;
- *planning,* which is a two-part process of identifying goals and the client's desired outcomes to address the assessed health and wellness needs along with the selection of appropriate nursing interventions to assist the client in attaining the outcomes;
- *implementation* or putting the plan of care into action; and
- *evaluation* by determining the client's progress toward attaining the identified outcomes and the client's response to and the effectiveness of the selected nursing interventions for the purpose of altering the plan as indicated.

Because these five steps are central to nursing actions in any setting, the nursing process is now included in the conceptual framework of nursing curricula and is accepted as part of the legal definition of nursing in the Nurse Practice Acts of most states.

When a client enters the healthcare system, whether as an inpatient, a clinic outpatient, or a home-care client, the nursing process steps are set into motion. The nurse collects data, identifies client needs (nursing diagnoses), establishes goals, creates measurable outcomes, and selects nursing interventions to assist the client in achieving these outcomes and goals. Finally, after the interventions have been implemented, the nurse evaluates the client's responses and the effectiveness of the plan of care in reaching the desired outcomes and goals to determine whether or not the needs or problems have been resolved and the client is ready to be discharged from the care setting. If the identified needs or problems remain unresolved, further assessment, additional nursing diagnoses, alteration of outcomes and goals, or changes of interventions are required.

Although we use the terms *assessment, diagnosis, planning, implementation,* and *evaluation* as separate, progressive steps, in reality they are interrelated. Together these steps form a continuous circle of thought and action, which recycles throughout the client's contact with the healthcare system. Figure 1.1 depicts a model for visualizing this process. You can see that the nursing process uses the nursing diagnosis which is the clinical judgment product of critical thinking. Based on this judgment, nursing interventions are selected and implemented. Figure 1.1 also shows how the progressive steps of the nursing process create an understandable model of both the products and the processes of critical thinking contained within the nursing process. The model graphically emphasizes both the dynamic and cyclic characteristics of the nursing process.

Application of the Nursing Process

The scientific method of problem-solving introduced in the previous section is used almost instinctively by most people, without conscious awareness.

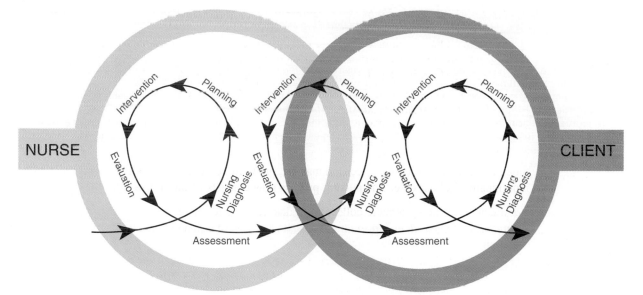

NURSE | CLIENT

Intervention · Planning · Evaluation · Nursing Diagnosis · Assessment

●Figure 1.1 Diagram of the nursing process. The steps of the nursing process are interrelated, forming a continuous circle of thought and action that is both dynamic and cyclic.

FOR EXAMPLE While studying for your semester finals, you snack on pepperoni pizza. After going to bed, you are awakened by a burning sensation in the center of your chest. You are young and in good health and note no other symptoms (assessment). You decide that your pain is the result of the spicy food you have eaten (diagnosis). You then determine that before you can return to sleep, you need to relieve the discomfort with an over-the-counter preparation (planning). You take a liquid antacid for your discomfort (implementation). Within a few minutes, you note the burning sensation is relieved, and you return to bed without further concern (evaluation)

As you see, this is a process you routinely use to solve problems in your life that can be readily applied to client-care situations. You need only to learn the new terms describing the nursing process, rather than having to think about each step (assessment, diagnosis/need identification, planning, implementation, and evaluation) in an entirely new way.

To effectively use the nursing process, the nurse needs to possess and apply some basic abilities. Particularly important is a thorough knowledge of science and theory, not only as applied in nursing but also in other related disciplines such as medicine and psychology. Creativity is needed in the application of nursing knowledge, as is adaptability in handling change and the many unexpected happenings that occur. As a nurse, you must make a commitment to practice your profession in the best possible way, trusting in yourself and your ability to do your job well and displaying the necessary leadership to organize and supervise as your position requires. In addition, intelligence, well-developed interpersonal skills, and competent technical skills are essential.

FOR EXAMPLE A diabetic client's irritable behavior could be the result of low serum glucose or the effects of excessive caffeine intake. However, it could also arise from a sense of helplessness regarding life events. A single behavior may have varied causes. It is important that your nursing assessment skills identify the underlying etiology to provide appropriate care.

The practice responsibilities presented in the definitions of nursing and the nursing process are explained in detail in the publication *Nursing: Scope & Standards of Practice*.[18] The standards provide workable guidelines to ensure that the practice of nursing can be carried out by each nurse. Table 1.1 presents an abbreviated description of the standards of clinical practice. With the ultimate goal of quality healthcare, the effective use of the nursing process will result

TABLE 1.1 **ANA Standards of Nursing Practice**

Standards of Practice

Describes a competent level of nursing care as demonstrated by the nursing process that encompasses all significant actions taken by the nurse in providing care and forms the foundation of clinical decision making.

1. Assessment: The registered nurse (RN) collects comprehensive data pertinent to the patient's health or situation.
2. Diagnosis: The RN analyzes the assessment data to determine the diagnoses or issues.
3. Outcome Identification: The RN identifies expected outcomes for a plan individualized to the patient or the situation.
4. Planning: The RN develops a plan that prescribes strategies and alternatives to attain expected outcomes.
5. Implementation: The RN implements the identified plan.
   a. Coordination of Care: The RN coordinates care delivery.
   b. Health Teaching and Health Promotion: The RN employs strategies to promote health and a safe environment.
   c. Consultation: The advanced practice RN and the nursing role specialist provide consultation to influence the identified plan, enhance the abilities of others, and effect change.
   d. Prescriptive Authority and Treatment: The advanced practice RN uses prescriptive authority, procedures, referrals, treatments, and therapies in accordance with state and federal laws and regulations.
6. Evaluation: The RN evaluates progress toward attainment of outcomes.

Standards of Professional Performance

Describes roles expected of all professional nurses appropriate to their education, position, and practice setting.

7. Quality of Practice: The RN systematically enhances the quality and effectiveness of nursing practice.
8. Education: The RN attains knowledge and competency that reflects current nursing practice.
9. Professional Practice Evaluation: The RN evaluates one's own nursing practice in relation to professional practice standards and guidelines, relevant statutes, rules, and regulations.
10. Collegiality: The RN interacts with and contributes to the professional development of peers and colleagues.
11. Collaboration: The RN collaborates with patient, family, and others in the conduct of nursing practice.
12. Ethics: The RN integrates ethical provisions in all areas of practice.
13. Research: The RN integrates research findings into practice.
14. Resource Utilization: The RN considers factors related to safety, effectiveness, cost, and impact on practice in the planning and delivery of nursing services.
15. Leadership: The RN provides leadership in the professional practice setting and the profession.

Source: American Nurses Association. (2004). *Nursing: Scope & Standards of Practice*. Silver Spring, MD: Nursesbooks.org.

in a viable nursing-care system that is recognized and accepted as nursing's body of knowledge and that can be shared with other healthcare professionals.

Advantages of Using the Nursing Process

There are many advantages to the use of the nursing process:

- The nursing process provides an organizing framework for meeting the individual needs of the client, the client's family/significant other(s), and the community.
- The steps of the nursing process focus the nurse's attention on the "individual" human responses of a client or group to a given health situation, resulting in a holistic plan of care addressing the specific needs of the client or group.
- The nursing process provides an organized, systematic method of problem-solving (while still allowing for creative solutions) that may minimize dangerous errors or omissions in caregiving and avoid time-consuming repetition in care and documentation.
- The use of the nursing process promotes the active involvement of clients in their healthcare, enhancing consumer satisfaction. Such participation increases clients' sense of control over what is happening to them, stimulates problem-solving, and promotes personal responsibility, all of which strengthen the client's commitment to achieving the identified goals.

- The use of the nursing process enables you as a nurse to have more control over your practice. This enhances the opportunity for you to use your knowledge, expertise, and intuition constructively and dynamically to increase the likelihood of a successful client outcome. This, in turn, promotes greater job satisfaction and your professional growth.
- The use of the nursing process provides a common language (nursing diagnosis) for practice, unifying the nursing profession. Using a system that clearly communicates the plan of care to coworkers and clients enhances continuity of care, promotes achievement of client goals, provides a vehicle for evaluation, and aids in the development of nursing standards. In addition, the structure of the process provides a format for documenting the client's response to all aspects of the planned care.
- The use of the nursing process provides a means of assessing nursing's economic contribution to client care. The nursing process supplies a vehicle for the quantitative and qualitative measurement of nursing care that meets the goal of cost-effectiveness and still promotes holistic care.

Summary

Nursing is continuing to evolve into a well-defined profession with a more clearly delineated definition and phenomena of concern. Fundamental philosophical beliefs and qualities have been identified that are important for the nurse to possess in order to provide quality care.

The nursing profession has developed a body of knowledge that contributes to the growth and well-being of the individual and the community, the prevention of illness, and the maintenance and/or restoration of health, or relief of pain and provision of support when a return to health is not possible. The nursing process is the basis of all nursing actions and is the essence of nursing, providing a flexible, orderly, logical problem-solving approach for administering nursing care so that client (whether individual, community, or population) needs for such care are met comprehensively and effectively. It can be applied in any healthcare or educational setting, in any theoretical or conceptual framework, and within the context of any nursing philosophy.

Each step of the nursing process builds on and interacts with the other steps, ensuring an effective practice model. Inclusion of the standards of clinical nursing practice provides additional information to reinforce understanding and opportunities to apply knowledge.

Please note, the term *client* rather than *patient* is used in this book to reflect the philosophy that the individuals or groups you work with are legitimate members of the decision-making process with some degree of control over the planned regimen and as able, active participants in the planning and implementation of their care.[4]

Next, we introduce the language described in the nursing process. This includes NANDA International's classification of nursing diagnoses,[19] the Iowa Intervention and Outcome Projects: Nursing Interventions Classification (NIC),[20] and the Nursing Outcomes Classification (NOC).[21] NANDA-I, NIC, and NOC have combined their classification systems (NNN Alliance) to provide a comprehensive nursing language.

References

1. Merriam-Webster Online Dictionary. Retrieved May 7, 2003 from www.m-w.com/dictionary.htm.
2. Nightingale, F. (1859). *Notes on Nursing: What It Is and What It Is Not.* Facsimile edition. Philadelphia: J. B. Lippincott, 1946.

3. Jacobi, E. M. (1976). Foreword. In Flanigan, L. (ed). *One Strong Voice: The Story of the American Nurses' Association*. Kansas City, MO: American Nurses Association.

4. Erickson, H. C., Tomlin, E. M., Swain, M. A. (1983). *Modeling and Role-Modeling: A Theory and Paradigm for Nursing*. Englewood Cliffs, NJ: Prentice-Hall.

5. Kikuchi, J. F. (1999). Clarifying the nature of conceptualizations about nursing. *Canadian J Nurs Res*, 30(4), 115–128.

6. American Nurses Association. (1980). *Nursing: A Social Policy Statement*. Kansas City, MO: Author.

7. American Nurses Association. (1995). *Nursing's Social Policy Statement*. Washington, DC: American Nurses Publishing.

8. Maslow, A. H. (1970). *Motivation and Personality*. 2d ed. New York: Harper & Row.

9. American Nurses Association. (2003). *Nursing's Social Policy Statement*. Washington, DC: Nursesbooks.org.

10. American Nurses Association. (2001). *Code of Ethics for Nurses*. Washington, DC: American Nurses Publishing.

11. Stolley, P. D., Lasky, T. (1995). *Investigating Disease Patterns: The Science of Epidemiology* (Scientific American Library, no. 57). New York: WH Freeman.

12. Barnsteiner, J., Provost, S. (2002). How to implement evidence-based practice: Some tried and true pointers. *Reflect Nurs Leadersh*, 28(2), 18.

13. Amarsi, Y. (2002). Evidence-based nursing: Perspective from Pakistan. *Reflect Nurs Leadersh*, 28(2), 28.

14. Shore, L. S. (1988). *Nursing Diagnosis: What It Is and How to Do It, a Programmed Text*. Richmond, VA: Medical College of Virginia Hospitals.

15. Peplau, H. E. (1952). *Interpersonal Relations in Nursing: A Conceptual Frame of Reference for Psychodynamic Nursing*. New York: Putnam.

16. King, L. (1971). *Toward a Theory for Nursing: General Concepts of Human Behavior*. New York: Wiley.

17. Yura, H., Walsh, M. B. (1988). *The Nursing Process: Assessing, Planning, Implementing, Evaluating*. 5th ed. Norwalk, CT: Appleton & Lange.

18. American Nurses Association. (2004). *Nursing: Scope & Standards of Practice*. Silver Spring, MD: Nursesbooks.org.

19. North American Nursing Diagnosis Association. (2001). *Nursing Diagnoses: Definitions & Classification*. Philadelphia: Author.

20. McCloskey, J. C., Bulecheck, G. M. (2000). *Nursing Interventions Classification (NIC)*. 3d ed. St. Louis, MO: Mosby.

21. Johnson, M., Maas, M., Moorhead, S. (2000). *Nursing Outcomes Classification (NOC)*. 2d ed. St. Louis, MO: Mosby.

CHAPTER 2

The Language of Nursing: NANDA, NIC, NOC, and Other Standardized Nursing Languages

In this chapter, we look at the process and progress of describing the work of nursing because, as Lang has stated, "If we cannot name it, we cannot control it, practice it, teach it, finance it, or put it into public policy."[1] At first glance, nursing seems a simple task. However, over many years, the profession has struggled, in part, as a result of changes in healthcare delivery and financing, the expansion of nursing's role, and the dawning of the computer age. Gordon reminds us that classification system development parallels knowledge development in a discipline.[2] As theory development and research have begun to define nursing, it has become necessary for nursing to find a common language to describe what nursing is, what nursing does, and how to codify it. Thus, the terms "classification systems" and "standardized language" were embraced, and the work continues.

Changes in the healthcare system occur at an ever-increasing rate. One of these changes is the movement toward a paperless (computerized or electronic) client record. The use of electronic healthcare information systems is rapidly expanding, and the focus has shifted from its original uses—financial and personnel management functions—to the efficient documentation of the client encounter, whether that is a single office visit or a lengthy hospitalization. The move to electronic documentation is being fueled by changes in healthcare delivery and reimbursement as well as the advent of alternative healthcare settings (outpatient surgeries, home health, rehabilitation or subacute units, extended or long-term care facilities, etc.), all of which increase the need for a commonality of communication to ensure continuity of care for the client, who moves from one setting or level of care to another.

These changes in the business and documentation of healthcare require the industry to generate data about its operations and outcomes. Evaluation and improvement of provided services are important to the delivery of cost-effective client care. Therefore, providers and consumers interested in outcomes of care benefit from accurate documentation of the care provided and the client's response. With the use of language or terminology that can be coded, healthcare information can be recorded in terms that are universal and easily entered into an electronic database and that can generate meaningful reporting data about its operation and outcomes. In short, standardized language is required.

A standardized language contains formalized terms that have definitions and guidelines for use. For example, if the impact of nursing care on financial and clinical outcomes is to be analyzed, coding of this information is essential. While it has been relatively easy to code medical procedures, nursing is more of an enigma, because its work has not been so clearly defined.

Since the 1970s, nursing leaders have been working to define the profession of nursing and to develop a commonality of words describing practice (a framework of communication and documentation) so that nursing's contribution to healthcare is captured, is visible in healthcare databases, and is thereby recognized as essential. Therefore, the focus of the profession has been on the effort to classify tasks and to develop standardized nursing languages (SNLs) to better demonstrate what nursing is and what nursing does.

Around the world, nursing researchers continue their efforts to identify and label people's experiences with (and responses to) health and illness as they relate to the scope of nursing practice. The use of universal nursing terminology directs our focus to the central content and process of nursing care by identifying, naming, and standardizing the "what" and "how" of the work of nursing—including both direct and indirect activities. This wider application for a standardized language has spurred its development.

A recognized pioneer in SNL is NANDA International's "nursing diagnosis."[3] Simply stated, a nursing diagnosis is defined as a clinical judgment about individual, family, or community responses to actual or potential health problems and life processes. Nursing diagnoses provide the basis for selecting nursing interventions to achieve outcomes for which the nurse is accountable.[4] NANDA-I nursing diagnoses currently include 206 labels with definitions, defining characteristics, and related or risk factors used to define a client need or problem. Once the client's need is defined, outcomes can be developed and nursing interventions chosen to achieve the desired outcomes.

The linkage of client problems or nursing diagnoses to specific nursing interventions and client outcomes has led to the development of several other SNLs, including Clinical Care Classification (CCC; originally Home Health Care Classification[5]),[6] Nursing Interventions Classification (NIC),[7] Nursing Outcomes Classification (NOC),[8] Omaha System-Community Health Classification System (OS),[9] Patient Care Data Set (PCDS; now retired),[10] and Perioperative Nursing Data Set (PNDS).[11]

Whereas some of these languages (e.g., OS and PNDS) are designed for a specific client population, the NANDA-I, NIC, and NOC languages are comprehensively designed for use across systems and settings and at individual, family, and community or population levels.[12]

NIC is a comprehensive standardized language providing 542 direct and indirect intervention labels (Table 2.1) with definitions. A list of activities a nurse might choose to carry out each intervention is also provided and can be modified as necessary to meet the specific needs of the client. These research-based interventions address general practice and specialty areas.

TABLE 2.1	Nursing Interventions Classification Labels
Abuse Protection Support	Admission Care
Abuse Protection Support: Child	Airway Insertion and Stabilization
Abuse Protection Support: Domestic Partner	Airway Management
Abuse Protection Support: Elder	Airway Suctioning
Abuse Protection Support: Religious	Allergy Management
Acid-Base Management	Amnioinfusion
Acid-Base Management: Metabolic Acidosis	Amputation Care
Acid-Base Management: Metabolic Alkalosis	Analgesic Administration
Acid-Base Management: Respiratory Acidosis	Analgesic Administration: Intraspinal
Acid-Base Management: Respiratory Alkalosis	Anaphylaxis Management
Acid-Base Monitoring	Anesthesia Administration
Active Listening	Anger Control Assistance
Activity Therapy	Animal-Assisted Therapy
Acupressure	Anticipatory Guidance

TABLE 2.1   continued

Anxiety Reduction
Area Restriction
Aromatherapy
Art Therapy
Artificial Airway Management
Aspiration Precautions
Assertiveness Training
Asthma Management
Attachment Promotion
Autogenic Training
Autotransfusion

Bathing
Bed Rest Care
Bedside Laboratory Testing
Behavior Management
Behavior Management: Overactivity/Inattention
Behavior Management: Self-Harm
Behavior Management: Sexual
Behavior Modification
Behavior Modification: Social Skills
Bibliotherapy
Biofeedback
Bioterrorism Preparedness
Birthing
Bladder Irrigation
Bleeding Precautions
Bleeding Reduction
Bleeding Reduction: Antepartum Uterus
Bleeding Reduction: Gastrointestinal
Bleeding Reduction: Nasal
Bleeding Reduction: Postpartum Uterus
Bleeding Reduction: Wound
Blood Products Administration
Body Image Enhancement
Body Mechanics Promotion
Bottle Feeding
Bowel Incontinence Care
Bowel Incontinence Care: Encopresis
Bowel Irrigation
Bowel Management
Bowel Training
Breast Examination
Breastfeeding Assistance

Calming Technique
Capillary Blood Sample
Cardiac Care
Cardiac Care: Acute
Cardiac Care: Rehabilitation
Cardiac Precautions
Caregiver Support
Care Management
Cast Care: Maintenance
Cast Care: Wet
Cerebral Edema Management
Cerebral Perfusion Promotion

Cesarean Section Care
Chemical Restraint
Chemotherapy Management
Chest Physiotherapy
Childbirth Preparation
Circulatory Care: Arterial Insufficiency
Circulatory Care: Mechanical Assist Device
Circulatory Care: Venous Insufficiency
Circulatory Precautions
Circumcision Care
Code Management
Cognitive Restructuring
Cognitive Stimulation
Communicable Disease Management
Communication Enhancement: Hearing Deficit
Communication Enhancement: Speech Deficit
Communication Enhancement: Visual Deficit
Community Disaster Preparedness
Community Health Development
Complex Relationship Building
Conflict Mediation
Constipation/Impaction Management
Consultation
Contact Lens Care
Controlled Substance Checking
Coping Enhancement
Cost Containment
Cough Enhancement
Counseling
Crisis Intervention
Critical Path Development
Culture Brokerage
Cutaneous Stimulation

Decision-Making Support
Delegation
Delirium Management
Delusion Management
Dementia Management
Dementia Management: Bathing
Deposition/Testimony
Developmental Care
Developmental Enhancement: Adolescent
Developmental Enhancement: Child
Dialysis Access Maintenance
Diarrhea Management
Diet Staging
Discharge Planning
Distraction
Documentation
Dressing
Dying Care
Dysreflexia Management
Dysrhythmia Management

Ear Care
Eating Disorders Management

(table continues on page 12)

TABLE 2.1 **Nursing Interventions Classification Labels** (continued)

Electroconvulsive Therapy Management
Electrolyte Management
Electrolyte Management: Hypercalcemia
Electrolyte Management: Hyperkalemia
Electrolyte Management: Hypermagnesemia
Electrolyte Management: Hypernatremia
Electrolyte Management: Hyperphosphatemia
Electrolyte Management: Hypocalcemia
Electrolyte Management: Hypokalemia
Electrolyte Management: Hypomagnesemia
Electrolyte Management: Hyponatremia
Electrolyte Management: Hypophosphatemia
Electrolyte Monitoring
Electronic Fetal Monitoring: Antepartum
Electronic Fetal Monitoring: Intrapartum
Elopement Precautions
Embolus Care: Peripheral
Embolus Care: Pulmonary
Embolus Precautions
Emergency Care
Emergency Cart Checking
Emotional Support
Endotracheal Extubation
Energy Management
Enteral Tube Feeding
Environmental Management
Environmental Management: Attachment Process
Environmental Management: Comfort
Environmental Management: Community
Environmental Management: Home Preparation
Environmental Management: Safety
Environmental Management: Violence Prevention
Environmental Management: Worker Safety
Environmental Risk Protection
Examination Assistance
Exercise Promotion
Exercise Promotion: Strength Training
Exercise Promotion: Stretching
Exercise Therapy: Ambulation
Exercise Therapy: Balance
Exercise Therapy: Joint Mobility
Exercise Therapy: Muscle Control
Eye Care

Fall Prevention
Family Integrity Promotion
Family Integrity Promotion: Childbearing Family
Family Involvement Promotion
Family Mobilization
Family Planning: Contraception
Family Planning: Infertility
Family Planning: Unplanned Pregnancy
Family Presence Facilitation
Family Process Maintenance
Family Support
Family Therapy
Feeding

Fertility Preservation
Fever Treatment
Financial Resource Assistance
Fire-Setting Precautions
First Aid
Fiscal Resource Management
Flatulence Reduction
Fluid/Electrolyte Management
Fluid Management
Fluid Monitoring
Fluid Resuscitation
Foot Care
Forensic Data Collection
Forgiveness Facilitation

Gastrointestinal Intubation
Genetic Counseling
Grief Work Facilitation
Grief Work Facilitation: Perinatal Death
Guided Imagery
Guilt Work Facilitation

Hair Care
Hallucination Management
Health Care Information Exchange
Health Education
Health Literacy Enhancement
Health Policy Monitoring
Health Screening
Health System Guidance
Heat/Cold Application
Heat Exposure Treatment
Hemodialysis Therapy
Hemodynamic Regulation
Hemofiltration Therapy
Hemorrhage Control
High-Risk Pregnancy Care
Home Maintenance Assistance
Hope Inspiration
Hormone Replacement Therapy
Humor
Hyperglycemia Management
Hypervolemia Management
Hypnosis
Hypoglycemia Management
Hypothermia Induction
Hypothermia Treatment
Hypovolemia Management

Immunization/Vaccination Management
Impulse Control Training
Incident Reporting
Incision Site Care
Infant Care
Infection Control
Infection Control: Intraoperative
Infection Protection

TABLE 2.1 continued

Insurance Authorization
Intracranial Pressure (ICP) Monitoring
Intrapartal Care
Intrapartal Care: High-Risk Delivery
Intravenous (IV) Insertion
Intravenous (IV) Therapy
Invasive Hemodynamic Monitoring

Journaling

Kangaroo Care

Labor Induction
Labor Suppression
Laboratory Data Interpretation
Lactation Counseling
Lactation Suppression
Laser Precautions
Latex Precautions
Learning Facilitation
Learning Readiness Enhancement
Leech Therapy
Limit Setting
Lower Extremity Monitoring

Malignant Hyperthermia Precautions
Massage
Mechanical Ventilation Management: Invasive
Mechanical Ventilation Management: Noninvasive
Mechanical Ventilatory Weaning
Medication Administration
Medication Administration: Ear
Medication Administration: Enteral
Medication Administration: Eye
Medication Administration: Inhalation
Medication Administration: Interpleural
Medication Administration: Intradermal
Medication Administration: Intramuscular (IM)
Medication Administration: Intraosseous
Medication Administration: Intraspinal
Medication Administration: Intravenous (IV)
Medication Administration: Nasal
Medication Administration: Oral
Medication Administration: Rectal
Medication Administration: Skin
Medication Administration: Subcutaneous
Medication Administration: Vaginal
Medication Administration: Ventricular Reservoir
Medication Management
Medication Prescribing
Medication Reconciliation
Meditation Facilitation
Memory Training
Milieu Therapy
Mood Management
Multidisciplinary Care Conference

Music Therapy
Mutual Goal Setting

Nail Care
Nausea Management
Neurologic Monitoring
Newborn Care
Newborn Monitoring
Nonnutritive Sucking
Normalization Promotion
Nutrition Management
Nutrition Therapy
Nutritional Counseling
Nutritional Monitoring

Oral Health Maintenance
Oral Health Promotion
Oral Health Restoration
Order Transcription
Organ Procurement
Ostomy Care
Oxygen Therapy

Pacemaker Management: Temporary
Pacemaker Management: Permanent
Pain Management
Parent Education: Adolescent
Parent Education: Childbearing Family
Parent Education: Infant
Parenting Promotion
Pass Facilitation
Patient Contracting
Patient Controlled Analgesia (PCA) Assistance
Patient Rights Protection
Peer Review
Pelvic Muscle Exercise
Perineal Care
Peripheral Sensation Management
Peripherally Inserted Central (PIC) Catheter Care
Peritoneal Dialysis Therapy
Pessary Management
Phlebotomy: Arterial Blood Sample
Phlebotomy: Blood Unit Acquisition
Phlebotomy: Cannulated Vessel
Phlebotomy: Venous Blood Sample
Phototherapy: Mood/Sleep Regulation
Phototherapy: Neonate
Physical Restraint
Physician Support
Pneumatic Tourniquet Precautions
Positioning
Positioning: Intraoperative
Positioning: Neurologic
Positioning: Wheelchair
Postanesthesia Care
Postmortem Care

(table continues on page 14)

TABLE 2.1 **Nursing Interventions Classification Labels** (continued)

Postpartal Care
Preceptor: Employee
Preceptor: Student
Preconception Counseling
Pregnancy Termination Care
Premenstrual Syndrome (PMS) Management
Prenatal Care
Preoperative Coordination
Preparatory Sensory Information
Presence
Pressure Management
Pressure Ulcer Care
Pressure Ulcer Prevention
Product Evaluation
Program Development
Progressive Muscle Relaxation
Prompted Voiding
Prosthesis Care
Pruritus Management

Quality Monitoring

Radiation Therapy Management
Rape-Trauma Treatment
Reality Orientation
Recreation Therapy
Rectal Prolapse Management
Referral
Relaxation Therapy
Religious Addiction Prevention
Religious Ritual Enhancement
Relocation Stress Reduction
Reminiscence Therapy
Reproductive Technology Management
Research Data Collection
Resiliency Promotion
Respiratory Monitoring
Respite Care
Resuscitation
Resuscitation: Fetus
Resuscitation: Neonate
Risk Identification
Risk Identification: Childbearing Family
Risk Identification: Genetic
Role Enhancement

Seclusion
Security Enhancement
Seduction Management
Seizure Management
Seizure Precautions
Self-Awareness Enhancement
Self-Care Assistance
Self-Care Assistance: Bathing/Hygiene
Self-Care Assistance: Dressing/Grooming
Self-Care Assistance: Feeding
Self-Care Assistance: IADL

Self-Care Assistance: Toileting
Self-Care Assistance: Transfer
Self-Efficacy Enhancement
Self-Esteem Enhancement
Self-Hypnosis Facilitation
Self-Modification Assistance
Self-Responsibility Facilitation
Sexual Counseling
Shift Report
Shock Management
Shock Management: Cardiac
Shock Management: Vasogenic
Shock Management: Volume
Shock Prevention
Sibling Support
Skin Care: Donor Site
Skin Care: Graft Site
Skin Care: Topical Treatments
Skin Surveillance
Sleep Enhancement
Smoking Cessation Assistance
Social Marketing
Socialization Enhancement
Specimen Management
Spiritual Growth Facilitation
Spiritual Support
Splinting
Sports-Injury Prevention: Youth
Staff Development
Staff Supervision
Subarachnoid Hemorrhage Precautions
Substance Use Prevention
Substance Use Treatment
Substance Use Treatment: Alcohol Withdrawal
Substance Use Treatment: Drug Withdrawal
Substance Use Treatment: Overdose
Suicide Prevention
Supply Management
Support Group
Support System Enhancement
Surgical Assistance
Surgical Precautions
Surgical Preparation
Surveillance
Surveillance: Community
Surveillance: Late Pregnancy
Surveillance: Remote Electronic
Surveillance: Safety
Sustenance Support
Suturing
Swallowing Therapy

Teaching: Disease Process
Teaching: Foot Care
Teaching: Group
Teaching: Individual
Teaching: Infant Nutrition 0–3 Months

TABLE 2.1   continued

Teaching: Infant Nutrition 4–6 Months	Transport: Intrafacility
Teaching: Infant Nutrition 7–9 Months	Trauma Therapy: Child
Teaching: Infant Nutrition 10–12 Months	Triage: Disaster
Teaching: Infant Safety 0–3 Months	Triage: Emergency Center
Teaching: Infant Safety 4–6 Months	Triage: Telephone
Teaching: Infant Safety 7–9 Months	Truth Telling
Teaching: Infant Safety 10–12 Months	Tube Care
Teaching: Infant Stimulation 0–4 Months	Tube Care: Chest
Teaching: Infant Stimulation 5–8 Months	Tube Care: Gastrointestinal
Teaching: Infant Stimulation 9–12 Months	Tube Care: Umbilical Line
Teaching: Preoperative	Tube Care: Urinary
Teaching: Prescribed Activity/Exercise	Tube Care: Ventriculostomy/Lumbar Drain
Teaching: Prescribed Diet	
Teaching: Prescribed Medication	Ultrasonography: Limited Obstetric
Teaching: Procedure/Treatment	Unilateral Neglect Management
Teaching: Psychomotor Skill	Urinary Bladder Training
Teaching: Safe Sex	Urinary Catheterization
Teaching: Sexuality	Urinary Catheterization: Intermittent
Teaching: Toddler Nutrition 13–18 Months	Urinary Elimination Management
Teaching: Toddler Nutrition 19–24 Months	Urinary Habit Training
Teaching: Toddler Nutrition 25–36 Months	Urinary Incontinence Care
Teaching: Toddler Safety 13–18 Months	Urinary Incontinence Care: Enuresis
Teaching: Toddler Safety 19–24 Months	Urinary Retention Care
Teaching: Toddler Safety 25–36 Months	
Teaching: Toilet Training	Validation Therapy
Technology Management	Values Clarification
Telephone Consultation	Vehicle Safety Promotion
Telephone Follow-Up	Venous Access Device (VAD) Maintenance
Temperature Regulation	Ventilation Assistance
Temperature Regulation: Intraoperative	Visitation Facilitation
Therapeutic Play	Vital Signs Monitoring
Therapeutic Touch	Vomiting Management
Therapy Group	
Thrombolytic Therapy Management	Weight Gain Assistance
Total Parenteral Nutrition (TPN) Administration	Weight Management
Touch	Weight Reduction Assistance
Traction/Immobilization Care	Wound Care
Transcutaneous Electrical Nerve Stimulation (TENS)	Wound Care: Burns
Transfer	Wound Care: Closed Drainage
Transport: Interfacility	Wound Irrigation

Source: Bulecheck, G., Butcher, H. K., Dochterman, J. (2008). *Nursing Interventions Classifications (NIC)*. 5th ed. St. Louis, MO: Mosby.

NOC is also a comprehensive standardized language providing 330 outcome labels (Table 2.2) with definitions; a set of indicators describing specific client, caregiver, family, or community states related to the outcome; and a 5-point Likert-type scale that facilitates tracking clients across care settings and that can demonstrate client progress even when outcomes are not fully met. The outcomes are research-based and are applicable in all care settings and clinical specialties.

TABLE 2.2   Nursing Outcomes Classification Labels

Abuse Cessation
Abuse Protection
Abuse Recovery
Abuse Recovery: Emotional
Abuse Recovery: Financial
Abuse Recovery: Physical
Abuse Recovery: Sexual
Abusive Behavior Self-Restraint
Acceptance: Health Status
Activity Tolerance
Acute Confusion Level
Adaptation to Physical Disability
Adherence Behavior
Adherence Behavior: Healthy Diet
Aggression Self-Control
Agitation Level
Alcohol Abuse Cessation Behavior
Allergic Response: Localized
Allergic Response: Systemic
Ambulation
Ambulation: Wheelchair
Anxiety Level
Anxiety Self-Control
Appetite
Aspiration Prevention
Asthma Self-Management

Balance
Blood Coagulation
Blood Glucose Level
Blood Loss Severity
Blood Transfusion Reaction
Body Image
Body Mechanics Performance
Body Positioning: Self-Initiated
Bone Healing
Bowel Continence
Bowel Elimination
Breastfeeding Establishment: Infant
Breastfeeding Establishment: Maternal
Breastfeeding Maintenance
Breastfeeding Weaning
Burn Healing
Burn Recovery

Cardiac Disease Self-Management
Cardiac Pump Effectiveness
Cardiopulmonary Status
Caregiver Adaptation to Patient Institutionalization
Caregiver Emotional Health
Caregiver Home Care Readiness
Caregiver Lifestyle Disruption
Caregiver-Patient Relationship
Caregiver Performance: Direct Care
Caregiver Performance: Indirect Care
Caregiver Physical Health
Caregiver Role Endurance
Caregiver Stressors

Caregiver Well-Being
Child Adaptation to Hospitalization
Child Development: 1 Month
Child Development: 2 Months
Child Development: 4 Months
Child Development: 6 Months
Child Development: 12 Months
Child Development: 2 Years
Child Development: 3 Years
Child Development: 4 Years
Child Development: Preschool
Child Development: Middle Childhood
Child Development: Adolescence
Circulation Status
Client Satisfaction
Client Satisfaction: Access to Care Resources
Client Satisfaction: Caring
Client Satisfaction: Case Management
Client Satisfaction: Communication
Client Satisfaction: Continuity of Care
Client Satisfaction: Cultural Needs Fulfillment
Client Satisfaction: Functional Assistance
Client Satisfaction: Pain Management
Client Satisfaction: Physical Care
Client Satisfaction: Physical Environment
Client Satisfaction: Protection of Rights
Client Satisfaction: Psychological Care
Client Satisfaction: Safety
Client Satisfaction: Symptom Control
Client Satisfaction: Teaching
Client Satisfaction: Technical Aspects of Care
Cognition
Cognitive Orientation
Comfort Status
Comfort Status: Environment
Comfort Status: Physical
Comfort Status: Psychospiritual
Comfort Status: Sociocultural
Comfortable Death
Communication
Communication: Expressive
Communication: Receptive
Community Competence
Community Disaster Readiness
Community Disaster Response
Community Health Status
Community Health Status: Immunity
Community Risk Control: Chronic Disease
Community Risk Control: Communicable Disease
Community Risk Control: Lead Exposure
Community Risk Control: Violence
Community Violence Level
Compliance Behavior
Compliance Behavior: Prescribed Diet
Compliance Behavior: Prescribed Medication
Concentration
Coordinated Movement
Coping

TABLE 2.2   continued

Decision-Making
Depression Level
Depression Self-Control
Development: Late Adulthood
Development: Middle Adulthood
Development: Young Adulthood
Diabetes Self-Management
Dignified Life Closure
Discharge Readiness: Independent Living
Discharge Readiness: Supported Living
Discomfort Level
Distorted Thought Self-Control
Drug Abuse Cessation Behavior

Electrolyte and Acid/Base Balance
Elopement Occurrence
Elopement Propensity Risk
Endurance
Energy Conservation

Fall Prevention Behavior
Falls Occurrence
Family Coping
Family Functioning
Family Health Status
Family Integrity
Family Normalization
Family Participation in Professional Care
Family Physical Environment
Family Resiliency
Family Social Climate
Family Support During Treatment
Fatigue Level
Fear Level
Fear Level: Child
Fear Self-Control
Fetal Status: Antepartum
Fetal Status: Intrapartum
Fluid Balance
Fluid Overload Severity

Gastrointestinal Function
Grief Resolution
Growth

Health Beliefs
Health Beliefs: Perceived Ability to Perform
Health Beliefs: Perceived Control
Health Beliefs: Perceived Resources
Health Beliefs: Perceived Threat
Health Orientation
Health-Promoting Behavior
Health Seeking Behavior
Hearing Compensation Behavior
Heedfulness of Affected Side
Hemodialysis Access

Hope
Hydration
Hyperactivity Level

Identity
Immobility Consequences: Physiological
Immobility Consequences: Psycho-Cognitive
Immune Hypersensitivity Response
Immune Status
Immunization Behavior
Impulse Self-Control
Infection Severity
Infection Severity: Newborn
Information Processing

Joint Movement: Ankle
Joint Movement: Elbow
Joint Movement: Fingers
Joint Movement: Hip
Joint Movement: Knee
Joint Movement: Neck
Joint Movement: Passive
Joint Movement: Shoulder
Joint Movement: Spine
Joint Movement: Wrist

Kidney Function
Knowledge: Arthritis Management
Knowledge: Asthma Management
Knowledge: Body Mechanics
Knowledge: Breastfeeding
Knowledge: Cancer Management
Knowledge: Cancer Threat Reduction
Knowledge: Cardiac Disease Management
Knowledge: Child Physical Safety
Knowledge: Conception Prevention
Knowledge: Congestive Heart Failure Management
Knowledge: Depression Management
Knowledge: Diabetes Management
Knowledge: Diet
Knowledge: Disease Process
Knowledge: Energy Conservation
Knowledge: Fall Prevention
Knowledge: Fertility Promotion
Knowledge: Health Behavior
Knowledge: Health Promotion
Knowledge: Health Resources
Knowledge: Hypertension Management
Knowledge: Illness Care
Knowledge: Infant Care
Knowledge: Infection Management
Knowledge: Labor and Delivery
Knowledge: Medication
Knowledge: Multiple Sclerosis Management
Knowledge: Ostomy Care
Knowledge: Pain Management

(table continues on page 18)

TABLE 2.2 **Nursing Outcomes Classification Labels** (continued)

Knowledge: Parenting
Knowledge: Personal Safety
Knowledge: Postpartum Maternal Health
Knowledge: Preconception Maternal Health
Knowledge: Pregnancy
Knowledge: Pregnancy & Postpartum Sexual Functioning
Knowledge: Prescribed Activity
Knowledge: Preterm Infant Care
Knowledge: Sexual Functioning
Knowledge: Substance Abuse Control
Knowledge: Treatment Procedure(s)
Knowledge: Treatment Regimen
Knowledge: Weight Management

Leisure Participation
Loneliness Severity

Maternal Status: Antepartum
Maternal Status: Intrapartum
Maternal Status: Postpartum
Mechanical Ventilation Response: Adult
Mechanical Ventilation Weaning Response: Adult
Medication Response
Memory
Mobility
Mood Equilibrium
Motivation
Multiple Sclerosis Self-Management

Nausea and Vomiting Control
Nausea and Vomiting: Disruptive Effects
Nausea and Vomiting Severity
Neglect Cessation
Neglect Recovery
Neurological Status
Neurological Status: Autonomic
Neurological Status: Central Motor Control
Neurological Status: Consciousness
Neurological Status: Cranial Sensory/Motor Function
Neurological Status: Peripheral
Neurological Status: Spinal Sensory/Motor Function
Newborn Adaptation
Nutritional Status
Nutritional Status: Biochemical Measures
Nutritional Status: Energy
Nutritional Status: Food & Fluid Intake
Nutritional Status: Nutrient Intake

Oral Hygiene
Ostomy Self-Care

Pain: Adverse Psychological Response
Pain Control
Pain: Disruptive Effects
Pain Level
Parent-Infant Attachment
Parenting: Adolescent Physical Safety

Parenting: Early/Middle Childhood Physical Safety
Parenting: Infant/Toddler Physical Safety
Parenting Performance
Parenting: Psychological Safety
Participation in Healthcare Decisions
Personal Autonomy
Personal Health Status
Personal Resiliency
Personal Safety Behavior
Personal Well-Being
Physical Aging
Physical Fitness
Physical Injury Severity
Physical Maturation: Female
Physical Maturation: Male
Play Participation
Postpartum Maternal Health Behavior
Post-Procedure Recovery
Prenatal Health Behavior
Pre-Procedure Readiness
Preterm Infant Organization
Psychomotor Energy
Psychosocial Adjustment: Life Change

Quality of Life

Respiratory Status
Respiratory Status: Airway Patency
Respiratory Status: Gas Exchange
Respiratory Status: Ventilation
Rest
Risk Control
Risk Control: Alcohol Use
Risk Control: Cancer
Risk Control: Cardiovascular Health
Risk Control: Drug Use
Risk Control: Hearing Impairment
Risk Control: Hyperthermia
Risk Control: Hypothermia
Risk Control: Infectious Process
Risk Control: Sexually Transmitted Diseases (STD)
Risk Control: Sun Exposure
Risk Control: Tobacco Use
Risk Control: Unintended Pregnancy
Risk Control: Visual Impairment
Risk Detection
Role Performance

Safe Home Environment
Safe Wandering
Seizure Control
Self-Care Status
Self-Care: Activities of Daily Living (ADL)
Self-Care: Bathing
Self-Care: Dressing
Self-Care: Eating
Self-Care: Hygiene

TABLE 2.2 continued

Self-Care: Instrumental Activities of Daily Living (IADL)
Self-Care: Non-Parenteral Medications
Self-Care: Oral Hygiene
Self-Care: Parenteral Medication
Self-Care: Toileting
Self Direction of Care
Self-Esteem
Self-Mutilation Restraint
Sensory Function
Sensory Function: Cutaneous
Sensory Function: Hearing
Sensory Function: Proprioception
Sensory Function: Taste and Smell
Sensory Function: Vision
Sexual Functioning
Sexual Identity
Skeletal Function
Sleep
Smoking Cessation Behavior
Social Interaction Skills
Social Involvement
Social Support
Spiritual Health
Stress Level
Student Health Status
Substance Addiction: Consequences
Substance Withdrawal Severity
Suffering Severity
Suicide Self-Restraint
Swallowing Status
Swallowing Status: Esophageal Phase
Swallowing Status: Oral Phase

Swallowing Status: Pharyngeal Phase
Symptom Control
Symptom Severity
Symptom Severity: Perimenopause
Symptom Severity: Premenstrual Syndrome
Systemic Toxic Clearance: Dialysis

Thermoregulation
Thermoregulation: Newborn
Tissue Integrity: Skin and Mucous Membranes
Tissue Perfusion: Abdominal Organs
Tissue Perfusion: Cardiac
Tissue Perfusion: Cellular
Tissue Perfusion: Cerebral
Tissue Perfusion: Peripheral
Tissue Perfusion: Pulmonary
Transfer Performance
Treatment Behavior: Illness or Injury

Urinary Continence
Urinary Elimination

Vision Compensation Behavior
Vital Signs

Weight: Body Mass
Weight Gain Behavior
Weight Loss Behavior
Weight Maintenance Behavior
Will to Live
Wound Healing: Primary Intention
Wound Healing: Secondary Intention

Source: Moorhead, S., Johnson, M., Maas, M. L., Swanson, E. (eds.). (2008). *Nursing Outcomes Classifications (NOC)*. 4th ed. St. Louis, MO: Mosby.

In addition, NIC and NOC have been linked to the Omaha System problems, to resident assessment protocols (RAPs) used in extended/long-term care settings, and to NANDA-I. This last linkage created the NANDA, NIC, NOC (NNN) Taxonomy of Nursing Practice. The combination of NANDA-I nursing diagnoses, NOC outcomes, and NIC interventions in a common unifying structure provides a comprehensive nursing language recognized by the American Nurses Association (ANA) that is coded in the Systematized Nomenclature of Medicine (SNOMED), a multidisciplinary terminology supporting the electronic client record.

Having an SNL entered into international coded terminology allows nursing to describe the care received by the client and to document the effects of that care on client outcomes, and it facilitates the comparison of nursing care across worldwide settings and diverse databases. In addition, it supports research by comparing client care delivered by nurses with that delivered by other providers, which is essential if nursing's contribution is to be recognized and nurses are to be reimbursed for the care they provide.

The 13 versions of SNLs (consisting of two data element sets and 10 terminologies) recognized by the ANA have been submitted to the National Library of Medicine for inclusion in the Unified Medical Language System Metathesaurus. The Metathesaurus provides a uniform, integrated distribution format from over 100 biomedical vocabularies and classifications (the majority in English and some in multiple languages), and it links many different names for the same concepts, establishing new relationships among terms from different source vocabularies.

Indexing of the entire medical record supports disease management activities (including decision support systems), research, and analysis of outcomes for quality improvement for all healthcare disciplines. Coding also supports telehealth (the use of telecommunications technology to provide medical information and healthcare services over distance) and facilitates access to healthcare data across care settings and different computer systems.

So, to those who stated, "Nursing will thrive as a unique and valued profession when nurses present a theory and rationalistic model for their practice . . . and actively participate in processes for change,"[13] we answer, "We are actively participating in processes for change, and as a profession, we will continue to grow."

References

1. Clark, J., Lang, N. (1992). Nursing's next advance: An internal classification for nursing practice. *Int Nurs Rev*, 39, 109–111, 128.
2. Gordon, M. (1998). Nursing nomenclature and classification system development. *Online J Issues Nurs*. Retrieved 2004 from http://nursingworld.org/ojin/tpc7/tpc7_1.htm.
3. NANDA International. (2003). *Nursing Diagnoses: Definitions & Classifications 2003–2004*. Philadelphia: Author.
4. Carroll-Johnson, R. M. (ed). (1991). *Classification of Nursing Diagnoses: Proceedings of the Ninth Conference*. Philadelphia: J. B. Lippincott.
5. Saba, V. K. (1994). *Home Health Care Classification (HHCC) of Nursing Diagnoses and Interventions* (Revised). Washington, DC: Author.
6. Saba, V. K. (2007). *Clinical Care Classification (CCC) System Manual: A Guide to Nursing Documentation*. New York: Springer.
7. McCloskey, J. C., Bulechek, G. M. (eds). (2004). *Nursing Interventions Classification (NIC)*. 4th ed. St. Louis, MO: Mosby.
8. Moorhead, S., Johnson, M., Maas, M. (eds). (2004). *Nursing Outcomes Classification (NOC)*. 3d ed. St. Louis, MO: Mosby.
9. Martin, K. S., Scheet, N. J. (1992). *The Omaha System: Applications for Community Health Nursing*. Philadelphia: W. B. Saunders.
10. Ozboldt, J. G. (1996). From minimum data to maximum impact: Using clinical data to strengthen patient care. *Adv Pract Nurs Q*, 1, 62–69.
11. Beyea, S. (2002). *Perioperative Nursing Data Set (PNDS)*. 2d ed. Denver: AORN.
12. Johnson, M., et al. (2001). *Nursing Diagnoses, Outcomes, and Interventions: NANDA, NOC, and NIC Linkages*. St. Louis, MO: Mosby.
13. Erickson, H. C., Tomlin, E. M., Swain, M. A. P. (1983). *Modeling and Role-Modeling*. Englewood Cliffs, NJ: Prentice-Hall.

CHAPTER 3

The Assessment Process: Developing the Client Database

The *Nursing: Scope & Standards of Practice*[1] addresses the assessment process. The standard stipulates that the data-collection process is systematic and ongoing. The nurse collects client health data from the client, significant others, and healthcare providers when appropriate. The priority of the data-collection activities is determined by the client's immediate condition or needs. Pertinent data are collected using appropriate assessment techniques and instruments. Relevant data are documented in a retrievable form.

The Client Database

The assessment step of the nursing process is focused on eliciting a profile of the client that allows the nurse to identify client problems or needs and corresponding nursing diagnoses, to plan care, to implement interventions, and to evaluate outcomes. This profile, or *client database*, supplies a sense of the client's overall health status, providing a picture of the client's physical, psychological, sociocultural, spiritual, cognitive, and developmental levels; economic status; functional abilities; and lifestyle. It is a combination of data gathered from the history-taking interview (a method of obtaining SUBJECTIVE information by talking with the client or significant others and listening to their responses), from the physical examination (a "hands-on" means of obtaining OBJECTIVE information), and from the results of laboratory tests and diagnostic studies. To be more specific, subjective data are what the client/significant others perceive and report, and objective data are what the nurse observes and gathers from other sources.

Assessment involves three basic activities:

- Systematically gathering data
- Organizing or clustering the data collected
- Documenting the data in a retrievable format

Gathering Data—The Interview

Information in the client database is obtained primarily from the client (who is the most important or primary source) and then from family members/significant others (secondary sources), as appropriate, through conversation and by observation during a structured interview. Clearly, the interview involves more than simply exchanging and processing data. Nonverbal communication is as important as the client's choice of words in providing the data. The ability to collect data that are meaningful to the client's health concerns depends heavily on the nurse's knowledge base; on the choice and sequence of questions; and on the ability to give meaning to the client's responses, integrate the data gathered, and prioritize the resulting information. Insight into the nature and behavior of the client is essential as well.

The nurse's initial responsibility is to observe, collect, and record data without drawing conclusions or making judgments or assumptions. Self-awareness is a crucial factor in the interaction, because perceptions, judgments, and assumptions can easily color the assessment findings unless they are recognized.

The quality of a history improves with experience with the interviewing process. Tips for obtaining a meaningful history include the following:

• Be a good listener.
• Listen carefully and attentively for whole thoughts and ideas, not merely isolated facts.
• Use skills of active listening, silence, and acceptance to provide ample time for the person to respond. Be as objective as possible.
• Identify only the client's or significant others' contributions to the history.

The interview question is the major tool used to acquire information. How the question is phrased is a skill that is important in obtaining the desired results and in getting the information necessary to make accurate nursing diagnoses. *Note:* Some questioning strategies to avoid include closed-ended and leading questions, probing, and agreeing or disagreeing that implies the client is "right" or "wrong." It is important to remember, too, that the client has the right to refuse to answer any question, no matter how reasonably phrased.

Nine effective data-collection questioning techniques include the following:

1. Open-ended questions allow clients maximum freedom to respond in their own way, impose no limitations on how the question may be answered, and can produce considerable information.
2. Hypothetical questions pose a situation and ask the client how it might be handled.
3. Reflecting or "mirroring" responses is a useful technique in getting at underlying meanings that might not be verbalized clearly.
4. Focusing consists of eye contact (within cultural limits), body posture, and verbal responses.
5. Giving broad openings encourages the client to take the initiative in what is to be discussed.
6. Offering general leads encourages the client to continue.
7. Exploring pursues a topic in more depth.
8. Verbalizing the implied gives voice to what has been suggested.
9. Encouraging evaluation helps clients to consider the quality of their own experiences.

The client's medical diagnosis can provide a starting point for gathering data. Knowledge of the anatomy and physiology of the specific disease process and severity of the condition also helps in choosing and prioritizing precise portions of the assessment. For example, when examining a client with severe chest pain, it may be wise to evaluate the pain and the cardiovascular system in a focused assessment before addressing other areas, possibly at a later time. Likewise, the duration and length of any assessment depend on circumstances such as the client's condition and the situation's urgency.

The data collected about the client or significant others contain a vast amount of information, some of which may be repetitive. However, some of it will be valuable for eliciting information that was not recalled or volunteered previously. Enough material needs to be noted in the history so that a complete picture is presented, and yet not so much that the information will not be read or used.

Gathering Data—The Physical Examination

The physical examination is performed to gather objective information and serves as a screening device. Four common methods used during the physical examination are inspection, palpation, percussion, and auscultation. These techniques incorporate the senses of sight, hearing, touch, and smell. For the data collected during the physical examination to be meaningful, it is vital to know the normal physical and emotional characteristics of humans well enough to be able to recognize deviations. To gain as much information as possible from the assessment procedure, the same format should be used each time a physical examination is performed to lessen the possibility of omissions.

Gathering Data—Laboratory Tests/Diagnostic Procedures

Laboratory and other diagnostic studies are a part of the information-gathering stage providing supportive evidence. These studies aid in the management, maintenance, and restoration of health. In reviewing and interpreting laboratory tests, it is important to remember that the origin of the test material does not always correlate to an organ or body system (e.g., a urine test to detect the presence of bilirubin and urobilinogen could indicate liver disease, biliary obstruction, or hemolytic disease). In some cases, the results of a test are *nonspecific,* because they indicate only a disorder or abnormality and not the location of the cause of the problem (e.g., an elevated erythrocyte sedimentation rate suggests the presence but not the location of an inflammatory process).

In evaluating laboratory tests, it is advisable to consider which medications (e.g., heparin, promethazine) are being administered to the client, including over-the-counter and herbal supplements (e.g., vitamin E), because these have the potential to alter, blur, or falsify results, creating a misleading diagnostic picture.

Documenting and Clustering the Data

Data gathered during the interview and physical examination, and from other records/sources, are organized and recorded in a concise, systematic way and clustered into similar categories. Various formats have been used to accomplish this, including a review of body systems. This approach has been utilized by both medicine and nursing for many years but was initially developed to aid the physician in making medical diagnoses. Currently, nursing is developing and fine-tuning its own tools for recording and clustering data. Several nursing models available to guide data collection include Doenges and Moorhouse Diagnostic Divisions (Table 3.1),[2,3] Gordon's Functional Health Patterns,[4] and Guzzetta's Clinical Assessment Tool.[5]

TABLE 3.1 **General Assessment Tool**

This is a suggested guideline/tool applicable in most care settings for creating a client database. It provides a nursing focus (Doenges & Moorhouse's Diagnostic Divisions of Nursing Diagnoses) that will facilitate planning client care. Although the sections are alphabetized here for ease of presentation, they can be prioritized or rearranged to meet individual needs.

Adult Medical/Surgical Assessment Tool

General Information

Name: _____ Age: _____ DOB: _____ Gender: _____ Race: _____
Admission Date: _____ Time: _____ From: _____
Reason for this visit/admission (primary concern): _____
Source of information: _____ Reliability (1–4 with 4 = very reliable): _____

Activity/Rest

Subjective (Reports)
Occupation: _____ Able to participate in usual activities/hobbies: _____ Leisure time/diversional activities: _____
Ambulatory: _____ Gait (describe): _____ Activity level (sedentary to very active): _____ Daily exercise (type): _____
Changes in muscle mass/tone/strength: _____
History of problems/limitations imposed by condition (e.g., immobility, transfer difficulties, weakness, breathlessness): _
_____
Feelings (e.g., exhaustion, restlessness, boredom, dissatisfaction): _____
Developmental factors (e.g., delayed/age): _____
Sleep: Hours: _____ Naps: _____ Aids: _____ Insomnia: _____ Related to: _____
  Difficulty falling asleep: _____ Difficulty staying asleep: _____
  Rested on awakening: _____ Excessive grogginess: _____ Bedtime rituals: _____
  Relaxation techniques: _____ Sleeps on more than one pillow: _____
Use of oxygen (type): _____ When used: _____
Medications or herbals for/affecting sleep: _____
Objective (Exhibits)
Observed response to activity: Heart rate: _____ Rhythm (reg/irreg): _____ Blood pressure: _____ Respiratory rate: _____
  Pulse oximetry: _____
Mental status (e.g., cognitive impairment, withdrawn/lethargic): _____
Neuromuscular assessment: Muscle mass/tone: _____ Posture (e.g., normal, stooped, curved spine): _____
  Tremors (location): _____ ROM: _____
  Strength: _____ Deformity: _____
Mobility aids (list): _____

Circulation

Subjective (Reports)
History of/treatment date: High blood pressure: ___ Brain injury: ___ Stroke: ___ Heart condition/surgery: ___ Rheumatic
  fever: ___ Palpitations: ___ Syncope: ___ Pain in legs: ___ Ankle/leg edema: ___ Blood clots: ___ Bleeding tendencies: ___
  Spinal cord injury/dysreflexia episodes (describe): _____
Slow/delayed healing (describe): _____
Extremities: Numbness (location): _____ Tingling (location): _____
Cough (describe)/hemoptysis: _____
Change in frequency/amount of urine: _____
Medications/herbals: _____
Objective (Exhibits)
Color (e.g., pale, cyanotic, jaundiced, mottled, ruddy): Skin: _____ Mucous membranes: _____ Lips: _____ Nailbeds: _____
  Conjunctiva: _____ Sclera: _____
Skin moisture (e.g., dry, diaphoretic): _____
BP (R & L): Lying: _____ Sitting: _____ Standing: _____ Pulse pressure: _____ Auscultatory gap: _____
Pulses (palpated 1–4 strength): Carotid: _____ Temporal: _____ Jugular: _____ Radial: _____ Femoral: _____ Popliteal: _____
  Posttibial: _____ Dorsalis pedis: _____
Cardiac (palpation): Thrill: _____ Heaves: _____
Heart sounds (auscultation): Rate: _____ Rhythm: _____ Quality: _____ Friction rub: _____
  Murmur (describe location/sounds): _____

TABLE 3.1 continued

Vascular bruit (location): _____ Jugular vein distention: _____

Breath sounds (describe location & sounds): _____

Extremities. Temperature: ___ Color: ___ Capillary refill (1–3 sec): ___ Edema (+1 to +4): ___ Homans sign (+ or –): ___

Varicosities (location): _____ Nail abnormalities: _____ Distribution/quality of hair: _____ Trophic skin changes: _____

Ego Integrity

Subjective (Reports)

Relationship status: _____

Expressed concerns (e.g., financial, relationships, recent or anticipated lifestyle/role changes): _____

Stress factors: _____ Usual ways of handling stress: _____

Expression of feelings of: Anger: _____ Anxiety: _____ Fear: _____ Grief: _____ Helplessness: _____ Hopelessness: _____

Powerlessness: _____

Cultural factors/ethnic ties: _____

Religious affiliation: _____ Active/practicing: _____ Practices prayer/meditation: _____

Religious/spiritual concerns: _____ Desires clergy visit: _____

Expression of sense of connectedness/harmony with self and others: _____

Medications/herbals: _____

Objective (Exhibits)

Emotional status (check those that apply):

Calm: _____ Anxious: _____ Angry: _____ Withdrawn: _____ Fearful: _____ Irritable: _____ Restive: _____ Euphoric: _____

Observed body language: _____ Observed physiological responses (e.g., crying, change in voice quality/volume): _____

Changes in energy field: Temperature: _____ Color: _____ Distribution: _____ Movement: _____ Sounds: _____

Elimination

Subjective (Reports)

Usual bowel elimination pattern: ___ Character of stool (e.g., hard, soft, liquid): ___ Stool color (e.g., brown, black, yellow, clay colored, tarry): _____ Last BM/Character of stool: _____ Constipation (acute/chronic): _____

Diarrhea (acute/chronic): _____ Bowel incontinence: _____ History of bleeding: _____ Hemorrhoids/fistula: _____

Laxative use: _____ How often: _____ Enema/suppository: _____ How often: _____

Usual voiding pattern and character of urine. _____

Difficulty voiding: _____ Urgency: _____ Frequency: _____ Retention: _____ Bladder spasms: _____

Pain/burning: _____

Urinary incontinence (type & time of day usually occurs): _____

History of kidney/bladder disease: _____

Diuretic use: _____ Other medications/herbals: _____

Objective (Exhibits)

Abdomen (auscultation): Bowel sounds (location/type): ___ Abdomen (palpation): Soft/firm: ___ Tenderness/pain (quadrant location): _____ Distention: _____ Palpable mass: _____ Size/girth: _____

CVA tenderness: _____

Bladder palpable: _____ Residual (per scan): _____ Overflow voiding: _____

Rectal sphincter tone (describe): _____ Hemorrhoids/fistulas: _____

Stool in rectum: _____ Impaction: _____ Occult blood: (+ or –): _____

Presence/use of catheter or continence devices: _____ Ostomy appliances (describe appliance and location): _____

Food/Fluid

Subjective (Reports)

Usual diet (type): ___ Calorie/carbohydrate/protein/fat (g/day): ___ # of meals daily: ___ Snacks (# daily, time consumed, type): _____

Last meal consumed/content: ___ _____

Food preferences: _____ Food allergies/intolerances: _____

Cultural or religious food preparation concerns/prohibitions: _____

Usual appetite: _____ Change in appetite: _____

Usual weight: _____ Unexpected/undesired weight loss or gain: _____

Nausea/vomiting: _____ related to? _____ Heartburn/indigestion: _____ related to? _____ relieved by? _____

(table continues on page 26)

TABLE 3.1 **General Assessment Tool** (continued)

Chewing/swallowing problems: _____ Gag/swallow reflex (present): _____
Facial injury/surgery: _____ Stroke/other neurologic deficit: _____
Teeth: Normal: _____ Dentures (full/partial): _____ Loose/absent teeth: _____ Sore mouth/gums: _____
Dental hygiene practices: _____ Professional dental care/frequency: _____
Diabetes/type: _____ Controlled with diet/pills/insulin: _____
Vitamin/food supplement use: _____ Medications/herbals: _____

Objective (Exhibits)
Current weight: _____ Height: _____ Body build: _____ Body fat %: _____
Skin turgor (e.g., firm, supple, dehydrated): _____ Mucous membranes (moist/dry): _____
Edema (describe): Generalized: _____ Dependent: _____ Feet/ankles: _____ Periorbital: _____ Abdominal/ascites: _____
Jugular vein distention: _____
Breath sounds (auscultation)/location: Normal: _____ Diminished: _____ Crackles: _____ Wheezes: _____
Condition of teeth/gums: _____ Appearance of tongue: _____ Mucous membranes: _____
Bowel sounds (quadrant location/type): _____ Hernia/masses: _____
Urine S/A or Chemstix: _____ Serum glucose (Glucometer): _____

Hygiene

Subjective (Reports)
Ability to carry out activities of daily living: Independent/dependent (level 1, *no assistance needed*, to level 4, *completely dependent*):
Mobility: _____ Needs assistance (describe): _____ Assistance provided by: _____
Equipment/prosthetic devices required: _____
Feeding: _____ Needs assistance preparing/eating (describe): _____ Assistive devices: _____
Bathing: _____ Needs assistance setup/regulating water temp/washing body parts (describe): _____ Preferred time of personal care/bath: _____
Dressing: _____ Needs assistance selecting clothing/dressing self (describe): _____
Toileting: _____ Needs assistance transferring/cleaning self (describe): _____

Objective (Exhibits)
General appearance: Manner of dress: _____ Grooming/personal habits: _____
Condition of hair/scalp: _____
Body odor: _____ Presence of vermin (e.g., lice, scabies): _____

Neurosensory

Subjective (Reports)
History of brain injury, trauma, stroke (residual effects): _____
Fainting spells/dizziness: _____ Headaches (location/type/frequency): _____
Tingling/numbness/weakness (location): _____
Seizures: _____ History/onset: _____ Type (e.g., generalized, partial): _____ Frequency: _____ Aura (describe): _____
Postictal state: _____ How controlled: _____
Vision loss/changes: ____ Glasses/contacts: ____ Last exam: ____ Glaucoma: ____ Cataract: ____ Eye surgery (type/date): ____
Hearing loss: _____ Sudden/gradual: _____ Hearing aids: _____ Last exam: _____
Sense of smell (changes): _____ Epistaxis: _____
Sense of taste (changes): _____
Other: _____

Objective (Exhibits)
Mental status (note duration of change):
Oriented: Time: _____ Place: _____ Person: _____ Situation: _____
Check all that apply: Alert: _____ Drowsy: _____ Lethargic: _____ Stuporous: _____ Comatose: _____
Cooperative: _____ Follows commands: _____ Agitated/restless: _____ Combative: _____
Delusions (describe): _____ Hallucinations (describe): _____
Affect (describe): _____ Speech: _____
Memory: Recent: _____ Remote: _____
Pupil shape: _____ Size/reaction: R/L: _____ Accommodation: _____
Facial droop: _____ Swallowing: _____
Handgrasp/release, R: _____ L: _____

TABLE 3.1   continued

Coordination: _____ Balance: _____ Walking: ___ _____
Deep tendon reflexes (present/absent/location): _____ Tremors: _____ Posturing: _____ Paralysis (L/R): _____

Pain/Discomfort

Subjective (Reports)
Primary focus: Location: _____ Intensity (use pain scale/pictures): _____
 Quality (e.g., stabbing, aching, burning): _____ Radiation: _____ _____
 Frequency: _____ Duration: _____
Precipitating/aggravating factors: _____
How relieved: OTC/prescription: _____ Nonpharmaceuticals/therapies: ___ _____
Associated symptoms (e.g., nausea, sleep problems, photosensitivity): _____
Effect on daily activities: _____ Relationships: _____ Job: _____ Enjoyment of life: _____
Additional pain focus/describe: _____
Cultural expectations regarding pain perception and expression: _____

Objective (Exhibits)
Facial grimacing: _____ Guarding affected area: _____ Posturing: _____ Behaviors: _____ Narrowed focus: _____
Emotional response (e.g., crying, withdrawal, anger): _____
Vital sign changes (acute pain): BP: _____ Pulse: _____ Respirations: _____

Respiration

Subjective (Reports)
Dyspnea/related to: _____ Precipitating factors: _____ Relieving factors: _____
Airway clearance (e.g., spontaneous/device): _____
Cough (e.g., hard, persistent, croupy): _____ Sputum color/character: _____ Requires suctioning: _____
History of/date: Bronchitis: _____ Emphysema: _____ Tuberculosis: _____ Recurrent pneumonia: _____ Exposure to noxious
fumes/allergens, infectious agents/diseases, poisons: _____
Smoker: _____ packs/day: _____ # of pack years: _____ Cigar use: _____ Smokeless: _____
Use of respiratory aids: _____ Oxygen (type & frequency): _____
Medications/herbals: _____ _____

Objective (Exhibits)
Respirations (spontaneous/assisted): _____ Rate: _____ Depth: _____ Chest excursion (e.g., equal/symmetrical): _____ Use of
 accessory muscles: _____ Nasal flaring: _____ Fremitus: _____
Breath sounds (describe): _____ Egophony: _____
Skin/mucous membrane color (e.g., pale, cyanotic): _____ Clubbing of fingers: _____
Sputum characteristics: _____
Mentation (e.g., calm, anxious, restless): _____ _____
Pulse oximetry: _____

Safety

Subjective (Reports)
Allergies/sensitivity (medications, foods, environment, latex): _____
 Type of reaction: _____
Blood transfusion/number: _____ Date: _____ Reaction (describe): ___ _____
Exposure to infectious diseases (e.g., measles, influenza, pink eye): _____
Exposure to pollution, toxins, poisons/pesticides, radiation (describe reactions): _____ _____
Geographic areas lived in/recent travel: _____ _____
Immunization history/date: Tetanus: _____ MMR: _____ Polio: _____ Hepatitis: _____ Pneumonia: _____ Influenza: _____ HPV: ___
Altered/suppressed immune system (list cause): ___ _____
History of sexually transmitted disease (date/type): _____ Testing: _____
High-risk behaviors (specify): _____
Uses seat belt regularly: _____ Uses bike helmet: _____ Other safety devices: _____
Work place safety/health issues (describe): _____ Occupation: _____ Currently working: _____ Rate working conditions (e.g.,
safety, noise, heating, water, ventilation): _____ _____
History of accidental injuries: ___ _____ Fractures/dislocations: _____

(table continues on page 28)

TABLE 3.1 **General Assessment Tool** (continued)

Arthritis/unstable joints: _____ Back problems: _____

Skin problems (e.g., rashes, lesions, moles, breast lumps, enlarged nodes)/describe: _____

Delayed healing (describe): _____

Cognitive limitations (e.g., disorientation, confusion): _____

Sensory limitations (e.g., impaired vision/hearing, detecting heat/cold, taste, smell, touch): _____

Prosthesis: _____ Ambulatory devices: _____

Violence (episodes or tendencies): _____

Objective (Exhibits)

Body temperature/method (e.g., oral, rectal, tympanic): _____

Skin integrity (mark location on diagram): Scars: _____ Rashes: _____ Lacerations: _____ Ulcerations: _____ Bruises: _____

Blisters: _____ Drainage: _____ Burns (degree/% of body surface): _____

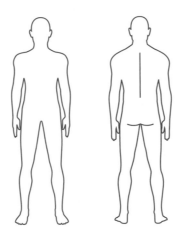

Musculoskeletal: General strength: _____ Muscle tone: _____ Gait: _____ ROM: _____ Paresthesia/paralysis: _____

Results of testing (e.g., cultures, immune function, TB, hepatitis): _____

Sexuality (Component of Social Interaction)

Subjective (Reports)

Sexually active: _____ Monogamous/committed relationship: _____ Use of condoms: _____

Birth control method: _____

Sexual concerns/difficulties: _____ Recent change in frequency/interest: _____ Pain/discomfort: _____

Objective: (Exhibits)

Comfort level with subject matter: _____

Female: Subjective (Reports)

Menstruation: Age at menarche: ___ Length of cycle: ___ Duration: ___ Number of pads/tampons used/day: ___ Last menstrual period: ___ Bleeding between periods: ___ Menopausal: ___ Last period: ___ Hysterectomy (type/date): ___ Problems with: Hot flashes: _____ Night sweats: _____ Vaginal lubrication: _____ Vaginal discharge: _____

Gynecological/breast surgery (type and date): _____

Infertility concerns: _____ Type of therapy: _____

Pregnant now: _____ Para: _____ Gravida: _____ Due date: _____

Practices breast self-examination: _____ Last mammogram: _____ Last Pap smear/results: _____

Hormonal therapy: _____ Supplemental calcium: _____ Other medications/herbals: _____

Objective (Exhibits)

Breast examination: _____

Genitalia: _____ Warts/lesions: _____ Vaginal bleeding/discharge: _____

Test results: _____ Pap: _____ Mammogram: _____ STD: _____

Male: Subjective (Reports)

Penis: Circumcised: _____ Lesions/discharge: _____ Vasectomy: _____

Prostate disorder/voiding difficulties: _____

TABLE 3.1 continued

Practice self examination. Breast: _____ Testicles: _____
Last proctoscopic/prostate examination: _____ Last PSA: _____
Medications/herbals: _____

Objective (Exhibits)
Genitalia: Penis: _____ Warts/lesions: _____ Bleeding/discharge: _____ Testicles (e.g., descended, lumps): _____
Prostate: _____
Breast examination: _____
Test results: _____ STD: _____ PSA: _____

Social Interactions

Subjective (Reports)
Relationship status: Single: _____ Married: _____ Living with partner: _____ Divorced: _____ Widowed: _____
  Years in relationship: _____ Perception of relationship: _____ Concerns/stresses: _____
Role within family structure: _____ Number/age of children: _____
  Individuals living in home: _____ Caregiver (to whom & how long): _____
Extended family/availability: _____ Other support person(s): _____
Perception of relationship with family members: _____
Ethnic/cultural affiliation: _____ Strength of ethnic identity: _____ Lives in ethnic community: _____
Feelings of (describe): Mistrust: _____ Rejection: _____ Unhappiness: _____ Loneliness/isolation: _____
Problems related to illness/condition: _____
Difficulties with communication (e.g., speech, another language, brain injury): _____
  Use of communication aids (list): _____ Requires interpreter: _____
Genogram: (complete on separate form)
Objective (Exhibits)
Communication/speech: Clear: _____ Slurred: _____ Unintelligible: _____ Aphasic: _____
  Unusual speech pattern/impairment: _____ Laryngectomy present: _____
  Use of speech/communication aids: _____
Verbal/nonverbal communication with family/SO(s): _____
  Family interaction (behavioral) pattern: _____

Teaching/Learning

Subjective (Reports)
Communication: Dominant language (specify): _____ Second language: _____
  Literate (reading/writing): _____
Education level: _____ Learning disabilities (specify): _____ Cognitive limitations: _____
Culture/ethnicity: _____ Where born: _____ If immigrant, how long in this country: _____
Health and illness beliefs/practices/customs: _____
  Which family member makes healthcare decisions/is spokesperson for client: _____
Presence of Advance Directives: _____ Code status: _____ Durable Medical Power of Attorney: _____ Designee: _____
Health goals: _____
Current health problem: _____ Client understanding of problem: _____
Special healthcare concerns (e.g., impact of religious/cultural practices, healthcare decisions, family involvement): _____
Familial risk factors (indicate relationship): Diabetes: _____ Thyroid (specify): _____ Tuberculosis: _____ Heart disease: _____
  Stroke: _____ High BP: _____
  Epilepsy/seizures: _____ Kidney disease: _____ Cancer: _____ Mental illness/depression: _____ Other: _____
Prescribed medications (list each separately):
  Drug: _____ Dose: _____ Times (circle last dose): _____
  Take regularly: _____ Purpose: _____ Side effects/problems: _____
Nonprescription drugs/frequency:
  OTC drugs: _____ Vitamins: _____ Herbals: _____ Street drugs: _____
Alcohol (amount/frequency): _____ Tobacco: _____ Smokeless tobacco: _____
Admitting diagnosis per provider: _____
Reason for hospitalization/visit per client: _____
  History of current problem/concern: _____
  Client expectations of this hospitalization/visit: _____

(table continues on page 30)

TABLE 3.1 **General Assessment Tool** (continued)

Will admission cause any lifestyle changes (describe): _____
Previous illnesses and/or hospitalizations/surgeries: _____
Evidence of failure to improve: _____
Last complete physical examination: _____

Discharge Plan Considerations

Projected length of stay (hours/days): _____ Anticipated date of discharge: _____
  Date information obtained: _____ Source: _____
Resources available: Persons: _____ Financial: _____ Community supports: _____ Groups: _____
Areas that may require alteration/assistance: Food preparation: ____ Shopping: ____ Transportation: ____ Ambulation: ____
  Self-care (specify): _____ Socialization: _____
  Medication/IV therapy: _____ Treatments: _____ Wound care: _____ Supplies: _____
  Homemaker/maintenance(specify): _____ Physical layout of home (specify): _____
Anticipated changes in living situation after discharge: _____ Living facility other than home (specify): _____
Referrals (date/source/services): Social services: _____ Rehabilitation: _____
Dietary: _____ Home care: _____ Resp/O_2: _____ Equipment: _____ Supplies: _____ Other: _____

The use of a nursing model as a framework for data collection (rather than a body-systems approach [assessing the heart, moving on to the lungs] or the commonly known head-to-toe approach) has the advantage of focusing data collection on the nurse's phenomena of concern—the human responses to health, illness, and life processes.[6] This facilitates the identification and validation of *nursing* diagnosis labels to describe the data accurately.

Reviewing and Validating Findings

The nurse's initial responsibility is to observe, collect, and record data without drawing conclusions or making judgments or assumptions. Self-awareness is a crucial factor in this interaction, because perceptions, judgments, and assumptions can easily color the assessment findings.

Validation is an ongoing process that occurs during the data-collection phase and upon its completion, when the data are reviewed and compared. The nurse should review the data to be sure that the recordings are factual, to identify errors of omission, and to compare the objective and subjective data for congruencies or inconsistencies that require additional investigation or a more focused assessment. Data that are grossly abnormal are rechecked, and any temporary factors that may affect the data are identified and noted. Validation is particularly important when the data are conflicting, when the data's source may be unreliable, or when serious harm to the client could result from any inaccuracies. Validating the information reduces the possibility of making wrong inferences or conclusions that could result in inaccurate nursing diagnoses, incorrect outcomes, or inappropriate nursing actions. This can be done by sharing the assumptions with the individuals involved (e.g., client, significant other/family) and having them verify the accuracy of those conclusions. Sharing pertinent data with other healthcare professionals, such as the physician, dietician, or physical therapist, can aid in collaborative planning of care. Data given in confidence should not be shared with other individuals (unless withholding that information would hinder appropriate evaluation or care of the client).

Summary

The assessment step of the nursing process emphasizes and should provide a holistic view of the client. The generalized assessment done during the overall data-gathering creates a profile of the client. A focused, or more detailed, assessment may be warranted given the client's condition or emergent time constraints, or it may be done to obtain more information about a specific issue that needs expansion or clarification. Both types of assessments provide important data that complement each other. A successfully completed assessment creates a picture of clients' states of wellness, their response to health concerns or problems, and individual risk factors—this is the foundation for identifying appropriate nursing diagnoses, developing client outcomes, and choosing relevant interventions necessary for providing individualized care.

References

1. American Nurses Association. (2004). *Nursing: Scope & Standards of Practice*. Silver Spring, MD: Nursesbooks.org.
2. Doenges, M. E., Moorhouse, M. F., Murr, A. C. (2010). *Nurse's Pocket Guide: Diagnoses, Interventions, and Rationales*. 12th ed. Philadelphia: F. A. Davis.
3. Doenges, M. E., Moorhouse, M. F., Murr, A. C. (2010). *Nursing Care Plans: Guidelines for Individualizing Client Care Across the Lifespan*. 8th ed. Philadelphia: F. A. Davis.
4. Gordon, M. (2008). *Assess Notes: Nursing Assessment and Diagnostic Reasoning*. Philadelphia: F. A. Davis.
5. Guzzetta, C. E., et al. (1989). *Clinical Assessment Tools for Use with Nursing Diagnoses*. St. Louis, MO: Mosby
6. American Nurses Association. (1995). *Nursing's Social Policy Statement*. Washington, DC: Author.

CHAPTER 4

Concept Mapping to Create and Document the Plan of Care

The plan of care may be recorded on a single page or in a multiple-page format, with one page for each nursing diagnosis or client diagnostic statement. The format for documenting the plan of care is determined by agency policy. As a practicing professional, you might use a computer with a plan-of-care database, preprinted standardized care plan forms, or clinical pathways. Whichever form you use, the plan of care enables visualization of the nursing process and must reflect the basic nursing standards of care; personal client data; nonroutine care; and qualifiers for interventions and outcomes, such as time, frequency, and amount.

As students, you are asked to develop plans of care that often contain more detail than what you see in the hospital plans of care. This is to help you learn how to apply the nursing process and create individualized client care plans. However, even though much time and energy may be spent focusing on filling the columns of traditional clinical care plan forms, some students never develop a holistic view of their clients and fail to visualize how each client need interacts with other identified needs. A new technique or learning tool has been developed to assist you in visualizing the linkages, to enhance your critical thinking skills, and to facilitate the creative process of planning client care.

Concept Mapping Client Care

Have you ever asked yourself whether you are more right-brained or left-brained? Those who naturally use their left brains are more linear in their thinking. Right-brain thinkers see more in pictures and illustrations. It is best for nurses to use the whole brain (right and left) when thinking about providing the broad scope of nursing care to clients.

No More Columns!

Traditional nursing care plans are linear—that is, they are designed in columns. They speak almost exclusively to the left brain. The traditional nursing care plan is organized according to the nursing process, which guides us in problem-solving the nursing care we give. However, the linear nature of the traditional plan does not facilitate interconnecting data from one "row" to another or between parts in a column. Concept mapping allows us to show the interconnections among various client symptoms, interventions, and problems as they impact each other.

You can keep the parts that are great about traditional care plans (problem-solving and categorizing) but change the linear or columnar nature of the plan to a design that uses the whole brain—bringing left-brained, linear problem-solving together with the freewheeling, interconnected, creative right brain. Joining concept mapping and care planning enables you to create a whole picture of a client with all the interconnections identified.

There are several diverse and innovative ways to mind map or to concept map nursing care plans.[1] The examples in this chapter use mind mapping and require placing the client at the center, with all ideas on one page (for a whole picture); the examples also use color-coding and creative energy.[2,3] When doing a large mapped plan of care, a light posterboard is often used so that all ideas fit on one page.

Components of a Concept Map

Tony Buzan developed the idea of concept mapping, a way to depict how ideas about a main subject are related. Mapping represents graphically the relationships and interrelationships of ideas and concepts.[4] It fosters and encourages critical thinking through brainstorming about a particular subject.

Instead of starting at the top of the page, concept mapping starts at the page's center. The main concept of our thinking goes in this center stage place.

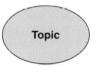

From that central thought, simply begin thinking of other main ideas that relate to the central topic. These ideas radiate out from the central idea likes spokes of a wheel (see subsequent discussion); however, they do not have to be added in a balanced manner; the "wheel" does not have to be round.

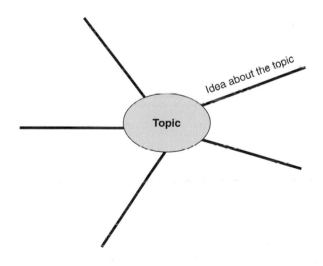

You will generate further ideas related to each spoke (see subsequent discussion); and your mind will race with even more ideas from those thoughts, which can be represented through pictures or words.

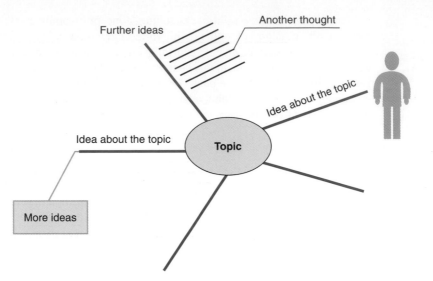

As you think of new ideas, write them down immediately. This may require going back and forth from one area of the page to another. Writing your concept map by hand allows you to move faster. Avoid using a computer to generate a map because it hinders the fast-paced process. You can group different concepts together by color-coding or by placement on the page (see subsequent discussion).

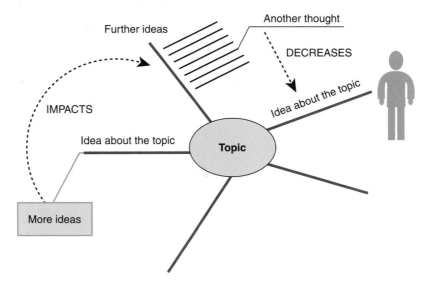

As you see connections and interconnections among groups of ideas, use arrows or lines to connect those concepts (refer to the dotted lines). You can also add defining phrases that explain how the interconnected thoughts relate to one another, as in the figure above.

Some left-brain thinkers find it very difficult to start their ideas in the middle of a page. If you are this type of thinker, try starting at the top of the page (see subsequent discussion), but you must still represent your ideas in illustration form, not in paragraphs.

Concept maps created by different people look different. They are unique to the mind's eye picture, so do not expect your map to be the same as someone else's.

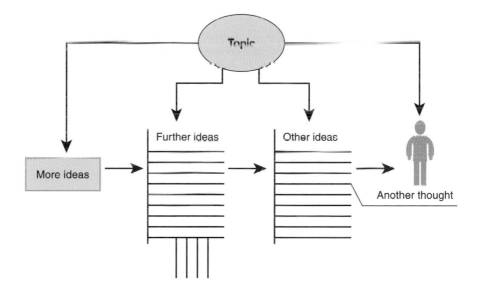

Concept Mapping a Plan of Care

Concept mapping is an exciting alternative format for illustrating a written plan of care. A mapped care plan will look very different from traditional plans of care, which are usually completed on linear forms.

To begin mapping a client plan of care, you must begin with the central topic—the client. Now you are thinking like a nurse. Create a shape that signifies "client" to you, and place it at your map's center. If your hand just cannot start at the center, then put the shape at the top. This will help you remember that the client, not the medical diagnosis or condition, is the focus of your plan. All other pieces of the map will be connected in some manner to the client. Many different pieces of information about the client can be connected directly to the client. For example, each of the following pieces of critical client data could stem from the center:

- 78-year-old widower
- No family in the state
- Obese
- Medical diagnosis of recurrent community-acquired pneumonia

Now, you must do a bit of thinking about how you think. To create the rest of your map, ask yourself how *you* plan client care. For example, which of these items do you see first or think of first as the basis for your plan: the clustered assessment data, nursing diagnoses, or outcomes? Whichever piece you choose becomes your first layer of connections. Suppose when thinking about a plan of care for a female client with heart failure, you think first in terms of all the nursing diagnoses about that woman and her condition. Your map would start with the diagnoses featured as the first "branches," each one listed separately in some way on the map.

Completing the map then becomes a matter of adding the rest of the pieces of the plan using the nursing process and your own way of thinking or planning as your guide. If you began your map using nursing diagnoses, you might think, "What signs and symptoms or data support these diagnoses?" Then, you would connect clusters of supporting data to the related nursing diagnosis. Or you might think, "What client outcomes am I trying to achieve when I address this nursing diagnosis?" In that case, you would next connect client outcomes (or NOC labels) to the nursing diagnoses.

To keep your map clear, as suggested previously, use different colors and maybe a different shape, spoke, or line for each piece of the care plan that you add. For example:

• Red for signs and symptoms (to signify danger)
• Yellow for nursing diagnoses (for "stop and think what this is")
• Green for nursing interventions or NIC labels (for "go")
• Blue (or some other color) for outcomes or NOC labels

When all the pieces of the nursing process are represented, each branch of the map is complete. There should be a nursing diagnosis (supported by subjective and objective assessment data), nursing interventions, desired client outcome(s), and any evaluation data, all connected in a manner that shows there is a relationship among them.

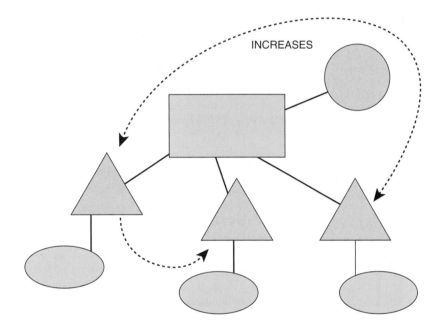

It is critical to understand that there is no preset order for the pieces, because one cluster is not more or less important than another (or one is not "subsumed" under another). It is important, however, that those pieces within a branch be in the same order in each branch.

So, you might ask, how is this different from writing out information in a linear manner? What makes mapping so special? One of the things you may have discovered about caring for clients is that the care you deliver is very interconnected. Taking care of one problem often results in the simultaneous correction of another. For example, if you resolve a fluid volume problem in a client with heart failure, you will also positively impact the client's gas exchange and decrease his or her anxiety. These kinds of interconnections cannot be shown on linear plans of care, yet they are what practicing nurses see in their mind's eye all the time. These interconnections can be represented on a map with arrows or dotted or dashed lines that tie related ideas together. Then, defining phrases that explain the nature of the interconnection can be added to further clarify the relationship, as shown in Figure 4.1.

In addition to the pieces of the nursing process, other components of care can be illustrated on a map. Nurses have certain responsibilities when clients have diagnostic tests (such as an

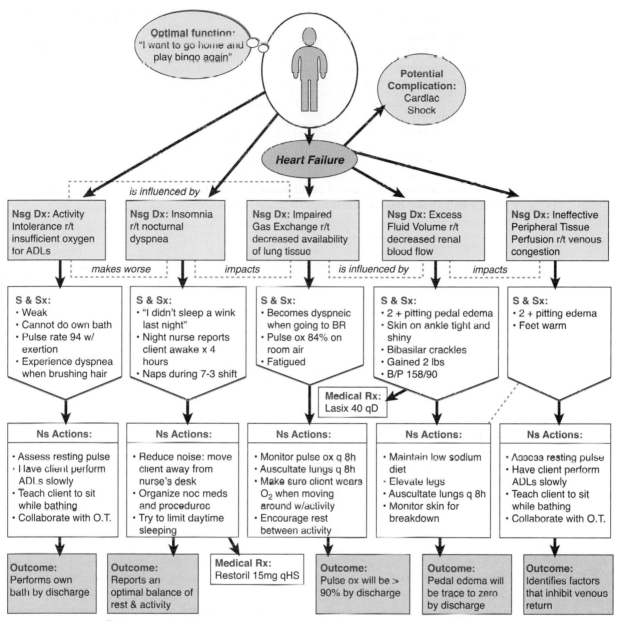

Figure 4.1 Concept map of a plan of care for a client with heart failure.

angiography or a bronchoscopy). These tests can be connected to the appropriate piece of your map, along with the correct nursing interventions related to those tests. Another item to be added is potential complications or collaborative problems.

Taking your clients' needs one step further, try asking every client you have (medical, surgical, or otherwise), "What is the most important thing to you now in relation to why you are here?" Obtaining this information builds an alliance between you and your client, and together you can work toward that desired outcome. Add it to your map and see how your plan of care becomes more client-centered (refer to Fig. 4.2).

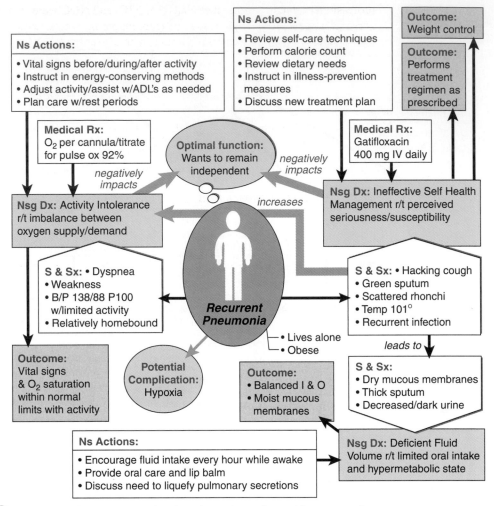

Ns Actions:

- Vital signs before/during/after activity
- Instruct in energy-conserving methods
- Adjust activity/assist w/ADL's as needed
- Plan care w/rest periods

Ns Actions:

- Review self-care techniques
- Perform calorie count
- Review dietary needs
- Instruct in illness-prevention measures
- Discuss new treatment plan

Outcome: Weight control

Outcome: Performs treatment regimen as prescribed

Medical Rx: O_2 per cannula/titrate for pulse ox 92%

Optimal function: Wants to remain independent

Medical Rx: Gatifloxacin 400 mg IV daily

negatively impacts

negatively impacts

Nsg Dx: Activity Intolerance r/t imbalance between oxygen supply/demand

Nsg Dx: Ineffective Self Health Management r/t perceived seriousness/susceptibility

increases

Recurrent Pneumonia

S & Sx: • Dyspnea
- Weakness
- B/P 138/88 P100 w/limited activity
- Relatively homebound

S & Sx: • Hacking cough
- Green sputum
- Scattered rhonchi
- Temp 101°
- Recurrent infection

leads to

• Lives alone
• Obese

Outcome: Vital signs & O_2 saturation within normal limits with activity

Potential Complication: Hypoxia

Outcome:
- Balanced I & O
- Moist mucous membranes

S & Sx:
- Dry mucous membranes
- Thick sputum
- Decreased/dark urine

Ns Actions:

- Encourage fluid intake every hour while awake
- Provide oral care and lip balm
- Discuss need to liquefy pulmonary secretions

Nsg Dx: Deficient Fluid Volume r/t limited oral intake and hypermetabolic state

Figure 4.2 Concept map of a plan of care for a client with pneumonia.

Summary

Concept maps allow you to do something that is different and creative. They require you to think (and learn), make connections, and use colors and shapes. They help you to focus on the client; and having the map on one page helps you to understand the "whole picture" better. Concept maps also help you to become better organized and to develop your own unique approach to "thinking like a nurse" much sooner.

A student who had written many traditional plans of care in her previous nursing program wrote the following about concept-mapped care plans:

Concept mapping is painting a picture using colors of the rainbow on blank paper to tell the story of your client using "NANDA" nursing diagnoses and the nursing process. Previously, I was a student in prison (my mind) who hated the words "CARE PLAN," writing page after page in narrative form. It was laborious to do and boring to read. There was no life or heartbeat.

Concept mapping opened the prison doors, and my care plan took on human form with a VOICE, a beating HEART, and COLOR while still incorporating the nursing process and standardized nursing language. My mind now took on the professional thought process that NANDA, NIC, and NOC were created to facilitate nursing; however, the magic was in concept mapping, which removed all my fears, and the client became a beautiful painting with a heartbeat.

References

1. Schuster, P. (2002). *Concept Mapping: A Critical-Thinking Approach to Care Planning*. Philadelphia: F. A. Davis.
2. Mueller, A., Johnston, M., Bligh, D. (2001). Mind-mapped care plans, a remarkable alternative to traditional nursing care plans. *Nurse Educ*, 26(2), 75–80.
3. Mueller, A., Johnston, M., Bligh, D. (2002). Viewpoint: Joining mind mapping and care planning to enhance student critical thinking and achieve holistic nursing care. *Nurs Diagn*, 13(1), 24–27.
4. Buzan, T. (1995). *The MindMap Book*. 2d ed. London: BBC Books.

CHAPTER 5

Nursing Diagnoses in Alphabetical Order

Activity Intolerance [specify level]

DEFINITION: Insufficient physiological or psychological energy to endure or complete required or desired daily activities

RELATED FACTORS

Generalized weakness
Sedentary lifestyle
Bedrest/immobility
Imbalance between oxygen supply and demand, [anemia]
[Cognitive deficits/emotional status; secondary to underlying disease process/depression]
[Pain, vertigo, dysrhythmias, extreme stress]

DEFINING CHARACTERISTICS

Subjective
Verbal report of fatigue, weakness
Exertional discomfort, dyspnea
[Verbalizes no desire for and/or lack of interest in activity]

Objective
Abnormal heart rate or blood pressure response to activity
Electrocardiographic changes reflecting arrhythmias or ischemia
[Pallor, cyanosis]

FUNCTIONAL LEVEL CLASSIFICATION[3] (GORDON, 1987):

Level I: Walk, regular pace, on level indefinitely; one flight or more but more short of breath than normally
Level II: Walk one city block [or] 500 ft on level; climb one flight slowly without stopping

---

Information that appears in brackets has been added by the authors to clarify and enhance the use of the nursing diagnoses.

Level III: Walk no more than 50 ft on level without stopping; unable to climb one flight of stairs without stopping
Level IV: Dyspnea and fatigue at rest

Sample Clinical Applications: Anemias, angina, aortic stenosis, bronchitis, emphysema, diabetes mellitus, dysmenorrhea, heart failure, HIV/AIDS, labor/preterm labor, leukemias, mitral stenosis, obesity, pain, pericarditis, peripheral vascular disease, rheumatic fever, thrombocytopenia, tuberculosis, uterine bleeding

DESIRED OUTCOMES/EVALUATION CRITERIA

Sample **NOC** linkages:
Activity Tolerance: Physiological response to energy-consuming movements with daily activities
Energy Conservation: Personal actions to manage energy for initiating and sustaining activity
Endurance: Capacity to sustain activity

Client Will (Include Specific Time Frame)
• Identify negative factors affecting activity tolerance and eliminate or reduce their effects when possible.
• Use identified techniques to enhance activity tolerance.
• Participate in necessary/desired activities.
• Report measurable increase in activity tolerance.
• Demonstrate a decrease in physiological signs of intolerance (e.g., pulse, respirations, and blood pressure remain within client's usual range).

ACTIONS/INTERVENTIONS

Sample **NIC** linkages:
Activity Therapy: Prescription of and assistance with specific physical, cognitive, social, and spiritual activities to increase the range, frequency, or duration of an individual's (or group's) activity
Energy Management: Regulating energy use to treat or prevent fatigue and optimize function
Exercise Promotion: Facilitation of regular physical activity to maintain or advance to a higher level of fitness and health

NURSING PRIORITY NO. 1

To identify causative/precipitating factors:

● Note presence of acute or chronic illness, such as heart failure, hypothyroidism, diabetes mellitus, AIDS, cancers, acute and chronic pain, etc. *Many factors cause or contribute to fatigue, but activity intolerance implies that the client cannot endure or adapt to increased energy or oxygen demands caused by an activity.*[1,8,9]
● Assess cardiopulmonary response to physical activity by measuring vital signs, noting heart rate and regularity, respiratory rate and work of breathing, and blood pressure before, during, and after activity. Note progression or accelerating degree of fatigue. *Dramatic changes in heart rate and rhythm, changes in usual blood pressure, and progressively worsening fatigue result from imbalance of oxygen supply and demand. These changes are potentially greater in the frail, elderly population.*[1,3,10,11]

- Note treatment-related factors such as side effects and interactions of medications. *Can influence presence and degree of fatigue.*
- Determine if client is receiving medications such as vasodilators, diuretics, or beta-blockers. *Orthostatic hypotension can occur with activity because of medication effects (vasodilation), fluid shifts (diuresis), or compromised cardiac pumping function.*[4]
- Note client reports of difficulty accomplishing tasks or desired activities. Evaluate current limitations or degree of deficit in light of usual status and what the client perceives causes, exacerbates, and helps the problem. *Provides comparative baseline, influences choice of interventions, and may reveal causes that the client is unaware of affecting energy, such as sleep deprivation, smoking, poor diet, depression, or lack of support.*[2,10,11]
- Ascertain ability to sit, stand, and move about as desired. Note degree of assistance necessary and/or use of assistive equipment. *Helps to differentiate between problems relating to movement and problems with oxygen supply and demand characterized by fatigue and weakness.*[2,8,9,11]
- Identify activity needs versus desires (e.g., client barely able to walk up stairs but states would like to play racquetball). *Assists caregiver in dealing with reality of situation as well as the feasibility of goals client wants to achieve when developing activity plan.*[4]
- Assess emotional or psychological factors affecting the current situation. *Stress and/or depression may be exacerbating the effects of an illness, or depression may be the result of therapy and/or limitations.*

NURSING PRIORITY NO. 2

To assist client to deal with contributing factors and manage activities within individual limits:

- Monitor vital signs before and during activity, watching for changes in blood pressure, heart and respiratory rate, as well as postactivity vital sign response. *Vital signs increase during activity and should return to baseline within 5 to 7 minutes after activity if response to activity is normal.*[1]
- Observe respiratory rate, noting breathing pattern, breath sounds, skin color, and mental status. *Pallor and/or cyanosis, presence of respiratory distress, or confusion may be indicative of need for oxygen during activities, especially if respiratory infection or compromise is present.*[4]
- Plan care with rest periods between activities *to reduce fatigue.*
- Assist with self-care activities. Adjust activities or reduce intensity level, or discontinue activities that cause undesired physiological changes. *Prevents overexertion.*
- Increase exercise/activity levels gradually; encourage stopping to rest for 3 minutes during a 10-minute walk, sitting down instead of standing to brush hair, and so forth. *Methods of conserving energy.*
- Encourage expression of feelings contributing to or resulting from condition. Provide positive atmosphere while acknowledging difficulty of the situation for the client. *Helps to minimize frustration, rechannel energy.*
- Involve client/significant others (SOs) in planning of activities as much as possible. *May give client opportunity to perform desired or essential activities during periods of peak energy.*
- Assist with activities and provide and monitor client's use of assistive devices. *Enables client to maintain mobility while protecting from injury.*
- Promote comfort measures and provide for relief of pain *to enhance client's ability and desire to participate in activities.*[9,11] (Refer to NDs acute Pain, chronic Pain.)
- Provide referral to collaborative disciplines such as exercise physiologist, psychological counseling/therapy, occupational/physical therapy, and recreation/leisure specialists. *May be needed to develop individually appropriate therapeutic regimens.*

🌐 Cultural 🤝 Collaborative 🏠 Community/Home Care ⟋ Diagnostic Studies ∞ Pediatric/Geriatric/Lifespan 💊 Medications

- Prepare for/assist with and monitor effects of exercise testing. *May be performed to determine degree of oxygen desaturation and/or hypoxemia that occurs with exertion or to optimize titration of supplemental oxygen when used.*[5,8]
- Implement graded exercise or rehabilitation program under direct medical supervision. *Gradual increase in activity avoids excessive myocardial workload and associated oxygen demand.*[4]
- Administer supplemental oxygen, medications, prepare for surgery, as indicated. *Type of therapy or medication is dependent on the underlying condition and might include medications (such as antiarryhthmics) or surgery (e.g., stents or coronary artery bypass graft [CABG]) to improve myocardial perfusion and systemic circulation. Other treatments might include iron preparations or blood transfusion to treat severe anemia or use of oxygen and bronchodilators to improve respiratory function.*[6,7]

NURSING PRIORITY NO. 3

To promote wellness (Teaching/Discharge Considerations):

- Review expectations of client/SOs/providers and explore conflicts or differences. *Helps to establish goals and to reach agreement for the most effective plan.*
- Assist or direct client/SOs to plan for progressive increase of activity level aiming for maximal activity within the client's ability. *Promotes improved or more normal activity level, stamina, and conditioning.*
- Instruct client/SOs in monitoring response to activity and in recognizing signs/symptoms that indicate need to alter activity level. *Assists in self-management of condition and in understanding of reportable problems.*[8,9]
- Give client information that provides evidence of daily or weekly progress to sustain motivation.
- Assist client to learn and demonstrate appropriate safety measures *to prevent injuries.*
- Provide information about proper nutrition to meet metabolic and energy needs, obtaining or maintaining normal body weight. *Energy is improved when nutrients are sufficient to meet metabolic demands.*[1]
- Encourage client to use relaxation techniques such as visualization or guided imagery as appropriate. *Useful in maintaining positive attitude and enhancing sense of well-being.*
- Encourage participation in recreation or social activities and hobbies appropriate for situation. (Refer to ND deficient Diversional Activity.)
- Monitor laboratory values (such as for anemia) and pulse oximetry.

DOCUMENTATION FOCUS

Assessment/Reassessment
- Level of activity as noted in Functional Level Classification.
- Causative or precipitating factors.
- Client reports of difficulty or change.

Planning
- Plan of care and who is involved in planning.
- Teaching plan.

Implementation/Evaluation
- Response to interventions, teaching, and actions performed.
- Modifications to plan of care.
- Attainment or progress toward desired outcome(s).

Discharge Planning
• Referrals to other resources.
• Long-term needs and who is responsible for actions.

References

1. Cox, H. C., et al. (2002). *Clinical Applications of Nursing Diagnosis: Adult, Child, Women's, Psychiatric, Gerontic, and Home Health Considerations.* 4th ed. Philadelphia: F. A. Davis, 231–237.
2. Blair, K. A. (1999). Immobility and activity intolerance in older adults. In Stanley, M., Beare, P. G. (eds). *Gerontological Nursing: A Health Promotion/Protection Approach.* 2d ed. Philadelphia: F. A. Davis, 193–202.
3. Gordon, M. (2002). *Manual of Nursing Diagnosis.* 10th ed. St. Louis, MO: Mosby, 223.
4. Hypertension: Severe; Heart failure: Chronic; Myocardial infarction; and Pneumonia: Microbial. In Doenges, M. E., Moorhouse, M. F., Geissler-Murr, A. C. (eds). (2002). *Nursing Care Plans: Guidelines for Individualizing Patient Care.* 6th ed. Philadelphia: F. A. Davis, 37, 51, 75, 133.
5. Exercise testing for evaluation of hypoxemia and/or desaturation: Revision & update. (2001). *Resp Care*, 46(5), 514–522.
6. Gibbons, R. J., et al. (1999). ACC/AHA/ACP-ASIM: Guidelines for the management of patients with chronic stable angina: A report of the American College of Cardiology/American Heart Association Task Force on Practice Guidelines. *J Am Coll Cardiol*, 33(7), 2092.
7. Congestive Heart Failure in Adults. (2002). Bloomington, MN: Institute for Clinical Systems Improvement (ICSI).
8. Michael, K. M., Allen, J. K., Macko, R. E. (2006). Fatigue after stroke: Relationship to mobility, fitness, ambulatory activity, social support, and falls efficacy. *Rehabil Nurs*, 31(5), 210–217.
9. Graf, C. (2006). Functional decline in hospitalized older adults. *Am J Nurs*, 106(1), 58–67.
10. Perry, A. (2005). Quality of life. *Rehabil Manage*, 18(7), 18–21.
11. Hurr, H. K., et al. (2005). Activity intolerance and impaired physical mobility in elders. *Int J of Nursing Terminologies and Classifications*, 16(3–4), 47–53.

risk for Activity Intolerance

DEFINITION: At risk of experiencing insufficient physiological or psychological energy to endure or complete required or desired daily activities

RISK FACTORS

History of previous intolerance
Presence of circulatory or respiratory problems, [dysrhythmias]
Deconditioned status; [aging]
Inexperience with the activity
[Diagnosis of progressive disease state or debilitating condition, anemia]
[Verbalized reluctance or inability to perform expected activity]

NOTE: A risk diagnosis is not evidenced by signs and symptoms as the problem has not occurred; rather, nursing interventions are directed at prevention.
Sample Clinical Applications: Anemias, angina aortic stenosis, bronchitis, emphysema, dysmenorrhea, heart failure, HIV/AIDS, labor/preterm labor, leukemias, mitral stenosis,

⊕ Cultural Collaborative Community/Home Care Diagnostic Studies ∞ Pediatric/Geriatric/Lifespan Medications

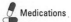

obesity, pain, pericarditis, peripheral vascular disease, rheumatic fever, thrombocytopenia, tuberculosis, uterine bleeding

DESIRED OUTCOMES/EVALUATION CRITERIA

Sample (NOC) linkages:
Endurance: Capacity to sustain activity
Energy Conservation: Personal actions to manage energy for initiating and sustaining activity
Circulation Status: Unobstructed, unidirectional blood flow at an appropriate pressure through large vessels of the systemic and pulmonary circuits

Client Will (Include Specific Time Frame)
• Verbalize understanding of potential loss of ability in relation to existing condition.
• Participate in conditioning or rehabilitation program to enhance ability to perform.
• Identify alternative ways to maintain desired activity level (e.g., if weather is bad, walking in a shopping mall could be an option).
• Identify conditions or symptoms that require medical reevaluation.

ACTIONS/INTERVENTIONS

Sample (NIC) linkages:
Energy Management: Regulating energy use to treat or prevent fatigue and optimize function
Exercise Promotion: Facilitation of regular physical activity to maintain or advance to a higher level of fitness and health
Pain Management: Alleviation of pain or a reduction in pain to a level of comfort that is acceptable to the client

NURSING PRIORITY NO. 1

To assess factors affecting current situation:

• Note presence of medical diagnosis and/or therapeutic regimens (e.g., AIDS, chronic obstructive pulmonary disease [COPD], cancer, heart failure or other cardiac problems, anemia, multiple medications or treatment modalities, extensive surgical interventions, musculoskeletal trauma, neurological disorders). *These have potential for interfering with client's ability to perform at a desired level of activity. Note: Many factors cause or contribute to fatigue, but activity intolerance implies that the individual cannot endure or adapt to increased energy or oxygen demands caused by an activity.*[1]
• Ask client/SO about usual level of energy *to identify potential problems and/or client's/ SO's perception of client's energy and ability to perform needed or desired activities.*
• Identify factors (e.g., age, functional decline, painful conditions, breathing problems, client resistive to efforts; vision or hearing impairments, climate or weather; unsafe areas to exercise; need for mobility assistance) *that could block or affect desired level of activity.*
• Determine current activity level and physical condition with observation, exercise tolerance testing, use of functional level classification system (e.g., Gordon's), as appropriate. *Provides baseline for comparison and opportunity to track changes.*

NURSING PRIORITY NO. 2

To develop/investigate alternative ways to remain active within the limits of the disabling condition/situation:

- Implement physical therapy or exercise program in conjunction with the client and other team members such as a physical and/or occupational therapist, exercise or rehabilitation physiologist. *Collaborative program with short-term achievable goals enhances likelihood of success and may motivate client to adopt a lifestyle of physical exercise for enhancement of health.*[2]
- Promote or implement conditioning program and support inclusion in exercise or activity groups to prevent or limit deterioration.
- Instruct client in proper performance of unfamiliar activities and/or alternate ways of doing familiar activities *to learn methods of conserving energy and promote safety in performing activities.*

NURSING PRIORITY NO. 3

To promote wellness (Teaching/Discharge Considerations):

- Discuss with client/SO relationship of illness or debilitating condition to inability to perform desired activity(ies). *Understanding these relationships can help with acceptance of limitations or reveal opportunity for changes of practical value.*[1,5]
- Provide information regarding factors, such as smoking when one has respiratory problems, weight management, lack of motivation or interest in exercise. *Education is essential to encourage modification of potential interferences to activity.*[3,4]
- Assist client/SO with planning for changes that may become necessary (e.g., shifting of family responsibilities, use of supplemental oxygen to improve client's ability to participate in desired activities). *Anticipatory guidance facilitates adaptation if symptoms occur.*[3,4] (Refer to ND Activity Intolerance.)
- Identify and discuss symptoms for which client needs to seek medical assistance or evaluation, *providing for timely intervention.*[3]
- Refer to appropriate sources for assistance (e.g., smoking cessation, dietary counseling) and/or equipment, as needed, *to sustain or improve activity level and to promote client safety.*

DOCUMENTATION FOCUS

Assessment/Reassessment
- Identified and potential risk factors for individual.
- Current level of activity tolerance and blocks to activity.

Planning
- Treatment options, including physical therapy or exercise program, other assistive therapies and devices.
- Lifestyle changes that are planned, who is to be responsible for each action, and monitoring methods.

Implementation/Evaluation
- Responses to interventions, teaching, and actions performed.
- Attainment or progress toward desired outcome(s).
- Modification of plan of care.

⊕ Cultural Collaborative Community/Home Care Diagnostic Studies ∞ Pediatric/Geriatric/Lifespan Medications

Discharge Planning
• Referrals for medical assistance and evaluation.

References

1. Cox, H. C., et al. (2002). *Clinical Applications of Nursing Diagnosis: Adult, Child, Women's, Psychiatric, Gerontic, and Home Health Considerations.* 4th ed. Philadelphia: F. A. Davis, 231–237.
2. Blair, K. A. (1999). Immobility and activity intolerance in older adults. In Stanley, M., Beare, P. G. (eds). *Gerontological Nursing: A Health Promotion/Protection Approach.* 2d ed. Philadelphia: F. A. Davis, 193–202.
3. Congestive Heart Failure in Adults. (2002). Bloomington, MN: Institute for Clinical Systems Improvement (ICSI).
4. Meleski, D. D. (2002). Families with chronically ill children. *Am J Nurs*, 102(5), 47.
5. Borroso, J. (2002). HIV-related fatigue. *Am J Nurs*, 102(5), 83.

ineffective Activity Planning

DEFINITION: Inability to prepare for a set of actions fixed in time and under certain conditions

RELATED FACTORS

Unrealistic perception of events or personal competence
Lack of family or friend support
Compromised ability to process information
Defensive flight behavior when faced with proposed solution
Hedonism [motivated by pleasure and/or pain]

DEFINING CHARACTERISTICS

Subjective
Verbalization of fear or worries toward a task to be undertaken
Excessive anxieties toward a task to be undertaken

Objective
Failure pattern of behavior
Lack of plan, resources, sequential organization
Procrastination
Unmet goals for chosen activity

Sample Clinical Applications: Depression, bipolar disorder, learning disabilities or dyslexia, chronic conditions (e.g., fibromyalgia, fatigue syndrome)

DESIRED OUTCOMES/EVALUATION CRITERIA

Sample NOC linkage:
Motivation: Inner urge that moves or promotes an individual to positive action(s)

(continues on page 48)

ineffective Activity Planning (continued)

Client Will (Include Specific Time Frame)
• Acknowledge difficulty with follow-through of activity plan.
• Identify negative factors affecting ability to plan activities.
• Willingly prepare to develop own plan for activity.
• Report lessened anxiety and fear toward planning.
• Be aware of and make plan to deal with procrastination.

ACTIONS/INTERVENTIONS

Sample (NIC) linkages:
Self-Awareness Enhancement: Assisting a patient to explore and understand his/her thoughts, feelings, motivations, and behaviors
Values Clarification: Assisting another to clarify her/his own values in order to facilitate effective decision making

NURSING PRIORITY NO. 1

To identify causative/precipitating factors:

● Determine individual problems with planning and follow-through with activity plan. *Identifies individual difficulties such as anxiety regarding what kind of activity to choose, lack of resources, lack of confidence in own ability.*[1]
● Perform complete physical examination. *May have underlying problems such as allergies, hypertension, asthma that contribute to fatigue and difficulty undertaking task.*[2]
● Review medication regimen. *Side effects may contribute to fatigue, affecting client's desire to get involved in any activity.*[2]
● Assess mental status; use Beck's Depression scale as indicated. *Anxieties and depression can interfere with client's ability and desire to be active.*[5]
● Identify client's personal values and perception of self, including strengths and weaknesses. *Provides information that will be helpful in planning care and choosing goals for this individual.*[1]
● Determine client's need to be in control, fear of dependency on others (although may need assistance from others), or belief he or she cannot do the task. *Indicative of external locus of control, where client sees others as having the control and ability.*[1]
● Identify cultural or religious issues that may affect how individual deals with issues of life. *Often person learns strict ideas in family of origin, such as rituals of Catholicism or the demands of prayers for Muslims, that affect how they see their ability to make choices or manage own life.*[1]
● Discuss awareness of procrastination, need for perfection or fear of failure. *Although client may not acknowledge it as a problem, this may be a factor in difficulty in planning for, choosing, and following through with activities that might be enjoyed.*[3]
● Assess client's ability to process information. *Low self-esteem, anxiety, and possibly difficulty with thinking ability may interfere with perception of the world.*[4]
● Discuss possibility that client is motivated by pleasure to avoid pain (hedonism). *Individual may seek activities that bring pleasure to avoid painful experiences and not realize he or she is using this to keep from completing tasks.*[4,7]
● Note availability and use of resources. *Client may have difficulty if family and friends are not supportive and other resources are not readily available.*[1]

NURSING PRIORITY NO. 2

To assist client to recognize and deal with individual factors and begin to plan appropriate activities:

- Encourage expression of feelings contributing to or resulting from situation. Maintain a positive atmosphere without being too cheerful. *Helps client to begin to be aware of frustration and redirect energy into productive actions.*[5]
- Discuss client's perception of self as worthless and not deserving of success and happiness. *This belief is common among individuals who are anxious and worried, believing anything they do is doomed to failure. Sometimes the underlying feelings are those of wanting to be perfect, and it is difficult to finish the task fearing it will not be perfect (perfectionism).*[3,4]
- Gently confront ambivalent, angry, or depressed feelings. *Client may react negatively and withdraw if these feelings are not dealt with in a sensitive manner.*[1]
- Help client learn how to reframe negative thoughts about self into a positive view of what is happening. *Reframing turns a negative thought into something positive to change how it affects the individual.*[1]
- Involve client/SOs in planning an activity. *Starting with one and having the support of family and nurse will help to promote success.*[1]
- Direct client to break down desired activity into specific steps. *Makes activity more manageable, and as each step is accomplished, individual feels more confident about ability to finish the task.*[1]
- Encourage client to recognize procrastinating behaviors and make a decision to change. *Procrastination is a learned behavior, possibly in the family of origin, and serves many purposes for the individual. It can be changed but may require intensive therapy.*[3]
- Accompany client to activity of own choosing, encouraging participation together if appropriate. *Support from caregiver may enable client to begin participating and gain confidence.*[1]
- Assist client to develop skills of relaxation, imagery or visualization and mindfulness. *Using these techniques can help the client learn to overcome stress and be able to manage life's difficulties more effectively.*[2,6]
- Assist client to investigate the idea that seeking pleasure (hedonism) is interfering with motivation to accomplish goals. *Some philosophers believe that pleasure is the only good for a person, and the individual does not see other aspects of life, interfering with accomplishments.*[7]

NURSING PRIORITY NO. 3

To promote wellness (Teaching/Discharge Criteria):

- Assist client to identify life goals and priorities. *Often individual has not thought about the possibility of these ideas and, when asked to do this, begins to think he or she can accomplish some goals.*[1]
- Review treatment goals and expectations of client and SOs. *Helps to clarify what has been discussed and decisions that have been made and provides an opportunity to change goals as needed.*[1]
- Discuss progress in learning to relax and deal productively with anxieties and fears. *As client sees that progress is being made, feelings of worthwhileness will be enhanced and individual will be encouraged to continue working toward goals.*[2,3]
- Identify community resources such as social services, senior center, or classes *to provide support and options for activities and change.*

⊛ • Refer for cognitive therapy. *This structured therapy can help the individuals identify, evaluate, and modify underlying assumptions and dysfunctional beliefs they may have and begin the process of change.*[5]

DOCUMENTATION FOCUS

Assessment/Reassessment
• Specific problems exhibited by client.
• Causative or precipitating factors.
• Client reports of difficulty making and following through with plans.

Planning
• Plan of care and who is involved in planning.
• Teaching plan.

Implementation/Evaluation
• Response to interventions, teaching, and actions performed.
• Attainment or progress toward desired outcome(s).

Discharge Planning
• Referrals to other resources.
• Long-term needs and who is responsible for actions.

References

1. Townsend, M. (2006). *Psychiatric Mental Health Nursing Concept of Care in Evidence-Based Practice*, 5th ed. Philadelphia: F. A. Davis.
2. Berczi, I. (1994). Stress and disease: The contributions of Hans Selye to neuroimmunology. In Berczi, I., Szélenyi, J. (eds.). *Advances in Psychoneuroimmunology*. New York: Plenum Press, 1–15.
3. Marano, H. E. (2003). Procrastination: Ten things to know. Retrieved March 2009 from www.psychologytoday.com/rss/pto-20030823-000001.html.
4. Ellis, A. (1965/1994). Showing people they are not worthless individuals. *Voices: The Art and Science of Psychotherapy*, 1(2), 74–77. Retrieved March 2009 from www.geocities.com/rebtus/worthless.html.
5. Butler, A. C., Beck, A. T. (1995). Cognitive therapy for depression. *Clin Psychol*, 48(3), 3–5.
6. Hopper, J. (revised 2008). Mindfulness and kindness, inner sources of freedom and happiness. Retrieved March 2009 from www.jimhopper.com/mindfulness/.
7. Moore, A. (2008). Hedonism. *The Stanford Encyclopedia of Philosophy*. March 2009 http://plato.stanford.edu/archives/fall2008/entries/hedonism.

(ineffective Airway Clearance)

DEFINITION: Inability to clear secretions or obstructions from the respiratory tract to maintain a clear airway

RELATED FACTORS

Environmental
Smoking; secondhand smoke; smoke inhalation

⊕ Cultural ⊛ Collaborative 🏠 Community/Home Care ⟋ Diagnostic Studies ∞ Pediatric/Geriatric/Lifespan ⚬ Medications

Obstructed airway
Retained secretions; secretions in the bronchi; exudate in the alveoli; excessive mucus; airway spasm; foreign body in airway; presence of artificial airway

Physiological
Chronic obstructive pulmonary disease (COPD); asthma; allergic airways; hyperplasia of the bronchial walls
Neuromuscular dysfunction
Infection

DEFINING CHARACTERISTICS

Subjective
Dyspnea

Objective
Diminished or adventitious breath sounds [rales, crackles, rhonchi, wheezes]
Cough, ineffective or absent; excessive sputum
Changes in respiratory rate and rhythm
Difficulty vocalizing
Wide-eyed; restlessness
Orthopnea
Cyanosis

Sample Clinical Applications: COPD, pneumonia, influenza, acute respiratory distress syndrome (ARDS), cancer of lung, cancer of head and neck, congestive heart failure (CHF), cystic fibrosis, neuromuscular diseases, inhalation injuries

DESIRED OUTCOMES/EVALUATION CRITERIA

Sample NOC linkages:
Respiratory Status: Airway Patency: Open, clear tracheobronchial passages for air exchange
Aspiration Control: Personal actions to prevent the passage of fluid and solid particles into the lung
Cognition: Ability to execute complex mental processes

Client Will (Include Specific Time Frame)
- Maintain airway patency.
- Expectorate or clear secretions readily.
- Demonstrate absence or reduction of congestion with breath sounds clear, respirations noiseless, improved oxygen exchange (e.g., absence of cyanosis, arterial blood gas [ABG] results within client norms).
- Verbalize understanding of cause(s) and therapeutic management regimen.
- Demonstrate behaviors to improve or maintain clear airway.
- Identify potential complications and how to initiate appropriate preventive or corrective actions.

(continues on page 52)

ineffective Airway Clearance (continued)
ACTIONS/INTERVENTIONS

Sample (NIC) linkages:
Airway Management: Facilitation of patency of air passages
Respiratory Monitoring: Collection and analysis of patient data to ensure airway patency and adequate gas exchange
Cough Enhancement: Promotion of deep inhalation by the patient with subsequent generation of high intrathoracic pressures and compression of underlying lung parenchyma for the forceful expulsion of air

NURSING PRIORITY NO. 1

To maintain adequate, patent airway:

- Identify client populations at risk. *Persons with impaired ciliary function (e.g., cystic fibrosis, status post-heart-lung transplantation); those with excessive or abnormal mucus production (e.g., asthma, emphysema, pneumonia, dehydration, bronchiectasis, mechanical ventilation); those with impaired cough function (e.g., neuromuscular diseases, such as muscular dystrophy; neuromotor conditions, such as cerebral palsy, spinal cord injury); those with swallowing abnormalities (e.g., poststroke, seizures, head/neck cancer, coma/sedation, tracheostomy, facial burns/trauma/surgery); those who are immobile (e.g., sedated individual, frail elderly, developmental delay); infant/child (e.g., feeding intolerance, abdominal distention, and emotional stressors that may compromise airway) are all at risk for problems with maintenance of open airways.*[1,2]
- Assess level of consciousness/cognition and ability to protect own airway. *Information essential for identifying potential for airway problems, providing baseline level of care needed, and influencing choice of interventions.*
- Evaluate respiratory rate/depth and breath sounds. *Tachypnea is usually present to some degree and may be pronounced during respiratory stress. Respirations may be shallow. Some degree of bronchospasm is present with obstruction in airways and may/may not be manifested in adventitious breath sounds, such as scattered moist crackles (bronchitis), faint sounds with expiratory wheezes (emphysema), or absent breath sounds (severe asthma).*[2]
- Position head appropriate for age and condition/disorder. *Repositioning head may, at times, be all that is needed to open or maintain open airway in at-rest or compromised individual, such as one with sleep apnea.*
- ∞ Insert oral airway, using correct size for adult or child, when indicated. Have appropriate emergency equipment at bedside (such as tracheostomy equipment, ambu-bag, suction apparatus) *to restore or maintain an effective airway.*[3,4]
- Evaluate amount and type of secretions being produced. *Excessive and/or sticky mucus can make it difficult to maintain effective airways, especially if client has impaired cough function, is very young or elderly, is developmentally delayed, has restrictive or obstructive lung disease, or is mechanically ventilated.*[5]
- Note ability to, and effectiveness of, cough. *Cough function may be weak or ineffective in diseases and conditions such as extremes in age (e.g., premature infant or elderly), cerebral palsy, muscular dystrophy, spinal cord injury (SCI), brain injury, postsurgery, and/or mechanical ventilation due to mechanisms affecting muscles of throat, chest, and lungs.*[5,6]
- ∞ Suction (nasal, tracheal, oral), when indicated, using correct-size catheter and suction timing for child or adult *to clear airway when secretions are blocking airways, client is unable to*

clear airway by coughing, cough is ineffective, infant is unable to take oral feedings because of secretions, or ventilated client is showing desaturation of oxygen by oximetry or ABGs.[2,5,7]

- Assist with or prepare for appropriate testing (e.g., pulmonary function test or sleep studies) *to identify causative or precipitating factors.*
- Assist with procedures (e.g., bronchoscopy, tracheostomy) *to clear or maintain open airway.*
- Keep environment free of smoke, dust, and feather pillows according to individual situation. *Precipitators of allergic type of respiratory reactions that can trigger/exacerbate acute episode.*[3]

NURSING PRIORITY NO. 2

To mobilize secretions:

- Elevate head of the bed or change position, as needed. *Elevation or upright position facilitates respiratory function by use of gravity; however, the client in severe distress will seek position of comfort.*[3]
- Position appropriately (e.g., head of bed elevated, side-to-side) and discourage use of oil-based products around nose *to prevent vomiting with aspiration into lungs.* (Refer to NDs risk for Aspiration, impaired Swallowing.)
- Encourage and instruct in deep-breathing and directed-coughing exercises; teach (presurgically) and reinforce (postsurgically) breathing and coughing while splinting incision *to maximize cough effort, lung expansion, and drainage, and to reduce pain impairment.*
- Mobilize client as soon as possible. *Reduces risk or effects of atelectasis, enhancing lung expansion and drainage of different lung segments.*[5]
- Administer analgesics, as indicated. *Analgesics may be needed to improve cough effort when pain is inhibiting. Note: Overmedication, especially with opioids, can depress respirations and cough effort.*
- Administer medications (e.g., expectorants, anti-inflammatory agents, bronchodilators, and mucolytic agents), as indicated, *to relax smooth respiratory musculature, reduce airway edema, and mobilize secretions.*[8]
- Increase fluid intake to at least 2000 mL/day within cardiac tolerance (may require IV in acutely ill, hospitalized client). Encourage or provide warm versus cold liquids, as appropriate. *Warm hydration can help liquefy viscous secretions and improve secretion clearance. Note: Individuals with compromised cardiac function may develop symptoms of CHF (crackles, edema, weight gain).*[4,5]
- Provide ultrasonic nebulizer or room humidifier, as needed, *to deliver supplemental humidification, helping to reduce viscosity of secretions.*
- Assist with use of respiratory devices and treatments (e.g., intermittent positive-pressure breathing [IPPB], incentive spirometer [IS], positive expiratory pressure [PEP] mask, mechanical ventilation, oscillatory airway device [flutter], assisted and directed cough techniques). *Various therapies/modalities may be required to maintain adequate airways, improve respiratory function and gas exchange.* (Refer to NDs ineffective Breathing Pattern, impaired Gas Exchange, impaired spontaneous Ventilation.)[3,11]
- Perform or assist client in learning airway clearance techniques, particularly when airway congestion is a chronic or long-term condition. *Numerous techniques may be used, including (but not limited to) postural drainage and percussion (CPT), flutter devices, high-frequency chest compression with an inflatable vest, intrapulmonary percussive ventilation administered by a percussinator, and active cycle breathing (ACB), as indicated. Many of these techniques are the result of research in treatments of cystic fibrosis and muscular dystrophy as well as other chronic lung diseases.*[1]

Nursing Diagnoses in Alphabetical Order

NURSING PRIORITY NO. 3

To assess changes, note complications:

- Auscultate breath sounds, noting changes in air movement *to ascertain current status and effects of treatments to clear airways.*
- Monitor vital signs, noting blood pressure or pulse changes. Observe for increased respiratory rate, restlessness or anxiety, and use of accessory muscles for breathing, *suggesting advancing respiratory distress.*
- Monitor and document serial chest radiographs, ABGs, pulse oximetry readings. *Identifies baseline status, influences interventions, and monitors progress of condition and/or treatment response.*
- Evaluate changes in sleep pattern, noting insomnia or daytime somnolence. *May be evidence of nighttime airway incompetence or sleep apnea.* (Refer to ND Insomnia.)
- Document response to drug therapy and/or development of adverse reactions or side effects with antimicrobial agents, steroids, expectorants, bronchodilators. *Pharmacological therapy is used to prevent and control symptoms, reduce severity of exacerbations, and improve health status. The choice of medications depends on availability of the medication and the client's decision making about medication regimen and response to any given medication.*[10]
- Observe for signs/symptoms of infection (e.g., increased dyspnea, onset of fever, increase in sputum volume, change in color or character) *to identify infectious process and promote timely intervention.*[10]
- Obtain sputum specimen, preferably before antimicrobial therapy is initiated, *to verify appropriateness of therapy. Note: The presence of purulent sputum during an exacerbation of symptoms is a sufficient indication for starting antibiotic therapy, but a sputum culture and antibiogram (antibiotic sensitivity) may be done if the illness is not responding to the initial antibiotic.*[10]

NURSING PRIORITY NO. 4

To promote wellness (Teaching/Discharge Considerations):

- Assess client's/caregiver's knowledge of contributing causes, treatment plan, specific medications, and therapeutic procedures *to determine educational needs.*
- Provide information about the necessity of raising and expectorating secretions versus swallowing them, *to note changes in color and amount.*
- Identify signs/symptoms to be reported to primary care provider. *Prompt evaluation and intervention is required to prevent/treat infection.*
- Demonstrate or assist client/SO in performing specific airway clearance techniques (e.g., forced expiratory breathing [also called "huffing"] or respiratory muscle strength training, chest percussion), if indicated.[11]
- Review breathing exercises, effective coughing techniques, and use of adjunct devices (e.g., IPPB or incentive spirometry) in preoperative teaching *to facilitate postoperative recovery, reduce risk of pneumonia.*
- Instruct client/SO/caregiver in use of inhalers and other respiratory drugs. Include expected effects and information regarding possible side effects and interactions of respiratory drugs with other medications, over-the-counter (OTC) medications, and herbals. Discuss symptoms requiring medical follow-up. *Client is often taking multiple medications that have similar side effects and potential for interactions. It is important to understand the difference between nuisance side effects (e.g., fast heartbeat after albuterol inhaler) and adverse effects (e.g., chest pain, hallucinations, or uncontrolled cardiac arrhythmia).*[9]

- Encourage and provide opportunities for rest; limit activities to level of respiratory tolerance. *Prevents or diminishes fatigue associated with underlying condition or efforts to clear airways.*
- Urge reduction or cessation of smoking. *Smoking is known to increase production of mucus and to paralyze (or cause loss of) cilia needed to move secretions to clear airway and improve lung function.*[10]
- Refer to appropriate support groups (e.g., smoking-cessation clinic, COPD exercise group, weight reduction, American Lung Association, Cystic Fibrosis Foundation, Muscular Dystrophy Association).
- Instruct in use of nocturnal positive pressure airflow for treatment of sleep apnea. (Refer to NDs Insomnia, Sleep Deprivation.)

DOCUMENTATION FOCUS

Assessment/Reassessment
- Related factors for individual client.
- Breath sounds, presence and character of secretions, use of accessory muscles for breathing.
- Character of cough and sputum.

Planning
- Plan of care and who is involved in planning.
- Teaching plan.

Implementation/Evaluation
- Client's response to interventions, teaching, and actions performed.
- Attainment or progress toward desired outcome(s).
- Modifications to plan of care.

Discharge Planning
- Long-term needs and who is responsible for actions to be taken.
- Specific referrals made.

References

1. Impaired Airway Clearance: Information for Patients and Information for Health Plans: The Vest Airway Clearance System. Advanced Respiratory, Inc. (2002). www.abivest.com.
2. Seay, S. J., Gay, S. L., Strauss, M. (2002). Tracheostomy emergencies. *Amer J Nurs,* 102(3), 59.
3. Doenges, M. E., Moorhouse, M. F., Geissler-Murr, A. C. (2002). *Nursing Care Plans: Guidelines for Individualizing Patient Care.* 6th ed. Philadelphia: F. A. Davis, 118–120.
4. Cox, H. C., et al. (2002). *Clinical Applications of Nursing Diagnosis: Adult, Child, Psychiatric, Gerontic, and Home Health Considerations.* 4th ed. Philadelphia: F. A. Davis, 244–249.
5. Fink, J. B., Hess, D. R. (2002). Secretion clearance techniques. In Hess, D. R., et al. (eds). *Respiratory Care: Principles and Practices.* Philadelphia: W. B. Saunders.
6. Blair, K. A. (1999). The aging pulmonary system. In Stanley, M., Beare, P. G. (eds). *Gerontological Nursing.* 2d ed. Philadelphia: F. A. Davis.
7. American Association for Respiratory Care (AARC). (1996). Suctioning of the patient in the home. Clinical Practice Guidelines. *Respir Care,* 41(7), 647–653.
8. Deglin, J. H., Vallerand, A. H. (2003). *Davis's Drug Guide for Nurses.* 8th ed. Bronchodilators: Pharmacologic Profile G56 Philadelphia: F. A. Davis.

9. Yngsdal-Krenz, R. (Spring 1999). Airway Clearance Techniques. Center Focus, newsletter of the University of Wisconsin, Madison.
10. Global strategy for the diagnosis, management, and prevention of chronic obstructive pulmonary disease. Developers: World Health Organization (WHO); National Heart, Lung and Blood Institute (NHLBI); Global Initative for Chronic Obstructive Lung Disease (GOLD). National Guideline Clearinghouse, May 2001. www.ngc.com.
11. McCool, F. D., Rosen, M. J. (2006). Nonpharmacologic airway clearance therapies. *Chest*, 129, 250S–259S.

latex Allergy Response

DEFINITION: A hypersensitive reaction to natural latex rubber products

RELATED FACTORS

Hypersensitivity to natural latex rubber protein

DEFINING CHARACTERISTICS

Subjective
Life-threatening reactions occurring <1 hour after exposure to latex proteins:
Tightness in chest; [feeling breathless]
Gastrointestinal characteristics: Abdominal pain; nausea
Orofacial characteristics: Itching of the eyes; nasal, facial, or oral itching; nasal congestion
Generalized characteristics: Generalized discomfort; increasing complaints of total body warmth
Type IV reactions occurring >1 hour after exposure to latex protein:
Discomfort reaction to additives such as thiurams and carbamates

Objective
Life-threatening reactions occurring <1 hour after exposure to latex proteins:
Contact urticaria progressing to generalized symptoms
Edema of the lips, tongue, uvula, or throat
Dyspnea; wheezing; bronchospasm; respiratory arrest
Hypotension; syncope; cardiac arrest
Orofacial characteristics: Edema of sclera or eyelids; erythema or tearing of the eyes; nasal or facial erythema; rhinorrhea
Generalized characteristics: Flushing; generalized edema; restlessness
Type IV reactions occurring >1 hour after exposure to latex protein:
Eczema; irritation; redness

Sample Clinical Applications: Multiple allergies, neural tube defects (e.g., spina bifida, myelomeningoceles), multiple surgeries at early age, chronic urological conditions (e.g., neurogenic bladder, exstrophy of bladder), spinal cord trauma

DESIRED OUTCOMES/EVALUATION CRITERIA

Sample NOC linkages:
Allergic Response: Localized: Severity of localized hypersensitive immune response to a specific environmental (exogenous) antigen

Allergic Response: Systemic: Severity of systemic hypersensitive immune response to a specific environmental (exogenous) antigen

Knowledge: Treatment Regimen: Extent of understanding conveyed about a specific treatment regimen

Client Will: (Include Specific Time Frame)
* Be free of signs of hypersensitive response.
* Verbalize understanding of individual risks and responsibilities in avoiding exposure.
* Identify signs/symptoms requiring prompt intervention.

ACTIONS/INTERVENTIONS

Sample (NIC) linkages:

Latex Precautions: Reducing the risk of a systemic reaction to latex

Allergy Management: Identification, treatment, and prevention of allergic responses to food, medications, insect bites, contrast material, blood, or other substances

Environmental Risk Protection: Preventing and detecting disease and injury in populations at risk from environmental hazards

NURSING PRIORITY NO. 1

To assess contributing factors:

* Identify persons in high-risk categories such as those with history of certain food allergies (e.g., banana, avocado, chestnut, kiwi, papaya, peach, nectarine); prior allergies, asthma, and skin conditions (e.g., eczema and other dermatitis); those occupationally exposed to latex products (e.g., healthcare workers, police, firefighters, emergency medical technicians [EMTs], food handlers, hairdressers, cleaning staff, factory workers in plants that manufacture latex-containing products); those with neural tube defects (e.g., spina bifida) or congenital urological conditions requiring frequent surgeries and/or catheterizations (e.g., exstrophy of the bladder). *Note: The most severe reactions tend to occur with latex proteins contacting internal tissues during invasive procedures and when they touch mucous membranes of the mouth, vagina, urethra, or rectum.*[9,10,11,13]
* Question client regarding latex allergy upon admission to healthcare facility, especially when procedures are anticipated (e.g., laboratory, emergency department, operating room, wound care management, one-day surgery, dentist). *Basic safety information to help healthcare providers prevent/prepare for safe environment for client and themselves while providing care.*[2,4,7]
* Discuss history of exposure: client works in environment where latex is manufactured or latex gloves are used frequently; child was blowing up balloons (may be an acute reaction to the powder); use of condoms (may affect either partner); individual requires frequent catheterizations. *Finding cause of reaction may be simple or complex but often requires diligent investigation and history-taking from multiple sources.*
* Administer or note presence of positive skin-prick test (SPT), when performed. *Sensitive, specific, and rapid test but should be used with caution in persons with suspected sensitivity, as it carries risk of anaphylaxis.*[10]
* Perform challenge or patch test, if appropriate, *to identify specific allergens in client with known type IV hypersensitivity.*
* Note response to radioallergosorbent test (RAST) or enzyme-linked latex-specific IgE (ELISA). *Performed to measure the quantity of IgE antibodies in serum after exposure to*

specific antigens and has generally replaced skin tests and provocation tests, which are inconvenient, often painful, and/or hazardous to the client.[1,10,11]

NURSING PRIORITY NO. 2

To take measures to reduce/limit allergic response/avoid exposure to allergens:

- Ascertain client's current symptoms, noting rash, hives, itching, eye symptoms, edema, diarrhea, nausea, and feeling of faintness. *Baseline for determining where the client is along a continuum of symptoms so that appropriate treatments can be initiated.*
- Determine time since exposure (e.g., immediate or delayed onset such as 24–48 hours).
- Assess skin (usually hands but may be anywhere) for dry, crusty, hard bumps, horizontal cracks caused by irritation from chemicals used in/on the latex item (e.g., latex or powder used in latex gloves, condoms). *Dry, itchy rash (contact irritation) is the most common response and is not a true allergic reaction but can progress to a delayed type of allergic contact dermatitis with oozing blisters and spread in a way similar to poison ivy.*[2–5,12]
- Assist with treatment of contact dermatitis/type IV reaction:
  Wash affected skin with mild soap and water.
  Wash hands between glove changes and after each glove removal.
  Avoid oil-based salves or lotions when using latex gloves.
  Consider application of topical steroid ointment.
  Inform client that the most common cause is latex gloves but that many other products contain latex and could aggravate condition.
  Monitor closely for signs of systemic reactions (e.g., difficulty breathing or swallowing; wheezing; hoarseness; stridor; hypotension; tremors; chest pain; tachycardia; dysrhythmias; edema of face, eyelids, lips, tongue, and mucous membranes). *Type IV response can progress to type I anaphylaxis.*
  Note behavior such as agitation, restlessness, and expressions of fearfulness in the presence of above listed symptoms. *Indicative of severe allergic response that can result in anaphylactic reaction and lead to respiratory or cardiac arrest.*[6]
- Administer treatment, as appropriate, if severe or life-threatening reaction occurs:
  Stop treatment or procedure, if needed.
  Support airway and administer 100% oxygen or mechanical ventilation, if needed.
  Administer emergency medications and treatments per protocol (e.g., antihistamines, epinephrine, corticosteroids, and IV fluids).
- Educate care providers in ways to prevent inadvertent exposure (e.g., post latex precaution signs in client's room, document allergy to latex in chart, routinely monitor client's environment for latex-containing products and remove them promptly) and in emergency treatment measures should they be needed.
- Ascertain that latex-safe environment (e.g., surgical suite, hospital room) and products are available according to recommended facility guidelines and standards, including equipment and supplies, (e.g., powder-free, low-protein latex products) and latex-free items (e.g., gloves, syringes, catheters, tubings, tape, thermometers, electrodes, oxygen cannulas, underpads, storage bags, diapers, feeding nipples), as appropriate.[2,9,10,13]
- Notify physicians, colleagues, and medical products suppliers of client's condition (e.g., pharmacy *so that medications can be prepared in latex-free environment,* home-care oxygen company *to provide latex-free cannulas*).
- Encourage client to wear medical ID bracelet *to alert providers to condition if client is unresponsive.*[3,4,7]

NURSING PRIORITY NO. 3

To promote wellness (Teaching/Learning):

- Instruct in signs of reaction and emergency treatment needs. *Reactions range from skin irritation to anaphylaxis. Reaction may be gradual but progressive, affecting multiple body systems, or may be sudden, requiring lifesaving treatment. Allergy can result in chronic illness, disability, career loss, hardship, and death. There is no cure except complete avoidance of latex.*

- Emphasize the critical importance of taking immediate action for type I reaction *to limit life-threatening symptoms.*

- Demonstrate equipment and injection procedure, and recommend client carry auto-injectable epinephrine *to provide timely emergency treatment, as needed.*

- Emphasize necessity of informing all new care providers of hypersensitivity *to reduce preventable exposures.*

- Instruct client/family/SO that latex exposure occurs through contact with skin or mucous membrane, by inhalation, parenteral injection, or wound inoculation.

- Instruct client/SO to survey and routinely monitor environment for latex-containing products and replace as needed.

- Provide printed lists or Web sites for identifying common household products that may contain latex (e.g., carpet backing, hoses, rubber grip utensils, diapers, undergarments, shoes, toys, pacifiers, computer mouse pads, erasers, rubber bands, and much more) and where to obtain latex-free products and supplies.[4,7]

- Provide resource and assistance numbers for emergencies. *When allergy is suspected or the potential for allergy exists, protection must begin with identification and removal of possible sources of latex.*

- Provide worksite review, where indicated, and recommendations to prevent exposure. *Latex allergy can be a disabling occupational disorder. Education about the problem promotes prevention of allergic reaction, facilitates timely intervention, and helps nurse to protect clients, latex-sensitive colleagues, and themselves.*[3,4]

- Recommend full medical workup for client presenting with hand dermatitis, especially if job tasks include use of latex.[8]

- Contact suppliers to verify that latex-free equipment, products, and supplies are available, including but not limited to low-allergen or powder-free synthetic gloves, airways, masks, stethoscope tubings, IV tubing, tape, thermometers, urinary catheters, stomach and intestinal tubes, electrodes, oxygen cannulas, pencil erasers, wrist name bands, and rubber bands.[7]

- Ascertain that procedures are in place to identify and resolve problems with medical devices relevant to allergic reactions or glove performance.[4]

- Refer to resources, including but not limited to ALERT (Allergy to Latex Education & Resource Team, Inc.), Latex Allergy News, Spina Bifida Association, National Institute for Occupational Safety and Health (NIOSH), Kendall's Healthcare Products (Web site), and Hudson RCI (Web site) *for further information about common latex products in the home, latex-free products, and assistance.*

DOCUMENTATION FOCUS

Assessment/Reassessment
- Assessment findings including type and extent of symptoms.
- Pertinent history of contact with latex products and frequency of exposure.

Planning
• Plan of care and interventions and who is involved in planning.
• Teaching plan.

Implementation/Evaluation
• Response to interventions, teaching, and actions performed.
• Attainment or progress toward desired outcome(s).
• Modifications to plan of care.

Discharge Planning
• Discharge needs, specific referrals made, additional resources available.

References

1. Cavanaugh, B. M. (1999). *Nurse's Manual of Diagnostic Tests*. 3d ed. Philadelphia: F. A. Davis.
2. Latex allergy: Protect yourself, protect your patients. Nursing World: Workplace Issues: Occupational Safety and Health. ANA Pub. No. WP-7, 1996.
3. Preventing allergic reactions to natural rubber latex in the workplace. National Institutes for Occupational Safety and Health (NIOSH) Alert. June 1997. DHHS (NIOSH) Pub. No. 97–135.
4. ANA Position Statement: Latex Allergy [online]. Effective September 1997. www.nursingworld.org.
5. Truscott, W., Roley, L. (1995). Glove-associated reactions: Addressing an increasing concern. *Dermatol Nurs*, 7(5), 283.
6. Urticaria and angioedema (1997). In Sommers, M. S., Johnson, S. A. (eds). *Davis's Manual of Nursing Therapeutics for Diseases and Disorders*. Philadelphia: F. A. Davis.
7. AANA Latex Protocol. Certified Registered Nurse Anesthetists (CRNA), American Association of Nurse Anesthetists. Developed 1993, Revised and Approved July 1998. www.aana.com.
8. Worthington, K., Wilburn, S. (2001). Latex allergy: What's the facility's responsibility and what's yours? *Amer J Nurs*, 101(7), 88.
9. Klotter, J. (2006) *Latex allergy prevention*. Townsend Letter for Doctors and Patients, May 1, 2006.
10. Behrman, A. J., Howarth, M. (2008). Latex allergy. Retrieved September 2009 from http://emedicine.medscape.com/article/756632-overview.
11. Allergy testing. Article for Lab Tests Online. Retrieved February 2007 from www.labtestsonline.
12. Haines, C. (2006). Learning about allergies to latex. Retrieved February 2007 from www.webmd.com/content/pages/10/1625.htm.
13. AORN Latex Guideline: 2004 standards, recommended practices, and guidelines. *AORN J*, 79(3), 653–672.

risk for latex Allergy Response

DEFINITION: Risk of hypersensitivity to natural latex rubber products

RISK FACTORS

History of reactions to latex
Allergies to bananas, avocados, tropical fruits, kiwi, chestnuts, poinsettia plants
History of allergies and asthma
Professions with daily exposure to latex

⊕ Cultural   Collaborative   Community/Home Care   Diagnostic Studies   ∞ Pediatric/Geriatric/Lifespan   Medications

Multiple surgical procedures, especially from infancy

NOTE: A risk diagnosis is not evidenced by signs and symptoms, as the problem has not occurred; rather, nursing interventions are directed at prevention.

Sample Clinical Applications: Multiple allergies, neural tube defects (e.g., spina bifida, myelomeningoceles), multiple surgeries at early age, chronic urological conditions (e.g., neurogenic bladder, exstrophy of bladder), spinal cord trauma

DESIRED OUTCOMES/EVALUATION CRITERIA

Sample (NOC) linkages:
Allergic Response: Localized: Severity of localized hypersensitive immune response to a specific environmental (exogenous) antigen
Risk Control: Personal actions to prevent, eliminate, or reduce modifiable health threats
Knowledge: Health Behavior: Extent of understanding conveyed about the promotion and protection of health

Client Will (Include Specific Time Frame)
• Identify and correct potential risk factors in the environment.
• Demonstrate appropriate lifestyle changes to reduce risk of exposure.
• Identify resources to assist in promoting a safe environment.
• Recognize need for and seek assistance to limit response or complications.

ACTIONS/INTERVENTIONS

Sample (NIC) linkages:
Latex Precautions: Reducing the risk of a systemic reaction to latex
Allergy Management: Identification, treatment, and prevention of allergic responses to food, medications, insect bites, contrast material, blood, or other substances
Risk Identification: Analysis of potential risk factors, determination of health risks, and prioritization of risk-reduction strategies for an individual or group

NURSING PRIORITY NO. 1

To assess causative/contributing factors:

● Identify persons in high-risk categories such as those with history of certain food allergies (e.g., banana, avocado, chestnut, kiwi, papaya, peach, nectarine), asthma, skin conditions (e.g., eczema); those occupationally exposed to latex products (e.g., healthcare workers, police/firefighters, emergency medical technicians [EMTs], food handlers, hairdressers, cleaning staff, factory workers in plants that manufacture latex-containing products); those with neural tube defects (e.g., spina bifida) or congenital urological conditions requiring frequent surgeries and/or catheterizations (e.g., exstrophy of the bladder). *Note: The most severe reactions tend to occur with latex proteins contacting internal tissues during invasive procedures and when they touch mucous membranes of the mouth, vagina, urethra, or rectum.*[5–7]
● Question client regarding latex allergy upon admission to healthcare facility, especially when procedures are anticipated (e.g., laboratory, emergency department, operating room, wound care management, one-day surgery, dentist). *Current information indicates that natural latex is found in thousands of medical supplies; however, many manufacturers are now using synthetic SB (styrene-butadiene) latex. These products have not been associated with allergic reactions, even among individuals who are sensitive to natural latex.*[1]

NURSING PRIORITY NO. 2

To assist in correcting factors that could lead to latex allergy:

- Ascertain that facilities have established policies and procedures. *Promotes awareness in the workplace to address safety and reduce risk to workers and clients.*[3]
- Create latex-safe environments in care setting (e.g., substitute nonlatex products, such as natural rubber gloves, PCV IV tubing, latex-free tape, thermometers, electrodes, oxygen cannulas). *Reduces risk of exposure.*[8,9]
- Promote good skin care when latex gloves may be preferred/required for barrier protection (e.g., in specific disease conditions such as HIV or during surgery). Use powder-free gloves, wash hands immediately after glove removal; refrain from use of oil-based hand cream. *Reduces dermal and respiratory exposure to latex proteins that bind to the powder in gloves.*[10]
- Discuss necessity of avoiding latex exposure. Recommend or assist client/family to survey environment and remove any medical or household products containing latex. *Avoidance of latex is the only way to prevent the allergic reaction.*[2]
- Provide worksite review, where indicated, and recommendations to prevent exposure. *Latex allergy can be a disabling occupational disorder. Education about the problem promotes prevention of allergic reaction, facilitates timely intervention, and helps nurse to protect clients, latex-sensitive colleagues, and themselves.*[1,4]

NURSING PRIORITY NO. 3

To promote wellness (Teaching/Discharge Considerations):

- Instruct client/care providers about types of potential reactions. *Reaction may be gradual and progressive (e.g., irritant contact rash with gloves); can be progressive, affecting multiple body systems; or may be sudden and anaphylactic requiring lifesaving treatment.*[1,3]
- Identify measures to take if reactions occur and ways to avoid exposure to latex products *to reduce risk of injury.* (Refer to ND latex Allergy Response.)
- Refer to allergist for testing as appropriate. *Testing may include challenge test with latex gloves, skin patch test, or blood test for IgE.*
- Encourage client to wear medical ID bracelet and emphasize importance of informing all new care providers of hypersensitivity *to reduce preventable exposures.*[1,4]
- Refer to resources (e.g., Latex Allergy News, National Institute for Occupational Safety and Health [NIOSH], Kendall's Healthcare Products [Web site], Hudson RCI [Web site]) *for further information about common latex products in the home, latex-free products, and assistance.*

DOCUMENTATION FOCUS

Assessment/Reassessment
- Assessment findings, pertinent history of contact with latex products, and frequency of exposure.

Planning
- Plan of care and who is involved in planning.
- Teaching plan.

Implementation/Evaluation
- Response to interventions, teaching, and actions performed.
- Attainment or progress toward desired outcome(s).
- Modifications to plan of care.

⊕ Cultural   Collaborative   🏠 Community/Home Care   ⬍ Diagnostic Studies   ∞ Pediatric/Geriatric/Lifespan   Medications

Discharge Planning
- Long-term needs and who is responsible for actions to be taken.
- Specific referrals made.

References

1. American Nurses Association (ANA). Position Statement: Latex Allergy [online]. Effective September 1997. www.nursingworld.org.
2. Statement on natural latex allergies and SB latex. Occupational Hazards. Retrieved February 11, 2003 from www.occupationalhazards.com.
3. Latex allergy: Protect yourself, protect your patients. Nursing World: Workplace Issues: Occupational Safety and Health. ANA Pub. No. WP-7, 1996.
4. Preventing allergic reactions to natural rubber in the workplace. National Institutes for Occupational Safety and Health (NIOSH) Alert. DHHS Pub. No. 97–135, June 1997.
5. Klotter, J. (2006) *Latex allergy prevention.* Townsend Letter for Doctors and Patients, May 1, 2006.
6. Behrman, A. J., Howarth, M. (2005). Latex allergy. Retrieved February 2007 from www.emedicine.com/emerg/topic814.htm.
7. Haines, C. (2006). Learning about allergies to latex. Retrieved February 2007 from www.webmd.com/allergies/guide/latex-allergies.
8. AORN latex guideline: 2004 standards, recommended practices, and guidelines. *AORN J,* 79(3), 653–672.
9. MoInlycke Health Care, US, LLC. (2006). Latex-safe is best gloving practice against latex allergy. PR Newswire. Retrieved February 2007 from www.biogellatexsafe.com/downloads/yahoo_finance_latex-safe.doc.
10. Centers for Disease Control and Prevention. (2000–2007). Latex allergy prevention. Article for National Institute for Occupational Safety and Health (NIOSH) Web site. Retrieved February 2007 from www.cdc.gov/niosh/98-113.html.

Anxiety [specify level: mild, moderate, severe, panic]

DEFINITION: Vague uneasy feeling of discomfort or dread accompanied by an autonomic response (the source often nonspecific or unknown to the individual); a feeling of apprehension caused by anticipation of danger. It is an alerting signal that warns of impending danger and enables the individual to take measures to deal with threat.

RELATED FACTORS

Unconscious conflict about essential [beliefs], goals and values of life
Situational or maturational crises
Stress
Familial association or heredity
Interpersonal transmission or contagion
Threat to self-concept [perceived or actual]; [unconscious conflict]
Threat of death [perceived or actual]
Threat to or change in health status [progressive/debilitating disease, terminal illness], interaction patterns, role function or status, environment [safety], economic status
Unmet needs
Exposure to toxins
Substance abuse

(continues on page 64)

Anxiety (continued)

[Positive or negative self-talk]

[Physiological factors, such as hyperthyroidism, pulmonary embolism, dysrhythmias, pheochromocytoma, drug therapy including steroids]

DEFINING CHARACTERISTICS

Subjective

Behavioral: Expressed concerns due to change in life events; insomnia

Affective: Regretful; scared; rattled; distressed; apprehensive; uncertain; fearful; feelings of inadequacy; jittery; worried; painful or persistent increased helplessness; [sense of impending doom]; [hopelessness]

Cognitive: Fear of unspecific consequences; awareness of physiological symptoms

Physiological: Shakiness

Sympathetic: Dry mouth, heart pounding; weakness; respiratory difficulties; anorexia; diarrhea

Parasympathetic: Tingling in extremities; nausea; abdominal pain; diarrhea; urinary frequency or hesitancy; faintness; fatigue; sleep disturbance; [chest, back, neck pain]

Objective

Behavioral: Poor eye contact, glancing about, scanning and vigilance, extraneous movement [e.g., foot shuffling, hand or arm movements, rocking motion]; fidgeting; restlessness; diminished productivity; [crying/tearfulness]; [pacing or purposeless activity]; [immobility]

Affective: Increased wariness; focus on self; irritability; overexcited; anguish

Cognitive: Preoccupation; impaired attention; difficulty concentrating; forgetfulness; diminished ability to problem-solve; diminished learning ability; rumination; tendency to blame others; blocking of thought; confusion; decreased perceptual field

Physiological: Voice quivering; trembling or hand tremors; increased tension; facial tension; increased perspiration

Sympathetic: Cardiovascular excitation; facial flushing; superficial vasoconstriction; increased pulse or respiration; increased blood pressure; pupil dilation; twitching; increased reflexes

Parasympathetic: Urinary urgency; decreased blood pressure or pulse

Sample Clinical Applications: Major life changes or events, hospital admissions, surgery, cancer, hyperthyroidism, drug intoxication or abuse, mental health disorders

DESIRED OUTCOMES/EVALUATION CRITERIA

Sample **NOC** linkages:

Anxiety Self-Control: Personal actions to eliminate or reduce feelings of apprehension, tension, or uneasiness from an unidentifiable source

Coping: Personal actions to manage stressors that tax an individual's resources

Impulse Self-Control: Self-restraint of compulsive or impulsive behaviors

Client Will (Include Specific Time Frame)
• Appear relaxed and report anxiety is reduced to a manageable level.
• Verbalize awareness of feelings of anxiety.
• Identify healthy ways to deal with and express anxiety.
• Demonstrate problem-solving skills.
• Use resources and support systems effectively.

ACTIONS/INTERVENTIONS

Sample **NIC** linkages:

Anxiety Reduction: Minimizing apprehension, dread, foreboding, or uneasiness related to an unidentified source or anticipated danger

Dementia Management: Provision of a modified environment for the patient who is experiencing a chronic confusional state

Calming Technique: Reducing anxiety in patient experiencing acute distress

NURSING PRIORITY NO. 1

To assess level of anxiety:

- Review familial and physiological factors, such as genetic depressive factors, psychiatric illness; active medical conditions (e.g., thyroid problems, metabolic imbalances, cardiopulmonary disease, anemia, dysrhythmias); recent or ongoing stressors (e.g., family member illness or death, spousal conflict or abuse, loss of job). *These factors can cause or exacerbate anxiety and anxiety disorders.*[7,13,14]
- Determine current prescribed medication regimen and recent drug history of prescribed or over-the-counter (OTC) medications (e.g., steroids, thyroid preparations, weight-loss pills, caffeine). *Can heighten feelings or sense of anxiety.*[13,14]
- Identify client's perception of the threat represented by the situation. *Distorted perceptions of the situation may magnify feelings. Understanding client's point of view promotes a more accurate plan of care.*[2]
- Note cultural factors that may influence anxiety. *Individual responses are influenced by the cultural values and beliefs, and culturally learned patterns of family of origin. (For example, Arab-Americans are very expressive about feelings, whereas Chinese are more reticent.)*[4]
- Monitor physical responses: for example, palpitations, rapid pulse, repetitive movements, pacing. *Changes in vital signs may suggest degree of anxiety client is experiencing or reflect the impact of physiological factors such as endocrine imbalances, medication effect.*[1,7]
- Observe behavior indicative of anxiety, *which can be a clue to the client's level of anxiety:*
  Mild
  Alert, more aware of environment, attention focused on environment and immediate events.
  Restless, irritable, wakeful, reports of insomnia.
  Motivated to deal with existing problems in this state.
  Moderate
  Perception narrower, concentration increased, and able to ignore distractions in dealing with problem(s).
  Voice quivers or changes pitch.
  Trembling, increased pulse or respirations.
  Severe
  Range of perception is reduced; anxiety interferes with effective functioning.
  Preoccupied with feelings of discomfort or sense of impending doom.
  Increased pulse or respirations with reports of dizziness, tingling sensations, headache, and so forth.
  Panic
  Ability to concentrate is disrupted; behavior is disintegrated; client distorts the situation and does not have realistic perceptions of what is happening.
  May be experiencing terror or confusion or be unable to speak or move (paralyzed with fear).

- Note own feelings of anxiety or uneasiness. *Feelings of anxiety are circular, and those in contact with the client may find themselves feeling more anxious.*[3]
- Note use of drugs (including alcohol and other drugs); insomnia or excessive sleeping, and limited or avoidance of interactions with others, *which may be behavioral indicators of use of drugs to deal with problems, or indicate withdrawal from drugs or substances.*[5]
- Review results of diagnostic tests (e.g., drug screens, cardiac testing, complete blood count [CBC], chemistry panel), *which can point to physiological sources of anxiety.*
- Review coping skills used in past. *Can determine those that might be helpful in current circumstances.*[6]

NURSING PRIORITY NO. 2

To assist client to identify feelings and begin to deal with problems:

- Establish a therapeutic relationship, conveying empathy and unconditional positive regard. *Enables client to become comfortable and to begin looking at feelings and dealing with situation.*[3]
- Be available to client for listening and talking. *Establishes rapport, promotes expression of feelings, and helps client/SO look at realities of the illness or treatment without confronting issues they are not ready to deal with.*[3]
- Encourage client to acknowledge and to express feelings—for example, crying (sadness), laughing (fear, denial), swearing (fear, anger)—using Active-listening, reflection techniques. *Often, acknowledging feelings enables client to accept and deal more appropriately with situation, thus relieving anxiety.*[8]
- Assist client to develop self-awareness of verbal and nonverbal behaviors. *Becoming aware helps client to control these behaviors and begin to deal with issues that are causing anxiety.*[9]
- Clarify meaning of feelings or actions by providing feedback and checking meaning with the client. *Validates meaning and ensures accuracy of communication.*[10]
- Acknowledge anxiety or fear. Do not deny or reassure client that everything will be all right. *Validates reality of feelings. False reassurances may be interpreted as lack of understanding or dishonesty, further isolating client.*[3]
- Be aware of defense mechanisms being used (e.g., denial, regression). *Use of defense mechanisms may be helpful coping mechanisms initially. However, continued use of such mechanisms diverts the energy that the client needs for healing, thus delaying the client from focusing and dealing with his actual problems.*[6]
- Identify coping skills the individual is using currently, such as anger, daydreaming, forgetfulness, eating, smoking, or lack of problem-solving. *These may be useful for the moment but may eventually interfere with resolution of current situation.*[6]
- Provide accurate information about the situation. *Helps client to identify what is reality based and provides opportunity for client to feel reassured.*[11]
- Respond truthfully, avoid bribing, and provide physical contact (e.g., hugging, rocking) when client is a child. *Soothes fears and provides assurance. Children need to recognize that their feelings are not different from others'.*[5]

NURSING PRIORITY NO. 3

To provide measures to comfort and aid client to handle problematic situations:

- Provide comfort measures (e.g., calm or quiet environment, soft music, warm bath, back rub: Therapeutic Touch). *Aids in meeting basic human need, decreasing sense of isolation, and assisting client to feel less anxious. Therapeutic Touch requires the nurse to have*

specific knowledge and experience to use the hands to correct energy field disturbances by redirecting human energies to help or heal.[3,11]

∞ • Modify procedures, as necessary (e.g., substitute oral for intramuscular medications, combine blood draws or use fingerstick method). *Limits degree of stress, avoids overwhelming child or anxious adult.*[2]

∞ • Manage environmental factors, such as harsh lighting, high traffic flow, excessive noise. *May be confusing or stressful to older individuals. Managing these factors can lessen anxiety, especially when client is in strange and unusual circumstances.*[2]

• Discuss the use of music and accommodate client's preferences. *Promotes calming atmosphere, helping to alleviate anxiety.*[3]

• Accept client as is. *The client may need to be where he or she is at this point in time, such as in denial after receiving the diagnosis of a terminal illness.*[3]

• Allow the behavior to belong to the client; do not respond personally. *Reacting personally can escalate the situation, promoting a nontherapeutic situation and increasing anxiety.*[1]

• Assist client to use anxiety for coping with the situation if helpful. *Moderate anxiety heightens awareness and can help client to focus on dealing with problems.*[9]

• Encourage awareness of negative self-talk and discuss replacing with positive statements, such as using "can" instead of "can't," etc. *Negative self-talk promotes feelings of anxiety and self-doubt. Becoming aware and replacing these thoughts can enhance sense of self-worth and reduce anxiety.*[9]

PANIC STATE

• Stay with client, maintaining a calm, confident manner. *Presence communicates caring and helps client to regain control and sense of calm.*[1]

• Speak in brief statements using simple words. *Client is not able to comprehend complex information at this time.*[1]

• Provide for nonthreatening, consistent environment or atmosphere. Minimize stimuli and monitor visitors and interactions with others. *Lessens effect of transmission of anxious feelings.*[1]

• Set limits on inappropriate behavior and help client to develop acceptable ways of dealing with anxiety.

• Provide safe controls and environment until client regains control. *Behavior may result in damage or injury that client will regret when control is regained, diminishing sense of self-worth.*[1]

• Gradually increase activities and involvement with others as anxiety is decreased. *Promotes sense of normalcy, helps control feelings of anxiety.*[1]

• Use cognitive therapy to focus on and correct faulty catastrophic interpretations of physical symptoms. *For example, thoughts of dying increase anxiety and feelings of panic. Controlling these thoughts allows client to look at situation more realistically and begin to deal appropriately with what is happening.*[1]

• Administer antianxiety agents or sedatives, as ordered. *Appropriate medication can be helpful in enabling the client to regain control.*[1]

NURSING PRIORITY NO. 4

To promote wellness (Teaching/Discharge Considerations):

• Assist client to identify and deal with precipitating factors, and learn new methods of coping with disabling anxiety. *Lessens possibility of repeat episodes.*[9]

• Review happenings, thoughts, and feelings preceding the anxiety attack. *Identifies factors that led to onset of attack, promoting opportunity to prevent recurrences.*[2]

- Identify actions and activities the client has previously used to cope successfully when feeling nervous or anxious. *Realizing that individual already has coping skills that can be applied in current and future situations can empower client.*[2]

- List helpful resources and people, including available hotline or crisis managers. *Provides ongoing and timely support.*[2]

- Encourage client to develop a regular exercise or activity program. *May be helpful in reducing level of anxiety by relieving tension and has been shown to raise endorphin levels to enhance sense of well-being.*[2]

- Assist in developing skills (e.g., awareness of negative thoughts, saying "Stop" and substituting a positive thought). *Eliminating negative self-talk can lead to feelings of positive self-esteem. (Note: Mild phobias seem to respond better to behavioral therapy.)*[10]

- Review such strategies as role-playing, use of visualizations to practice anticipated events, prayer or meditation. *These activities can help the client practice behaviors in a safe and supportive environment, enabling individual to manage anxiety-provoking situations.*[10]

- Review medication regimen and possible interactions, especially with OTC drugs, alcohol, herbal products. *Enhances understanding of reason for medication and can avoid untoward or harmful reactions from incompatible drugs.*[12]

- Discuss appropriate drug substitutions or changes in dosage or time of dose. *Ensures proper dosage and avoids untoward side effects. This is especially important in the elderly, who are particularly susceptible to multidrug complications.*[12]

- Refer to physician for drug management program or alteration of prescription regimen. *Drugs that often cause symptoms of anxiety include aminophylline, anticholinergics, dopamine, levodopa, salicylates, and steroids. Monitoring provides opportunity to correct possible undesirable effects of these drugs.*[12]

- Refer to individual and/or group therapy, as appropriate. *May be useful to help client deal with chronic anxiety states.*[2]

DOCUMENTATION FOCUS

Assessment/Reassessment
- Level of anxiety and precipitating or aggravating factors.
- Description of feelings (expressed and displayed).
- Awareness or ability to recognize and express feelings.
- Related substance use, if present.

Planning
- Treatment plan and individual responsibility for specific activities.
- Teaching plan.

Implementation/Evaluation
- Client involvement and response to interventions, teaching, and actions performed.
- Attainment or progress toward desired outcome(s).
- Modifications to plan of care.

Discharge Planning
- Referrals and follow-up plan.
- Specific referrals made.

References

1. Doenges, M., Moorhouse, M., Murr, A. (2002). *Nursing Care Plans: Guidelines for Individualizing Patient Care.* 6th ed. Philadelphia: F. A. Davis.

2. Doenges, M., Townsend, M., Moorhouse, M. (1998). *Psychiatric Care Plans: Guidelines for Individualizing Care.* 3d ed. Philadelphia: F. A. Davis.

3. Townsend, M. (2003). *Psychiatric Mental Health Nursing: Concepts of Care.* 4th ed. Philadelphia: F. A. Davis.

4. Lipson, J. G., Dibble, S. L., Minarik, P. A. (1996). *Culture & Nursing Care: A Pocket Guide. School of Nursing.* San Francisco: UCSF Nursing Press.

5. National Institute of Mental Health. (2000). Anxiety Disorders. NIH Pub. No. 00-3879. Rockville, MD: Author. www.nimh.nih.gov.anxiety/anxiety.cfm.

6. Stuart, G. W. (2001). Anxiety responses and anxiety disorders. In Stuart, G. W., Laraia, M. T. (eds). *Principles and Practice of Psychiatric Nursing,* 7th ed. St. Louis, MO: Mosby.

7. Kunert, P. K. (2002). Stress and adaptation. In Porth, C. M. (ed). *Pathophysiology: Concepts of Altered Health States.* Philadelphia: Lippincott.

8. Moller, M. D., Murphy, M. F. (1998). *Recovering from Psychosis: A Wellness Approach.* Nine Mile Falls, WA: Psychiatric Rehabilitation Nurses Inc.

9. Bohrer, G. J. (March 18, 2002). Anxiety, emotional and physical discomfort. *NurseWeek,* 3(1), 21–22. (Mountain West edition).

10. Burns, D. D. (1999). *Feeling Good: The New Mood Therapy.* New York: Avon.

11. Krieger, D. O. (1979). *The Therapeutic Touch: How to Use Your Hands to Heal.* Englewood Cliffs, NJ: Prentice Hall.

12. Townsend, M. (2001). *Nursing Diagnoses in Psychiatric Nursing: Care Plans and Psychotropic Medications.* 5th ed. Philadelphia: F. A. Davis.

13. Murphy, K. (2005). Anxiety: When is it too much? *Nursing Made Incredibly Easy!,* 3(5), 22–31.

14. Lamemch, T., Shah, A. M., Hsu, K. (2006). Anxiety. Retrieved January 2007 from www.emedicine.com/emerg/topic35.htm.

death Anxiety

DEFINITION: Vague uneasy feeling of discomfort or dread generated by perceptions of a real or imagined threat to one's existence

RELATED FACTORS

Anticipating pain; suffering; adverse consequences of general anesthesia; impact of death on others

Confronting reality of terminal disease; experiencing dying process; perceived proximity of death

Discussions on topic of death; observations related to death; near-death experience

Uncertainty of prognosis; nonacceptance of own mortality

Uncertainty about the existence of a higher power; life after death; an encounter with a higher power

DEFINING CHARACTERISTICS

Subjective
Reports fear of: developing a terminal illness; the process of dying; pain or suffering related to dying; loss of mental [or physical] abilities when dying; premature death; prolonged dying

Negative thoughts related to death and dying

(continues on page 70)

death Anxiety (continued)

Feeling powerlessness over dying

Worrying about the impact of one's death on significant others; [about meeting one's creator or feeling doubtful about the existence of God or higher being]

Concerns of overworking the caregiver

Sample Clinical Applications: Chronic debilitating health conditions, cancer, hospital admission, impending major surgery

DESIRED OUTCOMES/EVALUATION CRITERIA

Sample NOC linkages:

Dignified Life Closure: Personal actions to maintain control during approaching end of life

Fear Self-Control: Personal actions to eliminate or reduce disabling feelings of apprehension, tension, or uneasiness from an identifiable source

Acceptance: Health Status: Reconciliation to significant change in health circumstances

Client Will (Include Specific Time Frame)
- Identify and express feelings (e.g., sadness, guilt, fear) freely and effectively.
- Look toward or plan for the future one day at a time.
- Formulate a plan dealing with individual concerns and eventualities of dying.

ACTIONS/INTERVENTIONS

Sample NIC linkages:

Dying Care: Promotion of physical comfort and psychological peace in the final phase of life

Spiritual Support: Assisting the patient to feel balance and connection with a greater power

Grief Work Facilitation: Assistance with the resolution of a significant loss

NURSING PRIORITY NO. 1

To assess causative/contributing factors:

- Determine how client sees self in usual lifestyle role functioning and determine perception and meaning of anticipated loss to him or her and SO(s). *Provides information that can be compared to changes that are occurring. Understanding these factors are helpful for planning.*[1]
- Ascertain current knowledge of situation. *Identifies misconceptions, lack of information, and other pertinent issues and determines accuracy of knowledge. Healthcare providers may not be anticipating death at this time or in current situation.*[1]
- Determine client's role in family constellation. Observe patterns of communication in family and response of family/SO to client's situation and concerns. *In addition to identifying areas of need or concern, this also reveals strengths useful in addressing the current concerns.*[3]
- Assess impact of client reports of subjective experiences and experience with death (or exposure to death); for example, witnessed violent death or, as a child, viewed body in casket, and so forth. *Identifies possible feelings that may be affecting current situation, thus promoting accurate planning.*[2]
- Identify cultural factors or expectations and impact on current situation and feelings. *These factors affect client attitude toward events and impending loss. For instance, in Russia, the*

head of the family is informed first of the impending death, as they may not want the client to know, so he or she will have a peaceful death. Many cultures prefer to keep the client at home instead of in a long term care facility or hospital. Growth of the hospice movement in the United States provides palliative care and comfort during the client's final days in any setting.[4]

- Note age, physical and mental condition, and complexity of therapeutic regimen. *May affect ability to handle current situation. Younger people may handle stress of illness in more positive ways. Older people may be more accepting of possibility of death. Individuals of any age will deal with situation in own way, depending on diagnosis, condition, expectations, situation.*[1,8]
- Determine ability to manage own self-care, end-of-life decisions, and other affairs, as well as awareness and use of available resources. *Information will be necessary for determining needs, planning care.*[1,8]
- Observe behavior indicative of the level of anxiety present (mild to panic). *The level of anxiety affects client's/SO's ability to process information and participate in activities.*[5]
- Note use of drugs (including alcohol), presence of insomnia, excessive sleeping, avoidance of interactions with others. *Indicators of withdrawal and need for intervention to deal with symptoms or help client deal realistically with diagnosis or illness.*[6]
- Determine sense of futility, feelings of hopelessness, helplessness, lack of motivation to help self. *Indicators of depression and need for early intervention to help client acknowledge and deal with impending death.*[7,8]
- Listen for expressions of inability to find meaning in life or suicidal ideation. *Signs of depression indicating need for referral to therapist/psychiatrist and possible pharmacological treatment to help client deal with terminal illness or situation.*[7]

NURSING PRIORITY NO. 2

To assist client to deal with situation:

- Provide open and trusting relationship. *Promotes opportunity to explore feelings about impending death.*[2]
- Make time for nonjudgmental discussion of philosophical issues or questions about spiritual impact of illness or situation. *Can help client clarify own position on these issues.*[3]
- Respect client's desire or request not to talk. Provide hope within parameters of the individual situation. *Promotes open environment that encourages client to talk freely about thoughts and feelings. Client may not be ready to talk about situation or concerns about death, or may be denying reality of what is happening.*[1,8]
- Encourage expressions of feelings (anger, fear, sadness, etc.). Acknowledge anxiety or fear. Do not deny or reassure client that everything will be all right. Be honest when answering questions and providing information. *Enhances trust and therapeutic relationship.*[2]
- Use therapeutic communication skills of Active-listening. *Technique acknowledges reality of feelings and encourages client to find own solutions.*[2]
- Provide information about normalcy of feelings and individual grief reaction. *Most individuals question their reactions and whether they are normal or not, and information can provide reassurance for individual.*[3] (Refer to ND Grieving.)
- Identify coping skills currently used and how effective they are. Be aware of defense mechanisms being used by the client. *Provides a starting point to plan care and assists client to acknowledge reality and deal more effectively with what is happening.*[3]
- Review life experiences of loss, noting client strengths and successes. *Provides opportunity to identify and use previously successful skills.*[2]
- Provide calm, peaceful setting and privacy, as appropriate. *Promotes relaxation and enhances ability to deal with situation.*[1,8]

- Include family in discussions and decision making, as appropriate. *Involved family members can provide support and ideas for problem-solving.*[7]
- Note client's religious or spiritual orientation, involvement in religious or church activities, presence of conflicts regarding spiritual beliefs. *May benefit by referral to appropriate resource to help client resolve issues, if desired.*[7]
- Assist client to engage in spiritual growth activities, experience prayer or meditation, and forgiveness to heal past hurts. Provide information that anger with God is a normal part of the grief process. *May reduce feelings of guilt or conflict, allowing client to move forward toward resolution.*[1]
- Refer to therapists, spiritual advisors, or counselors, as appropriate. *Promotes facilitation of grief work.*[1]
- Refer to community agencies and resources. *Assists client/SO in planning for eventualities (legal issues, hospice home care, funeral plans, etc.).*[1]

NURSING PRIORITY NO. 3

To promote independence:

- Support client's efforts to develop realistic steps to put plans into action. *Provides sense of control over situation in which client does not have much control.*[1]
- Direct client's thoughts beyond present state, encouraging client to try to enjoy each day and look to the future, as appropriate. *Being in the moment can help client enjoy this time rather than dwelling on what is ahead.*[1]
- Provide opportunities for client to make simple decisions. *Enhances sense of control.*[1]
- Develop individual plan using client's locus of control. *Incorporating locus of control (internal or external) enhances success of plan by enabling client/family to manage situation more effectively.*[2]
- Treat expressed decisions and desires with respect and convey to others, as appropriate. *Expresses regard for the individual and enhances sense of control in situation that is not controllable.*[1]
- Assist with completion of Advance Directives and cardiopulmonary resuscitation (CPR) instructions. *Provides opportunity for client to understand options and express desires.*[1]
- Refer to palliative, hospice, or end-of-life care resources, as appropriate. *Provides support and assistance to client and SO/family through potentially complex and difficult process. Choice of type of care is dependent on timing of care (e.g., palliative care interfaces with curative treatment, which hospice does not allow).*[1]

DOCUMENTATION FOCUS

Assessment/Reassessment
- Assessment findings, including client's fears and signs/symptoms being exhibited.
- Responses and actions of family/SOs.
- Availability and use of resources.

Planning
- Plan of care and who is involved in planning.

Implementation/Evaluation
- Client's response to interventions, teaching, and actions performed.
- Attainment or progress toward desired outcome(s).
- Modifications to plan of care.

Cultural   Collaborative   Community/Home Care   Diagnostic Studies   Pediatric/Geriatric/Lifespan   Medications

Discharge Planning
• Identified needs and who is responsible for actions to be taken.
• Specific referrals made.

References

1. Doenges, M., Moorhouse, M., Murr, A. C. (2002). *Nursing Care Plans: Guidelines for Individualizing Patient Care*. 6th ed. Philadelphia: F. A. Davis.
2. Doenges, M., Townsend, M., Moorhouse, M. (1998). *Psychiatric Care Plans: Guidelines for Individualizing Care*. 3d ed. Philadelphia: F. A. Davis.
3. Townsend, M. (2003). *Psychiatric Mental Health Nursing: Concepts of Care*. 4th ed. Philadelphia: F. A. Davis.
4. Lipson, J. G., Dibble, S. L., Minarik, P. A. (1996). *Culture & Nursing Care: A Pocket Guide*. San Francisco: School of Nursing, UCSF Nursing Press.
5. Doenges, M., Moorhouse, M., Murr, A. C. (2004). *Nurse's Pocket Guide: Diagnoses, Interventions, and Rationales*. 9th ed. Philadelphia: F. A. Davis.
6. Bruera, E., et al. (1995). The frequency of alcoholism among patients with pain due to terminal cancer. *J Pain Symptom Manage*, 10(8), 599–603.
7. Paice, J. (2002). Managing psychological conditions in palliative care. *Amer J Nurs*, 102(11), 36–43.
8. Kouch, M. (2006). Managing symptoms for a "good death." *Nursing*, 36(11), 58–63.

risk for Aspiration

DEFINITION: At risk for entry of gastrointestinal secretions, oropharyngeal secretions, or [exogenous food] solids or fluids into tracheobronchial passages [due to dysfunction or absence of normal protective mechanisms]

RISK FACTORS

Reduced level of consciousness [sedation, anesthesia]
Depressed cough or gag reflexes
Impaired swallowing [inability of the epiglottis and true vocal cords to close off trachea]
Facial, oral, or neck surgery or trauma; wired jaws; [congenital malformations]
Situation hindering elevation of upper body [weakness, paralysis]
Incompetent lower esophageal sphincter [hiatal hernia or other esophageal disease affecting stomach valve function], delayed gastric emptying, decreased gastrointestinal (GI) motility, increased intragastric pressure, increased gastric residual
Presence of tracheostomy or endotracheal (ET) tube [inadequate or overinflation of tracheostomy/ET tube cuff]
[Presence of] GI tubes, tube feedings/medication administration

NOTE: A risk diagnosis is not evidenced by signs and symptoms, as the problem has not occurred; rather, nursing interventions are directed at prevention.
Sample Clinical Applications: Surgery, vomiting, bulimia nervosa, presence of nasogastric tube, brain injury, spinal cord injury, enteral feedings

(continues on page 74)

risk for Aspiration (continued)
DESIRED OUTCOMES/EVALUATION CRITERIA

Sample **NOC** linkages:
Aspiration Prevention: Personal actions to prevent the passage of fluid and solid particles into the lungs
Neurological Status: Ability of the peripheral and central nervous system to receive, process, and respond to internal and external stimuli
Respiratory Status: Airway Patency: Open, clear tracheobronchial passages for air exchange

Client Will (Include Specific Time Frame)
• Experience no aspiration as evidenced by noiseless respirations; clear breath sounds; clear, odorless secretions.
• Identify causative or risk factors.
• Demonstrate techniques to prevent and/or correct aspiration.

ACTIONS/INTERVENTIONS

Sample **NIC** linkages:
Aspiration Precautions: Prevention or minimization of risk factors in the patient at risk for aspiration
Artificial Airway Management: Maintenance of endotracheal and tracheostomy tubes and prevention of complications associated with their use
Postanesthesia Care: Monitoring and management of the patient who has recently undergone general or regional anesthesia

NURSING PRIORITY NO. 1

To assess causative/contributing factors:

● Identify at-risk client according to condition/disease process as listed in Risk Factors *to determine when more active observation and/or interventions may be required.*
● Assess for age-related risk factors, potentiating risk of aspiration (e.g., premature infant, elderly infirm).[13]
● Note level of consciousness or awareness of surroundings, cognitive impairment. *Aspiration is common in comatose clients, owing to inability to cough, to swallow well, and/or presence of artificial airway, mechanical ventilation, and tube feedings.*[1]
● Evaluate neuromuscular dysfunction, if present, noting muscle groups involved, degree of impairment, and whether acute or of a progressive nature (e.g., stroke, cerebral palsy, Parkinson's disease, Guillain-Barré syndrome, amyotrophic lateral sclerosis [ALS], psychiatric client following electric shock therapy). *May result in temporary or chronic, progressive impairment of protective muscle functions.*[12]
● Assess client's ability to swallow, strength of gag and cough reflex, and evaluate amount and consistency of secretions. *Helps to determine presence and effectiveness of protective mechanisms.*
● Observe for neck and facial edema; for example, client with head or neck surgery, tracheal or bronchial injury (upper torso burns, inhalation or chemical injury). *Problems with swallowing and maintenance of airways can be expected in this client, and the potential is high for aspiration and aspiration pneumonia.*

- Assess amount and consistency of respiratory secretions, breath sounds, and rate and depth of respirations as well as client's coughing and swallowing abilities. *Helps differentiate the potential cause for risk of aspiration. The major pathophysiological dysfunction is the inability of the epiglottis and true vocal cords to move to close the trachea (e.g., changes in the structures themselves or because messages to the brain are absent, decreased, or impaired). Problems with coughing (clearing airways) and swallowing (pooling of saliva, liquids) increase risk of aspiration and respiratory complications.*[2-4]
- Auscultate lung sounds periodically (especially in client who is coughing frequently or not coughing at all; ventilator client being tube-fed, immediately following extubation) and observe chest radiographs *to determine presence of aspirated food or secretions and "silent aspiration."*[5]
- Evaluate for/note presence of GI pathology and motility disorders. *Nausea with vomiting (associated with metabolic disorders, following surgery, certain medications) and gastroesophageal reflux disease (GERD) can be a cause for aspiration.*[3,6]
- Note administration of enteral feedings, which may be initiated when oral nutrition is not possible, such as in head injury, stroke or other neurological disorders, head and neck surgery, esophageal obstruction, and discontinuous GI tract. *Potential exists for regurgitation and aspiration, even with proper tube placement, necessitating the need for clients at high risk for aspiration associated with nasogastroenteral feedings to be evaluated for enteral feedings into the jejunum.*[7]
- Ascertain lifestyle habits (e.g., chronic use of alcohol and drugs, alcohol intoxication, tobacco, and other central nervous system [CNS] suppressant drugs). *Can affect awareness as well as impair gag and swallow mechanisms.*[5]
- Assist with and review diagnostic studies (e.g., video-fluoroscopy or fiber-optic endoscopy) *that may be done to assess for presence and degree of impairment.*[12]

NURSING PRIORITY NO. 2

To assist in correcting factors that can lead to aspiration:

- Place client in proper position for age and condition or disease affecting airways. *Adult and child should be upright for meals or placed on right side to decrease likelihood of drainage into trachea, and to reduce reflux and improve gastric emptying.*[2] *Prone position may provide shorter gastric emptying time and decreased incidence of regurgitation and subsequent aspiration in premature infants.*[8]
- Encourage client to cough, as able, to clear secretions. *May simply need to be reminded or encouraged to cough (such as might occur in elderly person with delayed gag reflex or in postoperative, sedated client).*[2]
- Provide close monitoring for use of oxygen masks in clients at risk for vomiting. Refrain from using oxygen mask for comatose individuals.
- Keep wire cutters or scissors with client at all times when jaws are wired or banded *to facilitate clearing airway in emergencies.*
- Assist with postural drainage and other respiratory therapies *to mobilize thickened secretions that may interfere with swallowing.*
- In client requiring suctioning to manage secretions:[2,9,10,15]
  Maintain operational suction equipment at bedside or chairside.
  Suction (oral cavity, nose, and ET/tracheostomy tube), as needed, using correct size of catheter and timing for adult or child *to clear secretions in client with more frequent or congested sounding cough; presence of coarse rhonchi and expiratory wheezing (audible with or without auscultation); visible secretions, increased peak pressures during volume-cycled ventilation; indication from client that suctioning is necessary; suspected*

aspiration of gastric or upper airway secretions; or otherwise unexplained increases in shortness of breath, respiratory rate, or heart rate.

Avoid triggering gag mechanism when performing suction or mouth care.

Avoid keeping client supine or flat when on mechanical ventilation (especially when also receiving enteral feedings). *Supine positioning and enteral feeding have been shown to be independent risk factors for the development of aspiration pneumonia.*

🏠 • For a verified swallowing problem:[3,5,12–14]

Provide a rest period prior to feeding time. *Rested person may have less difficulty with swallowing.*

Elevate client to highest or best possible position for eating and drinking.

Feed slowly, and instruct client to take small bites and to chew thoroughly.

Vary placement of food in client's mouth according to type of deficit (e.g., place food in right side of mouth if facial weakness present on left side). Use semisolid or soft foods that stick together and form a bolus (e.g., casseroles, puddings, stews), *which aids swallowing effort by improving client's ability to manipulate food with the tongue.*

Avoid pureed foods and mucus-producing foods (milk).

Determine food and liquid viscosity best tolerated by client. Add thickening agent to liquids, as appropriate. *Some individuals may swallow thickened liquids better than thin liquids.*

Offer very warm or very cold liquids *to activate temperature receptors in the mouth that help to stimulate swallowing.*

Avoid washing solids down with liquids *to prevent bolus of food pushing down too rapidly, increasing risk of aspiration.*

💊 • Provide oral medications in elixir form or crush, if appropriate. Have client self-medicate when possible. Time medications to coincide with meals when possible.

🔗 • Refer to physician *for medical and surgical interventions or speech therapist for specific exercises to strengthen muscles and techniques to enhance swallowing.*

• When feeding tube is in place:[3,11,15]

Note radiograph and/or measurement of aspirate pH following placement of feeding tube *to verify correct position.*

Ask client about feeling of fullness and/or measure residuals just prior to feeding and several hours after feeding, when appropriate, *to prevent overfeeding.*

Elevate head of bed 30 degrees during and for at least 30 minutes after bolus feedings.

Add food coloring (per protocol) to feeding *to identify regurgitation.*

∞ • Determine best position for infant/child (e.g., with the head of bed elevated 30 degrees and infant propped on right side after feeding). *Upper airway patency is facilitated by upright position, and turning to right side decreases likelihood of drainage into trachea.*

💊 • Provide oral medications in elixir form or crush, if appropriate.

💊 • Minimize use of sedatives/hypnotics when possible. *Agents can impair coughing and swallowing.*

NURSING PRIORITY NO. 3

To promote wellness (Teaching/Discharge Considerations):

🏠 • Review individual risk or potentiating factors with client/care provider.

🏠 • Provide information about the effects of aspiration on the lungs. *Note: Severe coughing and cyanosis associated with eating or drinking and voice change after swallowing indicates onset of respiratory symptoms associated with aspiration and requires intervention for actual presence of aspiration.*[13,14]

🏠 • Instruct in safety concerns when feeding orally or tube feeding. (Refer to ND impaired Swallowing.)

- Train client to suction self or train family members in suction techniques (especially if client has constant or copious oral secretions) *to enhance safety/self-sufficiency.*
- Instruct individual/family member to avoid or limit activities after eating that increase intra-abdominal pressure (straining, strenuous exercise, tight or constrictive clothing). *May slow digestion or increase risk of regurgitation.*

DOCUMENTATION FOCUS

Assessment/Reassessment
- Assessment findings and conditions that could lead to problems of aspiration.
- Verification of tube placement, observations of physical findings.

Planning
- Interventions to prevent aspiration or reduce risk factors and who is involved in the planning.
- Teaching plan.

Implementation/Evaluation
- Client's responses to interventions, teaching, and actions performed.
- Foods and fluids client handles with ease or difficulty.
- Amount and frequency of intake.
- Attainment or progress toward desired outcome(s).
- Modifications to plan of care.

Discharge Planning
- Long-term needs and who is responsible for actions to be taken.

References

1. Dimancescu, M. D. (Fall 1989). *Aspiration pneumonia* (Newsletter): Coma Recovery Institute.
2. Cox, H. C., et al. (2002). *Clinical Applications of Nursing Diagnosis: Adult, Child, Women's, Psychiatric, Gerontic, and Home Health Considerations.* 4th ed. Philadelphia: F. A. Davis.
3. Altered nutritional status. Clinical Practice Guidelines. Retrieved December 2002 from American Medical Directors Association (AMDA). www.amda.com.
4. American Gastroenterological Association. (1999). *Medical position statement: Management of oropharyngeal dysphagia*, 116(2), 452.
5. Galvan, T. J. (2001). Dysphagia: Going down and staying down. *Amer J Nurs*, 101(1), 37.
6. Clinical Consensus Statement: Managing Cough as a Defense Mechanism and as a Symptom. (1998). (Quick Reference Guide for Clinicians). Northbrook, IL: American College of Chest Physicians.
7. Eastern Association for the Surgery of Trauma (EAST). (March 1998). *Practice management guidelines for nutritional support of the trauma patient.* (EAST Web site).
8. Apnea of prematurity. Clinical Practice Guideline. (February 1999): National Association of Neonatal Nurses (NANN).
9. American Association for Respiratory Care (ARC). (April 1999). Removal of the endotracheal tube. *The ARC Clinical Practice Guidelines.* www.aarc.org.
10. American Association for Respiratory Care (ARC). (April 1999). Suctioning of the patient in the home. *The ARC Clinical Practice Guidelines.* www.aarc.org.
11. Metheny, N. A., Titler, M. G. (2001). Assessing placement of feeding tubes. *Amer J Nurs*, 101(5), 36.
12. Bowman, A., et al. (2005). Implementation of an evidence-based feeding protocol and aspiration risk reduction algorithm. *Crit Care Nurs Q*, 28(4), 324–333.
13. Goldstein, L. B. (2006). Cough and aspiration of food and liquids due to oral-pharyngeal dysphagia: ACCP evidence-based clinical practice guidelines. *Chest*, 129(1), 154S–168S.

14. Metheny, N. A. (2006). Preventing aspiration in older adults with dysphagia. *Medsurg Nurs,* 15(2).
15. McClave, S. A., et. al. (2005). Poor validity of residual volumes as a marker for risk of aspiration in critically ill patients. *Crit Care Med,* 33(2), 324–330.

risk for impaired Attachment

DEFINITION: Disruption of the interactive process between parent/significant other and child/infant that fosters the development of a protective and nurturing reciprocal relationship

RISK FACTORS

Inability of parents to meet personal needs
Anxiety associated with the parent role; [parents who themselves experienced altered attachment]
Premature infant or ill child who is unable to effectively initiate parental contact due to altered behavioral organization; parental conflict resulting from altered behavioral organization
Separation; physical barriers; lack of privacy
Substance abuse
[Difficult pregnancy and/or birth (actual or perceived)]
[Uncertainty of paternity; conception as a result of rape/sexual abuse]

NOTE: A risk diagnosis is not evidenced by signs and symptoms, as the problem has not occurred; rather, nursing interventions are directed at prevention.
Sample Clinical Applications: Prematurity, genetic or congenital conditions, autism, attention deficit disorder, developmental delay (parent or child), substance abuse (parent), bipolar disorder (parent)

DESIRED OUTCOMES/EVALUATION CRITERIA

Sample (NOC) linkages:
Parent-Infant Attachment: Parent and infant behaviors that demonstrate an enduring affectionate bond
Parenting Performance: Parental actions to provide a child a nurturing and constructive physical, emotional, and social environment
Child Development: [specify age group]: Milestones of physical, cognitive, and psychosocial progression by [specify] months/years of age

Parent Will (Include Specific Time Frame)
• Identify and prioritize family strengths and needs.
• Exhibit nurturing and protective behaviors toward child.
• Identify and use resources to meet needs of family members.
• Demonstrate techniques to enhance behavioral organization of the infant/child.
• Engage in mutually satisfying interactions with child.

🌐 Cultural 🔬 Collaborative 🏠 Community/Home Care ✏️ Diagnostic Studies ∞ Pediatric/Geriatric/Lifespan 💊 Medications

ACTIONS/INTERVENTIONS

Sample (NIC) linkages:
Attachment Promotion: Facilitation of the development of the parent-infant relationship
Parenting Promotion: Providing parenting information, support, and coordination of comprehensive services to high-risk families
Environmental Management: Attachment Process: Manipulation of the patient's surroundings to facilitate the development of the parent-infant relationship

NURSING PRIORITY NO. 1

To identify causative/contributing factors:

- Interview parents, noting their perception of situation, individual concerns. *Identifies problem areas and strengths to formulate appropriate plans to change situation that is currently creating problems for the parents.*[8]
- Assess parent/child interactions. *Identifies relationships, communication skills, and feelings about one another. The way in which a parent responds to a child and how the child responds to the parent largely determines how the child develops. Identifying the way in which the family responds to one another is crucial in determining the need for and type of interventions required.*[8]
- Ascertain availability and use of resources to include extended family, support groups, and finances. *Lack of support from or presence of extended family, lack of involvement in groups (e.g., church) or specific resources (e.g., La Leche League), and financial stresses can affect family negatively, interfering with ability to deal effectively with parenting responsibilities. Parents need support from both inside and outside of the family.*[9,12]
- Determine emotional and behavioral problems of the child. *Attachment-disordered children are unable to give and receive love and affection, defy parental rules and authority, and are physically and emotionally abusive, creating ongoing stress and turmoil in the family and in future relationships.*[12]
- Evaluate parents' ability to provide protective environment, participate in reciprocal relationship. *Parents may be immature, may be substance abusers, or may be mentally ill and unable or unwilling to assume the task of parenting. The ways in which the parent responds to the child is critical to the child's development, and interventions need to be directed at helping the parents to deal with own issues and learn positive parenting skills.*[1,7]
- Note attachment behaviors between parent and child(ren), recognizing cultural background. *For example, lack of eye contact and touching may indicate bonding problems. Behaviors such as eye-to-eye contact, use of en face position, talking to the infant in a high-pitched voice are indicative of attachment behaviors in American culture but may not be appropriate in another culture. Failure to bond effectively is thought to affect subsequent parent-child interaction.*[4,5]
- Assess parenting skill level, considering intellectual, emotional, and physical strengths and limitations. *Identifies areas of need for further education, skill training, and factors that might interfere with ability to assimilate new information.*[1,2]

NURSING PRIORITY NO. 2

To enhance behavioral organization of infant/child:

- Identify infant's strengths and vulnerabilities. *Each child is born with his or her own temperament that affects interactions with caregivers, and when these are known, actions can be taken to assist parents/caregivers to parent appropriately.*[2,7,11]

∞ • Educate parents regarding child growth and development, addressing parental perceptions. *Parents often have misconceptions about the abilities of their children, and providing correct information clarifies expectations and is more realistic.[6]*

∞ • Assist parents in modifying the environment. *The environment can be changed to provide appropriate stimulation; for example, to diminish stimulation before bedtime, to simplify when the environment is too complex to handle, and to provide life space where the child can play unrestricted, resulting in freedom for the child to meet his or her needs.[2,7]* (Refer to ND readiness for enhanced organized Infant Behavior.)

∞ • Model caregiving techniques that best support behavioral organization, such as attachment parenting. *Recognizing that the child deserves to have his or her needs taken seriously and responding to those needs in a loving fashion promotes trust, and children learn to model their behavior after what they have seen the parents do.[9,11]*

∞ • Respond consistently with nurturance to infant/child. *Babies come wired with an ability to signal their needs by crying, and when parents respond to these signals, they develop a sensitivity that in turn develops parental intuition, providing infants with gratification of their needs and trust in their environment.[10]*

NURSING PRIORITY NO. 3

To enhance best functioning of parents:

• Develop therapeutic nurse-client relationship. Provide a consistently warm, nurturant, and nonjudgmental environment. *Parents are often surprised to find that a tiny infant can cause so many changes in their lives and need help to adjust to this new experience. The warm, caring relationship of the nurse can help with this adjustment and provide the information and empathy they need at this time.[1]*

• Assist parents in identifying and prioritizing family strengths and needs. *Promotes positive attitude by looking at what they already do well and using those skills to address needs.[2]*

• Support and guide parents in process of assessing resources. *Outside support is important at this time, and making sure that parents receive the help they need will help them in this adjustment period.[12]*

∞ • Involve parents in activities with the infant/child that they can accomplish successfully. *Activities such as Baby Gymboree and baby yoga enable the parents to get to know their child and themselves, enhancing their confidence and self-concept.[12]*

• Recognize and provide positive feedback for nurturant and protective parenting behaviors. *Using I-messages to let parents know their behaviors are effective reinforces continuation of desired behaviors and promotes feelings of confidence in their abilities.[2,12]*

NURSING PRIORITY NO. 4

To support parent/child attachment during separation:

• Provide parents with telephone contact as appropriate. *Knowing there is someone they can call if they have problems provides a sense of security.[3]*

• Establish a routine time for daily phone calls or initiate calls as indicated when child is hospitalized. *Provides sense of consistency and control; allows for planning of other activities so parents can maintain contact and get information on a regular basis.[1]*

• Minimize number of professionals on team with whom parents must have contact. *Parents begin to know the individuals they are dealing with on a regular basis, fostering trust in these relationships and providing opportunities for modeling and learning.[3]*

• Invite parents to use resources, such as Ronald McDonald House, or provide a listing of a variety of local accommodations, restaurants. *When child is hospitalized out of town, parents need to have a place to stay so they can have ready access to the hospital and be able to rest and refresh from time to time.[5]*

- Arrange for parents to receive photos, progress reports from the child. *Provides information and comfort as the child progresses, allowing the parents to continue to have hope for a positive resolution.[3]*
- Suggest parents provide a photo and/or audiotape of themselves for the child. *Provides a connection during the separation, sustaining attachment between parent and child.[1]*
- Consider use of contract with parents. *Clearly communicating expectations of both family and staff serves as a reminder of what each person has committed to and serves as a tool to evaluate whether expectations are being maintained.[3]*
- Suggest parents keep a journal of infant/child progress. *Serves as a reminder of the progress that is being made, especially when they become discouraged and believe infant/child is "never" going to be better.[3]*
- Provide "homelike" environment for situations requiring supervision of visits. *An environment that is comfortable supports the family as they work toward resolving conflicts and promotes a sense of hopefulness, enabling them to experience success when family is involved with a legal situation.[12]*

NURSING PRIORITY NO. 5

To promote wellness (Teaching/Discharge Considerations):

- Refer to addiction counseling or treatment, individual counseling, or family therapies as indicated. *May need additional assistance when situation is complicated by drug abuse (including alcohol), mental illness, disruptions in caregiving, parents who are burned out with caring for child with attachment or other difficulties.[12,13]*
- Identify services for transportation, financial resources, housing, and so forth. *Assistance with these needs can help families focus on therapeutic regimen and on issues of parenting to improve family dynamics.[9]*
- Develop support systems appropriate to situation (e.g., extended family, friends, social worker). *Depending on individual situation, support from extended family, friends, social worker, or therapist can assist family to deal with attachment disorders.[10]*
- Explore community resources (e.g., church affiliations, volunteer groups, day/respite care). *Church affiliations, volunteer groups, day or respite care can help parents who are overwhelmed with care of a child with attachment or other disorder.[12]*

DOCUMENTATION FOCUS

Assessment/Reassessment
- Identified behaviors of both parents and child.
- Specific risk factors, individual perceptions and concerns.
- Interactions between parent and child.

Planning
- Plan of care and who is involved in planning.
- Teaching plan.

Implementation/Evaluation
- Parents'/child's responses to interventions, teaching, and actions performed.
- Attainment or progress toward desired outcomes.
- Modifications to plan of care.

Discharge Planning
• Long-term needs and who is responsible.
• Plan for home visits to support parents and to ensure infant/child safety and well-being.
• Specific referrals made.

References

1. Townsend, M. C. (2006). *Psychiatric Mental Health Nursing, Concepts of Care in Evidence-Based Practice.* 5th ed. Philadelphia: F. A. Davis.
2. Gordon, T. (2000). *Parent Effectiveness Training.* Updated ed. New York: Three Rivers Press.
3. Cox, H. C., et al. (2002). *Clinical Applications of Nursing Diagnosis: Adult, Child, Women's, Psychiatric, Gerontic, and Home Health Considerations.* 4th ed. Philadelphia: F. A. Davis.
4. Lipson, J. G., Dibble, S. L., Minarik, P. A. (1996). *Culture & Nursing Care. A Pocket Guide.* San Francisco: UCSF Nursing Press.
5. Doenges, M. E., Townsend, M. C., Moorhouse, M. F. (1998). *Psychiatric Care Plans Guidelines for Individualizing Care.* 3d ed. Philadelphia: F. A. Davis.
6. Gordon, T. (1989). *Teaching Children Self-Discipline: At Home and at School.* New York: Random House.
7. Gordon, T. (2000). *Family Effectiveness Training Video.* Solana Beach, CA: Gordon Training International.
8. Doenges, M. E., Moorhouse, M. F., Murr, A. C. (2008). *Nurse's Pocket Guide: Diagnoses, Interventions and Rationales.* 11th ed. Philadelphia: F. A. Davis.
9. Henningsen, M. (1996). *Attachment Disorder: Theory, Parenting and Therapy.* Evergreen, CO: Evergreen Family Counseling Center.
10. Sears, W. (1999). *Attachment Parenting: A Style That Works. Excerpted from Nighttime Parenting: How to Get Your Baby and Child to Sleep (La Leche International Book, revised edition).* New York: Plume.
11. Hunt, J. What Is Attachment Parenting? The Natural Child Project. Retrieved February 2004 from www.naturalchild.com/jan.hunt/attachmentparenting.html.
12. Corrective Attachment Parenting. Evergreen, CO: Evergreen Psychotherapy Center Attachment Treatment and Training Institute.
13. London, M. L., et al. (2007). *Maternal & Child Nursing Care.* Upper Saddle River, NJ: Pearson Prentice Hall.

Autonomic Dysreflexia

DEFINITION: Life-threatening, uninhibited sympathetic response of the nervous system to a noxious stimulus after a spinal cord injury (SCI) at T7 or above

RELATED FACTORS

Bladder or bowel distention; [catheter insertion, obstruction, irrigation]
Skin irritation
Deficient client and caregiver knowledge
[Sexual excitation; menstruation; pregnancy; labor and delivery]
[Environmental temperature extremes]

🌐 Cultural 🅐 Collaborative 🏠 Community/Home Care 🖊 Diagnostic Studies ∞ Pediatric/Geriatric/Lifespan 💊 Medications

DEFINING CHARACTERISTICS

Subjective
Headache (a diffuse pain in different portions of the head and not confined to any nerve distribution area)
Paresthesia, chilling, blurred vision, chest pain, metallic taste in mouth, nasal congestion

Objective
Paroxysmal hypertension (sudden periodic elevated blood pressure in which systolic pressure >140 mm Hg and diastolic >90 mm Hg)
Bradycardia or tachycardia
Diaphoresis (above the injury), red splotches on skin (above the injury), pallor (below the injury)
Horner's syndrome [contraction of the pupil, partial ptosis of the eyelid, enophthalmos and sometimes loss of sweating over the affected side of the face]; conjunctival congestion
Pilomotor reflex [gooseflesh formation when skin is cooled]

Sample Clinical Applications: Spinal cord injury

DESIRED OUTCOMES/EVALUATION CRITERIA

Sample (NOC) linkages:
Neurological Status: Autonomic: Ability of the autonomic nervous system to coordinate visceral and homeostatic function
Knowledge: Disease Process: Extent of understanding conveyed about a specific disease process
Symptom Severity: Severity of perceived adverse changes in physical, emotional, and social functioning

Client/Caregiver Will (Include Specific Time Frame)
• Identify specific precipitating factors.
• Recognize signs/symptoms of syndrome.
• Demonstrate corrective techniques.
• Experience no episodes of dysreflexia or will seek medical intervention in a timely manner.

ACTIONS/INTERVENTIONS

Sample (NIC) linkages:
Dysreflexia Management: Prevention and elimination of stimuli that cause hyperactive reflexes and inappropriate autonomic responses in a patient with a cervical or high thoracic cord lesion
Urinary Elimination Management [or] Bowel Management: Maintenance of an optimum urinary elimination pattern/establishment and maintenance of a regular pattern of bowel elimination
Anxiety Reduction: Minimizing apprehension, dread, foreboding, or uneasiness related to an unidentified source or anticipated danger

NURSING PRIORITY NO. 1

To assess precipitating risk factors:[1–3,7–9]

- Monitor for bladder distention, presence of bladder spasms or stones, or infection. *The most common stimulus for autonomic dysreflexia (AD) is bladder irritation or overstretch associated with urinary retention or infection; blocked catheter; overfilled collection bag; or noncompliance with intermittent catheterization.*
- Evaluate for bowel distention, fecal impaction, and problems with bowel management program. *Bowel irritation or overstretch is associated with constipation or impaction; digital stimulation, suppository or enema use during bowel program; hemorrhoids or fissures; and/or infection of gastrointestinal (GI) tract, such as might occur with ulcers or appendicitis.*
- Observe skin and tissue pressure areas, especially following prolonged sitting. *Skin and tissue irritants include direct pressure (e.g., object in chair or shoe, leg straps, abdominal support, orthotics; wounds (e.g., bruise, abrasion, lacerations, pressure ulcer); ingrown toenail; tight clothing; or sunburn or other burn.*
- Inquire about sexual activity and/or determine if reproductive issues are involved. *Overstimulation or vibration, sexual intercourse and ejaculation, scrotal compression, menstrual cramps, and/or pregnancy (especially labor and delivery) are known stimulants.*
- Inform client/care providers of additional precipitators during course of care. *Client is prone to physical conditions or treatments (e.g., intolerance to temperature extremes; deep vein thrombosis [DVT]; kidney stones; fractures or other trauma, surgical, dental, and diagnostic procedures) any of which can precipitate AD.*
- Monitor environmental temperature for extremes/drafts, *which can precipitate episode.*

NURSING PRIORITY NO. 2

To provide for early detection and immediate intervention:

- Investigate associated complaints/syndrome of symptoms (e.g., severe pounding headache, [blood pressure may be >200/100 mm Hg], chest pain, irregular heart rate or dysrhythmias, blurred vision, nausea, facial flushing, metallic taste, or severe anxiety; or minimal symptoms or expressed complaints in presence of significantly elevated blood pressure—silent AD]). *Body's reaction to misinterpreted sensations from below the injury site, resulting in an autonomic reflex, can cause blood vessels to constrict and increase blood pressure. This is a potentially life-threatening condition, requiring immediate and correct action.*[1–3,7,8]
- ∞ Note onset of crying, irritability, or somnolence in infant or child (may present with nonspecific symptoms; may not be able to verbalize discomforts).[1]
- Locate and eliminate causative stimulus, moving in stepwise fashion. (Cause can be anything that would normally cause pain or discomfort below level of injury.)[1–8]
  Assess for bladder distention *(most common cause of AD)*:
  Empty bladder by voiding or catheterization, applying local anesthetic ointment *to prevent exacerbation of AD by procedure.*
  Ascertain that urine is free-flowing if Foley or suprapubic catheter is in place, empty drainage bag, straighten tubing if kinked, and lower drainage bag if it is higher than bladder.
  Irrigate gently or change catheter, if not draining freely.
  Note color, character, and odor of urine; obtain specimen for culture as indicated *(infection can cause AD)*.
  Check for distended bowel *(if urinary problem is not causing AD)*:
  Perform digital stimulation, checking for constipation or impacted stool. (If symptoms first appear while performing digital stimulation, stop procedure.)

Apply local anesthetic ointment to rectum; remove impaction after symptoms subside *to remove causative problem without causing additional symptoms.*

Check for skin pressure or irritation *(if bowel problem is not causing AD):*

Perform a pressure release if sitting.

Check for tight clothing, straps, belts.

Note whether pressure sore has developed or changed.

Observe for bruising, signs of infection.

Check for ingrown toenail or other injury to skin, tissue (e.g., burns, sunburn) or fractured bones.

Check for other possible causes *(if skin pressure is not causing AD):*

Menstrual cramps, sexual activity, labor and delivery.

Abdominal conditions (e.g., colitis, ulcer).

Environmental temperature extremes.

- Take steps to reduce blood pressure, thereby *reducing potential for stroke (primary concern):*[1-8]

Elevate head of bed immediately, or place in sitting position with legs hanging down. *Lowers blood pressure by pooling of blood in legs.*

Loosen any clothing or restrictive devices. *May allow pooling of blood in abdomen and lower extremities.*

Monitor vital signs frequently during acute episode. *Blood pressure may fluctuate quickly due to impaired autonomic regulation.* Continue to monitor blood pressure at intervals during procedures to remove cause of AD and after acute episodic symptoms subside *to evaluate effectiveness of interventions and antihypertensives.*

- Administer medications, as indicated. *If an episode is particularly severe or persists after removal of suspected cause, antihypertensive medications with rapid onset and short duration (e.g., nifedipine, hydralazine, clonidine) may be used to block excessive autonomic nerve transmission, normalize heart rate, and reduce hypertension.*[1,4]

- Adjust dosage of antihypertensive medications carefully for child, elderly person, and pregnant woman. *Prevents complications, such as systemic hypotension or seizure activity, and maintains blood pressure within optimal range.*[1]

NURSING PRIORITY NO. 3

To promote wellness (Teaching/Discharge Considerations):

- Discuss with client/caregivers warning signs of AD, as listed previously. Be aware of client's communication abilities. *AD can occur at any age from infant to very old, and the individual may not be able to verbalize a pounding headache, which is often the first symptom during onset of AD.*[1,8]

- Ascertain that client/caregivers understand ways to avoid onset or treat syndrome as noted previously. Provide information card and instruct and periodically reinforce teaching, as needed, regarding:[1,2,5-8]

Maintaining indwelling catheter by keeping tubing free of kinks, bag empty and situated below bladder level, and checking daily for deposits (bladder grit) inside catheter.

Performing intermittent catheterization as often as necessary *to prevent overfilling or distention.*

Monitoring for adequate spontaneous voiding, noting frequency and amount.

Maintaining a regular and effective bowel evacuation program.

Performing routine skin assessments.

Monitoring all systems for signs of infection and reporting promptly *for timely medical treatment.*

Scheduling routine medical evaluations.

- Instruct family member/caregiver in proper blood pressure monitoring and discuss plan for monitoring hypertension during acute episodes. *A spinal cord–injured client's (both adult*

Nursing Diagnoses in Alphabetical Order

and child) baseline blood pressure is lower than that of a noninjured person, thus necessitating frequent measurements during acute episodes.

- Review proper use and administration of medications, when used. *Client may have medication(s) both for emergent situations and/or prevention of AD, and if so, should receive medication instructions as well as symptoms to report for immediate or emergent care, when blood pressure is not responsive.*[1,8]
- Refer for or advise treatment of sexual and reproductive concerns, as indicated.[9]
- Recommend wearing Medic Alert bracelet or necklace and carrying information card about signs/symptoms of AD and usual methods of treatment. *Provides vital information in emergency.*
- Assist client/family in identifying emergency referrals (e.g., physician, rehabilitation nurse/home-care supervisor). Place telephone number(s) in prominent place.

DOCUMENTATION FOCUS

Assessment/Reassessment
- Individual findings, noting previous episodes, precipitating factors, and individual signs/symptoms.

Planning
- Plan of care and who is involved in planning.
- Teaching plan.

Implementation/Evaluation
- Client's responses to interventions and actions performed, understanding of teaching.
- Attainment or progress toward desired outcome(s).
- Modifications to plan of care.

Discharge Planning
- Long-term needs and who is responsible for actions to be taken.

References

1. Consortium for Spinal Cord Medicine/Paralyzed Veterans of America. (2001). *Acute Management of Autonomic Dysreflexia: Individuals with Spinal Cord Injury Presenting to Health-Care Facilities*. Retrieved September 2003 from www.pva.org. Washington, DC: Paralyzed Veterans of America (PVA).
2. Acuff, M. (2005). Autonomic dysreflexia: What it is, what it does, and what to do if you experience it. *The Missouri Model Spinal Cord Injury System*. Columbia, MO: University of Missouri-Columbia, School of Health Professions.
3. Health: Autonomic dysreflexia. Retrieved January 2007 from Christopher & Dana Reeve Paralysis Resource Center: www.paralysis.org/site/c.erJMJUOxFmH/b.1338071/k.5E45/Autonomic_Dysreflexia.htm.
4. Deglan, J. H., Vallerand, A. H. (2003). *Davis's Drug Guide for Nurses*. 8th ed. Philadelphia: F. A. Davis.
5. Other complications of spinal cord injury: Autonomic dysreflexia (hyperreflexia) treatment. RehabTeamSite. Retrieved September 2009 from www.calder.med.miami.edu.
6. National Spinal Cord Injury Association (NSCIA). (2003). SCI complications resource. Retrieved 2003 from www.spinalcord.org.
7. Compagnolo, D. I. (2006). Autonomic dysreflexia in spinal cord injury. Retrieved January 2007 from www.emedicine.com/pmr/topic217.htm.
8. Cody, T., Zieroff, V. (2005). Autonomic dysreflexia. *Article for Northeast Rehabilitation Health Network*. Retrieved January 2007 from www.northeastrehab.com/Articles/dysreflexia.htm.
9. Ducharme, S. (2000). Sexuality and spinal cord injury. *Article for Paraplegia News*. Retrieved 2007 from www.stanleyducharme.com/resources/sex_spinalcord_injury.htm.

risk for Autonomic Dysreflexia

DEFINITION: At risk for life-threatening, uninhibited response of the sympathetic nervous system post-spinal shock, in an individual with a spinal cord injury [SCI] or lesion at T6 or above (has been demonstrated in clients with injuries at T7 and T8)

RISK FACTORS

An injury at T6 or above or a lesion at T6 or above AND at least one of the following noxious stimuli:

Musculoskeletal-Integumentary Stimuli
Cutaneous stimulations (e.g., pressure ulcer, ingrown toenail, dressing, burns, rash); sunburns; wounds
Pressure over bony prominences/genitalia; range-of-motion exercises; spasms
Fractures; heterotrophic bone

Gastrointestinal Stimuli
Constipation; difficult passage of feces; fecal impaction; bowel distention; hemorrhoids
Digital stimulation; suppositories; enemas
GI system pathology; esophageal reflux; gastric ulcers; gallstones

Urological Stimuli
Bladder distention or spasm
Detrusor sphincter dyssynergia
Catheterization; instrumentation; surgery
Urinary tract infection (UTI); cystitis; urethritis; epididymitis; calculi

Regulatory Stimuli
Temperature fluctuations; extreme environmental temperatures

Situational Stimuli
Positioning; surgical [or diagnostic] procedure
Constrictive clothing (e.g., straps, stockings, shoes)
Drug reactions (e.g., decongestants, sympathomimetics, vasoconstrictors); opioid withdrawal

Neurological Stimuli
Painful or irritating stimuli below the level of injury

Cardiac/Pulmonary Problems
Pulmonary emboli; deep-vein thrombosis

Reproductive Stimuli
Sexual intercourse; ejaculation; [vibrator overstimulation; scrotal compression]
Menstruation; pregnancy; labor and delivery; ovarian cyst

NOTE: A risk diagnosis is not evidenced by signs and symptoms, as the problem has not occurred; rather, nursing interventions are directed at prevention.
Sample Clinical Applications: Spinal cord injury

(continues on page 88)

risk for Autonomic Dysreflexia (continued)
DESIRED OUTCOMES/EVALUATION CRITERIA

Sample (NOC) linkages:
Risk Control: Personal actions to prevent, eliminate, or reduce modifiable health threats
Knowledge: Disease Process: Extent of understanding conveyed about a specific disease process
Caregiver Home Care Readiness: Extent of preparedness of a caregiver to assume responsibility for the healthcare of a family member in the home

Client Will (Include Specific Time Frame)
• Identify risk factors present.
• Demonstrate preventive or corrective techniques.
• Be free of episodes of dysreflexia.

ACTIONS/INTERVENTIONS

Sample (NIC) linkages:
Dysreflexia Management: Prevention and elimination of stimuli that cause hyperactive reflexes and inappropriate autonomic responses in a patient with a cervical or high thoracic cord lesion
Surveillance: Purposeful and ongoing acquisition, interpretation, and synthesis of patient data for clinical decision making
Medication Management: Facilitation of safe and effective use of prescription and over-the-counter (OTC) drugs

NURSING PRIORITY NO. 1

To assess risk factors present:

• Monitor for potential precipitating factors, including urological (e.g., bladder distention, UTIs, kidney stones); gastrointestinal—GI (e.g., bowel overdistention, hemorrhoids, digital stimulation); cutaneous (e.g., pressure ulcers, extreme external temperatures, dressing changes); reproductive (e.g., sexual activity, menstruation, pregnancy/delivery); and miscellaneous (e.g., pulmonary emboli, drug reaction, deep vein thrombosis [DVT]).[1,2,6,7]

NURSING PRIORITY NO. 2

To prevent occurrence:

∞ • Monitor vital signs routinely, noting changes in blood pressure, heart rate, and temperature, especially during times of physical stress *to identify trends and intervene in a timely manner. The baseline blood pressure in spinal cord-injured clients (adult and child) is lower than general population; therefore, an elevation of >15 mm Hg above baseline may be indicative of autonomic dysreflexia (AD).*[1,2,6,7]
• Instruct all caregivers in regularly timed or safe bowel and bladder or catheter care, and in interventions for long-term prevention of skin stress or breakdown (e.g., appropriate padding for skin and tissues, proper positioning with frequent pressure-relief actions, routine foot and toenail care) *to reduce risk of AD episode.*[1–7]
• Instruct client/caregivers in additional preventive interventions (e.g., temperature control; checking frequently for tight clothes or leg straps; sunburn and other burn prevention).[1–7]

- Administer antihypertensive medications, as indicated. *At-risk client may be placed on routine "maintenance dose," such as when noxious stimuli cannot be removed (e.g., presence of chronic sacral pressure ulcer, fracture, or acute postoperative pain).*[1]
- Refer to ND Autonomic Dysreflexia.

NURSING PRIORITY NO. 3

To promote wellness (Teaching/Discharge Considerations):

- Review warning signs of AD with client/caregiver (e.g., sudden, severe pounding headache; flushed, red face; increased blood pressure/acute hypertension; nasal congestion; anxiety; blurred vision; metallic taste in mouth; sweating and/or flushing above the level of SCI; goose bumps; bradycardia, cardiac irregularities). *AD can develop rapidly (in minutes), thus requiring quick intervention.*
- Be aware of client's communication abilities. *AD can occur at any age, from infant to very old, and the individual may not be able to verbalize a pounding headache, which is often the first symptom during onset of AD.*[1]
- Ascertain that client/caregiver understand ways to avoid onset of syndrome. Provide information card and instruct and periodically reinforce teaching, as needed, regarding the following:[1-7]
  Keeping indwelling catheter free of kinks, keeping bag empty and situated below bladder level, and checking daily for deposits (bladder grit) inside catheter.
  Catheterizing as often as necessary *to prevent overfilling.*
  Monitoring voiding patterns for adequate frequency and amount.
  Performing regular bowel evacuation program.
  Performing routine skin assessments.
  Monitoring all systems for signs/symptoms of infection and reporting promptly *for timely medical treatment.*
- Instruct family member/caregiver in proper blood pressure monitoring.
- Review use and administration of medications, when used. *Some clients are on medications routinely, and if so, should receive instructions for routine administration as well as symptoms to report for immediate or emergent care, when blood pressure is not responsive.*[1,6]
- Emphasize importance of regularly scheduled medical evaluations *to monitor status, identify developing problems.*
- Recommend wearing Medic Alert bracelet or necklace with information card about signs/symptoms of AD and usual methods of treatment. *Provides vital information in emergencies.*
- Assist client/family in identifying emergency referrals (e.g., physician, rehabilitation nurse or home-care supervisor). Place telephone number(s) in prominent place.

DOCUMENTATION FOCUS

Assessment/Reassessment
- Individual findings, noting previous episodes, precipitating factors, and individual signs/symptoms.

Planning
- Plan of care and who is involved in planning.
- Teaching plan.

Implementation/Evaluation
- Client's responses to interventions and actions performed, understanding of teaching.
- Attainment or progress toward desired outcome(s).
- Modifications to plan of care.

Discharge Planning
- Long-term needs and who is responsible for actions to be taken.

References

1. Consortium for Spinal Cord Medicine/Paralyzed Veterans of America. (2001). *Acute Management of Autonomic Dysreflexia: Individuals with Spinal Cord Injury Presenting to Health-Care Facilities.* Retrieved September 2003 from www.pva.org. Washington DC: Paralyzed Veterans of America (PVA).
2. Acuff, M. (2005). Autonomic dysreflexia: What it is, what it does, and what to do if you experience it. *The Missouri Model Spinal Cord Injury System.* Columbia, MO: University of Missouri-Columbia, School of Health Professions.
3. Christopher and Dana Reeve Paralysis Resource Center: Health: Autonomic Dysreflexia. Retrieved 2002 from www.paralysis.org/site/c.erJMJUOxFmH/b.1338071/k.5E45/Autonomic _Dysreflexia.htm.
4. Other complications of spinal cord injury: Autonomic dysreflexia (hyperreflexia) treatment. RehabTeam site. www.calder.med.miami.edu.
5. SCI Complications Resource: National Spinal Cord Injury Association (NSCIA). (Update January 2003) www.spinalcord.org.
6. Compagnolo, D. I. (2006). Autonomic dysreflexia in spinal cord injury. *Article for eMedicine Web site.* Retrieved January 2007 from www.emedicine.com/pmr/topic217.htm.
7. Cody, T., Zieroff, V. (2005). Autonomic dysreflexia. Article for Northeast Rehabilitation Health Network. Retrieved January 2007 from www.northeastrehab.com/Articles/dysreflexia.htm.

risk-prone health Behavior

DEFINITION: Inability to modify lifestyle/behavior in a manner that improves health status

RELATED FACTORS

Inadequate comprehension; low self-efficacy
Multiple stressors
Smoking; excessive alcohol
Inadequate social support; low socioeconomic status
Negative attitude toward healthcare

DEFINING CHARACTERISTICS

Subjective
Minimizes health status change
Fails to achieve optimal sense of control

Objective
Fails to take action that prevents health problems

Demonstrates nonacceptance of health status change

Sample Clinical Applications: New diagnosis/life changes for client, Alzheimer's disease, brain injury, personality or psychotic disorders, postpartum depression/psychosis, substance use/abuse

DESIRED OUTCOMES/EVALUATION CRITERIA

Sample **NOC** linkages:
Acceptance: Health Status: Reconciliation to significant change in health circumstances
Psychosocial Adjustment: Life Change: Adaptive psychosocial response of an individual to a significant life change
Treatment Behavior: Illness or Injury: Personal actions to palliate or eliminate pathology

Client Will (Include Specific Time Frame)
• Demonstrate increasing interest or participation in self-care.
• Develop ability to assume responsibility for personal needs when possible.
• Identify stress situations leading to difficulties in adapting to change in health status and specific actions for dealing with them.
• Initiate lifestyle changes that will permit adaptation to present life situations.
• Identify and use appropriate support systems.

ACTIONS/INTERVENTIONS

Sample **NIC** linkages:
Coping Enhancement: Assisting a patient to adapt to perceived stressors, changes, or threats that interfere with meeting life demands and roles
Counseling: Use of an interactive helping process focusing on the needs, problems, or feelings of the patient and significant others to enhance or support coping, problem-solving, and interpersonal relationships
Teaching: Disease Process: Assisting the patient to understand information related to a specific disease process

NURSING PRIORITY NO. 1

To assess degree of impaired function:

• Perform a physical and/or psychosocial assessment. *Determines the extent of the limitation(s) of the present condition.*[1]
• Listen to the client's perception of inability or reluctance to adapt to situations that are occurring at present. *Perceptions are reality to the client and need to be identified so they may be addressed and dealt with.*[3]
• Survey (with the client) past and present significant support systems (family, church, groups, and organizations). *Identifies helpful resources that may be needed in current situation or change in health status.*[2]
• Explore the expressions of emotions signifying impaired adjustment by client/SO(s). *Overwhelming anxiety, fear, anger, worry, passive or active denial can be experienced by the client who is having difficulty adjusting to change in health, feared diagnosis.*[4]

∞ ● Note child's interaction with parent/care provider. *Interactions can be indicative of problems when family is dealing with major health issues and change in family functioning. Development of coping behaviors is limited at this age, and primary caregivers provide support for the child and serve as role models.*[5]

∞ ● Determine whether child displays problems with school performance, withdraws from family/peers, or demonstrates aggressive behavior toward others/self. *Indicators of poor coping and need for specific interventions to help child deal with own health issues or what is happening in the family.*[6]

NURSING PRIORITY NO. 2

To identify the causative/contributing factors relating to the impaired adjustment:

● Listen to client's perception of factors leading to the present dilemma, noting onset, duration, presence or absence of physical complaints, social withdrawal. *Change often creates a feeling of disequilibrium, and the individual may respond with irrational or unfounded fears. Client may benefit from feedback that corrects misperceptions about how life will be with the change in health status.*[7]

● Note substance use or abuse (e.g., smoking, alcohol, prescription medications, street drugs) *that may be used as a coping mechanism, exacerbate health problem or impair client's comprehension of situation.*

● Identify possible cultural beliefs or values influencing client's response to change. *Different cultures deal with change of health issues, such as cancer, chronic obstructive pulmonary disease, diabetes mellitus, in different ways (i.e., Native Americans may believe they should be sick, quiet, and stoic; Chinese are often passive and expect the family to care for the client; Americans may be assertive and direct their care more frequently).*[14]

● Assess affective climate within family system and how it determines family members' response to adjustment to major health challenge. *Families who are high-strung and nervous may interfere with client's dealing with illness in a rational manner while those who are more sedate and phlegmatic may be more helpful to the client in accepting the current circumstances.*[2]

● Determine lack of or inability to use available resources. *The high degree of anxiety that usually accompanies a major lifestyle change often interferes with ability to deal with problems created by the change or loss. Helping client learn to use these resources enables him or her to take control of own illness.*[8]

● Discuss normalcy of anger as life is being changed and encourage channeling anger to healthy activities. *The increased energy of anger can be used to accomplish other tasks and enhance feelings of self-esteem.*[2]

● Review available documentation and resources, to determine actual life experiences (e.g., medical records, statements of SOs, consultants' notes). *In situations of great stress (physical or emotional), the client may not accurately assess occurrences leading to the present situation.*[9]

NURSING PRIORITY NO. 3

To assist client in coping/dealing with impairment:

● Organize a team conference (including client and ancillary services). *Individuals who are involved and knowledgeable can focus on contributing factors that are affecting client's adjustment to the current situation and can plan for management as indicated.*[11]

● Explain disease process or causative factors and prognosis as appropriate, promote questioning, and provide written and other resource materials. *Enhances understanding, clarifies information, and provides opportunity to review information at individual's leisure.*[10]

∞ • Share information with adolescent's peers with client's permission and involvement when illness or injury affects body image or function. *Peers are primary support for this age group, and sharing information promotes understanding and compassion.*[5]

• Provide an open environment encouraging communication. *Supports expression of feelings concerning impaired function so they can be dealt with realistically.*[2]

• Use therapeutic communication skills (e.g., Active-listening, acknowledgment, silence, I-statements). *Promotes open relationship in which client can explore possibilities and solutions for changing lifestyle situation.*[15]

• Acknowledge client's efforts to adjust: "You have done your best." *May reduce feelings of blame or guilt and defensive responses.*[12]

• Discuss and evaluate resources that have been useful to the client in adapting to changes in other life situations. *Vocational rehabilitation, employment experiences, psychosocial support services may be useful in current situation.*[12]

• Develop a plan of action with client to meet immediate needs (e.g., physical safety and hygiene, emotional support of professionals and SOs) and assist in implementation of the plan. *Provides a starting point to deal with current situation for moving ahead with plan for adjusting to change in life circumstances and for evaluation of progress toward goals.*[13]

• Reinforce structure in daily life. Include exercise as part of routine. *Routines help the client focus. Exercise improves sense of wellness and enhances immune response.*[10]

• Review with client coping skills used in previous life situations and role changes. *Identifies the strengths that may be used to facilitate adaptation to change or loss that has occurred.*[8]

• Refine or develop new coping strategies as appropriate. *Strengthens skills for dealing with change in health or lifestyle.*[10]

• Identify and problem-solve with the client frustrations in daily care. *Focusing on the smaller factors of concern gives the individual the ability to perceive the impaired function from a less threatening perspective (one-step-at-a-time concept). Also promotes sense of control over situation.*[10]

• Involve SO(s) in long-range planning for emotional, psychological, physical, and social needs. *Change that is occurring when illness is long term or permanent indicates that lifestyle changes will need to be dealt with on an ongoing basis, which may be difficult for client and family to adjust to.*[14]

• Refer for individual/family counseling as indicated. *May need additional assistance to cope with current situation.*[13]

NURSING PRIORITY NO. 4

To promote wellness (Teaching/Discharge Considerations):

• Identify strengths the client perceives in present life situation. Keep focus on the present. *Unknowns of the future may be too overwhelming when diagnosis or injury means permanent changes in lifestyle and long-term management.*[13]

• Assist SOs to learn methods of managing present needs. (Refer to NDs specific to client's deficits.) *Promotes internal locus of control and helps develop plan for long-term needs reflecting changes required by illness or changes in health status.*[2]

• Pace and time learning sessions to meet client's needs, providing for feedback during and after learning experiences (e.g., self-catheterization, range-of-motion exercises, wound care, therapeutic communication). Promotes skill and enhances retention, thereby improving confidence.[1]

• Refer to other resources in the long-range plan of care. *Long-term assistance may include such elements as home care, transportation alternatives, occupational therapy, or vocational rehabilitation that may be useful for making indicated changes in life, assisting with adjustment to new situation as needed.*[2]

🏠 • Assist client/SO(s) to see appropriate alternatives and potential changes in locus of control. *Often major change in health status results in loss of sense of control, and client needs to begin to look at possibilities for managing illness and what abilities can make life go on in a positive manner.*[10]

DOCUMENTATION FOCUS

Assessment/Reassessment
• Reasons for and degree of impairment.
• Client's/SO's perception of the situation.
• Effect of behavior on health status or condition.

Planning
• Plan for adjustments and interventions for achieving the plan and who is involved.
• Teaching plan.

Implementation/Evaluation
• Client responses to the interventions, teaching, and actions performed.
• Attainment or progress toward desired outcome(s).
• Modifications to plan of care.

Discharge Planning
• Resources that are available for the client and SO(s) and referrals that are made.

References

1. Doenges, M. E., Moorhouse, M. F., Geissler-Murr, A. C. (2002). *Nursing Care Plans: Guidelines for Individualizing Patient Care.* 6th ed. Philadelphia: F. A. Davis.
2. Doenges, M. E., Townsend, M. C., Moorhouse, M. F. (1998). *Psychiatric Care Plans: Guidelines for Individualizing Care.* 3d ed. Philadelphia: F. A. Davis.
3. Locher, J., et al. (2002). Effects of age and casual attribution to aging on health-related behaviors associated with urinary incontinence in older women. *Gerontologist*, 42(4), 515–521.
4. Cox, H., et al. (2002). *Clinical Applications of Nursing Diagnoses.* 4th ed. Philadelphia: F. A. Davis.
5. Pinhas-Hamiel, O., et al. (1996). Increased incidence of non-insulin-dependent diabetes mellitus among adolescents. *J Pediatr*, 128(8), 608.
6. Deckelbaum, R. J., Williams, C. L. (2001). Childhood obesity: The health issue. *Obesity Res*, 9(5), 239s.
7. Badger, J. M. (2001). Burns: The psychological aspect. *Am J Nurs*, 101(11), 38–41.
8. Bartol, T. (2002). Putting a patient with diabetes in the driver's seat. *Nursing*, 32(2), 53–55.
9. Konigova, R. (1992). The psychological problems of burned patients. The Rudy Hermans Lecture 1991. *Burns*, 18(3), 189–199.
10. Townsend, M. C. (2006). *Psychiatric Mental Health Nursing: Concepts of Care.* 3d ed. Philadelphia: F. A. Davis.
11. Grady, K. L. (2006). Management of heart failure in older adults. *J Cardiovasc Nurs*, 21(5 Suppl), S10–S14.
12. Rolland, J. S. (1994). *Families, Illness, and Disability.* New York: HarperCollins.
13. Wright, L. M., Leahey, M. (1987). *Families and Chronic Illness.* Springhouse, PA: Springhouse.
14. Lipson, J., Dibble, S., Minarik, P. (1996). *Culture & Nursing Care: A Pocket Guide.* San Francisco: UCSF Nursing Press.
15. Gordon, T. (2000). *Parent Effectiveness Training.* Updated ed. New York: Three Rivers Press.

risk for Bleeding

DEFINITION: At risk for decrease in blood volume that may compromise health

RISK FACTORS

Aneurysm, trauma, history of falls

Gastrointestinal (GI) disorders (e.g., gastric ulcer disease, polyps, varices)

Impaired liver function (e.g., cirrhosis, hepatitis)

Pregnancy related complications (e.g., placenta previa, molar pregnancy, abruption placenta); postpartum complications (e.g., uterine atony, retained placenta)

Inherent coagulopathies (e.g., thrombocytopenia, [hereditary hemorrhagic telangiectasia—HHT])

Treatment-related side effects (e.g., surgery, medications, administration of platelet deficient blood products, chemotherapy); circumcision

Disseminated intravascular coagulopathy

Deficient knowledge

NOTE: A risk diagnosis is not evidenced by signs and symptoms, as the problem has not occurred; rather, nursing interventions are directed at prevention

Sample Clinical Applications: Traumatic brain injury, femur fracture, aortic aneurysm, esophageal varices, pancreatitis, sickle cell anemia, use of anticoagulants such as Coumadin administration

DESIRED OUTCOMES/EVALUATION CRITERIA

Sample **NOC** linkages:

Blood Loss Severity: Severity of internal/external hemorrhage.

Blood Coagulation: Extent to which blood clots within normal period of time.

Risk Control: Personal actions to prevent, eliminate, or reduce modifiable health threats.

Client Will (Include Specific Time Frame)

• Be free of signs of active bleeding such as hemoptysis, hematuria, or hematemesis; or excessive blood loss as evidenced by stable vital signs, skin and mucous membranes free of pallor, usual mentation and urinary output.

• Display laboratory results for clotting times and factors within normal range for individual.

• Identify individual risks and engage in appropriate behaviors or lifestyle changes to prevent or reduce frequency of bleeding episodes.

ACTIONS/INTERVENTIONS

Sample **NIC** linkages:

Bleeding Precautions: Reduction of stimuli that may induce bleeding or hemorrhage in at-risk patients.

Bleeding Reduction [specify]: Limitation of the loss of blood volume during an episode of bleeding.

NURSING PRIORITY NO. 1

To assess causative/precipitating factors:

- Assess client risk. Note possible medical diagnoses or disease processes that may lead to bleeding as listed in Risk Factors, such as known or suspected major trauma, coagulopathies, gastric ulcers, liver disorders, pregnancy-related complications, malignancies, gram-negative sepsis, and so forth.
- Note type of injury(ies) present when client presents with trauma. *The pattern and extent of injury may or may not be readily determined. For example, unbroken skin can hide a significant injury with internal bleeding; or a puncture wound that appears superficial could nick an underlying blood vessel.*[1]
- Determine presence of hereditary factors, such as HHT, hemophilia, other factor deficiencies; thrombocytopenia; and so on. *Hereditary bleeding or clotting disorders predispose client to bleeding complications, either spontaneous bleeding as from pulmonary arteriovenous malformations or GI bleeding*[2] *or failure to clot in a timely manner.*[1]
- Obtain detailed history if a familial bleeding disorder is suspected. *Specialized testing may be needed, and/or referral to hematologist.*[1]
- Note client's gender. *While bleeding disorders are common in both men and women, women are affected more due to the increased risk of blood loss related to menstrual cycle and child delivery procedures.*[1,3]
- Note pregnancy-related factors, as indicated. *Many factors can occur, including overdistention of the uterus—pregnant with multiples, prolonged or rapid labor, lacerations occurring during vaginal delivery, or retained placenta that can place mother at risk for postpartum bleeding.*
- Evaluate client's medication regimen to note use of those predisposing to bleeding, such as nonsteroidal anti-inflammatory drugs (NSAIDs), anticoagulants, corticosteroids, and certain herbals such as ginkgo.[4]

NURSING PRIORITY NO. 2

To evaluate for potential bleeding:

- Monitor perineum and fundal height in postpartum client; wounds, dressings and tubes in client with trauma, surgery, or other invasive procedures *to identify active blood loss. Note: Hemorrhage may occur because of inability to achieve hemostasis in the setting of injury or result from the development of a coagulopathy.*[5] *Excessive bleeding may be defined by the individual client's physician or the facility's written policy—such as saturating two perineal pads/hour or >200 mL/chest tube drainage in 4 hours.*[6]
- Evaluate and mark boundaries of soft tissues in enclosed structures such as a leg or abdomen *to document expanding bruise or hematomas. Helps in identifying bleeding that may be occuring in a closed space, which renders client susceptible to complications, such as compartment syndrome or hypovolemia; permits earlier intervention.*
- Assess vital signs, including blood pressure, pulse (may be elevated initially), and respirations. Measure blood pressure lying, sitting, and standing as indicated *to evaluate for orthostatic hypotension*; and monitor invasive hemodynamic parameters when present (e.g., central venous pressure [CVP]) *to determine if intravascular fluid deficit exists. Note: Client could lose up to 2 liters of blood into chest, abdomen, or pelvis before hypotension signals the presence of a problem.*[7] *The American College of Surgeons Advanced Trauma Life Support (ATLS) lists 4 classes of hemorrhage, with class 1 involving up to 15% blood volume loss and little change in vital signs and class IV involving blood loss >40% of circulating volume and requiring aggressive resuscitation to prevent death.*[8]

- Hematest all secretions and excretions for occult blood *to more accurately determine possible source of bleeding when blood loss is occurring, and urgency of the situation.*
- Note client report of pain in specific areas, whether pain is increasing, diffuse, or localized. *Can help identify bleeding into tissues, organs, or body cavities.*
- Assess skin color and moisture, urinary output, level of consciousness or mentation. *Changes in these signs may be indicative of blood loss affecting systemic circulation or local organ function such as kidneys or brain.*
- Review laboratory data (e.g., complete blood count [CBC], including hemoglobin [Hb], platelet numbers and function; and other coagulation factors, which may be known by number—factor I, factor II, etc., or by name—prothrombin time [PT], partial thromboplastin time (PTT), fibrinogen, etc.) *to evaluate bleeding risk. An abrupt drop in Hb of 2 g/dLl can indicate active bleeding.*[9] *Note: When one or more of these factors are missing, produced in too small a quantity, or not functioning correctly, excessive bleeding can occur. Loss of factors may be due to acute blood loss, transfusion of factor-deficient blood, presence of inherited bleeding disorders, drugs that alter factors (e.g., warfarin, steroids, contraceptives, NSAIDs), or medical conditions affecting organs such as cirrhosis of the liver.*[10]
- Prepare client for, or assist with, diagnostic studies such as x-rays, computed tomography (CT) or magnetic resonance imaging (MRI) scans, ultrasound *to determine presence of injuries or disorders that could cause internal bleeding (e.g., ectopic pregnancy, damaged spleen following vehicle crash, epidural hemorrhage 2 days after a fall).*

NURSING PRIORITY NO. 3

To prevent bleeding/correct potential causes of excessive blood loss:

- Apply direct pressure and ice to bleeding site, insert nasal packing, or perform fundal massage as appropriate.
- Restrict activity, encourage bedrest or chair rest until bleeding abates.
- Maintain patency of vascular access *for fluid administration or blood replacement as indicated.*
- Assist with treatment of underlying conditions causing or contributing to blood loss, such as medical treatment of systemic infections or balloon tamponade of esophageal varices prior to sclerotherapy; use of proton pump inhibitor medications or antibiotics for gastric ulcer; surgery for internal abdominal trauma or retained placenta. *Treatment of underlying conditions may prevent or halt bleeding complications.*
- Provide special intervention in at-risk client (e.g., individual with bone marrow suppression, chemotherapy, uremia) *to prevent bleeding associated with tissue injury:*
  Monitor closely for overt bleeding.
  Observe for diffuse oozing from tubes, wounds, orifices with no observable clotting *to identify excessive bleeding and/or possible coagulopathy. Note: Client with certain conditions, such as obstetric complications, gram-negative sepsis, or massive trauma, may be predisposed to develop consumptive coagulopathy or disseminated intravascular coagulation (DIC), a potential lethal phenomena characterized by simultaneous clotting and continual bleeding.*[5]
  Maintain pressure or pressure dressings as indicated for longer period of time. *May be required to stop bleeding, such as pressure dressings over arterial puncture site or surgical dressings.*
  Hematest secretions and excretions for occult blood *for early identification of internal bleeding.*
  Protect client from trauma such as falls, accidental or intentional blows, or lacerations *that could cause bleeding.*
  Use soft toothbrush or toothettes for oral care *to reduce risk of injury to oral mucosa.*

- Collaborate in evaluating need for replacing blood loss or specific components and be prepared for emergency interventions. *Institution or physician may have specific guidelines for transfusion such as platelet count <20,000/mcL, or hemoglobin <6 g/dLl.*
- Be prepared to administer hemostatic agents such as desmopressin (DDAVP), *which promotes clotting and may stop bleeding by increasing coagulation factor VIII and von Willebrand factor;* or medications to prevent bleeding, such as proton pump inhibitors *to reduce risk of GI bleeding and need for replacement transfusion.*

NURSING PRIORITY NO. 4

To promote wellness (Teaching/Discharge Considerations):

- Provide information to client/family about hereditary or familial problems that predispose to bleeding complications.
- Instruct at-risk client and family regarding:

  Specific signs of bleeding requiring healthcare provider notification, such as active bright bleeding anywhere, prolonged epistaxis or trauma in client with known factor bleeding tendencies, black tarry stools, weakness, vertigo, syncope, and so forth.

  Need to inform healthcare providers when taking aspirin and other anticoagulants (e.g., Coumadin, Plavix), especially when elective surgery or other invasive procedure is planned. *These agents will most likely be withheld for a period of time prior to elective procedures to reduce potential for excessive blood loss.*

  Importance of periodic review of client's medication regimen *to identify medications which might cause or exacerbate bleeding problems. Note: Some prescriptions, over-the-counter (OTC) medications, and herbals (e.g., vitamin E, ginkgo, ginger, garlic, fish oils) promote bleeding.*[6]

  Necessity of regular medical and laboratory follow-up when on anticoagulants, such as Coumadin (Warfarin), *to determine needed dosage changes or client management issues requiring monitoring and/or modification.*

  Dietary measures to improve blood clotting, such as foods rich in vitamin K.

  Need to avoid alcohol in diagnosed liver disorders or seek treatment for alcoholism in presence of alcoholic varices.

  Techniques for postpartum client to check her own fundus and perform fundal massage as indicated, and to contact physician for postdischarge bleeding that is bright red or dark red with large clots. *May prevent blood loss complications, especially if client is discharged early from hospital.*

DOCUMENTATION FOCUS

Assessment/Reassessment
- Individual factors that may potentiate blood loss—type of injuries, obstetrical complications, etc.
- Baseline vital signs, mentation, urinary output, and subsequent assessments.
- Results of laboratory tests or diagnostic procedures.

Planning
- Plan of care and who is involved in the planning.
- Teaching plan.

Implementation/Evaluation
- Responses to interventions, teaching, and actions performed.
- Attainment or progress toward desired outcome(s).
- Modifications to plan of care.

Discharge Planning
- Long-term needs, identifying who is responsible for actions to be taken.
- Community resources or support for chronic problems.
- Specific referrals made.

References

1. Lambing, A. (2007). Bleeding disorders: Patient history key to diagnosis. *Nurs Pract*, 32(12), 16–24.
2. Ragsdale, J. A. (2007). Hereditary hemorrhagic telangiectasia from epistaxis to life-threatening GI bleeding. *Gastroenterol Nurs*, 30(4), 293–299.
3. Sommers, M. S., Johnson, S. A., Beery, T. A. (2007). *Diseases and Disorders: A Nursing Therapeutics Manual*. 3d ed. Philadelphia: F. A. Davis.
4. Ayers, D. M., Montgomery, M. (2009). Putting a stop to dysfunctional uterine bleeding. *Nursing*, 39(1), 44–50.
5. Lapointe, L. A. (2002). Coagulopathies in trauma patients. *AACN Clin Issues Crit Care Nurs*, 13(2), 192–203.
6. Beattie, S. (2007). Bedside emergency: Hemorrhage. *RN*, 70(8), 30–34.
7. Dutton, R. P. (2007). Current concepts in hemorrhagic shock. *Anesthesiol Clin North Am*, 25(1), 23–34.
8. Manning, J. E. (2004). Fluid and blood resuscitation. In Tintinalli, J. E. (ed.). *Emergency Medicine: A Comprehensive Study Guide*. New York: McGraw Hill.
9. Spahn, D. R., et al. (2006). Management of bleeding following major trauma: A European guideline. *Crit Care*, 11(1), R17.
10. Leeuwen, A. M., Kranpitz, T. R., Smith, L. (2006). *Davis Comprehensive Handbook of Diagnostic Tests with Nursing Implications*. 2d ed. Philadelphia: F. A. Davis.
11. Viscovsky, C. (2006). Interventions for clients with hematologic problems. In Ignatavicius, D. D., Workman, L. M. (eds.), *Medical-Surgical Nursing: Critical Thinking for Collaborative Care*, 5th ed. St. Louis, MO: Elsevier Saunders.
12. Steiner, M. E., Despotis, G. J. (2007). Transfusion algorithms and how they apply to blood conservation: The high-risk cardiac surgical patient. *Oncol Clin Nor Am*, 21(1), 177–184.

disturbed Body Image

DEFINITION: Confusion in [and/or dissatisfaction with] mental picture of one's physical self

RELATED FACTORS

Biophysical; illness; trauma; injury; surgery; [mutilation, pregnancy]
Illness treatment [change caused by biochemical agents (drugs), dependence on machine]
Psychosocial
Cultural; spiritual
Cognitive; perceptual
Developmental changes; [maturational changes]
[Significance of body part or functioning with regard to age, gender, developmental level, or basic human needs]

(continues on page 100)

disturbed Body Image (continued)
DEFINING CHARACTERISTICS

Subjective

Verbalization of feelings that reflect an altered view of one's body (e.g., appearance, structure, function)

Verbalization of perceptions that reflect an altered view of one's body in appearance

Verbalization of change in lifestyle

Fear of rejection or reaction by others

Focus on past strength, function, or appearance

Negative feelings about body (e.g., feelings of helplessness, hopelessness, or powerlessness); [depersonalization, grandiosity]

Preoccupation with change or loss

Refusal to verify actual change

Emphasis on remaining strengths; heightened achievement

Personalization of part or loss by name

Depersonalization of part or loss by impersonal pronouns

Objective

Behaviors of acknowledgment of one's body; avoidance of one's body; monitoring one's body

Nonverbal response to actual or perceived change in body (e.g., appearance, structure, function)

Missing body part

Actual change in structure or function

Not looking at or not touching body part

Trauma to nonfunctioning part

Change in ability to estimate spatial relationship of body to environment

Extension of body boundary to incorporate environmental objects

Intentional or unintentional hiding or overexposing of body part

Change in social involvement

[Aggression; low frustration tolerance level]

Sample Clinical Applications: Eating disorders (anorexia/bulimia nervosa), traumatic injuries, amputation, ostomies, aging process, arthritis, pregnancy, chronic renal failure, renal dialysis, burns

DESIRED OUTCOMES/EVALUATION CRITERIA

Sample **NOC** linkages:

Body Image: Positive perception of own appearance and body functions

Self-Esteem: Personal judgment of self-worth

Distorted Thought Self-Control: Self-restraint of disruption in perception, thought processes, and thought content

Client Will (Include Specific Time Frames)

• Verbalize acceptance of self in situation (e.g., chronic progressive disease, amputee, decreased independence, weight as is, effects of therapeutic regimen).

• Verbalize relief of anxiety and adaptation to altered body image.

• Verbalize understanding of body changes.

- Recognize and incorporate body image change into self-concept in accurate manner without negating self-esteem.
- Seek information and actively pursue growth.
- Acknowledge self as an individual who has responsibility for self.
- Use adaptive devices or prosthesis appropriately.

ACTIONS/INTERVENTIONS

Sample **NIC** linkages:

Body Image Enhancement: Improving a patient's conscious and unconscious perceptions and attitudes toward his or her body

Developmental Enhancement: Adolescent: Facilitating optimal physical, cognitive, social, and emotional growth of individuals during the transition from childhood to adulthood

Self-Esteem Enhancement: Assisting a patient to increase his or her personal judgment of self-worth

NURSING PRIORITY NO. 1

To assess causative/contributing factors:

- Discuss pathophysiology present or situation affecting the individual and refer to additional NDs, as appropriate. For example, when alteration in body image is related to neurological deficit (e.g., stroke), refer to ND unilateral Neglect; for presence of severe, ongoing pain, refer to ND chronic Pain; or in loss of sexual desire/ability, refer to ND Sexual Dysfunction.
- Determine whether condition is permanent with no hope for resolution. (May be associated with other NDs such as Self-Esteem [specify] or risk for impaired Attachment when child is affected.) *Identifies appropriate interventions based on reality of situation and need to plan for long- or short-term prognosis Note: There is always something that can be done to enhance acceptance, and it is important to hold out the possibility of living a good life with the disability.*[1]
- Assess mental and physical influence of illness or condition on the client's emotional state (e.g., diseases of the endocrine system, use of steroid therapy). *Some diseases can have a profound effect on one's emotions and need to be considered in the evaluation and treatment of the individual's behavior and reaction to the current situation.*[1,9]
- Evaluate level of client's knowledge of and anxiety related to situation. Observe emotional changes. *Provides information about starting point for providing information about illness. Emotional changes may indicate level of anxiety and need for intervention to lower anxiety before learning can take place.*[1]
- Recognize behavior indicative of overt preoccupation with body and its processes. *May interfere with ability to engage in therapy and indicate need to provide interventions to deal with concern before beginning therapy.*[2,3]
- Assume all individuals are sensitive to changes in appearance, but avoid stereotyping. *Not all individuals react to body changes in the same way, and it is important to determine how this person is reacting to changes.*[2,3]
- Have client describe self, noting what is positive and what is negative. Be aware of how client believes others see self. *Identifies self-image and whether there is a discrepancy between own view and how client believes others see him or her, which may have an effect on how client perceives changes that have occurred.*[3,4]
- ∞ Discuss meaning of loss or change to client. *A small (seemingly trivial) loss may have a big impact (such as the use of a urinary catheter or enema for bowel continence). A change in*

function (such as immobility) may be more difficult for some to deal with than a change in appearance. Permanent facial scarring of child may be difficult for parents to accept.[1]

- Use developmentally appropriate communication techniques for determining exact expression of body image in child (e.g., puppet play or constructive dialogue for toddler). *Developmental capacity must guide interaction to gain accurate information.*[4]
- Note signs of grieving or indicators of severe or prolonged depression. *May require evaluation of need for counseling or medications.*[3]
- Determine ethnic background and cultural or religious perceptions and considerations. *Understanding how these factors affect the individual in this situation and how they may influence how individual deals with what has happened is necessary to develop appropriate interventions.*[5]
- Identify social aspects of illness or disease. *Sexually transmitted diseases, sterility, or chronic conditions (e.g., vitiligo, multiple sclerosis) may affect how client views self and functions in social settings and how others view them.*[2,8]
- Observe interaction of client with SO(s). *Distortions in body image may be unconsciously reinforced by family members, or secondary gain issues may interfere with progress.*[2,8]

NURSING PRIORITY NO. 2.

To determine coping abilities and skills:

- Assess client's current level of adaptation and progress. *Client may have already adapted somewhat, and information provides starting point for developing plan of care.*[2]
- Listen to client's comments and note responses to the situation. *Different situations are upsetting to different people, depending on individual coping skills, severity of the perceived changes in body image, and past experiences with similar illnesses/conditions.*[2–4,8]
- Note withdrawn behavior and the use of denial. May be normal response to situation or may be indicative of mental illness (e.g., depression, schizophrenia).[6] (Refer to ND ineffective Denial.)
- Note dependence on prescription medications or use of addictive substances/alcohol. *May reflect dysfunctional coping as client turns to use of these substances to avoid dealing with changes that are occurring to body or ability to function in their accustomed manner.*[4]
- Identify previously used coping strategies and effectiveness. *Familiar coping strategies can be used to begin adaptation to current situation.*[2]
- Determine individual/family/community resources. *Can provide efficient assistance and support to enable the client to adapt to changing circumstances.*[4]

NURSING PRIORITY NO. 3

To assist client and SO(s) to deal with/accept issues of self-concept related to body image:

- Establish therapeutic nurse-client relationship. *Conveys an attitude of caring and develops a sense of trust in which client can discuss concerns and find answers to issues confronting him or her in new situation.*[4,8]
- Visit client frequently and acknowledge the individual as someone who is worthwhile. *Provides opportunities for listening to concerns and questions to promote dealing positively with individual situation and change in body image.*[1]
- Assist in correcting underlying problems when possible. *Promotes optimal healing and adaptation to individual situation (i.e., amputation, presence of colostomy, mastectomy, and impotence).*[1]
- Provide assistance with self-care needs or measures, as necessary, while promoting individual abilities and independence. *Client needs support to achieve the goal of independence and positive return to managing own life.*[4]

- Work with client's self-concept without moral judgments regarding client's efforts or progress (e.g., "You should be progressing faster; you're weak, lazy, not trying hard enough") *Such statements diminish self-esteem and are counterproductive to progress. Positive reinforcement encourages client to continue efforts and strive for improvement.*[2,8]
- Discuss concerns about fear of mutilation, prognosis, and rejection when client is facing surgery or potentially poor outcome of procedure or illness. *Addresses realities and provides emotional support to enable client to be ready to deal with whatever the outcome may be.*[1]
- Acknowledge and accept feelings of dependency, grief, and hostility. *Conveys a message of understanding.*[1]
- Encourage verbalization of anticipated conflicts *to enhance handling of potential situations. Provides an opportunity to imagine and practice how different situations can be dealt with, thus promoting confidence.*[4]
- Encourage client and SO(s) to communicate feelings to each other and discuss situation openly. *Enhances relationship, improving sense of self-worth and sense of support.*[2]
- Alert staff to be cognizant of own facial expressions and other nonverbal behaviors. *Important to convey acceptance and not revulsion, especially when the client's appearance is affected. Clients are very sensitive to reactions of those around them, and negative reactions will affect self-esteem and may retard adaptation to situation.*[1]
- Encourage family members to treat client normally and not as an invalid. *Helps client return to own routine and begin to gain confidence in ability to manage own life.*[1]
- Encourage client to look at and touch affected body part *to begin to incorporate changes into body image. Acceptance will enhance self-esteem and enable client to move forward in a positive manner.*[1,7]
- Allow client to use denial without participating (e.g., client may at first refuse to look at a colostomy; the nurse says, "I am going to change your colostomy now" and proceeds with the task). *Provides individual time to adapt to situation.*[4,9]
- Set limits on maladaptive behavior; assist client to identify positive behaviors. *Self-esteem will be damaged if client is allowed to continue behaviors that are destructive or not helpful, and adaptation to new image will be delayed.*[4,10]
- Provide accurate information, as desired or requested. Reinforce previously given information. *Accurate knowledge helps client make better decisions for the future.*[4]
- Discuss the availability of prosthetics, reconstructive surgery, and physical and occupational therapy or other referrals, as dictated by individual situation. *Provides hope that situation is not impossible and the future does not look so bleak.*[1,7,8]
- Help client to select and creatively use clothing or makeup *to minimize body changes and enhance appearance.*[1]
- Discuss reasons for infectious isolation and procedures when used, and make time to sit down and talk or listen to client while in the room. *Promotes understanding and decreases sense of isolation and loneliness.*[1]

NURSING PRIORITY NO. 4

To promote wellness (Teaching/Discharge Considerations):

- Begin counseling or other therapies (e.g., biofeedback or relaxation techniques) as soon as possible. *Provides early and ongoing sources of support to promote rehabilitation in a timely manner.*[1]
- Provide information at client's level of acceptance and in small segments. *Allows for easier assimilation.*[1,2,7]
- Clarify misconceptions and reinforce explanations given by other health team members. *Ensures client is hearing factual information to make the best decisions for own situation.*[1,2,7]

🏠 • Include client in decision-making process and problem-solving activities. *Promotes adherence to decisions and plans that are made.*[1]

🏠 • Assist client to incorporate therapeutic regimen into activities of daily living (ADLs) (e.g., specific exercises, housework activities). *Promotes continuation of program by helping client see that progress can be made within own daily activities.*[1]

🏠 • Identify and plan for alterations to home and work environment or activities when necessary. *Accommodates individual needs and supports independence.*[1,9]

🏠 • Assist client in learning strategies for dealing with feelings and venting emotions. *Helps individual move toward healing and optimal recuperation.*[1,2]

🏠 • Offer positive reinforcement for efforts made (e.g., wearing makeup, using prosthetic device). *Client needs to hear that what he or she is doing is helping.*[1,9]

🔘 • Refer to appropriate support groups. *May need additional help to adjust to new situation and life changes.*[1]

DOCUMENTATION FOCUS

Assessment/Reassessment
• Observations, presence of maladaptive behaviors, emotional changes, stage of grieving, level of independence.
• Physical wounds, dressings; use of life-support-type machine (e.g., ventilator, dialysis machine).
• Meaning of loss or change to client.
• Support systems available (e.g., SOs, friends, groups).

Planning
• Plan of care and who is involved in planning.
• Teaching plan.

Implementation/Evaluation
• Client's response to interventions, teaching, and actions performed.
• Attainment or progress toward desired outcome(s).
• Modifications of plan of care.

Discharge Planning
• Long-term needs and who is responsible for actions.
• Specific referrals made (e.g., rehabilitation center, community resources).

References

1. Doenges, M., Moorhouse, M., Murr, A. C. (2002). *Nursing Care Plans: Guidelines for Individualizing Patient Care.* 6th ed. Philadelphia: F. A. Davis.
2. Doenges, M., Townsend, M., Moorhouse, M. (1998). *Psychiatric Care Plans: Guidelines for Individualizing Care.* 3d ed. Philadelphia: F. A. Davis.
3. Townsend, M. (2003). *Psychiatric Mental Health Nursing: Concepts of Care.* 4th ed. Philadelphia: F. A. Davis.
4. Cox, H., et al. (2002). *Clinical Applications of Nursing Diagnosis: Adult, Child, Women's Psychiatric, Gerontic and Home Health Considerations.* 4th ed. Philadelphia: F. A. Davis.
5. Lipson, J. G., Dibble, S. L., Minarik, P. A. (1996). *Culture & Nursing Care: A Pocket Guide. School of Nursing.* San Francisco: UCSF Nursing Press.
6. Townsend, M. (2001). *Nursing Diagnoses in Psychiatric Nursing: Care Plans and Psychotropic Medications.* 5th ed. Philadelphia: F. A. Davis.
7. Aacovou, I. (2005). The role of the nurse in the rehabilitation of patients with radical changes in body image due to burn injuries. *Annals of Burns and Fire Disasters,* 18(2), 89–94.
8. Breakey, J. W. (1997). Body image: The inner mirror. *J Prosthet Orthot,* 9(3), 107–112.

9. Kater, K. (2006). Building healthy body esteem in a body toxic world. Retrieved June 2007 from www.bodyimagehealth.org.

10. Reasoner, R. The true meaning of self-esteem. Retrieved June 2007 from www.self-esteem -nase.org/whatisselfesteem.shtml.

risk for imbalanced Body Temperature

DEFINITION: At risk for failure to maintain body temperature within normal range

RISK FACTORS

Extremes of age or weight

Exposure to cold/cool or warm/hot environments; inappropriate clothing for environmental temperature

Dehydration

Inactivity; vigorous activity

Medications causing vasoconstriction or vasodilation; sedation; [use or overdose of certain drugs or exposure to anesthesia]

Illness or trauma affecting temperature regulation [e.g., infections, systemic or localized; neoplasms, tumors; collagen/vascular disease]; altered metabolic rate

NOTE: A risk diagnosis is not evidenced by signs and symptoms, as the problem has not occurred; rather, nursing interventions are directed at prevention.

Sample Clinical Applications: Any infectious process, surgical procedures, brain injuries, hypo-/hyperthyroidism, prematurity

DESIRED OUTCOMES/EVALUATION CRITERIA

Sample **NOC** linkages:

Risk Control: Personal actions to prevent, eliminate, or reduce modifiable health threats

Infection Severity: Severity of infection and associated symptoms

Hydration: Adequate water in the intracellular and extracellular compartments of the body

Client Will (Include Specific Time Frame)

• Maintain body temperature within normal range.

• Verbalize understanding of individual risk factors and appropriate interventions.

• Demonstrate behaviors for monitoring and maintaining appropriate body temperature.

ACTIONS/INTERVENTIONS

Sample **NIC** linkages:

Fever Treatment: Management of a patient with hyperpyrexia caused by nonenvironmental factors

Temperature Regulation: Attaining or maintaining body temperature within a normal range

Temperature Regulation: Intraoperative: Attaining or maintaining desired intraoperative body temperature

NURSING PRIORITY NO. 1

To identify causative/risk factors present:

- Note presence of condition that can affect body's heat production and heat dissipation (e.g., spinal cord injury [SCI]; burns or skin diseases; endocrine disorders; neurological disorders, such as Parkinson's disease; kidney disease; being significantly overweight or underweight).[3,4,7,8]
- Determine if present illness or condition results from exposure to environmental factors, surgery, infection, or trauma. *Helps to determine the scope of interventions that may be needed (e.g., simple addition of warm blankets after surgery or hypothermia therapy following brain trauma).*[1]
- Monitor laboratory values (e.g., tests indicative of infection, thyroid or other endocrine tests, drug screens) *to identify potential internal causes of temperature imbalances.*
- Note client's age (e.g., premature neonate, young child, or aging individual), *as it can directly impact ability to maintain or regulate body temperature and respond to changes in environment.*[2]
- Assess nutritional status *to determine metabolism effect on body temperature and to identify foods or nutrient deficits that affect metabolism.*[1,2]

NURSING PRIORITY NO. 2

To prevent occurrence of temperature alteration:

- Monitor temperature regularly (e.g., every 1–4 hr) measuring core body temperature whenever needed to observe this vital sign. *Traditionally, temperature measurements have been taken orally (good in alert, oriented adult), rectally (accurate but not always easy to obtain), or axillary (readings may be lower than core temperature), with each site offering advantages and disadvantages in terms of accuracy and safety. Newer technologies allow temperatures to be instantly and accurately measured. Tympanic temperature measurement is a noninvasive way to measure core temperature, as blood is supplied to the tympanic membrane by the carotid artery. This method is preferred by healthcare providers and parents, although some pediatricians may still prefer rectal temperature measurements in sick newborns or infants.*[3]
- Maintain comfortable ambient environment *to reduce risk of body-temperature alterations.*[1,2,4,6,7]
  Provide environmental heating or cooling measures, as needed, such as space heater or air conditioner or fans.
  Ascertain that cooling and warming equipment and supplies are available during or following procedures and surgery.
- Dress or discuss with client/caregivers appropriate dressing for client's condition.[6–8]
  Wear layers of clothing that can be removed or added as needed. Wear hat and gloves in cold weather; wear light, loose protective clothing in hot weather; and wear water-resistant outer gear *to protect from changes in weather or wet weather chill.*
  Cover infant's head with knit cap, use layers of lightweight blankets. Place newborn infant under radiant warmer. Teach parents to dress infant appropriately for weather and home environment. *Newborns/infants can have temperature instability with heat loss greatest through head and by evaporation and convection.*[5]
- Maintain adequate fluid intake. Offer cool or warm liquids, as appropriate. *Hydration assists in maintaining normal body temperature.*[1,2,4,7,8]

- Restore and maintain core temperature within client's normal range. (If temperature is below or above normal range, or parameters defined by physician, refer to NDs Hypothermia or Hyperthermia for additional interventions.)
- Recommend lifestyle changes, such as cessation of substance use, normalization of body weight, nutritious meals, or regular exercise *to maximize metabolism and general health.*[1,2]
- Refer at-risk persons to appropriate community resources (e.g., home care, social services, Foster Adult Care, housing agencies) *to provide assistance to meet individual needs.*[1]

NURSING PRIORITY NO. 3

To promote wellness (Teaching/Discharge Considerations):

- Review potential problem or individual risk factors with client/SO(s).
- Discuss effects of age and gender with client/caregiver, as appropriate. *Older or debilitated persons, infants, and young children typically feel more comfortable in higher ambient temperatures. Women notice feeling cool quicker than men, which may be related to body size or to differences in metabolism and the rate that blood flows to extremities to regulate body temperature.*[6,7]
- Instruct in measures to protect from identified risk factors. *Provides understanding for ways in managing lifestyle and environment (e.g., adding or removing clothing; adding or removing heat sources; evaluating home or shelter for ability to manage heat and cold; addressing nutritional and hydration status) and enhances self-care abilities.*[6]
- Review client's medications for possible thermoregulatory side effects (e.g., diuretics, certain sedatives and antipsychotic agents, some heart and blood pressure medications, or anesthesia).[1,2,7,8]
- Discuss with client using sympathomimetics (e.g., cocaine, methamphetamines) the effects of drug on body-temperature regulation.[1,2,7,8]
- Identify ways to prevent accidental thermoregulation problems. *For example, hypothermia can result from overzealous cooling to reduce fever, or maintaining too warm an environment when client has lost the ability to perspire can lead to hyperthermia.*

DOCUMENTATION FOCUS

Assessment/Reassessment
- Identified individual causative or risk factors.
- Record of core temperature, initially and prn.
- Results of diagnostic studies and laboratory tests.

Planning
- Plan of care and who is involved in planning.
- Teaching plan, including best ambient temperature and ways to prevent hypothermia or hyperthermia.

Implementation/Evaluation
- Response to interventions, teaching, and actions performed.
- Attainment or progress toward desired outcome(s).
- Modifications to plan of care.

Discharge Planning
- Long-term needs and who is responsible for actions.
- Specific referrals made.

References

1. Doenges, M. E., Moorhouse, M. F., Geissler-Murr, A. C. (2002). Surgical intervention. *Nursing Care Plans: Guidelines for Individualizing Patient Care*. 6th ed. Philadelphia: F. A. Davis.
2. Cox, H. C., et al. (2002). *Clinical Applications of Nursing Diagnosis: Adult, Child, Women's, Psychiatric, Gerontic, and Home Health Considerations*. 4th ed. Philadelphia: F. A. Davis.
3. Nicoll, L. H. (2002). Heat in motion: Evaluating and managing temperature. *Nursing*, 32(5), s1–s12.
4. American Academy of Pediatrics: Section on Anesthesiology. (1999). Guidelines for the pediatric perioperative anesthesia environment. *Pediatrics*, 103(2), 512–515.
5. Early discharge of the term newborn. (1999). Guideline from National Association of Neonatal Nurses. National Guideline Clearinghouse Web site. www.guideline.gov.
6. Beattie, S. (2006). In from the cold. *RN*, 69(11), 22–27.
7. Lien, C. A. Thermoregulation in the elderly. Syllabus on Geriatric Anesthesiology. Retrieved January 2007 from American Society of Anesthesiologists Web site. www.asahq.org/clinical/geriatrics/thermo.htm.
8. Hoppe, J., Sinert, R. (2006). Heat exhaustion and heatstroke. Retrieved March 2007 from www.emedicine.com/emerg/topic/236.htm.

Bowel Incontinence

DEFINITION: Change in normal bowel habits characterized by involuntary passage of stool

RELATED FACTORS

Toileting self-care deficit; environmental factors (e.g., inaccessible bathroom); impaired cognition; immobility
Dietary habits; medications; laxative abuse
Stress
Colorectal lesions; impaired reservoir capacity
Incomplete emptying of bowel; impaction; chronic diarrhea
General decline in muscle tone; abnormally high abdominal or intestinal pressure
Rectal sphincter abnormality; loss of rectal sphincter control; lower or upper motor nerve damage

DEFINING CHARACTERISTICS

Subjective
Recognizes rectal fullness but reports inability to expel formed stool
Urgency; inability to delay defecation
Self-report of inability to feel rectal fullness

Objective
Constant dribbling of soft stool
Fecal staining of clothing and/or bedding
Fecal odor
Red perianal skin
Inability to recognize or inattention to urge to defecate

 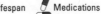

Sample Clinical Applications: Hemorrhoids, rectal prolapse, anal/gynecological surgery, childbirth injuries/uterine prolapse, spinal cord injury (SCI), stroke, multiple sclerosis (MS), ulcerative colitis, dementia

DESIRED OUTCOMES/EVALUATION CRITERIA

Sample NOC linkages:
Bowel Continence: Control of passage of stool from the bowel
Bowel Elimination: Formation and evacuation of stool
Neurological Status: Ability of the peripheral and central nervous system (CNS) to receive, process, and respond to internal and external stimuli

Client Will (Include Specific Time Frame)
• Verbalize understanding of causative or controlling factors.
• Identify individually appropriate interventions.
• Participate in therapeutic regimen to control incontinence.
• Establish and maintain as regular a pattern of bowel functioning as possible.

ACTIONS/INTERVENTIONS

Sample NIC linkages:
Bowel Incontinence Care: Promotion of bowel continence and maintenance of perineal skin integrity
Bowel Incontinence Care: Encopresis: Promotion of bowel continence in children
Bowel Training: Assisting the patient to train the bowel to evacuate at specific intervals

NURSING PRIORITY NO. 1

To assess causative/contributing factors:

● Identify pathophysiological conditions present (e.g., multiple sclerosis, acute or chronic cognitive impairments, spinal cord injury, stroke, ileus, ulcerative colitis).
● Determine historical aspects of incontinence with preceding or precipitating factors. *Common causes include (1) structural changes in the sphincter muscle (e.g., hemorrhoids, rectal prolapse, anal or gynecological surgery, childbirth injuries); (2) injuries to sensory nerves (e.g., SCI, trauma, stroke, tumor, radiation therapy, MS); (3) strong-urge diarrhea (e.g., ulcerative colitis, Crohn's disease, infectious diarrhea); (4) dementia (e.g., acute or chronic cognitive impairment, not necessarily related to sphincter control); (5) result of toxins (e.g., salmonella); and (6) effects of improper diet or type and rate of enteral feedings.*[1-6,8]
● Note client's age and gender. *Constipation from holding stool is more common in children Bowel incontinence is more common in children and elderly adults (difficulty responding to urge in a timely manner, problems walking or undoing zippers); more common in boys than girls, but more common in elderly women than elderly men.*[1-6]
● Review medication regimen, including over-the-counter (OTC) drugs. *Laxative abuse, drugs with side effects of diarrhea (e.g., antibiotics) or constipation (e.g., sedatives, hypnotics, opioids, muscle relaxants) may impact bowel control.*
● Perform physical evaluation. Palpate abdomen for masses and auscultate for presence and location and characteristics of bowel sounds.

is persistent and constant can interfere with breathing (such as can occur with asthma, acute bronchitis, cystic fibrosis, croup, whooping cough).[1,6–10] (Refer to ND ineffective Airway Clearance.)

- Assess client's awareness and cognition. *Affects ability to manage own airway and cooperate with interventions such as controlling breathing and managing secretions.*[2,8,9]
- Assist with and monitor results of diagnostic testing (e.g., pulmonary or cardiac function studies, neuromuscular evaluation, sleep studies) *to diagnose presence and severity of lung diseases and degree of respiratory compromise.*
- Review chest radiographs and laboratory data (e.g., ABGs, pulse oximetry at rest and activity, drug screens, white blood cell [WBC] count, blood and sputum culture tests for viruses and bacteria).

NURSING PRIORITY NO. 2

To provide for relief of causative factors promoting ease of breathing:[6–12]

- Assist in treatment of underlying conditions, administering medications and therapies as ordered.
- Suction airway to clear secretions as needed. (Refer to ND impaired Airway Clearance for additional interventions.)
- Maintain emergency equipment in readily accessible location, and include age and size appropriate airway, ET, and tracheostomy tubes (e.g., infant, child, adolescent, or adult).
- Administer oxygen (by cannula, mask, mechanical ventilation) at lowest concentration needed (per ABGs, pulse oximetry) *for underlying pulmonary condition and current respiratory problem.*[12–14] (Refer to ND impaired Gas Exchange for additional interventions.)
- Elevate head of bed, or have client sit up in chair; support with pillows *to prevent slumping and promote rest;* or place in position of comfort, as appropriate, *to promote maximal inspiration.* In ventilated client, place in prone position for short periods when indicated *to improve pulmonary perfusion and increase oxygen diffusion.*
- Reposition client frequently *to enhance respiratory effort and ventilation of all lung segments, especially if immobility is a factor.*
- Encourage early ambulation using assistive devices, as individually indicated. Involve client in program of exercise training *to prevent onset or reduce severity of respiratory complications, and to improve respiratory muscle strength.*[12]
- Direct client in breathing efforts as needed. Encourage slower and deeper respirations, use of pursed-lip technique, *to assist client in "taking control" of the situation, especially when condition is associated with anxiety and air hunger.*
- Coach client in effective coughing techniques. Place in appropriate position for clearing airways. Splint rib cage and surgical incisions as appropriate. Medicate for pain, as indicated. *Promotes breathing that is more effective, and airway management when client is guarding, as might occur with chest, rib cage, or abdominal injuries or surgeries.* (Refer to NDs acute Pain; chronic Pain for additional interventions.)
- Provide and assist with use of respiratory therapy adjuncts such as spirometry.
- Maintain calm attitude while working with client/SOs. Provide quiet environment, instruct and reinforce client in the use of relaxation techniques, and administer antianxiety medications as indicated *to reduce intensity of anxiety and deal with fear that may be present.* (Refer to NDs Fear; Anxiety for additional interventions.)
- Avoid overfeeding, such as might occur with young infant or client on tube feedings. *Abdominal distention can interfere with breathing as well as increase risk of aspiration.*
- Assist with bronchoscopy or chest tube insertion as indicated.

NURSING PRIORITY NO. 3

To promote wellness (Teaching/Discharge Considerations):

- Review with client/SO the type of respiratory condition, treatments, rehabilitation measures, and quality-of-life issues. *Many conditions with impaired breathing are associated with chronic conditions that require lifetime management by client and healthcare providers.*[9]
- Instruct and reinforce breathing retraining. *Education may include many measures, such as conscious control of respiratory rate, effective use of accessory muscles, breathing exercises (diaphragmatic, abdominal breathing, inspiratory resistive, and pursed-lip), assistive devices such as rocking bed.*[6]
- Discuss relationship of smoking to respiratory function. Stress importance of smoking cessation and smoke-free environment.
- Encourage client/SO(s) to develop a plan for smoking cessation. Provide appropriate referrals.
- Encourage self-assessment and symptom management:[6–12]
  Use of equipment to identify respiratory decompensation, such as peak flow meter.
  Appropriate use of oxygen (dosage, route, and safety factors).
  Medication regimen, including actions, side effects, and potential interactions of medications, over-the-counter (OTC) drugs, vitamins, and herbal supplements.
  Adhere to home treatments such as metered-dose inhalers (MDIs), compressor, nebulizer, chest physiotherapies.
  Dietary patterns and needs; access to foods and nutrients supportive of health and breathing.
  Management of personal environment, including stress reduction, rest and sleep, social events, travel, and recreation issues.
  Avoidance of known irritants, allergens, and sick persons.
  Immunizations against influenza and pneumonia.
  Early intervention when respiratory symptoms occur, and what symptoms require reporting to medical providers, seeking emergency care.
- Discuss benefits of exercise for endurance, muscle strengthening, and flexibility training *to improve general health and respiratory muscle function.*
- Refer to physical therapy and pulmonary rehabilitation programs and resources as indicated.[12,13]
- Review energy conservation techniques (e.g., sitting instead of standing to wash dishes, pacing activities, taking short rest periods between activities) *to limit fatigue and improve endurance.*
- Review environmental factors (e.g., exposure to dust, high pollen counts, severe weather, perfumes, animal dander, household chemicals, fumes, secondhand smoke; insufficient home support for safe care) *that may require avoidance/modification of lifestyle or environment to limit impact on client's breathing.*[13–15]
- Reinforce instruction in proper use and safety concerns for home oxygen therapy, and/or use of respirator or diaphragmatic stimulator, rocking bed, apnea monitor, when used. *Protects client's safety, especially when used in the very young, fragile elderly, or when cognitive or neuromuscular impairment present.*
- Discuss impact of respiratory condition on occupational performance, as well as work environment issues that affect client.
- Provide referrals as indicated by individual situation. *May include a wide variety of services and providers, including support groups, comprehensive rehabilitation program, occupational nurse, oxygen and durable medical equipment (DME) companies for supplies, home health services, occupational and physical therapy, transportation, assisted or alternate living facilities, local and national Lung Association chapters, and Web sites for educational materials.*

DOCUMENTATION FOCUS

Assessment/Reassessment
- Relevant history of problem.
- Respiratory pattern, breath sounds, use of accessory muscles.
- Laboratory values.
- Use of respiratory supports, ventilator settings, and so forth.

Planning
- Plan of care, specific interventions, and who is involved in the planning.
- Teaching plan.

Implementation/Evaluation
- Response to interventions, teaching, actions performed, and treatment regimen.
- Mastery of skills, level of independence.
- Attainment or progress toward desired outcome(s).
- Modifications to plan of care.

Discharge Planning
- Long-term needs, including appropriate referrals and action taken, available resources.
- Specific referrals provided.

References

1. Evidence-based clinical practice guideline of community-acquired pneumonia in children 60 days to 17 years of age. (2000). Retrieved September 2009 from Cincinnati Children's Hospital Medical Center www.guideline.gov/summary/summary.aspx?ss=15&doc_id=9690&nbr=5199.
2. Stanley, M., Beare, P. G. (1999). *Gerontological Nursing: A Health Promotion/Protection Approach.* 2d ed. Philadelphia: F. A. Davis.
3. Lung disease in minorities in 1999. Focus Asthma. Retrieved September 2009 from www.stateoftheair.org.
4. Purnell, L. D., Paulanka, B. J. (1998). *Transcultural Health Care: A Culturally Competent Approach.* Philadelphia: F. A. Davis.
5. Minority lung disease data—Major acute infections: Influenza and pneumonia. American Lung Association: State of the Air 2002. Retrieved September 2009 from www.stateoftheair.org.
6. Global Initiative for Chronic Obstructive Lung Disease (GOLD); World Health Organization; National Heart, Lung, and Blood Institute. (2008 update). Global strategy for the diagnosis, management, and prevention of chronic obstructive pulmonary disease. National Guideline Clearinghouse [NGC 2205]. Retrieved September 2009 from www.goldcopd.com.
7. Engel, J. (2002). *Mosby's Pocket Guide to Pediatric Assessment.* 4th ed. St. Louis, MO: Mosby.
8. Cox, H. C., et al. (2002). *Clinical Applications of Nursing Diagnosis: Adult, Child, Women's, Gerontic, and Home Health Considerations.* 4th ed. Philadelphia: F. A. Davis, 256–261.
9. Doenges, M. E., Moorhouse, M. F., Geissler-Murr, A. C. (2002). *Nursing Care Plans: Guidelines for Individualizing Patient Care.* 6th ed. Philadelphia: F. A. Davis, 167.
10. Irwin, R. S., et al. (1998). *Managing Cough as a Defense Mechanism and as a Symptom: A Clinical Reference Guide.* Northbrook, IL: American College of Chest Physicians (ACCP).
11. Marion, B. S. (2001). A turn for the better: "Prone positioning" of patients with ARDS. *Amer J Nurs,* 101(5), 26–33.
12. Ries, A. L., et al. (1997, revised 2007). Pulmonary rehabilitation: Joint ACCP/AACVPR evidence-based clinical practice guidelines. National Guideline Clearinghouse. Retrieved September 2009 from www.guideline.gov.
13. Bauldoff, G. S., Diaz, P. T. (2006). Improving outcomes for COPD patients. *Nurs Pract,* 31(8), 26–43.

🌐 Cultural   Collaborative   🏠 Community/Home Care   Diagnostic Studies   ∞ Pediatric/Geriatric/Lifespan   Medications

14. Pruitt, B. (2006). Weaning patients from mechanical ventilation. *Nursing*, 36(9), 36–41.
15. Saglimbeni, A. J. (2005). Exercise-induced asthma. Retrieved January 2007 from www.emedicine.com/SPORTS/topic155.htm.

decreased Cardiac Output

DEFINITION: Inadequate blood pumped by the heart to meet the metabolic demands of the body. [Note: In a hypermetabolic state, although cardiac output may be within normal range, it may still be inadequate to meet the needs of the body's tissues. Cardiac output and tissue perfusion are interrelated, although there are differences. When cardiac output is decreased, tissue perfusion problems will develop; however, tissue perfusion problems can exist without decreased cardiac output.]

RELATED FACTORS

Altered heart rate or rhythm [conduction]
Altered stroke volume
Altered preload [e.g., decreased venous return]
Altered afterload [e.g., systemic vascular resistance]
Altered contractility [e.g., ventricular-septal rupture, ventricular aneurysm, papillary muscle rupture, valvular disease]

DEFINING CHARACTERISTICS

Subjective
Altered Heart Rate/Rhythm: Palpitations
Altered Preload: Fatigue
Altered Afterload: [Feeling breathless]
Altered Contractility: Orthopnea or paroxysmal nocturnal dyspnea [PND]
Behavioral/Emotional: Anxiety

Objective
Altered Heart Rate/Rhythm: [Dysrhythmias], arrhythmias (tachycardia, bradycardia); EKG [ECG] changes
Altered Preload: Jugular vein distention; edema; weight gain; increased or decreased central venous pressure (CVP); increased or decreased pulmonary artery wedge pressure (PAWP); murmurs
Altered Afterload: Dyspnea; clammy skin; skin [and mucous membrane] color changes [cyanosis, pallor]; prolonged capillary refill; decreased peripheral pulses; variations in blood pressure readings; increased or decreased systemic vascular resistance (SVR); increased or decreased pulmonary vascular resistance (PVR); oliguria; [anuria]
Altered Contractility: Crackles; cough; decreased cardiac index; decreased ejection fraction; decreased stroke volume index (SVI) or left ventricular stroke work index (LVSWI), S3 or S4 sounds [gallop rhythm]
Behavioral/Emotional: Restlessness

Sample Clinical Applications: Myocardial infarction (MI), congestive heart failure (CHF), valvular heart disease, dysrhythmias, cardiomyopathy, cardiac contusions/trauma, pericarditis, ventricular aneurysm

(continues on page 134)

decreased Cardiac Output (continued)
DESIRED OUTCOMES/EVALUATION CRITERIA

Sample (NOC) linkages:
Cardiac Pump Effectiveness: Adequacy of blood volume ejected from the left ventricle to support systemic perfusion pressure
Circulation Status: Unobstructed, unidirectional blood flow at an appropriate pressure through large vessels of the systemic and pulmonary circuits
Energy Conservation: Personal actions to manage energy for initiating and sustaining activity

Client Will (Include Specific Time Frame)
• Display hemodynamic stability (e.g., blood pressure, cardiac output, urinary output, peripheral pulses).
• Report or demonstrate decreased episodes of dyspnea, angina, and dysrhythmias.
• Demonstrate an increase in activity tolerance.
• Verbalize knowledge of the disease process, individual risk factors, and treatment plan.
• Participate in activities that reduce the workload of the heart (e.g., stress management or therapeutic medication regimen program, weight reduction, balanced activity/rest plan, proper use of supplemental oxygen, cessation of smoking).
• Identify signs of cardiac decompensation, alter activities, and seek help appropriately.

ACTIONS/INTERVENTIONS

Sample (NIC) linkages:
Hemodynamic Regulation: Optimization of heart rate, preload, afterload, and contractility
Cardiac Care: Limitation of complications resulting from an imbalance between myocardial oxygen supply and demand for a patient with symptoms of impaired cardiac function
Circulatory Care: Mechanical Assist Devices: Temporary support of the circulation through the use of mechanical devices or pumps

NURSING PRIORITY NO. 1

To identify causative/contributing factors:

• Review clients at risk as noted in Related Factors and Defining Characteristics. *In addition to individuals obviously at risk with known cardiac problems, there is a potential for cardiac output problems in persons with trauma, hemorrhage, alcohol and other drug intoxication, chronic use, or overdose; pregnant women with hypertensive states; individuals with chronic renal failure; with brainstem trauma, or spinal cord injury (SCI) at T8 or above.*[1]

 • Note age and ethnic-related cardiovascular considerations. *In infants, failure to thrive with poor ability to suck and feed can be indications of heart problems. Children with poor cardiac function are tachypneic, exercise-intolerant, and may have episodes of syncope because of restricted ventricular outflow (such as might occur with aortic stenosis or abnormal vasomotor tone).*[2,3] *When in the supine position, pregnant women incur decreased vascular return during the second and third trimesters, potentially compromising cardiac output.*[4] *Contractile force is naturally decreased in the elderly with reduced ability to increase cardiac output in response to increased demand. Also, arteries are stiffer, veins more dilated, and heart valves less competent, often resulting in systemic hypertension and blood pooling.*[5] *Heart failure may affect as many as 1 in 10 elderly people.*[6] *Generally,*

higher-risk populations include African Americans (because of higher incidence of hypertension, obesity, and diabetes mellitus) and Latinos (higher incidence of obesity and diabetes mellitus).[7]

- Review diagnostic studies, including/not limited to: chest radiograph, cardiac stress testing, electrocardiogram (ECG), echocardiogram, cardiac output and ventricular ejection studies, and heart scan or catheterization. *For example, ECG may show previous or evolving MI, left ventricular hypertrophy, and valvular stenosis. Ventricular function studies with ejection fraction (EF) <40% is indicative of systolic dysfunction, and cardiac output <4 L/m is indicative of heart failure (HF). Additional cardiac studies (e.g., radionuclide scans or catheterization) may be indicated to assess left ventricular function, valvular function, and coronary circulation. Chest radiography may show enlarged heart, pulmonary infiltrates.*[8–10,14,15]

- Review laboratory data, including but not limited to complete blood count (CBC), electrolytes, arterial blood gases (ABGs), cardiac enzymes; kidney, thyroid, and liver function studies; cultures (e.g., blood, wound, or secretions), bleeding and coagulation studies *to identify imbalances, disease processes, and effects of interventions.*[1,8]

NURSING PRIORITY NO. 2

To assess degree of debilitation:

- Assess for signs of poor ventricular function or impending cardiac failure and shock:[1–5,9]
    Client reports or demonstrates extreme fatigue, intolerance for activity, sudden or progressive weight gain, swelling of extremities, and progressive shortness of breath.
    Client reports chest pain. *May indicate evolving heart attack; can also accompany congestive heart failure. Chest pain may be atypical in women experiencing an MI and is often atypical in the elderly owing to altered pain perception.*
    Mental status changes. *Confusion, agitation, decreased cognition and coma may occur due to decreased brain perfusion.*
    Changes in heart rate or rhythm: Tachycardia at rest, bradycardia, atrial fibrillation, or multiple dysrhythmias may be noted. *Heart irritability is common, reflecting conduction defects and/or ischemia.*
    Heart sounds may be distant, with irregular rhythms; murmurs-systolic *(valvular stenosis and shunting)* and diastolic *(aortic or pulmonary insufficiency)* or gallop rhythm (S3, S4) noted *when heart failure is present and ventricles are stiff.*
    Peripheral pulses may be weak and thready, *reflecting hypotension, vasoconstriction, shunting, and venous congestion.*
    Changes in skin color, moisture, temperature, and capillary refill time. *Pallor or cyanosis, cool moist skin, and slow capillary refill time may be present because of peripheral vasoconstriction and decreased oxygen saturation. Note: Children with chronic heart failure and adults with chronic obstructive pulmonary disease (COPD) often show clubbing of fingertips.*
    Blood pressure changes. *Hypertension may be chronic or blood pressure elevated initially in client with impending cardiogenic, hypovolemic, or septic shock. Later, as cardiac output decreases, profound hypotension can be present, often with narrowed pulse pressure.*
    Breath sounds may reveal bilateral crackles and wheezing *associated with congestion. Respiratory distress and failure often occurs as shock progresses.*
    Edema with neck vein distention is often present, and pitting edema is noted in extremities and dependent portions of body *because of impaired venous return. Other veins in trunk and extremities can be prominent, owing to venous congestion.*

∞ Urinary output may be decreased or absent *reflecting poor perfusion of kidneys. Note: Output <30 mL/hr (adult) or <10 mL/hr (child) indicates inadequate renal perfusion.*

NURSING PRIORITY NO. 3

To minimize/correct causative factors, maximize cardiac output:

Acute/severe phase[1–3,9–12,14,17]

- Keep client on bed or chair rest in position of comfort. In congestive state, semi-Fowler's position is preferred. May raise legs 20 to 30 degrees in shock situation. *Decreases oxygen consumption and demand, reducing myocardial workload and risk of decomposition.*
- Administer supplemental oxygen, as indicated (by cannula, mask, endotracheal [ET] or tracheostomy tube with mechanical ventilation) *to improve cardiac function by increasing available oxygen and reducing oxygen consumption. Critically ill client may be on ventilator to support cardiopulmonary function.*[14]
- Monitor vital signs frequently *to evaluate response to treatments and activities.* Perform periodic hemodynamic measurements, as indicated (e.g., arterial, CVP, PAWP , and left atrial pressure [LAP]; cardiac output and cardiac index [CO/CI], and oxygen saturation). *These measurements (via central line monitoring) are commonly used in the critically ill to provide continuous, accurate assessment of cardiac function and response to inotropic and vasoactive medications that affect cardiac contractility and systemic circulation (preload and afterload).*[17]
- Monitor cardiac rhythm continuously *to note changes, and evaluate effectiveness of medications and devices (e.g., implanted pacemaker/defibrillator).*
- Administer or restrict fluids, as indicated. *Replacement of blood and large amounts of IV fluids may be needed if low output state is due to hypovolemia.* Use infusion pumps for IVs *to monitor IV rates closely to prevent bolus or exacerbation of fluid overload.*
- Assess hourly or periodic urinary output and daily weight, noting 24-hr total fluid balance *to evaluate kidney function and effects of interventions, as well as to allow for timely alterations in therapeutic regimen.*
- Administer medications as indicated (e.g., inotropic drugs *to enhance cardiac contractility,* antiarrhythmics *to improve cardiac output,* diuretics *to reduce congestion by improving urinary output,* vasopressors, and/or dilators as indicated *to manage systemic effects of vasoconstriction and low cardiac output*; pain medications and antianxiety agents *to reduce oxygen demand and myocardial workload*; anticoagulants *to improve blood flow and prevent thromboemboli).*
- Note reports of anorexia or nausea and limit or withhold oral intake as indicated. *Symptoms may be systemic reaction to low cardiac output, visceral congestion, or reaction to medications or pain.*
- Assist with preparations for and monitor response to support procedures or devices as indicated (e.g., cardioversion, pacemaker, angioplasty, coronary artery bypass graft [CABG] or valve replacement, intra-aortic balloon pump [IABP], left ventricular assist device [LVAD]). *Any number of interventions may be required to correct a condition causing heart failure or to support a failing heart during recovery from myocardial infarction, while awaiting transplantation, or for long-term management of chronic heart failure.*
- Promote rest *to reduce catecholamine-induced stress response and cardiac workload*:[1,13,17]
  Decrease stimuli, providing quiet environment.
  Schedule activities and assessments *to maximize sleep periods.*
  Assist with or perform self-care activities for client.
  Avoid the use of restraints whenever possible, especially if client is confused.

- Use sedation and analgesics, as indicated, with caution *to achieve desired rest state without compromising hemodynamic responses.*

Postacute/chronic phase[1]

- Provide for adequate rest, positioning client for maximum comfort.
- Encourage changing positions slowly, dangling legs before standing *to reduce risk of orthostatic hypotension.*
- Increase activity levels gradually as permitted by individual condition, noting vital sign response to activity.
- Administer medications, as appropriate, and monitor cardiac responses.
- Encourage relaxation techniques *to reduce anxiety, muscle tension.*
- Refer for nutritional needs assessment and management *to provide for supportive nutrition while meeting diet restrictions (e.g., IV nutrition or total parenteral nutrition [TPN], sodium-restricted or other type diet with frequent small feedings).*
- Monitor intake/output and calculate 24-hour fluid balance. Provide or restrict fluids, as indicated, *to maximize cardiac output and improve tissue perfusion.*[17]

NURSING PRIORITY NO. 4

To enhance safety/prevent complications:[1,4,16,17]

- Wash hands before and after client contact, maintain aseptic technique during invasive procedures, and provide site care, as indicated, *to prevent nosocomial infection.* (Refer to ND risk for Infection for additional interventions.)
- Provide antipyretics and fever control actions as indicated. Adjust ambient environmental temperature *to maintain body temperature in near-normal range.*
- Maintain patency of invasive intravascular monitoring and infusion lines and tape connections *to prevent exsanguination or air embolus.*
- Minimize activities that can elicit Valsalva response (e.g., rectal straining, vomiting, spasmodic coughing with suctioning, prolonged breath-holding during pushing stage of labor) and encourage client to breathe deeply in and out during activities that increase risk of Valsalva effect. *Valsalva response to breath-holding causes increased intrathoracic pressure, reducing cardiac output and blood pressure.*[16]
- Avoid prolonged sitting position for all clients, and supine position for sleep or exercise for gravid clients (second and third trimesters) *to maximize vascular return.*[4,17]
- Elevate legs when in sitting position and edematous extremities when at rest. Apply antiembolic hose or sequential compression devices when indicated, being sure they are individually fitted and appropriately applied. *Limits venous stasis, improves venous return, and reduces risk of thrombophlebitis.* (Refer to ND ineffective peripheral tissue Perfusion for additional interventions.)
- Provide skin care, special bed or mattress (e.g., air, water, gel, foam) and assist with frequent position changes *to prevent the development of pressure sores.*
- Provide psychological support *to reduce anxiety and its adverse effects on cardiac function:* Maintain calm attitude and limit stressful stimuli.
  Provide and encourage use of relaxation techniques, such as massage therapy, soothing music, or quiet activities.
  Promote visits from family/SO(s) *to provide positive social interaction.*
  Provide information about testing procedures and client participation.
  Explain limitations imposed by condition and dietary and fluid restrictions.
  Share information about positive signs of improvement.

NURSING PRIORITY NO. 5

To promote wellness (Teaching/Discharge Considerations):[1,13,18]

- Provide information to clients/caregivers on individual condition, therapies, and expected outcomes. Use various forms of teaching according to client needs, desires, and learning style.
- Direct client and/or caregivers to resources for emergency assistance, financial help, durable medical supplies, and psychosocial support and respite, especially when client has impaired functional capabilities or requires supporting equipment (e.g., pacemaker, LVAD, or 24-hour oxygen).
- Emphasize importance of regular medical follow-up care *to monitor client's condition and response to treatment and provide most effective care.*
- Educate client/caregivers about drug regimen, including indications, dose and dosing schedules, potential adverse side effects, or drug/drug interactions. *Client is often on multiple medications, which can be difficult to manage, thus increasing potential that medications can be missed or incorrectly used.*
- Emphasize reporting of adverse and nuisance side effects of medications *so that adjustments can be made in dosing or another class of medication considered.*
- Discuss significant signs/symptoms that need to be reported to healthcare provider, such as *unrelieved or increased chest pain, dyspnea, fever, swelling of ankles, and sudden unexplained cough—these are all "danger signs" that require immediate evaluation and possible change of usual therapies.*[18]
- Provide instruction for home monitoring of weight, pulse, and blood pressure, as appropriate, *to detect change and allow for timely intervention.*
- Recommend seasonal influenza or other flu and pneumonia vaccination.
- Discuss individual's particular risk factors (e.g., smoking, stress, obesity, recent MI) and specific resources for assistance (e.g., written information sheets, direction to helpful Web sites, formalized rehabilitation programs, and home interventions) for management of identified factors for:
  Smoking cessation
  Stress management techniques
  Energy conservation techniques
  Nutrition education regarding specific needs (e.g., to improve general health status, reduce or gain weight, lower blood fat levels, manage sodium)
  Exercise and activity plan *to systematically increase endurance*
- Refer to NDs Activity Intolerance, deficient Diversional Activity, ineffective Coping, compromised family Coping, Sexual Dysfunction, acute/chronic Pain, imbalanced Nutrition (specify), deficient/excess Fluid Volume, as indicated.

DOCUMENTATION FOCUS

Assessment/Reassessment
- Baseline and subsequent findings and individual hemodynamic parameters, heart and breath sounds, ECG pattern, presence and strength of peripheral pulses, skin and tissue status, renal output, and mentation.

Planning
- Plan of care and who is involved in planning.
- Teaching plan.

Implementation/Evaluation
* Client's responses to interventions, teaching, and actions performed.
* Status and disposition at discharge.
* Attainment or progress toward desired outcome(s).
* Modifications to plan of care.

Discharge Planning
* Discharge considerations and who will be responsible for carrying out individual actions.
* Long-term needs.
* Specific referrals made.

References

1. Doenges, M. E., Moorhouse, M. F., Geissler-Murr, A. C. (2002). *Nursing Care Plans: Guidelines for Individualizing Patient Care*. 6th ed. Philadelphia: F. A. Davis.
2. Cox, H. C., et al. (2002). *Clinical Applications of Nursing Diagnosis: Adult, Child, Women's Psychiatric, Gerontic, and Home Health Considerations*. 4th ed. Philadelphia: F. A. Davis, 262–269.
3. Pathophysiologic interpretation of cardiac symptoms and signs. *Pediatric Cardiology for Parents and Patients, Rush Children's Heart Center*. Retrieved September 2009 from http://pediatriccardiology.uchicago.edu/MP/Cardiac-H&P/Cardiac-H&P.
4. Ladewig, P., et al. (2002). *Contemporary Maternal-Newborn Nursing Care*. 5th ed. Upper Saddle River, NJ: Prentice Hall.
5. Stanley, M., Beare, P. G. (1999). *Gerontological Nursing: A Health Promotion/Protection Approach*. 2d ed. Philadelphia: F. A. Davis.
6. Heidenreich, P. A., Ruggerico, C. M., Massie, B. M. (2000). Effect of a home-based monitoring system on hospitalization and resource use for patients with heart failure. Pilot study supported by Agency for Healthcare Research and Quality (National Research Service Award Training Grant T32 HS00028). Retrieved January 2007 from www.ahrq.gov.
7. Purnell, L. D., Paulanka, B. J. (1998). *Transcultural Health Care: A Culturally Competent Approach*. Philadelphia: F. A. Davis.
8. Cavanaugh, B. M. (1999). *Nurse's Manual of Laboratory and Diagnostic Tests*. 3d ed. Philadelphia: F. A. Davis, 654–659.
9. Heart failure. (2002). *Clinical Practice Guideline*. Columbia, MD: American Medical Directors Association (AMDA), NGC, 2529.
10. The pharmacologic management of chronic heart failure. (2001). Washington, DC: Department of Veterans Affairs, Veterans Health Administration.
11. Bond, A. E., et al. (2003). The left ventricular assist device. *Am J Nurs*, 103(1), 33–40.
12. Gawlinski, A., McAtee, M. E. (May 2002). Biventricular pacing: New treatment for patients with heart failure: Important nursing implications. *Am J Nurs Suppl. Critical Care Update*, 102(5), 4–7.
13. Clinical practice guidelines: Cardiac rehabilitation guidelines. (October 1995). Cosponsored by the National Heart, Lung, and Blood Institute and Agency for Healthcare Policy and Research (AHCPR). Retrieved January 2007 from www.ahrq.gov.
14. Brandler, E. S., Sinert, R., Hostetler, M. A. (2006). Shock, cardiogenic. Retrieved January 2007 from www.emedicine.com/emerg/topic530.htm.
15. Olade, R., Safi, A., Kesari, S. (2006). Cardiac catheterization (left heart). Retrieved January 2007 from www.emedicine.com/emerg/topic2958.htm.
16. Bernardi, L., Saviolo, R., Sodick, D. H. (1989). Do hemodynamic responses to the Valsalva maneuver reflect myocardial dysfunction? *Chest*, 95(5), 986–991.
17. Cheever, K. H. (2005). An overview of pulmonary arterial hypertension: Risks, pathogenesis, clinical manifestations, and management. *J Cardiovasc Nurs*, 20(2), 108–116.

18. Purgason, K. (2006). Broken hearts: Differentiating stress-induced cardiomyopathy from acute myocardial infarction in the patient presenting with acute coronary syndrome. *Dimens Crit Care Nurs*, 25(6), 247–253.

Caregiver Role Strain

DEFINITION: Difficulty in performing caregiver role

RELATED FACTORS

Care receiver health status
Illness severity or chronicity
Unpredictability of illness course; instability of care receiver's health
Increasing care needs; dependency
Problem behaviors; psychological or cognitive problems
Addiction; codependency

Caregiving activities
Discharge of family member to home with significant care needs [e.g., premature birth, congenital defect, frail elder poststroke]
Unpredictability of care situation; 24-hour care responsibilities; amount or complexity of activities; years of caregiving
Ongoing changes in activities

Caregiver health status
Physical problems; psychological or cognitive problems
Inability to fulfill one's own/others' expectations; unrealistic expectations of self
Marginal coping patterns
Addiction; codependency

Socioeconomic
Competing role commitments
Alienation or isolation from others
Insufficient recreation

Caregiver–care receiver relationship
Unrealistic expectations of caregiver by care receiver
History of poor relationship
Mental status of elder inhibits conversation
Presence of abuse or violence

Family processes
History of marginal family coping or family dysfunction

Resources
Inadequate physical environment for providing care (e.g., housing, temperature, safety)
Inadequate equipment for providing care; inadequate transportation
Insufficient finances

Inexperience with caregiving; insufficient time; physical energy; emotional strength; lack of support

Lack of caregiver privacy

Deficient knowledge about or difficulty accessing community resources; inadequate community services (e.g., respite services, recreational resources)

Formal or informal assistance or support

Caregiver is not developmentally ready for caregiver role

DEFINING CHARACTERISTICS

Subjective

Caregiving activities: Apprehension about possible institutionalization of care receiver; the future regarding care receiver's health or caregiver's ability to provide care; care receiver's care if caregiver unable to provide care

Caregiver health status—physical:

GI upset; weight change

Headaches; fatigue; rash

Hypertension; cardiovascular disease; diabetes

Caregiver health status—emotional:

Feeling depressed; anger; stress; frustration; increased nervousness

Disturbed sleep

Lack of time to meet personal needs

Caregiver health status—socioeconomic: Changes in leisure activities; refuses career advancement

Caregiver-care receiver relationship:

Difficulty watching care receiver go through the illness

Grief/uncertainty regarding changed relationship with care receiver

Family processes: Concerns about family members

Objective

Caregiving activities:

Difficulty performing or completing required tasks

Preoccupation with care routine

Dysfunctional change in caregiving activities

Caregiver health status—emotional:

Impatience; increased emotional lability; somatization

Impaired individual coping

Caregiver health status—socioeconomic: Low work productivity; withdraws from social life

Family processes: Family conflict

[NOTE: The presence of this problem may encompass other numerous problems/high-risk concerns, such as deficient Diversional Activity, Insomnia, Fatigue, Anxiety, ineffective Coping, compromised family Coping or disabled family Coping, decisional Conflict, ineffective Denial, Grieving, Hopelessness, Powerlessness, Spiritual Distress, ineffective Health Maintenance, impaired Home Maintenance, Sexual Dysfunction or ineffective Sexuality Pattern, readiness for enhanced family Coping, interrupted Family Processes, Social Isolation. Careful attention to data-gathering will identify and clarify the client's specific needs, which can then be coordinated under this single diagnostic label.]

(continues on page 142)

Caregiver Role Strain (continued)
Sample Clinical Applications: Chronic conditions (e.g., severe brain injury, spinal cord injury [SCI], severe developmental delay), progressive debilitating conditions (e.g., muscular dystrophy, multiple sclerosis [MS], dementia or Alzheimer's disease, end-stage chronic obstructive pulmonary disease [COPD], renal failure, renal dialysis), substance abuse, end-of-life care, psychiatric conditions (e.g., schizophrenia, personality disorders)

DESIRED OUTCOMES/EVALUATION CRITERIA

Sample **NOC** linkages:
Caregiver Role Endurance: Severity of disturbances in the lifestyle of a family member due to caregiving
Caregiver Stressors: Severity of biopsychosocial pressure on a family care provider caring for another over an extended period of time
Caregiver Well-Being: Extent of positive perception of primary care provider's health status and life circumstances

Caregiver Will (Include Specific Time Frame)
• Identify resources within self to deal with situation.
• Provide opportunity for care receiver to deal with situation in own way.
• Express more realistic understanding and expectations of the care receiver.
• Demonstrate behavior or lifestyle changes to cope with or resolve problematic factors.
• Report improved general well-being, ability to deal with situation.

ACTIONS/INTERVENTIONS

Sample **NIC** linkages:
Caregiver Support: Provision of the necessary information, advocacy, and support to facilitate primary patient care by someone other than a healthcare professional
Family Involvement Promotion: Facilitating family participation in the emotional and physical care of the patient
Parenting Promotion: Providing parenting information, support, and coordination of comprehensive services to high-risk families

NURSING PRIORITY NO. 1

To assess degree of impaired function:

• Inquire about and observe physical condition of care receiver and surroundings as appropriate. *Important to determine factors that may indicate problems that can interfere with ability to continue caregiving.*[4]
• Assess caregiver's current state of functioning (e.g., hours of sleep, nutritional intake, personal appearance, demeanor). *Provides basis for determining needs that indicate caregiver is having difficulty dealing with role.*[4]
• Determine use of prescription, over-the-counter (OTC), or illicit drugs, alcohol. *Caregiver may turn to using these substances to deal with situation.*[1]
• Identify safety issues concerning caregiver and receiver. *The stress and anxiety of caregiving situations can lead to inattention, and by identifying these issues, an opportunity is provided to correct problems before injury occurs.*[1]

- Assess current actions of caregiver and how they are received by care receiver. *Caregiver may be trying to be helpful but is not perceived as helpful; may be too protective or may have unrealistic expectations of care receiver's abilities, which can lead to misunderstanding and conflict.*[4]
- Note choice and frequency of social involvement and recreational activities. *Caregiver needs to take time away from situation to maintain own sense of self and ability to continue in role.*[1]
- Determine use and effectiveness of resources and support systems. *May not be aware of what is available or may need help in using them to the best advantage.*[4]

NURSING PRIORITY NO. 2

To identify the causative/contributing factors relating to the impairment:

- Note presence of high-risk situations. *Elderly client with total self-care dependence or caregiver with several small children with one child requiring extensive assistance due to physical condition or developmental delays may necessitate role reversal resulting in added stress or placing excessive demands on parenting skills.*[4]
- Determine current knowledge of the situation, noting misconceptions, lack of information. *May interfere with caregiver/care receiver's response to situation.*[2]
- Identify relationship of caregiver to care receiver (e.g., spouse/lover, parent/child, sibling, friend). *Close relationships may make it more difficult to remain separate when caring for care receiver.*[2]
- Ascertain proximity of caregiver to care receiver. *Caregiver could be living in the home of care receiver (e.g., spouse or parent of disabled child), or could be adult child stopping by to check on elderly parent each day, providing support, food preparation, shopping, assistance in emergencies. Note: There is added stress in maintaining own life and responsibilities when caregiver has to travel some distance to provide care.*[4,10]
- Note care receiver's physical and mental condition, as well as the complexity of therapeutic regimen. *Caregiving activities can be complex, requiring hands-on care, problem-solving skills, clinical judgment, organizational and communication skills that can tax the caregiver, increasing likelihood of burnout.*[7,10]
- Determine caregiver's level of involvement in and preparedness for the responsibilities of caring for the client, and anticipated length of care. *Information needed to develop plan of care that takes into consideration who will provide care, timing, and any other factors to maintain coverage for situation.*[4]
- Ascertain physical and emotional health, developmental level and abilities, and additional responsibilities of caregiver (e.g., job, raising family). *Provides clues to potential stressors and possible supportive interventions.*[1,10,11]
- Assess caregiver as appropriate, using tool such as Burden Interview or Caregiver Reaction Assessment *to further determine caregiver's stressors and abilities providing additional information to aid in planning.*[17,18]
- Identify individual cultural factors and impact on caregiver. *Helps clarify expectations of caregiver and receiver, family, and community. Many cultures, such as Native American, Cuban, believe strongly in keeping care receiver in the home and caring for them.*[5]
- Identify presence and degree of conflict between caregiver/care receiver/family. *Stressful situations can exacerbate underlying feelings of anger and resentment, resulting in difficulty managing caregiving needs.*[2]
- Determine preillness and current behaviors that may be interfering with the care or recovery of the care receiver. *Underlying personality of care receiver may create situation in which old conflicts interfere with current treatment regimen.*[2]
- Note codependency needs and enabling behaviors of caregiver. *These behaviors can interfere with competent caregiving and contribute to caregiver burnout.*[2]

NURSING PRIORITY NO. 3

To assist caregiver to identify feelings and begin to deal with problems:

- Establish a therapeutic relationship, conveying empathy and unconditional positive regard. *A compassionate approach blending the nurse's expertise in healthcare with the caregiver's firsthand knowledge of the care receiver can provide encouragement, especially in a long-term difficult situation.*[2,10,12]
- Acknowledge difficulty of the situation for the caregiver/family. *Research shows that the two greatest predictors of caregiver strain are poor health, and the feeling that there is no choice but to take on additional responsibilities.*[10]
- Discuss caregiver's view of and concerns about situation. *Important to identify issues so planning and solutions can be developed.*[7]
- Encourage caregiver to acknowledge and express negative feelings. Discuss normalcy of the reactions without using false reassurance. *There are no bad feelings, and individual needs to understand that all are acceptable to be expressed, dealt with, but not acted on in the situation.*[2]
- Discuss caregiver's life goals, perceptions, and expectations of self. *Clarifies unrealistic thinking and identifies potential areas of flexibility or compromise.*[4]
- Discuss caregiver's perception of impact of and ability to handle role changes necessitated by situation. *May not initially realize the changes that will be encountered as situation develops, and it helps to identify and plan for changes before they arise.*[1]

NURSING PRIORITY NO. 4

To enhance caregiver's ability to deal with current situation:

- Identify strengths of caregiver and care receiver. *Bringing these to the individual's awareness promotes positive thinking and helps with problem-solving to deal more effectively with circumstances.*[4]
- Discuss strategies to coordinate caregiving tasks and other responsibilities (e.g., employment, care of children/other dependents, housekeeping activities). *Managing these tasks will reduce the stress associated with performing the activities of daily living.*[1]
- Facilitate family conference to share information and develop plan for involvement in care activities as appropriate. *Involving everyone promotes sense of control and ownership of plan and willingness to follow through on responsibilities.*[1]
- Identify classes or needed specialists (e.g., first aid and cardiopulmonary resuscitation [CPR] classes, enterostomal specialist, physical therapist). *Provides information needed to manage tasks of caregiving more effectively, giving individuals more sense of control.*[1]
- Determine need for and sources of additional resources (e.g., financial, legal, respite care, educational, social, spiritual). *Can help to resolve problems that arise in the course of caregiving that are out of the knowledge or abilities of the individual. Solving these issues can relieve caregiver of anxiety and concern.*[4,13]
- Provide information or demonstrate techniques for dealing with acting out, violent, or disoriented behavior. *Presence of dementia necessitates learning these techniques or skills to enhance safety of caregiver and receiver.*[2]
- Identify equipment needs and resources, appropriate adaptive aids. *Enhances the independence and safety of the care receiver and makes the task of caregiving easier.*[1]
- Provide contact person or case manager to partner with care provider(s) in coordinating care, providing physical and social support, and to assist with problem-solving as needed or desired. *Promotes more effective caregiving, thereby preventing burnout.*[2,10,14]

NURSING PRIORITY NO. 5

To promote wellness (Teaching/Discharge Considerations):

* Advocate for and assist caregiver to plan for and implement changes that may be necessary (e.g., home-care providers, adult day care, eventual placement in long-term care facility). *As caregiving tasks become more difficult, other options need to be considered, and planning ahead can promote acceptance of necessary changes.*[8,11,15]

* Encourage attention to own needs (e.g., eating and sleeping regularly, setting realistic goals, talking with trusted friend, periodic respite from caregiving), accepting own feelings, acknowledging frustrations and limitations, and being realistic about loved one's condition. *Supports and enhances caregiver's general well-being and coping ability.*[15,16]

* Review signs of burnout (e.g., emotional or physical exhaustion, changes in appetite and sleep, withdrawal from friends/family or life interests). *Recognition of developing problem allows for timely intervention.*

* Discuss and demonstrate stress management techniques and importance of self-nurturing (e.g., pursuing self-development interests, hobbies, social activities, spiritual enrichment). *Being involved in activities such as these can prevent caregiver burnout.*[4,15]

* Encourage involvement in caregiver support group. *Having others to share concerns and fears is therapeutic; provides ideas for different ways to manage problems, helping caregivers deal more effectively with the situation.*[1]

* Refer to classes or other therapies as indicated. *Provides additional information as needed.*[1]

* Identify available 12-step program when indicated *to provide tools to deal with enabling or codependent behaviors that impair level of function. Provides a more structured environment to learn how to deal with problems of caregiving situation.*[2]

* Refer to counseling or psychotherapy as needed. *Intensive treatment may be needed in highly stressful situations.*[2]

* Provide bibliotherapy of appropriate references and Web sites for self-paced learning and encourage discussion of information. *Further information can help individuals understand what is happening and manage more effectively.*[9]

DOCUMENTATION FOCUS

Assessment/Reassessment
* Assessment findings, functional level and degree of impairment, caregiver's understanding and perception of situation.
* Identified risk factors.

Planning
* Plan of care and individual responsibility for specific activities.
* Identification of inner resources, behavior or lifestyle changes to be made.
* Needed resources, including type and source of assistive devices and durable equipment.
* Teaching plan.

Implementation/Evaluation
* Caregiver's/receiver's response to interventions, teaching, and actions performed.
* Attainment or progress toward desired outcome(s).
* Modifications to plan of care.

Discharge Planning
* Plan for continuation or follow-through of needed changes.
* Referrals for assistance and evaluation.

References

1. Doenges, M., Moorhouse, M., Murr, A. (2002). *Nursing Care Plans: Guidelines for Individualizing Patient Care.* 6th ed. Philadelphia: F. A. Davis.
2. Doenges, M., Townsend, M., Moorhouse, M. (1998). *Psychiatric Care Plans: Guidelines for Individualizing Care.* 3d ed. Philadelphia: F. A. Davis.
4. Cox, H., et al. (2002). *Clinical Applications of Nursing Diagnosis: Adult, Child, Women's, Psychiatric, Gerontic, and Home Health Considerations.* 4th ed. Philadelphia: F. A. Davis.
5. Lipson, J. G., Dibble, S. L., Minarik, P. A. (1996). *Culture & Nursing Care: A Pocket Guide.* San Francisco: UCSF Nursing Press.
7. Hareven, T. K., Adams, K. J. (eds). (1982). *Aging and Life Course Transitions: An Interdisciplinary Perspective.* New York: Guilford.
8. Liken, M. A. (2001). Caregivers in crisis: Moving a relative with Alzheimer's to assisted living. *Clin Nurs Res,* 10(1), 53–69.
9. Liken, M. A. (2001). Experiences of family caregivers of a relative with Alzheimer's disease. *J Psychosoc Nurs,* 39(12), 32–37.
10. Schumacher, K., Beck, C. A., Marren, J. M. (2006). Family caregivers: Caring for older adults, working with their families. *Am J Nurs,* 106(8), 40–49.
11. Weiss, B. (2005). When a family member requires your care. *RN,* 68(4), 63–65.
12. O'Donnell, R. P., et al. (2005). The health and well-being of caregivers of children with cerebral palsy. *Pediatrics,* 115(6), e626–e636.
13. Spurlock, W. R. (2005). Spiritual well-being and caregiver burden in Alzheimer's caregivers. *Geriatr Nurs,* 26(3), 154–161.
14. Haigler, D. H., Bauer, L. J., Travis, S. S. (2006). "Caring for you, caring for me": A ten-year caregiver educational initiative of the Rosalynn Carter Institute for Human Development. *Health Soc Work,* 31(2), 149–152.
15. Haines, C. (2005). Heart failure: Recognizing caregiver burnout. Retrieved February 2007 from www.webmd.com/content/Article/51/40695.htm.
16. Boyles, S. (2005). Spouse caregivers most likely to be abusive. Retrieved February 2007 from www.webmd.com/content/Article/100/105831.htm.
17. Given, C. W., et al. (1992). The caregiver reaction assessment (CRA) for caregivers to persons with chronic physical and mental impairments. *Res Nurs Health,* 15, 271–283.
18. Zarit, S. H., Todd, P. A., Zarit, J. M. (1986). Subjective burden of husbands and wives as caregivers: A longitudinal study. *Gerontologist,* 26, 260–266.

risk for Caregiver Role Strain

DEFINITION: Caregiver is vulnerable for felt difficulty in performing the family caregiver role

RISK FACTORS

Illness severity of the care receiver; psychological or cognitive problems in care receiver; addiction or codependency

Discharge of family member with significant home-care needs; premature birth, congenital defect

Unpredictable illness course or instability in the care receiver's health

Duration of caregiving required; inexperience with caregiving; complexity/amount of caregiving tasks; caregiver's competing role commitments

Caregiver health impairment

Caregiver is female, spouse

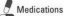

Caregiver not developmentally ready for caregiver role [e.g., a young adult needing to provide care for middle-aged parent]; developmental delay or retardation of the care receiver or caregiver

Presence of situational stressors that normally affect families (e.g., significant loss, disaster or crisis, economic vulnerability, major life events [such as birth, hospitalization, leaving home, returning home, marriage, divorce, change in employment, retirement, death])

Inadequate physical environment for providing care (e.g., housing, transportation, community services, equipment)

Family or caregiver isolation

Lack of respite or recreation for caregiver

Marginal family adaptation or dysfunction prior to the caregiving situation

Marginal caregiver's coping patterns

Past history of poor relationship between caregiver and care receiver

Care receiver exhibits deviant, bizarre behavior

Presence of abuse or violence

NOTE: A risk diagnosis is not evidenced by signs and symptoms, as the problem has not occurred; rather, nursing interventions are directed at prevention.

Sample Clinical Applications: Chronic conditions (e.g., severe brain injury, spinal cord injury [SCI], severe developmental delay), progressive debilitating conditions (e.g., muscular dystrophy, multiple sclerosis [MS], dementia/Alzheimer's disease, end-stage chronic obstructive pulmonary disease [COPD], renal failure, renal dialysis), substance abuse, end-of-life care, psychiatric conditions (e.g., schizophrenia, personality disorders)

DESIRED OUTCOMES/EVALUATION CRITERIA

Sample **NOC** linkages:

Caregiver Home Care Readiness: Extent of preparedness of a caregiver to assume responsibility for the healthcare of a family member in the home

Caregiver Stressors: Severity of biopsychosocial pressure on a family care provider caring for another over an extended period of time

Family Resiliency: Positive adaptation and function of the family system following significant adversity or crisis

Caregiver Will (Include Specific Time Frame)
• Identify individual risk factors and appropriate interventions.
• Demonstrate or initiate behaviors or lifestyle changes to prevent development of impaired function.
• Use available resources appropriately.
• Report satisfaction with current situation.

ACTIONS/INTERVENTIONS

Sample **NIC** linkages:

Caregiver Support: Provision of the necessary information, advocacy, and support to facilitate primary patient care by someone other than a healthcare professional

Family Support: Promotion of family values, interests, and goals

Parenting Promotion: Providing parenting information, support, and coordination of comprehensive services to high-risk families

NURSING PRIORITY NO. 1

To assess factors affecting current situation:

- ∞ • Note presence of high-risk situations (e.g., elderly client with total self-care dependence or several small children with one child requiring extensive assistance due to physical condition or developmental delays). *May necessitate role reversal resulting in added stress, or places excessive demands on parenting skills. Identification of high-risk situations can help in planning and resolving problems before they can become unmanageable.*[1]

- Identify relationship and proximity of caregiver to care receiver (e.g., spouse/lover, parent/child, friend). *There is added stress in maintaining own life and responsibilities when caregiver has to travel some distance to provide care.*[4] *Close relationships may create problems of codependency and identification that can be counterproductive to caregiving.*[3]

- Determine current knowledge of the situation, noting misconceptions, lack of information. *May interfere with caregiver/care receiver's response to situation.*[2]

- Compare caregiver's and receiver's view of situation. *Different views need to be openly expressed so each person understands how other sees situation.*[1]

- Note complexity of therapeutic regimen and physical and mental status of care receiver to ascertain potential areas of need (e.g., teaching, direct care support, respite). *Knowledge of these factors is necessary for planning adequate care for the individual. Plans for additional help may be necessary to prevent caregiver role strain.*[1]

- Determine caregiver's level of responsibility, involvement in care, and anticipated length of care. *Information that may indicate level of stress that could be anticipated for the situation. Progressive debilitation taxes caregiver and may alter ability to meet client's and own needs.*[1]

- 🌐 • Identify individual cultural factors and impact on caregiver. *Helps clarify expectations of caregiver/receiver, family, and community. Many cultures, such as Native American, Cuban, believe strongly in keeping care receiver in the home and caring for them.*[5]

- Ascertain caregiver's physical and emotional health, developmental level and abilities, as well as additional responsibilities of caregiver (e.g., job, raising family). *Provides information indicative of ability of the individual to take on the task of caregiver, as well as clues to potential stressors and possible supportive interventions.*[4,11,12]

- Assess caregiver as appropriate using tool such as Burden Interview or Caregiver Reaction Assessment *to further determine caregiver's stressors and abilities providing additional information to aid in planning.*[6,7]

- Identify strengths and weaknesses of caregiver and care receiver. *Caregiver may not be aware of demands that will be expected. Knowing these factors helps to determine how to use them to advantage in planning and delivering care.*

- Note any codependency needs of caregiver and plan for dealing appropriately with them. *Can contribute to burnout unless identified and dealt with.*[2]

- 🏠 • Verify safety of caregiver/receiver. *Identifying and correcting unsafe situations is crucial so both individuals can be assured of safety in dealing with difficult situation.*[2]

- 🏠 • Determine available supports and resources currently used. *Helpful to identify if they are being used effectively.*[4]

NURSING PRIORITY NO. 2

To enhance caregiver's ability to deal with current situation:

- Establish a therapeutic relationship, conveying empathy and unconditional positive regard. *Promotes positive environment in which needs and concerns can be discussed and proactive solutions identified.*[2]

- Discuss strategies to coordinate care and other responsibilities (e.g., employment, care of children/dependents, housekeeping activities). *Such planning can prevent chaos and resultant burnout.*[8]
- Facilitate family conference as appropriate to share information and develop plan for involvement in care activities. *When everyone is involved and listened to, each person is more likely to carry out his or her responsibilities.*[4]
- Refer to classes and/or specialists (e.g., first aid and cardiopulmonary resuscitation [CPR] classes, enterostomal specialist, physical therapist) for special training as indicated. *Additional information that can help individuals involved feel more competent and able to deal with situation more effectively.*[1]
- Identify additional resources to include financial, legal, respite care. *Can help to resolve problems that arise in the course of caregiving that are out of the knowledge or abilities of the individual. Solving these issues can relieve caregiver of associated anxiety and concern.*[4]
- Identify equipment needs and resources, and appropriate adaptive aids. *Enhances the independence and safety of the care receiver and reduces chances for untoward incidents.*[1]
- Identify contact person or case manager as needed to coordinate care, provide support, assist with problem-solving. *Assistance with planning minimizes problems that could arise.*[10]
- Provide information or demonstrate techniques for dealing with acting out, violent, or disoriented behavior. *Planning ways to deal with these behaviors before they occur promotes safety and enhances positive outcomes.*[2]
- Assist caregiver to recognize codependent behaviors (i.e., doing things for others that others are able to do for themselves) and how these behaviors affect the situation. *Provides options for changing behaviors in ways that enhance the caregiving situation.*[2]

NURSING PRIORITY NO. 3

To promote wellness (Teaching/Discharge Considerations):

- Review signs of burnout (e.g., emotional or physical exhaustion, changes in appetite and sleep, withdrawal from friends/family or life interests). *Recognition of developing problem allows for timely intervention.*[13]
- Discuss and demonstrate stress management techniques and importance of self-nurturing (e.g., meeting personal needs, pursuing self-development interests, hobbies, social activities, spiritual enrichment). *Improves or maintains quality of life for caregiver. May provide care provider with options to protect self.*[4,6,13]
- Encourage involvement in caregiver or other specific support group(s). *Opportunity to be with others in similar situations, and discussing different ways to handle problems helps caregiver deal with difficult role in positive ways.*[3]
- Provide bibliotherapy of appropriate references and Web sites and encourage discussion of information. *Promotes retention of new information that can help caregiver manage more effectively.*[3]
- Advocate for and assist caregiver to plan for and implement changes that may become necessary for the care receiver (e.g., home-care providers, eventual placement in long-term care facility, use of palliative or hospice services). *Getting information and thinking about possibilities will help with decision making. As caregiving tasks become more difficult, other options need to be considered, and planning ahead can promote acceptance of necessary changes.*[8,12,13]
- Refer to classes and other therapists as indicated. *May need additional support and information.*[3]

🏠 • Identify available 12-step program when indicated to provide tools *to deal with codependent behaviors that impair level of function. Provides a more structured environment to learn how to deal with problems of caregiving situation in positive ways.*[1,2]

🔗 • Refer to counseling or psychotherapy as needed. *May need additional help to resolve issues that are interfering with caregiving responsibilities.*[4]

DOCUMENTATION FOCUS

Assessment/Reassessment
• Identified risk factors and caregiver perceptions of situation.
• Reactions of care receiver/family.

Planning
• Treatment plan and individual responsibility for specific activities.
• Teaching plan.

Implementation/Evaluation
• Caregiver/receiver response to interventions, teaching, and actions performed.
• Attainment or progress toward desired outcome(s).
• Modifications to plan of care.

Discharge Planning
• Long-term needs and who is responsible for actions to be taken.
• Specific referrals provided for assistance and evaluation.

References

1. Doenges, M., Moorhouse, M., Murr, A. (2002). *Nursing Care Plans: Guidelines for Individualizing Patient Care.* 6th ed. Philadelphia: F. A. Davis.
2. Doenges, M., Townsend, M., Moorhouse, M. (1998). *Psychiatric Care Plans: Guidelines for Individualizing Care.* 3d ed. Philadelphia: F. A. Davis.
3. Townsend, M. (2003). *Psychiatric Mental Health Nursing: Concepts of Care.* 4th ed. Philadelphia: F. A. Davis.
4. Cox, H., et al. (2002). *Clinical Applications of Nursing Diagnosis: Adult, Child, Women's, Psychiatric, Gerontic, and Home Health Considerations.* 4th ed. Philadelphia: F. A. Davis.
5. Lipson, J. G., Dibble, S. L., Minarik, P. A. (1996). *Culture & Nursing Care: A Pocket Guide.* San Francisco: UCSF Nursing Press.
6. Given, C. W., et al. (1992). The caregiver reaction assessment (CRA) for caregivers to persons with chronic physical and mental impairments. *Res Nurs Health,* 15, 271–83.
7. Zarit, S. H., Todd, P. A., Zarit, J. M. (1986). Subjective burden of husbands and wives as caregivers: A longitudinal study. *Gerontologist,* 26, 260–266.
8. Liken, M. A. (2001). Caregivers in crisis: Moving a relative with Alzheimer's to assisted living. *Clin Nurs Res,* 10(1), 53–69.
9. Liken, M. A. (2001). Experiences of family caregivers of a relative with Alzheimer's disease. *J Psychosoc Nurs,* 39(12), 33–37.
10. Halper, J., et al. (2000). *Multiple Sclerosis: Best Practices in Nursing Care (monograph).* Columbia, MD: Medicalliance.
11. Schumacher, K., Beck, C. A., Marren, J. M. (2006). Family caregivers: Caring for older adults, working with their families. *Am J Nurs,* 106(8), 40–49.
12. Weiss, B. (2005). When a family member requires your care. *RN,* 68(4), 63–65.
13. Haines, C. (2005). Heart failure: Recognizing caregiver burnout. Retrieved February 2007 from www.webmd.com/content/Article/51/40695.htm.

readiness for enhanced Childbearing Process

DEFINITION: A pattern of preparing for, maintaining, and strengthening a healthy pregnancy and childbirth process and care of newborn

RELATED FACTORS

To be developed by nurse researchers and submitted to NANDA

DEFINING CHARACTERISTICS

During Pregnancy

Subjective
Reports appropriate prenatal lifestyle (e.g., diet, elimination, sleep, bodily movement, exercise, personal hygiene), a realistic birth plan, appropriate physical preparations, availability of support systems
Reports managing unpleasant symptoms of pregnancy

Objective
Has regular prenatal health visits
Demonstrates respect for unborn baby; prepares necessary newborn care items
Seeks necessary knowledge (e.g., of labor and delivery, newborn care)

During Labor and Delivery

Subjective
Reports lifestyle (e.g., diet, elimination, sleep, bodily movement, personal hygiene that is appropriate for the stage of labor)

Objective
Responds appropriately to onset of labor
Is proactive in labor and delivery; uses relaxation techniques appropriate for stage of labor; utilizes support systems appropriately
Demonstrates attachment behavior to the newborn baby

After Birth

Subjective
Reports appropriate postpartum lifestyle (e.g., diet, elimination, sleep, bodily movement, exercise, personal hygiene)

Objective
Demonstrates attachment behavior to the baby, basic baby care techniques, appropriate baby feeding techniques
Provides safe environment for the baby
Utilizes support systems appropriately
Demonstrates appropriate breast care

Sample Clinical Applications: First, second, and third trimesters of pregnancy; labor and delivery; postpartum; newborn

(continues on page 152)

readiness for enhanced Childbearing Process (continued)
DESIRED OUTCOMES/EVALUATION CRITERIA

Sample **NOC** linkages:
Knowledge: Pregnancy: Extent of understanding conveyed about promotion of a healthy pregnancy and prevention of complications
Knowledge: Labor & Delivery: Extent of understanding conveyed about labor and vaginal delivery
Knowledge: Infant Care: Extent of understanding conveyed about caring for a baby from birth to first birthday

Client Will (Include Specific Time Frame)
• Demonstrate healthy pregnancy free of preventable complications.
• Engage in activities to prepare for birth process and care of newborn.
• Experience complication-free labor and childbirth.
• Display culturally appropriate bonding behaviors.
• Verbalize understanding of care requirements to promote health of self and infant.

ACTIONS/INTERVENTIONS

Sample **NIC** linkages:
Childbirth Preparation: Providing information and support to facilitate childbirth and to enhance the ability of an individual to develop and perform the parental role

NURSING PRIORITY NO. 1

To determine individual needs:

PRENATAL
● Evaluate current knowledge and cultural beliefs regarding normal physiological and psychological changes of pregnancy, as well as beliefs about activities, self-care, and so on. *Provides information to assist in identifying needs and creating individual plan of care.*[2,3]
● Determine degree of motivation for learning. *Client may have difficulty learning unless the need for it is clear.*[3]
● Identify who provides support/instruction within the clients culture (e.g., grandmother, other family member, curandero or doula, other cultural healer). Work with support person(s) when possible, using interpreter as needed. *Helps ensure quality and continuity of care because support person(s) may be more successful than the healthcare provider in communicating information.*[1,2,4]
● Determine client's commitments to work, family, community, and self; and roles and responsibilities within family unit, and use of supportive resources. *Helps in setting realistic priorities to assist client in making adjustments, such as changing work hours, shifting of household chores and responsibilities, prioritizing and curtailing some outside commitments, and so on.*[12,17]
● Evaluate the client's/couple's response to pregnancy, individual and family stressors, and cultural implications of pregnancy and childbirth. *The client's/couple's ability to adapt positively depends on support systems, cultural beliefs, resources, and effective coping mechanisms developed in dealing with past stressors. Initially, even if the pregnancy is planned, the expectant mother may feel ambivalent toward the pregnancy because of personal or professional goals, financial concerns, and possible role changes that a child will necessitate.*[1,2]

- Determine client's/couple's perception of fetus as a separate entity and extent of preparations being made for this infant. *Activities such as choosing a name or nicknaming the baby in utero and home preparations indicate completion of psychological tasks of pregnancy. Note: Cultural or familial beliefs may limit visible preparations out of concern that bad outcome may result.*[2]
- Assess economic situation and financial needs. Note use of available resources. *Impact of pregnancy on family with limited resources can create added stress and result in limited prenatal care and preparation for newborn.*
- Determine usual pregravid weight and dietary patterns. *Research studies have found a positive correlation between pregravid maternal obesity and increased perinatal morbidity rates (e.g., hypertension and gestational diabetes) associated with preterm births and macrosomia.*[16]

LABOR AND DELIVERY

- Ascertain client's understanding and expectations of the labor process. *The client's/couple's coping skills are most challenged during the active and transition phases as contractions become increasingly intense. Lack of knowledge, misconceptions, or unrealistic expectations can have a negative impact on coping abilities.*
- Review birth plan developed by client/partner. Note cultural expectations/preferences. *Verifies that choices made are amenable to the specific care setting, accommodate individual wishes, and reflect client/fetal status. Note: Some cultures or personal values may limit male involvement in the delivery process, necessitating the identification of other support person(s).*[1,6,10]

POSTPARTUM/NEWBORN CARE

- Determine plan for discharge after delivery and home care support and needs. *Early planning can facilitate discharge and help ensure that client/infant needs will be met.*[3]
- Ascertain client's perception of labor and delivery, length of labor, and client's fatigue level. *There is a correlation between length of labor and the ability of some clients to assume responsibility for self-care/infant care tasks and activities.*
- Assess mother's strengths and needs, noting age, marital status or relationship, presence and reaction of siblings and other family, available sources of support, and cultural background. *Identifies potential risk factors and sources of support, which influence the client's/couple's ability to assume role of parenthood. For example, the adolescent may still be formulating goals and an identity. She may have difficulty accepting the infant as a person and coping with full-time parenting responsibility. The single parent who lacks support systems may have difficulty assuming sole responsibility for parenting. Cultures in which the extended family members live together may provide more emotional and physical support, facilitating adoption of the new role.*[1,6]
- Appraise level of parents' understanding of infant's physiological needs and adaptation to extrauterine life associated with maintenance of body temperature, nutrition, respiratory needs, and bowel and bladder functioning. *Identifies areas of concern/need, which could require additional information and/or demonstration of care activities.*[3,12]
- Evaluate nature of emotional and physical parenting that client/couple received during their childhood. *Parenting role is learned, and individuals use their own parents as role models. Those who experienced a negative upbringing or poor parenting may require additional support to meet the challenges of effective parenting.*
- Note father's/partner's response to birth and to parenting role. *Client's ability to adapt positively to parenting may be strongly influenced by the father's/partner's reaction.*

Nursing Diagnoses in Alphabetical Order

- Assess client's readiness and motivation for learning. Assist client/couple in identifying needs. *The postpartal period provides an opportunity to foster maternal growth, maturation, and competence. However, the client needs time to move from a "taking-in" to a "taking-hold" phase, in which her receptiveness and readiness is heightened and she is emotionally and physically ready for learning new information to facilitate mastery of her new role.*[4]

NURSING PRIORITY NO. 2

To promote maximum participation in childbearing process:

PRENATAL

- Maintain open attitude toward beliefs of client/couple. *Acceptance is important to developing and maintaining relationship and supporting independence.*[2]
- Explain office visit routine, rationale for ongoing screening and close monitoring (e.g., urine testing, blood pressure monitoring, weight, fetal growth). Emphasize importance of keeping regular appointments. *Reinforces relationship between health assessment and positive outcome for mother/baby.*[12]
- Suggest father/siblings attend prenatal office visits and listen to fetal heart tones (FHT) as appropriate. *Promotes a sense of involvement and helps make baby a reality for family members.*
- Provide information about need for additional laboratory studies, diagnostic tests or procedure(s). Review risks and potential side effects. *Aids in making informed decisions.*[8,12]
- Discuss any medications that may be needed to control or treat medical conditions. *Helpful in choosing treatment options because need must be weighed against possible harmful effects on the fetus.*[12]
- Provide anticipatory guidance, including discussion of nutrition, regular moderate exercise, comfort measures, rest, employment, breast care, sexual activity, and health habits and lifestyle. *Information encourages acceptance of responsibility and promotes self-care:*

  Review nutrition requirements and optimal prenatal weight gain to support maternal-fetal needs. *Dietary focus should be on balanced nutrients and calories to produce appropriate weight gain and to supply adequate vitamins and minerals for healthy fetus. Inadequate prenatal weight gain and/or below normal prepregnancy weight increases the risk of intrauterine growth restriction (IUGR) in the fetus and delivery of a low-birth-weight (LBW) infant.*[8,12]

   Encourage moderate exercise such as walking, or non-weight-bearing activities (e.g., swimming, bicycling) in accordance with client's physical condition and cultural beliefs. *Nonendurance, antepartal exercise regimens tend to shorten labor, increase likelihood of a spontaneous vaginal delivery, and decrease need for oxytocin augmentation.*[4,5] *In some cultures, inactivity may be viewed as a protection for mother/child.*[1,6]

  Recommend a consistent sleep and rest schedule (e.g., 1 to 2 hour daytime nap and 8 hours of sleep each night) in a dark, cool room. *Provides rest to meet metabolic needs associated with growth of maternal/fetal tissues.*[12]

  Identify anticipatory adaptations for SO/family necessitated by pregnancy. *Family members will need to be flexible in adjusting own roles and responsibilities in order to assist client to meet her needs related to the demands of pregnancy, both expected and unplanned, such as prolonged nausea, fatigue, and emotional lability.*[12]

  Provide or reinforce information about potential teratogens, such as alcohol, nicotine, illicit drugs, STORCH group of viruses (**s**yphilis, **t**oxoplasmosis, **o**ther, **r**ubella, **c**ytomegalovirus [CMV], **h**erpes simplex), and HIV. *Helps client make informed decisions and choices about behaviors and environment that can promote healthy offspring. Note: Research* *supports the fact that alcohol and recreational drug use can lead to a wide range of negative effects in the neonate. Smoking negatively affects placental circulation; even smoking fewer than 10 cigarettes per day is associated with an increased risk of fetal death, damage in utero, abruptio placentae, placenta previa, and low birth weights.*[4,8,13–15]

- Use various methods for learning, including pictures, to discuss fetal development. *Visualization enhances reality of child and strengthens learning process.*[4]
- Discuss signs of labor onset; how to distinguish between false and true labor, when to notify healthcare provider and to leave for hospital or birth center; and stages of labor and delivery. *Helps client to recognize onset of labor, to ensure timely arrival, and to cope with labor and delivery process.*[12]
- Review signs/symptoms requiring evaluation by primary provider during prenatal period (e.g., excessive vomiting, fever, unresolved illness of any kind, decreased fetal movement). *Allows for timely intervention.*[12]

LABOR AND DELIVERY

- Identify clients support person/coach and ascertain that the individual is providing support that client requires. *Coach may be clients husband or significant other or doula, and support can take the form of physical and emotional support for the mother, and aid in initiation of bonding with the neonate.*[4]
- Demonstrate or review behaviors and techniques (e.g., breathing, focused imagery, music, other distraction; aromatherapy; abdominal effleurage, back and leg rubs, sacral pressure, repositioning, back rest; oral and perineal care, linen changes; shower or hot tub use) partner can use to assist with pain control and relaxation. *Enhances feeling of well-being. May block pain impulses within the cerebral cortex through conditioned responses and cutaneous stimulation, facilitating progression of normal labor.*[4]
- Discuss available analgesics, usual responses and side effects (client and fetal), and duration of analgesic effect in light of current situation. *Allows client to make informed choice about means of pain control and can allay client's fears or anxieties about medication use. Note: If conservative measures are not effective and increasing muscle tension impedes progress of labor, judicious use of medication can enhance relaxation, shorten labor, limit fatigue, and prevent complications.*[4]
- Support client's decision about the use or nonuse of medication in a nonjudgmental manner. Continue encouragement for efforts and use of relaxation techniques. *Enhances client sense of control and may prevent or decrease need for medication. Note: Continued support may be needed to help reduce feelings of failure in the client/couple who may have anticipated an unmedicated birth and did not follow through with that plan.*[12]

POSTPARTUM/NEWBORN CARE

- Initiate early breast- or oral feeding according to hospital protocol. *Initial feeding for breastfed infants usually occurs in the delivery room. Otherwise, 5 to 15 mL of sterile water may be offered in the nursery to assess effectiveness of sucking, swallowing, gag reflexes, and patency of esophagus. If aspirated, sterile water is easily absorbed by pulmonary tissues.*[7,9]
- Note frequency and amount and length of feedings. Encourage demand feedings instead of "scheduled" feedings. *Hunger and length of time between feedings vary from feeding to feeding.*[7,9] Note frequency, amount, and appearance of regurgitation. *Excessive regurgitation increases feeding needs.*
- Evaluate neonate/maternal satisfaction following feedings. *Provides opportunity to answer client questions, offer encouragement for efforts, identify needs, and problem-solve solutions.*[7,9]

Nursing Diagnoses in Alphabetical Order

- Demonstrate and supervise infant care activities related to feeding and holding; bathing, diapering, and clothing; care of circumcised male infant; and care of umbilical cord stump. Provide written and pictorial information for parents to refer to after discharge. *Promotes understanding of principles and techniques of newborn care; fosters parents' skills as caregivers.*[3,12]

- Provide information about newborn interactional capabilities, states of consciousness, and means of stimulating cognitive development. *Helps parents recognize and respond to infant cues during interactional process; fosters optimal interaction, attachment behaviors, and cognitive development in infant. The state of consciousness can be divided into the sleep and the wake states, involving separate and predictable behavioral characteristics.*[12]

- Promote sleep and rest. *Reduces metabolic rate and allows nutrition and oxygen to be used for healing process rather than for energy needs.*[12]

- Provide for unlimited participation for father and siblings. Ascertain whether siblings attended an orientation program. *Facilitates family development and ongoing process of acquaintance and attachment. Helps family members feel comfortable caring for newborn.*

- Monitor and document the client's/couple's interactions with infant. Note presence of bonding (acquaintance) behaviors (e.g., making eye contact, using high-pitched voice and en face [face-to-face] position as culturally appropriate, calling infant by name, and holding infant closely).[2,12]

NURSING PRIORITY NO. 3

To enhance optimal well-being:

PRENATAL

- Emphasize importance of maternal well-being. *Fetal well-being is directly related to maternal well-being, especially during the first trimester, when developing organ systems are most vulnerable to injury from environmental or hereditary factors.*

- Review physical changes to be expected during each trimester. *Questions will continue to arise as new changes occur, regardless of whether changes are expected or unexpected, and knowledge of "what's normal" can be reassuring. Also prepares client/couple for managing common discomforts associated with pregnancy.*[4,12]

- Explain psychological reactions including ambivalence, introspection, stress reactions, and emotional lability as characteristic of pregnancy. *Helps client/couple understand mood swings and may provide opportunities for partner to offer support/affection at these times.*[4]

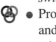 • Provide necessary referrals (e.g., dietitian, social services, food stamps or Women, Infants, and Children [WIC] food programs) as indicated. *May need additional assistance with nutritional choices; may have budget or financial constraints. Supplemental federally funded food program helps promote optimal maternal, fetal and infant nutrition.*[12]

- Identify reportable danger signals of pregnancy, such as bleeding, cramping, acute abdominal pain, backache, edema, visual disturbance, headaches, and pelvic pressure. *Helps client to distinguish normal from abnormal findings, thus assisting her in seeking timely, appropriate healthcare.*[12]

- Encourage attendance at prenatal and childbirth classes. Provide information about father/ sibling or grandparent participation in classes and delivery as client desires. *Knowledge gained helps reduce fear of unknown and increases confidence that couple can manage the preparation for the birth of their child. Helps family members to realize they are an integral part of the pregnancy and delivery.*[11,12]

- Provide list of appropriate reading materials for client, couple, and siblings regarding adjusting to newborn. *Information helps individual realistically analyze changes in family structure, roles, and behaviors.*[3]

LABOR AND DELIVERY

- Monitor labor progress, maternal and fetal well-being per protocol. Provide continuous intrapartal professional support or doula. *Fear of abandonment can intensify as labor progresses. The client may experience increased anxiety and/or loss of control when left unattended. Doulas can provide client with emotional, physical, and informational support as an adjunct to primary nurse.*[2,8]
- Reinforce use of positive coping mechanisms. *Enhances feelings of competence and fosters self-esteem.*[12]

POSTPARTUM/NEWBORN CARE

- Provide information about self-care, including perineal care and hygiene; physiological changes, including normal progression of lochial discharge; needs for sleep and rest; importance of progressive postpartal exercise program; role changes. *Helps prevent infection, fosters healing and recuperation, and contributes to positive adaptation to physical and emotional changes enhancing feelings of general well-being.*[12]
- Review normal psychological changes and needs associated with the postpartal period. *Client's emotional state may be somewhat labile at this time and often is influenced by physical well-being. Anticipating such changes may reduce the stress associated with this transition period that necessitates learning new roles and taking on new responsibilities.*[4,8,12]
- Discuss sexuality needs and plans for contraception. Provide information about available methods, including advantages and disadvantages. *Couple may need clarification regarding available contraceptive methods and the fact that pregnancy could occur even prior to the 4- to 6-week postpartum visit.*[8]
- Reinforce importance of postpartal examination by healthcare provider and interim follow-up as appropriate. *Follow-up visit is necessary to evaluate recovery of reproductive organs, healing of episiotomy or laceration repair, general well-being, and adaptation to life changes.*[12]
- Provide oral and written information about infant care and development, feeding, and safety issues. Offer appropriate references. Elicit cultural beliefs. *Helps prepare for new caretaking role, acquiring necessary items of furniture, clothing, and supplies; helps prepare for breastfeeding and/or bottle feeding.*[8,12]
- Discuss physiology and benefits of breastfeeding, nipple and breast care, special dietary needs, factors that facilitate or interfere with successful breastfeeding, use of breast pump and appropriate suppliers. *Helps ensure adequate milk supply, prevents nipple cracking and soreness, facilitates comfort, and establishes role of breastfeeding mother.*[8]
- Refer client to support groups (e.g., La Leche League International, Lact-Aid) or lactation consultant. *Provides ongoing help to promote a successful breastfeeding outcome.*[7,9]
- Identify available community resources as indicated (e.g., WIC program). *WIC and other federal programs support well-being through client education and enhanced nutritional intake for infant.*[12]
- Discuss normal variations and characteristics of infant, such as caput succedaneum, cephalhematoma, pseudomenstruation, breast enlargement, physiologic jaundice, and milia. *Helps parents to recognize normal variations and may reduce anxiety.*[4,12]
- Emphasize newborn's need for follow-up evaluation by healthcare provider and timely immunizations. *Ongoing evaluation is important for monitoring growth and development. Immunizations are necessary to protect the infant from childhood diseases with associated serious complications.*[12]
- Identify manifestations of illness and infection and the times at which a healthcare provider should be contacted. Demonstrate proper technique for taking temperature, administering oral medications, or providing other care activities as required. *Early recognition of illness and prompt use of healthcare facilitate treatment and positive outcome.*[12]

Nursing Diagnoses in Alphabetical Order

● Refer client/couple to community postpartal parent groups. *Increases parents knowledge of child rearing and child development, and provides supportive atmosphere while parents incorporate new roles.*

DOCUMENTATION FOCUS

Assessment/Reassessment
• Assessment findings, general health, previous pregnancy experience.
• Cultural beliefs and expectations.
• Specific birth plan and individuals to be involved in delivery.
• Arrangements for postpartal recovery period.
• Response to newborn.

Planning
• Plan of care and who is involved in planning.
• Teaching plan.

Implementation/Evaluation
• Response to interventions, teaching, and actions performed.
• Attainment or progress toward desired outcome(s).
• Modifications to plan of care.

Discharge Planning
• Long-term needs and who is responsible for actions to be taken.
• Available resources, specific referrals made.

References

1. Lauderdale, J. (2007). Transcultural perspectives in childbearing. In Andrews, M. M., Boyle, J. S. (eds.), *Transcultural Concepts in Nursing Care*, 5th ed. Philadelphia: Wolters Kluwer Health, Lippincott Williams & Wilkins.
2. Purnell, L. D., Paulanka, B. J. (2008). *Transcultural Health Care: Culturally Competent Approach*. 3d ed. Philadelphia: F. A. Davis.
3. Bastable, S. B. (2005). *Essentials of Patient Education*. Sudbury, MA: Jones and Bartlett.
4. Editorial Staff. (2008). Complications and high-risk conditions of the prenatal period. In *Straight A's in Maternal-Neonatal Nursing*. 2nd ed. Philadelphia: Wolters Kluwer, Lippincott Williams & Wilkins.
5. American College of Obstetricians and Gynecologists (ACOG), Committee on Obstetric Practice. (2002). Exercise during pregnancy and the postpartum period. ACOG Committee Opinion 267. *Obst Gynecol*, 99(1), 171–173.
6. Editorial Staff. (2007). Cultural childbearing practices. Monograph in *Lippincott Manual of Nursing Practice Pocket Guides: Maternal-Neonatal Nursing*, Philadelphia: Lippincott Williams & Wilkins.
7. Meek, J. (ed). (2002). *The American Academy of Pediatrics New Mothers Guide to Breastfeeding*. New York: Bantam.
8. Holloway, B., Moredich, C., Aduddell, K. (2006). *OB Peds Women's Health Notes: Nurses Clinical Pocket Guide*. Philadelphia: F. A. Davis.
9. American Academy of Family Physicians. Breastfeeding, family physicians supporting (position paper). Retrieved April 2009 from www.aafp.org/online/en/home/policy/policies/b/breastfeedingpositionpaper.html.
10. Murry, M. (2008). What is a birth plan and why do I need one? Retrieved April 2009 from www.mayoclinic.com/health/birth-plan/MY00052.
11. Mayo Clinic Staff. (2007). Childbirth education: Get ready for labor and delivery. Retrieved April 2009 from www.mayoclinic.com/health/pregnancy/PR00119.

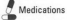

12. Ricci, S. S., Kyle, T. (2008). *Maternity and Pediatric Nursing*. Philadelphia: Lippincott Williams & Wilkins.
13. Surgeon General. (2005, revised 2007). Surgeon General's advisory on alcohol use in pregnancy. Retrieved March 2009 from www.surgeongeneral.gov/pressreleases/sg02222005.html.
14. March of Dimes. (2006). Fact sheets: Illicit drug use during pregnancy. Retrieved March 2009 from www.marchofdimes.com/professionals/14332_1169.asp.
15. Dharan, V. B. Parvianen, E. L. K. (2009). Psychosocial and environmental pregnancy risks. Retrieved March 2009 from http://emedicine.medscape.com/article/259346-overview.
16. Ehrenberg, H. M. (2009). Maternal obesity, uterine activity, and the risk of spontaneous preterm birth. *Obstet Gynecol*, 113(1), 48–52.
17. March of Dimes. Work and pregnancy. Retrieved April 2009 from www.marchofdimes.com/pnhec/159_11488.asp.

(impaired Comfort)

DEFINITION: Perceived lack of ease, relief and transcendence in physical, psychospiritual, environmental and social dimensions

RELATED FACTORS

To be developed by nurse researchers and submitted to NANDA

DEFINING CHARACTERISTICS

Subjective
Reports: distressing symptoms, lack of contentment or ease in situation, hunger, itching, being uncomfortable, cold, hot
Disturbed sleep pattern, inability to relax
Anxiety, fear
Illness-related symptoms, treatment-related side effects (e.g., medication, radiation)
Insufficient resources (e.g., financial, social support)
Lack of privacy

Objective
Restlessness, irritability, moaning, crying
Lack of environmental control

Sample Clinical Applications: Presence of chronic physical or psychological conditions

DESIRED OUTCOMES/EVALUATION CRITERIA

Sample **NOC** linkages:
Comfort Level: Overall physical, psychospiritual, sociocultural, and environmental ease and safety of an individual
Personal Well-Being: Extent of positive perception of one's health status
Quality of life: Extent of positive perception of current life circumstances

Client Will (Include Specific Time Frame)
Engage in behaviors or lifestyle changes to increase level of ease.
Verbalize sense of comfort and contentment.
Participate in desirable and realistic health-seeking behaviors.

(continues on page 160)

---

impaired Comfort (continued)
ACTIONS/INTERVENTIONS

Sample NIC linkages:
Self-Modification: Reinforcement of self-directed change initiated by the patient to achieve personally important goals
Relaxation Therapy: Use of techniques to encourage and elicit relaxation for the purpose of decreasing undesirable signs and symptoms such as pain, muscle tension, or anxiety
Self-Awareness Enhancement: Assisting a patient to explore and understand his/her thoughts, feelings, motivations, and behaviors

NURSING PRIORITY NO. 1

To assess etiology/precipitating contributory factors:

- Determine the type of discomfort client is experiencing such as physical pain, feeling of discontent, lack of ease in social settings, or inability to rise above one's problems or pain (lack of transcendence).[1]
- Note cultural or religious beliefs and values that impact perceptions and expectations of comfort.
- Ascertain locus of control. *Presence of external locus of control may hamper efforts to achieve sense of peace or contentment.*
- Discuss concerns with client and Active-listen to identify underlying issues (e.g., physical and/or emotional stressors; and/or external factors such as environmental surroundings, social interactions) that could impact client's ability to control own well-being. *Helps to determine client's specific needs, ability to change own situation.*
- Establish context(s) in which lack of comfort is realized: physical—pertaining to bodily sensations; psychospiritual—pertaining to internal awareness of self and meaning in ones life, relationship to a higher order or being; environmental—pertaining to external surroundings, conditions and influences; sociocultural—pertaining to interpersonal, family and societal relationships:[1]

PHYSICAL
- Determine how client is managing pain and pain components. *Lack of control may be related to other issues or emotions such as fear, loneliness, anxiety, noxious stimuli, anger.*[1]
- Ascertain what has been tried or is required for comfort or rest (e.g., head of bed up or down, music on or off, white noise, rocking motion, certain person or thing).[2]

PSYCHOSPIRITUAL
- Determine how psychological and spiritual indicators overlap (e.g., meaningfulness, faith, identity, self-esteem) for client.[1]
- Ascertain if client/SO desires support regarding spiritual enrichment, including prayer, meditation, or access to spiritual counselor of choice.[3]

ENVIRONMENTAL
- Determine that clients environment respects privacy, and provides natural lighting and readily accessible view to outdoors—*an aspect that can be manipulated to enhance comfort.*[1,3]

SOCIAL

- Ascertain meaning of comfort in context of interpersonal, family, and cultural values and societal relationships.[4]
- Validate client/SO understanding of clients situation and ongoing methods of managing condition, as appropriate and/or desired by client. *Considers client/family needs in this area and shows appreciation for their desires.*[4]

NURSING PRIORITY NO. 2

To assist client to alleviate discomfort:

- Review knowledge base and note coping skills that have been used previously to change behavior and promote well-being. *Brings these to client's awareness and promotes use in current situation.*[8]
- Acknowledge client's strengths in present situation, and build on those strengths in planning for future.

PHYSICAL

- Collaborate in treating and managing medical conditions involving oxygenation, elimination, mobility, cognitive abilities, electrolyte balance, thermoregulation, hydration, *to promote physical stability.*[2,5,6]
- Work with client to prevent pain, nausea, itching, thirst, and other physical discomforts.
- Review medications or treatment regimen *to determine possible changes or options to reduce side effects.*
- Suggest parent be present during procedures *to comfort child.*
- Provide age-appropriate comfort measures (e.g., back rub, change of position, cuddling, use of heat or cold) *to provide nonpharmacological pain management.*
- Discuss interventions and activities to promote ease such as Therapeutic Touch (TT), massage, healing touch, biofeedback, self-hypnosis, guided imagery, breathing exercises; play therapy, and humor *to promote relaxation and refocus attention.*
- Assist client to use and modify medication regimen *to make best use of pharmacological pain or symptom management.*
- Assist client/SO(s) to develop plan for activity and exercise within individual ability emphasizing necessity of allowing sufficient time to finish activities.
- Maintain open and flexible visitation with client's desired persons.
- Encourage and plan care to allow individually adequate rest periods *to prevent fatigue.* Schedule activities for periods when client has the most energy *to maximize participation.*
- Discuss routines to promote restful sleep.

PSYCHOSPIRITUAL

- Interact with client in therapeutic manner. *The nurse could be the most important comfort intervention for meeting clients needs. For example assuring client that nausea can be treated successfully with both pharmacologic and nonpharmacologic methods may be more effective than simply administering antiemetic without reassurance and comforting presence.*[1]
- Encourage verbalization of feelings and make time for listening and interacting.
- Identify ways (e.g., meditation, sharing oneself with others, being out in nature or garden, other spiritual activities) to achieve connectedness or harmony with self, others, nature, higher power.
- Establish realistic activity goals with client. *Enhances commitment to promoting optimal outcomes.*

- Involve client/SO(s) in schedule planning and decisions about timing and spacing of treatments *to promote relaxation and reduce sense of boredom.*
- Encourage client to do whatever possible (e.g., self-care, sit up in chair, walk). *Enhances self-esteem and independence.*
- Use distraction with music, chatting, texting with family/friends, watching TV or videos, playing computer games *to limit dwelling on and transcend unpleasant sensations and situations.*
- Encourage client to develop assertiveness skills, prioritizing goals and activities, and to make use of beneficial coping behaviors. *Promotes sense of control and improves self-esteem.*
- Offer or identify opportunities for client to participate in experiences that enhance control and independence.

ENVIRONMENTAL
- Provide quiet environment, calm activities.
- Provide for periodic changes in the personal surroundings when client is confined. Use the individuals input in creating the changes (e.g., seasonal bulletin boards, color changes, rearranging furniture, pictures).
- Suggest activities, such as bird feeders or baths for bird-watching, a garden in a window box or terrarium, or a fish bowl or aquarium, *to stimulate observation as well as involvement and participation in activity.*

SOCIAL
- Encourage age-appropriate diversional activities (e.g., TV, radio, computer games, playtime, socialization or outings with others).
- Avoid overstimulation or understimulation (cognitive and sensory).
- Make appropriate referrals to available support groups, hobby clubs, service organizations.

NURSING PRIORITY NO. 3

To promote wellness (Teaching/Discharge Considerations):

- Provide information about condition, health risk factors, or concerns in desired format (e.g., pictures, TV programs, articles, handouts, audio/visual materials; classes, group discussions, Internet Web sites, and other databases) as appropriate. *Use of multiple modalities enhances acquisition and retention of information and gives client choices for accessing and applying information.*

PHYSICAL
- Promote overall health measures (e.g., nutrition, adequate fluid intake, appropriate vitamin or iron supplementation).
- Discuss potential complications and possible need for medical follow-up or alternative therapies. *Timely recognition and intervention can promote wellness.*
- Assist client/SO(s) to identify and acquire necessary equipment (e.g., lifts, commode chair, safety grab bars, personal hygiene supplies) to meet individual needs.

PSYCHOSPIRITUAL
- Collaborate with others when client expresses interest in lessons, counseling, coaching and/or mentoring *to meet or enhance emotional and spiritual comfort.*
- Encourage client's contributions toward meeting realistic goals.
- Recommend client take time to be introspective in the search for contentment or transcendence.

ENVIRONMENTAL
- Create a compassionate, supportive and therapeutic environment incorporating clients cultural and age and developmental factors.
- Correct environmental hazards that could influence safety and negatively affect comfort.
- Arrange for home visit and evaluation as needed.
- Discuss long-term plan for taking care of environmental needs.

SOCIAL
- Advocate for growth-promoting environment in conflict situations, and consider issues from client/family perspective.
- Identify resources or referrals (e.g., knowledge and skills, financial resources and assistance; personal or psychological support group; social activities).

DOCUMENTATION FOCUS

Assessment/Reassessment
- Individual findings including client's description of current status or situation, and factors impacting sense of comfort.
- Pertinent cultural or religious beliefs and values.
- Medication use and nonpharmacological measures.

Planning
- Plan of care, specific interventions, and who is involved in planning.
- Teaching plan.

Implementation/Evaluation
- Responses to interventions, teaching, and actions performed.
- Attainment or progress toward desired outcome(s).
- Modifications to plan of care.

Discharge Planning
- Long-term needs and who is responsible for actions to be taken.
- Specific referrals made.

References

1. Kolcaba, K. Y., Fisher E. M. (1996). A holistic perspective on comfort care as an advance directive. *Crit Care Nurs Q*, 18(4), 66–67.
2. Kolcaba, K., DiMarco, M. A. (2005). Comfort theory and its application to pediatric nursing. *Pediatr Nurs*, 31(3), 187–194.
3. Barclay, L., Lie, D. (2007). New guidelines issued for family support in patient-centered ICU. CME/CE for Medscape Web site. Retrieved February 2009 from www.medscape/viewarticle/551738.
4. Malinowski, A., Stamler, L. L. (2002). Comfort: Exploration of the concept in nursing. *J Adv Nurs*, 39(6), 599–606.
5. Kolcaba, K. (2006). FAQs (Frequently Asked Questions). Retrieved January 2009 from www.thecomfortline.com/FAQ.htm.
6. Kaplow, R. (2003). AACN synergy model for patient care: A framework to optimize outcomes. *Crit Care Nurse Suppl* (Feb), 27–30.
7. Wilson, L., Kolcaba, K. (2004). Practical application of comfort theory in the perianesthesia setting. *J Perianesth Nurs Online*, 19(3), 135–224.
8. Townsend, M. C. (2003). *Psychiatric Mental Health Nursing Concepts of Care*. 4th ed. Philadelphia: F. A. Davis.

readiness for enhanced Comfort

DEFINITION: A pattern of ease, relief, and transcendence in physical, psychospiritual, environmental, or social dimensions that can be strengthened

RELATED FACTORS

To be developed by nurse researchers and submitted to NANDA

DEFINING CHARACTERISTICS

Subjective
Expresses desire to enhance comfort or feeling of contentment
Expresses desire to enhance relaxation
Expresses desire to enhance resolution of complaints

Objective
[Appears relaxed, calm]
[Participates in comfort measures of choice]

Sample Clinical Applications: Presence of chronic physical or psychological conditions, or any individual seeking improved quality of life

DESIRED OUTCOMES/EVALUATION CRITERIA

Sample NOC linkages:
Comfort Status: Overall physical, psychospiritual, sociocultural, and environmental ease and safety of an individual
Personal Well-Being: Extent of positive perception of one's health status
Quality of Life: Extent of positive perception of current life circumstances

Client Will (Include Specific Time Frame)
• Verbalize sense of comfort or contentment.
• Demonstrate behaviors of optimal level of ease.
• Participate in desirable and realistic health-seeking behaviors.

ACTIONS/INTERVENTIONS

Sample NIC linkages:
Self-Modification Assistance: Reinforcement of self-directed change initiated by the patient to achieve personally important goals
Relaxation Therapy: Use of techniques to encourage and elicit relaxation for the purpose of decreasing undesirable signs and symptoms such as pain, muscle tension, or anxiety
Self-Awareness Enhancement: Exploration and understanding of patient's thoughts, feelings, motivations, and behaviors

NURSING PRIORITY NO. 1

To determine current level of comfort/motivation for growth:

- Determine the type of comfort client is experiencing: (1) relief—as from pain; (2) ease—a state of calm or contentment; or (3) transcendence—state in which one rises above one's problems or pain.[1]
- Note cultural or religious beliefs and values that impact perceptions of comfort.
- Ascertain motivation and expectations for change. *Motivation to improve and high expectations can encourage client to make changes that will improve his or her life. However, presence of external locus of control or unrealistic expectations may hamper efforts.*
- Discuss concerns with client and Active-listen to identify underlying issues (e.g., physical or emotional stressors, or external factors such as environmental surroundings, social interactions) that could impact client's ability to control own well-being. *Helps to determine client's level of satisfaction with current situation and readiness for change.*
- Establish context(s) in which comfort is realized: (1) physical—pertaining to bodily sensations; (2) psychospiritual—pertaining to internal awareness of self and meaning in one's life; relationship to a higher order or being; (3) environmental—pertaining to external surroundings, conditions, and influences; (4) sociocultural—pertaining to interpersonal, family, and societal relationships:[1]

PHYSICAL

- Verify that client is managing pain and pain components effectively. *Success in this arena usually addresses other issues or emotions (e.g., fear, loneliness, anxiety, noxious stimuli, anger).*[1]
- Ascertain what is used or required for comfort or rest (e.g., head of bed up or down, music on or off, white noise, rocking motion, certain person or thing).[2]

PSYCHOSPIRITUAL

- Determine how psychological and spiritual indicators overlap (e.g., meaningfulness, faith, identity, self-esteem) for client in enhancing comfort.[1]
- Ascertain that client/SO has received desired support regarding spiritual enrichment, including prayer, meditation, or access to spiritual counselor of choice.[3]

ENVIRONMENTAL

- Determine that client's environment respects privacy and provides natural lighting and readily accessible view to outdoors *(an aspect that can be manipulated to enhance comfort).*[1,3]

SOCIAL

- Ascertain meaning of comfort in context of interpersonal, family, and cultural values and societal relationships.[4]
- Validate client/SO understanding of client's situation and ongoing methods of managing condition, as appropriate or desired by client. *Considers client/family needs in this area and shows appreciation for their desires.*[4]

NURSING PRIORITY NO. 2

To assist client in developing plan to improve comfort:

- Review knowledge base and note coping skills that have been used previously to change behavior and promote well-being. *Brings these to client's awareness and promotes use in current situation.*[8]
- Acknowledge client's strengths in present situation and build on in planning for future.

PHYSICAL

- Collaborate in treating or managing medical conditions involving oxygenation, elimination, mobility, cognitive abilities, electrolyte balance, thermoregulation, hydration *to promote physical stability.*[2,5,6]
- Work with client to prevent pain, nausea, itching, thirst, other physical discomforts.
- Suggest parent be present during procedures *to comfort child.*
- Provide age-appropriate comfort measures (e.g., back rub, change of position, cuddling, use of heat or cold) *to provide nonpharmacological pain management.*
- Review interventions and age-appropriate activities that promote ease such as Therapeutic Touch (TT), biofeedback, self-hypnosis, guided imagery, breathing exercises, play therapy, and humor *to promote relaxation and refocus attention.*
- Assist client to use and modify medication regimen *to make best use of pharmacological pain management.*
- Assist client/SO(s) to develop plan for activity and exercise within individual ability, emphasizing necessity of allowing sufficient time to finish activities.
- Maintain open and flexible visitation with client's desired persons.
- Encourage and plan care to allow individually adequate rest periods *to prevent fatigue.* Schedule activities for periods when client has the most energy *to maximize participation.*
- Discuss routines to promote restful sleep.

PSYCHOSPIRITUAL

- Interact with client in therapeutic manner. *The nurse could be the most important comfort intervention for meeting client's needs. For example, assuring client that nausea can be treated successfully with both pharmacological and nonpharmacological methods may be more effective than simply administering an antiemetic without reassurance and comforting presence.*[7]
- Encourage verbalization of feelings and make time for listening and interacting.
- Identify ways (e.g., meditation, sharing oneself with others, being out in nature or garden, other spiritual activities) to achieve connectedness or harmony with self, others, nature, higher power.
- Establish realistic activity goals with client. *Enhances commitment to promoting optimal outcomes.*
- Involve client/SO(s) in schedule planning and decisions about timing and spacing of treatments *to promote relaxation and reduce sense of boredom.*
- Encourage client to do whatever possible (e.g., self-care, sit up in chair, walk). *Enhances self-esteem and independence.*
- Use distraction with music, chatting or texting with family/friends, watching TV, playing video or computer games *to limit dwelling on and transcend unpleasant sensations and situations.*
- Encourage client to develop assertiveness skills, prioritizing goals and activities, and to make use of beneficial coping behaviors. *Promotes sense of control and improves self-esteem.*
- Offer and identify opportunities for client to participate in experiences that enhance control and independence.

ENVIRONMENTAL

- Provide quiet environment, calm activities.
- Provide for periodic changes in the personal surroundings when client is confined. Use the individual's input in creating the changes (e.g., seasonal bulletin boards, color changes, re-arranging furniture, pictures).
- Suggest activities, such as bird feeders or baths for bird-watching, a garden in a window box or terrarium, or a fishbowl or aquarium, *to stimulate observation as well as involvement and participation in activity.*

SOCIAL

- Encourage age-appropriate diversional activities (e.g., TV, radio, playtime, socialization or outings with others).
- Avoid overstimulation or understimulation (cognitive and sensory).
- Make appropriate referrals to available support groups, hobby clubs, or service organizations.

NURSING PRIORITY NO. 3

To promote optimum wellness (Teaching/Discharge Considerations):

- Provide information about condition or health risk factors, or concerns in desired format (e.g., pictures, TV programs, articles, handouts, audio/visual materials, classes, group discussions, Web sites, and other databases), as appropriate. *Use of multiple modalities enhances acquisition and retention of information and gives client choices for accessing and applying information.*

PHYSICAL

- Promote overall health measures (e.g., nutrition, adequate fluid intake, appropriate vitamin and iron supplementation).
- Discuss potential complications and possible need for medical follow-up or alternative therapies. *Timely recognition and intervention can promote wellness.*
- Assist client/SO(s) to identify and acquire necessary equipment (e.g., lifts, commode chair, safety grab bars, personal hygiene supplies) to meet individual needs.

PSYCHOSPIRITUAL

- Collaborate with others when client expresses interest in lessons, counseling, coaching, or mentoring to meet or enhance emotional and spiritual comfort.
- Promote client's contributions toward meeting realistic goals.
- Encourage client to take time to be introspective in the search for contentment or transcendence.

ENVIRONMENTAL

- Create a compassionate, supportive, and therapeutic environment that incorporates client's cultural and age and developmental factors.
- Correct environmental hazards that could influence safety or negatively affect comfort.
- Arrange for home visit and evaluation, as needed.
- Discuss long-term plan for taking care of environmental needs.

Nursing Diagnoses in Alphabetical Order

SOCIAL

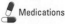 • Advocate for growth-promoting environment in conflict situations and consider issues from client/family perspective.

• Support client/SO access to resources (e.g., knowledge and skills, financial resources or assistance, personal or psychological support, social systems).

DOCUMENTATION FOCUS

Assessment/Reassessment

• Individual findings, including client's description of current status or situation.
• Motivation and expectations for change.
• Pertinent cultural or religious beliefs and values.
• Medication use and nonpharmacological measures.

Planning

• Plan of care, specific interventions, and who is involved in planning.
• Teaching plan.

Implementation/Evaluation

• Responses to interventions, teaching, and actions performed.
• Attainment or progress toward desired outcome(s).
• Modifications to plan of care.

Discharge Planning

• Long-term needs and who is responsible for actions to be taken.
• Specific referrals made.

References

1. Kolcaba, K. Y., Fisher, E. M. (1996). A holistic perspective on comfort care as an advance directive. *Crit Care Nurs Quarterly*, 18(4), 66–67.
2. Kolcaba, K., DiMarco, M. A. (2005). Comfort theory and its application to pediatric nursing. *Pediatr Nurse*, 31(3), 187–194.
3. Barclay, L., Lie, D. (2007). New guidelines issued for family support in patient-centered ICU. Retrieved February 2007 from CME/CE for Medscape Web site. www.medscape/viewarticle/551738.
4. Malinowski, A., Stamler, L. L. (2002). Comfort: Exploration of the concept in nursing. *J Adv Nurs*, 39(6), 599–606.
5. Kolcaba, K. (2006). FAQs (Frequently Asked Questions). Retrieved February 2007 from On the Comfort Line. Web site devoted to the Concept of Comfort in Nursing. www.thecomfortline.com/FAQ.htm.
6. Kaplow, R. (2003). AACN synergy model for patient care: A framework to optimize outcomes. *Crit Care Nurse Suppl (Feb)*, 27–30.
7. Wilson, L., Kolcaba, K. (2004). Practical application of comfort theory in the perianesthesia setting. *J of Perianesth Nurs Online*. Retrieved February 2007 from www.aspan.org/JOPAN/comfot_theory.htm.
8. Townsend, M. C. (2003). *Psychiatric Mental Health Nursing Concepts of Care*. 4th ed. Philadelphia: F. A. Davis.

impaired verbal Communication

DEFINITION: Decreased, delayed, or absent ability to receive, process, transmit, and use a system of symbols

RELATED FACTORS

Decrease in circulation to brain, brain tumor
Anatomical deficit (e.g., cleft palate, alteration of the neurovascular visual system, auditory system, or phonatory apparatus)
Difference related to developmental age
Physical barrier (tracheostomy, intubation)
Physiological conditions [e.g., dyspnea]; alteration of central nervous system (CNS); weakening of the musculoskeletal system
Psychological barriers (e.g., psychosis, lack of stimuli); emotional conditions [depression, panic, anger]; stress
Environmental barriers
Cultural difference
Lack of information
Side effects of medication
Alteration of self-esteem or self-concept
Altered perceptions
Absence of SO(s)

DEFINING CHARACTERISTICS

Subjective
[Reports of difficulty expressing self]

Objective
Inability to speak dominant language
Speaks or verbalizes with difficulty; stuttering; slurring
Does not or cannot speak; willful refusal to speak
Difficulty forming words or sentences (e.g., aphonia, dyslalia, dysarthria)
Difficulty expressing thoughts verbally (e.g., aphasia, dysphasia, apraxia, dyslexia)
Inappropriate verbalization, [incessant, loose association of ideas; flight of ideas]
Difficulty in comprehending or maintaining usual communication pattern
Absence of eye contact; difficulty in selective attending; partial or total visual deficit
Inability or difficulty in use of facial or body expressions
Dyspnea
Disorientation to person, space, time
[Inability to modulate speech]
[Message inappropriate to content]
[Use of nonverbal cues (e.g., pleading eyes, gestures, turning away)]
[Frustration, anger, hostility]

Sample Clinical Applications: Brain injury or stroke, facial trauma, head or neck cancer, radical neck surgery, laryngectomy, cleft lip/palate, dementia, Tourette's syndrome, autism, schizophrenia

(continues on page 170)

---

impaired verbal Communication (continued)
DESIRED OUTCOMES/EVALUATION CRITERIA

Sample **NOC** linkages:
Communication: Reception, interpretation, and expression of spoken, written, and nonverbal messages
Communication: Expressive: Expression of meaningful verbal or nonverbal messages
Information Processing: Ability to acquire, organize, and use information

Client Will (Include Specific Time Frame)
• Verbalize or indicate an understanding of the communication difficulty and plans for ways of handling.
• Establish method of communication in which needs can be expressed.
• Participate in therapeutic communication (e.g., using silence, acceptance, restating reflecting, Active-listening, and I-messages).
• Demonstrate congruent verbal and nonverbal communication.
• Use resources appropriately.

ACTIONS/INTERVENTIONS

Sample **NIC** linkages:
Communication Enhancement: Speech Deficit: Assistance in accepting and learning alternative methods for living with impaired speech
Communication Enhancement: Hearing Deficit: Assistance in accepting and learning alternative methods for living with diminished hearing
Active Listening: Attending closely to and attaching significance to a patient's verbal and nonverbal messages

NURSING PRIORITY NO. 1

To assess causative/contributing factors:

• Identify physiological or neurological conditions impacting speech such as severe shortness of breath, cleft palate, facial trauma, neuromuscular weakness, stroke, brain tumors or infections, dementia, brain trauma, deafness or hard of hearing.
• Review results of diagnostic studies (e.g., speech, language, and hearing evaluations, neurological testing or brain function studies—such as electroencephalogram [EEG], computed tomography [CT] scan, psychological evaluations) *to assess and delineate underlying conditions affecting verbal communication.*
• Note new onset or diagnosis of deficits that will progress or permanently affect speech.
• Note presence of physical barriers, including tracheostomy/intubation, wired jaws; or problem resulting in failure of voice production or "problem voice" *(pitch, loudness, or quality calls attention to voice rather than what speaker is saying as might occur with electronic voice box or "talking valves" when tracheostomy in place).*[7,8]
• Determine age and developmental considerations: (1) child too young for language or has developmental delays affecting speech and language skills or comprehension; (2) autism or other mental impairments; (3) older client doesn't or isn't able to speak, verbalizes with difficulty, has difficulty hearing or comprehending language or concepts.[1–3]
• Obtain history of hearing and speech-related pathophysiology or trauma (e.g., cleft lip/palate, traumatic brain injury, shaken baby syndrome, frequent ear infections affecting hearing, or sensorineural changes associated with aging).

- Identify dominant language spoken. *Knowing the language spoken and fluency in English is important to understanding. While some individuals may be fluent in English, they may still have limited understanding of the language, especially the language of health professionals, and may have difficulty answering questions, describing symptoms, or following directions.*[17]
- Ascertain whether client is recent immigrant, country of origin and what cultural, ethnic group client identifies as own *(e.g., recent immigrant may identify with home country and its people, beliefs, and healthcare practices).*[6]
- Determine cultural factors affecting communication such as beliefs concerning touch and eye contact. *Certain cultures may prohibit client from speaking directly to healthcare provider; some Native Americans, Appalachians, or young African Americans may interpret direct eye contact as disrespectful, impolite, an invasion of privacy, or aggressive; Latinos, Arabs, and Asians may shout and gesture when excited;*[4] *silence and tone of voice has various meanings, and slang words can cause confusion or misunderstandings;*[5] and conditions or factors of high prevalence in certain groups and populations *(e.g., middle-ear infection high among Native Americans with potential for hearing deficits).*
- Identify environmental barriers: recent or chronic exposure to hazardous noise in home, job, recreation, and healthcare setting (e.g., rock music, jackhammer, snowmobile, lawn mower, truck traffic or busy highway, heavy equipment, medical equipment). Noise not only affects hearing, but it also increases blood pressure and breathing rate, can have negative cardiovascular effects, disturbs digestion, increases fatigue, causes irritability, and reduces attention to tasks.[9]
- Investigate client reports of problems such as constantly raising voice to be heard, can't hear someone 2 feet away, conversation in room sounds muffled or dull, too much energy required to listen, or pain or ringing in ears after exposure to noise.[9]
- Determine if client with communication impairment has a speech or language problem, or both. *When a speech problem is present, the language code can be correct, but words might be garbled, person may stutter, or there may be problems with voice. Language and speech problems can exist together or by themselves. Language is a code made up of rules (e.g., what words mean, how to make new words, combine words, and what combinations work in what situations). When a person cannot understand the language code, there is a receptive problem.*[10]
- Determine presence of psychological or emotional barriers: history or presence of psychiatric conditions (e.g., manic-depressive illness, schizoid or affective behavior); high level of anxiety, frustration, or fear; presence of angry, hostile behavior. Note effect on speech and communication.[1,4]
- Identify information barriers such as lack of knowledge or misunderstanding of terms related to client's medical conditions, procedures, treatments, and equipment.[4]
- Assess level of understanding in a sensitive manner. *Individual may be reluctant to say they don't understand or may be embarrassed to ask for help. Head nodding and smiles do not always mean comprehension.*[17]

NURSING PRIORITY NO. 2

To assist client to establish a means of communication to express needs, wants, ideas, and questions:

- Ascertain that you have client's attention before communicating.
- Establish rapport with client, initiate eye contact, shake hands, address by preferred name, meet family members present; ask simple questions, smile, engage in brief social conversation if appropriate. *Helps establish a trusting relationship with client/family, demonstrating caring about the client as a person.*[2–4,19]

- Advise other care providers of client's communication deficits (e.g., deafness, aphasia, mechanical ventilations strategies) and needed means of communication (e.g., writing pad, signing, yes/no responses, gestures, picture board) *to minimize client's frustration and promote understanding.*[20]
- Provide and encourage use of glasses, hearing aids, dentures, electronic speech devices as needed *to maximize sensory perception and improve speech patterns.*[2,4]
- Maintain a calm, unhurried manner, sit at client's eye level if possible. Provide sufficient time for client to respond. *Sitting down conveys that nurse has time and interest in communicating.*
- Pay attention to speaker. Be an active listener.
- Begin conversation with elderly individual with casual and familiar topics (e.g., weather, happenings with family members) *to convey interest and stimulate conversation and reminiscence.*[2,15]
- Reduce environmental distractions and background noise (e.g., close the door, turn down the radio or television).[15,21,22]
- Refrain from shouting when directing speech to confused, deaf, or hearing-impaired client. Speak slowly and clearly, pitching voice low *to increase likelihood of being understood.*[2,16,21,22]
- Be honest and let speaker know when you have difficulty understanding. Repeat part of message that you do understand, *so speaker does not have to repeat entire message.*[11]
- Clarify type and special features of aphasia, when present. *Aphasia is a temporary, permanent, or progressive impairment of language, affecting production or comprehension of speech and the ability to read or write. Some people with aphasia have problems primarily with expressive language (what is said), others with receptive language (what is understood). Aphasia can also be global (person understands almost nothing that is said and says little or nothing).*[4,11]
- Note diagnosis of apraxia *(impairment in carrying out purposeful movements affecting rhythm and timing of speech)*, dysarthria *(language code can be correct but the right body parts do not move at the right time to produce the right message)*, or dementia *(defect is in decline in mental functions, including memory, attention, intellect, and personality) to help clarify individual needs, appropriate interventions.*[11,12]
- Determine meaning of words used by the client and congruency of communication and nonverbal messages.
- Evaluate the meaning of words that are used/needed to describe aspects of healthcare (e.g., pain) and ascertain how to communicate important concepts.[5]
- Observe body language, eye movements, and behavioral clues *For example, client may react with tears, grimacing, stiff posture, turning away, angry outbursts when pain present.*[14]
- Use confrontation skills, when appropriate, within an established nurse-client relationship *to clarify discrepancies between verbal and nonverbal cues.*[4,16]
- Point to objects or demonstrate desired actions when client has difficulty with language. *Speaker's own body language can be used to assist client's understanding.*
- Validate meaning of nonverbal communication; do not make assumptions, *because they may be wrong.* Be honest; if you do not understand, seek assistance from others.[19]
- Work with confused, brain-injured, mentally disabled, or sensory-deprived client *to correctly interpret his or her environment.* Establish understanding and convey to others meaning of symbolic speech *to reduce frustration.* Teach basic signs such as "eat," "toilet," "more," "finished" *to communicate basic needs.*[4,16]
- Provide reality orientation by responding with simple, straightforward, honest statements. Associate words with objects using repetition and redundancy *to improve communication patterns.*[2,4,16]

- Assess psychological response to communication impairment, willingness to find alternative means of communication.
- Identify family member who can speak for client and who is the family decision maker regarding healthcare decisions.[5,17]
- Note SO's/parents'/caregiver's speech patterns and interactive manner of communicating with client, including gestures.[21]
- Obtain interpreter with language or signing abilities and preferably with medical knowledge when needed. *Federal law mandates that interpretation services be made available. Trained, professional interpreter who translates precisely and possesses a basic understanding of medical terminology and healthcare ethics is preferred (over a family member) to enhance client and provider interactions.*[6,18]
- Evaluate ability to read, write, and musculoskeletal status, including manual dexterity (e.g., ability to hold a pen and write); and need or desire for pictures or written communications and instructions as part of treatment plan.
- Plan for and provide alternative methods of communication:[2–4,18]
  Provide pad and pencil, slate board *when client is able to write but cannot speak.*
  Use letter or picture board *when client can't write and picture concepts are understandable to both parties.*
  Establish hand or eye signals *when client can understand language but cannot speak or has physical barrier to writing.*
  Remove isolation mask *when client is deaf and reads lips.*
  Obtain or provide access to typewriter or computer *if communication impairment is long-standing or client is used to this method.*
- Consider form of communication when placing IV. *IV positioned in hand or wrist may limit ability to write or sign.*
- Answer call bell promptly. Anticipate needs and avoid leaving client alone with no way to summon assistance. *Reduces fear, conveys caring to client, and protects nurse from problems associated with failure to provide due care.*[13]
- Refer for appropriate therapies and support services. *Client and family may have multiple needs (e.g., sources for further examinations and rehabilitation services, local community or national support groups and services for disabled, financial assistance with obtaining necessary aids for improving communication).*[4,13]

NURSING PRIORITY NO. 3

To promote wellness (Teaching/Discharge Considerations):

- Encourage family presence and use of touch. Involve them in plan of care as much as possible. *Enhances participation and commitment to plan, assists in normalizing family role patterns, and provides support and encouragement when learning new patterns of communicating.*[4]
- Review information about condition, prognosis, and treatment with client/SOs, reinforcing that loss of speech does not imply loss of intelligence.
- Teach client and family the needed techniques for communication, whether it be speech or language techniques, or alternate modes of communicating. Encourage family to involve client in family activities using enhanced communication techniques. *Reduces stress of difficult situation and promotes earlier return to more normal life patterns.*[4]
- Assess family for possible role changes resulting from client's impairment. Discuss methods of dealing with impairment.
- Use and assist client/SOs to learn therapeutic communication skills of acknowledgment, Active-listening, and I-messages. *Improves general communication skills, emphasizes acceptance, and conveys respect.*

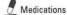

- Discuss ways to provide environmental stimuli as appropriate *to maintain contact with reality; or reduce environmental stimuli or noise. Unwanted sound affects physical health, increases fatigue, reduces attention to tasks, and makes speech communication more difficult.*[9,15]
- Refer to appropriate resources (e.g., speech or language therapist, support groups [e.g., stroke club], individual/family and/or psychiatric counseling) *to address long-term needs, enhance coping skills.*
- Refer to NDs ineffective Coping; disabled family Coping; Anxiety; Fear for additional interventions.

DOCUMENTATION FOCUS

Assessment/Reassessment
- Assessment findings, pertinent history information (i.e., physical, psychological, or cultural concerns).
- Meaning of nonverbal cues, level of anxiety client exhibits.

Planning
- Plan of care and specific interventions (e.g., type of alternative communication, translator).
- Teaching plan.

Implementation/Evaluation
- Response to interventions, teaching, and actions performed.
- Attainment or progress toward desired outcomes.
- Modifications to plan of care.

Discharge Planning
- Discharge needs, referrals made, additional resources available.

References

1. Szymanski, L., King, B. (1999). Practice parameters for the assessment and treatment of children, adolescents, and adults with mental retardation and comorbid mental disorders. American Academy of Child and Adolescent Psychiatry (AACAP) Working Group on Quality Issues. *J Am Acad Child Adolesc Psychiatry*, 38(12 suppl).
2. Stanley, M., Beare, P. G. (1999). *Gerontological Nursing: A Health Promotion Approach.* 2d ed. Philadelphia: F. A. Davis.
3. Cox, H. C., et al. (2002). *Clinical Applications of Nursing Diagnosis: Adult, Child, Women's, Psychiatric, Gerontic, and Home Health Considerations.* 4th ed. Philadelphia: F. A. Davis.
4. Doenges, M. E., Moorhouse, M. F., Geissler-Murr, A. C. (2002). *Nurse's Pocket Guide: Diagnoses, Interventions, and Rationales.* 8th ed. Philadelphia: F. A. Davis, 134–138.
5. Purnell, L., Paulanka, B. (1998). *Transcultural Health Care: A Culturally Diverse Approach.* 2d ed. Philadelphia: F. A. Davis.
6. Enslein, J., et al. (2002). Evidence-based protocol. Interpreter facilitation for persons with limited English proficiency. Retrieved September 2003 from National Guidelines Clearinghouse. www.guideline.gov/browse/gawithdrawn.aspx?st=U: University of Iowa Gerontological Nursing Interventions Research Center.
7. Questions/Answers about Voice Problems. Retrieved September 2003 from (Information sheet). American Speech-Language-Hearing Association (ASHA). www.asha.org.
8. American Speech-Language-Hearing Association (ASHA). Speech for patients with tracheostomies or ventilators (information sheet). Retrieved September 2003 from www.asha.org.
9. American Speech-Language-Hearing Association (ASHA). Noise (information sheet). Retrieved September 2003 from www.asha.org.

⊕ Cultural ⟳ Collaborative 🏠 Community/Home Care ⟋ Diagnostic Studies ∞ Pediatric/Geriatric/Lifespan ⚕ Medications

10. American Speech-Language-Hearing Association (ASHA). What is language? What is speech? Retrieved September 2003 from www.asha.org.
11. National Aphasia Association (NAA). (Revised June 1999). Aphasia fact sheet. Retrieved September 2003 from www.aphasia.org.
12. National Aphasia Association. (Revised January 2001). Understanding primary progressive aphasia. Retrieved September 2003 from www.aphasia.org.
13. Doenges, M. E., Moorhouse, M. F., Geissler-Murr, A. C. (2002). *Nursing Care Plans: Guidelines for Individualizing Patient Care*. 6th ed. Philadelphia: F. A. Davis.
14. Hahn, J. (1999). Cueing in to patient language. *Reflections*, 25(1), 8–11.
15. American Speech-Language-Hearing Association (ASHA). (2000). Tip sheet. "I can hear, but I can't understand what's being said." Retrieved September 2003 from www.asha.org.
16. Research Dissemination Core: Acute Confusion/Delirium. (1998). Iowa City: University of Iowa Gerontological Nursing Interventions Research Center.
17. Lipson, J. G., Dibble, S. L., Minarik, P. A. (1996). *Culture & Nursing Care: A Pocket Guide*. San Francisco: UCSF Nursing Press.
18. Harquez-Rebello, M. C., Tornel-Costa, M. C. (1997). Design of a non-verbal method of communication using cartoons. *Rev Neurol*, 25(148), 2027–2045.
19. Understanding transcultural nursing. (2005). *Nursing*, 35(1), 14–23. Supplement Career Directory.
20. Jacobs, D. H. (2005). Aphasia. Retrieved February 2007 from www.emedicine.com/NEURO/topic437.htm.
21. Wallhagen, M. I., Pettengill, E., Whiteside, M. (2006). Sensory impairment in older adults part 1: Hearing loss. *Am J Nurs*, 106(10), 40–49.
22. Sommer, K. D., Sommer, N. W. (2002). When your patient is hearing impaired. *RN*, 65(12), 28–32.

readiness for enhanced Communication

DEFINITION: A pattern of exchanging information and ideas with others that is sufficient for meeting one's needs and life goals and can be strengthened

RELATED FACTORS

To be developed by nurse researchers and submitted to NANDA

DEFINING CHARACTERISTICS

Subjective
Expresses willingness to enhance communication
Expresses thoughts or feelings
Expresses satisfaction with ability to share information or ideas with others

Objective
Able to speak or write a language
Forms words, phrases, sentences
Uses or interprets nonverbal cues appropriately

Sample Clinical Applications: Brain injury or stroke, head or neck cancer, facial trauma, cleft lip/palate, Tourette's syndrome, autism, foreign born individual communicating in second language

(continues on page 176)

readiness for enhanced Communication (continued)
DESIRED OUTCOMES/EVALUATION CRITERIA

Sample **NOC** linkages:
Communication: Reception, interpretation, and expression of spoken, written, and nonverbal messages
Information Processing: Ability to acquire, organize, and use information

Client/SO/Caregiver Will (Include Specific Time Frame)
• Verbalize or indicate an understanding of the communication process.
• Identify ways to improve communication.

ACTIONS/INTERVENTIONS

Sample **NIC** linkages:
Communication Enhancement: Speech Deficit: Assistance in accepting and learning alternative methods for living with impaired speech
Communication Enhancement: Hearing Deficit: Assistance in accepting and learning alternative methods for living with diminished hearing
Active Listening: Attending closely to and attaching significance to a patient's verbal and nonverbal messages

NURSING PRIORITY NO. 1

Assess how client is managing communication and potential difficulties:

• Identify circumstances that result in client's desire to improve communication. *Many factors are involved in communication, and identifying specific needs and expectations helps in developing realistic goals and determining likelihood of success.*
• Ascertain motivation and expectations for change. *Motivation to improve and high expectations can encourage client to make changes that will improve his or her life. However, presence of external locus of control or unrealistic expectations may hamper efforts.*
• Evaluate mental status. *Disorientation, psychotic conditions may be affecting speech and the communication of thoughts, needs, and desires.*
• Determine client's developmental level of speech and language comprehension. *Provides baseline information for developing plan for improvement.*
• Determine ability to read and write preferred language. *Evaluating grasp of language as well as musculoskeletal states, including manual dexterity (e.g., ability to hold a pen and write) provides information about nature of client's situation.* Educational plan can address language skills. Neuromuscular deficits require individual physical or occupational therapeutic program to improve.
• Determine country of origin, dominant language, whether client is recent immigrant, and what cultural or ethnic group client identifies as own. *Recent immigrant may identify with home country and its people, language, beliefs, and healthcare practices affecting desire to learn language skills and ability to improve interactions in new country.*[1]
• Ascertain if interpreter is needed or desired. *Law mandates that interpretation services be made available. Trained, professional interpreter who translates precisely and possesses a basic understanding of medical terminology and healthcare ethics is preferred over family member to enhance client and provider interaction and sharing of information.*[1]

- Determine comfort level in expression of feelings and concepts in nonproficient language. *Concern about language skills can impact perception of own ability to communicate effectively.*
- Note any physical challenges to effective communication (e.g., hearing impairment, talking tracheostomy apparatus, wired jaws) or physiological or neurological conditions (e.g., severe shortness of breath, neuromuscular weakness, stroke, brain trauma, deafness, cleft palate, facial trauma). *Client may be dealing with speech or language comprehension, or have voice production problems (pitch, loudness or quality), which calls attention to voice rather than what speaker is saying. These barriers may need to be addressed to enable client to improve communication skills.*[2,3]
- Clarify meaning of words used by the client to describe important aspects of life and health or well-being (e.g., pain, sorrow, anxiety). *Words can easily be misinterpreted when sender and receiver have different ideas about their meanings. This can affect the way both client and caregivers communicate important concepts. Restating what one has heard can clarify whether an expressed statement has been understood or misinterpreted.*[4]
- Determine presence of emotional lability or frequency of unstable behaviors. *Emotional or psychiatric issues can affect communication and interfere with understanding.*
- Evaluate congruency of verbal and nonverbal messages. *Communication is enhanced when verbal and nonverbal messages are congruent.*[5]
- Determine lack of knowledge or misunderstanding of terms related to client's specific situation. *Indicators of need for additional information, clarification to help client improve ability to communicate.*
- Evaluate need or desire for pictures or written communications and instructions as part of treatment plan. *Alternative methods of communication can help client feel understood and promote feelings of satisfaction with interaction.*

NURSING PRIORITY NO. 2

To improve client's ability to communicate thoughts, needs, and ideas:

- Maintain a calm, unhurried manner. Provide sufficient time for client to respond. *An atmosphere in which client is free to speak without fear of criticism provides the opportunity to explore all the issues involved in making decisions to improve communication skills.*[10]
- Pay attention to speaker. Be an active listener. *The use of Active-listening communicates acceptance and respect for the client, establishing trust and promoting openness and honest expression. It communicates a belief that the client is a capable and competent person.*
- Sit down, maintain eye contact, preferably at client's level, and spend time with the client. *Conveys message that the nurse has time and interest in communicating.*[10]
- Encourage client to express feelings and clarify meaning of nonverbal clues. *Client may be reluctant to share dissatisfaction with events.*
- Help client identify and learn to avoid use of nontherapeutic communication. *These barriers are recognized as detriments to open communication, and learning to avoid them maximizes the effectiveness of communication between client and others.*
- Obtain interpreter with language or signing abilities as needed. *May be needed to enhance understanding of words and language concepts to ascertain that interpretation of communication is accurate.*[6,10]
- Encourage use of pad and pencil, slate board, letter or picture board when interacting or to interface in new situations, as indicated. *When client has physical impairments that interfere with spoken communication, alternative means can provide concepts that are understandable to both parties.*[4,10]

- Obtain or provide access to voice-enabled computer. *Use of these devices may be more helpful when communication challenges are long standing or when client is used to using them.*[1]
- Respect client's cultural communication needs. *Different cultures can dictate beliefs of what is normal or abnormal, (i.e., in some cultures, eye-to-eye contact is considered disrespectful, impolite, or an invasion of privacy; silence and tone of voice have various meanings, and slang words can cause confusion).*[4]
- Provide or encourage use of glasses, hearing aids, dentures, electronic speech devices, as needed. *These devices maximize sensory perception and can improve understanding and enhance speech patterns.*[7]
- Reduce distractions and background noises (e.g., close the door, turn down the radio or television). *A distracting environment can interfere with communication, limiting attention to tasks, and makes speech and communication more difficult. Reducing noise can help both parties hear clearly, improving understanding.*[8]
- Associate words with objects using repetition and redundancy, point to objects, or demonstrate desired actions. *Speaker's own body language can be used to enhance client's understanding when neurological conditions result in difficulty understanding language.*[9]
- Use confrontation skills carefully, when appropriate, within an established nurse-client relationship. *Can be used to clarify discrepancies between verbal and nonverbal cues, enabling client to look at areas that may require change.*[10]

NURSING PRIORITY NO. 3

To promote optimum communication:

- Discuss with family/SO and other caregivers effective ways in which the client communicates. *Identifying positive aspects of current communication skills enables family members to learn and move forward in desire to enhance ways of interacting.*[10]
- Encourage client and family to familiarize themselves with and use new or developing communication technologies. *Enhances family relationships and promotes self-esteem for all members, as they are able to communicate regardless of problems (e.g., progressive neurological disorder) that could interfere with ability to interact.*[10]
- Reinforce client's/SO's learning and use of therapeutic communication skills of acknowledgment, Active-listening, and I-messages. *Improves general communication skills, emphasizes acceptance, and conveys respect, enabling family relationships to improve.*
- Refer to appropriate resources (e.g., speech therapist, language classes, individual/family or psychiatric counseling). *May need further assistance to overcome challenges as family reaches toward desired goal of enhanced communication.*

DOCUMENTATION FOCUS

Assessment/Reassessment
- Assessment findings, pertinent history information (i.e., physical, psychological, or cultural concerns).
- Meaning of nonverbal cues, level of anxiety client exhibits.
- Motivation and expectations for change.

Planning
- Plan of care and specific interventions (e.g., type of alternative communication, translator).
- Teaching plan.

Implementation/Evaluation
• Progress toward desired outcome(s).
• Modifications to plan of care.

Discharge Planning
• Discharge needs, referrals made, additional resources available.

References

1. Enslein, J., et al. (2002). Evidence-based protocol. Interpreter facilitation for persons with limited English proficiency. University of Iowa Gerontological Nursing Interventions Research Center. National Guidelines Clearinghouse. Retrieved September 2003 from www.guideline.gov/browse/gawithdrawn.aspx?st=U.
2. American Speech-Language-Hearing Association (ASHA). Questions/answers about voice problems (information sheet). Retrieved September 2003 from www.asha.org.
3. American Speech-Language-Hearing Association (ASHA). Speech for patients with tracheostomies or ventilators (information sheet). Retrieved September 2003 from www.asha.org.
4. Purnell, L., Paulanka, B. (1998). *Transcultural Health Care: A Culturally Diverse Approach.* 2d ed. Philadelphia: F. A. Davis.
5. Hahn, J. (1999). Cueing in to client language. *Reflections,* 25(1), 8–11.
6. American Speech-Language-Hearing Association (ASHA). What is language? What is speech? Retrieved September 2003 from www.asha.org.
7. Stanley, M., Beare, P. G. (1999). *Gerontological Nursing: A Health Promotion Approach.* 2d ed. Philadelphia: F. A. Davis.
8. American Speech-Language-Hearing Association (ASHA). Noise (information sheet). Retrieved September 2003 from www.asha.org.
9. Acute Confusion/Delirium. (1998). Iowa City: Research Dissemination Core, University of Iowa Gerontological Nursing Interventions Research Center.
10. Cox, H. C., et al. (2002). *Clinical Applications of Nursing Diagnosis: Adult, Child, Women's, Psychiatric, Gerontic, and Home Health Considerations.* 4th ed. Philadelphia: F. A. Davis.

decisional Conflict [specify]

DEFINITION: Uncertainty about course of action to be taken when choice among competing actions involves risk, loss, or challenge to values and beliefs

RELATED FACTORS

Unclear personal values or beliefs; perceived threat to value system
Lack of experience or interference with decision making
Lack of relevant information, multiple or divergent sources of information
Moral obligations that require performing/not performing actions
Moral principles, rules, or values that support mutually inconsistent courses of action
Support system deficit
[Age, developmental state]
[Family system, sociocultural factors]
[Cognitive, emotional, behavioral level of functioning]

(continues on page 180)

decisional Conflict (continued)
DEFINING CHARACTERISTICS

Subjective
Verbalizes uncertainty about choices; undesired consequences of alternative actions being considered
Verbalizes feeling of distress while attempting a decision
Questions moral principles, rules, values or personal values or beliefs while attempting a decision

Objective
Vacillates between alternative choices; delayed decision making
Self-focusing
Physical signs of distress or tension (e.g., increased heart rate, increased muscle tension, restlessness)

Sample Clinical Applications: Therapeutic options with undesired side effects (e.g., amputation, visible scarring) or conflicting with belief system (e.g., blood transfusion, termination of pregnancy); chronic disease states, dementia, Alzheimer's disease, terminal or end-of-life situations

DESIRED OUTCOMES/EVALUATION CRITERIA

Sample NOC linkages:
Decision-Making: Ability to choose between two or more alternatives
Health Beliefs: Personal convictions that influence health behaviors
Psychosocial Adjustment: Life Change: Psychosocial adaptation of an individual to a life change

Client Will (Include Specific Time Frame)
• Verbalize awareness of positive and negative aspect of choices and alternative actions.
• Acknowledge and ventilate feelings of anxiety and distress associated with choice or related to making difficult decision.
• Identify personal values and beliefs concerning issues.
• Make decision(s) and express satisfaction with choices.
• Meet psychological needs as evidenced by appropriate expression of feelings, identification of options, and use of resources.
• Display relaxed manner, calm demeanor, and free of physical signs of distress.

ACTIONS/INTERVENTIONS

Sample NIC linkages:
Decision-Making Support: Providing information and support for a person who is making a decision regarding healthcare
Values Clarification: Assisting another to clarify patient's own values in order to facilitate effective decision making
Coping Enhancement: Assisting a patient to adapt to perceived stressors, changes, or threats that interfere with meeting life demands and roles

NURSING PRIORITY NO. 1

To assess causative/contributing factors:

∞ • Determine usual ability to manage own affairs. Clarify who has legal right to intervene on behalf of child/developmentally delayed adult (e.g., parent, other relative, or court-appointed guardian/advocate). *Family disruption or conflicts can complicate decision-making process. All adults have the right to make their own decisions unless a legal court has ruled the individual is incompetent and a guardian appointed.*[4]

• Note expressions of indecision, dependence on others, availability and involvement of support persons (e.g., lack of or conflicting advice). *Care providers need to be sensitive to the physical, cognitive, and emotional effects of illness on decision-making capabilities and whether the individual wants to be involved in making the decision.*[6]

• Ascertain dependency of other(s) on client and/or issues of codependency. *Influence of others may lead client to make decision that is not what is really wanted or in his or her best interest.*[1]

• Active-listen, identify reason for indecisiveness. *Helps client to clarify problem and begin looking for resolution. May talk about uncertainty—and alternative choices that can lead to risky, uncertain outcomes—and the need to make value judgments about losses versus the gains.*[2,6]

• Identify cultural values and beliefs or moral obligations and principles that may be creating conflict for client and complicating decision-making process. *These issues must be addressed before client can be at peace with the decision that is made.*[5]

• Determine effectiveness of current problem-solving techniques. *Provides information about client's ability to make decisions that are needed or desired.*[1]

• Note presence and intensity of physical signs of anxiety (e.g., increased heart rate, muscle tension). *Client may be conflicted about the decision that is required and may need help to deal with anxiety to begin to deal with reality of situation. Different treatment decisions may have more uncertainty and generate more conflict in client.*[2,6]

• Listen for expressions of inability to find meaning in life or reason for living, feelings of futility, or alienation from God and others around them. (Refer to ND Spiritual Distress, as indicated.) *May need to talk about reasons for feelings of alienation to resolve concerns and may engage in questioning about own values.*[6,7]

• Review information client has to support the decision to be made. *Inaccurate or incomplete information and misinterpretations complicate the process and may result in a poor outcome.*[8,9]

NURSING PRIORITY NO. 2

To assist client to develop/effectively use problem-solving skills:

• Promote safe and hopeful environment, as needed. *Client needs to be protected and supported while he or she regains inner control.*[8]

• Encourage verbalization of conflicts and concerns. *Helps client to clarify these issues so he or she can come to a resolution of the situation.*[8,9]

• Accept verbal expressions of anger or guilt. Set limits on maladaptive behavior. *Verbalization of feelings enables client to sift through feelings and begin to deal with situation. Behavior that is inappropriate is not helpful for dealing with the situation and will lead to feelings of guilt and low self-worth.*[2]

• Clarify and prioritize individual goals, noting where the subject of the "conflict" falls on this scale. *Helps to identify importance of problems client is addressing, enabling realistic problem-solving.*[2]

- Identify strengths and use of positive coping skills (e.g., use of relaxation techniques, willingness to express feelings). *Helpful for developing solutions to current situation.*[1]
- Identify positive aspects of this experience and assist client to view it as a learning opportunity. *Reframing the situation can help the client see things in a different light, enabling client to develop new and creative solutions.*[1]
- Correct misperceptions client may have and provide factual information, as needed. *Promotes understanding and enables client to make better decisions for own situation.*[1,6]
- Provide opportunities for client to make simple decisions regarding self-care and other daily activities. Accept choice not to do so. Advance complexity of choices, as tolerated. *Acceptance of what client wants to do, with gentle encouragement to progress, enhances self-esteem and ability to try more. Providing individualized decision support can help the client move to more difficult decisions.*[1,6]
- ∞ Encourage child to make developmentally appropriate decisions concerning own care. *Fosters child's sense of self-worth and enhances ability to learn and exercise coping skills.*[4]
- Discuss time considerations, setting time line for small steps and considering consequences related to not making or postponing specific decisions to facilitate resolution of conflict. *When time is a factor in making a decision, these strategies can promote movement toward solution.*[4]
- Have client list some alternatives to present situation or decisions, using a brainstorming process. Include family in this activity, as indicated (e.g., placement of parent in long-term care facility, use of intervention process with addicted member). Refer to NDs interrupted Family Processes; dysfunctional Family Processes; compromised family Coping; Moral Distress. *Involving family and looking at different options can promote successful resolution of decision to be made.*[8,9]
- Practice use of problem-solving process with current situation and decision. *Promotes identification of different possibilities that may not have been thought of otherwise.*[1]
- ⊕ Discuss and clarify spiritual concerns, accepting client's values in a nonjudgmental manner. *Client will be willing to consider own situation when accepted as an individual of worth.*[5]

NURSING PRIORITY NO. 3

To promote wellness (Teaching/Discharge Considerations):

- 🏠 Promote opportunities for using conflict-resolution skills, identifying steps as client does each one. *Learning this process can help to solve current dilemma and provide the person with skills they can use in the future.*[3]
- Provide positive feedback for efforts and progress noted. *Client needs to hear he or she is doing well, and feedback promotes continuation of efforts.*[2]
- 🏠 Encourage involvement of family/SO(s), as desired or available. *Provides support for the client and facilitates resolution.*[10]
- Support client for decisions made, especially if consequences are unexpected or difficult to cope with. *Positive feedback promotes feelings of success even when difficult situations occur or outcome is less than desired.*[10]
- ⊛ Encourage attendance at stress-reduction or assertiveness classes. *Learning these skills can help client achieve lowered stress level that can promote ability to make decisions.*[4]
- ⊛ Refer to other resources, as necessary (e.g., clergy, psychiatric clinical nurse specialist or psychiatrist, family or marital therapist, addiction support groups). *May need this additional help to deal with complicated problems and facilitate problem-solving and decision making.*[2]

DOCUMENTATION FOCUS

Assessment/Reassessment
- Assessment findings, behavioral responses, degree of impairment in lifestyle functioning.
- Individuals involved in the conflict.
- Personal values and beliefs.

Planning
- Plan of care, specific interventions, and who is involved in the planning process.
- Teaching plan.

Implementation/Evaluation
- Client's and involved individuals' responses to interventions, teaching, and actions performed.
- Ability to express feelings and identify options.
- Use of resources.
- Attainment or progress toward desired outcome(s).
- Modifications to plan of care.

Discharge Planning
- Long-term needs, actions to be taken, and who is responsible for doing.
- Specific referrals made.

References

1. Doenges, M., Moorhouse, M., Murr, A. (2002). *Nursing Care Plans: Guidelines for Individualizing Patient Care.* 6th ed. Philadelphia: F. A. Davis.
2. Doenges, M., Townsend, M., Moorhouse, M. (1998). *Psychiatric Care Plans: Guidelines for Individualizing Care.* 3d ed. Philadelphia: F. A. Davis.
3. Townsend, M. (2003). *Psychiatric Mental Health Nursing: Concepts of Care.* 4th ed. Philadelphia: F. A. Davis.
4. Cox, H., et al. (2002). *Clinical Applications of Nursing Diagnosis: Adult, Child, Women's, Psychiatric, Gerontic, and Home Health Considerations.* 4th ed. Philadelphia: F. A. Davis.
5. Lipson, J. G., Dibble, S. L., Minarik, P. A. (1996). *Culture & Nursing Care: A Pocket Guide.* San Francisco: UCSF Nursing Press.
6. Llewelllyn-Thomas, H. (2004). Helping patients make health care decisions. Evaluative Clinical Sciences Dartmouth Medical School. Retrieved July 2007 from www.dartmouthatlas.org/atlases/DecisionSupport.pdf.
7. Hareven, T. K., Adams, K. J. (eds). (1982). *Aging and Life Course Transitions: An Interdisciplinary Perspective.* New York: Guilford.
8. Liken, M. A. (2001). Caregivers in crisis: Moving a relative with Alzheimer's to assisted living. *Clin Nurs Res,* 10(1), 53–69.
9. Liken, M. A. (2001). Experiences of family caregivers of a relative with Alzheimer's disease. *J Psychosoc Nurs,* 39(12), 33–37.
10. Halper, J., et al. *Multiple Sclerosis: Best Practices in Nursing Care (monograph).* Columbia, MD: Medicalliance.

parental role Conflict

DEFINITION: Parent experience of role confusion and conflict in response to crisis

RELATED FACTORS

Separation from child due to chronic illness [or disability]

Intimidation with invasive modalities (e.g., intubation); restrictive modalities (e.g., isolation); specialized care centers

Home care of a child with special needs [e.g., apnea monitoring, postural drainage, hyperalimentation]

Change in marital status, [conflicts of the role of the single parent]

Interruptions of family life due to home-care regimen (e.g., treatments, caregivers, lack of respite)

DEFINING CHARACTERISTICS

Subjective

Parent(s) express(es) concerns or feeling of inadequacy to provide for child's needs (e.g., physical and emotional)

Parent(s) express(es) concerns about changes in parental role; about family (e.g., functioning, communication, health)

Express(es) concern about perceived loss of control over decisions relating to their child

Verbalize(s) feelings of guilt or frustration; anxiety; fear

[Verbalizes concern about role conflict of wanting to date while having responsibility of child care]

Objective

Demonstrates disruption in caretaking routines

Reluctant to participate in usual caretaking activities even with encouragement and support

Sample Clinical Applications: Prematurity, genetic or congenital conditions, chronic illness (parent/child)

DESIRED OUTCOMES/EVALUATION CRITERIA

Sample (NOC) linkages:

Parenting Performance: Parental actions to provide a child nurturing and constructive physical, emotional, and social environment

Role Performance: Congruence of an individual's role behavior with role expectations

Caregiver Home Care Readiness: Preparedness to assume responsibility for the health-care of a family member or significant other in the home

Parent(s) Will (Include Specific Time Frame)

• Verbalize understanding of situation and expected parent's/child's role.
• Express feelings about child's illness or situation and effect on family life.
• Demonstrate appropriate behaviors concerning parenting role.
• Assume caretaking activities, as appropriate.
• Handle family disruptions effectively.

ACTIONS/INTERVENTIONS

Sample (NIC) linkages:
Parenting Promotion: Providing parenting information, support, and coordination of comprehensive services to high-risk families
Role Enhancement: Assisting a patient, significant other, or family to improve relationships by clarifying and supplementing specific role behaviors
Family Process Maintenance: Minimization of family process disruption effects

NURSING PRIORITY NO. 1

To assess causative/contributory factors:

- Assess individual situation and parent's perception of and concern about what is happening and expectations of self as caregiver. *Identifies needs of the family to deal realistically with the current situation and what interventions are necessary to work toward identified goals.*[5]
- Note parental status, including age and maturity, stability of relationship, single parent, other responsibilities. *Young parents may lack the necessary maturity to deal with unexpected illness of infant or child. Single parent may feel overwhelmed in trying to balance work and caretaking responsibilities. Increasing numbers of elderly individuals who were expecting retirement and a simpler life are providing full-time care for young grandchildren whose parents are unavailable or unable to provide care.*[1]
- Ascertain parent's understanding of child's developmental stage and expectations for the future to identify misconceptions and strengths. *Parents often have no information regarding developmental stages and have unrealistic expectation of abilities of the child. Identifying what the parents know and providing information can help them deal more realistically with the situation.*[1]
- Note coping skills currently used by each individual as well as how problems have been dealt with in the past. *Provides basis for comparison and reference for client's coping abilities in current situation.*[1]
- Determine use of substances (e.g., alcohol, other drugs, including prescription medications). *May interfere with individual's ability to cope/problem-solve and manage current illness/ situation and indicates need for additional interventions.*[8]
- Determine availability and use of resources, including extended family, support groups, and financial. *Factors that may affect ability to manage illness, unexpected expenses, caregiving activities, and so forth.*[1]
- Perform testing such as Parent-Child Relationship Inventory (PCRI) for further evaluation as indicated. *Provides information on which to develop plan of care and appropriate interventions.*[1]
- Determine cultural or religious influences on parenting expectations of self and child, sense of success or failure. *Parenting is one of the most important jobs individuals will have and one for which they are least prepared. Family of origin practices and beliefs will influence parents in how they parent, and this information is crucial to developing a plan of care that meets their needs.*[4]

NURSING PRIORITY NO. 2

To assist parents to deal with current crisis:

- Encourage free verbal expression of feelings (including negative feelings of anger and hostility), setting limits on inappropriate behavior. *Verbalization of feelings enables parent(s) to sift through situation and begin to deal with reality of what is happening. Inappropriate behavior is not helpful for dealing with the situation and will lead to feelings of guilt and low self-worth.*[2]

- Acknowledge difficulty of situation and normalcy of feeling overwhelmed and helpless. Encourage contact with parents who experienced similar situation with child and had positive outcome. *Parents feel listened to when feelings are acknowledged, and hearing how other parents have dealt with situation can give them hope.*[2]
- Provide information in an honest and forthright manner at level of understanding of the client, including technical information when appropriate. *Helping client understand what is happening corrects misconceptions and helps to make decisions that meet individual needs.*[3]
- Promote parental involvement in decision making and care as much as possible or desired. *When family members are involved in the process, it enhances their sense of control, and they are more likely to follow through on plans that are made.*[2]
- Encourage interaction and facilitate communication between parent(s) and child. *Sometimes people who find themselves in difficult or distressful situations tend to withdraw because they do not know what to do. Encouraging these interactions enables them to connect with one another to facilitate dealing with situation.*[2]
- Discuss problems of attachment disorder when diagnosed in an adopted child . *Children who have been adopted often suffer from problems of believing they will not be loved, and parents need to learn reasons behind problems as well as skills to deal with them.*[9,10]
- Promote use of assertiveness, relaxation skills. *Providing information and helping individuals learn these skills will help them to deal more effectively with situation or crisis.*[6]
- Instruct parent in proper administration of medications and treatments as indicated. *May need to be involved in care, and knowing how to do these activities enhances their sense of control and comfort in their ability to handle situation.*[5]
- Provide for and encourage use of respite care, parent time off. *Parents may believe they are being "selfish" if they take time out for themselves, that they have to remain with the child. However, parents are important, children are important, and the family is important, and when parents take time for themselves, it enhances their emotional well-being and promotes ability to deal with ongoing situation.*[7,11]
- Help single parent distinguish between parental love and partner love. *New focus of parent's attention or love may result in neglect of relationship with child. Attention needs to be given to both individuals for the relationships to flourish.*[9]

NURSING PRIORITY NO. 3

To promote wellness (Teaching/Discharge Considerations):

- Provide anticipatory guidance relevant to the situation and long-term expectations of the illness. *Encourages making plans for future needs, provides feelings of hope, and promotes sense of control over difficult situation.*[3]
- Encourage parents to set realistic and mutually agreed-on goals. *As family members work together, they can feel empowered and more apt to follow through on decisions that they are involved in making.*[2,12]
- Discuss infant attachment behaviors such as breastfeeding on cue, co-sleeping, and baby-wearing (carrying baby around on chest or back) as appropriate. *Dealing with ill child and home-care pressures can strain the bond between parent/child. Activities such as these encourage secure relationships.*[12]
- Provide and identify learning opportunities specific to needs. *Activities such as parenting classes, information about equipment use, and methods of troubleshooting can enhance knowledge and ability to deal with situation.*[3]

- Refer to community resources, as appropriate (e.g., visiting nurse, respite care, social services, psychiatric care or family therapy, well-baby clinics, special needs support services). *Provides additional assistance, as needed, to handle individual situation or illness.*[5]
- Refer to ND impaired Parenting for additional interventions.

DOCUMENTATION FOCUS

Assessment/Reassessment
- Findings, including specifics of individual situation, parental concerns, perceptions, expectations.

Planning
- Plan of care and who is involved in the planning.
- Teaching plan.

Implementation/Evaluation
- Parent's responses to interventions, teaching, and actions performed.
- Attainment or progress toward desired outcome(s).
- Modifications to plan of care.

Discharge Planning
- Long-term needs and who is responsible for each action to be taken.
- Specific referrals made.

References

1. Townsend, M. C. (2003). *Psychiatric Mental Health Nursing Concepts of Care.* 4th ed. Philadelphia: F. A. Davis.
2. Gordon, T. (2000). *Parent Effectiveness Training.* Updated edition New York: Three Rivers Press.
3. Cox, H. C., et al. (2002). *Clinical Applications of Nursing Diagnosis: Adult, Child, Women's, Psychiatric, Gerontic, and Home Health Considerations.* 4th ed. Philadelphia: F. A. Davis.
4. Lipson, J. G., Dibble, S. L., Minarik, P. A. (1996). Culture & Nursing Care: A Pocket Guide. San Francisco: UCSF Nursing Press.
5. Doenges, M. E., Townsend, M. C., Moorhouse, M. F. (1998). *Psychiatric Care Plans Guidelines for Individualizing Care.* 3d ed. Philadelphia: F. A. Davis.
6. Gordon, T. (1989). *Teaching Children Self-Discipline: At Home and at School.* New York: Random House.
7. Gordon, T. (2000). *Family Effectiveness Training Video.* Solana Beach, CA: Gordon Training International.
8. Townsend, M. (2001). *Nursing Diagnoses in Psychiatric Nursing: Care Plans and Psychotropic Medications.* 5th ed. Philadelphia: F. A. Davis.
9. Pickhardt, C. (2002). *Role Conflict of the Single Parent.* Mesa, AZ: Adoption Media, LLC.
10. Breazeale, T. (2001). Attachment parenting: A practical approach for the reduction of attachment disorders and the promotion of emotionally secure children. Master's thesis submitted to the faculty of Bethel College.
11. Walant, K. (September 2000). A little self-care goes a long way. Attachment Parenting International News. Retrieved July 2007 from www.attachmentparenting.org/artselfcare.shtml.
12. Sands, S. (September 1, 2004). Some call it alternative parenting; they call it traditional. Gazette. Retrieved July 2007 from www.attachmentparenting.org/gazettearticle.shtml.

acute Confusion

DEFINITION: Abrupt onset of reversible disturbances of consciousness, attention, cognition, and perception that develop over a short period of time

RELATED FACTORS

Alcohol abuse; drug abuse; [medication reaction/interaction; anesthesia, surgery; metabolic imbalances]
Fluctuation in sleep-wake cycle
Over 60 years of age
Delirium [including febrile epilepticum (following or instead of an epileptic attack), toxic and traumatic]
Dementia
[Exacerbation of a chronic illness, hypoxemia]
[Severe pain]

DEFINING CHARACTERISTICS

Subjective
Hallucinations [visual or auditory]
[Exaggerated emotional responses]

Objective
Fluctuation in cognition or level of consciousness
Fluctuation in psychomotor activity [tremors, body movement]
Increased agitation or restlessness
Misperceptions, [inappropriate responses]
Lack of motivation to initiate or follow through with purposeful behavior
Lack of motivation to initiate or follow through with goal-directed behavior

Sample Clinical Applications: Brain injury or stroke, respiratory conditions with hypoxia, medication adverse reactions, drug or alcohol intoxication, hyperthermia, infectious processes, malnutrition, eating disorders, fluid and electrolyte imbalances, chemical exposure

DESIRED OUTCOMES/EVALUATION CRITERIA

Sample NOC linkages:
Cognition: Ability to execute complex mental processes
Information Processing: Ability to acquire, organize, and use information
Distorted Thought Self-Control: Self-restraint of disruption in perception, thought processes, and thought content

Client Will (Include Specific Time Frame)
• Regain and maintain usual reality orientation and level of consciousness.
• Verbalize understanding of causative factors when known.
• Initiate lifestyle or behavior changes to prevent or minimize recurrence of problem.

ACTIONS/INTERVENTIONS

Sample (NIC) linkages:
Delirium Management: Provision of a safe and therapeutic environment for the patient who is experiencing an acute confusional state
Reality Orientation: Promotions of patient's awareness of personal identity, time, and environment
Surveillance: Safety: Purposeful and ongoing collection and analysis of information about the client and the environment for use in promoting and maintaining patient safety

NURSING PRIORITY NO. 1

To assess causative/contributing factors:

- Identify factors present such as recent trauma/fall; use of large numbers of medications or polypharmacy; intoxication, substance use or abuse; history or current seizure activity, episodes of fever, pain, presence of acute infection (especially urinary tract infection [UTI] in elderly client), exposure to toxic substances, traumatic events; person with dementia experiencing sudden change in environment, unfamiliar surroundings or people. *Acute confusion is a symptom associated with numerous causes (e.g., hypoxia, abnormal metabolic conditions, ingestion of toxins or medications, electrolyte abnormalities, sepsis, systemic infections, nutritional deficiencies, endocrine disorders, central nervous system [CNS] infections, other neurological pathology, acute psychiatric disorders). Note: Elderly persons may be more affected by toxic or metabolic insults than younger people.*[1,11,12]

- Assess mental status. *Typical symptoms of delirium include anxiety, disorientation, tremors, hallucinations, delusions, and incoherence. Onset is usually sudden, developing over a few hours or days.*[2]

- Evaluate vital signs. *Signs of poor tissue perfusion (i.e., hypotension, tachycardia, tachypnea, or fever) may identify underlying cardiovascular or infectious cause for mental status changes.*[2]

- Determine current medications and drug use (especially antianxiety agents, barbiturates, lithium, methyldopa, disulfiram, cocaine, alcohol, amphetamines, hallucinogens, opiates). *Use, misuse, overdose, and withdrawal of many drugs is associated with high risk of confusion, disorientation, and delirium.*[1,11]

- Investigate possibility of alcohol or illicit drug withdrawal or medication interactions. *Noncompliance with regimen, sudden discontinuation or overuse of substances, and certain drug combinations increase risk of toxic reactions and adverse reactions or interactions.*[1,2,12]

- Evaluate for exacerbation of psychiatric conditions (e.g., mood disorder, dissociative disorders, dementia). *Identification of the presence of mental illness provides opportunity for correct treatment and medication.*[10,11]

- Assess diet and nutritional status to identify possible deficiencies of essential nutrients and vitamins. *Failure to eat (forgetfulness or lack of food) can lead to deficiencies (e.g., vitamin B_{12}, folate, thiamine, iron) that could affect mental status.*[2,11]

- Evaluate sleep and rest status, noting deprivation or oversleeping. *Discomfort, worry, and lack of sleep and rest can cause or exacerbate confusion.* (Refer to ND Insomnia, as appropriate.)

- Monitor laboratory values (e.g., complete blood count [CBC], blood cultures, oxygen saturation, electrolytes, thyroid, ammonia levels, liver function studies, serum glucose, urinalysis, toxicology, and drug levels [including peak and trough, as appropriate]).[1-7,11]

- Review results of diagnostic studies (e.g., brain scans or imaging studies, electroencephalogram [EEG], lumbar puncture and cerebrospinal fluid [CSF] studies).[11]

NURSING PRIORITY NO. 2

To determine degree of impairment:

- Talk with client/SOs to determine client's physical, functional, cognitive, and behavioral baseline, observed changes, and onset and precipitator of changes *to understand and clarify the current situation.*[1]
- Collaborate with medical and psychiatric providers *to evaluate extent of impairment in orientation, attention span, ability to follow directions, send and receive communication, appropriateness of response.*[1]
- Note occurrence and timing of agitation, hallucinations, and violent behaviors *(e.g., delirium may occur as early as 1 or 2 days after last drink in an alcoholic; or "sundown syndrome" may occur in intensive care unit [ICU], with client oriented during daylight hours but confused during night).*[1,3]
- Determine threat to safety of client/others. *Delirium can cause client to become verbally and physically aggressive, resulting in behavior threatening to safety of self and others.*

NURSING PRIORITY NO. 3

To maximize level of function, prevent further deterioration:

- Assist with treatment of underlying problem (e.g., establish and maintain normal fluid and electrolyte balance and oxygenation, treat infectious process or pain, detoxify from alcohol and other drugs, provide psychological interventions).[1–7,9,11,12,14]
- Monitor and adjust medication regimen and note response. Determine which medications can be changed or eliminated when polypharmacy, side effects, or adverse reactions are determined to be associated with current condition.
- Implement helpful communication measures, such as:[1–7,9,11,14]
  Use short, simple sentences. Speak slowly and clearly.
  Call client by name and identify yourself at each contact.
  Tell client what you want done, not what to do.
  Orient client to surroundings, staff, and necessary activities as often as needed.
  Acknowledge client's fears and feelings. *Confusion can be very frightening, especially when client knows thinking is not normal.*
  Listen to what client says and try to identify message and emotion or need being communicated.
  Limit choices and decisions until client is able to make them.
  Give simple directions. Allow sufficient time for client to respond, to communicate, and to make decisions.
  Present reality concisely and briefly and avoid challenging illogical thinking. *Defensive reactions may result.*
  Refer to ND impaired verbal Communication for additional interventions.
- Manage environment, using the following measures:[1–7,9,11,14]
  Provide undisturbed rest periods. Eliminate extraneous noise and stimuli. *Preventing overstimulation can help client relax and can result in reduced level of confusion.*[10]
  Provide calm and comfortable environment with good lighting. Encourage client to use vision or hearing aids, when needed, *to reduce disorientation and discomfort from sensory overload or deprivation.*

Observe client on regular basis, informing client of this schedule.

Provide adequate supervision (may need one-to-one during severe episode); remove harmful objects from environment; provide siderails, seizure precautions; place call bell and position needed items within reach, clear traffic paths; ambulate with devices to meet client's safety needs.

Provide clear feedback on appropriate and inappropriate behavior.

Remove client from situation; provide time-out, seclusion, as indicated, *for protection of client/others.*

Encourage family/SO(s) to participate in reorientation and provide ongoing normal life input (e.g., current news and family happenings). Provide normal levels of essential sensory and tactile stimulation—include personal items and pictures. *Client may respond positively to well-known person and familiar items.*

- Note behavior that may be indicative of potential for violence and take appropriate actions to prevent injury to client/caregiver. (Refer to ND risk for self-/other-directed Violence.)
- Administer medication cautiously to control restlessness, agitation, and hallucinations. *In acute confusion, the short-term goal is to calm the person down quickly. Sedation with conventional antipsychotic agent (e.g., haloperidol, lorazepam) may be used, although many other medications can be used, depending on the underlying cause of the delirium.*[1,5–7]
- Assist with treatment of alcohol or drug intoxication and/or withdrawal, as indicated.[11,12,14]
- Avoid or limit use of restraints. *May worsen agitation, increase likelihood of untoward complications including injury or death.*[5,12]
- Mobilize elderly client (especially after orthopedic injury) as soon as possible. *Older person with low level of activity prior to crisis is at particular risk for acute confusion and may fare better when out of bed.*[4,14]
- Establish and maintain elimination patterns. *Disruption of elimination may be a cause for confusion, or changes in elimination may also be a symptom of acute confusion.*[5]
- Consult with psychiatric clinical nurse specialist or psychiatrist for additional interventions related to disruptive behaviors, psychosis, and unresolved symptoms.
- Refer to NDs disturbed Thought Processes and disturbed Sensory Perception for additional interventions.

NURSING PRIORITY NO. 4

To promote wellness (Teaching/Discharge Considerations):

- Explain reason for confusion, if known. *Acute confusion usually subsides over time as client recovers from underlying cause or adjusts to situation, but can be frightening to client/ SO. Information about cause and treatment to improve condition may be helpful in managing sense of fear and powerlessness.*[13,14]
- Educate SO/caregivers to monitor client at home for sudden change in cognition and behavior. *An acute change is a classic presentation of delirium and should be considered a medical emergency. Early intervention can often prevent long-term complications.*[8]
- Discuss need for ongoing medical review of client's medications to limit possibility of misuse and/or potential for dangerous side effects or interactions. *Medications are frequent precipitants of acute confusion, especially in very young or old.*[8,9]
- Stress importance of keeping vision and hearing aids in good repair *to improve client's interpretation of environmental stimuli and communication.*
- Provide appropriate referrals. *Additional assistance may be required for client with confusion (e.g., cognitive retraining, substance abuse support groups, medication monitoring program, Meals on Wheels, home health, and adult day care).*[1]

DOCUMENTATION FOCUS

Assessment/Reassessment
- Nature, duration, frequency of problem.
- Current and previous level of function, effect on independence and lifestyle (including safety concerns).

Planning
- Plan of care and who is involved in planning.
- Teaching plan.

Implementation/Evaluation
- Response to interventions and actions performed.
- Attainment or progress toward desired outcomes.
- Modifications to plan of care.

Discharge Planning
- Long-term needs and who is responsible for actions to be taken.
- Available resources and specific referrals.

References

1. Doenges, M. E., Moorhouse, M. F., Geissler-Murr, A. C. (2002). *Nurse's Pocket Guide: Diagnoses, Interventions and Rationales.* 8th ed. Philadelphia: F. A. Davis, 142–145.
2. Delirium and Acute Problematic Behavior in the Long-Term Care Setting (complete summary). (1998, update 2008). Retrieved September 2009 from National Guideline Clearinghouse www.guideline.gov. Columbia, MD: American Medical Directors Association (AMDA).
3. Stanley, M., Bear, P. G. (1999). *Gerontological Nursing: A Health Promotion/Protection Approach.* 2d ed. Philadelphia: F. A. Davis, 342–349.
4. Matthiesen, V., et al. (1994). Acute confusion: Nursing intervention in older patients. *Orthop Nurs*, 13, 25.
5. Rapp, C. G., Titler, M. G. (1997). In Iowa Veterans Affairs Nursing Research Consortium, et al. (eds). *Acute Confusion/Delirium.* Iowa City: University of Iowa.
6. American Psychiatric Association. . Practice guideline for the treatment of patients with delirium. (1999). *Am J Psychiatry*, 156(5 Suppl), 1–20.
7. Expert Consensus Guideline Series. Agitation in older persons with dementia: A guide for families and caregivers. (2005). Retrieved September 2009 from www.psychguides.com/gahe.php.
8. Ackley, B. J., Ladwig, G. B. (2002). *Nursing Diagnosis Handbook: A Guide to Planning Care.* 5th ed. St. Louis, MO: Mosby.
9. Cox, H. C., et al. (2002). *Clinical Applications of Nursing Diagnosis: Adult, Child, Women's, Psychiatric, Gerontic, and Home Health Considerations.* 4th ed. Philadelphia: F. A. Davis, 391–397.
10. Doenges, M. E., Townsend, M. C., Moorhouse, M. F. (1999). *Psychiatric Care Plans Guidelines for Individualizing Care.* 3d ed. Philadelphia: F. A. Davis.
11. Jacobs, D. H. (2006). Confusional states and acute memory disorders. Retrieved January 2007 from www.emedicine.com/neuro/topic435.htm.
12. Jenninngs-Ingle, S. (2007). The sobering facts about alcohol withdrawal syndrome. *Nursing Made Incredibly Easy!*, 5(1), 50–60.
13. McCaffrey, R., Rozzano, L. (2006). The effect of music on pain and acute confusion in older adults undergoing hip and knee surgery. *Holist Nurs Pract*, 20(5), 218–224.
14. Naylor, M. D., et al. (2005). Cognitively impaired older adults. *Am J Nurs*, 105(2), 52–61.

Cultural   Collaborative   Community/Home Care   Diagnostic Studies   Pediatric/Geriatric/Lifespan   Medications

chronic Confusion

DEFINITION: Irreversible, long-standing, and/or progressive deterioration of intellect and personality characterized by decreased ability to interpret environmental stimuli; decreased capacity for intellectual thought processes; and manifested by disturbances of memory, orientation, and behavior

RELATED FACTORS

Alzheimer's disease
Korsakoff's psychosis
Multi-infarct dementia
Cerebral vascular attack
Head injury

DEFINING CHARACTERISTICS

Objective
Clinical evidence of organic impairment
Altered interpretation
Altered response to stimuli
Progressive or long-standing cognitive impairment
No change in level of consciousness
Impaired socialization
Impaired short-term or long-term memory
Altered personality

Sample Clinical Applications: Brain injury or stroke, dementia/Alzheimer's disease, medication adverse reactions, drug or alcohol abuse, malnutrition, eating disorders, chemical exposure

DESIRED OUTCOME/EVALUATION CRITERIA

Sample **NOC** linkages:
Physical Injury Severity: Severity of injuries from accidents and trauma
Cognitive Orientation: Ability to identify person, place, and time accurately

Client Will (Include Specific Time Frame)
• Remain safe and free from harm.
• Maintain usual level of orientation.

Family/SO Will (Include Specific Time Frame)
• Verbalize understanding of disease process and prognosis, and client's needs.
• Identify and participate in interventions to deal effectively with situation.
• Provide for maximal independence while meeting safety needs of client.
Knowledge: Disease Process: Extent of understanding conveyed about a specific disease process

(continues on page 194)

chronic Confusion (continued)
ACTIONS/INTERVENTIONS

Sample NIC linkages:
Dementia Management: Provision of a modified environment for the patient who is experiencing a chronic confusional state
Calming Technique: Reducing anxiety in patient experiencing acute distress
Surveillance: Purposeful and ongoing acquisition, interpretation, and synthesis of patient data for clinical decision making

NURSING PRIORITY NO. 1

To assess degree of impairment:

- Determine the underlying cause for chronic confusion, as noted in Related Factors. *Helps to sort out possible causes and likelihood for improvement, as well as helping to identify potentially useful interventions and therapies.*[1]
- Review and evaluate responses on diagnostic examinations (e.g., cognitive, functional capacity, behavior, memory impairments, reality orientation, attention span, quality of life). *A combination of tests (e.g., Confusion Assessment Method [CAM], Mini-Mental State Examination [MMSE], Alzheimer's Disease Assessment Scale [ADAS-cog], Brief Dementia Severity Rating Scale [BDSRS], Neuropsychiatric Inventory [NPI], Functional Assessment Questionnaire [FAQ], Clinical Global Impression of Change [CGIC]) is often needed to complete an evaluation of client's overall condition relating to chronic or irreversible condition.*[2,8]
- Talk with SO(s) regarding baseline behaviors, length of time since onset or progression of problem, their perception of prognosis, and other pertinent information and concerns for client. *The client's SO/primary caregiver is an invaluable and essential source of information, regarding history and current situation, as both cognitive and behavioral symptoms tend to change over time and are often variable from day to day. If history reveals a gradual and insidious decline over months to years and if memory loss is a prominent part of the confusion, dementia is likely. Conditions that permanently damage brain structure and tissue (e.g., vascular, traumatic, infectious or demyelinating conditions) can lead to dementia in person of any age.*[1–4,9,10]
- Obtain information regarding recent changes or disruptions in client's health or routine. *Decline in physical health or disruption in daily living situation (e.g., hospitalization, change in medications, or moving to new home) can exacerbate agitation or bring on acute confusion.* (Refer to ND acute Confusion.)
- Evaluate client's response to primary care providers as well as receptiveness to interventions. *Awareness of these dynamics is helpful for evaluation of ongoing needs for both client and caregiver as client becomes increasingly dependent on caregivers or resistant to interventions.*
- Determine client and caregiver anxiety level in relation to situation. Note behavior that may be indicative of potential for violence. *The diagnosis of irreversible condition, the organic brain changes, and the day-to-day problems of living with it causes great stress and can potentiate violence.*[3]

NURSING PRIORITY NO. 2

To limit effects of deterioration/maximize level of function:

- Monitor for treatable conditions (e.g., depression, infections, malnutrition, electrolyte imbalances, and adverse medication reactions) *that may contribute to or exacerbate distress, discomfort, and agitation.*[1–6]

- Implement behavioral and environmental management interventions to promote orientation, provide opportunity for client interaction using current cognitive skills, and preserve client's dignity and safety:[2-6]

  Ascertain interventions previously used or tried and evaluate effectiveness.

  Provide calm environment, eliminate extraneous noise and stimuli *that may increase client's level of agitation or confusion.*

  Introduce yourself at each contact, if needed. Call client by preferred name.

  Use touch judiciously. Tell client what is being done before touching *to reduce sense of surprise or negative reaction.*

  Be supportive and sensitive to fears, misperceived threats, and frustration with expressing what is wanted.

  Be open and honest when discussing client's disease, abilities, and prognosis.

  Maintain continuity of caregivers and care routines as much as possible.

  Use positive statements, offer guided choices between two options.

  Avoid speaking in loud voice, crowding, restraining, shaming, demanding, or condescending actions toward client.

  Set limits on acting-out behavior *for safety of client/others.*

  Remove from stressors and agitation triggers or danger; move client to quieter place; offer privacy.

  Simplify client's tasks and routines *to reduce agitation associated with multiple options or demands.*

  Provide for or assist with daily care activities, including bathing, dressing, grooming, toileting, exercise. *Client may "forget" how to perform activities of daily living (ADLs).*

  Monitor and assist with meeting nutritional needs, feeding and fluid intake; monitor weight. Provide finger food if client has problems with eating utensils or is unable to sit to eat.

  Assist with toileting and perineal care, as needed. Provide incontinence supplies.

  Allow adequate rest between stimulating events.

  Use lighting and visual aids *to reduce confusion.*

  Encourage family/SO(s) to provide ongoing orientation/input to include current news and family happenings.

  Maintain reality-oriented relationship and environment (e.g., clocks, calendars, personal items, seasonal decorations).

  Encourage participation in resocialization groups.

  Allow client to reminisce or exist in own reality if not detrimental to well-being.

  Avoid challenging illogical thinking because defensive reactions may result.

  Provide appropriate safety measures. *Client who is confused needs close supervision. Safety measures (such as use of identification bracelet and alarms on unlocked exits; lockup of toxic substances and medication; supervision of outdoor activities and wandering; removal of car or car keys; and lowered temperature on hot water tank) can prevent injuries.*[5]
- Avoid use of restraints as much as possible. Use vest (instead of wrist) restraints when required. Provide pants with hip pad insert. *Although restraints can prevent falls, they can increase client's agitation and distress, resulting in injury or even death.*[8,10]
- Administer medications (e.g., antidepressants, anxiolytics, antipsychotics), as ordered, at lowest possible therapeutic dose. Monitor for expected and/or adverse responses, side effects, and interactions. *May be used to manage symptoms of psychosis and aggressive behavior but need to be used cautiously.*[5]
- Implement complementary therapies (e.g., music therapy, hand massage, Therapeutic Touch—if touch is tolerated—aromatherapy, bright-light treatment), as ordered or desired *Use of alternative therapies can be calming and provide relaxation, thus allowing care to be provided with less difficulty.*[7]

● Refer to NDs acute Confusion, impaired Memory, disturbed Thought Processes, impaired verbal Communication for additional interventions.

NURSING PRIORITY NO. 3

To assist SO(s) to develop coping strategies:

● Determine family dynamics, cultural values, resources, availability, and willingness to participate in meeting client's needs. Evaluate SO's attention to own needs, including health status, grieving process, and respite. *Primary caregiver and other members of family will suffer from the stress that accompanies caregiving and will require ongoing information and support.*
● Discuss caregiver burden, if appropriate. Provide educational materials and list of available resources, help lines, Web sites, and so forth, as desired, *to assist SO(s) in dealing and coping with long-term care issues.*[5,8] (Refer to NDs Caregiver Role Strain, risk for Caregiver Role Strain.)
● Involve SO(s) in care and discharge planning. Maintain frequent interactions with SOs *in order to relay information, to change care strategies, try different responses, or implement other problem-solving solutions.*[6]
 ● Identify appropriate community resources (e.g., Alzheimer's Disease and Related Disorders Association [ADRDA], stroke or other brain injury support groups, senior support groups, respite care, clergy, social services, therapists, attorney services for advance directives, and durable power of attorney) *to provide support for client and SOs and assist with problem-solving.*[5]

NURSING PRIORITY NO. 4

To promote wellness (Teaching/Discharge Considerations):

● Discuss how client's condition may progress, ongoing age-appropriate treatment needs, and appropriate follow-up. *Intermittent evaluations are needed to determine client's general health, any deterioration in cognitive function, or required adjustment in medication regimen to help the client maintain the highest possible level of functioning.*[6]
● Review medications with SO/caregiver(s), including dosage, route, action, expected and reportable side effects, and potential drug interactions *to prevent or limit complications associated with multiple psychiatric and CNS medications.*[5]
● Develop plan of care with family to meet client's and SO's individual needs. *The individual plan is dependent on cultural and belief patterns as well as family (personal, emotional, and financial) resources.*[6]
● Instruct SO/caregivers to share information about client's condition, functional status, and medications whenever encountering new providers. *Clients often have multiple doctors, each of whom may prescribe medications with potential for adverse effects and overmedication.*[7]
● Provide appropriate referrals (e.g., Meals on Wheels, adult day care, home-care agency, nursing home placement, respite care for family member). *May need additional assistance to maintain the client in the home setting or make arrangements for placement if necessary.*[6]

DOCUMENTATION FOCUS

Assessment/Reassessment
• Individual findings, including current level of function, recent changes, and rate of anticipated changes.
• Client/caregiver response to situation.
• Results of diagnostic testing.

Cultural   Collaborative   Community/Home Care   Diagnostic Studies   Pediatric/Geriatric/Lifespan   Medications

Planning
• Plan of care and who is involved in planning.

Implementation/Evaluation
• Response to interventions and actions performed.
• Attainment or progress toward desired outcomes.
• Modifications to plan of care.

Discharge Planning
• Long-term needs and who is responsible for actions to be taken.
• Available resources, specific referrals made.

References

1. Bostwick, J. M. (2000). The many faces of confusion: Timing and collateral history often holds the key to diagnosis. *Postgrad Med*, 108(6), 60–72.
2. Alzheimer's Disease and Related Disorders Association (ADRDA). (2003, update 2009). About Alzheimer's. Retrieved September 2009 from Physicians and professional care professionals site: Various educational materials. www.alz.org.
3. Doenges, M. E., Moorhouse, M. F., Geissler-Murr, A. C. (2002). *Nurse's Pocket Guide: Diagnoses, Interventions, and Rationales*. 8th ed. Philadelphia: F. A. Davis, 145–147.
4. Agitation in older persons with dementia: A guide for families and caregivers. (April 1998). Expert Consensus Guideline Series. Expert Knowledge Systems, LLC. Ross Editorial Services. www.psychguides.com/gahe.php.
5. Sommers, M. S., Johnson, S. A. (1997). Alzheimer's disease and delirium/dementia. *Davis's Manual of Nursing Therapeutics for Diseases and Disorders*. Philadelphia: F. A. Davis.
6. Kovach, C. R., Wilson, S. A. (1999). Dementia in older adults. In Stanley, M., Beare, P. G. (eds). *Gerontological Nursing: A Health Promotion/Protection Approach*. 2d ed. Philadelphia: F. A. Davis.
7. Burns, A., Byrne, J., Ballard, C. (2002). Sensory stimulation in dementia: An effective option for managing behavioral problems. *Br Med J*, 325, 1312–1313. Summarized on Dementia Center Health and Age Web site: www.healthandage.com.
8. Naylor, M. D., et al. (2005). Cognitively impaired older adults. *Am J Nurs*, 105(2), 52–61.
9. Borbasi, S., et al. (2006). Health professionals' perspective of providing care to people with dementia in the acute setting: Toward better practice. *Geriatr Nurs*, 27(5), 300–308.
10. Jacobs, D. H. (2006). Confusional states and acute memory disorders. Retrieved January 2007 from www.emedicine.com/neuro/topic435.htm.

(risk for acute Confusion)

DEFINITION: At risk for reversible disturbances of consciousness, attention, cognition, and perception that develop over a short period of time

RELATED FACTORS

Alcohol use; substance abuse
Infection; urinary retention
Pain
Fluctuation in sleep-wake cycle
Medication/drugs: Anesthesia; anticholinergics; diphenhydramine; opioids; psychoactive drugs; multiple medications

(continues on page 198)

● Provide appropriate referrals (e.g., medication monitoring program, nutritionist, substance abuse treatment, support groups, home health and adult day care).[1,2]

DOCUMENTATION FOCUS

Assessment/Reassessment
- Existing conditions and risk factors for individual.
- Current level of function, effect on independence and ability to meet own needs, including food and fluid intake and medication use.

Planning
- Plan of care and who is involved in planning.
- Teaching plan.

Implementation/Evaluation
- Response to interventions and actions performed.
- Attainment or progress toward desired outcomes.
- Modifications to plan of care.

Discharge Planning
- Long-term needs and who is responsible for actions to be taken.
- Available resources and specific referrals.

References

1. Acute confusion. In Doenges, M. E., Moorhouse, M. F., Geissler-Murr, A. C. (eds). (2005). *Nursing Diagnosis Manual: Planning, Individualizing and Documentation Client Care*. Philadelphia: F. A. Davis, 150–154.
2. Jacobs, D. H. (2006). Confusional states and acute memory disorders. Article for eMedicine Web site. Retrieved January 2007 from www.emedicine.com/neuro/topic435.htm.
3. Naylor, M. D., et al. (2005). Cognitively impaired older adults. *Am J Nurs*, 105(2), 52–61.
4. Jennings-Ingle, S. (2007). The sobering facts about alcohol withdrawal syndrome. *Nursing Made Incredibly Easy!*, 5(1), 50–60.
5. *Delirium and Acute Problematic Behavior in the Long-Term Care Setting* (complete summary). (1998, update 2008). Retrieved September 2009 from National Guideline Clearinghouse www.guideline.gov. Columbia, MD: American Medical Directors Association (AMDA).

Constipation

DEFINITION: Decrease in normal frequency of defecation accompanied by difficult or incomplete passage of stool and/or passage of excessively hard, dry stool

RELATED FACTORS

Functional
Irregular defecation habits; inadequate toileting (e.g., timeliness, positioning for defecation, privacy)
Insufficient physical activity; abdominal muscle weakness
Recent environmental changes
Habitual denial or ignoring of urge to defecate

🌐 Cultural   Collaborative 🏠 Community/Home Care 🔬 Diagnostic Studies ∞ Pediatric/Geriatric/Lifespan 💊 Medications

Psychological
Emotional stress; depression; mental confusion

Pharmacological
Antilipemic agents; laxative overdose; calcium carbonate; aluminum-containing antacids; nonsteroidal anti-inflammatory agents; opiates; anticholinergics; diuretics; iron salts; pheno-thiazines; sedatives; sympathomimetics; bismuth salts; antidepressants; calcium channel blockers; anticonvulsants

Mechanical
Hemorrhoids; pregnancy; obesity
Rectal abscess, ulcer, or prolapse; rectal anal fissures or strictures; rectocele
Prostate enlargement; postsurgical obstruction
Neurological impairment; Hirschsprung's disease; tumors
Electrolyte imbalance

Physiological
Poor eating habits; change in usual foods or eating patterns; insufficient fiber or fluid intake; dehydration
Inadequate dentition or oral hygiene
Decreased motility of gastrointestinal tract

DEFINING CHARACTERISTICS

Subjective
Change in bowel pattern; unable to pass stool; decreased frequency; decreased volume of stool
Increased abdominal pressure; feeling of rectal fullness or pressure
Abdominal pain; pain with defecation; nausea; vomiting; headache; indigestion; generalized fatigue

Objective
Hard, formed stool
Straining with defecation
Hypoactive or hyperactive bowel sounds; borborygmi
Distended abdomen; abdominal tenderness with/without palpable muscle resistance; palpable abdominal or rectal mass
Percussed abdominal dullness
Presence of soft pastelike stool in rectum; oozing liquid stool; bright red blood with stool
Severe flatus; anorexia
Atypical presentations in older adults (e.g., change in mental status, urinary incontinence, unexplained falls, elevated body temperature)

Sample Clinical Applications: Abdominal surgeries, hemorrhoids, anal lesions, irritable bowel syndrome, diverticulitis, spinal cord injury (SCI), multiple sclerosis (MS), enteral or parenteral feedings, hypothyroidism, iron deficiency anemia, uremia, renal dialysis, Alzheimer's disease/dementia

(continues on page 202)

Constipation (continued)
DESIRED OUTCOMES/EVALUATION CRITERIA

Sample **NOC** linkages:
Bowel Elimination: Formation and evacuation of stool
Nutritional Status: Nutrient Intake: Adequacy of usual pattern of nutrient intake
Self-Care: Non-Parenteral Medications: Ability to administer oral and topical medications to meet therapeutic goals independently with or without assistive device

Client Will (Include Specific Time Frame)
• Establish or regain normal pattern of bowel functioning.
• Verbalize understanding of etiology and appropriate interventions or solutions for individual situation.
• Demonstrate behaviors or lifestyle changes to prevent recurrence of problem.
• Participate in bowel program, as indicated.

ACTIONS/INTERVENTIONS

Sample **NIC** linkages:
Constipation/Impaction Management: Prevention and alleviation of constipation/impaction
Bowel Management: Establishment and maintenance of a regular pattern of bowel elimination
Ostomy Care: Maintenance of elimination through a stoma and care of surrounding tissue

NURSING PRIORITY NO. 1

To identify causative/contributing factors:

● Review medical/surgical history *to identify conditions commonly associated with constipation, including problems with colon or rectum (e.g., obstruction, scar tissue or stricture, diverticulitis, irritable bowel syndrome, tumors, anal fissure), metabolic or endocrine disorders (e.g., diabetes mellitus, hypothyroidism, uremia), limited physical activity (e.g., bedrest, poor mobility, chronic disability), chronic pain problems (especially when client is on pain medications), pregnancy and childbirth, recent abdominal or perianal surgery, and neurological disorders (e.g., Parkinson's disease, MS, spinal cord abnormalities).*[1,2,4,5,7–12]

∞ ● Note client's age. *Constipation is more likely to occur in individuals older than 55 years of age*[1,13] *but can occur in any age from infant to elderly. A bottle-fed infant is more prone to constipation than breastfed infant, especially when formula contains iron.*[2,5] *Toddlers are at risk because of developmental factors (e.g., too young, too interested in other things, rigid schedule during potty training), and children and adolescents are at risk because of unwillingness to take break from play, poor eating and fluid intake habits, and withholding because of perceived lack of privacy.*[3] *Many older adults experience constipation as a result of duller nerve sensations, incomplete emptying of the bowel, or failing to attend to signals to defecate.*[4]

● Review daily dietary regimen, noting if diet is deficient in fiber. *Imbalanced nutrition influences the amount and consistency of feces.*[2] *Inadequate dietary fiber (vegetable, fruits, and whole grains) and highly processed foods contribute to poor intestinal function.*[1,4,5,8]

● Assess general oral and dental health. *Dental problems can impact dietary intake (e.g., loss of teeth can force individuals to eat soft foods, mostly lacking in fiber).*[1,4]

- Determine fluid intake to note deficits. *Most individuals do not drink enough fluids, even when healthy, reducing the speed at which stool moves through the colon. Active fluid loss through sweating, vomiting, diarrhea, or bleeding can greatly increase chances for constipation.*[1,2,4,5,7–10]
- Evaluate medication or drug usage *for agents that could slow passage of stool and cause or exacerbate constipation (e.g., narcotic pain relievers, antidepressants, anticonvulsants, aluminum-containing antacids, chemotherapy, iron, contrast media, steroids).*[1,2,4,5,7–11]
- Note energy and activity level, and exercise pattern. *Lack of physical activity or regular exercise is often a factor in constipation.*[1–4,7,8,10,13]
- Identify areas of life changes or stressors. *Factors such as pregnancy, travel, traumas, changes in personal relationships, occupational factors, or financial concerns can cause or exacerbate constipation.*[7,10]
- Determine access to bathroom, privacy, and ability to perform self-care activities.
- Investigate reports of pain with defecation. *Hemorrhoids, fissures, skin breakdown, or other abnormal findings may be hindering passage of stool or causing client to hold stool.*[1,5–8]
- Discuss laxative and enema use. Note signs or reports of laxative abuse or overuse of stimulant laxatives. *This is most common among older adults preoccupied with having daily bowel movement.*[5,7,13]
- Auscultate abdomen for presence, location, and characteristics of bowel sounds *reflecting bowel activity.*
- Palpate abdomen for hardness, distention, and masses, *indicating possible obstruction or retention of stool.*
- Perform digital rectal examination, as indicated, *to evaluate rectal tone and detect tenderness, blood, or fecal impaction.*
- Assist with medical workup (e.g., x-rays, abdominal imaging, colonoscopy, proctosigmoidoscopy, colonic transit studies, stool sample tests) *for identification of possible causative factors.*[11–13]

NURSING PRIORITY NO. 2

To determine usual pattern of elimination:

- Discuss customary elimination habits (e.g., normal urge time [client unable to eliminate unless in own home, passing hard stool after prolonged effort, and anal pain]). *Helps to identify and clarify client's perception of problem. For example, constipation has been defined as not only infrequent stools (less than three per week), but also straining with bowel movements, hard stools, unproductive urges, and feeling of incomplete evacuation.*[8]
- Ascertain presence of associated symptoms. *Bloating, abdominal pain, loss of appetite, and feeling of being unwell often accompany constipation and are present between infrequent stools.*[8]
- Note factors that usually stimulate bowel activity and any interferences present. *Client may describe having to sit in a particular position or needing to apply perineal pressure or digital stimulation to start stool. Interferences can include not wanting to use a particular facility or not wanting to interrupt play or an activity.*[8]

NURSING PRIORITY NO. 3

To assess current pattern of elimination:

- Note color, odor, consistency, amount, and frequency of stool following each bowel movement during assessment phase. *Provides a baseline for comparison, promoting recognition of changes. If usual number of weekly bowel movements is decreased, stool is hard formed, or client is straining, constipation is likely present.*[2,10]

- Ascertain duration of current problem and client's degree of concern. *Long-standing condition that client has "lived with" may not cause undue concern, while an acute postsurgical constipation can cause great distress. Client's response may/may not be congruent with the severity of condition.*[10]
- Note interventions client has tried to relieve current situation (e.g., dietary supplements/fiber pills, laxatives, suppositories, enemas), and document success/lack of effectiveness.

NURSING PRIORITY NO. 4

To facilitate return to usual/acceptable pattern of elimination:

- Review client's current medication regime with physician *to determine if drugs contributing to constipation can be discontinued or changed.*
- Promote lifestyle changes:[1–10]
  Instruct in and encourage balanced fiber and bulk in diet (e.g., fruits, vegetables, and whole grains) and fiber supplements (e.g., wheat bran, psyllium) *to improve consistency of stool and enhance passage through colon. Note: Improvement in elimination as a result of dietary changes takes time and is not a treatment for acute constipation.*[11]
  Limit foods with little or no fiber (e.g., ice cream, cheese, meat, and processed foods).
  Promote adequate fluid intake, including water, high-fiber fruit, and vegetable juices. Suggest drinking warm, stimulating fluids (e.g., decaffeinated coffee, hot water, tea) *to promote moist, soft feces and facilitate passage of stool.*
  Encourage daily activity and exercise within limits of individual ability *to stimulate contractions of the intestines.*
  Encourage client to not ignore urge. Provide privacy and routinely scheduled time for defecation (bathroom or commode preferable to bedpan) *to promote psychological readiness and comfort.*
- Administer medications, as indicated: stool softeners *(to provide moisture to stool)*, mild stimulants *(to cause rhythmic muscle contractions)*, lubricants *(to enable stool to move more easily)*, saline or hyperosmolar laxatives *(to draw water into colon)*, or bulk-forming agents *(to absorb water in intestine)*, as prescribed or routinely when appropriate (e.g., client receiving opiates, decreased level of activity or immobility).[1–3,7–10]
- Administer enemas or suppositories, as indicated. Digitally remove impacted stool, when necessary, after applying lubricant and anesthetic ointment to anus *to soften impaction and decrease rectal pain.*[7,8]
- Provide sitz bath before stools *to relax sphincter* and after stools *for soothing effect to rectal area.*[5,10]
- Establish bowel program *to provide predictable and effective elimination and reduce evacuation problems when long-term or permanent bowel dysfunction is present (such as with SCI).* Include dietary and fluid management, use of particular position for defecation, abdominal massage, Valsalva maneuver, deep breathing, ingestion of warm fluids, digital stimulation, and medications or enemas.[9,10]
- Support treatment of underlying medical cause where appropriate (e.g., surgery to repair rectal prolapse, thyroid treatment) *to improve body and bowel function.*[1–10]

NURSING PRIORITY NO. 5

To promote wellness (Teaching/Discharge Considerations):[1,8,10]

- Discuss client's particular anatomy and physiology of bowel and acceptable variations in elimination.[1,8,10]
- Provide information and resources to client/SO about relationship of diet, exercise, fluid, and appropriate use of laxatives, as indicated.[1,8,10]

🏠 • Provide social and emotional support *to help client manage actual or potential disabilities associated with long-term bowel management.* Discuss rationale for and encourage continuation of successful interventions.[1,8,10]

🏠 • Encourage client to maintain elimination diary, if appropriate, *to facilitate monitoring of long-term problem and choice of interventions.*[1,8,10]

🏠 • Design bowel management program to be easily replicated in home and community setting.[1,8,10]

⚕ • Identify specific actions to be taken if problem does not resolve *to promote timely intervention, thereby enhancing client's independence.*[1,8,10]

DOCUMENTATION FOCUS

Assessment/Reassessment
• Usual and current bowel pattern, duration of the problem, and interventions used.
• Characteristics of stool.
• Individual contributing factors.

Planning
• Plan of care, specific interventions or changes in lifestyle necessary to correct individual situation, and who is involved in planning.
• Teaching plan.

Implementation/Evaluation
• Responses to interventions, teaching, and actions performed.
• Change in bowel pattern, character of stool.
• Attainment or progress toward desired outcomes.
• Modifications to plan of care.

Discharge Planning
• Individual long-term needs, noting who is responsible for actions to be taken.
• Recommendations for follow-up care.
• Specific referrals made.

References

1. Hert, M., Huseboe, J. (2001). Management of constipation. University of Iowa Gerontological Nursing Interventions Research Center. Iowa City. Available at www.nursing.uiowa.edu/products_services/evidence_based.htm.

2. Cox, H. C., et al. (2002). *Clinical Applications of Nursing Diagnosis: Adult, Child, Women's, Psychiatric, Gerontic, and Home Health Considerations.* 3d ed. Philadelphia: F. A. Davis, 192–205.

3. Streeter, B. L. (2002). Teenage constipation: A case study. *Gastroenterol Nurs,* 25(6), 253–256.

4. Stanley, M. (1999). The aging gastrointestinal system, with nutritional considerations. In Stanley, M., Beare , P. G. (eds) *Gerontological Nursing: A Health Promotion/Protection Approach.* 7th ed. Philadelphia: F. A. Davis, 180–181.

5. Constipation in children. Retrieved September 2009 from NIH Pub. No. 02–4633, October 2001, National Digestive Diseases Information Clearinghouse (NDDIC), Bethesda, MD. http://digestive.niddk.nih.gov/ddiseases/pubs/constipationchild/index.htm.

6. Functional constipation and soiling in children. [NCG 1011]. (2008). Retrieved September 2009 from www.guideline.gov. Ann Arbor: University of Michigan Medical Center.

7. Constipation. Retrieved September 2009 from National Digestive Diseases Information Clearinghouse (NDDIC) http://digestive.niddk.nih.gov/ddiseases/pubs/constipation/.

8. Locke, G. R., Pemberton, J. H., Phillips, S. F. (2000). American Gastroenterological Association: Medical position statement: Guidelines on constipation. *Gastroenterology*, 119(6), 1761–1766.

9. Neurogenic Bowel Management in Adults with Spinal Cord Injury. Consortium for Spinal Cord Medicine, Paralyzed Veterans of America. Washington, DC: Consortium of Spinal Medicine.

10. Doenges, M. E., Moorhouse, M. F., Geissler-Murr, A. C. (2002). *Nurse's Pocket Guide: Diagnoses, Interventions, and Rationales*. 8th ed. Philadelphia: F. A. Davis, 151.

11. Marks, J. W. (2006). Constipation. Retrieved January 2007 from www.medicinenet.com.

12. Holson, D., Gathers, S. (2006). Constipation. Retrieved January 2007 from www.emedicine.com/emerg/topic111.htm.

13. Aazer, S. A. (2005). Constipation in adults. Retrieved January 2007 from www.emedicinehealth.com.

perceived Constipation

DEFINITION: Self-diagnosis of constipation and abuse of laxatives, enemas, and suppositories to ensure a daily bowel movement

RELATED FACTORS

Cultural or family health beliefs
Faulty appraisal [long-term expectations or habits]
Impaired thought processes

DEFINING CHARACTERISTICS

Subjective
Expectation of a daily bowel movement
Expected passage of stool at same time every day
Overuse of laxatives, enemas, or suppositories

Sample Clinical Applications: Irritable bowel, confused states/dementia, hypochondriasis

DESIRED OUTCOMES/EVALUATION CRITERIA

Sample **NOC** linkages:
Health Beliefs: Personal convictions that influence health behaviors
Bowel Elimination: Formation and evacuation of stool
Knowledge: Health Behavior: Extent of understanding conveyed about the promotion and protection of health

Client Will (Include Specific Time Frame)
- Verbalize understanding of physiology of bowel function.
- Identify acceptable interventions to promote adequate bowel function.
- Decrease reliance on laxatives and/or enemas.
- Establish individually appropriate pattern of elimination.

ACTIONS/INTERVENTIONS

Sample **NIC** linkages:

Bowel Management: Establishment and maintenance of a regular pattern of bowel elimination

Counseling: Use of an interactive helping process focusing on the needs, problems, or feelings of the patient and SOs to enhance or support coping, problem-solving, and interpersonal relationships

Medication Management: Facilitation of safe and effective use of prescription and over-the-counter drugs

NURSING PRIORITY NO. 1

To identify factors affecting individual beliefs:

- Determine client's understanding of a "normal" bowel pattern. Compare with client's current bowel functioning. *Helps to identify areas for discussion or intervention. For example, what is considered "normal" varies with the individual, cultural, and familial factors with differences in expectations and dietary habits.*[1] *In addition, individuals can think they are constipated when, in fact, their bowel movements are regular and soft, possibly revealing a problem with thought processes or perception. Some people believe they are constipated, or irregular, if they do not have a bowel movement every day, because of ideas instilled from childhood.*[2] *The elderly client may believe that laxatives or purgatives are necessary for elimination, when in fact the problem may be long-standing habits (e.g., insufficient fluids, lack of exercise and/or fiber in the diet).*[3]
- Discuss client's use of laxatives. *Perceived constipation typically results in self-medicating with various laxatives. Although laxatives may correct the acute problem, chronic use leads to habituation, requiring ever-increasing doses that result in drug dependency and, ultimately, a hypotonic laxative colon.*[5]
- Identify interventions used by client to correct perceived problem *to establish needed changes or interventions or points for discussion and teaching.*

NURSING PRIORITY NO. 2

To promote wellness (Teaching/Discharge Considerations):

- Discuss the following with client/SO/caregiver *(to clarify issues regarding actual and perceived bowel functioning, and to provide support during behavior modification/bowel retraining):*[3,4]
  Review anatomy and physiology of bowel function and acceptable variations in elimination.
- Identify detrimental effects of habitual laxative or enema use, and discuss alternatives.
  Provide information about relationship of diet, hydration, and exercise to improved elimination.
  Encourage client to maintain elimination calendar or diary, if appropriate.
  Provide support by Active-listening and discussing client's concerns or fears.
  Provide social and emotional support *to help client manage actual or potential disabilities associated with long-term bowel management.*
  Encourage use of stress-reduction activities and refocusing of attention while client works to establish individually appropriate pattern.
- Offer educational materials and resources for client/SO to peruse at home *to assist them in making informed decisions regarding constipation and management options.*
- Refer to ND Constipation for additional interventions, as appropriate.

DOCUMENTATION FOCUS

Assessment/Reassessment
• Assessment findings, client's perceptions of the problem.
• Current bowel pattern, stool characteristics.

Planning
• Plan of care, specific interventions, and who is involved in the planning.
• Teaching plan.

Implementation/Evaluation
• Client's responses to interventions, teaching, and actions performed.
• Changes in bowel pattern, character of stool.
• Attainment or progress toward desired outcome(s).
• Modifications to plan of care.

Discharge Planning
• Referral for follow-up care.

References

1. Pieken, S. R. (2004). Constipation. *Gastrointestinal Health: A Self-Help Nutritional Program to Prevent, Cure, or Alleviate Irritable Bowel Syndrome, Ulcers, Heartburn, Gas, Constipation.* 3d ed. New York: HarperCollins, 99–104.
2. Constipation (HIH Pub. No. 95–2745, July 1995). Bethesda, MD: National Digestive Diseases Information Clearinghouse (NDDIC).
3. Stanley, M. (1999). The aging gastrointestinal system with nutritional considerations. In Stanley, M., Beare, P. G. (eds). *Gerontological Nursing: A Health Promotion/Protection Approach.* 7th ed. Philadelphia: F. A. Davis, 180–181.
4. Hert, M., Huseboe, J. (1998). Management of constipation. Research Dissemination Core: [NGC 543]. Retrieved June 2003 from www.guideline.gov/browse/gawithdrawn.aspx?st=U. Iowa City: University of Iowa Gerontological Nursing Interventions Research Center.
5. Brasson, M. D. (2007). Constipation. Retrieved June 2007 from www.emedicine.com/med/topic2833.htm.

risk for Constipation

DEFINITION: At risk for a decrease in normal frequency of defecation accompanied by difficult or incomplete passage of stool and/or passage of excessively hard, dry stool

RISK FACTORS

Functional
Irregular defecation habits; inadequate toileting (e.g., timeliness, positioning for defecation, privacy)
Insufficient physical activity, abdominal muscle weakness
Recent environmental changes
Habitual denial or ignoring of urge to defecate

Psychological
Emotional stress, depression, mental confusion

Physiological

Change in usual foods or eating patterns, insufficient fiber or fluid intake, dehydration, poor eating habits

Inadequate dentition or oral hygiene

Decreased motility of gastrointestinal tract

Pharmacological

Phenothiazines; nonsteroidal anti-inflammatory agents; sedatives; aluminum-containing antacids; laxative overuse; bismuth salts; iron salts; anticholinergics; antidepressants; anticonvulsants; antilipemic agents; calcium channel blockers; calcium carbonate; diuretics; sympathomimetics; opiates

Mechanical

Hemorrhoids, pregnancy; obesity

Rectal abscess or ulcer, anal stricture or fissures, rectal prolapse, rectocele

Prostate enlargement, postsurgical obstruction

Neurological impairment; Hirschsprung's disease; tumors

Electrolyte imbalance

NOTE: A risk diagnosis is not evidenced by signs and symptoms, as the problem has not occurred; rather, nursing interventions are directed at prevention.

Sample Clinical Applications: Abdominal surgeries, hemorrhoids/anal lesions, irritable bowel syndrome, diverticulitis, spinal cord injury (SCI), multiple sclerosis (MS), enteral/parenteral feedings, hypothyroidism, iron deficiency anemia, uremia/renal dialysis, Alzheimer's disease/dementia

DESIRED OUTCOMES/EVALUATION CRITERIA

Sample NOC linkages:

Bowel Elimination: Formation and evacuation of stool

Risk Control: Personal actions to prevent, eliminate, or reduce modifiable health threats

Knowledge: Medication: Extent of understanding conveyed about the safe use of medication

Client/Caregiver Will (Include Specific Time Frame)

• Maintain effective pattern of bowel functioning.

• Verbalize understanding of risk factors and appropriate interventions or solutions related to individual situation.

• Demonstrate behaviors or lifestyle changes to prevent developing problem.

ACTIONS/INTERVENTIONS

Sample NIC linkages:

Constipation/Impaction Management: Prevention and alleviation of constipation/impaction

Bowel Management: Establishment and maintenance of a regular pattern of bowel elimination

Medication Management: Facilitation of safe and effective use of prescription and over-the-counter (OTC) drugs

NURSING PRIORITY NO. 1

To identify individual risk factors/needs:

- Review medical/surgical history *to identify conditions commonly associated with constipation, including problems with colon or rectum (e.g., obstruction, scar tissue or stricture, diverticulitis, irritable bowel syndrome, tumors, anal fissure), metabolic or endocrine disorders (e.g., diabetes mellitus, hypothyroidism, uremia), limited physical activity (e.g., bedrest, poor mobility, chronic disability), chronic pain problems (especially when client is on pain medications), pregnancy and childbirth, recent abdominal or perianal surgery, neurological disorders (e.g., Parkinson's, MS, spinal cord abnormalities).*[1,2,4-11]
- Note client's age. *Constipation is more likely to occur in individuals older than 55 years of age*[1] *but can occur in any age from infant to elderly. A bottle-fed infant is more prone to constipation than a breastfed infant, especially when formula contains iron.*[2,5] *Toddlers are at risk because of developmental factors (e.g., too young, too interested in other things, rigid schedule during potty training), and children and adolescents are at risk because of unwillingness to take break from play, poor eating and fluid intake habits, and withholding because of perceived lack of privacy.*[3] *Many older adults experience constipation as a result of blunted nerve sensations, incomplete emptying of the bowel, or failing to attend to signals to defecate.*[4]
- Discuss usual elimination pattern and use of laxatives *to establish baseline and identify possible areas for intervention or instruction.*
- Ascertain client's beliefs and practices about bowel elimination, such as "must have a bowel movement every day or I need an enema." *These factors reflect familial or cultural thinking about elimination, which affect client's lifetime patterns.*
- Review daily dietary regimen. *Imbalanced nutrition influences the amount and consistency of feces.*[2] *Inadequate dietary fiber (vegetable, fruits, and whole grains) highly processed foods contribute to poor intestinal function.*[1,4,6]
- Assess general oral and dental health. *Dental problems can impact dietary intake (e.g., loss of teeth can force individuals to eat soft foods, mostly lacking in fiber).*[1,4]
- Determine fluid intake *to note deficits. Most individuals do not drink enough fluids, even when healthy, reducing the speed at which stool moves through the colon. Active fluid loss through sweating, vomiting, diarrhea, or bleeding can greatly increase chances for constipation.*[1,2,4,5,8]
- Evaluate medication or drug usage *for agents that could slow passage of stool and increase risk of constipation (e.g., narcotic pain relievers, antidepressants, anticonvulsants, aluminum-containing antacids, chemotherapy, iron, contrast media, steroids).*[1,2,4-8]
- Note energy and activity level and exercise pattern. *Lack of physical activity or regular exercise is often a factor in constipation.*[1-6,8]
- Identify areas of life changes or stressors. *Factors such as pregnancy, travel, traumas, and changes in personal relationships, occupational factors, or financial concerns can cause or exacerbate constipation.*[5,8]
- Auscultate abdomen for presence, location, and characteristics of bowel sounds *reflecting bowel activity.*

NURSING PRIORITY NO. 2

To facilitate normal bowel function:

- Promote healthy lifestyle for elimination:[1-11]
  Instruct in and encourage balanced fiber and bulk (e.g., fruits, vegetables, and whole grains) in diet and fiber supplements (e.g., wheat bran, psyllium) *to improve consistency of stool and facilitate passage through colon.*

Limit foods with little or no fiber (e.g., ice cream, cheese, meat, and processed foods).

Promote adequate fluid intake, including water, high-fiber fruit and vegetable juices. Suggest drinking warm, stimulating fluids (e.g., decaffeinated coffee, hot water, tea) *to promote moist, soft feces and facilitate passage of stool.*

Encourage daily activity and exercise within limits of individual ability to stimulate contractions of the intestines.

Encourage client to not ignore urge. Provide privacy and routinely scheduled time for defecation (bathroom or commode preferable to bedpan) to promote psychological readiness and comfort.

- Administer medications (stool softeners, mild stimulants, or bulk-forming agents) prn and/or routinely when appropriate *to prevent constipation (e.g., client taking pain medications, especially opiates, or who is inactive, immobile, or unconscious).*[11]

NURSING PRIORITY NO. 3

Promote wellness (Teaching/Discharge Considerations):

- Discuss physiology and acceptable variations in elimination. *May help reduce concerns and anxiety about situation.*[1,6,8]
- Review individual risk factors or potential problems and specific interventions for prevention of constipation.[1,6,8]
- Encourage treatment of underlying medical causes where appropriate *to improve organ function, including the bowel.*[1,6,8]
- Educate client/SO about safe and risky practices for managing constipation. *Information can assist client to make beneficial choices when need arises.*[1,6,8]
- Encourage client to maintain elimination diary if appropriate *to help monitor bowel pattern.*[1,6,8]
- Discuss client's current medication regime with physician *to determine if drugs that may contribute to constipation can be discontinued or changed.*[11]
- Refer to NDs Constipation; perceived Constipation for additional interventions as appropriate.

DOCUMENTATION FOCUS

Assessment/Reassessment
- Current bowel pattern, characteristics of stool, medications.
- Individual risk factors.

Planning
- Plan of care and who is involved in planning.
- Teaching plan.

Implementation/Evaluation
- Responses to interventions, teaching, and actions performed.
- Attainment or progress toward desired outcomes.
- Modifications to plan of care.

Discharge Planning
- Individual long-term needs, noting who is responsible for actions to be taken.
- Specific referrals made.

References

1. Hert, M., Huseboe, J. (2001). Management of constipation. Retrieved from www.nursing.uiowa .edu/products_services/evidence_based.htm. Iowa City: University of Iowa Gerontological Nursing Interventions Research Center.

2. Cox, H. C., et al. (2002). *Clinical Applications of Nursing Diagnosis: Adult, Child, Women's, Psychiatric, Gerontic, and Home Health Considerations*. 3d ed. Philadelphia: F. A. Davis, 192–205.

3. Streeter, B. L. (2002). Teenage constipation: A case study. *Gastroenterol Nurs*, 25(6), 253–256.

4. Stanley, M. (1999). The aging gastrointestinal system, with nutritional considerations. In Stanley, M., Beare, P. G. (eds). *Gerontological Nursing: A Health Promotion/Protection Approach*. 7th ed. Philadelphia: F. A. Davis, 180–181.

5. Constipation (NIH Pub. no. 95–2754, July 1995). Retrieved from http://nddic@info.niddk.nih.gov. Bethesda, MD: National Digestive Diseases Information Clearinghouse (NDDIC).

6. Locke, G. R., Pemberton, J. H., Phillips, S. F. (2000). American Gastroenterological Association: Medical position statement: Guidelines on constipation. *Gastroenterology*, 119(6), 1761–1766.

7. Consortium for Spinal Cord Medicine, Paralyzed Veterans of America. (1998). *Neurogenic Bowel Management in Adults with Spinal Cord Injury*. Washington, DC: Consortium for Spinal Cord Medicine.

8. Doenges, M. E., Moorhouse, M. F., Geissler-Murr, A. C. (2002). *Nurse's Pocket Guide: Diagnoses, Interventions, and Rationales*. 8th ed. Philadelphia: F. A. Davis, 151.

9. Marks, J. W. (2006). Constipation. Retrieved January 2007 from www.medicinenet.com.

10. Holson, D., Gathers, S. (2006). Constipation. Retrieved January 2007 from www.emedicine.com/emerg/topic111.htm.

11. Wooten, J. M. (2006). OTC laxatives aren't all the same. Retrieved January 2007 from www.rnweb.com/rnweb/author/authorDetail.jsp?id=6733.

Contamination

DEFINITION: Exposure to environmental contaminants in doses sufficient to cause adverse health effects

RELATED FACTORS

External
Chemical contamination of food or water; presence of atmospheric pollutants
Inadequate municipal services (trash removal, sewage treatment facilities)
Geographic area (living in area where high level of contaminants exist)
Playing in outdoor areas where environmental contaminants are used
Personal or household hygiene practices
Living in poverty (increases potential for multiple exposure, lack of access to healthcare, and poor diet)
Use of environmental contaminants in the home (e.g., pesticides, chemicals, environmental tobacco smoke)
Lack of breakdown of contaminants once indoors (breakdown is inhibited without sun and rain exposure)
Flooring surface (carpeted surfaces hold contaminant residue more than hard floor surfaces)
Flaking, peeling paint or plaster in presence of young children
Paint, lacquer, in poorly ventilated areas or without effective protection
Inappropriate use or lack of protective clothing
Unprotected contact with heavy metals or chemicals (e.g., arsenic, chromium, lead)
Exposure to radiation (occupation in radiography, employment in nuclear industries and electrical generating plants, living near nuclear industries and electrical generation plants)
Exposure to disaster (natural or man-made); exposure to bioterrorism

Internal

Age (children less than 5 years, older adults); gestational age during exposure; developmental characteristics of children

Female gender; pregnancy

Nutritional factors (e.g., obesity, vitamin and mineral deficiencies)

Preexisting disease states; smoking

Concomitant exposures; previous exposures

DEFINING CHARACTERISTICS

(Defining characteristics are dependent on the causative agent. Agents cause a variety of individual organ responses as well as systemic responses.)

Subjective/Objective

Pesticides: (Major categories of pesticides: insecticides, herbicides, fungicides, antimicrobials, rodenticides; major pesticides: organophosphates, carbamates, organochlorines, pyrethrum, arsenic, glycophosphates, bipyridyis, chlorophenoxy)

Dermatological, gastrointestinal, neurological, pulmonary, or renal effects of pesticide

Chemicals: (Major chemical agents: petroleum-based agents, anticholinesterases; type I agents act on proximal tracheobronchial portion of the respiratory tract, type II agents act on alveoli, type III agents produce systemic effects)

Dermatological, gastrointestinal, immunological, neurological, pulmonary, or renal effects of chemical exposure

Biologicals: Dermatological, gastrointestinal, neurological, pulmonary, or renal effects of exposure to biologicals (toxins from living organisms [bacteria, viruses, fungi])

Pollution: (Major locations: air, water, soil; major agents: asbestos, radon, tobacco [smoke], heavy metal, lead, noise, exhaust)

Neurological or pulmonary effects of pollution exposure

Waste: (Categories of waste: trash, raw sewage, industrial waste)

Dermatological, gastrointestinal, hepatic, or pulmonary effects of waste exposure

Radiation: (Categories: Internal—ingestion of radioactive material [e.g., food or water contamination]; external—exposure through direct contact with radioactive material)

Immunological, genetic, neurological, or oncological effects of radiation exposure

Sample Clinical Applications: *Escherichia coli* infection, plague, hantavirus, asthma, botulism, cholera, lead or other heavy metal poisoning, chemical burns, asbestosis, carbon monoxide poisoning, radiation sickness

DESIRED OUTCOMES/EVALUATION CRITERIA

Sample NOC linkages:

Symptom Severity: Severity of perceived adverse changes in physical, emotional, and social functioning

Knowledge: Personal Safety: Extent of understanding conveyed about prevention of unintentional injuries

Risk Control: Personal actions to prevent, eliminate, or reduce modifiable health threats

(continues on page 214)

Contamination (continued)

Client Will (Include Specific Time Frame)
- Be free of injury.
- Verbalize understanding of individual factors that contributed to injury and plans for correcting situation(s) where possible.
- Modify environment, as indicated, to enhance safety.

Sample NOC linkages:
Community Health Status: General state of well-being of a community or population
Community Risk Control: Lead Exposure: Community actions to reduce lead exposure and poisoning
Community Disaster Readiness: Community preparedness to respond to a natural or man-made calamitous event

Client/Community Will (Include Specific Time Frame)
- Identify hazards that led to exposure or contamination.
- Correct environmental hazards, as identified.
- Demonstrate necessary actions to promote community safety.

ACTIONS/INTERVENTIONS

In reviewing this ND, it is apparent there is overlap with other diagnoses. We have chosen to present generalized interventions. Although there are commonalities to Contamination situations, we suggest that the reader refer to other primary diagnoses, as indicated, such as ineffective Airway Clearance, ineffective Breathing Pattern, impaired Gas Exchange, ineffective Home Maintenance, risk for Infection, risk for Injury, risk for Poisoning, impaired/risk for impaired Skin Integrity, risk for Suffocation, ineffective tissue Perfusion (specify), and Trauma.

Sample NIC linkages:
Risk Identification: Analyzing potential risk factors, determining health risks, and prioritizing risk-reduction strategies for an individual or group
Community Health Development: Assisting members of a community to identify a community's health concerns, mobilize resources, and implement solutions
Environmental Risk Protection: Preventing and detecting disease and injury in populations at risk from environmental hazards

NURSING PRIORITY NO. 1

To evaluate degree/source of exposure:

- Ascertain (1) type of contaminant(s) to which client has been exposed (e.g., chemical, biological, air pollutant); (2) manner of exposure (e.g., inhalation, ingestion, topical); (3) whether exposure was accidental or intentional; and (4) immediate or delayed reactions. *Determines course of action to be taken by all emergency and other care providers. Note: Intentional exposure to hazardous materials requires notification of law enforcement for further investigation and possible prosecution.*[1-6]
- Note age and gender. *Children (less than 5 years of age) are at greater risk for adverse effects from exposure to contaminants because (1) smaller body size causes them to receive a more concentrated "dose" than adults; (2) they spend more time outside than most adults, increasing exposure to air and soil pollutants; (3) young children spend more time on the floor, increasing exposure to toxins in carpets and low cupboards; (4) they consume*

🌐 Cultural 🔄 Collaborative 🏠 Community/Home Care ✏️ Diagnostic Studies ∞ Pediatric/Geriatric/Lifespan   Medications *more water and food per pound than adults, increasing their body-weight-to-toxin ratio; and (5) development of fetal, infant, and young children's organ systems can be disrupted. Older adults have a normal decline in function of immune, integumentary, cardiac, renal, hepatic, and pulmonary systems, an increase in adipose tissue mass, and a decline in lean body mass. Females in general have a greater proportion of body fat than men, increasing the chance of accumulating more lipid soluble toxins.[1-6]*

- Ascertain geographic location (e.g., home, work) where exposure occurred. *Individual and/or community intervention may be needed to modify or correct problem.*
- Note socioeconomic status and availability and use of resources. *Living in poverty increases potential for multiple exposures, delayed or lack of access to healthcare, and poor general health, potentially increasing the severity of adverse effects of exposure.[6]*
- Determine factors associated with particular contaminant:

    Pesticides: Determine if client has ingested contaminated foods (e.g., fruits, vegetables, commercially raised meats) or inhaled agent (e.g., aerosol bug sprays, in vicinity of crop spraying).[2,3,9]

    Chemicals: Ascertain if client uses environmental contaminants in the home or at work (e.g., pesticides, chemicals, chlorine household cleaners) and fails to use or inappropriately uses protective clothing.[2,3,9]

    Pollution air/water: Determine if client has been exposed and is sensitive to atmospheric pollutants (e.g., radon, benzene [from gasoline], carbon monoxide, automobile emissions [numerous chemicals], chlorofluorocarbons [refrigerants, solvents], ozone or smog, particles [acids, organic chemicals, particles in smoke], commercial plants [e.g., pulp and paper mills]).[7]

    Investigate possibility of home-based exposure to air pollution—carbon monoxide (e.g., poor ventilation, especially in the winter months [poor heating systems, use of charcoal grill indoors, car left running in garage]; cigarette or cigar smoke indoors; ozone (spends a lot of time outdoors such as playing children, adults participating in moderate to strenuous work or recreational activities).[7]

    Biologicals: Determine if client may have been exposed to biological agents (bacteria, viruses, fungi) or bacterial toxins (e.g., botulinum, ricin). *Exposure occurring as a result of an act of terrorism would be rare; however, individuals may be exposed to bacterial agents or toxins through contaminated or poorly prepared foods.*

    Waste: Determine if client lives in area where trash and garbage accumulates, or is exposed to raw sewage or industrial wastes that can contaminate soil and water.

    Radiation: Ascertain if client/household member experienced accidental exposure (e.g., occupation in radiography, living near or working in nuclear industries, or electrical generating plants).

- Observe for signs and symptoms of infective agent and sepsis, such as fatigue, malaise, headache, fever, chills, diaphoresis, skin rash, and altered level of consciousness. *Initial symptoms of some diseases may mimic influenza and be misdiagnosed if healthcare providers do not maintain an index of suspicion.*
- Note presence and degree of chemical burns and initial treatment provided.
- Assist with diagnostic studies, as indicated. *Provides information about type and degree of exposure and organ involvement or damage.*
- Identify psychological response (e.g., anger, shock, acute anxiety, confusion, denial) to accidental or mass exposure incident. *Although these are normal responses, they may recycle repeatedly and result in post-trauma syndrome if not dealt with adequately.*
- Alert proper authorities to presence/exposure to contamination, as appropriate. *Depending on agent, there may be reporting requirements to local, state, and national agencies such as the local health department and Centers for Disease Control and Prevention (CDC).*

NURSING PRIORITY NO. 2

To assist in treating effects of exposure:

- Implement a coordinated decontamination plan (e.g., removal of clothing, showering with soap and water, other initial decontamination procedures) following consultation with medical toxicologist, hazardous materials team, industrial hygiene, and safety officer *to prevent further harm to client and to protect healthcare providers.*[8]
- Insure availability and proper use of personal protective equipment (PPE) (e.g., high-efficiency particulate air [HEPA] filter masks, special garments, and barrier materials, including gloves and face shield) *to protect from exposure to biological, chemical, and radioactive hazards.*[10]
- Provide for isolation or group/cohort individuals with same diagnosis or exposure, as resources require. *Limited resources may dictate open ward-like environment; however, the need to control spread of infection still exists. Only plague, smallpox, and viral hemorrhagic fevers require more than standard infection control precautions.*
- Provide therapeutic interventions, as individually appropriate. *Specific needs of the client and the level of care available at a given time and location determine response.*
- Refer pregnant client for individually appropriate diagnostic procedures or screenings. *Helpful in determining effects of teratogenic exposure on fetus allowing for informed choices and preparations.*[14]
- Screen breast milk in lactating client following radiation exposure. *Depending on type and amount of exposure, breastfeeding may need to be briefly interrupted or occasionally terminated.*[12,13]
- Cooperate with and refer to appropriate agencies (e.g., CDC; U.S. Army Medical Research Institute of Infectious Diseases [USAMRIID]; Federal Emergency Management Agency [FEMA]; Department of Health and Human Services [DHHS]; Office of Emergency Preparedness [OEP]; and Environmental Protection Agency [EPA]) *to prepare for and manage mass casualty incidents.*[9,10]

NURSING PRIORITY NO. 3

To promote wellness (Teaching/Discharge Considerations):

CLIENT/CAREGIVER
- Identify individual safety needs and injury or illness prevention in home, community, and work setting.
- Install carbon monoxide monitors and a radon detector in home, as appropriate.
- Review individual nutritional needs, appropriate exercise program, and need for rest. *Essentials for well-being and recovery.*
- Repair, replace, or correct unsafe household items and situations (e.g., storage of solvents in soda bottles, flaking or peeling paint or plaster, filtering unsafe tap water).
- Stress importance of supervising infant/child or individuals with cognitive limitations.
- Encourage removal of or proper cleaning of carpeted floors, especially for small children and persons with respiratory conditions. *Carpets hold up to 100 times as much fine particle material as a bare floor and can contain metals, pesticides.*[1]
- Identify commercial cleaning resources, if appropriate, *for safe cleaning of contaminated articles and surfaces.*
- Install dehumidifier in damp areas *to retard growth of molds.*[1]
- Encourage timely cleaning or replacement of air filters on furnace and air-conditioning unit. *Good ventilation cuts down on indoor air pollution from carpets, machines, paints, solvents, cleaning materials, and pesticides.*

- Discuss protective actions for specific "bad air" days (e.g., limiting or avoiding outdoor activities), especially in sensitive groups (e.g., children who are active outdoors, adults involved in moderate or strenuous outdoor activities, persons with respiratory diseases).[6]
- Review effects of secondhand smoke and importance of refraining from smoking in home and car where others are likely to be exposed.
- Recommend periodic inspection of well water and tap water *to identify possible contaminants.*
- Encourage client/caregiver to develop a personal or family disaster plan, to gather needed supplies to provide for self/family during a community emergency, and to learn how specific public health threats might affect client and actions *to reduce the risk to health and safety.*
- Instruct client to always refer to local authorities and health experts for specific up-to-date information for community, and to follow their advice.
- Refer to counselor or support groups for ongoing assistance in dealing with traumatic incident and aftereffects of exposure.
- Provide bibliotherapy including written resources and appropriate Web sites *for later review and self-paced learning.*
- Refer to smoking-cessation program, as needed.

COMMUNITY
- Promote community education programs in different modalities, languages, cultures, and educational levels geared *to increasing awareness of safety measures and resources available to individuals/community.*
- Review pertinent job-related health department and Occupational Safety and Health Administration (OSHA) regulations.
- Refer to resources that provide information about air quality (e.g., pollen index, "bad air days").
- Encourage community members/groups to engage in problem-solving activities.
- Verify presence or participate in developing a comprehensive disaster plan for the community that includes a chain of command, equipment, communication, training, decontamination area(s), and safety and security plans *to ensure an effective response to any emergency (e.g., flood, toxic spill, infectious disease outbreak, radiation release).*[11]

DOCUMENTATION FOCUS

Assessment/Reassessment
- Details of specific exposure, including location and circumstances.
- Client's/caregiver's understanding of individual risks/safety concerns.

Planning
- Plan of care and who is involved in planning.
- Teaching plan.

Implementation/Evaluation
- Individual responses to interventions, teaching, and actions performed.
- Specific actions and changes that are made.
- Attainment or progress toward desired outcome(s).
- Modifications to plan of care.

Discharge Planning
- Long-term plans for discharge needs, lifestyle and community changes, and who is responsible for actions to be taken.
- Specific referrals made.

References

1. McElgunn, V. (1990). Environmental hazards and child health and development: Advances in research and policy. Presentation in the Linking Research to Practice: Second Canadian Forum Proceedings Report and published by the Canadian Child Care Federation. Retrieved February 2007 from www.cfc-efc.ca/cccf.
2. Chemical toxins safety. (1999). Fact sheet for Resources for Child Care Givers. All Family Resources Web site. Retrieved February 2007 from www.familymanagement.com/childcare/facility/chemical.toxins.safety.html.
3. Rajen, M. (2006). Toxins everywhere. *New Straits Times*. Retrieved February 2007 from www.redorbit.com/news/health/786618/toxins_everywhere/index.html.
4. Stabin, M. G., Breitz, H. (2000). Breast milk secretion of radiopharmaceuticals; mechanisms, findings, and radiation dosimetry. *J Nuclear Med*, 41(5), 863–873.
5. Environmental Protection Agency. (1998). *The EPA Children's Environmental Health Yearbook, Chapter 1*. Washington, DC: U.S. Department of Health and Human Services.
6. Wilkinson, R., Marmot, M. (2003). *Social Determinants of Health: The Solid Facts*. 2d ed. Copenhagen, Denmark: World Health Organization.
7. Smog—Who does it hurt? What you need to know about ozone and your health. (1999). *Public information brochure*. Washington, DC: U.S. Environmental Protection Agency.
8. Jagminas, L. (2005). CBRN-Evaluation of a biological warfare victim. Retrieved February 2007 from www.emedicime.com/emerg/topic891.htm.
9. Jagminas, L., Erdman, D. P. (2006). CBRNE—Chemical decontamination. Retrieved February 2007 from www.emedicime.com/emerg/topic893.htm.
10. Arnold, J. L. (2006). Personal protective equipment. Article for patient education. Retrieved February 2007 from www.emedicinehealth.com.
11. Bauer, J., Steinhauer, R. (2002). A readied response: The emergency plan. *RN*, 65(6), 40.
12. When should a mother avoid breastfeeding? (August 2006). Centers for Disease Control and Prevention. Retrieved February 2007 from www.cdc.gov/breastfeeding/disease/contraindicators.htm.
13. Breastfeeding guidelines following radiopharmaceutical administration. Retrieved February 2007 from http://nuclearpharmacy.uams.edu/resources/breastfeeding.asp.
14. American Academy of Family Physicians: Breastfeeding (Position paper). Retrieved February 2007 from www.aafp.org/online/en/home/policy/policies/b/breastfeedingpositionpaper.html.

risk for Contamination

DEFINITION: Accentuated risk of exposure to environmental contaminants in doses sufficient to cause adverse health effects

RISK FACTORS

External
Chemical contamination of food or water; presence of atmospheric pollutants
Inadequate municipal services (trash removal, sewage treatment facilities)
Geographic area (living in area where high level of contaminants exist)
Playing in outdoor areas where environmental contaminants are used
Personal or household hygiene practices
Living in poverty (increases potential for multiple exposure, lack of access to healthcare, and poor diet)
Use of environmental contaminants in the home (e.g., pesticides, chemicals, environmental tobacco smoke)

Cultural   Collaborative   Community/Home Care   Diagnostic Studies   Pediatric/Geriatric/Lifespan   Medications

Lack of breakdown of contaminants once indoors (breakdown is inhibited without sun and rain exposure)

Flooring surface (carpeted surfaces hold contaminant residue more than hard floor surfaces)

Flaking, peeling paint or plaster in presence of young children

Paint, lacquer, and so forth, in poorly ventilated areas or without effective protection

Inappropriate use or lack of protective clothing

Unprotected contact with heavy metals or chemicals (e.g., arsenic, chromium, lead)

Exposure to radiation (occupation in radiography, employment in nuclear industries and electrical generating plants, living near nuclear industries and electrical generation plants)

Exposure to disaster (natural or man-made); exposure to bioterrorism

Internal

Age (children less than 5 years, older adults); gestational age during exposure; developmental characteristics of children

Female gender; pregnancy

Nutritional factors (e.g., obesity, vitamin and mineral deficiencies)

Preexisting disease states; smoking

Concomitant exposure; previous exposures

NOTE: A risk diagnosis is not evidenced by signs and symptoms, as the problem has not occurred; rather, nursing interventions are directed at prevention.

Sample Clinical Applications: *Escherichia coli* infection, plague, hantavirus, asthma, botulism, cholera, lead or other heavy metal poisoning, chemical burns, asbestosis, carbon monoxide poisoning, radiation sickness

DESIRED OUTCOMES/EVALUATION CRITERIA

Sample **NOC** linkages:

Knowledge: Personal Safety: Extent of understanding conveyed about prevention of unintentional injuries

Risk Control: Personal actions to prevent, eliminate, or reduce modifiable health threats

Client Will (Include Specific Time Frame)
- Verbalize understanding of individual factors that contribute to possibility of injury and take steps to correct situation(s).
- Demonstrate behaviors, lifestyle changes to reduce risk factors and protect self from injury.
- Modify environment as indicated to enhance safety.
- Be free of injury.
- Support community activities for disaster preparedness.

Sample **NOC** linkages:

Community Health Status: General state of well-being of a community or population

Community Risk Control: Lead Exposure: Community actions to reduce lead exposure and poisoning

Community Disaster Readiness: Community preparedness to respond to a natural or man-made calamitous event

Community Will (Include Specific Time Frame)
- Identify hazards that could lead to exposure or contamination.
- Correct environmental hazards as identified.
- Demonstrate necessary actions to promote community safety and disaster preparedness.

ACTIONS/INTERVENTIONS

Sample **NIC** linkages:

Risk Identification: Analysis of potential risk factors, determination of health risks, and prioritization of risk-reduction strategies for an individual or group

Community Health Development: Assisting members of a community to identify a community's health concerns, mobilize resources, and implement solutions

Environmental Risk Protection: Preventing and detecting disease and injury in populations at risk from environmental hazards

NURSING PRIORITY NO. 1

To evaluate degree/source of risk inherent in the home, community, and work site:

- Ascertain type of contaminant(s) and exposure routes posing a potential hazard to client or community (e.g., air, soil, or water pollutants; food source, chemical, biological, radiation) as listed in Risk Factors. *Determines course of action to be taken by client/community/care providers.*
- Note age and gender of client(s) or community base (e.g., community health clinic serving primarily poor children or elderly; school near large industrial plant, family living in smog-prone area). *Young children, frail elderly, and females have been found to be at higher risk for effects of exposure to toxins.*[1,2] (Refer to ND Contamination.)
- Ascertain client's geographic location at home or work (e.g., lives where crop spraying is routine; works in nuclear plant; contract worker or soldier returning from combat area). *Individual and/or community intervention may be needed to reduce risks of accidental or intentional exposures.*
- Note socioeconomic status and availability and use of resources. *Living in poverty increases the potential for multiple exposures, delayed or lack of access to healthcare, and poor general health.*[3]
- Determine client's/SO's understanding of potential risk and appropriate protective measures.

NURSING PRIORITY NO. 2

To assist client to reduce or correct individual risk factors:

- Assist client to develop plan to address individual safety needs and injury or illness prevention in home, community, and work setting.
- Repair, replace, or correct unsafe household items or situations (e.g., flaking or peeling paint or plaster, filtering unsafe tap water).
- Review effects of secondhand smoke and importance of refraining from smoking in home or car *where others are likely to be exposed.*
- Encourage removal or proper cleaning of carpeted floors, especially for small children, persons with respiratory conditions. *Carpets hold up to 100 times as much fine-particle material as a bare floor and can contain metals, pesticides.*[1]
- Encourage timely cleaning or replacement of air filters on furnace and air-conditioning unit. *Good ventilation cuts down on indoor air pollution from carpets, machines, paints, solvents, cleaning materials, and pesticides.*
- Recommend periodic inspection of well water and tap water *to identify possible contaminants.*
- Encourage client to install carbon monoxide monitors and a radon detector in home as appropriate.
- Recommend placing dehumidifier in damp areas *to retard growth of molds.*

🌐 Cultural 😊 Collaborative 🏠 Community/Home Care 🧪 Diagnostic Studies ∞ Pediatric/Geriatric/Lifespan 💊 Medications

- Review proper handling of household chemicals:[4,5]
  Read chemical labels *to be aware of primary hazards (especially in commonly used house-hold cleaning and gardening products)*.
  Follow directions printed on product label (e.g., avoid use of certain chemicals on food preparation surfaces, refrain from spraying garden chemicals on windy days).
  Choose least hazardous products for the job, preferably multiuse products *to reduce number of different chemicals used and stored*. Use products labeled "nontoxic" wherever possible.
  Use form of chemical that most reduces risk of exposure (e.g., cream instead of liquid or aerosol).
  Wear protective clothing, gloves, and safety glasses when using chemicals. Avoid mixing chemicals at all times, and use in well-ventilated areas.
  Store chemicals in locked cabinets. Keep chemicals in original labeled containers and do not pour into other containers.
- Place safety stickers on chemicals *to warn of harmful contents*.
- Review proper food-handling, storage, and cooking techniques.
- Stress importance of pregnant or lactating women following fish or wildlife consumption guidelines provided by state, U.S. territorial, or Native American tribes. *Ingestion of non-commercial fish or wildlife can be a significant source of pollutants.*[8]

NURSING PRIORITY NO. 3

To promote wellness (Teaching/Discharge Considerations):

HOME

- Discuss general safety concerns with client/SO.
- Stress importance of supervising infant/child or individuals with cognitive limitations.
- Post emergency and poison control numbers in a visible location.
- Encourage learning cardiopulmonary resuscitation (CPR) and first aid.
- Discuss protective actions for specific "bad air" days (e.g., limiting/avoiding outdoor activities).
- Review pertinent job-related safety regulations. Stress necessity of wearing appropriate protective equipment.
- Encourage client/caregiver develop a personal/family disaster plan, to gather needed supplies to provide for self/family during a community emergency; to learn how specific public health threats might affect client and actions to promote preparedness and reduce the risk to health and safety.
- Provide information and refer to appropriate resources about potential toxic hazards and protective measures. Provide bibliotherapy including written resources and appropriate Web sites *for client review and self-paced learning*.
- Refer to smoking-cessation program as needed.

COMMUNITY

- Promote education programs geared toward increasing awareness of safety measures and resources available to individuals/community.
- Review pertinent job-related health department and Occupational Safety and Health Administration (OSHA) regulations to safeguard the workplace and the community.
- Verify presence or participate in developing a comprehensive disaster plan for the community that includes a chain of command, equipment, communication, training, decontamination area(s), safety and security plans *to ensure an effective response to any emergency (e.g., flood, toxic spill, infectious disease outbreak, radiation release).*[6]
- Refer to appropriate agencies (e.g., Centers for Disease Control and Prevention [CDC], U.S. Army Medical Research Institute of Infectious Diseases [USAMRIID]; Federal Emergency Management Agency [FEMA]; Department of Health and Human Services [DHHS], Office of Emergency Preparedness [OEP]; EPA) *to prepare for and manage mass casualty incidents.*[7]

DOCUMENTATION FOCUS

Assessment/Reassessment
• Client's/caregiver's understanding of individual risks and safety concerns.

Planning
• Plan of care and who is involved in planning.
• Teaching plan.

Implementation/Evaluation
• Individual responses to interventions, teaching, and actions performed.
• Specific actions and changes that are made.
• Attainment or progress toward desired outcome(s).
• Modifications to plan of care.

Discharge Planning
• Long-term plans, lifestyle and community changes, and who is responsible for actions to be taken.
• Specific referrals made.

References

1. McElgunn, V. (1990). Environmental hazards and child health and development: Advances in research and policy. Presentation in the Linking Research to Practice: Second Canadian Forum Proceedings Report and published by the Canadian Child Care Federation. Retrieved February 2007 from www.cfc-efc.ca/cccf.
2. Environmental Protection Agency. (1998). *The EPA Children's Environmental Health Yearbook, Chapter 1*. Washington, DC: U.S. Department of Health and Human Services.
3. Wilkinson, R., Marmot, M. (2003). *Social Determinants of Health: The Solid Facts*. 2d ed. Copenhagen, Denmark: World Health Organization.
4. Rajen, M. (2006). Toxins everywhere. *New Straits Times*. Retrieved February 2007 from www.redorbit.com/news/health/786618/toxins_everywhere/index.html.
5. Chemical toxins safety. (1999). Fact sheet for Resources for Child Care Givers. All Family Resources Web site. Retrieved February 2007 from www.familymanagement.com/childcare/facility/chemical.toxins.safety.html.
6. Bauer, J., Steinhauer, R. (2002). A readied response: The emergency plan. *RN*, 65(6), 40.
7. Jagminas, L., Erdman, D. P. (2006). CBRNE-Chemical decontamination. Retrieved February 2007 from www.emedicime.com/emerg/topic893.htm.
8. American Academy of Family Physicians: Breastfeeding (Position paper). Retrieved February 2007 from www.aafp.org/online/en/home/policy/policies/b/breastfeedingpositionpaper.html.

compromised family Coping

DEFINITION: Usually supportive primary person (family member or close friend [SO]) provides insufficient, ineffective, or compromised support, comfort, assistance, or encouragement that may be needed by the client to manage or master adaptive tasks related to his or her health challenge

RELATED FACTORS

Coexisting situations affecting the significant person
Developmental or situational crises the significant person may be facing

🌐 Cultural ⚛ Collaborative 🏠 Community/Home Care ⬚ Diagnostic Studies ∞ Pediatric/Geriatric/Lifespan ⚗ Medications

Prolonged disease [or disability progression] that exhausts the supportive capacity of SO(s)
Exhaustion of supportive capacity of significant people
Inadequate or incorrect understanding of information by a primary person
Lack of reciprocal support; little support provided by client, in turn, for primary person;
[unrealistic expectations of client/SO(s) or each other]
Temporary preoccupation by a significant person
Temporary family disorganization or role changes
[Lack of mutual decision-making skills]
[Diverse coalitions of family members]

DEFINING CHARACTERISTICS

Subjective
Client expresses a complaint or concern about significant other's response to health problem
SO expresses an inadequate knowledge base or understanding, which interferes with effective supportive behaviors
SO describes preoccupation with personal reaction (e.g., fear, anticipatory grief, guilt, anxiety) to client's need

Objective
SO attempts assistive or supportive behaviors with less-than-satisfactory results
SO displays protective behavior disproportionate to the client's abilities or need for autonomy
SO enters into limited personal communication with client
SO withdraws from client
[SO displays sudden outbursts of emotions or emotional lability, or interferes with necessary nursing/medical interventions]

Sample Clinical Applications: Chronic conditions (e.g., chronic obstructive pulmonary disease [COPD], AIDS, Alzheimer's disease, pain, renal failure), substance abuse, cancer, depression, hypochondriasis

DESIRED OUTCOMES/EVALUATION CRITERIA

Sample (NOC) linkages:
Family Coping: Family actions to manage stressors that tax family resources
Family Normalization: Capacity of the family system to develop strategies for optimal functioning when a member has a chronic illness or disability
Family Social Climate: Supportive milieu as characterized by family member relationships and goals

Family Will (Include Specific Time Frame)
• Identify resources within themselves to deal with the situation.
• Interact appropriately with the client, providing support and assistance, as indicated.
• Provide opportunity for client to deal with situation in own way.
• Verbalize knowledge and understanding of illness, disability, or condition.
• Express feelings honestly.
• Identify need for outside support and seek such.

(continues on page 224)

---

compromised family Coping (continued)
ACTIONS/INTERVENTIONS

Sample (NIC) linkages:
Family Involvement Promotion: Facilitating family participation in the emotional and physical care of the patient
Family Support: Promotion of family values, interests, and goals
Family Mobilization: Utilization of family strengths to influence patient's health in a positive direction

NURSING PRIORITY NO. 1

To assess causative/contributing factors:

- Identify underlying situation(s) that may contribute to the inability of family to provide needed assistance to the client. *Circumstances may have preceded the illness and now have a significant effect (e.g., client had a heart attack during sexual activity, mate is afraid of repeating).*[1]
- Note cultural factors related to family relationships that may be involved in problems of caring for member who is ill. *Family composition and structure, methods of decision making, and gender issues and expectations will affect how family deals with stress of illness/ negative prognosis. Depending on role the ill client has in the family (e.g, mother or father) other members may have difficulty assuming authoritative role and managing the family.*[6]
- Note the length of illness or condition (e.g., cancer, multiple sclerosis [MS]), and/or other long-term situations that may exist. *Chronic or unresolved illness, accompanied by changes in role performance or responsibility, often exhausts supportive capacity and coping abilities of SO/family.*[1]
- Assess information available to and understood by the family/SO(s). *Access to and understanding of information regarding the specific illness or condition, treatment, and prognosis is essential to family cooperation and care of the client.*[2,3]
- Discuss family perceptions of situation. *Expectations of client and family members may/may not be realistic and may interfere with ability to cope with situation.*[1]
- Identify role of the client in family and how illness has changed the family organization. *Illness affects how client performs usual functions in the family and affects how others in the family take over those responsibilities. These changes may result in dysfunctional behaviors, anger, hostility, and hopelessness.*[1]
- Note factors (beside the client's illness) that are affecting abilities of family members to provide needed support. *Individual members' preoccupation with own needs and concerns can interfere with providing needed care or support during stresses of long-term illness. Additionally, caregivers may incur decreased or lost income, or risk losing own health insurance if they alter their work hours to care for client.*[1]

NURSING PRIORITY NO. 2

To assist family to reactivate/develop skills to deal with current situation:

- Listen to client's/SO's comments, remarks, and expression of concern(s). Note nonverbal behaviors and responses and congruency. *Provides information and promotes understanding of client's view of the illness and needs related to current situation.*[1]
- Encourage family members to verbalize feelings openly and clearly. *Promotes understanding of feelings in relationship to current events, and helps them to hear what other person is saying, leading to more appropriate interactions.*[5]

- Discuss underlying reasons for client's behavior. *Helps family/SO understand and accept or deal with client behaviors that may be triggered by emotional or physical effects of illness.*[4]
- Assist the family and client to understand "who owns the problem" and who is responsible for resolution. Avoid placing blame or guilt. *When these boundaries are defined, each individual can begin to take care of own self and stop taking care of others in inappropriate ways.*[3,4]
- Encourage client and family to develop problem-solving skills to deal with the situation. *Use of these skills enables each member of the family to identify what he or she sees as the problem to be dealt with and contribute ideas for solutions that are acceptable to them, promoting more effective interactions among the family members.*[4]

NURSING PRIORITY NO. 3

To promote wellness (Teaching/Discharge Considerations):

- Provide information for family/SO(s) about specific illness/condition. *Promotes better understanding of need for following therapeutic regimen to provide maximum benefit.*[8]
- Involve client and family in planning care as often as possible. *When family members are knowledgeable and understand needs, commitment to plan is enhanced.*[7,8]
- Promote assistance of family in providing client care, as appropriate. *Identifies ways of demonstrating support while maintaining client's independence (e.g., providing favorite foods, engaging in diversional activities).*[5]
- Refer to appropriate resources for assistance, as indicated (e.g., counseling, psychotherapy, financial, spiritual). *May need additional help, and getting to the appropriate resource provides accurate help for individual situation (e.g., family counseling, financial planning).*[7,8]
- Refer to NDs Anxiety, death Anxiety, ineffective Coping, readiness for enhanced family Coping, disabled family Coping, Fear, Grieving, as appropriate.

DOCUMENTATION FOCUS

Assessment/Reassessment
- Assessment findings, including current and past coping behaviors, emotional response to situation and stressors.
- Availability and use of support systems.

Planning
- Plan of care, who is involved in planning and areas of responsibility.
- Teaching plan.

Implementation/Evaluation
- Responses of family members/client to interventions, teaching, and actions performed.
- Attainment or progress toward desired outcome(s).
- Modifications to plan of care.

Discharge Planning
- Long-term plans and who is responsible for actions.
- Specific referrals made.

References

1. Doenges, M., Moorhouse, M., Geissler-Murr, A. (2002). *Nursing Care Plans: Guidelines for Individualizing Patient Care.* 6th ed. Philadelphia: F. A. Davis.
2. Bluman, I. G., et al. (1999). Attitudes, knowledge, and risk perceptions of women with breast and/or ovarian cancer considering testing for BRCA1 and BRCA2. *J Clin Oncol,* 17(3), 1040–1046.

3. Doenges, M., Townsend, M., Moorhouse, M. (1998). *Psychiatric Care Plans: Guidelines for Individualizing Care*. 3d ed. Philadelphia: F. A. Davis.
4. Townsend, M. (2006). *Psychiatric Mental Health Nursing: Concepts of Care*. 5th ed. Philadelphia: F. A. Davis.
5. Cox, H., et al. (2002). *Clinical Applications of Nursing Diagnosis: Adult, Child, Women's, Psychiatric, Gerontic, and Home Health Considerations*. 4th ed. Philadelphia: F. A. Davis.
6. Lipson, J. G., Dibble, S. L., Minarik, P. A. (1996). *Culture & Nursing Care: A Pocket Guide*. San Francisco: UCSF Nursing Press.
7. Hareven, T. K., Adams, K. J. (eds). (1982). *Aging and Life Course Transitions: An Interdisciplinary Perspective*. New York: Guilford.
8. Ammon, S. (2001). Managing patients with heart failure. *Am J Nurs*, 101(12), 34–40.

defensive Coping

DEFINITION: Repeated projection of falsely positive self-evaluation based on a self-protective pattern that defends against underlying perceived threats to positive self-regard

RELATED FACTORS

Conflict between self-perception and value system; uncertainty
Fear of failure, humiliation, or repercussions; low level of self confidence
Low level of confidence in others; deficient support system
Unrealistic expectations of self
Lack of resilience
Low level of confidence in others

DEFINING CHARACTERISTICS

Subjective
Denial of obvious problems or weaknesses
Projection of blame or responsibility
Hypersensitive to slight or criticism
Grandiosity
Rationalizes failures
[Refuses or rejects assistance]

Objective
Superior attitude toward others
Difficulty establishing or maintaining relationships; [avoidance of intimacy]
Hostile laughter; ridicule of others; [aggressive behavior]
Difficulty in perception of reality testing or reality distortion
Lack of follow-through in treatment or therapy
Lack of participation in treatment or therapy
[Attention-seeking behavior]

Sample Clinical Applications: Eating disorders, substance abuse, chronic illness; bipolar, adjustment, or dissociative disorders

🌐 Cultural   Collaborative   🏠 Community/Home Care   Diagnostic Studies   ∞ Pediatric/Geriatric/Lifespan   Medications

DESIRED OUTCOMES/EVALUATION CRITERIA

Sample (NOC) linkages:
Self-Esteem: Personal judgment of self-worth
Coping: Actions to manage stressors that tax an individual's resources
Social Interaction Skills: An individual's use of effective interaction behaviors

Client Will (Include Specific Time Frame)
• Verbalize understanding of own problems and stressors.
• Identify areas of concern or problems.
• Demonstrate acceptance of responsibility for own actions, successes, and failures.
• Participate in treatment program or therapy.
• Maintain involvement in relationships.

ACTIONS/INTERVENTIONS

Sample (NIC) linkages:
Self-Awareness Enhancement: Assisting a patient to explore and understand his or her thoughts, feelings, motivations, and behaviors
Coping Enhancement: Assisting a patient to adapt to perceived stressors, changes, or threats that interfere with meeting life demands and roles
Counseling: Use of an interactive helping process focusing on the needs, problems, or feelings of the patient and significant others to enhance or support coping, problem-solving, and interpersonal relationships

NURSING PRIORITY NO. 1

To determine degree of impairment:

● Assess ability to comprehend current situation, developmental level of functioning. *Crucial to planning care for this individual. Client will have difficulty functioning in these circumstances.*[1]
● Determine level of anxiety and effectiveness of current coping mechanisms. *Severe anxiety will interfere with ability to cope, and client will need to assess what is working and develop new ways to deal with current situation.*[2]
● Perform or review results of testing, such as Taylor Manifest Anxiety Scale (T-MAS) and Marlowe-Crowne Social Desirability Scale (MCSDS), as indicated. *Helps to identify coping styles, enabling more accurate therapeutic interventions.*
● Determine coping mechanisms used (e.g., projection, avoidance, rationalization) and purpose of coping strategy (e.g., may mask low self-esteem). *Provides information about how these behaviors affect current situation.*[3]
● Assist client to identify and consider need to address problem differently. *Until client is willing to consider different approaches to dealing with situation, little progress can be expected.*[1]
● Describe all aspects of the problem through the use of therapeutic communication skills such as Active-listening. *Provides an opportunity for the client to clarify the situation and begin to look at options for problem-solving.*[2]
● Observe interactions with others. *Noting difficulties and ability to establish satisfactory relationships can provide clues to client behaviors that interfere with interactions with others.*[2]

- Note availability of family/friends support for client in current situation. *SOs may not be supportive when person is denying problems or exhibiting unacceptable behaviors.*
- Note expressions of grandiosity in the face of contrary evidence (e.g., "I'm going to buy a new car" when the individual has no job or available finances). *Evidence of distorted thinking and possibility of mental illness.*[3]
- Assess physical condition. *Defensive coping style has been connected with physical well-being and illnesses, especially chronic health concerns (e.g., congestive heart failure [CHF], diabetes, chronic fatigue syndrome).*[5]

NURSING PRIORITY NO. 2

To assist client to deal with current situation:

- Provide explanation of rules of the treatment program, and discuss consequences of lack of cooperation. Encourage client participation in setting of consequences and agreement to them. *Promotes understanding and possibility of cooperation on the part of the client, especially when they have been involved in the decisions.*[2]
- Set limits on manipulative behavior; be consistent in enforcing consequences when rules are broken and limits tested. *Providing clear information and following through on identified consequences reduces the ability to manipulate staff or therapist and environment.*[3]
- Develop therapeutic relationship to enable client to test new behaviors in a safe environment. Use positive, nonjudgmental approach and I-messages. *Promotes sense of self-esteem and enhances sense of control.*[1]
- Encourage control in all situations possible; include client in decisions and planning. *Preserves autonomy, enabling realization of sense of self-worth.*[1]
- Acknowledge individual strengths and incorporate awareness of personal assets and strengths in plan. *Promotes use of positive coping behaviors and progress toward effective solutions.*[4]
- Convey attitude of acceptance and respect (unconditional positive regard). *Avoids threatening client's self-concept, preserving existing self-esteem.*[2]
- Encourage identification and expression of feelings. *Provides opportunity for client to learn about and accept self and feelings as normal.*[2]
- Provide or encourage use of healthy outlets for release of hostile feelings (e.g., punching bags, pounding boards). Involve in outdoor recreation program when available. *Promotes acceptable expression of these feelings, which, when unexpressed, can lead to development of undesirable behaviors and make situation worse.*[4]
- Provide opportunities for client to interact with others in a positive manner. *Promotes self-esteem and encourages client to learn how to develop and enhance relationships.*[4]
- Assist client with problem-solving process. Identify and discuss responses to situation, maladaptive coping skills. Suggest alternative responses to situation. *Helps client select more adaptive strategies for coping.*[2]
- Use confrontation judiciously *to help client begin to identify defense mechanisms (e.g., denial, projection) that are hindering development of satisfying relationships.*[2]
- Assist with treatments for physical illnesses as appropriate. *Taking care of physical self will enable client to deal with emotional and psychological issues more effectively.*[4]

NURSING PRIORITY NO. 3

To promote wellness (Teaching/Discharge Considerations):

- Use cognitive-behavioral therapy. *Helps change negative thinking patterns when rigidly held beliefs are used by client to defend the individual against low self-esteem.*[3]

Cultural Collaborative Community/Home Care Diagnostic Studies Pediatric/Geriatric/Lifespan Medications

- Encourage client to learn and use relaxation techniques, guided imagery, and positive affirmation of self. *Enables client to incorporate and practice new behaviors to deal with stressors and view or respond to situation in a more realistic and positive manner.*[4]
- Promote involvement in activities or classes as appropriate. *Client can practice new skills, develop new relationships, and learn new and positive ways of interacting with others.*[1]
- Refer to additional resources (e.g., substance rehabilitation, family or marital therapy), as indicated. *Can be useful in making desired changes and developing new coping skills.*[2]
- Refer to ND ineffective Coping for additional interventions.

DOCUMENTATION FOCUS

Assessment/Reassessment
- Assessment findings, client perception of the present situation, presenting behaviors.
- Usual coping methods, degree of impairment.
- Health concerns.

Planning
- Plan of care, specific interventions, and who is involved in development of the plan.
- Teaching plan.

Implementation/Evaluation
- Response to interventions, teaching, and actions performed.
- Attainment or progress toward desired outcome(s).
- Modifications to plan of care.

Discharge Planning
- Referrals and follow-up programming.

References

1. Doenges, M., Moorhouse, M., Murr, A. (2004). *Nursing Care Plans: Guidelines for Individualizing Patient Care*. 7th ed. Philadelphia: F. A. Davis.
2. Doenges, M., Townsend, M., Moorhouse, M. (1998). *Psychiatric Care Plans: Guidelines for Individualizing Care*. 3d ed. Philadelphia: F. A. Davis.
3. Townsend, M. (2006). *Psychiatric Mental Health Nursing: Concepts of Care*. 5th ed. Philadelphia: F. A. Davis.
4. Cox, H., et al. (2002). *Clinical Applications of Nursing Diagnosis: Adult, Child, Women's, Psychiatric, Gerontic, and Home Health Considerations*. 4th ed. Philadelphia: F. A. Davis.
5. Creswell, C., Chalder, T. (2001). Defensive coping styles in chronic fatigue syndrome. *J Psychosom Res*, 51(4), 607–610.

disabled family Coping

DEFINITION: Behavior of significant person (family member or other primary person) that disables his or her capacities and the client's capacities to effectively address tasks essential to either person's adaptation to the health challenge

RELATED FACTORS

Significant person with chronically unexpressed feelings (e.g., guilt, anxiety, hostility, despair)
Dissonant coping styles for dealing with adaptive tasks by the significant person and client among significant people
Highly ambivalent family relationships
Arbitrary handling of family's resistance to treatment [that tends to solidify defensiveness as it fails to deal adequately with underlying anxiety]
[High-risk family situations, such as single or adolescent parent, abusive relationship, substance abuse, acute or chronic disabilities, member with terminal illness]

DEFINING CHARACTERISTICS

Subjective
[Expresses despair regarding family reactions or lack of involvement]

Objective
Psychosomaticism
Intolerance; rejection; abandonment; desertion; agitation; aggression; hostility; depression
Carrying on usual routines without regard for client's needs; disregarding client's needs
Neglectful care of the client in regard to basic human needs or illness treatment
Neglectful relationships with other family members.
Family behaviors that are detrimental to well-being
Distortion of reality regarding the client's health problem
Impaired restructuring of a meaningful life for self, impaired individualization, prolonged overconcern for client
Taking on illness signs of client
Client's development of dependence

Sample Clinical Applications: Chronic conditions (e.g., chronic obstructive pulmonary disease [COPD], AIDS, Alzheimer's disease, chronic pain, renal failure, brain/spinal cord injury [SCI]), substance abuse, cancer, genetic conditions (e.g., Down syndrome, sickle cell disease, Huntington's disease), depression, hypochondriasis

DESIRED OUTCOMES/EVALUATION CRITERIA

Sample NOC linkages:
Family Normalization: Capacity of the family system to develop strategies for optimal functioning when a member has a chronic illness or disability
Family Coping: Family actions to manage stressors that tax family resources
Family Social Climate: Supportive milieu as characterized by family member relationships and goals

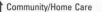

> **Family Will (Include Specific Time Frame)**
> • Verbalize more realistic understanding and expectations of the client.
> • Visit or contact client regularly.
> • Participate positively in care of client, within limits of family's abilities and client's needs.
> • Express feelings and expectations openly and honestly as appropriate.
>
> **ACTIONS/INTERVENTIONS**
>
> Sample **NIC** linkages:
> **Family Therapy:** Assisting family members to move their family toward a more productive way of living
> **Family Support:** Promotion of family values, interests, and goals
> **Family Involvement Promotion:** Facilitating family participation in the emotional and physical care of the patient

NURSING PRIORITY NO. 1

To assess causative/contributing factors:

- Ascertain preillness behaviors and interactions of the family. *Provides comparative baseline for developing plan of care and determining interventions needed.*[4,8]
- Identify current behaviors of the family members (e.g., withdrawal or not visiting, brief visits, or ignoring client when visiting; anger and hostility toward client and others; ways of touching between family members; expressions of guilt). *Indicators of extent of problems existing within family. Relationships among family members before and after current illness affect ability to deal with problems of caretaking and lengthy illness.*[1,8]
- Discuss family perceptions of situation. *Expectations of client and family members may not be realistic and may interfere with ability to deal with situation.*[6]
- Note cultural factors related to family relationships that may be involved in problems of caring for member who is ill. *Family composition and structure, methods of decision making, gender issues, and expectations will affect how family perceives situation and deals with stress of illness, negative prognosis.*[7]
- Note other factors that may be stressful for the family (e.g., financial difficulties or lack of community support, as when illness occurs when out of town). *Appropriate referrals can be made to provide information and assistance as needed. If not addressed, these problems can lead to caregiver burnout and compassion fatigue.*[6]
- Determine readiness of family members to be involved with care of the client. *Family members are involved in their lives, jobs, and families and may find it difficult to manage tasks necessary for helping with care of the client.*[5,6]

NURSING PRIORITY NO. 2

To provide assistance to enable family to deal with the current situation:

- Establish rapport with family members who are available. *Promotes therapeutic relationship and support for problem-solving solutions.*[1]
- Acknowledge difficulty of the situation for the family. *Communicates understanding of family's feelings and can reduce blaming and guilt feelings.*[2]
- Active-listen concerns, note both overconcern and lack of concern. *Identifies accuracy of client's information and measure of concern, which may interfere with ability to resolve situation.*[2]

- Allow free expression of feelings, including frustration, anger, hostility, and hopelessness while placing limits on acting out or inappropriate behaviors. *Provides opportunity to identify accuracy and validate appropriateness of feelings. Limits or minimizes risk of violent behavior.*[4]
- Give accurate information to SO(s) from the beginning. *Establishes trust and promotes opportunity for clarification and correction of misunderstandings.*[4]
- Act as liaison between family and healthcare providers. *Establishes single contact to provide explanations and clarify treatment plan, enhancing reliability of information.*[4]
- Provide brief, simple explanations about use and alarms when equipment (such as a ventilator) is required. Identify appropriate professional(s) for continued support and problem-solving. *Having information and ready access to appropriate resources can reduce feelings of helplessness and promote sense of control.*[1]
- Provide time for private interaction between client and family/SO(s). *Individuals need to talk about what is happening and process new and frightening information to learn to deal with situation or diagnosis within family relationships.*[3]
- Accompany family when they visit client. *Being available for questions, concerns, and support promotes trusting relationship in which family feels free to learn all they can about situation or diagnosis.*[3]
- Assist SO(s) to initiate therapeutic communication with client. *Learning to use new methods of communication (Active-listening and I-messages) can enhance relationships and promote effective problem-solving for the family.*[3]
- Include SO(s) in the plan of care. Provide instruction and demonstrate necessary skills. *Promotes family's ability to provide care and develop a sense of control over difficult situation.*[3,5]
- Refer client to protective services as necessitated by risk of physical harm or neglect. *Removing client from home enhances individual safety. May reduce stress on family to allow opportunity for therapeutic intervention.*[3]

NURSING PRIORITY NO. 3

To promote wellness (Teaching/Discharge Considerations):

- Assist family to identify coping skills being used and how these skills are or are not helping them deal with situation. *When family members know this information, they can begin to enhance those skills that are more effective in promoting healthy family functioning in difficult times.*[3]
- Answer family's questions patiently and honestly. Reinforce information provided by other providers. *Continues trusting relationship with family members and promotes understanding of the situation/prognosis so family members can deal more effectively with what is happening.*[1]
- Reframe negative expressions into positive whenever possible. *A positive frame contributes to supportive interactions and can lead to better outcomes.*[3]
- Respect family needs for withdrawal and intervene judiciously. *Situation may be overwhelming, and time away can be beneficial to continued participation. A brief respite can refresh family members who are serving as caregivers and permit renewed ability to manage situation.*[1]
- Encourage family to deal with the situation in small increments rather than trying to deal with the whole picture. *Reduces likelihood of individual being overwhelmed by possibilities that may face them in potentially disabling or fatal outcomes.*[1]
- Assist the family to identify familiar things that would be helpful to the client (e.g., a family picture on the wall), especially when hospitalized for long time, such as in hospice or

long-term care. *Reinforces and maintains orientation and provides a sense of home and family for client.*[1,5]

🏠 ● Refer family to appropriate resources as needed (e.g., family therapy, financial counseling, spiritual advisor). *May need additional help to deal with difficult situation or illness.*[6]

● Refer to ND Grieving as appropriate.

DOCUMENTATION FOCUS

Assessment/Reassessment
• Assessment findings, current and past behaviors, family members who are directly involved and support systems available.
• Emotional response(s) to situation or stressors.
• Specific health and therapy challenges.

Planning
• Plan of care, specific interventions, and who is involved in planning.
• Teaching plan.

Implementation/Evaluation
• Responses of individuals to interventions, teaching, and actions performed.
• Attainment or progress toward desired outcome(s).
• Modifications to plan of care.

Discharge Planning
• Ongoing needs, available resources, other follow up recommendations, and who is responsible for actions.
• Specific referrals made.

References

1. Doenges, M., Moorhouse, M., Murr, A. (2002). *Nursing Care Plans: Guidelines for Individualizing Patient Care.* 6th ed. Philadelphia: F. A. Davis.
2. Doenges, M., Townsend, M., Moorhouse, M. (1998). *Psychiatric Care Plans: Guidelines for Individualizing Care.* 3d ed. Philadelphia: F. A. Davis.
3. Townsend, M. (2003). *Psychiatric Mental Health Nursing: Concepts of Care.* 4th ed. Philadelphia: F. A. Davis.
4. Cox, H., et al. (2002). *Clinical Applications of Nursing Diagnosis: Adult, Child, Women's, Psychiatric, Gerontic, and Home Health Considerations.* 4th ed. Philadelphia: F. A. Davis.
5. Hareven, T. K., Adams, K. J. (eds). (1982). *Aging and Life Course Transitions. An Interdisciplinary Perspective.* New York: Guilford.
6. Sims, D. D. (1993). *If I Could Just See Hope: Finding Your Way Through Grief.* Louisville, KY: Grief.
7. Lipson, J. G., Dibble, S. L., Minarik, P. A. (1996). *Culture & Nursing Care: A Pocket Guide.* San Francisco: UCSF Nursing Press.
8. Defensive Functioning Scale, Brandies University Psychological Counseling Center. (2002). Retrieved July 2007 from www.brandeis.edu/pcc/coping.html.

ineffective Coping

DEFINITION: Inability to form a valid appraisal of the stressors, inadequate choices of practiced responses, or inability to use available resources

RELATED FACTORS

Situational or maturational crises

High degree of threat

Inadequate opportunity to prepare for stressor; disturbance in pattern of appraisal of threat

Inadequate level of confidence in ability to cope; inadequate level of perception of control; uncertainty

Inadequate resources available; inadequate social support created by characteristics of relationships

Disturbance in pattern of tension release

Inability to conserve adaptive energies

Gender differences in coping strategies

[Work overload, too many deadlines]

[Impairment of nervous system; cognitive, sensory, or perceptual impairment, memory loss]

[Severe or chronic pain]

DEFINING CHARACTERISTICS

Subjective

Verbalization of inability to cope or ask for help

Sleep disturbance; fatigue

Abuse of chemical agents

[Reports of muscular or emotional tension, lack of appetite]

Objective

Lack of goal-directed behavior or resolution of problem, including inability to attend to and difficulty with organizing information; [lack of assertive behavior]

Use of forms of coping that impede adaptive behavior [including inappropriate use of defense mechanisms, verbal manipulation]

Inadequate problem-solving

Inability to meet role expectations or basic needs [including skipping meals, little or no exercise, no time for self, no vacations]

Decreased use of social support

Poor concentration

Change in usual communication patterns

High illness rate [including high blood pressure, ulcers, irritable bowel, frequent headaches or neck pain]

Risk taking

Destructive behavior toward self [including overeating, excessive smoking or drinking, overuse of prescribed or over-the-counter (OTC) medications, illicit drug use]; destructive behavior toward self

[Behavioral changes (e.g., impatience, frustration, irritability, discouragement)]

Sample Clinical Applications: New diagnosis of major illness, chronic conditions, major depression, substance abuse, eating disorders, bipolar disorder, social anxiety disorder, pregnancy, parenting

DESIRED OUTCOMES/EVALUATION CRITERIA

Sample (NOC) linkages:
Coping: Personal actions to manage stressors that tax an individual's resources
Impulse Self-Control: Self-restraint of compulsive or impulsive behaviors
Decision-Making: Ability to make judgments and choose between two or more alternatives

Client Will (Include Specific Time Frame)
• Assess the current situation accurately.
• Identify ineffective coping behaviors and consequences.
• Verbalize awareness of own coping abilities.
• Verbalize feelings congruent with behavior.
• Meet psychological needs as evidenced by appropriate expression of feelings, identification of options, and use of resources.

ACTIONS/INTERVENTIONS

Sample (NIC) linkages:
Coping Enhancement: Assisting a patient to adapt to perceived stressors, changes, or threats that interfere with meeting life demands and roles
Decision-Making Support: Providing information and support for a person who is making a decision regarding healthcare
Impulse Control Training: Assisting the patient to mediate impulsive behavior through application of problem-solving strategies to social and interpersonal situations

NURSING PRIORITY NO. 1

To determine degree of impairment:

● Identify individual stressors (e.g., family, social, work environment, life changes or nursing/healthcare management). *Helps define problem(s), providing a starting point for intervention.*[1]

● Evaluate ability to understand events, provide realistic appraisal of situation. *Necessary information for developing workable plan of care.*[2]

● Identify developmental level of functioning. *People tend to regress to a lower developmental stage during illness or crisis, and recognition of client's level enables more appropriate interventions to be implemented.*[2]

● Assess current functional capacity and note how it is affecting the individual's coping ability. *Promotes identification of strategies that will be helpful in current situation.*[4]

● Determine alcohol intake, drug use, smoking habits, sleeping and eating patterns. *Substance abuse impairs ability to deal with what is happening in current situation. Identification of impaired sleeping and eating patterns provides clues to extent of anxiety and impaired coping.*[2,3,16]

● Ascertain impact of illness on sexual needs and relationship. *Illnesses, medications, and many treatment regimens can affect sexual functioning, further stressing coping ability.*[2,3]

● Assess level of anxiety and coping on an ongoing basis. *Identifies changes in ability to cope and worsening of ability to understand at an early stage where intervention can be most effective.*[4]

- Note speech and communication patterns. Be aware of negative or catastrophizing thinking. *Identifies existing problems and assesses ability to understand situation and communicate needs.*[7,15]
- Observe and describe behavior in objective terms. Validate observations. *Promotes accuracy and assures correctness of conclusions to arrive at the best possible solutions.*[7]

NURSING PRIORITY NO. 2

To assess coping abilities and skills:

- Ascertain client's understanding of current situation and its impact on life and work. *Client may not understand situation, and being aware of these factors is necessary to planning care and identifying appropriate interventions.*[8]
- Active-listen and identify client's perceptions of what is happening and effectiveness of coping techniques. *Reflecting client's thoughts can provide a forum for understanding perceptions in relation to reality for planning care and determining accuracy of interventions needed.*[2,3]
- Discuss cultural background and whether some beliefs from family may contribute to difficulties coping with situation. *Family of origin can have a positive or negative effect on individual's ability to deal with stressful situations.*[5]
- Evaluate client's decision-making ability. *When ability to make decisions is impaired by illness or treatment regimen, it is important to take this into consideration when planning care to maximize participation and positive outcomes.*[9]
- Determine previous methods of dealing with life problems. *Identifies successful techniques that can be used in current situation. Often client is preoccupied by current concerns and does not think about previous successful skills.*[8]

NURSING PRIORITY NO. 3

To assist client to deal with current situation:

- Call client by name. Ascertain how client prefers to be addressed. *Using client's name enhances sense of self and promotes individuality and self-esteem.*[2]
- Encourage communication with staff/SOs. *Developing positive interactions between staff, SO(s) and client ensures that everyone has the same understanding.*[8]
- Use reality orientation (e.g., clocks, calendars, bulletin boards) and make frequent references to time, place as indicated. Place needed and familiar objects within sight for visual cues. *Often client can be disoriented by changes in routine, anxiety about illness and treatment regimens, and these measures help the client maintain orientation and a sense of reality.*[9]
- Provide for continuity of care with same personnel taking care of the client as often as possible. *Developing relationships with same caregivers promotes trust and enables client to discuss concerns and fears freely.*[9]
- Explain disease process, procedures, or events in a simple, concise manner. Devote time for listening. *May help client to express emotions, grasp situation, and feel more in control.*[10]
- Discuss use of medications as needed. *Short-term use of anti-anxiety medication or antidepressants may be helpful for lifting mood and encouraging individual to develop new coping skills.*[6]
- Provide for a quiet environment, position equipment out of view as much as possible. *Anxiety is increased by noisy surroundings.*[8]
- Schedule activities so periods of rest alternate with nursing care. Increase activity slowly. *Client is weakened by illness and failure to cope with situation. Ensuring rest can promote ability to cope.*[8]

- Assist client in use of diversion, recreation, relaxation techniques. *Learning new skills can be helpful for reducing stress and will be useful in the future as the client learns to cope more successfully.*[8]
- Emphasize positive body responses to medical conditions, but do not negate the seriousness of the situation (e.g., stable blood pressure during gastric bleed or improved body posture in depressed client). *Acknowledging the reality of the illness while accurately stating the facts can provide hope and encouragement.*[8]
- Encourage client to try new coping behaviors and gradually master situation. *Practicing new ways of dealing with what is happening leads to being more comfortable and can promote a positive outcome as client relaxes and handles illness and treatment regimen more successfully.*[9]
- Confront client when behavior is inappropriate, pointing out difference between words and actions. *Provides external locus of control, enhancing safety while client learns self-control.*[2]
- Assist in dealing with change in concept of body image as appropriate. (Refer to ND disturbed Body Image.) *New view of self may be negative, and client needs to incorporate change in a positive manner to enhance self-image.*[11]

NURSING PRIORITY NO. 4

To provide for meeting psychological needs:

- Treat the client with courtesy and respect. Converse at client's level, providing meaningful conversation while performing care. *Enhances therapeutic relationship.*[2]
- Take advantage of teachable moments. *Individuals learn best and are open to new information when they feel accepted and are in a comfortable environment.*[11]
- Allow client to react in own way without judgment by staff/caregivers. Provide support and diversion as indicated. *Unconditional positive regard and support promotes acceptance, enabling client to deal with difficult situation in a positive way.*[8]
- Encourage verbalization of fears and anxieties and expression of feelings of denial, depression, and anger. *Free expression allows for dealing with these feelings, and when the client knows that these are normal reactions, he or she can deal with them better.*[11]
- Help client to learn how to substitute positive thoughts for negative ones (i.e., "I can do this; I am in charge of myself"). *The mind plays a significant role in one's response to stressors, and negative thoughts can actually increase the impact of the stressor.*[15]
- Provide opportunity for expression of sexual concerns. *Important aspect of person that may be difficult to express. Providing an opening for discussion by asking sensitive questions allows client to talk about concerns.*[11]
- Help client to set limits on acting-out behaviors and learn ways to express emotions in an acceptable manner. *Enables client to gain sense of self-esteem, promoting internal locus of control.*[2]

NURSING PRIORITY NO. 5

To promote wellness (Teaching/Discharge Considerations):

- Give updated or additional information needed about events, cause (if known), and potential course of illness as soon as possible. *Knowledge helps reduce anxiety or fear, allows client to deal with reality.*[8]
- Provide and encourage an atmosphere of realistic hope. *Promotes optimistic outlook, energizing client to address situation. Client needs to hear positive things while undergoing difficult circumstances.*[8]

- Give information about purposes and side effects of medications and treatments. *Client feels included (promoting sense of control), enabling client to cope with situation in a more positive manner.*[8]

- Emphasize importance of follow-up care. *Checkups verify that regimen is being followed accurately and that healing is progressing to promote a satisfactory outcome.*[8]

- Encourage and support client in evaluating lifestyle, occupation, and leisure activities. *Helps client to look at difficult areas that may contribute to anxiety and ability to cope, to make changes gradually without undue or debilitating anxiety.*[8,16]

- Discuss effects of stressors (e.g., family, social, work environment, or nursing/healthcare management) and ways to deal with them. *Addressing these factors will enable client to develop strategies to make changes needed to promote wellness.*[8]

- Provide for gradual implementation and continuation of necessary behavior or lifestyle changes. *Change is difficult, and beginning slowly enhances commitment to plan.*[8]

- Discuss or review anticipated procedures and client concerns, as well as postoperative expectations when surgery is recommended. *Knowledge allays fears and helps client to understand procedures and treatments and expected results. When client has prior information about what to expect during postoperative course, he or she will remain calm, anxiety will be reduced, and client will cope more effectively with situation.*[11,14]

- Refer to outside resources and professional therapy as indicated or ordered. *May be necessary to assist with long-term improvement.*[11]

- Determine desire for religious representative or spiritual counselor and facilitate arrangements for visit. *Spiritual needs are an integral part of being human, and determining and meeting individual preferences helps client deal with concerns, and desires for discussion or assistance in this area.*[12]

- Provide information or consultation as indicated for sexual concerns. Provide privacy when client is not in home. *Individuals are sexual beings, and concerns about role in family/relationship, ability to function are often not readily expressed. Discussion opens opportunity for clarification and understanding, and helps to meet need for intimacy.*[11]

- Refer to other NDs as indicated (e.g., Anxiety, impaired verbal Communication, acute/chronic Pain, risk for self-/other-directed Violence). *Provides further assistance in area of identified need.*[13]

DOCUMENTATION FOCUS

Assessment/Reassessment
- Baseline findings, degree of impairment, and client's perceptions of situation.
- Coping abilities and previous ways of dealing with life problems.

Planning
- Plan of care, specific interventions, and who is involved in planning.
- Teaching plan.

Implementation/Evaluation
- Client's responses to interventions, teaching, and actions performed.
- Medication dose, time, and client's response.
- Attainment or progress toward desired outcome(s).
- Modifications to plan of care.

Discharge Planning
- Long-term needs and actions to be taken.
- Support systems available, specific referrals made, and who is responsible for actions to be taken.

References

1. Doenges, M., Moorhouse, M., Murr, A. (2002). *Nursing Care Plans, Guidelines for Individualizing Patient Care.* 6th ed. Philadelphia: F. A. Davis.
2. Doenges, M., Townsend, M., Moorhouse, M. (1998). *Psychiatric Care Plans: Guidelines for Individualizing Care.* 3d ed. Philadelphia: F. A. Davis.
3. Townsend, M. (2003). *Psychiatric Mental Health Nursing: Concepts of Care.* 4th ed. Philadelphia: F. A. Davis.
4. Cox, H., et al. (2002). *Clinical Applications of Nursing Diagnosis: Adult, Child, Women's Psychiatric, Gerontic, and Home Health Considerations.* 3d ed. Philadelphia: F. A. Davis.
5. Lipson, J. G., Dibble, S. L., Minarik, P. A. (1996). *Culture & Nursing Care: A Pocket Guide.* San Francisco: UCSF Nursing Press.
6. Townsend, M. (2001). *Nursing Diagnoses in Psychiatric Nursing: Care Plans and Psychotropic Medications.* 5th ed. Philadelphia: F. A. Davis.
7. Hareven, T. K., Adams, K. J. (eds). (1982). *Aging and Life Course Transitions: An Interdisciplinary Perspective.* New York: Guilford.
8. Cherif, M., Younis, E. I. (2000). Liver transplantation. *Clin Fam Prac*, 2(1), 117.
9. Liken, M. A. (2001). Caregivers in crisis: Moving a relative with Alzheimer's to assisted living. *Clin Nurs Res*, 10(1), 53–69.
10. HIV/AIDS Treatment Information Service. (2001). Guidelines for the use of antiretroviral agents in HIV-infected adults and adolescents. Retrieved November 2001 from www.hivatis.org/guidelines/adult/aug13_01/pdf/aaaug13s.pdf.
11. Tan, G., Waldman, K., Bostick, R. (Winter 2002). Psychosocial issues, sexuality, and cancer. *Sexuality Disabil*, 20(4), 297–318.
12. Geiter, H. (2002). The spiritual side of nursing. *RN*, 65(5), 43–44.
13. Doenges, M., Moorhouse, M., Murr, A. (2004). *Nurse's Pocket Guide: Diagnoses, Interventions, and Rationales.* 9th ed. Philadelphia: F. A. Davis.
14. Dispatcher stress—Actively coping with stress. Retrieved July 2007 from www.headsets911.com/activecoping.htm.
15. Coping with stress. (2000). Retrieved July 2007 from www.hubbynet.com/stresscoping.htm.
16. Franke, J. (1999). Stress, burnout, and addiction. *Tex Med*, 95(3), 43–52.

(ineffective community Coping)

DEFINITION: Pattern of community activities for adaptation and problem-solving that is unsatisfactory for meeting the demands or needs of the community

RELATED FACTORS

Deficits in community social support services or resources
Inadequate resources for problem-solving
Ineffective or nonexistent community systems (e.g., lack of emergency medical system, transportation system, or disaster planning systems)
Natural or man-made disasters

DEFINING CHARACTERISTICS

Subjective
Community does not meet its own expectations
Expressed vulnerability; community powerlessness
Stressors perceived as excessive

(continues on page 240)

ineffective community Coping (continued)

Objective
Deficits of community participation
Excessive community conflicts
High illness rates
Increased social problems (e.g., homicide, vandalism, arson, terrorism, robbery, infanticide, abuse, divorce, unemployment, poverty, militancy, mental illness)

Sample Clinical Applications: High rate of illness, injury, or violence in community

DESIRED OUTCOMES/EVALUATION CRITERIA

Sample (NOC) linkages:
Community Competence: Capacity of a community to collectively problem-solve to achieve goals
Community Health Status: General state of well-being of a community or population
Community Disaster Readiness: Community preparedness to respond to a natural or man-made calamitous event

Community Will (Include Specific Time Frame)
• Recognize negative and positive factors affecting community's ability to meet its demands or needs.
• Identify alternatives to inappropriate activities for adaptation and problem-solving.
• Report a measurable increase in necessary or desired activities to improve community functioning.

ACTIONS/INTERVENTIONS

Sample (NIC) linkages:
Community Health Development: Facilitating members of a community to identify a community's health concerns, mobilize resources, and implement solutions
Environmental Management: Community: Monitoring and influencing of the physical, social, cultural, economic, and political conditions that affect the health of groups and communities
Community Disaster Preparedness: Preparing for an effective response to a large-scale disaster

NURSING PRIORITY NO. 1

To identify causative or precipitating factors:

🏠 • Evaluate community activities as related to meeting collective needs within the community itself and between the community and the larger society. *Determines what activities are currently available and what needs are not being met, either by the local or county/state entities. Provides information on which to base the steps needed to begin planning for desired changes.*[1]

🏠 • Note community reports of community functioning (e.g., immunization status, transportation, water supply, financing), including areas of weakness or conflict. *Community is responsible for identifying needed changes for possible action.*[1]

🏠 • Identify effects of Related Factors on community activities. Note immediate needs (e.g., healthcare, food, shelter, funds). *Provides a baseline to determine community needs, and*

identifying factors that are pertinent to the community allows community to deal with current concerns.[1,5]

• Plan for the possibility of a disaster when determined by current circumstances. *In relation to threats, terrorist activities, and natural disasters, actions need to be coordinated between the local and the larger community.*[5]

• Determine availability and use of resources. *Helpful to begin planning to correct deficiencies that have been identified. Sometimes even though resources are available, they are not being used appropriately or fully.*[2]

• Identify unmet demands or needs of the community. *Determining where the deficiencies are is a crucial step to beginning to make an accurate plan for correction. Sometimes elected bodies see the problems differently from the general population and conflict can arise; therefore, it is important for communication to resolve the issues that are in question.*[2]

NURSING PRIORITY NO. 2

To assist the community to reactivate/develop skills to deal with needs:

• Determine community strengths. *Promotes understanding of ways in which community is already meeting identified needs, and once identified, they can be built on to develop plan to improve community.*[1]

• Identify and prioritize community goals. *Goals enable the identification of actions to direct the changes that are needed to improve the community. Prioritizing enables actions to be taken in order of importance.*[1]

• Encourage community members/groups to engage in problem-solving activities. *Individuals who are involved in the problem-solving process and make a commitment to the solutions have an investment and are more apt to follow through on their commitments.*[3]

• Develop a plan jointly with community to deal with deficits in support. *Working together will enhance efforts and help to meet identified goals.*[3]

NURSING PRIORITY NO. 3

To promote wellness as related to community health:

• Create plans managing interactions within the community itself and between the community and the larger society. *These activities will meet collective needs.*[1]

• Assist the community to form partnerships within the community and between the community and the larger society. *Promotes long-term development of the community to deal with current and future problems.*[1]

• Provide channels for dissemination of information to the community as a whole—for example, print media; radio and TV reports, and community bulletin boards; speakers' bureau; reports to committees, councils, advisory boards on file and accessible to the public. *Having information readily available for everyone provides opportunity for all members of the community to know what is being planned and have input into the planning. Keeping community informed promotes understanding of needs and plans and probability of follow-through to successful outcomes.*[1]

• Make information available in different modalities and geared to differing educational levels and cultural and ethnic populations of the community. *Assures understanding by all members of the community and promotes cooperation with planning and follow-through.*[1]

• Seek out and evaluate underserved populations, including the homeless. *These members of the community deserve to be helped to become productive citizens and be involved in the changes that are occurring.*[3]

Nursing Diagnoses in Alphabetical Order

🏠 • Work with community members to identify lifestyle changes that can be made to meet the goals identified to improve community deficits. *Changing lifestyles can promote a sense of power and encourage members to become involved in improving their community.*[4]

DOCUMENTATION FOCUS

Assessment/Reassessment
• Assessment findings, including perception of community members regarding problems.
• Availability of resources.

Planning
• Plan of care and who is involved in planning.
• Teaching plan.

Implementation/Evaluation
• Response of community entities to plan, interventions, and actions performed.
• Attainment or progress toward desired outcome(s).
• Modifications to plan of care.

Discharge Planning
• Long-term plans and who is responsible for actions to be taken.

References

1. Higgs, Z. R., Gustafson, D. (1985). *Community as a Client: Assessment and Diagnosis*. Philadelphia: F. A. Davis.
2. Hunt, R. (1998). Community-based nursing. *Am J Nurs*, 98(10), 44.
3. Schaeder, C., et al. (1997). Community nursing organizations: A new frontier. *Am J Nurs*, 97(1), 63.
4. Lai, S. C., Cohen, M. N. (1999). Promoting lifestyle changes. *Am J Nurs*, 99(4), 63.
5. Doenges, M., Moorhouse, M., Geissler-Murr, A. (2002). *Nursing Care Plans: Guidelines for Individualizing Patient Care*. 6th ed. Philadelphia: F. A. Davis.

readiness for enhanced Coping

DEFINITION: A pattern of cognitive and behavioral efforts to manage demands that is sufficient for well-being and can be strengthened

RELATED FACTORS

To be developed by nurse researchers and submitted to NANDA

DEFINING CHARACTERISTICS

Subjective
Defines stressors as manageable
Seeks social support or knowledge of new strategies
Acknowledges power
Acknowledges possible environmental changes

Objective
Uses a broad range of problem-oriented or emotion-oriented strategies
Uses spiritual resources

Sample Clinical Applications: Chronic health conditions (e.g., asthma, diabetes mellitus, arthritis, systemic lupus, multiple sclerosis [MS], AIDS), mental health concerns (e.g., seasonal affective disorder, attention deficit disorder, Down syndrome)

DESIRED OUTCOMES/EVALUATION CRITERIA

Sample NOC linkages:
Coping: Personal actions to manage stressors that tax an individual's resources
Quality of Life: Extent of positive perception of current life circumstances
Hope: Optimism that is personally satisfying and life-supporting

Client Will (Include Specific Time Frame)
• Assess current situation accurately.
• Identify effective coping behaviors currently being used.
• Verbalize feelings congruent with behavior.
• Meet psychological needs as evidenced by appropriate expression of feelings, identification of options, and use of resources.

ACTIONS/INTERVENTIONS

Sample NIC linkages:
Coping Enhancement: Assisting a patient to adapt to perceived stressors, changes, or threats that interfere with meeting life demands and roles
Self-Awareness Enhancement: Assisting a patient to explore and understand his or her thoughts, feelings, motivations, and behaviors
Teaching: Individual: Planning, implementation, and evaluation of a teaching program designed to address a patient's particular needs

NURSING PRIORITY NO. 1

To determine needs and desire for improvement:

● Evaluate client's understanding of situation and ability to provide realistic appraisal of situation. Provides information about client's perception, cognitive ability, and whether the client is aware of the facts of the situation, which reveals essential information for planning care.[1]

● Determine stressors that may be affecting client. *Accurate identification of situation that client is dealing with provides information for planning interventions to enhance coping abilities.*[1]

● Ascertain motivation and expectations for change. *Motivation to improve and high expectations can encourage client to make changes that will improve his or her life. However, presence of external locus of control or unrealistic expectations may hamper efforts.*

● Identify social supports available to client. *Available support systems, such as family/friends, can provide client with ability to handle current stressful events, and "talking it out" with an empathic listener will help client move forward to enhance coping skills.*[1]

- Review coping strategies client is aware of and currently using. *The desire to improve one's coping ability is based on an awareness of the status of the stressful situation.*[1]
- Determine use of alcohol or other drugs and smoking habits during times of stress. *Recognition of potential for substituting these actions or old habits to deal with anxiety increases individual's awareness of opportunity to choose new ways to cope with life stressors.*[2]
- Assess level of anxiety and coping on an ongoing basis. *Provides baseline to develop plan of care to improve coping abilities.*[2]
- Note speech and communication patterns. *Assesses ability to understand and provides information necessary to help client make progress in desire to enhance coping abilities.*[2]
- Evaluate client's decision-making ability. *Understanding client's ability provides a starting point for developing plan and determining what information client needs to develop more effective coping skills.*[1]

NURSING PRIORITY NO. 2

To assist client to develop enhanced coping skills:

- Active-listen and clarify client's perceptions of current status. *Reflecting client's statements and thoughts can provide a forum for understanding perceptions in relation to reality for planning care and determining accuracy of interventions needed.*[3]
- Review previous methods of dealing with life problems. *Enables client to identify successful techniques used in the past, promoting feelings of confidence in own ability.*[2]
- Discuss desire to improve ability to manage stressors of life. *Understanding client's decision to seek new information to enhance life will help client determine what is needed to learn new coping skills.*[1]
- Discuss understanding of concept of knowing what can and cannot be changed. *Acceptance of reality that some things cannot be changed allows client to focus energies on dealing with things that can be changed.*[1]
- Help client strengthen problem-solving skills. *Learning the process for problem-solving will promote successful resolution of potentially stressful situations that arise.*[4]

NURSING PRIORITY NO. 3

To promote optimal well-being (Teaching/Learning Considerations):

- Discuss predisposing factors related to any individual's response to stress. *Understanding that genetic influences, past experiences, and existing conditions determine whether a person's response is adaptive or maladaptive will give client a base on which to continue to learn what is needed to improve life.*[1]
- Encourage client to develop a stress-management program. *An individualized program of relaxation, meditation, and so forth, enhances sense of balance in life and strengthens client's ability to manage challenging situations.*[1]
- Recommend involvement in activities of interest, such as exercise/sports, music, and art. *Individuals must decide for themselves what coping strategies are adaptive for them. Most people find enjoyment and relaxation in these kinds of activities.*[1]
- Discuss possibility of doing volunteer work in an area of the client's choosing. *Many individuals report satisfaction in giving of themselves—involvement with caring for others/pets, and client may find sense of fulfillment in service to others.*[1]
- Refer to classes and/or reading material and Web sites, as appropriate. *May be helpful to further learning and pursuing goal of enhanced coping ability.*[1]

DOCUMENTATION FOCUS

Assessment/Reassessment
- Baseline information, client's perception of need to enhance abilities.
- Coping abilities and previous ways of dealing with life problems.
- Motivation and expectation for change.

Planning
- Plan of care, specific interventions, and who is involved in planning.
- Teaching plan.

Implementation/Evaluation
- Client's responses to interventions, teaching, and actions performed.
- Attainment or progress toward desired outcome(s).
- Modifications to plan of care.

Discharge Planning
- Long-term needs and actions to be taken.
- Support systems available, specific referrals made, and who is responsible for actions to be taken.

References

1. Townsend, M. (2003). *Psychiatric Mental Health Nursing Concepts of Care*. 4th ed. Philadelphia: F. A. Davis.
2. Doenges, M. E., Moorhouse, M. F., Murr, A. C. (2004). *Nurse's Pocket Guide: Diagnoses, Interventions, and Rationales*. 9th ed. Philadelphia: F. A. Davis.
3. Doenges, M., Townsend, M., Moorhouse, M. (1998). *Psychiatric Care Plans: Guidelines for Individualizing Care*. 3d ed. Philadelphia: F. A. Davis.
4. Gordon, T. (2000). *Parent Effectiveness Training*. Updated ed. New York: Three Rivers Press.

readiness for enhanced community Coping

DEFINITION: Pattern of community activities for adaptation and problem-solving that is satisfactory for meeting the demands or needs of the community but can be improved for management of current and future problems/stressors

RELATED FACTORS

Social supports available
Resources available for problem-solving
Sense of power to manage stressors

DEFINING CHARACTERISTICS

One or more characteristics that indicate effective coping

Subjective
Agreement that community is responsible for stress management

(continues on page 246)

readiness for enhanced community Coping (continued)

Objective
Active planning by community for predicted stressors
Active problem-solving by community when faced with issues
Positive communication among community members
Positive communication between community and aggregates and larger community
Programs available for recreation or relaxation
Resources sufficient for managing stressors

Sample Clinical Applications: Reduced rates of illness, injury, or violence

DESIRED OUTCOMES/EVALUATION CRITERIA

Sample (NOC) linkages:
Community Competence: Capacity of a community to collectively problem-solve to achieve goals
Community Health Status: General state of well-being of a community or population
Community Disaster Readiness: Community preparedness to respond to a natural or man-made calamitous event

Community Will (Include Specific Time Frame)
- Identify positive and negative factors affecting management of current and future problems/stressors.
- Have an established plan in place to deal with identified problems and stressors.
- Describe management of challenges in characteristics that indicate effective coping.
- Report a measurable increase in ability to deal with problems and stressors.

ACTIONS/INTERVENTIONS

Sample (NIC) linkages:
Program Development: Planning, implementing, and evaluating a coordinated set of activities designed to enhance wellness, or to prevent, reduce, or eliminate one or more health problems of a group or community
Environmental Management: Community: Monitoring and influencing of the physical, social, cultural, economic, and political conditions that affect the health of groups and communities
Health Policy Monitoring: Surveillance and influence of government and organization regulations, rules, and standards that affect nursing systems and practices to ensure quality care of patients

NURSING PRIORITY NO. 1

To determine existence of and deficits or weaknesses in management of current and future problems/stressors:

- Review community plan for dealing with problems and stressors, untoward events such as natural disaster or terrorist activity. *Provides a baseline for comparisons of preparedness with other communities and developing plan to address concerns.*[5]
- Assess effects of Related Factors on management of problems and stressors. *Identifying social supports available and awareness of the power of the community can enhance the plans needed to improve the community.*[1]

🌐 Cultural   ♻ Collaborative   🏠 Community/Home Care   ✏ Diagnostic Studies   ∞ Pediatric/Geriatric/Lifespan   💊 Medications

- Identify limitations in current pattern of community activities, such as transportation, water needs, and roads. *Recognition of the factors that can be improved through adaptation and problem-solving will make it easier for the community to proceed with planning to make necessary improvements.*[4]
- Evaluate community activities as related to management of problems and stressors within the community itself and between the community and the larger society. *Disasters occurring in a community (or in the country as a whole) affect the local community, and need to be recognized and addressed.*[5]

NURSING PRIORITY NO. 2

To assist the community in adaptation and problem-solving for management of current and future needs/stressors:

- Define and discuss current needs and anticipated or projected concerns. *Agreement on scope and parameters of needs is essential for effective planning.*[2]
- Determine community's strengths. *Plan can build on strengths to address areas of weakness.*[2]
- Identify and prioritize goals to facilitate accomplishment. *Helps to bring the community together to meet a common concern or threat, maintain focus, and facilitate accomplishment.*[5]
- Identify and interact with available resources (e.g., persons, groups, financial, governmental, as well as other communities) *Promotes cooperation. Major catastrophes, such as earthquakes, floods, and terrorist activity, affect more than the local community, and communities need to work together to deal with and accomplish reconstruction and future growth.*[6]
- Make a joint plan with the community and the larger community to deal with adaptation and problem-solving. *Promotes management of problems and stressors to enable most effective solution for identified concern.*[3]
- Seek out and involve underserved and at-risk groups within the community, including the homeless. *Supports communication and commitment of community as a whole.*[3]

NURSING PRIORITY NO. 3

To promote optimal well-being of community:

- Assist the community to form partnerships within the community and between the community and the larger society. *Promotes long-term developmental growth of the community.*[5]
- Support development of plans for maintaining these interactions.
- Establish mechanism for self-monitoring of community needs and evaluation of efforts. *Facilitates proactive—rather than reactive—responses by the community.*
- Use multiple formats to disseminate information, such as TV, radio, print media, billboards, as well as computer bulletin boards, speakers' bureau, and reports to community leaders and groups on file and accessible to the public. *Keeps community informed regarding plans, needs, outcomes to encourage continued understanding and participation.*[6]

DOCUMENTATION FOCUS

Assessment/Reassessment
- Assessment findings and community's perception of situation.
- Identified areas of concern, community strengths and weaknesses.

Planning
- Plan and who is involved and responsible for each action.
- Teaching plan.

Implementation/Evaluation
- Response of community entities to the actions performed.
- Attainment or progress toward desired outcomes.
- Modifications to plan.

Discharge Planning
- Short- and long-term plans to deal with current, anticipated, and potential problems and who is responsible for follow-through.
- Specific referrals made, coalitions formed.

References

1. Higgs, Z. R., Gustafson, D. (1985). *Community as a Client: Assessment and Diagnosis*. Philadelphia: F. A. Davis.
2. Hunt, R. (1998). Community-based nursing. *Am J Nurs*, 98(10), 44.
3. Schaeder, C., et al. (1997). Community nursing organizations: A new frontier. *Am J Nurs*, 97(1), 63.
4. Lai, S. C., Cohen, M. N. (1999). Promoting lifestyle changes. *Am J Nurs*, 99(4), 63.
5. Doenges, M., Moorhouse, M., Geissler-Murr, A. (2002). *Nursing Care Plans: Guidelines for Individualizing Patient Care*. 6th ed. Philadelphia: F. A. Davis.
6. Stanhope, M., Lancaster, J. (2000). *Community and Public Health Nursing*. 5th ed. St. Louis, MO: Mosby.

readiness for enhanced family Coping

DEFINITION: Effective managing of adaptive tasks by family member involved with the patient's health challenge, who now exhibits desire and readiness for enhanced health and growth in regard to self and in relation to the patient

RELATED FACTORS

Needs are sufficiently gratified to enable goals of self-actualization to surface
Adaptive tasks effectively addressed to enable goals of self-actualization to surface
[Developmental stage, situational crises and supports]

DEFINING CHARACTERISTICS

Subjective
Family member attempts to describe growth impact of crisis [on his or her own values, priorities, goals, or relationships]
Individual expresses interest in making contact with others who have experienced a similar situation

Objective
Family member moves in direction of health-promotion or enriching lifestyle
Chooses experiences that optimize wellness

Sample Clinical Applications: Genetic disorders (e.g., Down syndrome, cystic fibrosis, neural tube defects), traumatic injury (e.g., amputation, spinal cord), chronic conditions (e.g., asthma, AIDS, Alzheimer's disease)

Cultural Collaborative Community/Home Care Diagnostic Studies Pediatric/Geriatric/Lifespan Medications

DESIRED OUTCOMES/EVALUATION CRITERIA

Sample (NOC) linkages:
Family Participation in Professional Care: Family involvement in decision making, delivery, and evaluation of care provided by healthcare personnel
Family Coping: Family actions to manage stressors that tax family resources
Family Functioning: Capacity of the family system to meet the needs of its members during developmental transitions

Family Will (Include Specific Time Frame)
• Express willingness to look at own role in the family's growth.
• Verbalize desire to undertake tasks leading to change.
• Report feelings of self-confidence and satisfaction with progress being made.

ACTIONS/INTERVENTIONS

Sample (NIC) linkages:
Normalization Promotion: Assisting parents and other family members of children with chronic diseases or disabilities in providing normal life experiences for their children and families
Family Support: Promotion of family values, interests, and goals
Family Involvement Promotion: Facilitating family participation in the emotional and physical care of the patient

NURSING PRIORITY NO. 1

To assess situation and adaptive skills being used by the family members:

• Determine individual situation and stage of growth family is experiencing and demonstrating. *Essential elements needed to identify family needs and develop plan of care for improving communication and interactions. Changes that are occurring may help family adapt, grow, and thrive when faced with these transitional events.*[1,7]

• Ascertain motivation and expectations for change. *Motivation to improve and high expectations can encourage individuals to make changes that will improve their lives; however, presence of external locus of control or unrealistic expectations may hamper efforts.*

• Observe communication patterns of family. Listen to family's expressions of hope, planning, effect on relationships and life. *Provides clues to difficulties that individuals may have in expressing themselves effectively to others. Beginning to plan for the future with hope promotes changes in relationships that can enhance living for those involved.*[3]

• Note expressions such as "Life has more meaning for me since this has occurred." *Such statements identify change in values that may occur with the diagnosis or stress of a serious or potentially fatal illness.*[1]

• Identify cultural or religious health beliefs and expectations. *For example: Navajo parents may define family as nuclear, extended, or clan, and it is important to identify who are the primary child-rearing persons. Beliefs about causes of condition may affect how family interacts with client (e.g., African Americans may believe the condition is punishment for improper behavior and may react with anger and statements of condemnation).*[6]

NURSING PRIORITY NO. 2

To assist family to develop/strengthen potential for growth:

- Provide time to talk with family to discuss their views of the situation. *Provides an opportunity to hear family's understanding and determine how realistic their ideas are for planning how they are going to deal with situation in the most positive manner.*[3]
- Establish a relationship with family/client. *Therapeutic relationships foster growth and enable family to identify skills needed for coping with difficult situation or illness.*[3]
- Provide a role model with whom the family may identify. *Setting a positive example can be a powerful influence in changing behavior, and as family members learn more effective communication skills, consideration for others, warmth and understanding, family relationships will be enhanced.*[2]
- Discuss importance of open communication and of not having secrets. *Functional communication is clear, direct, open, and honest, with congruence between verbal and nonverbal. Dysfunctional communication is indirect, vague, controlled, with many double-bind messages. Awareness of this information can enhance relationships among family members.*[3]
- Demonstrate techniques such as Active-listening, I-messages, and problem-solving. *Learning these skills can facilitate effective communication and improve interactions within the family.*[2]
- Establish social goals of achieving and maintaining harmony with oneself, family, and community. *Enables client to interact with others in positive ways.*[3]

NURSING PRIORITY NO. 3

To promote optimum family well-being (Teaching/Discharge Considerations):

- Assist family to support the client in meeting own needs within ability or constraints of the illness or situation. *Family members may do too much for client or may not do enough, believing client "wants to be babied." With information and support, they can learn to allow client to take the lead in doing what he or she is able to do.*[3]
- Provide experiences for the family to help them learn ways of assisting and supporting client. *Learning is enhanced when individual participates in hands-on opportunities to try out new activities.*[4]
- Discuss cultural beliefs and practices that may impact family members' interaction with client and dealing with condition. *Preconceived biases may interfere with efforts toward positive growth.*[6]
- Identify other individuals/groups with similar conditions and assist client/family to make contact (groups such as Reach for Recovery, CanSurmount, Al-Anon, and so on). *Provides ongoing support for sharing common experiences, problem-solving, and learning new behaviors.*[5]
- Assist family members to learn new, more effective ways of dealing with feelings and reactions. *Growth process is essential to reach the goal of enhancing the family relationships.*[3]
- Encourage family members to pursue personal interests, hobbies, or leisure activities *to promote individual well-being and strengthen coping abilities.*[7]

DOCUMENTATION FOCUS

Assessment/Reassessment
- Adaptive skills being used, stage of growth.
- Family communication patterns.
- Motivation and expectations for change.

Cultural · Collaborative · Community/Home Care · Diagnostic Studies · Pediatric/Geriatric/Lifespan · Medications

Planning
- Plan of care, specific interventions, and who is involved in planning.
- Teaching plan.

Implementation/Evaluation
- Client's responses to interventions, teaching, and actions performed.
- Attainment or progress toward desired outcome(s).
- Modifications to plan of care.

Discharge Planning
- Identified needs for follow-up care, support systems.
- Specific referral made.

References

1. Doenges, M., Moorhouse, M., Murr, A. (2002). *Nursing Care Plans: Guidelines for Individualizing Patient Care*. 6th ed. Philadelphia: F. A. Davis.
2. Doenges, M., Townsend, M., Moorhouse, M. (1998). *Psychiatric Care Plans: Guidelines for Individualizing Care*. 3d ed. Philadelphia: F. A. Davis.
3. Townsend, M. (2003). *Psychiatric Mental Health Nursing: Concepts of Care*. 4th ed. Philadelphia: F. A. Davis.
4. Cox, H., et al. (2002). *Clinical Applications of Nursing Diagnosis: Adult, Child, Women's Psychiatric, Gerontic, and Home Health Considerations*. 4th ed. Philadelphia: F. A. Davis.
5. Sims, D. (1993). *If I Could Just See Hope*. Louisville, KY: Grief.
6. Lipson, J. G., Dibble, S. L., Minarik, P. A. (1996). *Culture & Nursing Care: A Pocket Guide*. San Francisco: UCSF Nursing Press.
7. Beckett, C. (2000). Family theory as a framework for assessment. Retrieved September 2009 from www.jan.ucc.nau.edu/~nur350-c/class/2_family/theory/lesson2-1-3.html.

risk for sudden infant Death Syndrome

DEFINITION: Presence of risk factors for sudden death of an infant under 1 year of age [Sudden infant death syndrome (SIDS) is the sudden death of an infant under 1 year of age, which remains unexplained after a thorough case investigation, including performance of a complete autopsy, examination of the death scene, and review of the clinical history. SIDS is a subset of sudden unexpected death in infancy (SUDI) that is the sudden and unexpected death of an infant due to natural or unnatural causes.]

RISK FACTORS

Modifiable
Delayed or lack of prenatal care
Infants placed to sleep in the prone or side-lying position
Soft underlayment (loose articles in the sleep environment)
Infant overheating or overwrapping
Prenatal or postnatal smoke exposure

(continues on page 252)

risk for sudden infant Death Syndrome (continued)

Potentially Modifiable
Young maternal age
Low birth weight; prematurity

Nonmodifiable
Male gender
Ethnicity (e.g., African American, Native American)
Seasonality of SIDS deaths (higher in winter and fall months)
Infant age of 2 to 4 months

NOTE: A risk diagnosis is not evidenced by signs and symptoms, as the problem has not occurred; rather, nursing interventions are directed at prevention.
Sample Clinical Applications: Any child during first year of life

DESIRED OUTCOMES/EVALUATION CRITERIA

Sample NOC linkages:
Risk Detection: Activities taken to identify personal health threats
Risk Control: Actions to eliminate or reduce actual, personal, and modifiable health threats
Knowledge: Infant Care: Extent of understanding conveyed about caring for a baby up to 12 months

Parent Will (Include Specific Time Frame)
• Verbalize knowledge of modifiable factors.
• Make changes in environment to prevent death occurring from other factors.
• Follow medically recommended regimen for prenatal and postnatal care.

ACTIONS/INTERVENTIONS

Sample NIC linkages:
Risk Identification: Analysis of potential risk factors, determination of health risks, and prioritization of risk-reduction strategies for an individual or group
Parent Education: Infant: Instruction on nurturing and physical care during the first year of life
Teaching: Infant Safety [specify age]: Instruction on safety during first year of life

NURSING PRIORITY NO. 1

To assess causative/contributing factors:

• Identify individual risk factors pertaining to situation. *Determines modifiable or potentially modifiable factors that can be addressed and treated. SIDS is the most common cause of unexplained death between 1 month and 1 year of age, with peak incidence occurring between the second and fourth month.*[1,7]

 • Determine ethnicity, cultural background of family. *Although the overall rate of SIDS in the United States has declined by more than 50% since 1990, rates have declined less among non-Hispanic black and American Indian/Alaska Native infants.*[7–9]

• Note whether mother smoked during pregnancy or is currently smoking. *Many risk factors for SIDS also apply to non-SIDS deaths as well, and smoking is known to negatively affect the fetus prenatally as well as the infant after birth.*[1,2,10] *Some reports indicate an increased risk of SIDS in babies of smoking mothers.*[3,10]

Cultural   Collaborative   Community/Home Care   Diagnostic Studies   Pediatric/Geriatric/Lifespan   Medications

- Assess extent of prenatal care, how early begun, extent to which mother followed recommended care measures. *Prenatal care is important for all pregnancies to afford the optimal opportunity for all infants to have a healthy start to life.*[4]
- Determine client's knowledge of premature labor and actions to be taken in the event they occur. *Prompt action can prevent early delivery and the complications of prematurity.*[4]
- Note use of alcohol or other drugs (including prescribed medications) during and after pregnancy. *While these are not known to affect the occurrence of SIDS, a healthy baby will be less apt to have problems. Note: Studies have shown that Native American infants whose mothers drank any amount of alcohol 3 months before conception through the first trimester had six times the risk of SIDS as those whose mothers did not drink. Mothers who consumed five or more drinks at one sitting during the first trimester had eight times the risk as those whose mothers did not binge drink.*[5]

NURSING PRIORITY NO. 2

To promote use of activities to minimize risk of SIDS:

- Stress importance of placing infant on his or her back to sleep, both at nighttime and nap time. *Research confirms that fewer babies die of SIDS when they sleep on their backs and that side-lying position is not to be used.*[6,8]
- Advise all formal child care providers as well as grandparents, babysitters, neighbors, or anyone who will have responsibility for the care of the child during sleep to maintain correct sleeping position. *The recommendation is to always place the infant on the back until he or she can roll over; then repositioning is not required.*[1,7,10]
- Encourage parents to schedule "tummy time" only while infant is awake. *This activity promotes strengthening of back and neck muscles while parents are close and baby is not sleeping.*[1]
- Encourage early and medically recommended prenatal care and continue with well-baby checkups and immunizations after birth. *Prematurity presents many problems for the newborn, and keeping babies healthy prevents problems that could put the infant at risk for SIDS. Immunizing infants prevents many illnesses that can be life-threatening.*[1,4]
- Encourage breastfeeding, if possible. *Breastfeeding has many advantages (immunological, nutritional, and psychosocial), promoting a healthy infant. While this does not preclude the occurrence of SIDS, healthy babies are less prone to many illnesses and health problems.*[1,4]
- Discuss issues of bedsharing or co-sleeping and the concerns regarding sudden unexpected infant deaths from accidental entrapment under a sleeping adult or suffocation by becoming wedged in a couch or cushioned chair. *While co-sleeping is controversial, there are concerns about problems of accidental death from suffocation. Bedsharing or putting infant to sleep on an unsafe surface results in dangerous sleep environments that place infants at substantial risk for SUDI.*[6]
- Note cultural beliefs about bedsharing. *Bedsharing is more common among breastfed infants, young, unmarried, low income, or those from a minority group. Additional study is needed to better understand bedsharing practices and its associated risks and benefits.*[6]

NURSING PRIORITY NO. 3

To promote wellness (Teaching/Discharge Considerations):

- Discuss known facts about SIDS with parents. *SIDS is not preventable, although research indicates that SIDS deaths have reduced since back-sleeping position policy was implemented. It is not contagious or hereditary and is not an unusual disease. The cause, while not known, is not suffocation, aspiration, or regurgitation.*[1,7]

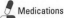 ● Recommend attention to factors below that may help in reducing risk:

Avoid overdressing or overheating infants during sleep. *Baby should be kept warm, but not too warm. Too many layers of clothing or blankets can overheat the infant. Room temperature that is comfortable for an adult will be comfortable for the baby. Note: Infants who were dressed in two or more layers of clothes as they slept had six times the risk of SIDS as those dressed in fewer layers.*[1,4,10]

Place infant on a firm mattress in an approved crib. *Avoiding soft mattresses, sofas, cushions, waterbeds, other soft surfaces, while not known to prevent SIDS, will minimize chance of suffocation.*[1]

Remove fluffy and loose bedding from sleep area, making sure baby's head and face are not covered during sleep. *Using only sleep clothing without a blanket, or if a blanket is used, making sure it is below baby's face and tucked in at the foot of the bed minimizes possibility of suffocation.*[1]

Verify that day-care center/provider(s) are trained in observation and modifying risk factors (e.g., sleeping position) *to reduce risk of death while infant in their care.*

Discourage excessive checking of the infant. *Since there is nothing that can currently be done (beyond proper sleep positioning) to reduce the occurrence of SIDS, excessive checking only tires the parents and creates an atmosphere of tension and anxiety.*[1,2]

● Discuss the use of apnea monitors. *Apnea monitors are not recommended to prevent SIDS but may be used to monitor other medical problems. Only a small percentage of infants who died of SIDS were known to have prolonged apnea episodes, and monitors are also not medically recommended for subsequent siblings.*[1,2,10]

● Recommend contacting public health nurse for visit to new mother at least once or twice following discharge. *Researchers found that Native American infants whose mothers received such visits were 80% less likely to die from SIDS than those who were never visited.*[4]

● Refer parents to local SIDS programs and resources for learning (e.g., National SIDS/Infant Death Resource Center and similar Web sites). *Provides reassurance and information for self-paced learning.*[1]

● Encourage consultation with primary care provider if baby shows any signs of illness or behaviors that concern parent. *Promotes timely evaluation and intervention for treatable problems.*[1]

DOCUMENTATION FOCUS

Assessment/Reassessment
• Baseline findings, degree of parental anxiety or concern.
• History of infant deaths within family.

Planning
• Plan of care, specific interventions, and who is involved in planning.
• Teaching plan.

Implementation/Evaluation
• Parent's responses to interventions, teaching, and actions performed.
• Attainment or progress toward desired outcome(s)
• Modifications to plan of care.

Discharge Planning
• Long-term needs and actions to be taken.
• Support systems available, specific referrals made, and who is responsible for actions to be taken.

References

1. Epidemiology/risk reduction. (2008). Angel Eyes (The Colorado SIDS Program). Retrieved May 2009 from www.angeleyes.org/index_2.html.
2. Beers, M. H., Berkow, R. (1999). *The Merck Manual of Diagnosis and Therapy*. 17th ed. Whitehouse Station, NJ: Merck Research Laboratories.
3. Phillips, C. R. (1996). *Family-Centered Maternity and Newborn Care*. 4th ed. St. Louis, MO: Mosby.
4. London, M., et al. (2003). *Maternal Newborn & Child Nursing; Family-Centered Care*. Upper Saddle River, NJ: Prentice Hall.
5. Iyasu, S., et al. (2002). Risk factors for sudden infant death syndrome among Northern Plains Indians. *JAMA*, 288(21), 2717.
6. American Academy of Pediatrics, Task Force on Sleep Position and SIDS. (2000). Changing concepts of sudden infant death syndrome: Implications for infant sleep environment and position. *Pediatrics*, 105, 650–656.
7. National SIDS/Infant Death Resource Center. (2005). What is SIDS? U.S. Dept of Health and Human Services-Health Resources and Services Administration (HRSA). Retrieved February 2009 from www.sidscenter.org/documents/SIDRC/WhatIsSIDS.pdf.
8. The changing concept of sudden infant death syndrome: Diagnostic coding shifts, controversies regarding the sleeping environment, and new variations to consider in reducing risk. (2005). *Pediatrics*, 116(5), 1245–1255.
9. CDC Office of Minority Health and Health Disparities (OMHD). (2006). Eliminate disparities in infant mortality. Retrieved May 2009 from www.cdc.gov/omhd/AMH/factsheets/infant.htm.
10. Carroll, J. L., Siska, E. S. (1998). SIDS: Counseling parents to reduce the risk. *American Family Physicians*, 57(7), 1566–1572.

readiness for enhanced Decision Making

DEFINITION: A pattern of choosing courses of action that are sufficient for meeting short- and long-term health-related goals and can be strengthened

RELATED FACTORS

To be developed by nurse researchers and submitted to NANDA

DEFINING CHARACTERISTICS

Subjective
Expresses desire to enhance:
Decision making
Congruency of decisions with personal sociocultural values and goals
Risk-benefit analysis of decisions
Understanding of choices for decision making
Understanding of the meaning of choices
Use of reliable evidence for decisions

Sample Clinical Applications: Any acute or chronic condition, or healthy individual looking to improve well-being

(continues on page 256)

NURSING PRIORITY NO. 1

To assess causative/contributing factors:

- Identify situational crisis or problem and client's perception of the situation. *Identification of both reality and client's perception, which may not be the same as the reality, are necessary for planning care accurately.*[1]
- Ascertain cultural values or religious beliefs affecting perception of situation, sense of personal responsibility for crisis. *Knowing that lifestyle or choices may have caused or contributed to current situation may limit client's ability to accept outcome or view event realistically, and make choices regarding therapeutic regimen or lifestyle changes.*[5]
- Determine stage and degree of denial. *These factors will help identify whether the client is in early stages of denial and may be more amenable to intervention than those who are well entrenched in their beliefs. Treatment needs to begin where the client is and progress from there.*[1,6]
- Compare client's description of symptoms or conditions to reality of clinical picture and impact of illness or problem on lifestyle. *Identifies extent of discrepancy between the two and where treatment needs to start to help client accept reality.*[1]

NURSING PRIORITY NO. 2

To assist client to deal appropriately with situation:

- Develop nurse-client relationship using therapeutic communication skills of Active-listening and I-messages. *Promotes trust in which client can begin to look at reality of situation and deal with it in a positive manner.*[2]
- Provide safe, nonthreatening environment. *Allows client to feel comfortable enough to talk freely without fear of judgment and to deal with issues realistically.*[2]
- Encourage expressions of feelings, accepting client's view of the situation without confrontation. Set limits on maladaptive behavior *to promote safety. Helps client to work through and understand feelings. Unacceptable behavior is counterproductive to making progress, as client will view self negatively.*[2]
- Present accurate information as appropriate, without insisting that the client accept what has been presented. *Avoids confrontation, which may further entrench client in denial. Open manner permits client to begin to accept reality.*[2]
- Discuss client's behaviors in relation to illness (e.g., diabetes mellitus, alcoholism, terminal cancer) and point out the results of these behaviors. *Information can help client accept reality and opt to change behaviors.*[3]
- Encourage client to talk with SO(s)/friends. *May clarify concerns and reduce isolation and withdrawal. Constructive feedback from others facilitates understanding.*[4]
- Involve in group sessions. *Promotes discussion and feedback to enhance learning. Client can hear other views of reality and test own perceptions.*[4]
- Avoid agreeing with inaccurate statements or perceptions. *Prevents perpetuating false reality.*[2]
- Provide positive feedback for constructive moves toward independence. *Promotes repetition of desired behavior.*[4]

NURSING PRIORITY NO. 3

To promote wellness (Teaching/Discharge Considerations):

- Provide written information about illness or situation for client and family. *Provides client/family with reminders and resources they can refer to as they consider options.*[1]

- Involve family members/SO(s) in long-range planning. *Provides support, helps to identify and meet individual needs for the future.*[4]
- Refer to appropriate community resources (e.g., Diabetes Association, MS Society, Alcoholics Anonymous). *May be needed to help client with long-term adjustment.*[2]
- Refer to ND ineffective Coping.

DOCUMENTATION FOCUS

Assessment/Reassessment
- Assessment findings, degree of personal vulnerability and denial.
- Impact of illness or problem on lifestyle.

Planning
- Plan of care and who is involved in the planning.
- Teaching plan.

Implementation/Evaluation
- Client's response to interventions, teaching, and actions performed.
- Use of resources.
- Attainment or progress toward desired outcome(s).
- Modifications to plan of care.

Discharge Planning
- Long-term needs and who is responsible for actions taken.
- Specific referrals made.

References

1. Doenges, M. E., Moorhouse, M. F., Geissler-Murr, A. (2002). *Nursing Care Plans: Guidelines for Individualizing Patient Care.* 6th ed. Philadelphia: F. A. Davis.
2. Doenges, M. E., Townsend, M. C., Moorhouse, M. F. (1998). *Psychiatric Care Plans.* 3d ed. Philadelphia: F. A. Davis.
3. Burgess, E. (1994). Denial and terminal illness. *Am J Hosp Palliat Care,* 11(2), 46–48.
4. Robinson, A. W. (1999). Getting to the heart of denial. *Amer J Nurs,* 99(5), 38–42.
5. Lipson, J. G., Dibble, S. L., Minarik, P. A. (1996). *Culture & Nursing Care: A Pocket Guide.* San Francisco: UCSF Nursing Press.
6. Roberto, D. (2007). Man in denial. Retrieved September 2009 from www.robdiego.com/denial.htm.

impaired Dentition

DEFINITION: Disruption in tooth development/eruption patterns or structural integrity of individual teeth

RELATED FACTORS

Dietary habits; nutritional deficits
Selected prescription medications; chronic use of tobacco, coffee, tea, or red wine
Ineffective oral hygiene; sensitivity to heat or cold; chronic vomiting
Deficient knowledge regarding dental health; excessive intake of fluorides or use of abrasive cleaning agents
Barriers to self-care; lack of access or economic barriers to professional care
Genetic predisposition; bruxism
[Traumatic injury, surgical intervention]

DEFINING CHARACTERISTICS

Subjective
Toothache

Objective
Halitosis
Tooth enamel discoloration; erosion of enamel; excessive plaque
Worn down or abraded teeth; crown or root caries; tooth fracture(s); loose teeth; missing teeth; absence of teeth
Premature loss of primary teeth; incomplete eruption for age (may be primary or permanent teeth)
Excessive calculus
Malocclusion or tooth misalignment; asymmetrical facial expression

Sample Clinical Applications: Facial trauma or surgery, malnutrition, eating disorders, head or neck cancer, seizure disorder

DESIRED OUTCOMES/EVALUATION CRITERIA

Sample NOC linkages:
Oral Hygiene: Condition of the mouth, teeth, gums, and tongue
Self-Care: Oral Hygiene: Ability to care for own mouth and teeth independently with or without assistive device
Knowledge: Health Behavior: Extent of understanding conveyed about the promotion and protection of health

Client/SO Will (Include Specific Time Frame)
• Display healthy gums and mucous membranes and teeth in good repair.
• Report adequate nutritional and fluid intake.
• Verbalize understanding of appropriate oral hygiene regimen.
• Demonstrate effective dental hygiene skills.
• Follow through on referrals for appropriate dental care.

ACTION/INTERVENTIONS

Sample (NIC) linkages:
Oral Health Maintenance: Maintenance and promotion of oral hygiene and dental health for the patient at risk for developing oral or dental lesions
Oral Health Restoration: Promotion of healing for a patient who has an oral mucosa or dental lesion
Referral: Arrangement for services by another care provider or agency

NURSING PRIORITY NO. 1

To assess causative/contributing factors:

- Inspect oral cavity. Note presence or absence and intactness of teeth or dentures and appearance of gums. *Provides baseline for planning and interventions in terms of safety, nutritional needs, and aesthetics.*[1]
- Evaluate current status of dental hygiene and oral health *to determine need for instruction or coaching, assistive devices, and/or referral to dental care providers.*[1]
- Note presence of halitosis. *Bad breath may be result of numerous local or systemic conditions, including smoking, periodontal disease, dehydration, malnutrition, ketoacidosis, infections, or some antiseizure medications. Management can include simple mouth care or treatment of underlying conditions.*[2]
- Document age, developmental and cognitive status, and manual dexterity. Evaluate nutritional and health state, noting presence of conditions such as bulimia or chronic vomiting; musculoskeletal impairments; or problems with mouth (e.g., bleeding disorders, cancer lesions, abscesses, facial trauma). *Factors affecting client's dental health and ability to provide own dental care.*[1]
- Note current situation that will affect dental health (e.g., presence of airway/endotracheal [ET] intubation, facial fractures, jaw surgery, new braces, and use of anticoagulants or chemotherapy) that require special mouth care activities.[1,7]
- Document (photograph) facial injuries before treatment *to provide "pictorial baseline" for future comparison and evaluation.*

NURSING PRIORITY NO. 2

To treat/manage dental care needs:

- Ascertain client's usual method of oral care *to provide continuity of care or to build on client's existing knowledge base and current practices in developing plan of care.*[1]
- Assist with or provide oral care, as indicated:[1,8,9]
  Offer tap water or saline rinses, diluted alcohol-free mouthwashes.
  Provide gentle gum massage and tongue brushing with soft toothbrush, using fluoride toothpaste *to manage tartar buildup, if appropriate.*
  Use foam sticks *to swab gums and oral cavity when brushing not possible or inadvisable.*
  Assist with brushing and flossing when client is unable to do self-care.
  Demonstrate and assist with electric or battery-powered mouth care devices (e.g., toothbrush, plaque remover) as indicated.
  Assist with or provide denture care when indicated (e.g., remove and clean after meals and at bedtime).
- Remind client to brush teeth as indicated. *Cues may be needed if client is young, elderly, or cognitively or emotionally impaired.*

- Reposition endotracheal tubes and airway adjuncts routinely, carefully padding and protecting teeth and prosthetics.[7]
- Suction as needed, if client is unable to manage secretions.
- Maintain good jaw and facial alignment when fractures are present.
- Provide appropriate diet for optimal nutrition, considering client's ability to chew (e.g., liquids or soft foods), and offering low-sugar, low-starch foods and snacks *to minimize tooth decay.*
- Avoid thermal stimuli when teeth are sensitive. Recommend use of specific toothpastes designed *to reduce sensitivity of teeth.*
- Administer antibiotics as needed *to treat oral or gum infections that may be present and to prevent nosocomial infection in critically ill client whose teeth may be colonized by significant bacteria.*[3]
- Recommend use of analgesics and topical analgesics as needed *when dental pain is present.*
- Administer prophylactic antibiotic therapy prior to some dental procedures in susceptible individuals (e.g., presence of prosthetic heart valve, prior infective endocarditis, certain congenital heart defects, cardiac transplant with subsequent valvulopathy) *to reduce risk of infective endocarditis resulting from manipulation of gingival tissue or the periapical region of teeth, or procedures that will perforate the oral mucosa.*[10]
- Direct client to notify dental care provider when bleeding disorder present or anticoagulant therapy (including aspirin) being used. *May impact choice of procedure or technique in order to prevent excess bleeding.*
- Refer to appropriate care providers (e.g., dental hygienists, dentists, periodontist, oral surgeon).

NURSING PRIORITY NO. 3

To promote wellness (Teaching/Discharge Considerations):

- Instruct client/caregiver to inspect oral cavity and in home-care interventions *to provide good oral care, and prevent tooth decay and periodontal disease.*[4]
- Review or demonstrate proper toothbrushing techniques (i.e., brushing with bristles perpendicular to teeth surfaces) after meals and flossing daily. Suggest brushing with fluoride-containing toothpaste if client able to swallow and manage oral secretions. *This is the most effective way of reducing plaque formation and preventing periodontal disease.*[8]
- Discuss dental and oral health needs, both as client perceives needs and according to professional standards. *Client's perceptions are shaped by self-image, family, and cultural expectations or conditions created by disease or trauma. Current healthcare practices and education are geared toward practices that improve client's appearance and health, including reduced consumption of refined sugars, optimal fluoridation, access to preventative and restorative dental care, prevention of oral cancers and prevention of craniofacial injuries.*[4]
- Recommend that clients of all ages decrease sugary and high-carbohydrate foods in diet and snacks *to reduce buildup of plaque and risk of cavities caused by acids associated with the breakdown of sugar and starch.*[4]
- Instruct older client and caregiver(s) concerning their special needs and importance of regular dental care. *Elderly are prone to (1) experience decay around older fillings (also have more fillings in mouth); (2) receding gums, exposing root surfaces, which decay easily; (3) have reduced production of saliva, and use multiple medications that can cause dry mouth with loss of tooth and gum protection; and (4) loosening of teeth or poorly fitting dentures associated with gum or bone loss. These factors (often compounded by disease conditions and lack of funds) affect nutrient intake, chewing, swallowing, and oral cavity health.*[5]

∞ ● Advise mother regarding age-appropriate concerns:[1,4-6]

Instruct mother to refrain from allowing baby to fall asleep with bottle containing formula, milk, or sweetened beverages. Suggest use of water and pacifier during night *to prevent bottle tooth decay.*

Determine pattern of tooth appearance and tooth loss and compare to norms for primary and secondary teeth.

Discuss tooth discoloration and needed follow-up. *Brown or black spots on teeth usually indicates decay; gray tooth color may indicate nerve injury; multiple cavities in adolescent could be caused from repeated vomiting or bulimia.*

Discuss pit and fissure sealants. *Painted-on tooth surface sealants are becoming widely available to reduce number of cavities and sometimes are available through community dental programs.*

Determine if school dental health programs are available or recommend regular professional dental examinations as child grows.

Discuss with children/parents problems associated with oral piercing, if individual is contemplating piercing or needs to know what to watch for after piercing. *Common symptoms that occur with piercing of lips, gums, and tongue include pain, swelling, infection, increased flow of saliva, and chipped or cracked teeth requiring diligent oral care or more frequent dental examination to prevent complications.*

Discuss use of or need for safety devices (e.g., helmets, face mask, mouth guards) *to prevent or limit severity of sports-related facial injuries and tooth damage or loss*

∞ ● Discuss with pregnant women special needs and regular dental care. *Pregnant women need additional calcium and phosphorus to maintain good dental health and provide for strong teeth and bones in fetal development. Many women avoid dental care during pregnancy whether because of concerns for fetal health or other reasons (including lack of financial resources). However, one research study of 400 women suggests that pregnant women who receive treatment for periodontal disease can reduce their risk of giving birth to low-birth-weight or preterm baby.*[4]

● Review resources that are needed and available for the client to perform adequate dental hygiene care (e.g., toothbrush, paste, clean water, referral to dental care providers, access to financial assistance, personal care assistant).

● Encourage cessation of tobacco (especially smokeless) and enrolling in smoking cessation classes *to reduce risk of oral cancers and other health problems.*

● Discuss advisability of dental checkup and care prior to instituting chemotherapy or radiation *to minimize oral, dental, or tissue damage.*

DOCUMENTATION FOCUS

Assessment/Reassessment
- Individual findings, including individual factors influencing dentition problems.
- Baseline photos and description of oral cavity or structures.

Planning
- Plan of care and who is involved in planning.
- Teaching plan.

Implementation/Evaluation
- Responses to interventions, teaching, and actions performed.
- Attainment or progress toward desired outcome(s).
- Modifications to plan of care.

Discharge Planning

• Individual long-term needs, noting who is responsible for actions to be taken.

• Specific referrals made.

References

1. Doenges, M. E., Moorhouse, M. F., Murr, A. C. (2004). *Nurse's Pocket Guide: Diagnoses, Interventions, and Rationales*. 9th ed. Philadelphia: F. A. Davis.
2. Ayers, K. M., Colquhoun, A. N. (1998). Halitosis: causes, diagnosis, and treatment. *N Z Dent J*, 94(418), 156–160.
3. Scannapieco, F. A., Stewart, E. M., Mylotte, J. M. (1992). Colonization of dental plaque by respiratory pathogens in medical intensive care patients. *Crit Care Med*, 20, 740.
4. Retrieved July 2003 from public education pamphlets from the American Dental Association: Your diet and dental health; Oral changes with age; Sealants; Oral piercing; National Academy of Sciences panel reaffirms effectiveness of fluoride; Periodontal treatment can reduce risk of some pregnancy complications: study. (Original study from the University of Chile was published in *J Periodontology*, August 2002.) Pamphlets published at various times on the ADA.org Web site. www.ada.org/public/media.
5. How to keep a healthy smile for life. (2008). Retrieved September 2009 from American Academy of Periodontology. www.perio.org/consumer/smileforlife.htm.
6. Engel, J. (2002). *Moby's Pocket Guide to Pediatric Assessment*. 4th ed. St. Louis, MO: Mosby.
7. Truman, B. I., et al. (July 2002). Recommendations on selected interventions to prevent dental caries, oral and pharyngeal cancers, and sports-related craniofacial injuries. *Am J Prev Med*, 23(1 Suppl), 21–54.
8. Stiefel, K. A., et al. (2000). Improving oral hygiene for the seriously ill patient: Implementing research-based practice. *Medsurg Nurs*, 9(1), 40.
9. Tooth Decay: Prevention. (2005). Retrieved February 2007 from www.webmd.com/hw/dental/hw/172611.asp.
10. Stiles, S., Vega, C. P. (April 24, 2007). AHA updates recommendations for antibiotic prophylaxis for dental procedures. Retrieved July 2007 from www.medscape.com/viewarticle/555596.

risk for delayed Development

DEFINITION: At risk for delay of 25% or more in one or more of the areas of social or self-regulatory behavior or cognitive, language, gross, or fine motor skills

RISK FACTORS

Prenatal

Maternal age <15 years or >35 years

Unplanned or unwanted pregnancy; lack of, late, or poor prenatal care

Inadequate nutrition; poverty; illiteracy

Genetic or endocrine disorders; infections; substance abuse

Individual

Prematurity; congenital or genetic disorders

Vision or hearing impairment; frequent otitis media

Inadequate nutrition; failure to thrive

Chronic illness; chemotherapy; radiation therapy

Brain damage (e.g., hemorrhage in postnatal period, shaken baby, abuse, accident); seizures

⊕ Cultural 🅐 Collaborative 🏠 Community/Home Care ✐ Diagnostic Studies ∞ Pediatric/Geriatric/Lifespan 🗴 Medications

Positive drug screening(s); substance abuse; lead poisoning
Foster or adopted child
Behavior disorders
Technology-dependent
Natural disaster

Environmental
Poverty
Violence

Caregiver
Mental retardation; severe learning disability
Abuse
Mental illness

NOTE: A risk diagnosis is not evidenced by signs and symptoms, as the problem has not occurred; rather, nursing interventions are directed at prevention.

Sample Clinical Applications: Congenital or genetic disorders, prematurity, infection, nutritional problems (malnutrition, anorexia, failure to thrive), toxic exposures (e.g., lead), substance abuse, endocrine disorders, abuse or neglect, developmental delay

DESIRED OUTCOMES/EVALUATION CRITERIA

Sample **NOC** linkage:
Child Development: [specify age]: Milestones of physical, cognitive, and psychosocial progression by [specify] months or years of age

Client Will (Include Specific Time Frame)
• Perform motor, social, self-regulatory behavior, cognitive and language skills appropriate for age or within scope of present capabilities.

Sample **NOC** linkages:
Knowledge: Infant Care: Extent of understanding conveyed about caring for a baby from birth to first birthday
Parenting Performance: Parental actions to provide a child a nurturing and constructive physical, emotional, and social environment

Parent/Caregiver Will (Include Specific Time Frame)
• Verbalize understanding of age-appropriate development and expectations.
• Identify individual risk factors for developmental delay or deviation.
• Formulate plan(s) for prevention of developmental deviation.
• Initiate interventions or lifestyle changes promoting appropriate development.

ACTIONS/INTERVENTIONS

Sample **NIC** linkages:
Developmental Enhancement: Child [or] Adolescent: Facilitating or teaching parents/caregivers to facilitate the optimal gross motor, fine motor, language, cognitive, social, and emotional growth of preschool and school-age children during the transition from childhood to adulthood
Risk Identification: Analysis of potential risk factors, determination of health risks, and prioritization of risk-reduction strategies for an individual or group

---

NURSING PRIORITY NO. 1

To assess causative/contributing factors:

- Identify condition(s) that could contribute to developmental deviations as listed in Risk Factors (e.g., extremes of maternal age; prenatal substance abuse, fetal alcohol syndrome; brain injury or damage, especially that occurring before or at time of birth; prematurity; family history of developmental disorders; chronic severe illness, brain infections; mental illness or retardation; shaken baby syndrome abuse; family violence; failure to thrive; poverty; inadequate nutrition). *Developmental delay occurs when a child fails to achieve one or more developmental milestones and may be the result of one or multiple factors.*[1]

- Participate in multidisciplinary evaluation to assess client's development, including neurological exams or assessment tools such as Draw-a-Person, Denver Developmental Screening Test, Bender's Visual Motor Gestalt Test, Early Language Milestone (ELM) Scale 2, and developmental language disorders (DLD). *Delays may affect speech and language, fine or gross motor skills, or personal and social skills requiring a coordinated treatment approach based on client's specific needs.*[1,8–10]

- Obtain information from variety of sources. *Parents are often the first ones to think that there is a problem with their baby's development and should be encouraged to have routine well-baby checkups and screening for developmental delays. Teachers, family members, physicians, and others interacting with a client (older than infant) may have valuable input regarding behaviors that may indicate problems or developmental issues.*[1,2]

- Identify cultural beliefs, norms, and values, as they may impact parent/caregiver view of situation. *What is considered normal or abnormal development may be based on cultural beliefs or expectations.*[3]

- Ascertain nature of required parent/caregiver activities and evaluate caregiver's abilities to perform needed activities.

- Note severity and pervasiveness of situation (e.g., potential for long-term stress leading to abuse or neglect versus situational disruption during period of crisis or transition that may eventually level out). *Situations require different interventions in terms of the intensity and length of time that assistance and support may be critical to the parent/caregiver. A crisis can produce great change within a family, some of which can be detrimental to the individual or family unit.*[4–6]

- Evaluate environment in which long-standing care will be provided. *The physical, emotional, financial, and social needs of a family are impacted and intertwined with the needs of the client. Changes may be needed in the physical structure of the home or family roles, resulting in disruption and stress, placing everyone at risk.*[4,6]

NURSING PRIORITY NO. 2

To assist in preventing or limiting developmental delays:

- Note chronological age and review expectations for "normal development" *to help determine developmental expectations (e.g., when child should roll over, sit up alone, speak first words, attain a certain weight or height), and how the expectations may be altered by child's condition. Note: Pediatrician may screen with a motor quotient (MQ, which is child's age calculated by milestones met divided by chronological age and multiplied by 100). A MQ between 50 and 70 requires further evaluation and intervention.*[1,7]

- Review expected skills/activities, using authoritative text (e.g., Gesell, Musen/Congor), reports of neurological exams, or assessment tools. *Provides guide for evaluation of growth and development, and for comparative measurement of individual's progress.*[2,4]

- Describe realistic, age-appropriate patterns of development to parent/caregiver and promote activities and interactions that support developmental tasks where client is at this time. *Important in planning interventions in keeping with the individual's current status and potential. Each child will have own unique strengths and challenges.*[1-3]
- Collaborate with related professional resources (e.g., physical, occupational, rehabilitation, or speech therapists; home health agencies; social services, nutritionist; special-education teacher, family therapists; technological and adaptive equipment specialists; vocational counselor). *Multidisciplinary team care increases likelihood of developing a well-rounded plan of care that meets client/family's specialized and varied needs.*[4,10]

NURSING PRIORITY NO. 3

To promote wellness (Teaching/Discharge Considerations):

- Engage in and encourage prevention strategies (e.g., abstinence from drugs, alcohol and tobacco for pregnant women/child, referral for treatment programs, referral for violence prevention counseling, anticipatory guidance for potential handicaps [vision, hearing, failure to thrive]). *Promoting wellness starts with preventing complications and/or limiting severity of anticipated problems. Such strategies can often be initiated by nurses where the potential is first identified, in the community setting.*[1,4]
- Evaluate client's progress on continual basis. Identify target symptoms requiring intervention *to make referrals in a timely manner and/or to make adjustments in plan of care, as indicated.*[2]
- Emphasize importance of follow-up appointments as indicated *to promote ongoing evaluation, support, or management of situation.*[2]
- Discuss proactive wellness actions to take (e.g., periodic laboratory studies to monitor nutritional status or getting immunizations on schedule to prevent serious infections) *to avoid preventable complications.*[2]
- Maintain positive, hopeful attitude. Encourage setting of short-term realistic goals for achieving developmental potential. *Small, incremental steps are often easier to deal with, and successes enhance hopefulness and well-being.*[6]
- Provide information as appropriate, including pertinent reference materials, reliable Web sites. *Bibliotherapy provides opportunity to review data at own pace, enhancing likelihood of retention.*[1,2]
- Encourage attendance at educational programs (e.g., parenting classes, infant stimulation sessions; food buying, cooking, and nutrition; home and family safety, anger management, seminars on life stresses, aging process) *to address specific learning need or desires and interact with others with similar life challenges.*[2]
- Identify available community and national resources as appropriate (e.g., early intervention programs, gifted and talented programs, sheltered workshop, crippled children's services, medical equipment and supplier, caregiver support and respite services). *Provides additional assistance to support family efforts and can help identify community responsibilities (e.g., services required to be provided to school-age child).*[1]

DOCUMENTATION FOCUS

Assessment/Reassessment
- Assessment findings, individual needs, including developmental level.
- Caregiver's understanding of situation and individual role.

Planning
- Plan of care and who is involved in the planning.
- Teaching plan.

Implementation/Evaluation
- Client's response to interventions, teaching, and actions performed.
- Caregiver response to teaching.
- Attainment or progress toward desired outcome(s).
- Modifications to plan of care.

Discharge Planning
- Identified long-term needs and who is responsible for actions to be taken.
- Specific referrals made, sources for assistive devices, educational tools.

References

1. Developmental delays: A pediatrician's guide to your children's health and safety. Retrieved September 2009 from www.keepkidshealthy.com/welcome/conditions/developmentaldelays .html.
2. Volkmar, F., et al. American Academy of Child and Adolescent Psychiatry Working Group on Quality Issues. (1999). Practice parameters for the assessment and treatment of children, adolescents, and adults with autism and other pervasive developmental disorders. *J Am Acad Child Adolesc Psychiatry*, 38(12 suppl), 32s–54s.
3. Leininger, M. M. (1996). *Transcultural Nursing: Theories, Research and Practices*. 2d ed. Hilliard, OH: McGraw-Hill.
4. Doenges, M. E., Moorhouse, M. F., Geissler Murr, A. C. (2004). ND: Growth and development, delayed. *Nurse's Pocket Guide: Diagnoses, Interventions, and Rationales*. 9th ed. Philadelphia: F. A. Davis, 266–271.
5. Engel, J. (2002). *Mosby's Pocket Guide to Pediatric Assessment*. St. Louis, MO: Mosby.
6. Cox, H. C., et al. (2002). *Clinical Applications of Nursing Diagnosis: Adult, Child, Women's, Psychiatric, Gerontic, and Home Health Considerations*. 4th ed. Philadelphia: F. A. Davis.
7. Greenstein, D. B. Caring for children with special needs—Developmental delays. The National Network for Child Care. Retrieved September 2009 from www.ces.ncsu.edu/depts/fcs/pdfs/NC12.pdf.
8. Schiffman, R. F. (2004). Drug and substance use in adolescents. *MCN Am J Matern Child Nurs*, 29(1), 21–27.
9. Grenz, K., et al. (2005). Preventive services for children and adolescents. Institute for Clinical Systems Improvement [ICSI]. Article for National Guideline Clearinghouse Web site. Retrieved February 2007 from www.guideline.gov.
10. Blann, L. E. (2005). Early intervention for children and families with special needs. *MCN Am J Matern Child Nurs*, 30(4), 263–267.

(Diarrhea)

DEFINITION: Passage of loose, unformed stools

RELATED FACTORS

Psychological
High stress levels; anxiety

Situational
Laxative or alcohol abuse; toxins; contaminants
Adverse effects of medications; radiation
Tube feedings
Travel

Physiological
Inflammation; irritation
Infectious processes; parasites
Malabsorption

DEFINING CHARACTERISTICS

Subjective
Abdominal pain
Urgency, cramping

Objective
Hyperactive bowel sounds
At least three loose liquid stools per day

Sample Clinical Applications: Inflammatory bowel disease, gastritis, enteral feedings, alcohol abuse, antibiotic use, food allergies or contamination, AIDS, radiation, parasites

DESIRED OUTCOMES/EVALUATION CRITERIA

Sample NOC linkages:
Bowel Elimination: Formation and evacuation of stool
Hydration: Adequate water in the intracellular and extracellular compartments of the body
Knowledge: Illness Care: Extent of understanding conveyed about illness-related information needed to achieve and maintain optimal health

Client Will (Include Specific Time Frame)
• Reestablish and maintain normal pattern of bowel functioning.
• Verbalize understanding of causative factors and rationale for treatment regimen.
• Demonstrate appropriate behavior to assist with resolution of causative factors (e.g., proper food preparation or avoidance of irritating foods).

ACTIONS/INTERVENTIONS

Sample NIC linkages:
Diarrhea Management: Management and alleviation of diarrhea
Fluid Monitoring: Collection and analysis of patient data to regulate fluid balance
Perineal Care: Maintenance of perineal skin integrity and relief of perineal discomfort

NURSING PRIORITY NO. 1

To assess causative factors/etiology:

∞ • Evaluate client's/caregiver's perception of symptoms. *People perceive having diarrhea in many different ways, but generally if client is having loose watery stools occurring more*

---

than three times a day for 3 days or more, the diagnosis of diarrhea can be made. The condition can affect people of all ages, although its effect is more dangerous for infants and frail elderly (due to risk of dehydration).[1-3]

- Obtain comprehensive history of symptoms to help in identifying cause and treatment needs:[1,2,4-6,13,14]

  Ascertain onset and pattern of diarrhea, noting whether acute or chronic. **Acute diarrhea** *caused by (1) viral, bacterial, or parasitic infections (e.g., Norwalk virus, rotavirus; salmonella, shigella; and giardia, amebiasis, respectively); (2) bacterial food-borne toxins (e.g.,* Staphylococcus aureus, Escherichia coli*); (3) medications (e.g., antibiotics, chemotherapy agents, colchicine, laxatives); and (4) enteral tube feedings lasting a few days up to a week.* **Chronic diarrhea** *caused by irritable bowel syndrome; infectious diseases; inflammatory bowel disease; colon cancer and treatments; severe constipation; malabsorption disorders; laxative abuse; certain endocrine disorders (e.g., hyperthyroidism, Addison's disease) almost always lasts more than 3 weeks.*

  Review history and observe stools for **characteristics** (e.g., soft to watery stools, bloody, greasy), **frequency** (e.g., more than normal number of stools/day), **time of day** (e.g., after meals), **volume**, and **duration**.

  Identify any **associated signs/symptoms** (e.g., fever/chills, abdominal cramping, emotional upset, weight loss), **aggravating factors** (e.g., stress, foods), or **mitigating factors** (e.g., changes in diet, use of prescription or OTC medications).

  Note reports of abdominal or rectal pain. *Pain is often present with inflammatory bowel disease, irritable bowel syndrome, and mesenteric ischemia.*

- Note client's age. *Diarrhea in infant/young child and older or debilitated client can cause complications of dehydration and electrolyte imbalances.*
- Determine recent travel to developing countries or foreign environments; change in drinking water or food intake, consumption of unsafe food; swimming in untreated surface water; similar illness of family members/others close to client *that may help identify causative environmental factors.*[2,4-6]
- Review medications, noting side effects, possible interactions. *Many drugs (e.g., antibiotics, digitalis, angiotensin-converting enzyme [ACE] inhibitors, nonsteroidal anti-inflammatory drugs [NSAIDs], hypoglycemia agents, cholesterol-lowering drugs) can cause or exacerbate diarrhea, particularly in the elderly. Beginning antibiotic therapy often causes changes in bowel habits.*[1,2,6-8]
- Evaluate diet history and note nutritional, fluid, and electrolyte status *that may be causing or exacerbating diarrhea.*
- Auscultate abdomen for presence, location, and characteristics of bowel sounds. *High-pitched, rapidly occurring, loud or tinkling bowel sounds often accompany diarrhea.*[9]
- Determine if incontinence is present. *May indicate presence of fecal impaction, particularly in elderly, where impaction may be accompanied by diarrhea.*[3] (Refer to ND Bowel Incontinence.)
- Review results of laboratory testing on stool specimens. *Can reveal presence of bacterial or viral infection, parasites, fat, blood, offending drugs, metabolic disorder, malabsorption syndrome, gastroenteritis, colitis, and so forth.*[1,2,4-6]
- Assist with/prepare for additional evaluation as indicated. *Chronic diarrhea may require more invasive testing, including upper and/or lower gastrointestinal (GI) radiographs, ultrasound, endoscopic evaluations, biopsy, and so forth.*[12]

NURSING PRIORITY NO. 2

To alleviate/limit condition:

- Assist with treatment of underlying conditions (e.g., infections, malabsorption syndrome, cancer) and complications of diarrhea. *Treatments are varied and may be as simple as allowing time for recovery from a self-limiting gastroenteritis, or may require complex treatments, including antimicrobials and rehydration, or community health interventions for contaminated food or water sources.*[14]

- Encourage bedrest during acute episode. *Rest reduces intestinal motility and metabolic rate when infection or hemorrhage is a complication.*[1–6,8,10]
- Restrict solid food intake, if indicated. *May help on short-term to allow for bowel rest and reduced intestinal workload, especially if cause of diarrhea is under investigation or vomiting is present. Note: Child's preferred or usual diet may be continued to prevent or limit dehydration, with the possible limitation of fruit, fruit juices, or milk, if these factors are exacerbating the diarrhea.*[5,9]
- Limit caffeine and high-fat (e.g., butter, fried foods) or high-protein (e.g., meats) and foods known to cause or aggravate diarrhea (e.g., extremely hot or cold foods, chili), milk, and fruits or fruit juices as appropriate.[1–6,8,10]
- Adjust strength and/or rate of enteral tube feedings; change formula as indicated *when diarrhea is associated with tube feedings.*[1–6,8,10]
- Consider change in infant formula. *Diarrhea may be result of or aggravated by intolerance to specific formula.*[9,10]
- Change medications as appropriate (e.g., stopping magnesium-containing antacid or antibiotic causing diarrhea).[7,8]
- Promote the use of relaxation techniques (e.g., progressive relaxation exercise, visualization techniques) *to decrease stress and anxiety.*[1–6,8,10]
- Administer medications *to treat or limit diarrhea, as indicated, depending on cause. May include use of antidiarrheals, anti-infectives, antispasmodics, and so forth.*[1–6,8,10,14]
- Assist client to manage situation:[12]
  Respond to call for assistance promptly.
  Place bedpan in bed with client (if desired) or commode chair near bed *to provide quick access and reduce need to wait for assistance of others.*
  Provide privacy; remove stool promptly; use room deodorizers *to reduce noxious odors, limit embarrassment.*
  Use incontinence pads, depending on the severity of the problem.
  Provide emotional and psychological support. *Diarrhea can be source of great embarrassment and can lead to social isolation and feeling of powerlessness. Intimate relationship and sexual activity may be affected and need specific interventions to resolve.*
- Maintain skin integrity:[12]
  Assist as needed with pericare after each bowel movement *to prevent skin excoriation and breakdown.*
  Provide prompt diaper or incontinence pad change and gentle cleansing, *because skin breakdown can occur quickly with diarrhea.*
  Apply lotion or skin barrier ointment as needed.
  Provide dry linen as necessary.
  Expose perineum and buttocks to air or use heat lamp with caution if needed *to keep area dry*
  Refer to ND impaired Skin Integrity.

NURSING PRIORITY NO. 3

To restore/maintain hydration/electrolyte balance:

- Note reports of thirst, less frequent or absent urination, dry mouth and skin, weakness, light-headedness, headache. *Signs/symptoms of dehydration and need for rehydration.*[1,3,5,6,10]

∞ • Observe for or question parents about young child crying with no tears, fever, decreased urination, or no wet diapers for 6 to 8 hours, listlessness or irritability, sunken eyes, dry mouth and tongue, and suspected or documented weight loss. *Child needs urgent or emergency treatment for dehydration if these signs are present and child is not taking fluids.*[1–3,5,6,10]

∞ • Note presence of low blood pressure or postural hypotension, tachycardia, poor skin hydration or turgor. *Presence of these factors indicates severe dehydration and electrolyte imbalance. The frail elderly can progress quickly to this point, especially when vomiting is present or client's normal food and fluid intake is below requirements.*[1–3,5,6,10]

• Monitor total intake and output, including stool output as possible. *Provides estimation of fluid needs.*[1,3,5,6,10]

∞ • Weigh infant's diapers to determine output.[1–3,5,6,10]

• Offer and encourage water, plus broth or soups that contain sodium, and fruit juices or soft fruits or vegetables that contain potassium *to replace water and electrolytes.*[1–3,5,6,10]

• Recommend oral intake of beverages such as Gatorade, Pedialyte, Infalyte, Smart Water. *Commercial rehydration solutions containing electrolytes may prevent or correct imbalances.*[1–3,5,6,10]

⊛ • Administer enteral or parenteral feedings and IV and electrolyte fluids as indicated. *Intravenous fluids may be needed either short-term to restore hydration status (e.g., acute gastroenteritis) or long-term (severe osmotic diarrhea). Enteral or parenteral nutrition is reserved for clients unable to maintain adequate nutritional status because of long-term diarrhea (e.g., wasting syndrome, malnutrition states).*[1–3,5,6,10]

NURSING PRIORITY NO. 4

To promote return to normal bowel functioning:

• Encourage intake of nonirritating liquids, increasing intake as tolerated and gradually returning to normal diet.[1,2,4–6,10,11]

• Recommend products such as natural fiber, plain natural yogurt, Lactinex *to restore normal bowel flora.*[1,2,4–6,10,11]

💊 • Administer medications as ordered *to treat infectious process, decrease motility, and/or absorb water.*[1,2,4–6,10,11]

NURSING PRIORITY NO. 5

To promote wellness (Teaching/Discharge Considerations):

🏠 • Review individual's causative factors and appropriate interventions *to prevent recurrence.*

💊 • Discuss medication regimen, including prescription and over-the-counter (OTC) drugs, *especially when client has multiple medications with potential for diarrhea as side effect or interaction.*[12]

🏠 • Instruct clients planning to travel outside the United States about traveler's diarrhea and ways to prevent or limit food- and waterbourne illness *(e.g., do not drink tap water, use tap water ice cubes, or brush your teeth with tap water; avoid raw fruits and vegetables, unless they can be peeled; avoid raw or rare meat or fish; discuss destination with local health department for particular recommendations, such as advisability of use of protective antibiotics).*[12]

🏠 • Assess home or living environment, if indicated. *Discussion with client/caregivers may be needed regarding (1) sanitation and hygiene (e.g., hand hygiene and laundry practices), (2) safe food storage and preparation (to reduce risk of food-borne infections), and (3) particular risks in select populations (e.g., persons with chronic liver disease should avoid*

shellfish; persons with impaired immune defenses are at increased risk for diarrhea associated with raw dairy products or unheated deli meats; pregnant women should avoid undercooked meats [infectious diarrhea]).[12]

- Emphasize importance of hand hygiene *to prevent spread of infectious causes of diarrhea such as* Clostridium difficile, *S. aureus, and so forth.*[15]
- Instruct parent/caregiver in signs of dehydration and importance of fluid and electrolyte replacement, as well as simple food and fluids to provide rehydration.

DOCUMENTATION FOCUS

Assessment/Reassessment
- Assessment findings, including characteristics and pattern of elimination.

Planning
- Plan of care and who is involved in planning.
- Teaching plan.

Implementation/Evaluation
- Client's response to treatment, teaching, and actions performed.
- Attainment or progress toward desired outcome(s).
- Modifications to plan of care.

Discharge planning
- Recommendations for follow-up care.

References

1. Hogan, C. M. (1998). The nurse's role in diarrhea management. *Oncol Nurs Forum*, 25(5), 879–885.
2. Diarrhea. National Digestive Diseases Information Clearinghouse. (NDDIC). National Institutes of Health Pub. No. 01–2749 January 2001.
3. Carnaveli, D. L., Patrick, M. (1993). *Nursing Management for the Elderly*. 3d ed. Philadelphia: J. B. Lippincott.
4. Evidence-based clinical guideline for acute gastroenteritis (AGE) in children in children aged 2 months through 5 years. (2006). Cincinnati Children's Hospital Medical Center. Retrieved September 2009 from www.guideline.gov.
5. American Gastroenterological Association medical position statement: Guidelines for the evaluation of chronic diarrhea. (1999). Retrieved July 2003 from www.guideline.gov.
6. Guerrant, R. L., et al. (2001). Practice guidelines for the management of infectious diarrhea. *Clin Infect Dis*, 32(3), 331–351.
7. Ratnaike, R. N. (2000). Drug-induced diarrhea in older persons. *Clin Geriatr*, 8(1), 67–76.
8. Vogel, L. C. (1995). Antibiotic-induced diarrhea. *Orthop Nurs*, 14, 38–41.
9. Engel, J. (2002). *Mosby's Pocket Guide to Pediatric Assessment*. 4th ed. St. Louis, MO: Mosby.
10. Larson, C. E. (2000). Evidence-based practice: Safety and efficacy of oral rehydration therapy for the treatment of diarrhea and gastroenteritis in pediatrics. *Pediatr Nurs*, 26(2), 177–179.
11. Peikin, R. (1999). *Diarrhea in Gastrointestinal Health*. New York: HarperCollins.
12. Doenges, M. E., Moorhouse, M. F., Geissler-Murr, A. C. (2002). ND Diarrhea, risk for in gastrointestinal disorders. *Nursing Care Plans: Guidelines for Individualizing Patient Care*. 6th ed. Philadelphia: F. A. Davis.
13. Marks, J. W., Lee, D. (2004). Diarrhea. Article for MedicineNet Web site. Retrieved February 2007 from www.medicinenet.com.
14. Diskin, A. (2006). Gastroenteritis. Retrieved February 2007 from www.emedicine.com/emerg/topic213.htm.

15. DeNoon, D. (2006). C. Diff: New threat from old bug: Epidemic gut infection causing rapid rise in life-threatening disease. Retrieved February 2007 from www.medicinenet.com.

risk for compromised human Dignity

DEFINITION: At risk for perceived loss of respect and honor

RISK FACTORS

Loss of control of body functions; exposure of the body
Perceived humiliation or invasion of privacy
Disclosure of confidential information; stigmatizing label; use of undefined medical terms
Perceived dehumanizing treatment or intrusion by clinicians
Inadequate participation in decision making
Cultural incongruity

NOTE: A risk diagnosis is not evidenced by signs and symptoms, as the problem has not occurred; rather, nursing interventions are directed at prevention.
Sample Clinical Applications: Chronic conditions (e.g., multiple sclerosis [MS], stroke, quadriplegia, amyotrophic lateral sclerosis [ALS])

DESIRED OUTCOMES/EVALUATION CRITERIA

Sample NOC linkages:
Client Satisfaction: Protection of Rights: Extent of positive perception of protection of a patient's legal and moral rights provided by nursing staff
Client Satisfaction: Cultural Needs Fulfillment: Extent of positive perception of integration of cultural beliefs, values, and social structures into nursing care

Client Will (Include Specific Time Frame)
• Verbalize awareness of specific problem.
• Identify positive ways to deal with situation.
• Demonstrate problem-solving skills.
• Express sense of dignity in situation.

ACTIONS/INTERVENTIONS

Sample NIC linkages:
Cultural Brokerage: The deliberate use of culturally competent strategies to bridge or mediate between the patient's culture and the biomedical healthcare system
Patient Rights Protection: Protection of healthcare rights of a patient, especially a minor, incapacitated, or incompetent patient unable to make decisions
Emotional Support: Provision of reassurance, acceptance, and encouragement during times of stress

NURSING PRIORITY NO. 1

To determine individual situation as perceived by client:

- Determine client's perception and specific factors that could lead to sense of loss of dignity. *Human dignity is a totality of the individual's uniqueness—mind, body, and spirit, and all components must be considered.*[4]
- Note names or labels, or items used by staff, friends/family that stigmatize the client. *Human dignity is threatened by insensitive as well as inadequate healthcare and lack of client participation in care decisions.*[4]
- Identify cultural beliefs or values and degree of importance to client. *Individuals cling to their basic beliefs and values, especially during times of stress, which may result in conflict with current circumstances.*[7]
- Identify client's/SO's healthcare goals and expectations. *Clarifies client's (or SO's/family's) vision, provides framework for planning care, identifies possible conflicts.*[2]
- Note availability of support systems. *Client will feel loved and valued and will be able to manage difficult circumstances better when the support of family and friends surrounds individual.*[2]
- Ascertain response of family/SOs to client's situation. *It is important that family supports and values client to enable him or her to manage situation. If they are not supportive or conflicts arise, client may need to separate self from family members who are negative.*[3]

NURSING PRIORITY NO. 2

To assist client to deal with situation in positive ways:

- Ask client by what name he or she would like to be addressed. *Name is important to a person's identity and recognizes his or her individuality. Many older people prefer to be addressed in a formal manner (e.g., Mr. or Mrs.).*[2,7]
- Active-listen feelings, encouraging client to verbalize concerns. Be available for support and assistance. *Helps client to discover underlying reasons for feelings and discuss solutions.*[5]
- Respect the client's needs and wishes for quiet, privacy, talking, or silence. *Conveys respect and concern for client's dignity.*[3]
- Provide for privacy when discussing sensitive or personal issues. *Demonstrates respect for client and promotes sense of safe environment for free exchange of thoughts and feelings.*[3]
- Use understandable terms when talking to client/family about the medical condition, procedures, and treatments. *Most lay people do not understand medical terms and may be hesitant to ask what is meant.*[6]
- Encourage family/SO(s) to treat client with respect and understanding, especially when the client is older and may be irritable and difficult to deal with. *Everyone needs to be treated with respect and dignity, regardless of individual abilities or frailty.*[4]
- Include client and family in decision making, especially regarding end-of-life issues. *Helps the individual feel respected or valued and involved in the care process.*[2]
- Involve facility or local ethics committee as appropriate *to facilitate mediation or resolution of conflicts between client/family and staff, or client and family members.*
- Protect client's privacy when providing personal care and during procedures. Assure client is covered adequately when care is being given. *Prevents embarrassment over unnecessary exposure and conveys a message of caring.*[6]
- Clean client immediately when vomiting, bleeding, or incontinence occurs. Speak in a gentle voice. *Assures client that these things cannot be helped and that nurses are glad to take care of the problem.*

NURSING PRIORITY NO. 3

To promote wellness (Teaching/Discharge Considerations):

- 🏠 • Discuss client's rights as an individual. *While hospitals and other care settings have a Client's Bill of Rights, a broader view of human dignity is stated in the U.S. Constitution.*[1,6]
- 🏠 • Assist with planning for the future, taking into account client's desires and rights. *As the client plans for the future, the needs of the self as a human who has dignity are considered and incorporated to preserve that dignity.*[4]
- 🌐 • Incorporate familial, religious, and cultural factors that have meaning for client in planning process. *When these issues are addressed and incorporated in plan of care, they add to the feelings of inclusion for the client.*[4,7]
- ♨ • Refer to other resources (e.g., pastoral care, counseling, organized support groups, classes), as appropriate. *May need additional assistance to deal with illness/situation.*[6]

DOCUMENTATION FOCUS

Assessment/Reassessment
- Assessment findings, including individual risk factors, client's perceptions, and concerns about involvement in care.
- Individual cultural or religious beliefs and values, healthcare goals.
- Responses and involvement of family/SOs.

Planning
- Plan of care and who is involved in planning.
- Teaching plan.

Implementation/Evaluation
- Client's response to interventions, teaching, and actions performed.
- Attainment or progress toward desired outcome(s).
- Modifications to plan of care.

Discharge Planning
- Long-term needs and who is responsible for actions to be taken.
- Specific referrals made.

References

1. Champion aspirations for human dignity. Retrieved March 2007 from The White House historical material, www.georgewbush-whitehouse.archives.gov/nsc/nss/2006/sectionII.html.
2. Schulman, A. (2005). Bioethics and the question of human dignity. Human Dignity and Bioethics: Essays Commissioned by the Presidents' Council on Bioethics. Retrieved March 2007 from www.bioethics.gov/reports/human_dignity/chapter1.html.
3. Cheshire, W. P., Jr. (2007). Grey matters when eloquence is inarticulate. *Ethics & Medicine: An International Journal of Bioethics*, 22(3). Retrieved March 2007 from Center for Bioethics and Human Dignity www.cbhd.org/resources/neuroethics/cheshire_2007-01-26.htm.
4. The Center for Ethics and Advocacy in Healthcare. Mission statement: Our beliefs. Retrieved March 2007 from www.healthcare-ethics.org/about/.
5. Gordon, T. (2000). *Parent Effectiveness Training.* New York: Three Rivers Press.
6. Doenges, M., Moorhouse, M., Murr, A. (2002). *Nursing Care Plans: Guidelines for Individualizing Patient Care.* 6th ed. Philadelphia: F. A. Davis.
7. Lipson, J. G., Dibble, S. L., Minarik, P. A. (1996). *Culture & Nursing Care: A Pocket Guide.* San Francisco: UCSF Nursing Press.

moral Distress

DEFINITION: Response to the inability to carry out one's chosen ethical/moral decision/action

RELATED FACTORS

Conflict among decision makers, [e.g., client/family, healthcare providers, insurance payers, regulatory agencies]
Conflicting information guiding moral or ethical decision making; cultural conflicts
Treatment decisions; end-of-life decisions; loss of autonomy
Time constraints for decision making; physical distance of decision maker

DEFINING CHARACTERISTICS

Subjective
Expresses anguish (e.g., powerlessness, guilt, frustration, anxiety, self-doubt, fear) over difficulty of acting on one's moral choice

DESIRED OUTCOMES/EVALUATION CRITERIA

Sample NOC linkages:
Decision-Making: Ability to make judgments and choose between two or more alternatives
Client Satisfaction: Protection of Rights: Extent of positive perception of a patient's legal and moral rights provided by nursing staff
Participation in Healthcare Decision: Personal involvement in selecting and evaluating healthcare options to achieve desired outcome

Client Will (Include Specific Time Frame)
• Verbalize understanding of causes for conflict in own situation.
• Be aware of own moral values conflicting with desired or required course of action.
• Identify positive ways or actions necessary to deal with own self and situation.
• Express sense of satisfaction with or acceptance of resolution.

ACTIONS/INTERVENTIONS

Sample NIC linkages:
Values Clarification: Assisting another to clarify her or his own values in order to facilitate effective decision making
Decision-Making Support: Providing information and support for a patient who is making a decision regarding healthcare
Mutual Goal-Setting: Collaborating with a patient to identify and prioritize care goals, then developing a plan of care for achieving those goals

NURSING PRIORITY NO. 1

To identify cause/situation in which moral distress is occurring:

• Note situations or individuals at high risk for conflict. *For example, family members may not agree on proper course of action for comatose loved one, parents faced with expectation of taking ventilator-dependent child home and effect on family as a whole,[8] care providers discontinuing life-support measures for preterm infant are likely to encounter some degree of distress with decision making but may be silent about their discomfort. Recognizing potential for moral distress allows for timely intervention and support for involved parties.*

- Determine client's perceptions and specific factors resulting in a sense of distress, and all parties involved in situation. *Conflict may be personal or job related. Moral conflict centers around lessening the amount of harm suffered, with the involved individuals usually struggling with decisions such as what "can be done" to prevent, improve, or cure a medical condition or what "ought to be done" in a specific situation, often within financial constraints or scarcity of resources.[6]*

- Note use of sarcasm, avoidance, apathy, crying, reports of depression or loss of meaning. *Individuals may not understand their feelings of uneasiness or distress or know that the emotional basis for moral distress is anger.[4]*

- Ascertain response of family/SOs to client's situation/healthcare choices. *May provide clues to emotional or conflictual problems individual is experiencing.*

- Identify healthcare goals and expectations. *New treatment options and technology can prolong life, or postpone death based on the individual's personal viewpoint, increasing the possibility of conflict with others, including healthcare providers.[2]*

- Ascertain cultural beliefs and values, and degree of importance to client. *Cultural diversity may lead to disparate views and expectations between client, SO/family members, and healthcare providers. When tensions between conflicting values cannot be resolved, persons experience moral distress.[2]*

- Note attitudes and expressions of dissatisfaction of caregivers/staff. *Client may feel pressure or disapproval if own views are not congruent with expectations of those perceived to be more knowledgeable or in "authority." Furthermore, healthcare providers may themselves feel moral distress in carrying out or refraining from performing requested interventions.[7]*

- Determine degree of emotional and physical distress (e.g., fatigue, headaches, forgetfulness, anger, guilt, resentment) individual(s) are experiencing and impact on ability to function. *Moral distress can be very destructive, affecting one's ability to carry out daily tasks and care for self or others, and may lead to a crisis of faith.[5]*

- Assess sleep habits of involved parties. *Evidence suggests that sleep deprivation can harm a person's physical and emotional well-being, hindering the ability to integrate emotion and cognition to guide moral judgment.[5]*

- Perform or review results of moral distress test, such as the Moral Distress Assessment questionnaire (MDAQ) or Moral Distress Scale, *to help measure degree of involvement and identify possible actions to improve situation.[3,10]*

- Note availability of family/friends/coworkers. *Provides support and encouragement for difficult situation.[4]*

NURSING PRIORITY NO. 2

To assist client/involved individuals to develop/effectively use problem-solving skills:

- Encourage involved individuals to recognize and name the experience, resulting in moral sensitivity. *Brings concerns out in the open so they can be dealt with.[1]*

- Provide time for nonjudgmental discussion of philosophical issues or questions about impact of conflict leading to moral questioning of current situation. *Moral issues have been discussed and studied for many years (e.g., philosophers, such as Piaget [1932] with his early work in developmental moral psychology, discussed what is the basis for moral reasoning). It is not possible to accurately read another's mind, and open discussion helps those involved in conflict to better understand the situation and begin to look at options.[9]*

- Use skills such as Active-listening, I-messages, and problem-solving *to clarify feelings of anxiety and conflict. Helps to understand what the ethical dilemmas are that lead to moral distress (e.g., family members ignoring advanced directives of loved one, providing lifesaving care to a death-row inmate, terminally ill individual requesting assistance to die, families living with the moral experience of caring for a ventilator-assisted child in the home).*[8]
- Provide privacy when discussing sensitive personal issues. *Shows regard and concern for individual's self-worth* [2]
- Ascertain coping behaviors client has used successfully in the past that may be used in the current situation. *When encouraged, individuals can recall past situations where they had a positive experience and used successful coping skills.*[4]
- Identify role models (e.g., other individuals who have experienced similar problems in their lives). *Sharing of experiences, identifying options can be helpful to deal with current situation.*[1]
- Involve facility or local ethics committee, or ethicist as appropriate *to educate, make recommendations, and facilitate mediation or resolution of issues.*[3]

NURSING PRIORITY NO. 3

To promote wellness (Teaching/Discharge Considerations):

- Engage all parties, as appropriate, in developing plan to address conflict. *Resolving one's moral distress requires making changes or compromises while preserving one's integrity and authenticity.*[4]
- Incorporate identified familial, religious, and cultural factors that have meaning for client. *Can provide comfort for the person.*[7]
- Refer to appropriate resources for support/guidance (e.g., pastoral care, counseling, organized support groups, classes) as indicated. *These resources can help client as they pursue the search for moral resolution.*[8]
- Assist individual to recognize that if she or he follows their moral decisions, they may clash with the legal system, and refer to appropriate resource for legal opinion/options.[3]
- Encourage the work organization to provide better support resources and structures. Discuss changes in the healthcare system that have resulted in more complex healthcare decisions. *The complexity of healthcare choices, expectations of clients/families, increasing costs or limitations in resources has resulted in increased pressures on healthcare providers and has led to ethics becoming a required component of clinical practice. Acknowledging reality of potential areas of conflict and providing proactive discussions for staff as well as support for involved individuals when making difficult decisions can decrease moral distress for staff and families.*[2,8]

DOCUMENTATION FOCUS

Assessment/Reassessment
- Individual findings, including nature of moral conflict, individuals involved in conflict.
- Physical and emotional responses to conflict.
- Individual cultural or religious beliefs and values, healthcare goals.
- Responses and involvement of family/SOs or coworkers.

Planning
- Plan of care and who is involved in planning.
- Teaching plan.

Implementation/Evaluation
- Responses to interventions and teaching.
- Effects of participation in classes or mediation activities.
- Attainment or progress toward desired outcome(s).
- Modifications to plan of care.

Discharge Planning
- Long-term needs and who is responsible for actions to be taken.
- Available resources.
- Specific referrals made.

References

1. Elpern, E. H., Covert, B., Kleinpell, R. (2005). Moral distress of staff nurses in a medical intensive care unit. *Am J Crit Care*, 14, 523–539.
2. Kalvemark, S., et al. (2004). Living with conflicts—Ethical dilemmas and moral distress in the health care system. *Soc Sci Med*, 58(6), 1075–1084. Dept. of Public Health and Caring Sciences, Uppsala University, Uppsala, Sweden.
3. Hanna, D. R. (2002). Moral distress redefined: The lived experience of moral distress of nurses who participated in legal, elective, surgically induced abortions. Retrieved July 2007 from www.escholarship.bc.edu/dissertations/AAI3053658/.
4. Cheshire, W. P. (2007). Grey matters when eloquence is inarticulate. Ethics & Medicine: An International Journal of Bioethics, 22(3). Retrieved July 2007 from Center for Bioethics and Human Dignity www.cbhd.org/resources/neuroethics/cheshire_2007-02-26.htm.
5. Preidt, R. (2007). Sleeplessness clouds moral choices. American Academy of Sleep Medicine. Retrieved July 2007 from www.ktvotv3.com/Global/story.asp?S=6170132&nav=menu124_5.
6. Kopala, B., Burkhart, L. (2005). Ethical dilemma and moral distress: Proposed new NANDA diagnoses. *In J Nurs Terminol Classif*, 16(1).
7. Nichols, S. (2002). Mindreading and the core architecture of moral psychology. *Cognition*, 84, 221–236.
8. Carnevale, F. A., Alexander, E., Renneck, J. (2006). Daily living with distress and enrichment: The moral experience of families with ventilator-assisted children at home. *Pediatrics*, 117(1), e48–e60.
9. Piaget, J. (1932). In Gabain, M. (ed). *The Psychology of Moral Development: The Nature and Validity of Moral Stages* (Translation published 1965). New York: Free Press.
10. Corley, M. (1993). Moral distress of critical care nurses. *Am J Crit Care Nurs*, 4(4), 280–285.

risk for Disuse Syndrome

DEFINITION: At risk for deterioration of body systems as the result of prescribed or unavoidable musculoskeletal inactivity

Note: Complications from immobility can include pressure ulcer, constipation, stasis of pulmonary secretions, thrombosis, urinary tract infection and/or retention, decreased strength or endurance, orthostatic hypotension, decreased range of joint motion, disorientation, body image disturbance, and powerlessness.

RISK FACTORS

Severe pain; [chronic pain]
Paralysis; [other neuromuscular impairment]
Mechanical or prescribed immobilization

Altered level of consciousness
[Chronic physical or mental illness]

NOTE: A risk diagnosis is not evidenced by signs and symptoms, as the problem has not occurred; rather, nursing interventions are directed at prevention.

Sample Clinical Applications: Multiple sclerosis (MS), cerebral palsy, muscular dystrophy, postpolio syndrome, brain injury or stroke, spinal cord injury (SCI), arthritis, osteoporosis, fractures, amputation, dementia

DESIRED OUTCOMES/EVALUATION CRITERIA

Sample NOC linkages:
Immobility Consequences: Physiological: Severity of compromise in physiological functioning due to impaired physical mobility
Risk Control: Personal actions to prevent, eliminate, or reduce modifiable health threats
Immobility Consequences: Psycho-Cognitive: Severity of compromise in psycho-cognitive functioning due to impaired physical mobility

Client Will (Include Specific Time Frame)
- Display intact skin and tissues or achieve timely wound healing.
- Maintain or reestablish effective elimination patterns.
- Be free of signs/symptoms of infectious processes.
- Demonstrate absence of pulmonary congestion with breath sounds clear.
- Demonstrate adequate peripheral perfusion with stable vital signs, skin warm and dry, palpable peripheral pulses.
- Maintain usual reality orientation.
- Maintain or regain optimal level of cognitive, neurosensory, and musculoskeletal functioning.
- Express sense of control over the present situation and potential outcome.
- Recognize and incorporate change into self-concept in accurate manner without negative self-esteem.

ACTIONS/INTERVENTIONS

Sample NIC linkages:
Energy Management: Regulating energy use to treat or prevent fatigue and optimize function
Environmental Management: Manipulation of the patient's surroundings for therapeutic benefit
Exercise Promotion: Facilitation of regular physical exercise to maintain or advance to a higher level of fitness and health

NURSING PRIORITY NO. 1

To evaluate probability of developing complications:

- Identify underlying conditions/pathology (e.g., cancer, trauma; fractures with casting, immobilization devices; surgery, chronic disease conditions, malnutrition; neurological conditions [e.g., stroke, brain or SCI, postpolio syndrome, MS]; chronic pain conditions; use of predisposing medications [e.g., steroids]) that cause or exacerbate problems associated with inactivity and immobility.

- Identify potential concerns, including cognition, mobility, and exercise status. *Disuse syndrome can be a complication of and cause for bedridden state. The syndrome can include muscle and bone atrophy, stiffening of joints, brittle bones, reduction of cardiopulmonary function, loss of red blood cells (RBCs), decreased sex hormones, decreased resistance to infections, increased proportion of body fat in relation to muscle mass and chemical changes in the brain, which adversely impact client's activities of daily living (ADLs), social life, and quality of life.*[1,2]

- Note client's age. *Age-related physiological changes accompanied by chronic illness predispose older adults to functional decline related to inactivity and immobility.*[3,8]

- Determine if client's condition is acute/short-term or whether it may be a long-term/permanent condition. *Relatively short-term conditions (e.g., simple fracture treated with cast) may respond quickly to rehabilitative efforts. Long-term conditions (e.g., stroke, aged person with dementia, cancers, demyelinating or degenerative diseases, SCI, and psychological problems such as depression or learned helplessness) have a higher risk of complications for the client and caregiver.*

- Assess and document (ongoing) client's functional status, including cognition, vision, and hearing, social support, psychological well-being, abilities in performance of ADLs *for comparative baseline, to evaluate response to treatment and to identify preventative interventions or necessary services.*[8]

- Evaluate client's risk for injury. *Risk is greater in client with cognitive problems, lack of safe or stimulating environment, inadequate mobility aids, and/or sensory-perception problems.*[3]

- Ascertain attitudes of individual/SO about condition (e.g., cultural values, stigma). Note misconceptions. The client may be influenced (positively or negatively) by peer group and family role expectations.

- Evaluate client's/family's understanding and ability to manage care for prolonged period. Ascertain availability and use of support systems. *Caregivers may be influenced by their own physical or emotional limitations, degree of commitment to assisting the client toward optimal independence, or available time.*[3]

- Review psychological assessment of client's emotional status. *Potential problems that may arise from presence of condition need to be identified and dealt with to avoid further debilitation.*[3]

NURSING PRIORITY NO. 2

To identify/provide individually appropriate preventive or corrective interventions:

Skin:[6,7]

- Inspect skin on a frequent basis, noting changes. Monitor skin over bony prominences.
- Reposition frequently as individually indicated *to relieve pressure.*
- Provide skin care daily and prn, drying well and using gentle massage and lotion *to stimulate circulation.*
- Keep skin, clothing, and area clean and dry *to prevent skin irritation and breakdown.*
- Initiate use of padding devices (e.g., foam, egg-crate/gel/water/air mattress or cushions) *to reduce pressure on and enhance circulation to compromised tissues.*
- Review nutritional status and promote diet with adequate protein, calorie, and vitamin and mineral intake *to aid in healing and promote general good health of skin and tissues.*
- Refer to NDs impaired Skin Integrity, impaired Tissue Integrity for additional interventions.

Elimination:[6–8]

- Observe elimination pattern, noting changes and potential problems.

- Encourage balanced diet, including fruits and vegetables high in fiber and with adequate fluids *for optimal stool consistency and to facilitate passage through colon.*
- Provide or encourage adequate fluid intake, include water and cranberry juice *to reduce risk of urinary infections.*
- Maximize mobility at earliest opportunity.
- Evaluate need for stool softeners, bulk-forming laxatives.
- Implement consistent bowel management or bladder training programs, as indicated.
- Monitor urinary output and characteristics *to identify changes associated with infection.*
- Refer to NDs Constipation, Diarrhea, Bowel Incontinence, impaired Urinary Elimination, Urinary Retention for additional interventions.

Respiration:[6,7]

- Monitor breath sounds and characteristics of secretions *for early detection of complications (e.g., atelectasis, pneumonia).*
- Encourage ambulation and upright position. Reposition, cough, deep-breathe on a regular schedule *to facilitate clearing of secretions and prevent atelectasis.*
- Encourage use of incentive spirometry. Suction as indicated *to clear airways.*
- Demonstrate techniques and assist with postural drainage when indicated for long-term airway clearance difficulties.
- Assist with and instruct family and caregivers in quad coughing techniques or diaphragmatic weight training *to maximize ventilation (in presence of SCI).*
- Discourage smoking. Refer for smoking cessation program as indicated.
- Refer to NDs ineffective Airway Clearance, ineffective Breathing Pattern, impaired Gas Exchange, impaired spontaneous Ventilation for additional interventions.

Vascular (tissue perfusion):[6-8]

- Assess cognition and mental status (ongoing). *Changes can reflect state of cardiac health, cerebral oxygenation impairment, or be indicative of a mental or emotional state that could adversely affect safety and self-care.*
- Determine core and skin temperature. Investigate development of cyanosis, changes in mentation *to identify changes in oxygenation status.*
- Routinely evaluate circulation and nerve function of affected body parts. *Changes in temperature, color, sensation, and movement can be the effect of immobility, disease, aging, or injury.*
- Encourage or provide adequate fluid *to prevent dehydration and circulatory stasis.*
- Monitor blood pressure before, during, and after activity—sitting, standing, and lying if possible *to ascertain response to and tolerance of activity.*
- Assist with position changes as needed. Raise head gradually. Institute use of tilt table or sitting upright on side of bed and arising slowly where appropriate to reduce incidence of injury that may occur as a result of orthostatic hypotension.
- Maintain proper body position; avoid use of constricting garments and restraints *to prevent vascular congestion.*
- Provide range-of-motion exercise. Refer for and assist with physical therapy exercises *for strengthening, restoration of optimal range of motion, and prevention of circulatory problems related to disuse.*[4]
- Ambulate as quickly and as often as possible, using mobility aids and frequent rest stops to assist client in continuing activity. *Upright position and weight bearing helps maintain bone strength, increases circulation, and prevents postural hypotension.*[8]
- Institute peripheral vascular support measures (e.g., elastic hose, Ace wraps, sequential compression devices) *to enhance venous return and reduce incidence of thrombophlebitis.*

- Refer to NDs risk for Activity Intolerance; decreased Cardiac Output; risk for Peripheral Neurovascular Dysfunction; ineffective peripheral tissue Perfusion for additional interventions.

🏠 **Musculoskeletal (mobility, range of motion, strength, and endurance):**[5–8]

- Perform or assist with range-of-motion exercises and involve client in active exercises with physical or occupational therapy *to promote bone health, muscle strengthening, flexibility, optimal conditioning, and functional ability.*
- Have client do exercises in bed if not contraindicated. *In-bed exercises help maintain muscle strength and tone.*
- Maximize involvement in self-care *to restore or maintain strength and functional abilities.*
- Intersperse activity with rest periods. Pace activities as possible *to increase strength and endurance in a gradual manner and reduce failure of planned exercise because of exhaustion or overuse of weak muscles or injured area.*
- Identify need and use of supportive devices (e.g., cane, walker, or functional positioning splints) as appropriate *to assist with safe mobility and functional independence.*
- Evaluate role of pain in mobility problem. Implement pain management program as individually indicated.
- Avoid or monitor closely the use of restraints, and immobilize client as little as possible *to reduce possibility of agitation and injury.*
- Refer to NDs Activity Intolerance; risk for Falls; impaired physical Mobility; acute Pain; chronic Pain; impaired Walking for additional interventions.

🏠 **Sensory-perception:**[6–8]

- Orient client as necessary to time, place, person, and situation. Provide cues for orientation (e.g., clock, calendar). *Disturbances of sensory interpretation and thought processes are associated with immobility as well as aging, being ill, disease processes/treatments, and medication effects.*
- Provide appropriate level of environmental stimulation (e.g., music, TV, radio, personal possessions, and visitors). *Needs vary depending on the client, the nature of the current problem, and whether client is at home or in a healthcare facility. Having normal life cues can help with mental stimulation and restoration of health.*
- Encourage participation in recreational or diversional activities and regular exercise program (as tolerated) *to decrease the sensory deprivation associated with immobility and isolation.*
- Promote regular sleep hours, use of sleep aids, and usual presleep rituals *to promote normal sleep and rest cycle.*
- Refer to NDs chronic Confusion, deficient Diversional Activity, Insomnia, disturbed Sensory Perception for additional interventions.

Self-Esteem, Powerlessness, Hopelessness, Social Isolation:[6,7]

- 🏠 Determine factors that may contribute to impairment of client's self-esteem and social interactions. *Many factors can be involved, including the client's age, relationship status, usual health state; presence of disabilities, including pain; or financial, environmental, and physical problems; current situation causing immobility and client's state of mind concerning the importance of the current situation in regard to the rest of client's life and desired lifestyle.*
- Ascertain if changes in client's situation are likely to be short-term, temporary; or long-term, or permanent. *Can affect both the client and care provider's coping abilities and willingness to engage in activities that prevent or limit effects of immobility.*

- Assess living situation (e.g., lives with spouse, parents, alone) and determine factors that may positively or adversely affect client's progress, roles, and/or safety.
- Explain or review all care procedures and plans. *Improves knowledge and facilitates decision making. Involves client in own care, enhances sense of control, and promotes independence.*
- Encourage questions and verbalization of feelings. *Aids in reducing anxiety and promotes learning about condition and specific needs.*
- Acknowledge concerns; provide presence and encouragement.
- Refer for mental, psychological, or spiritual services as indicated *to provide counseling, support, and medications.*
- Provide for and assist with mutual goal-setting, involving SO(s). *Promotes sense of control and enhances commitment to goals.*
- Ascertain that client can communicate needs adequately (e.g., call light, writing tablet, picture or letter board, interpreter).
- Refer to NDs impaired verbal Communication, Powerlessness, ineffective Role Performance, Self-Esteem [specify], impaired Social Interaction for additional interventions.

Body Image:[6,7]

- Evaluate for presence or potential for emotional, mental, and behavioral conditions that may contribute to isolation and degeneration. *Disuse syndrome often affects those individuals who are already isolated for one reason or another (e.g., serious illness or injury with disfigurement, frail elderly living alone, individual with severe depression, person with unacceptable behavior or without support system).*
- Orient to body changes through discussion and written information *to promote acceptance and understanding of needs.*
- Promote interactions with peers and normalization of activities within individual abilities.
- Refer to NDs disturbed Body Image, disturbed personal Identity, situational low Self-Esteem, Social Isolation for additional interventions.

NURSING PRIORITY NO. 3

To promote wellness (Teaching/Discharge Considerations):

- Assist client/caregivers in development of individualized plan of care *to best meet the client's potential, enhance safety, and prevent or limit affects of disuse.*
- Provide information about individual needs and areas of concerns (e.g., client's mental status, living environment, nutritional needs). *Information can help client and care providers to understand what long-term goals could be attained, what barriers may need to be overcome, and what constitutes progress or lack of progress requiring further evaluation and intervention.*[6]
- Review therapeutic regimen. *Treatment may be required for underlying condition(s), stress management, medications, therapies, and needed lifestyle changes.*
- Encourage involvement in regular exercise program, including isometric or isotonic activities, active or assistive range of motion to limit consequences of disuse and maximize level of function.[2]
- Promote self-care and SO-supported activities *to gain or maintain independence.*
- Recommend suitable balanced nutrition as well as use of supplements if needed *to provide energy for healing and maximal organ function.*
- Refer to appropriate community health providers and resources *to provide necessary assistance (e.g., help with meal preparation, financial help for groceries, dietitian or nutritionist).*[7]

Nursing Diagnoses in Alphabetical Order

- Review signs/symptoms requiring medical evaluation/follow-up *to promote timely interventions and limit adverse effects of situation.*[6]
- Identify community support services (e.g., financial, counseling, home maintenance, respite care, transportation).
- Refer to appropriate rehabilitation or home-care and support resources *to help client/care providers learn more about specific condition and acquire needed assistance, adaptive devices and necessary equipment.*

DOCUMENTATION FOCUS

Assessment/Reassessment
- Assessment findings, noting individual areas of concern, functional level, degree of independence, support systems and available resources.

Planning
- Plan of care and who is involved in planning.
- Teaching plan.

Implementation/Evaluation
- Client's response to interventions, teaching, and actions performed.
- Changes in level of functioning.
- Attainment or progress toward desired outcome(s).
- Modifications to plan of care.

Discharge Planning
- Long-term needs and who is responsible for actions to be taken.
- Specific referrals made, resources for specific equipment needs.

References

1. Disuse syndrome. (1999). Retrieved August 2003 from Department for the Care of the Aged: Laboratory of Rehabilitation Research National Institute for Longevity Sciences Web site. www.nils.go.jp/organ/dca/lrr/reh-e.html.
2. Hanson, R. W. (2000). Physical exercise, in self-management of chronic pain. Retrieved July 2007 from Patient Handbook. www.long-beach.med.va.gov/Our_Services/Patient_Care/cpmpbook/cpmp-11.html.
3. Blair, K. A. (1999). Immobility and activity intolerance in older adults. In Stanley, M., Beare, P. G. (eds). *Gerontological Nursing: A Health Promotion/Protection Approach.* 2d ed. Philadelphia: F. A. Davis.
4. Jiricka, M. K. (1994). Alterations in activity intolerance. In Port, C. M. (ed). *Pathophysiology: Concepts of Altered Health States.* Philadelphia: J. B. Lippincott.
5. Metzlar, D. J., Harr, J. (1996). Positioning your patient properly. *Am J Nurs*, 96, 33–37.
6. Doenges, M. E., Moorhouse, M. F., Geissler-Murr, A. C. (2004). *Nurse's Pocket Guide: Diagnoses, Interventions, and Rationales.* 9th ed. Philadelphia: F. A. Davis.
7. Cox, H. C., et al. (2002). *Clinical Applications of Nursing Diagnosis: Adult, Child, Women's, Psychiatric, Gerontic, and Home Health Considerations.* 4th ed. Philadelphia: F. A. Davis.
8. Graf, C. (2006). Functional decline in hospitalized older adults. *Am J Nurs*, 106(1), 58–67.

Cultural Collaborative Community/Home Care Diagnostic Studies Pediatric/Geriatric/Lifespan Medications

deficient Diversional Activity

DEFINITION: Decreased stimulation from (or interest or engagement in) recreational or leisure activities [Note: Internal/external factors may or may not be beyond the individual's control.]

RELATED FACTORS

Environmental lack of diversional activity [e.g., long-term hospitalization; frequent, lengthy treatments; homebound]
[Physical limitations, bedridden, fatigue, pain]
[Situational, developmental problem, lack of sources]
[Psychological condition such as depression]

DEFINING CHARACTERISTICS

Subjective
Client's statements regarding boredom (e.g., wish there were something to do, to read)
Usual hobbies cannot be undertaken in hospital [home or other care setting]
[Changes in abilities or physical limitations]

Objective
[Flat affect, disinterest, inattentiveness]
[Restlessness, crying]
[Lethargy, withdrawal]
[Hostility]
[Overeating or lack of interest in eating; weight loss or gain]

Sample Clinical Applications: Traumatic injuries, chronic pain, prolonged recovery (e.g., postoperative, complicated fractures), cancer therapy, chronic/debilitating conditions (e.g., congestive heart failure [CHF], chronic obstructive pulmonary disease [COPD], renal failure, multiple sclerosis [MS]), awaiting organ transplantation

DESIRED OUTCOMES/EVALUATION CRITERIA

Sample NOC linkages:
Leisure Participation: Use of relaxing, interesting, and enjoyable activities to promote well-being
Social Involvement: Social interactions with persons, groups, or organizations
Health Promoting Behavior: Personal actions to sustain or increase wellness

Client Will (Include Specific Time Frame)
• Recognize own psychological response (e.g., hopelessness and helplessness, anger, depression) and initiate appropriate coping actions.
• Engage in satisfying activities within personal limitations.

(continues on page 290)

deficient Diversional Activity (continued)
ACTIONS/INTERVENTIONS

Sample (NIC) linkages:
Recreation Therapy: Purposeful use of recreation to promote relaxation and enhancement of social skills
Activity Therapy: Prescription of and assistance with specific physical, cognitive, social, and spiritual activities to increase the range, frequency, or duration of an individual's (or group's) activity
Exercise Promotion: Facilitation of regular physical exercise to maintain or advance to a higher level of fitness and health

NURSING PRIORITY NO. 1

To assess precipitating/etiological factors:

● Assess client's physical, cognitive, emotional, and environmental status. *Validates reality of diversional deprivation when it exists, or identifies the potential for loss of desired diversional activity, in order to plan for prevention or early intervention where possible.*
● Observe for restlessness, flat facial expression, withdrawal, hostility, yawning, or statements of boredom as noted above, especially in individual likely to be confined either temporarily or long-term. *May be indicative of need for diversional interventions.*[1]
● Note potential impact of current disability or illness on lifestyle (e.g., young child with leukemia, elderly person with fractured hip, individual with severe depression). *Provides comparative baseline for assessments and interventions.*[9]
● Be aware of age and developmental level, gender, cultural factors, and the importance of a given activity in client's life. *When illness interferes with individual's ability to engage in usual activities, such as a lifelong dancer with incapacitating osteoporosis, a woman with strong cultural expectations who is unable to take care of her family, the person may have difficulty engaging in meaningful substitute activities.*
● Determine client's actual ability to participate in available activities, noting attention span, physical limitations and tolerance, level of interest or desire, and safety needs. *Presence of depression or disinterest in life, problems of immobility, protective isolation, and lack of stimulation, developmental delay, or sensory deprivation may interfere with desired activity. However, lack of involvement may not reflect client's actual abilities, but may rather be a matter of misperception about abilities.*[9]

NURSING PRIORITY NO. 2

To motivate and stimulate client involvement in solutions:

● Institute or continue appropriate actions to deal with concomitant conditions such as anxiety, depression, grief, dementia, physical injury, isolation and immobility, malnutrition, acute or chronic pain, and so forth. *These conditions interfere with the individual's ability to engage in meaningful activities that will stimulate his or her interest.*
● Introduce activities at client's current level of functioning, progressing to more complex activities, as tolerated. *Provides opportunity for client to experience successes, reaffirming capabilities and enhancing self-esteem.*[8]
● Establish therapeutic relationship, acknowledging reality of situation and client's feelings. *May be feeling sense of loss when unable to participate in usual activities or to interact socially as desired.*[8]

- Accept hostile expressions while limiting aggressive acting-out behavior. *Permission to express feelings of anger, hopelessness allows for beginning resolution. However, destructive behavior is counterproductive to self-esteem and problem-solving.*[8]
- Involve client and parent/SO/caregiver in determining client's needs, desires, and available resources. *Helps ensure that plan is attentive to client's interests and resources, increasing likelihood of client participation.*[2]
- Encourage parent/caregiver of young child to engage in play with confined child. *Reduces child's boredom, and play is essential to young child's development.*[3]
- Review history of lifelong activities and hobbies client has enjoyed. Discuss reasons client is not doing these activities now, and whether client can or would like to resume these activities. *Diversional activities can provide positive and productive avenues into which client can channel thoughts and time.*[4]
- Assist client/caregiver to set realistic goals for diversional activities, communicating hope and patience. *Can help client realize that this situation is not hopeless, that there are choices for improving the current situation, and that the future can hold the promise for improvement.*
- Provide instruction in relaxation techniques (e.g., meditation, sharing experiences, reminiscence, soft music, guided visualization) *to enhance coping skills.*[8]
- Participate in decisions about timing and spacing of visitors, leisure and care activities to promote relaxation and reduce sense of boredom as well as prevent overstimulation and exhaustion.[8]
- Encourage client to assist in scheduling required and optional activity choices. *For example, client may want to watch favorite television show at bath time; if bath can be rescheduled later, client's sense of control is enhanced.*[8]
- Encourage mix of desired activities/stimuli (e.g., music, news, educational presentations, movies, computer or Internet access, books or other reading materials, visitors, games, arts and crafts, sensory enrichment [e.g., massage, aromatherapy], grooming and beauty care, cooking, social outings, gardening, discussion groups, as appropriate). *Activities need to be personally meaningful and not physically/ emotionally overwhelming for client to derive the most benefit.*[4,10]
- Refrain from making changes in schedule without discussing with client. *It is important for staff to be sensitive and responsible in making and following through on commitments to client.*[8]
- Provide change of scenery (indoors and out where possible). Provide for periodic changes in the personal environment when client is confined inside, eliciting the client's input for likes and desires. *Change (e.g., new pictures on the wall, seasonal colors/flowers, altering room furniture, or outdoor light and air) can provide positive sensory stimulation, reduce client's boredom, improve sense of normalcy and control.*[5]
- Suggest activities such as bird feeders/baths for bird-watching, a garden in a window box or terrarium, or a fishbowl or aquarium *to stimulate observation as well as involvement and participation in activity (e.g., bird identification, picking out feeders and seeds).*[8]
- Involve recreational, occupational, play, music, or movement therapists as appropriate *to help identify enjoyable activities for client; to procure assistive devices or modify activities for individual situation. Assists client to express needs and feelings, share experiences, escape healthcare routines, and participate in self-healing.*[1,6,7]

NURSING PRIORITY NO. 3

To promote wellness (Teaching/Discharge Considerations):

- Explore options for useful activities using the person's strengths/abilities and interests to engage the client/SO.

- Make appropriate referrals to available resources (e.g., exercise groups, senior activities, hobby clubs, volunteering, companion and service organizations) *to introduce or continue diversional activities in community/home settings.*
- Refer to NDs ineffective Coping; Hopelessness; Powerlessness; Social Isolation for additional interventions.

DOCUMENTATION FOCUS

Assessment/Reassessment
- Specific assessment findings, including blocks to desired activities.
- Individual choices for activities.

Planning
- Plan of care, specific interventions, and who is involved in planning.

Implementation/Evaluation
- Client's responses to interventions, teaching, and actions performed.
- Attainment or progress toward desired outcome(s).
- Modifications to plan of care.

Discharge Planning
- Long-term needs and who is responsible for actions to be taken.
- Referrals made and available community resources.

References

1. Radziewicz, R. M. (1992). Using diversional activities to enhance coping. *Cancer Nurs*, 15(4), 293.
2. Cox, H. C., et al. (2002). *Clinical Applications of Nursing Diagnosis: Adult, Child, Women's, Psychiatric, Gerontic, and Home Health Considerations.* 4th ed. Philadelphia: F. A. Davis, 275–278.
3. Engel, J. (2002). *Mosby's Pocket Guide to Pediatric Assessment.* 4th ed. St. Louis, MO: Mosby.
4. Harley, K., et al. (2002). *Making each moment count: Developing a diversional therapies program for patients with hematologic malignancies* (Abstract from Oncology Nursing Society Convention).
5. Dossey, B. M. (1998). Holistic modalities & healing moments. *Am J Nurs*, 98(6), 44–47.
6. Williams, M. A. (1988). The physical environment and patient care. *Am Rev Nurs Res*, 6, 61.
7. Coaten, R. (2002). Movement matters. *National Healthcare J,* (5), 53.
8. Doenges, M. E., Moorhouse, M. F., Geissler-Murr, A. C. (2002). Psychosocial aspects of care. *Nursing Care Plans: Guidelines for Individualizing Patient Care.* 6th ed. Philadelphia: F. A. Davis.
9. Heriot, C. S. (1999). Developmental tasks and development in the later years of life. In Stanley, M., Bear, P. G. (eds). *Gerontological Nursing: A Health Promotion/Protection Approach.* 2d ed. Philadelphia: F. A. Davis.
10. Wheeler, S. L., Houston, K. (2005). The role of diversional activities in the general medical hospital setting. *Holist Nurs Pract*, 19(2), 67–69.

risk for Electrolyte Imbalance

DEFINITION: At risk for change in serum electrolyte levels that may compromise health.

RISK FACTORS

Fluid imbalance (e.g., dehydration, water intoxication); diarrhea; vomiting
Endocrine dysfunction
Renal dysfunction
Impaired regulatory mechanisms (e.g., diabetes insipidus, syndrome of inappropriate secretion of antidiuretic hormone)
Treatment-related side effects (e.g., medications, drains)

NOTE: A risk diagnosis is not evidenced by signs and symptoms, as the problem has not occurred; rather, nursing interventions are directed at prevention.
Sample Clinical Applications: Renal failure, anorexia nervosa, diabetes mellitus, Crohn's disease; gastroenteritis, pancreatitis, traumatic brain injury, cancer, multiple trauma, burns, sickle cell disease

DESIRED OUTCOMES/EVALUATION CRITERIA

Sample (**NOC**) linkages:
Electrolyte & Acid Base Balance: Balance of electrolytes and nonelectrolytes in the intracellular and extracellular compartments of the body

Client Will (Include Specific Time Frame)
• Display laboratory results within normal range for individual.
• Be free of complications resulting from electrolyte imbalance.
• Identify individual risks and engage in appropriate behaviors or lifestyle changes to prevent or reduce frequency of electrolyte imbalances.
Sample (**NOC**) linkages:
Risk Control: Personal actions to prevent, eliminate, or reduce modifiable health threats

Client Will (Include Specific Time Frame)
• Identify individual risks and engage in appropriate behaviors or lifestyle changes to prevent or reduce frequency of electrolyte imbalances.

ACTIONS/INTERVENTIONS

Sample (**NIC**) linkages:
Electrolyte Monitoring: Collection and analysis of patient data to regulate electrolyte balance
Electrolyte Management: Promotion of electrolyte balance and prevention of complications resulting from abnormal or undesired serum electrolyte levels

NURSING PRIORITY NO. 1.

To assess causative/contributing factors:

● Identify client with current or newly diagnosed condition commonly associated with electrolyte imbalances, such as inability to eat or drink; febrile illness; active bleeding or other fluid loss, including vomiting, diarrhea, gastrointestinal drainage, burns.

- Assess specific client risk, noting chronic disease processes that may lead to electrolyte imbalance as listed in Risk Factors, including kidney disease, metabolic or endocrine disorders, chronic alcoholism, cancers or cancer treatments, conditions causing hemolysis such as massive trauma, multiple blood transfusions, sickle cell disease.[1] Electrolyte excesses are caused by factors that (1) increase electrolyte intake or absorption, (2) shift electrolytes from an electrolyte pool to the extracellular fluid, or (3) decrease electrolyte excretion.[4] Electrolyte deficits are caused by factors that (1) decrease electrolyte intake or absorption, (2) shift electrolytes from the extracellular fluid to an electrolyte pool, (3) increase electrolyte excretion, or (4) cause abnormal loss of electrolytes.[4]
- Review client's medications *for those associated with electrolyte imbalance, such as diuretics, laxatives, corticosteroids, barbiturates, some antibiotics and so forth.*

NURSING PRIORITY NO. 2.

To identify potential electrolyte deficit:

- Assess mental status, noting client/caregiver report of change—altered attention span, recall of recent events, other cognitive functions. *Altered mental status is the most common sign of hypernatremia.*[2]
- Monitor heart rate and rhythm by palpation and auscultation. *Weak pulse or thready pulse can be associated with hypokalemia; tachycardia, bradycardia, and other dysrhythmias are associated with various electrolyte imbalances, including potassium, calcium, and magnesium.*[1–3]
- Ascultate breath sounds, assess respirations noting rate and depth and ease of respiratory effort, observe color of nail beds and mucous membranes, and note pulse oximetry or blood gas measurement, as indicated. *Certain electrolyte imbalances, such as hypokalemia, can cause or exacerbate respiratory insufficiency.*[2]
- Review electrocardiogram (ECG). *The ECG reflects electrophysiological, anatomical, metabolic, and hemodynamic alterations and is routinely used for the diagnosis of electrolyte and metabolic disturbances, as well as myocardial ischemia, cardiac dysrhythmias, structural changes of the myocardium, and drug effects.*[1–4]
- Assess gastrointestinal symptoms, noting presence, absence, and character of bowel sounds; presence of acute or chronic diarrhea; persistent vomiting, high nasogastric tube output. *Any disturbance of gastrointestinal (GI) functioning carries with it the potential for electrolyte imbalances.*[4,5]
- Review client's food intake. Note presence of anorexia, vomiting, or recent fad or unusual diet; look for chronic malnutrition. *Can point to potential electrolyte imbalances, either deficiencies or excesses, such as high sodium content.*[5]
- Evaluate motor strength and function. *Neuromuscular function, including steadiness of gait, handgrip strength, reactivity of reflexes, can provide clues to electrolyte imbalances, including sodium, potassium, and calcium.*[2,4]
- Assess fluid intake and output. *Many factors, such as inability to drink, large diuresis, chronic kidney failure, trauma, or surgery affect individual's fluid balance, thereby disrupting electrolyte transport, function, and excretion.*[1–5]
- Review laboratory results for abnormal findings. *Electrolytes include sodium, potassium, calcium, chloride, bicarbonate (carbon dioxide), and magnesium. These chemicals are absolutely essential in many bodily functions, including fluid balance, movement of fluid within and between body compartments,*[6] *nerve conduction, muscle contraction—including the heart; blood clotting and pH balance. Excitable cells, such as nerve and muscle, are particularly sensitive to electrolyte imbalances.*[4]

- Assess for specific imbalances:

Sodium (Na⁺)

Dominant extracellular cation and cannot freely cross the cell membrane.[6]

Review laboratory results—normal range in adults is 135 to 145 mEq/L. *Elevated sodium (hypernatremia) can occur if client has an overall deficit of total body water which occurs via two mechanisms: (1) inadequate fluid intake and (2) water loss;[7,8] and can be associated with low potassium, metabolic acidosis, and hypoglycemia.[2]*

Monitor for physical or mental disorders impacting fluid intake. *Impaired thirst sensation, inability to express thirst or obtain needed fluids may lead to hypernatremia.[7,8]*

Note presence of medical conditions that may impact sodium level. *Congestive heart failure (CHF), liver and kidney failure, pneumonia, metabolic acidosis, intestinal conditions resulting in prolonged GI suction are associated with hyponatremia.[4,6,9] Hypernatremia can result from simple conditions such as febrile illness causing fluid loss and/or restricted fluid intake or from complicated conditions such as kidney and endocrine diseases affecting sodium intake or excretion.*

Note presence of cognitive dysfunction such as confusion, restlessness, abnormal speech *(which may be cause or effect of sodium imbalance); orthostatic blood pressure changes, tachycardia, low urine output; or other clinical findings such as generalized weakness, swollen tongue, weight loss, seizures. Signs suggesting hypernatremia.[7,8]*

Assess for nausea, malaise, lethargy, orthostatic blood pressure changes—if fluid volume is also depleted; confusion, decreased level of consciousness, or headache. *Signs and symptoms suggestive of hyponatremia, which can lead to seizures and coma if untreated.[6]*

Assess for nausea, abdominal cramping, lethargy, orthostatic blood pressure changes—if fluid volume is also depleted; confusion, decreased level of consciousness, or headache. *Signs and symptoms suggestive of hyponatremia which can lead to seizures and coma if untreated.*

Review drug regimen. *Drugs such as anabolic steroids, angiotensin, cisplatin, mannitol may increase sodium level. Drugs such as diuretics, laxatives, theophylline, triamterene can decrease sodium level.[4]*

Potassium (K⁺)

Most abundant intracellular cation, obtained through diet, excreted via kidneys.[6]

Review laboratory results—normal range in adults is 3.5 to 5.0 mEq/L.

Obtain ECG as indicated.

Identify at-risk population. *Extremes of age (premature or elderly); ingestion of unusual diet with high-potassium, low-sodium foods; clients receiving IV potassium boluses or transfusions of whole blood or packed cells; use of potassium supplements, including over-the-counter (OTC) herbals or salt substitutes increase possibility of hyperkalemia.*

Note presence of medical conditions that may impact potassium level. *Metabolic acidosis, burn or crush injuries, massive hemolysis, diabetes, kidney disease/renal failure, cancer, sickle cell trait are associated with hyperkalemia.[6] Situations that may lead to hypokalemia are those that decrease potassium intake—excessive fluid resuscitation, fasting, or unbalanced diet; shift potassium from the extracellular fluid into cells—alkalosis, some malignancies; or increase potassium loss through diuresis or renal disorders such as acute tubular necrosis (ATN), nasogastric suction, diarrhea.[10,11]*

Evaluate reports of abdominal cramping, fatigue, hyperactive bowel motility, muscle twitching and cramps followed by muscle weakness. Note presence of depressed reflexes, ascending flaccid paralysis of legs and arms. *Signs/symptoms suggesting hyperkalemia.[2,6,10]*

Note presence of anorexia, abdominal distention, diminished bowel sounds, postural hypotension, muscle weakness, flaccid paralysis. *May be manifestations of hypokalemia.[11]*

Review drug regimen. *Use of potassium-sparing diuretics, other medications, such as NSAIDs, angiotensin-converting enzyme (ACE) inhibitors, certain antibiotics such as pentamidine may increase potassium level.[6,10,11] Medications such as albuterol, terbutaline, or some diuretics may cause hypokalemia.[10]*

Calcium (Ca^{2+})

Most abundant cation in the body participates in almost all vital processes, working with sodium to regulate depolarization and the generation of action potentials. Disruption of these processes causes cellular irritability and dysfunction.[2,4,11]

Laboratory results—normal range for adults is 8.5 to 10.5 mg/dL. *Elevated calcium (hypercalcemia) associated with excessive urination (polyuria), constipation, lethargy, muscle weakness, anorexia, headache, coma. Hypocalcemia can lead to cardiac dysrhythmias, hypotension, and heart failure; muscle cramps, facial spasms (positive Chvostek's sign); numbness and tingling sensations, muscle twitching (positive Trousseau's sign); seizures; or tetany. Low serum albumin levels, and vitamin D deficiency may also be associated with hypocalcemia.[4,12]*

Note presence of medical conditions impacting calcium level. *Acidosis, Addison's disease, cancers (e.g., bone, lymphoma, leukemias), hyperparathyroidism, lung disease (e.g., tuberculosis, histoplasmosis), thyrotoxicosis, polycythemia may lead to increased calcium level. Chronic diarrhea, intestinal disorders such as Crohn's disease; pancreatitis, alcoholism, renal failure, or renal tubular disease; recent orthopedic surgery or bone healing; history of thyroid surgery or irradiation of upper middle chest and neck; and psychosis may result in hypocalcemia. [2,4,12]*

Review drug regimen. *Drugs such as anabolic steroids, some antacids, lithium, oral contraceptives, vitamins A and D, amoxapine can increase calcium levels. Drugs such as albuterol, anticonvulsants, glucocorticoids, insulin; laxative overuse; phosphates, trazodone, or long-term anticonvulsant therapy can decrease calcium levels.[4]*

Magnesium (Mg^{2+})

Second-most abundant intracellular cation after potassium, magnesium controls absorption or function of sodium, potassium, calcium, and phosphorus. [2,4,10]

Review laboratory results—normal range in adults is 1.5 to 2.0 mEq/L. *Excess magnesium (hypermagnesemia) occurs rarely but affects the central nervous, neuromuscular, and cardiopulmonary systems.*

Note GI and renal function. *Main controlling factors of magnesium are GI absorption and renal excretion.[13] Low levels of potassium, calcium, phosphorus, and magnesium may be manifest at the same time if GI absorption is impaired.[15] High levels of magnesium, calcium, phosphate, and potassium often occur together in setting of kidney disease.[14,15]*

Note presence of medical condition impacting magnesium level. *Diabetic acidosis, multiple myeloma, renal insufficiency, eclampsia, asthma, certain cardiac dysrhythmias, tumor lysis syndrome, GI hypomotility, adrenal insufficiency, neoplasms with skeletal muscle involvement, extensive soft tissue injury or necrosis, shock, sepsis, severe burns, cardiac arrest are associated with hypermagnesemia.[4,13,14] Conditions resulting in decreased intake (e.g., starvation, alcoholism, parenteral feeding); excess gastrointestinal losses (e.g., diarrhea, vomiting, nasogastric suction, malabsorption); renal losses (e.g., inherited renal tubular defects among others); or miscellaneous other causes including calcium abnormalities, chronic metabolic acidosis, diabetic ketoacidosis can lead to hypomagnesemia.[2,4,13]*

Monitor for symptoms of hypermagnesemia. *Presence of nausea, vomiting, weakness, vasodilation suggest mild to moderate elevation of magnesium level (>3.5−5.0 mEq/L), while the presence of heart blocks, ventilatory failure, and stupor are associated with severe hypermagnesemia (>10.0 mEq/L), which can lead to coma and death.[14]*

Note muscular weakness, tremors, seizures, paresthesia, hypertension, and cardiac abnormalities. *Signs of hypomagnesemia that may lead to potentially fatal complications, including ventricular dysrhythmias, coronary artery vasospasm, sudden death.*[10,13]

Review drug regimen. *Drugs such as aspirin and progesterone may increase magnesium level; albuterol, digoxin, diuretics, oral contraceptives, aminoglycosides, proton-pump inhibitors, immunosuppressants, cisplatin, cyclosporines are some of the medications that may decrease magnesium levels.* [4]

NURSING PRIORITY NO. 3.

To prevent imbalances:

- Collaborate in treatment of underlying conditions *to prevent or limit effects of electrolyte imbalances caused by disease or organ dysfunction.*
- Observe and intervene with elderly hospitalized person upon admission and during facility stay. *Elderly are more prone to electrolyte imbalances related to fluid imbalances, use of multiple medications including diuretics, heart and blood pressure medications, lack of appetite or interest in eating or drinking; lack of appropriate dietary and/or medication supervision at home, and so forth.*[2]
- Provide balanced nutrition to hospitalized client, using best route for feeding and monitoring intake, weight, and bowel function. *Obtaining and utilizing electrolytes and other minerals depends on client receiving them in a readily available route, preferably by oral ingestion, or by GI tube or parenteral route.*
- Measure and report all fluid losses, including emesis, diarrhea, wound or fistula drainage. *Loss of fluids rich in electrolytes can lead to imbalances.*
- Maintain fluid balance *to prevent dehydration and shifts of electrolytes.*
- Use pump or controller device when administering IV electrolyte solutions *to provide medication at desired rate and prevent untoward effects of excessive or too rapid delivery.*

NURSING PRIORITY NO. 4.

To promote wellness (Teaching/Discharge Considerations):

- Discuss ongoing concerns for client with chronic health problems, such as kidney disease, diabetes, cancer; individuals taking multiple medications; and/or client deciding to take medications or OTC drugs differently than prescribed. *By addressing these issues during each clinic visit, it may be possible to identify client at risk for electrolyte imbalances. Early intervention can help prevent serious complications.*
- Consult with dietitian or nutritionist for specific teaching needs. *Learning how to incorporate foods that increase electrolyte intake or identifying food or condiment alternatives when client is taking in too much of an electrolyte (such as client with renal failure not receiving dialysis curtailing high-potassium foods) increases client's self-sufficiency and likelihood of success.*
- Teach client/caregiver to take or administer drugs as prescribed—especially diuretics, antihypertensives, and cardiac drugs *to reduce potential of complications associated with medication-induced electrolyte imbalances.*
- Instruct client/caregiver in reportable symptoms. *For example, sudden change in mentation or behavior 2 days after starting a new diuretic could indicate hyponatremia, or elderly person taking digitalis for atrial fibrillation and a diuretic may by hypokalemic.*[2]
- Provide information regarding calcium supplements, as indicated. *It is popular wisdom to instruct people, women in particular, to take calcium for prevention of osteoporosis. However, calcium absorption cannot take place without vitamins D and K and magnesium. Client taking calcium may need additional information or resources.*[17]

- Review client's medications at each visit *for possible change in dosage or drug choice based on client's response, change in condition, or development of side-effects.*
- Discuss medications with primary care provider *to determine if different pharmaceutical intervention is appropriate. For example, changing to potassium-sparing diuretic or withholding a diuretic in presence of may correct imbalance.*[16]

DOCUMENTATION FOCUS

Assessment/Reassessment
- Identified or potential risk factors for individual.
- Assessment findings, including vital signs, mentation, muscle strength and reflexes, presence of fatigue, respiratory distress.
- Results of laboratory tests and diagnostic studies.

Planning
- Plan of care, specific interventions, and who is involved in the planning.
- Teaching plan.

Implementation/Evaluation
- Client's responses to treatment, teaching, and actions performed.
- Attainment or progress toward desired outcome(s).
- Modifications to plan of care.

Discharge Planning
- Long-term needs, identifying who is responsible for actions to be taken.
- Specific referrals made.

References

1. Lederer, E., Ouseph, R., Yazel, L. (2007). Hypokalemia. Retrieved January 2009 from http://emedicine.medscape.com/article/242008-overview.
2. Workman, M. L. (2006). Interventions for clients with electrolyte imbalances. In Ignatavicius, D. D., Workman, M. L. (eds). *Medical-Surgical Nursing: Critical Thinking for Collaborative Care.* 5th ed. St. Louis, MO: Elsevier Saunders.
3. Wung, S., Kozik, T. (2008). Electrocardiographic evaluation of cardiovascular status. *J Cardiovasc Nurs*, 23(2), 169–174.
4. Leeuwen, A. M., Kranpitz, T. R., Smith, L. (2006). *Davis's Comprehensive Handbook of Diagnostic Tests with Nursing Implications.* 2d ed. Philadelphia: F. A. Davis.
5. Lyman, B. (2002). Metabolic complications associated with parenteral nutrition. *J Infus Nurs*, 25(1), 36–44.
6. Simon, E. E., Hamrahian, S. M Hyponatremia. Retrieved January 2009 from http://emedicine.medscape.com/article/242166-overview.
7. Elgart, H. N. (2004). Assessment of fluids and electrolytes. *AACN Clin Issues*, 15(4), 607–621.
8. Pham, T. Q Hypernatremia. Retrieved January 2009 from http://emedicine.medscape.com/article/241094-overview.
9. Sonnenblick, M., Friedlander, Y., Rosin, A. J. (1993). Diuretic-induced severe hyponatremia: Review and analysis of 129 reported patients. *Chest*, 103(2), 601–606.
10. Lederer, E., et al. Hyperkalemia. Retrieved January 2009 from http://emedicine.medscape.com/article/240903-overview.
11. Muller, A. C., Bell, A. E. (2008). Diagnostic update: Electrolyte update: Potassium, chloride and magnesium. *Crit Care Nurs*, 3(1), 5–7.
12. Felver, L., Kirkhorn, M. J. (2005). Fluid, electrolyte, and acid-base homeostatis. In Copstead, L. E. C., Banasik, J. L. (eds). *Pathophysiology.* 2d ed. St. Louis, MO: Elsevier Saunders.

⊕ Cultural   Collaborative   🏠 Community/Home Care   Diagnostic Studies   ∞ Pediatric/Geriatric/Lifespan   Medications

13. Suneja, M., Muster, H. A. (2008). Hypocalcemia. Retrieved January 2009 from http://emedicine.medscape.com/article/241893-overview.
14. Fulop, T., et al. (2007). Hypomagesemia. Retrieved January 2009 from http://emedicine.medscape.com/article/246366-overview.
15. Novello, N. P., Blumstein, H. A Hypermagnesemia. Retrieved January 2009 from http://emedicine.medscape.com/article/7666604-overview.
16. Moe, S. M. (2008). Disorders involving calcium, phosphorus, and magnesium. *Prim Care*, 35(2), 215–237.
17. Stark, J. (2006). The renal system. In Alspach, J. G. (ed). *Core Curriculum for Critical Care Nursing*. St. Louis, MO: Saunders.
18. Brown, S. E Bone health: The calcium myth. Retrieved January 2009 from www.womentowomen.com/bonehealth/calciummyth.aspx.

disturbed Energy Field

DEFINITION: Disruption of the flow of energy [aura] surrounding a person's being that results in a disharmony of the body, mind, or spirit

RELATED FACTORS

Slowing or blocking of energy flow secondary to:
Pathophysiological factors: Illness, pregnancy, injury
Treatment-related factors: Immobility, labor and delivery, perioperative experience, chemotherapy
Situational factors: Pain, fear, anxiety, grieving
Maturational factors: Age-related developmental difficulties or crisis

DEFINING CHARACTERISTICS

Objective
Perception of changes in patterns of energy flow, such as:
Movement (wave, spike, tingling, dense, flowing)
Sounds (tone, words)
Temperature change (warmth, coolness)
Visual changes (image, color)
Disruption of the field (deficient, hole, spike, bulge, obstruction, congestion, diminished flow in energy field)

Sample Clinical Applications: Illness, trauma, cancer, pain, impaired immune system, fatigue, surgical procedures

DESIRED OUTCOMES/EVALUATION CRITERIA

Sample **NOC** linkages:
Personal Well-Being: Extent of positive perception of one's health status
Coping: Personal actions to manage stressors that tax an individual's resources
Symptom Severity: Severity of perceived adverse changes in physical, emotional, and social functioning

(continues on page 300)

disturbed Energy Field (continued)

Client Will (Include Specific Time Frame)
• Acknowledge feelings of anxiety and distress.
• Verbalize sense of relaxation and well-being.
• Display reduction in severity and/or frequency of symptoms.

ACTIONS/INTERVENTIONS

Sample NIC linkages:
Therapeutic Touch: Attuning to the universal healing field, seeking to act as an instrument for healing influence, and using the natural sensitivity of the hands to gently focus and direct the intervention process
Meditation Facilitation: Facilitating a person to alter his or her level of awareness by focusing specifically on an image or thought
Pain Management: Alleviation of pain or a reduction in pain to a level of comfort that is acceptable to the patient

NURSING PRIORITY NO. 1

To determine causative/contributing factors:

● Review current situation and concerns of client. Encourage client to talk about condition, past history, emotional state, or other relevant information. Note body gestures, tone of voice, words chosen to express feelings and issues. *Recent studies reported that Therapeutic Touch (TT) produced positive outcomes by decreasing levels of anxiety and pain perception and improving sense of well-being and quality of life; TT may also be beneficial in reducing behavioral symptoms of dementia (e.g., manual manipulation/restlessness, vocalization, pacing).*[8,10–14]

● Determine client's motivation and desire for treatment. *Following explanation of TT process and expected results, client may have unrealistic expectations or may understand purpose and believe process will be helpful.*[2] *Although attitude can affect success of therapy, TT is often successful even when the client is skeptical.*[11]

● Note use of medications, other drug use (e.g., alcohol). *May affect client's ability to relax and take full advantage of the TT process.*[4] *However, TT may be helpful in reducing anxiety level in individuals undergoing alcohol withdrawal.*[9]

● Perform or review results of testing, as indicated, such as the State-Trait Anxiety Inventory (STAI) or the Affect Balance Scale. *Provides measure of the client's anxiety to evaluate need for treatment or intervention.*[3]

NURSING PRIORITY NO. 2

To evaluate energy field:

● Develop therapeutic nurse-client relationship, initially accepting role of healer or guide as client desires. *This relationship is one in which both participants recognize each other as unique and important human beings and in which mutual learning occurs. The role of the nurse and the use of self as a therapeutic tool is recognized.*[3]

● Place client in sitting or supine position with legs and arms uncrossed. Place pillows or other supports *to enhance comfort. Promotes relaxation and feelings of peace, calm, and security, preparing the client to derive the most benefit from the procedure.*[1]

🏠 ● Center self physically and psychologically. *A quiet mind and focused attention turns to the healing intent.*[6]

🏠 ● Move hands slowly over the client at level of 2 to 6 inches above skin. *Assesses state of energy field and flow of energy within the system. The feelings that may be noted are tingling, warmth, coolness, comfort, peace, calm, and security.*[5]

🏠 ● Identify areas of imbalance or obstruction in the field. *Areas of asymmetry; feelings of heat or cold, tingling, congestion or pressure, decreased or disrupted energy flow, pulsation, congestion, heaviness, decreased flow may be identified.*[7]

NURSING PRIORITY NO. 3

To provide therapeutic intervention:

🏠 ● Explain the process of TT and answer questions as indicated *to prevent unrealistic expectation. TT is the knowledgeable and purposeful patterning of the client environmental energy field to relieve discomfort and anxiety. Providing information that the fundamental focus of TT is on healing and wholeness, not curing signs/symptoms of disease, helps the client to understand the process.*[6]

🏠 ● Discuss findings of evaluation with client. *Including the client in the process by sharing the findings of the nurse combined with sensations the client experienced provides the best opportunity to derive benefit from the procedure.*[2]

🏠 ● Assist client with exercises to promote "centering." *Deep breathing, guided imagery, and the process of centering increases the potential to self-heal, enhance comfort, reduce anxiety.*[2]

🏠 ● Perform unruffling process, keeping hands 2 to 6 inches from client's body and sweeping them downward and out of the field from head to toe, concentrating on areas of congestion. *Dissipates impediments to free flow of energy within the system and between nurse and client, promoting the reception of healing energy and allowing the client to use own resources for self-healing.*[6]

🏠 ● Focus on areas of disturbance identified, holding hands over or on skin, or place one hand in back of body with other hand in front. At the same time, concentrate on the intent to help the client heal. *This move allows the client's body to pull or repattern energy as needed and corrects energy imbalances.*[1]

∞ ● Shorten duration of treatment 2 to 3 minutes as appropriate. *Children, elderly individuals, those with head injuries, and others who are severely debilitated are generally more sensitive to overloading energy fields.*[1,2]

🏠 ● Make coaching suggestions in a soft voice. *Pleasant images or other visualizations, deep breathing enhance feelings of relaxation and help to relieve anxiety.*[1,2]

🏠 ● Use hands-on massage or apply pressure to acupressure points as appropriate during process. *The addition of these methods can enhance the relaxation and benefit client receives from TT.*[6]

🏠 ● Note changes in energy sensations as session progresses. Stop when the energy field is symmetrical and there is a change to feelings of peaceful calm. *Signifies energy is balanced, further intervention is not necessary, and client is ready to rest.*[1,2]

🏠 ● Hold client's feet for a few minutes at end of session. *Assists in "grounding" the body energy, completing the session.*[1]

🏠 ● Provide client time for a period of peaceful rest following procedure. *TT promotes feelings of peace and comfort, relieving anxiety and promoting self-healing.*[1]

NURSING PRIORITY NO. 4

To promote wellness (Teaching/Discharge Considerations):

- • Allow period of client dependency, as appropriate. *Period of dependency permits client to strengthen own inner resources at his or her own pace.*[1]
- • Encourage ongoing practice of the therapeutic process. *Helping client and family members to learn skill of TT will promote feelings of control of illness and health. It can be used anytime, anywhere, and with friends and family.*[4]
- • Instruct in use of stress-reduction activities (e.g., centering/meditation, relaxation exercises, guided imagery). *Continuous use of these activities can promote harmony among mind-body-spirit.*[2]
- • Discuss importance of integrating techniques into daily activity plan, for sustaining or enhancing sense of well-being. *Helps client to understand that making these a way of life will help them in dealing with challenges of illness and promote a healthy lifestyle.*[1]
- • Have client practice each step and demonstrate the complete TT process following the session. *Client displays readiness to assume responsibilities for self-healing as he or she learns the TT process.*[1,2]
- • Promote attendance at a support group where members can help each other practice and learn the techniques of TT. *The support of others helps the client to become proficient in new skill.*[2]
- • Reinforce that TT is a complementary intervention and stress importance of seeking timely evaluation and continuing other prescribed treatment modalities as appropriate. *Failure to follow prescribed therapeutic regimen may result in poor outcome and worsening of condition.*
- • Refer to other resources as identified (e.g., psychotherapy, clergy, medical treatment of disease processes, hospice). *Encourages the individual to address total well-being and facilitate peaceful death.*[6]

DOCUMENTATION FOCUS

Assessment/Reassessment
- Assessment findings, including characteristics and differences in the energy field.
- Client's perception of problem and need for treatment.

Planning
- Plan of care and who is involved in planning.
- Teaching plan.

Implementation/Evaluation
- Changes in energy field.
- Client's response to interventions, teaching, and actions performed.
- Attainment or progress toward desired outcomes.
- Modifications to plan of care.

Discharge Planning
- Long-term needs and who is responsible for actions to be taken.
- Specific referrals made.

References

1. Krieger, D. (1979). *The Therapeutic Touch: How to Use Your Hands to Heal.* Englewood Cliffs, NJ: Prentice Hall.

2. Buguslawski, M. (1980). Therapeutic touch: A facilitator of pain relief. *Top Clin Nurs, 2,* 27–37.
3. Townsend, M. C. (2003). *Psychiatric Mental Health Nursing Concepts of Care.* 4th ed. Philadelphia: F. A. Davis.
4. Daglish, S. (1999). Therapeutic touch in an acute care community hospital. *Can Nurse,* 95(3), 57–58.
5. Hayes, J., Cox, C. (1999). The experience of therapeutic touch from a nursing perspective. *Br J Nurs,* 8(18), 1249–1254.
6. Meehan, T. (1998). Therapeutic touch as a nursing intervention. *J Adv Nurs,* 28(1), 117–125.
7. Marnhinweg, G. (1996). Energy field disturbance validation study. *Healing Touch Newsletter,* 6(11).
8. Woods, D. L., Craven, R. F., Whitney, J. (2005). The effect of therapeutic touch on behavioral symptoms of persons with dementia. *Altern Ther Health Med,* 11(1), 66–74.
9. Larden, C. N., Palmer, M. L., Janssen, P. (2004). Efficacy of therapeutic touch in treating pregnant inpatients who have a chemical dependency. *J Holist Nurs,* 22(4), 320–332.
10. Woods, D. L., Dimond, M. (2002). The effect of therapeutic touch on agitated behavior and cortisol in persons with Alzheimer's disease. *Biol Res Nurs,* 4(2), 104–114.
11. Denison, B. (2004). Touch the pain away: New research on therapeutic touch and persons with fibromyalgia syndrome. *Holist Nurs Pract,* 18(3), 142–151.
12. Smith, D. W., et al. (2002). Effects of integrating therapeutic touch into a cognitive behavioral pain treatment program. Report of a pilot clinical trial. *J Holist Nurs,* 20(4), 367–387.
13. Samarel, N., et al. (1998). Effects of dialogue and therapeutic touch on preoperative and postoperative experiences of breast cancer surgery: An exploratory study. *Oncol Nurs Forum,* 25(8), 1369–1376.
14. Giasson, M., Bouchard, L. (1998). Effect of therapeutic touch on the well-being of persons with terminal cancer. *J Holist Nurs,* 16(3), 383–398.

impaired Environmental Interpretation Syndrome

DEFINITION: Consistent lack of orientation to person, place, time, or circumstances over more than 3 to 6 months, necessitating a protective environment

RELATED FACTORS

Dementia [Alzheimer's disease, multi-infarct, Pick's disease, AIDS dementia]
Huntington's disease
Depression

DEFINING CHARACTERISTICS

Objective
Consistent disorientation
Chronic confusional states
Inability to follow simple directions
Inability to reason or concentrate; slow in responding to questions
Loss of occupation or social functioning

Sample Clinical Applications: Dementia (e.g., Alzheimer's, AIDS, alcoholism), depression, brain injury, Huntington's disease

(continues on page 304)

impaired Environmental Interpretation Syndrome (continued)
DESIRED OUTCOMES/EVALUATION CRITERIA

Sample NOC linkages:
Physical Injury Severity: Severity of injuries from accidents and trauma
Cognitive Orientation: Ability to identify person, place, and time accurately

Client Will (Include Specific Time Frame)
• Be free of harm.
• Sustain/demonstrate improvement in cognition.
Safe Home Environment: Physical arrangements to minimize environmental factors that might cause physical harm or injury in the home

Caregiver Will (Include Specific Time Frame)
• Identify individual client safety concerns and needs.
• Modify activities and environment to provide for safety.

ACTIONS/INTERVENTIONS

Sample NIC linkages:
Environmental Management: Manipulation of the patient's surroundings for therapeutic benefit
Reality Orientation: Promotions of patient's awareness of personal identity, time, and environment
Surveillance: Purposeful and ongoing acquisition, interpretation, and synthesis of patient data for clinical decision making
(Refer to NDs acute Confusion, chronic Confusion; impaired Memory; disturbed Thought Processes, for additional relevant assessment and interventions.)

NURSING PRIORITY NO. 1

To assess causative/precipitating factors:

● Determine presence of conditions or behaviors leading to client's current problem. (*Note:* It is possible that there is no identifiable event.) *Can provide clues for likelihood for improvement as well as help to identify potentially useful interventions and therapies.*[1]
● Note presence or reports of client's misinterpretation of environmental information (e.g., sensory, cognitive, or social cues), history and progression of condition, length of time since onset, future expectations, and incidents of injury or accidents. *Identifies specific areas of concern, potential risks.*
● Review client's behavioral changes with client/SO(s) regarding baseline behaviors, length of time since onset or progression of problem, their perception of prognosis; identify additional impairments. *The client's SO/primary caregiver is an invaluable and essential source of information regarding past history and current situation, as both cognitive and behavioral symptoms tend to change over time and are often variable from day to day.*[1]
● Obtain information regarding recent changes or disruptions in client's health (e.g., decreased agility, loss of balance, decline in visual acuity, failure to eat, loss of interest in personal grooming, forgetfulness resulting in unsafe actions) or routine (e.g., hospitalization,

change in medications, or moving to new home). *Decline in physical health or disruption in daily living situation can exacerbate symptoms, causing agitation or delirium.*[1]

- Test ability to receive and send effective communication. *Client may be nonverbal or require assistance with or interpretation of verbalizations.*
- Determine anxiety level in relation to situation. Note behavior that may be indicative of potential for violence. *Places both client and SO at risk and requires prompt intervention for safety of all*
- Evaluate client's response to primary care providers as well as receptiveness to interventions. *Awareness of these dynamics is helpful for evaluation of ongoing needs for both client and caregiver, as client becomes increasingly dependent on caregivers or resistant to interventions.*[3]
- Identify potential environmental dangers and evaluate client's level of awareness (if any) of threat. *Highlights problems that may impact client care and safety or add to client's difficulties in interpretation of sensory input.*
- Evaluate responses on diagnostic examinations (e.g., memory impairments, reality orientation, attention span, calculations). *A combination of tests, including (but not limited to) magnetic resonance imaging (MRI)/brain scan; Confusion Assessment Method (CAM); Mini-Mental State Examination (MMSE); Brief Dementia Severity Rating Scale (BDSRS); Alzheimer's Disease Assessment Scale, cognitive subsection (ADAS-cog); Functional Assessment Questionnaire (FAQ); Clinical Global Impression of Change (CGIC); Neuropsychiatric Inventory (NPI), is often needed to determine client's overall condition relating to chronic or irreversible condition.*[2,11]

NURSING PRIORITY NO. 2

To provide/promote safe environment:

- Collaborate in management of treatable conditions (e.g., infections, malnutrition, electrolyte imbalances, and adverse medication reactions) *that may contribute to or exacerbate confusion.*
- Include SO(s)/caregivers in planning process. Identify previous/usual patterns for activities, such as sleeping, eating, self-care, and so forth, *to incorporate into plan of care to the extent possible and lessen confusion.*
- Implement behavioral and environmental management interventions, *to promote orientation, provide opportunity for client interaction using current cognitive skills, preserve client's dignity and safety:*[1–6]
  Provide calm environment, eliminate extraneous noise or stimuli.
  Introduce yourself at each contact if needed. Call client by preferred name.
  Keep communication and questions simple. Use concrete terms. Use symbols instead of words when hearing or other impaired *to improve communication.*
  Avoid speaking in loud voice, crowding, restraining, shaming, demanding, or condescending actions toward client.
  Use touch judiciously. Tell client what is being done before touching.
  Simplify client's tasks and routines, limit number of decisions or choices client needs to make at one time, offer guided choices between two options.
  Promote and structure activities and rest periods, allow adequate rest between stimulating events.
  Recommend limiting number of visitors client interacts with at one time.
  Avoid challenging illogical thinking *because defensive reactions may result.*
  Redirect client's attention when behavior is agitated or dangerous. Set limits on acting-out behavior.

Remove from stressors and agitation triggers or danger; move client to quieter place; offer privacy.

Use lighting and visual aides *to reduce confusion about surroundings.*

Maintain continuity of caregivers, care routines, and surroundings as much as possible.

Provide simple orientation measures, such as one-number calendar, personal items, seasonal decorations, and so forth.

Be supportive and sensitive to fears, misperceived threats, and frustration with expressing what is wanted.

- Be open and honest when discussing client's disease, abilities, and prognosis. Use positive statements. *Promotes trust without diminishing hope in ability to deal with situation.*
- Provide safety measures (e.g., close supervision, alarms on exits, locking doors to unprotected areas or stairwells, toxic substances and medication lockup, supervision of outdoor activities and wandering, removal of car or car keys, lowered temperature on hot water tank); discourage or supervise smoking, monitor activities of daily living (ADLs) (e.g., use of stove, sharp knives, choice of clothing in relation to environment and season). *Impaired judgment and inattention to detail place client at increased risk for injury to self and others.*
- Place identity tags in clothes and belongings, provide bracelet or necklace *to facilitate identification and safe return if client wanders away or gets lost.*
- Avoid use of restraints. Use vest (instead of wrist) restraints if restraints required. *Although restraints can prevent falls, they can increase client's agitation and distress and possibly cause entrapment and death.*[12]
- Administer medications to manage symptoms and maximize abilities. Use lowest possible therapeutic dose and monitor for expected or adverse responses, side effects, and interactions.
- Implement complementary therapies as indicated or desired, such as music therapy, hand massage (if touch is tolerated), Therapeutic Touch, aromatherapy, bright-light treatment. *May help client relax, refocus attention, stimulate memories.*[7]
- Refer to NDs impaired verbal Communication; acute Confusion; chronic Confusion; impaired Memory; disturbed Sensory Perception; disturbed Thought Processes; risk for Trauma; Wandering for additional interventions.

NURSING PRIORITY NO. 3

To assist caregiver to deal with situation:

- Determine family dynamics, cultural values, resources, availability, and willingness to participate in meeting client's needs.
- Evaluate SO's attention to own needs, including health status, grieving process, and respite. Discuss caregiver burden, if appropriate. *Primary caregiver and other members of family will suffer from the stress that accompanies caregiving and require information and support.*[2–6,9,10] (Refer to ND risk for Caregiver Role Strain for additional interventions.)
- Involve SO(s) in care and discharge planning. Maintain frequent interactions with SOs *to relay information, change care strategies, try different responses, or implement other problem-solving solutions.*
- Provide educational materials reflecting SO/family needs and learning styles and lists of available resources, such as newsletters, books, reliable Web sites, telephone help lines, and so forth. *Reduces sense of overload, allows individuals to review or refer to resources as needed on their own time frame.*
- Review safety measures regarding client's environmental impairments. *Client not only can lose items but also can get lost in familiar places, requiring special attention to client's*

possessions, as well as to physical safety in the home and community. The client may believe that caregivers are stealing the "lost" items; or the client may leave home and be unable to get back.[8]

- Avoid leaving client alone in home. Suggest installation of home security system or motion detectors. Register client with Safe Return program of Alzheimer's Association. Talk with neighbors and police if client is prone to wander. *If the general public is on alert for a person with dementia who may need help, the chances of finding that person are greatly enhanced.*[8]

- Identify appropriate community resources (e.g., Alzheimer's Disease and Related Disorders Association [ADRDA]; stroke or other brain injury support groups; senior support groups, respite care, clergy, social services, therapists, attorney services for advance directives and durable power of attorney) *to provide support for client and SOs, and assist with problem-solving, decision making.*

NURSING PRIORITY NO. 4

To promote wellness (Teaching/Discharge Considerations):

- Provide specific information about disease process, prognosis, and client's particular needs. *Client usually requires more social and behavioral support than medical management, although intermittent medical evaluations are needed to determine client's general health, any deterioration in cognitive function, requiring adjustment in medication regimen, and so forth.*[13]

- Develop plan of care with family to meet client's and SO's specific needs. *Success of the individual plan is dependent on cultural and belief patterns, as well as family (personal, emotional, and financial) resources.*

- Perform home assessment *to identify specific safety issues and appropriate solutions, including using keyed locks for exterior doors to prevent client from wandering off while SO engaged in other household activities, locking up matches or smoking material, removing knobs from the stove so client does not turn on burner and leave it unattended, securing sharp knives and firearms.*

- Instruct SO/caregivers to share information about client's condition, functional status, and medications whenever encountering new providers. *Clients often have multiple doctors, each of whom may prescribe medications, with potential for adverse effects and overmedication.*[3,7]

- Investigate local resources; provide appropriate referrals (e.g., case managers, counselors, support groups, financial services, Meals on Wheels, adult day care, adult foster care, respite care for family, home-care agency, nursing home placement). *Individuals are generally not capable of carrying alone the heavy burdens of caring for a relative with this problem. Caregivers need help and support (whether or not they are trying to provide total care) to deal with exhaustion and unresolved feelings.*[9,10]

- Discuss need for or appropriateness of genetic testing and counseling for family members. *Diagnosis of dementias such as early onset Alzheimer's or Huntington's disease necessitate additional support for family members who may be at risk themselves.*

DOCUMENTATION FOCUS

Assessment/Reassessment
- Assessment findings, including degree of impairment.
- Involvement and availability of family members to provide care.

Planning
- Plan of care and who is involved in planning.
- Teaching plan.

Implementation/Evaluation
- Response to treatment plan, interventions, and actions performed.
- Attainment or progress toward desired outcomes.
- Modifications to plan of care.

Discharge Planning
- Long-term needs, who is responsible for actions to be taken.
- Specific referrals made

References

1. Bostwick, J. M. (2000). The many faces of confusion: Timing and collateral history often holds the key to diagnosis. *Postgrad Med*, 108(6), 60–72.
2. Alzheimer's Disease and Related Disorders Association (ADRDA). (2003). About Alzheimer's. Physicians and Care Professionals, Various Educational Materials. Retrieved 2003 from www.alz.org.
3. Doenges, M. E., Moorhouse, M. F., Geissler-Murr, A. C. (2002). *Nurse's Pocket Guide: Diagnoses, Interventions, and Rationales*. 8th ed. Philadelphia: F. A. Davis, 145–147.
4. Expert Consensus Guideline Series: Agitation in older persons with dementia: A guide for families and caregivers. (1998). Expert Knowledge Systems, LLC. Ross Editorial Services. Retrieved 2003 from www.psychguides.com.
5. Sommers, M. S., Johnson, S. A. (1997). Alzheimer's disease and delirium/dementia. *Davis's Manual of Nursing Therapeutics for Diseases and Disorders*. Philadelphia: F. A. Davis.
6. Kovach, C. R., Wilson, S. A., (1999). Dementia in older adults. In Stanley, M., Beare, P. G. (eds). *Gerontologic Nursing: A Health Promotion/Protection Approach*. 2d ed. Philadelphia: F. A. Davis .
7. Burns, A., Byrne, J., Ballard, C. (2002). Sensory stimulation in dementia: An effective option for managing behavioral problems. *Br Med J*, 325, 1312–1313.
8. Rowe, M. A. (2003). People with dementia who become lost. *Am J Nurs*, 103(7), 32.
9. Brynes, G. (2000). *Dealing with dementia: Help for relatives, friends and caregivers. Information brochure*. Baltimore: Northern County Psychiatric Associates.
10. The mid stage of Alzheimer's disease: Tips for dealing with dementia sufferers. Retrieved August 2003 from www.dementia.com.
11. Naylor, M. D., et al. (2005). Cognitively impaired older adults. *Am J Nurs*, 105(2), 52–61.
12. Jacobs, D. H. (2006). Confusional states and acute memory disorders. Retrieved January 2007 from www.emedicine.com/neuro/topic435.htm.
13. Beatty, G. E. (2006). Shedding light on Alzheimer's. *Am J Prim Health Care*, 31(9), 32–43.

adult Failure to Thrive

DEFINITION: Progressive functional deterioration of a physical and cognitive nature; individual's ability to live with multisystem diseases, cope with ensuing problems, and manage his or her care are remarkably diminished

RELATED FACTORS

Depression
[Major disease, degenerative condition]
[Aging process]

DEFINING CHARACTERISTICS

Subjective
Expresses loss of interest in pleasurable outlets
Altered mood state
Verbalizes desire for death

Objective
Inadequate nutritional intake; consumption of minimal to no food at most meals (i.e., consumes less than 75% of normal requirements); anorexia
Unintentional weight loss (e.g., 5% in 1 month, 10% in 6 months)
Physical decline (e.g., fatigue, dehydration, incontinence of bowel and bladder)
Cognitive decline (e.g., problems with responding to environmental stimuli; demonstrated difficulty in reasoning, decision making, judgment, memory, concentration; decreased perception)
Apathy
Decreased participation in activities of daily living (ADLs); self-care deficit; neglect of home environment or financial responsibilities
Decreased social skills or social withdrawal
Frequent exacerbations of chronic health problems

Sample Clinical Applications: Chronic debilitating conditions (e.g., AIDS, Alzheimer's disease, multiple sclerosis [MS]), cancer, terminal illnesses, major depression

DESIRED OUTCOMES/EVALUATION CRITERIA

Sample **NOC** linkages:
Will to Live: Desire, determination, and effort to survive

Client Will (Include Specific Time Frame)
• Express sense of optimism for future.

Sample **NOC** linkages:
Psychosocial Adjustment: Life Change: Adaptive psychosocial response of an individual to a significant life change
Physical Aging: Normal physical changes that occur with the natural aging process

(continues on page 310)

---

adult Failure to Thrive (continued)

Client/Caregiver Will (Include Specific Time Frame)
• Acknowledge presence of factors affecting well-being.
• Identify corrective/adaptive measures for individual situation.
• Demonstrate behaviors/lifestyle changes necessary to enhance functional status.

ACTIONS/INTERVENTIONS

Sample NIC linkages:
Mood Management: Providing for safety, stabilization, recovery, and maintenance of a patient who is dysfunctionally depressed or elevated mood
Hope Inspiration: Enhancing the belief in one's capacity to initiate and sustain actions
Self-Care Assistance: Assisting another to perform activities of daily living
Refer to NDs Activity Intolerance; risk prone health Behaviors; chronic Confusion; ineffective Coping; impaired Dentition; risk for Falls; complicated Grieving; risk for Loneliness; imbalanced Nutrition: less than body requirements; Relocation Stress Syndrome; Self-Care Deficit (specify); chronic low Self-Esteem; risk for Spiritual Distress; impaired Swallowing, as appropriate, for additional relevant interventions.

NURSING PRIORITY NO. 1

To identify causative/contributing factors:

● Assess client's/SO's perception of factors leading to present condition, noting onset, duration of decline. *Adult failure to thrive (FTT) is characterized by malnutrition associated with consistent weight loss; loss of physical, cognitive, and social functioning; impaired immune function; and depression.[1] The condition may be diagnosed when client is hospitalized for such problems as urinary tract infection, decubitus ulcers, falls, and mental confusion. Although it can occur as a result of an acute health problem or elder abuse, FTT is most often associated with chronic health conditions, social isolation, and budgetary constraints.[2,10]*

● Note presence or absence of physical complaints (e.g., fatigue, weight loss, others as noted in Defining Characteristics) and presence of conditions (e.g., heart disease, undetected diabetes mellitus, dementia, stroke, renal failure, terminal conditions). *These contributing factors may or may not be recognized by the client or SOs.*

● Assist with or review results of testing, as indicated (e.g., endocrine or metabolic testing, gastrointestinal endoscopy, psychiatric evaluation). *Aversion to eating and decline in mental function could reflect physical problem (e.g., gastric infection with* Helicobacter pylori) *or be the result of an emotional or psychological condition (e.g., depression).[9,11]*

● Identify cultural beliefs, norms, and values that are influencing client/caregiver understanding of dietary needs. *Although many cultures have their own distinct theories of nutritional practices for health promotion and disease prevention, the need for nutritional balance of a diet is almost universally recognized as essential for healing, general health, and sustaining a quality life.[3]*

● Review with client/SO previous and current life situations, including role changes, multiple losses (e.g., death of loved ones, change in living arrangements, finances, independence), social isolation, and grieving *to identify stressors that may be affecting current situation.*

● Determine nutritional status. *Malnutrition (e.g., weight loss and laboratory abnormalities) and factors contributing to failure to eat (e.g., chronic nausea, loss of appetite, no access to*

food or cooking, poorly fitting dentures, no one with whom to share meals, depression, financial problems) greatly impact health status and quality of life—especially for the elderly individual.[4–6,10,11]

- Evaluate client's level of adaptive behavior and client/caregiver knowledge and skills about health maintenance, environment, and safety *in order to instruct, intervene, and refer appropriately.*
- Ascertain safety of home environment and persons providing care *to identify potential for/presence of neglectful or abusive situations and/or need for referrals.*

NURSING PRIORITY NO. 2

To assess degree of impairment:

- Collaborate with multidisciplinary team to determine severity of client's nutritional and functional limitations. *Various scales may be used to determine the extent of problem, to implement treatment, and to make appropriate referrals. Note: FTT is a recognized diagnosis for admission to hospice care.*[7]
- Obtain current weight *to provide comparative baseline and evaluate response to interventions.*
- Active-listen client's/caregiver's perception of problem. *Conveys sense of confidence in client's ability to identify and solve current problems.*[8]
- Discuss individual concerns about feelings of loss/loneliness and relationship between these feelings and current decline in well-being. Note desire or willingness to change situation. *Motivation or lack thereof can impede or facilitate achieving desired outcomes.*[10]

NURSING PRIORITY NO. 3

To assist client to achieve/maintain general well-being:

- Assist with treatment of underlying medical or psychiatric conditions *that could positively influence current situation (e.g., resolution of infection, addressing depression).*
- Develop plan of action with client/caregiver *to meet immediate needs for nutrition, safety, and self-care and facilitate implementation of actions.*
- Refer to dietitian or nutritionist to assist in planning meals to meet client's specific needs, taste, and abilities. *Plans could include offering client's favorite food(s), attending social events (e.g., ice cream social, happy hour), or participating in family style meals. In addition, interventions may be geared toward treatment of depression, grief, or loss and cultural or environmental adaptation measures.*[11,12] (Refer to ND imbalanced Nutrition: less than body requirements for additional interventions.)
- Monitor caloric intake and weigh regularly, as indicated. Maintain food diary, as appropriate. *Provides data to evaluate effectiveness of interventions.*
- Explore strengths and successful coping skills the individual has previously used and apply to current situation. Refine or develop new strategies, as appropriate. *Incorporating these into problem-solving builds on past successes.*[8]
- Assist client to develop goals for dealing with life or illness situation. Involve SO in long range planning. *Promotes commitment to goals and plan, thereby maximizing outcomes.*

NURSING PRIORITY NO. 4

To promote wellness (Teaching/Discharge Considerations):

- Assist client/SO(s) to identify useful community resources (e.g., support groups, Meals on Wheels, social worker, home care or assistive care, placement services). *Enhances coping, assists with problem-solving, and may reduce risks to client and caregiver.*

Nursing Diagnoses in Alphabetical Order

● Encourage client to talk about positive aspects of life and to keep as physically active as possible *to reduce effects of dispiritedness (e.g., "feeling low," sense of being unimportant, disconnected).*[12]

 ● Introduce concept of mindfulness (living in the moment). *Promotes feeling of capability and belief that this moment can be dealt with.*

 ● Promote socialization within individual limitations *to provide additional stimulation, reduce sense of isolation.*

 ● Help client explore reasons for living or begin to deal with end-of-life issues and provide support for grieving. *Enhances hope and sense of control, providing opportunity for client to take charge of own future.*[8,12]

 ● Offer opportunities to discuss life goals and support client/SO in setting/attaining new goals for this time in their lives *to enhance hope for the future.*

 ● Assist client/SO/family to understand that FTT commonly occurs near the end of life and cannot always be reversed.[10]

● Refer to pastoral care, counseling or psychotherapy *for grief work.*

● Discuss appropriateness of and refer to palliative services or hospice care, as indicated.

DOCUMENTATION FOCUS

Assessment/Reassessment
• Individual findings, including current weight, dietary pattern, perceptions of self, food and eating, motivation for loss, support and feedback from SOs.
• Perception of losses or life changes.
• Ability to perform ADLs, participate in care, meet own needs.
• Motivation for change, support and feedback from SO(s).

Planning
• Plan of care, specific interventions, and who is involved in planning.
• Teaching plan.

Implementation/Evaluation
• Responses to interventions and actions performed, general well-being, weekly weight.
• Attainment or progress toward desired outcome(s).
• Modifications to plan of care.

Discharge Planning
• Long-term needs and who is responsible for actions to be taken.
• Community resources and support groups.
• Specific referrals made.

References

1. Groom, D. D. (1993). Elder care: A diagnostic model for failure to thrive. *J Gerontol Nurs,* 19, 6.
2. Stanley, M. (1999). The aging gastrointestinal system, with nutritional considerations. In Stanley, M., Beare, P. G. (eds). *Gerontological Nursing: A Health Promotion/Protection Approach.* 2d ed. Philadelphia: F. A. Davis.
3. Purnell's Model for Cultural Competence. (1998). In Purnell, L. D., Paulanka, B. J. (eds). *Transcultural Health Care: A Culturally Competent Approach.* Philadelphia: F. A. Davis, 34.
4. Wallace, J. I., Schwartz, R. S. (1997). Involuntary weight loss in elderly outpatients. *Clin Geriatr Med,* 13, 717.
5. Scott, D. D., Chase, M. (2003). Nutritional management in the rehabilitation setting. Retrieved July 2007 from www.emedicine.com/pmr/topic159.htm.

⊕ Cultural   Collaborative   🏠 Community/Home Care   ⟋ Diagnostic Studies   ∞ Pediatric/Geriatric/Lifespan   Medications

6. Karnofsky Performance Status Scale rating criteria. (1993). In Doyle, D., Hanks, G. W. C., MacDonald, N. (eds). *Oxford Textbook of Palliative Medicine*. New York: Oxford University Press.
7. Adult failure to thrive/debility, unspecified. (1993). *Medicare worksheet for determining prognosis*: Hospice of Southern Illinois.
8. Townsend, M. C. (2003). *Psychiatric Mental Health Nursing Concepts of Care*. 4th ed. Philadelphia: F. A. Davis.
9. Portnoi, V. A. (1997). *Helicobacter pylori infection and anorexia of aging. Arch Intern Med*, 157, 269.
10. Robertson, R. G., Montagnini, M. (2004). Geriatric failure to thrive. *Am Fam Physician*, 70(2), 343–350.
11. DiMaria-Ghalili, R. A., Amelia, E. (2005). Nutrition in older adults: Interventions and assessment can help curb the growing threat of malnutrition. *Am J Nurs*, 105(3), 4050.
12. Butcher, H. K., McGonigal-Kenney, M. (2005). Depression & dispiritedness in later life: A "gray drizzle of horror" isn't inevitable. *Am J Nurs*, 105(12), 52–61.

risk for Falls

DEFINITION: Increased susceptibility to falling that may cause physical harm

RISK FACTORS

Adults
History of falls
Wheelchair use; use of assistive devices (e.g., walker, cane)
Age 65 or over; lives alone
Lower-limb prosthesis

Physiological
Presence of acute illness; postoperative conditions
Visual/hearing difficulties
Arthritis
Orthostatic hypotension; faintness when turning/extending neck
Sleeplessness
Anemias; vascular disease
Neoplasms (i.e., fatigue/limited mobility)
Urgency; incontinence; diarrhea
Postprandial blood sugar changes; [hypoglycemia]
Impaired physical mobility; foot problems; decreased lower extremity strength
Impaired balance; difficulty with gait; proprioceptive deficits [e.g., unilateral neglect]
Neuropathy

Cognitive
Diminished mental status [e.g., confusion, delirium, dementia, impaired reality testing]

Medications
Antihypertensive agents; angiotensin-converting enzyme (ACE) inhibitors; diuretics; tricyclic antidepressants; antianxiety agents; hypnotics; tranquilizers; narcotics
Alcohol use

(continues on page 314)

risk for Falls (continued)

Environment
Restraints
Weather conditions (e.g., wet floors, ice)
Cluttered environment; throw or scatter rugs; no antislip material in bath or shower
Unfamiliar, dimly lit room

Children
<2 years of age; male gender when >1 year of age
Lack of gate on stairs, window guards, auto restraints
Unattended infant on elevated surface (e.g., bed or changing table); bed located near window
Lack of parental supervision

NOTE: A risk diagnosis is not evidenced by signs and symptoms, as the problem has not occurred; rather, nursing interventions are directed at prevention.
Sample Clinical Applications: Osteoporosis, seizure disorder, cerebrovascular disease, cataracts, dementia, paralysis, hypotension, cardiac dysrhythmias, amputation, inner ear infection, alcohol abuse or intoxication

DESIRED OUTCOMES/EVALUATION CRITERIA

Sample NOC linkages:
Physical Injury severity: Severity of injuries from accidents and trauma

Client Will (Include Specific Time Frame)
• Be free of injury.
Knowledge: Fall Prevention: Extent of understanding conveyed about prevention of falls
Fall Prevention Behavior: Personal or family caregiver actions to minimize risk factors that might precipitate falls in the personal environment

Client/Caregivers Will (Include Specific Time Frame)
• Verbalize understanding of individual risk factors that contribute to possibility of falls.
• Demonstrate behaviors, lifestyle changes to reduce risk factors and protect self from injury.
• Modify environment as indicated to enhance safety.

ACTIONS/INTERVENTIONS

Sample NIC linkages:
Fall Prevention: Instituting special precautions with patient at risk for injury from falling
Environmental Management: Safety: Manipulation of the patient's surroundings for therapeutic benefit
Risk Identification: Analysis of potential risk factors, determination of health risks, and prioritization of risk-reduction strategies for an individual or group

NURSING PRIORITY NO. 1

To evaluate source/degree of risk:

• Review client's general health status *noting factors that may affect safety such as chronic/ debilitating conditions, polypharmacy, recent trauma, prolonged bedrest or immobility, sedentary lifestyle.*

- Assess and document client's fall risk using a fall scale (e.g., Morse Fall Scale [MFS], Functional Ambulation Profile [FAP], Tinetti Balance and Gait Assessment) upon admission, change in status, transfer, and discharge. *Fall risk scales are widely used in acute care and long-term settings and include numbered rating scales for (1) history of falls, (2) secondary diagnosis, (3) use of ambulatory aid, (4) presence of IV, (5) gait and transfer abilities, and (6) mental status. An MFS score of >51 indicates the client is at high risk for falls and requires high fall-prevention interventions.*[1,2,7,8]
- Note client's age/developmental level, gender, decision-making ability, level of competence. *Infants, young children (e.g., climbing on objects, stairs), young adults (e.g., sports activities), and elderly (e.g., significant vision, cognitive, or mobility impairments; osteoporosis; or loss of muscle, fat, and subcutaneous tissue) are at greatest risk because of developmental issues or impaired/lack of ability to self-protect.*[2]
- Assess client's cognitive status (e.g., presence of brain injury, dementia, neurological disorders of multiple kinds). *Affects ability to perceive own limitations or recognize danger. If client is unable to protect self, responsibility falls upon primary care provider(s).*
- Evaluate client's muscle strength, balance, gross and fine motor coordination. Review history of past or current physical injuries (e.g., musculoskeletal injuries; orthopedic surgery) *that may be altering coordination, gait, and balance.*
- Assess mood, coping abilities, personality styles. *Individual's temperament, typical behavior, stressors, and level of self-esteem can affect attitude toward safety issues, resulting in carelessness or increased risk-taking without consideration of consequences.*[7,8]
- Determine client's/SO's level of knowledge about and attendance to safety needs. *May reveal lack of knowledge needed to provide for safety, or choice to make a different decision for some reason (e.g., "We can't hire a home assistant"; "I can't watch him every minute"; "It's not manly") or may not have resources to attend to safety issues in all settings.*[3]
- Evaluate client's use, misuse, or failure to use assistive aids when indicated. *Client may have assistive device but is at high risk for falls while adjusting to altered body state and use of unfamiliar device. Client might refuse to use devices for various reasons (e.g., waiting for help; just doesn't like it for whatever reason).*[7,8]
- Identify environmental hazards in the care setting, home or other environment. *Determining needs and deficits provides opportunities for intervention and instruction (e.g., concerning clearing of hazards, intensifying client supervision; obtaining safety equipment; referring for vision evaluation).*[7,8]
- Ascertain caregiver's expectations of client (whether child, cognitively impaired and/or elderly family member) and compare with actual abilities. *Reality of client's abilities and needs may be different than perception or desires of caregivers.*
- Note socioeconomic status and availability and use of resources in other circumstances. *Can affect current coping abilities.*

NURSING PRIORITY NO. 2

To assist client/caregiver to reduce or correct individual risk factors:

- Collaborate in treatment of disease or condition(s) (e.g., acute illness, dementia, incontinence, neurological or musculoskeletal conditions) *to improve client's overall health and thereby reduce potential for falls.*
- Review consequences of previously determined risk factors and client/SO response (e.g., client's current fall and hip fracture caused by failure to make safety provisions for client's impairments).[3]
- Recommend or implement needed interventions and safety devices *to manage conditions that could contribute to falling and to promote safe environment for individual and others:*[1–6]

Situate bed to enable client to exit toward his or her stronger side whenever possible.

Place bed in lowest possible position, use raised-edge mattress, pad floor at side of bed, or place mattress on floor as appropriate.

Use half side rail instead of full side rails or upright pole to assist individual in arising from bed.

Provide chairs with firm, high seats and lifting mechanisms when indicated.

Provide appropriate day or night lighting; evaluate vision, encourage use of prescription eyewear.

Assist with transfers and ambulation; show client/SO ways to move safely.

Provide and instruct in use of mobility devices and safety devices, like grab bars and call light or personal assistance systems.

Clear environment of hazards (e.g., obstructing furniture, small items on the floor, electrical cords, throw rugs).

Lock wheels on movable equipment (e.g., wheelchairs, beds).

Encourage use of treaded slippers, socks, and shoes, and maintain nonskid floors and floor mats.

Provide foot and nail care.

- Provide or encourage use of analgesics before activity if pain is interfering with desired activities. *Balance and movement can be impaired by pain associated with multiple conditions such as trauma or arthritis.*[1,2]

- Follow up with physician to review client's usual medication regimen (e.g., narcotics/opiates, psychotropics, antihypertensives, diuretics), *which can contribute to weakness, confusion, balance and gait disturbances. May benefit from dose adjustment, change in choice of medication prescribed, or time of administration.*[6-8]

- Refer to physical medicine specialist, physical or occupational therapist, recreation therapist as appropriate. *May require evaluation (e.g., balance, muscle strength) and exercises to improve client's balance, strength, or mobility, to improve or relearn ambulation, to identify and obtain appropriate assistive devices for mobility, environmental safety, or home modification.*

- Perform home visit when appropriate. *Useful in determining client's specific needs and available resources, or verifying that home safety issues are addressed, including supervision, access to emergency assistance, and client's ability to manage self-care in the home.*

NURSING PRIORITY NO. 3

To promote wellness (Teaching/Discharge Considerations):[1-6]

- Educate client/SO/caregivers in fall prevention; address the need for exercise balanced with need for client/care provider safety. *While fall prevention is necessary, the need to protect the client from harm must be balanced with preserving client's independence. If the client is overly afraid of falling, the lack of activity will result in deconditioning and an even greater risk of falling.*[3]

- Discuss importance of monitoring client/intervening in conditions (e.g., client fatigue; acute illness; depression; objects that block traffic patterns in home; insufficient lighting; unfamiliar surroundings; client attempting tasks that are too difficult for present level of functioning, inability to contact someone when help is needed) *that have been shown to contribute to occurrence of falls.*[7,8]

- Address individual environmental factors associated with falling and create or instruct in safe physical environment such as bed height, room lighting, removal of loose carpet or throw rugs, repair of uneven flooring, installing grab bars in bathrooms.

- Refer to community resources as indicated. Provide written material for review and reinforcement of learning. *Client/caregivers may need or desire information (now or later)*

about financial assistance, home modifications, referrals for counseling, home care, sources for safety equipment, or placement in extended care facility.

* Connect client/family with sources of assistance (e.g., neighbors, friends, support groups) *to check on client on regular basis, to assist elderly or handicapped individuals in providing such things as structural maintenance, clearing of snow, gravel, or ice from walks and steps, and so on.*

* Promote community awareness about the problems of design of buildings, equipment, transportation, and workplace accidents that contribute to falls.

DOCUMENTATION FOCUS

Assessment/Reassessment
* Individual risk factors noting current physical findings (e.g., bruises, cuts, anemia, and use of alcohol, drugs, and prescription medications).
* Client's/caregiver's understanding of individual risks and safety concerns.
* Caregiver's expectations of client's abilities.

Planning
* Plan of care and who is involved in planning.
* Teaching plan.

Implementation/Evaluation
* Individual responses to interventions, teaching, and actions performed.
* Specific actions and changes that are made.
* Attainment or progress toward desired outcomes.
* Modifications to plan of care.

Discharge Planning
* Long-term plans for discharge needs, lifestyle, home setting and community changes, and who is responsible for actions to be taken.
* Specific referrals made.

References

1. American Medical Directors Association (AMDA). (1999). Clinical practice guideline: Falls and fall risk. Retrieved July 2007 from www.amda.com/tools/cpg/falls.cfm.
2. VHA National Center for Patient Safety (NCPS) Fall Prevention and Management. Includes articles on Morse Fall Scale, standard and high risk fall prevention measures and safety education. Retrieved July 2007 from www.va.gov/ncps/CogAids/FallPrevention/index.html.
3. Henkel, G. (2002). Beyond the MDS. Team approach to falls assessment, prevention & management. *Caring for the Aged*, 3(4), 15–20.
4. Doenges, M. E., Moorhouse, M. F., Geissler-Murr, A. C. (2002). Nursing care plan: Extended care, falls, risk for. *Nursing Care Plans: Guidelines for Individualizing Patient Care* (CD-ROM). 6th ed. Philadelphia: F. A. Davis.
5. Daus, C. (1999). Maintaining mobility: Assistive equipment helps the geriatric population stay active and independent. *Rehabil Manage*, 12(5), 58–61.
6. Horn, L. B. (2000). Reducing the risk of falls in the elderly. *Rehabil Manage*, 13(3), 36–38.
7. Bright, L. (2005). Strategies to improve the patient safety outcome indicator: Preventing or reducing falls. *Home Healthcare Nurse*, 23(1), 29–36.
8. Poe, S. S., et al. (2005). An evidence-based approach to fall risk assessment, prevention, and management: Lessons learned. *J Nurs Care Qual*, 20(2), 107–116.

dysfunctional Family Processes

DEFINITION: Psychosocial, spiritual, and physiological functions of the family unit are chronically disorganized, which leads to conflict, denial of problems, resistance to change, ineffective problem-solving, and a series of self-perpetuating crises

RELATED FACTORS

Abuse of alcohol; [addictive substances]
Family history of alcoholism or resistance to treatment
Inadequate coping skills; addictive personality; lack of problem-solving skills
Biochemical influences; genetic predisposition

DEFINING CHARACTERISTICS

Subjective
Feelings
Anxiety, tension, distress; decreased self-esteem, worthlessness; lingering resentment
Anger, suppressed rage; frustration; shame, embarrassment; hurt; unhappiness; guilt
Emotional isolation, loneliness; powerlessness; insecurity; hopelessness; rejection
Responsibility for alcoholic's behavior; vulnerability; mistrust
Depression; hostility; fear; confusion; dissatisfaction; loss
Being different from other people; misunderstood
Emotional control by others; being unloved; lack of identity
Abandonment; confused love and pity; moodiness; failure
Roles and Relationships
Family denial; deterioration in family relationships; disturbed family dynamics; ineffective spouse communication; marital problems; intimacy dysfunction
Altered role function; disrupted family roles or rituals; inconsistent parenting; low perception of parental support; chronic family problems
Lack of skills necessary for relationships; lack of cohesiveness
Pattern of rejection; economic problems; neglected obligations

Objective
Feelings: Repressed emotions
Roles and relationships:
Closed communication systems
Triangulating family relationships; reduced ability of family members to relate to each other for mutual growth and maturation
Family does not demonstrate respect for individuality or autonomy of its members
Behavioral:
Alcohol abuse; substance abuse other than alcohol; nicotine addiction
Enabling to maintain drinking [or substance use]; inadequate understanding or deficient knowledge about alcoholism [or substance abuse]
Family special occasions are alcohol-centered
Rationalization; denial of problems; refusal to get help; inability to accept or receive help appropriately
Inappropriate expression of anger; blaming; criticizing; verbal abuse of children/spouse/parent

Lying; broken promises; lack of reliability; manipulation; dependency

Inability to express or accept wide range of feelings; difficulty with intimate relationships; diminished physical contact

Harsh self-judgment; difficulty having fun; self-blaming; isolation; unresolved grief; seeking approval or affirmation

Impaired communication; contradictory or paradoxical communication; controlling communication; power struggles

Ineffective problem-solving skills; lack of dealing with conflict; orientation toward tension relief rather than achievement of goals; agitation; escalating conflict; chaos

Disturbances in concentration; disturbances in academic performance in children; failure to accomplish developmental tasks; difficulty with life-cycle transitions

Inability to meet emotional, security, or spiritual needs of its members

Inability to adapt to change; immaturity; stress-related physical illnesses; inability to accept health; inability to deal constructively with traumatic experiences

Sample Clinical Applications: Alcohol abuse or withdrawal, prescription or illicit drug abuse, fetal alcohol syndrome

DESIRED OUTCOMES/EVALUATION CRITERIA

Sample **NOC** linkages:
Family Functioning: Capacity of the family system to meet the needs of its members during developmental transitions
Family Social Climate: Supportive milieu as characterized by family member relationships and goals
Substance Addiction Consequences: Severity of change in health status and social functioning due to substance addiction

Family Will (Include Specific Time Frame)
• Verbalize understanding of dynamics of codependence.
• Participate in individual/family treatment programs.
• Identify ineffective coping behaviors and consequences of choices or actions.
• Demonstrate and plan for necessary lifestyle changes.
• Take action to change self-destructive behaviors or alter behaviors that contribute to client's drinking or substance use.
• Demonstrate improvement in parenting skills.

ACTIONS/INTERVENTIONS

Sample **NIC** linkages:
Counseling: Use of an interactive helping process focusing on the needs, problems, or feelings of the patient and SOs to enhance or support coping, problem-solving, and interpersonal relationships
Substance Use Treatment: Supportive care of patient/family members with physical and psychosocial problems associated with the use of alcohol or drugs
Family Process Maintenance: Minimization of family process disruption effects

NURSING PRIORITY NO. 1

To assess contributing factors/underlying problem(s):

- Assess current level of functioning of family members. *Information necessary for planning care determines areas for focus, potential for change.*[2]
- Ascertain family's understanding of current situation; note results of previous involvement in treatment. *Family with a member who is addicted to alcohol has often had frequent hospitalizations in the past. Knowing what has brought about the current situation will determine a starting place for this treatment plan.*[2]
- Review family history, explore roles of family members and circumstances involving substance use. *Although one member may be identified as the client, all of the family members are participants in the problem and need to be involved in the solution.*[5]
- Determine history of accidents or violent behaviors within family and current safety issues. *Identifies family at risk and degree of concern or disregard of individual members to determine course of action to prevent further violence.*[2,4]
- Discuss current and past methods of coping. *Family members have developed coping skills to deal with behaviors of client, which may or may not be useful to changing the situation. Skills identified as useful can help to change the present situation. Those identified as not helpful (enabling behaviors) can be targeted for intervention to bring about desired changes and improve family functioning.*[1,2,5]
- Determine extent and understanding of enabling behaviors being evidenced by family members. *Family members may have developed behaviors that support the client continuing the pattern of addiction. Awareness, identification, and knowledge of these behaviors provide opportunity for individuals to begin the process of change.*[2,5]
- Identify sabotage behaviors of family members. *Issues of secondary gain (conscious or unconscious) may impede recovery. Even though family member(s) may verbalize a desire for the individual to become substance-free, the reality of interactive dynamics is that they may unconsciously not want the individual to recover because this would affect the family member(s) own role in the relationship.*[2]
- Note presence and extent of behaviors of family, client, and staff that might be "too helpful," such as frequent requests for assistance, excuses for not following through on agreed-on behaviors, feelings of anger or irritation with others. *Identification of specific behaviors (enabling) can help family members see what they do that complicates acceptance of situation by substance abuser and that need to be changed to facilitate resolution of problem.*[5]

NURSING PRIORITY NO. 2

To assist family to change destructive behaviors:

- Seek mutual agreement on behaviors and responsibilities for nurse and client/family members. *Maximizes understanding of what is expected of each person and minimizes opportunity for manipulation of each individual.*[5]
- Confront and examine denial and sabotage behaviors used by family members. *Identifies specific behaviors that individuals can be aware of and begin to change so they can move beyond blocks to recovery.*[6]
- Discuss use of anger, rationalization, or projection and ways in which these interfere with problem resolution. *Awareness of own feelings can lead to a decision to change, client then has to face the consequences of his or her own actions and may choose to get well.*[6]
- Encourage family to identify and deal with anger. Solve concerns and develop solutions. *Understanding what leads to anger and violence can lead to new behaviors and changes in the family for healthier relationships.*[3]

- Determine family strengths, areas for growth, individual/family successes. *Family members may not realize they have strengths, and as they identify these areas, they can choose to learn and develop new strategies for a more effective family structure.*[2]
- Remain nonjudgmental in approach to family members and to member who uses alcohol or drugs. *Individual already sees self as unworthy, and judgment on the part of caregivers to family will interfere with ability to be a change agent.*[5]
- Provide information regarding effects of addiction on mood and personality of the involved person. *Family members have been dealing with client's behavior for a time, and information can help them to understand and cope with negative behaviors without being judgmental or reacting angrily.*[2]
- Distinguish between destructive aspects of enabling behavior and genuine motivation to aid the user. *Family members often want to help but need distinguish between behavior that is helpful and that which is not, to begin to solve problems of addiction.*[6]
- Identify use of manipulative behaviors and discuss ways to avoid or prevent these situations. *The client often manipulates the people around him or her to maintain the status quo. When family begins to interact in a straightforward, honest manner, manipulation is not possible and healing can begin.*[2]

NURSING PRIORITY NO. 3

To promote wellness (Teaching/Discharge Considerations):

- Provide factual information to client/family about the effects of addictive behaviors on the family and what to expect after discharge from program. *Family may have unrealistic expectations about changes that have occurred in therapy, and having information will help them deal more effectively with the difficulties of continuing the changes as they return to their new life without alcohol or substance.*[5]
- Provide information about enabling behavior, addictive disease characteristics for both user and nonuser who is codependent. *Education is a prime ingredient in treatment of addiction and can assist family members to deal realistically with these issues.*[6]
- Discuss importance of restructuring life activities, work and leisure relationships. *Previous lifestyle and relationships supported substance use requiring change to prevent relapse.*[7]
- Encourage family to refocus celebrations to exclude alcohol use. *Because celebrations often include the use of alcohol, this is one area where change can be made that can reduce the risk of relapse.*[7]
- Provide support for family members; encourage participation in group work. *Support is essential to changing client and family behaviors. Participating in group provides an opportunity to practice new skills of communication and behavior.*[5]
- Encourage involvement with/refer to self-help groups, Al-Anon, AlaTeen, Narcotics Anonymous, family therapy groups. *Regular attendance at a group can provide support; help client see how others are dealing with similar problems; and learn new skills, such as problem solving, for handling family disagreements.*[7]
- Provide bibliotherapy including reliable Web sites, as appropriate. *Reading provides helpful information for making desired changes, especially when client/family members are dedicated to making change and willing to learn new ways of interacting within the family.*[7]
- Refer to NDs compromised/disabled family Coping, interrupted Family Processes as appropriate, for additional interventions.

DOCUMENTATION FOCUS

Assessment/Reassessment
- Assessment findings, including history of substance(s) that have been used, and family risk factors/safety concerns.
- Family composition and involvement.
- Results of previous treatment involvement.
- Cultural or religious beliefs and values.

Planning
- Plan of care and who is involved in planning.
- Teaching plan.

Implementation/Evaluation
- Responses of family members to treatment, teaching, and actions performed.
- Attainment or progress toward desired outcome(s).
- Modifications to plan of care.

Discharge Planning
- Long-term needs, who is responsible for actions to be taken.
- Specific referrals made.

References

1. Messina, J., Messina, C. (2007). Tools for handling control: Eliminating manipulation. Retrieved July 2007 from www.coping.org/control/manipul.htm.
2. Townsend, M. C. (2003). *Psychiatric Mental Health Nursing Concepts of Care*. 4th ed. Philadelphia: F. A. Davis.
3. Gordon, T. (2000). *Parent Effectiveness Training*. Updated ed. New York: Three Rivers Press.
4. Screening for family violence. Retrieved August 2007 from www.ahrq.gov/clinic/2ndcps/famviol.pdf.
5. American Nurses Association. (1987). *Task Force on Substance Abuse Nursing Practice: The care of clients with addictions; dimensions of nursing practice*. Kansas City, MO: American Nurses Association.
6. Nye, C. L., Zucker, R. A., Fitzgerald, H. E. (1999). Early family-based intervention in the path to alcohol problems, rationale and relationship between treatment process characteristics and child and parenting outcomes. *J Stud Alcohol Suppl*, 13, 10–21.
7. Sielhamer, R. A., Jacob, T., Dunn, N. J. (1993). The impact of alcohol consumption on parent-child relationships in families of alcoholics. *J Stud Alcohol*, 54, 189.

(interrupted Family Processes)

DEFINITION: Change in family relationships and/or functioning

RELATED FACTORS

Situational transition or crises
Developmental transition or crises
Shift in health status of a family member
Family roles shift; power shift of family members

⊕ Cultural Collaborative 🏠 Community/Home Care ✏ Diagnostic Studies ∞ Pediatric/Geriatric/Lifespan 💊 Medications

Modification in family finances or family social status
Interaction with community

DEFINING CHARACTERISTICS

Subjective
Changes in power alliances; satisfaction with family, expressions of conflict within family, effectiveness in completing assigned tasks, stress-reduction behaviors, expressions of conflict with or isolation from community resources, somatic complaints
[Family expresses confusion about what to do, verbalizes they are having difficulty responding to change]

Objective
Changes in assigned tasks, participation in problem-solving or decision making, communication patterns, mutual support, availability for emotional support or affective responsiveness, intimacy, patterns or rituals

Sample Clinical Applications: Chronic illness, cancer, surgical procedures, traumatic injury, substance abuse, Alzheimer's disease, pregnancy, adolescent rebellion, conduct disorder

DESIRED OUTCOMES/EVALUATION CRITERIA

Sample **NOC** linkages:
Family Functioning: Capacity of the family system to meet the needs of its members during developmental transitions
Family Normalization: Capacity of the family system to develop strategies for optimal functioning when a member has a chronic illness or disability
Family Social Climate: Supportive milieu as characterized by family member relationships and goals

Family Will (Include Specific Time Frame)
- Express feelings freely and appropriately.
- Demonstrate individual involvement in problem-solving processes directed at appropriate solutions for the situation or crisis.
- Direct energies in a purposeful manner to plan for resolution of the crisis.
- Verbalize understanding of illness/trauma, treatment regimen, and prognosis.
- Encourage and allow member who is ill to handle situation in own way, progressing toward independence.

ACTIONS/INTERVENTIONS

Sample **NIC** linkages:
Family Process Maintenance: Minimization of family process disruption effects
Family Integrity Promotion: Facilitating family participation in the emotional and physical care of the patient
Normalization Promotion: Assisting parents and other family members of children with chronic diseases or disabilities in providing normal life experiences for their children and families

---

NURSING PRIORITY NO. 1

To assess individual situation for causative/contributing factors:

- Determine pathophysiology, illness or trauma, developmental crisis present. *Identifies areas of need for planning care for this family.*[2]

- Identify family developmental stage (e.g., marriage, birth of a child, children leaving home, death of a spouse). *Developmental stage will affect family functioning; for instance, a couple who are newly married will be dealing with issues of learning how to live with each other; children leaving home may result in problems of "empty-nest syndrome"; or death of a spouse radically changes life for the survivor.*[2,8]

- Note components of family: parent(s), children, male/female, extended family available. *Affects how individuals deal with current stressors. Relationships among members may be supportive or strained.*[6]

- Observe patterns of communication in this family. Are feelings expressed? Freely? Who talks to whom? Who makes decisions? For whom? Who visits? When? What is the interaction between family members? *Identifies not only weakness and areas of concern to be addressed but also strengths that can be used for resolution of problem(s).*[6,9]

- Assess boundaries of family members. Do members share family identity and have little sense of individuality? Do they seem emotionally distant, not connected with one another? *These factors are critical to understanding family dynamics and developing strategies for change. Boundaries need to be clear so individual family members are free to be responsible for themselves.*[6]

- Ascertain role expectations of family members. Who is the ill member (e.g., nurturer, provider)? How does the illness affect the roles of others? *Each person may see the situation in own individual manner; clear identification and sharing of these expectations promotes understanding. Family members may expect client to continue to perform usual role or may not allow client to do anything (either action can create problems for the ill member). Realistic planning can provide positive sense of self for the client.*[2,8]

- Determine "family rules" (e.g., adult concerns such as finances, illness, and so on are kept from the children). *Rules may be imposed by adults rather than through a democratic process involving all family members, leading to conflict and angry confrontations. Setting positive family rules with all family members participating can promote a functional family.*[2,3]

- Identify parenting skills and expectations. *Ineffective parenting and unrealistic expectations may contribute to abuse. Understanding normal responses, progression of developmental milestones may help parent cope with changes necessitated by current crisis.*[2,3]

- Note energy direction. Are efforts at resolution/problem-solving purposeful or scattered? *Provides clues about interventions that may be appropriate to assist client and family in directing energies in a more effective manner.*[2,9]

- Listen for expressions of despair/helplessness (e.g., "I don't know what to do") to note degree of distress. *Such feelings may contribute to difficulty adjusting to situation (e.g., teenage independence, change in health status of household breadwinner, dependence of aging parent on grown child) and ability to cooperate with plan of care or treatment regimen required.*[4]

- Note cultural and/or religious beliefs and values affecting perceptions and expectations of family members. *These factors affect client/SO reactions and adjustment to situation, and may limit choice of interventions and potential for successful resolution. For example, Arab-American family relationships often include nuclear and extended family, with families making collective decisions. Men are expected to be responsible for carrying out decisions. Women are usually delegated care for daily needs of the family, while children may have little independence, and birth control may not be allowed for teenagers.*[7]

🏠 • Assess support systems available outside of the family. *Having these resources can help the family begin to pull together and deal with current situation and problems they are facing.*[2]

NURSING PRIORITY NO. 2

To assist family to deal with situation/crisis:

• Deal with family members in warm, caring, respectful way. *Provides feelings of empathy and promotes individual's sense of worth and competence in ability to handle current situation.*[2]

• Acknowledge difficulties and realities of the situation. *Communicates message of understanding and reinforces that some degree of conflict is to be expected and can be used to promote growth.*[3]

• Encourage expressions of anger. Avoid taking them personally. *Feelings of anger are to be expected when individuals are dealing with difficult situation. Appropriate expression enables progress toward resolution of the stages of the grieving process when indicated. Not taking their anger personally maintains boundaries between nurse and family.*[2,5]

• Stress importance of continuous, open dialogue between family members to facilitate ongoing problem-solving. *Promotes understanding and assists family members to maintain clear communication and resolve problems effectively.*[6,10]

• Provide information, verbal and written, and reinforce as necessary. *Promotes understanding and opportunity to review as needed.*[2]

• Assist family to identify and encourage their use of previously successful coping behaviors. *Most people have developed effective coping skills that when identified can be useful in current situation.*[6,10]

• Recommend contact by family members on a regular, frequent basis. *Promotes feelings of warmth and caring and brings family closer to one another, enabling them to manage current difficult situation.*[2]

⊘ • Arrange for and encourage family participation in multidisciplinary team conference or group therapy as appropriate. *Participation in family and group therapy for an extended period increases likelihood of success as interactional issues (e.g., marital conflict, scapegoating of children) can be addressed and dealt with. Involvement with others can help family members to experience new ways of interacting and gain insight into their behavior, providing opportunity for change.*[2,5]

⊘ • Involve family in social support and community activities of their interest and choice. *Involvement with others outside of family constellation provides opportunity to observe how others handle problems and deal with conflict.*[2,8]

NURSING PRIORITY NO. 3

To promote wellness (Teaching/Discharge Considerations):

🏠 • Encourage use of stress-management techniques (e.g., appropriate expression of feelings, relaxation exercises). *The relaxation response helps members think more clearly, deal more effectively with conflict, and promote more effective relationships to enhance family interactions.*[4]

🏠 • Provide educational materials and information. *Learning about the problems they are facing can assist family members in resolution of current crisis.*[2]

⊘ • Refer to classes (e.g., Parent Effectiveness, specific disease or disability support groups, self-help groups, clergy, psychological counseling or family therapy as indicated). *Can assist family to effect positive change and enhance conflict-resolution skills. Presence of substance abuse problems requires all family members to seek support and assistance in dealing with situation to promote a healthy outcome.*[2,3] (Refer to ND dysfunctional Family Processes for additional interventions as appropriate.)

• Assist family to identify situations that may lead to fear or anxiety (e.g., diagnosis of chronic debilitating condition, decline in mental functioning of aging spouse/parent, sexually active teenager). (Refer to NDs Anxiety, Fear.) *Promotes opportunity to provide anticipatory guidance.*[1,5]

 • Involve family in mutual goal-setting to plan for the future. *When all members of the family are involved, commitment to goals and continuation of plan are more likely to be maintained.*[3]

• Identify community agencies (e.g., Meals on Wheels, visiting nurse, trauma support group, American Cancer Society, Veterans Administration). *Provides both immediate and long-term support.*[6]

DOCUMENTATION FOCUS

Assessment/Reassessment
• Assessment findings, including family composition, developmental stage of family, and role expectations.
• Family communication patterns.
• Cultural or religious beliefs and values.

Planning
• Plan of care, specific interventions, and who is involved in planning.
• Teaching plan.

Implementation/Evaluation
• Each individual's response to interventions, teaching, and actions performed.
• Attainment or progress toward desired outcome(s).
• Modifications to plan of care.

Discharge Planning
• Long-term needs, noting who is responsible for actions to be taken.
• Specific referrals made.

References

1. Doenges, M. E., Moorhouse, M. F., Geissler-Murr, A. C. (2004). *Nurse's Pocket Guide: Diagnoses, Interventions, and Rationales.* 9th ed. Philadelphia: F. A. Davis.
2. Townsend, M. C. (2003). *Psychiatric Mental Health Nursing Concepts of Care.* 4th ed. Philadelphia: F. A. Davis.
3. Gordon, T. (2000). *Parent Effectiveness Training.* Updated ed. New York: Three Rivers Press.
4. Cox, H. C., et al. (2002). *Clinical Applications of Nursing Diagnosis: Adult, Child, Women's, Psychiatric, Gerontic, and Home Health Considerations.* 4th ed. Philadelphia: F. A. Davis.
5. Amato, P. R., Booth, A. (2000). *A Generation at Risk: Growing Up in an Era of Family Upheaval.* Cambridge, MA: Harvard University Press.
6. Wright, L., Leahey, M. (2000). *Nurses and Families: A Guide to Assessment and Intervention.* 3d ed. Philadelphia: F. A. Davis.
7. Lipson, J. G., Dibble, S. L., Minarik, P. A. (1996). *Culture & Nursing Care: A Pocket Guide.* San Francisco: UCSF Nursing Press.
8. Kearl's Guide to the Sociology of the Family. Retrieved September 2009 from www.trinity.edu/~mkearl/family.html.
9. Adams, L. (July 2008). How families resolve conflicts. *The Family Connection Newsletter.*
10. DaFo Whitehead, B., Popenoe, D. *The State of Our Unions: The Social Health of Marriage in America 2004.* Piscataway, NJ: Rutgers University National Marriage Project.

readiness for enhanced Family Processes

DEFINITION: A pattern of family functioning that is sufficient to support the well-being of family members and can be strengthened

RELATED FACTORS

To be developed by nurse researchers and submitted to NANDA

DEFINING CHARACTERISTICS

Subjective
Expresses willingness to enhance family dynamics
Communication is adequate
Relationships are generally positive; interdependent with community; family tasks are accomplished
Energy level of family supports activities of daily living (ADLs)
Family adapts to change

Objective
Family functioning meets needs of family members
Activities support the safety or growth of family members
Family roles are appropriate or flexible for developmental stages
Respect for family members is evident; boundaries of family members are maintained
Family resilience is evident
Balance exists between autonomy and cohesiveness

Sample Clinical Applications: Chronic health conditions (e.g., asthma, diabetes mellitus, arthritis, systemic lupus, multiple sclerosis [MS], AIDS), mental health concerns (e.g., seasonal affective disorder, attention deficit disorder, Down syndrome)

DESIRED OUTCOMES/EVALUATION CRITERIA

Sample NOC linkages:
Family Social Climate: Supportive milieu as characterized by family member relationships and goals
Family Health Status: Overall health and social competence of family unit
Family Resiliency: Positive adaptation and function of the family system following significant adversity or crisis

Client Will (Include Specific Time Frame)
• Express feelings freely and appropriately.
• Verbalizes understanding of desire for enhanced family dynamics.
• Demonstrate individual involvement in problem-solving to improve family communications.
• Acknowledges awareness of and respect for boundaries of family members.

(continues on page 328)

readiness for enhanced Family Processes (continued)
ACTIONS/INTERVENTIONS

Sample NIC linkages:
Family Support: Promotion of family values, interests, and goals
Parent Education: Childrearing Family: Assisting parents to understand and promote the physical, psychological, and social growth and development of their toddler, preschool, or school-age child/children
Normalization Promotion: Assisting parents and other family members of children with chronic illnesses or disabilities in providing normal life experiences for their children and families

NURSING PRIORITY NO. 1

To determine current status of family:

- Determine family composition: parent(s), children, male/female, extended family involved. *Many family forms exist in society today, such as biological, nuclear, single-parent, step-family, communal, and homosexual couple or family. A better way to determine a family may be to determine the attribute of affection, strong emotional ties, a sense of belonging, and durability of membership.*[1,6]
- Identify participating members of family: parent(s), children, male/female, extended family. *Identifies members of family who need to be involved and taken into consideration in developing plan of care to improve family functioning.*[1]
- Note stage of family development. *While the North American middle-class family stages may be described as single, young adult, newly married, family with young children, family with adolescents, grown children, later life, developmental tasks may vary greatly among cultural groups. This information provides a framework for developing a plan to enhance family processes.*[1]
- Ascertain motivation and expectations for change. *Motivation to improve and high expectations can encourage family to make changes that will improve their life. However, unrealistic expectations may hamper efforts.*[7]
- Observe patterns of communication in the family. Are feelings expressed freely? Who talks to whom? Who makes decisions? For whom? Who visits? When? What is the interaction between family members? *Identifies not only possible weakness or areas of concern to be addressed but also strengths that can be used for planning improvement in family communication. Effective communication is that in which verbal and nonverbal messages are clear, direct, and congruent.*[1,2]
- Assess boundaries of family members. Do members share family identity and have little sense of individuality? Do they seem emotionally connected with one another? *Individuals need to respect one another, and boundaries need to be clear so family members are free to be responsible for themselves.*[1,3]
- Identify "family rules" that are accepted in the family. *Families interact in certain ways over time and develop patterns of behavior that are accepted as the way "we behave" in this family. "Functional families'" rules are constructive and promote the needs of all family members.*[1]
- Note energy direction. *Efforts at problem-solving, resolution of different opinions, growth may be purposeful or may be scattered and ineffective.*[3]
- Determine cultural and/or religious factors influencing family interactions. *Expectations related to socioeconomic beliefs may be different in various cultures; for instance, traditional*

views of marriage and family life may be strongly influenced by Roman Catholicism in Italian-American and Latino-American families. In some cultures, the father is considered the authority figure and the mother is the homemaker. These beliefs may be functional or dysfunctional in any given family and may change with stressors/circumstances (e.g., financial, loss or gain of a family member, personal growth).[1,3,7]

- Note health of married individuals. *Recent reports have determined that marriage increases life expectancy by as much as 5 years.*[5]

NURSING PRIORITY NO. 2

To assist the family to improve family interactions:

- Establish nurse-family relationship. *Promotes a warm, caring atmosphere in which family members can share thoughts, ideas, and feelings openly and in a nonjudgmental manner.*[3]
- Acknowledge difficulties and realities of individual situation. *Reinforces that some degree of conflict is to be expected in family interactions that can be used to promote growth.*[1,3]
- Emphasize importance of continuous, open dialogue between family members. *Facilitates ongoing expression of open, honest feelings and opinions and effective problem-solving.*[1,4]
- Assist family to identify and encourage use of previously successful coping behaviors. *Promotes recognition of previous successes and confidence in own abilities to learn and improve family interactions.*[2,4]
- Acknowledge differences among family members with open dialogue about how these differences have occurred. *Conveys an acceptance of these differences among individuals and helps to look at how they can be used to strengthen the family process.*[3]
- Identify effective parenting skills already being used and additional ways of handling difficult behaviors that may develop. *Allows the individual family members to realize that some of what has been done already was helpful, and helps them to learn new skills to manage family interactions in a more effective manner.*[3]

NURSING PRIORITY NO. 3

To promote optimum well-being (Teaching/Discharge Considerations):

- Discuss and encourage use of stress-management techniques. *Relaxation exercises, visualization, and similar skills can be useful for promoting reduction of anxiety and ability to manage stress that occurs in their lives.*[1]
- Encourage participation in learning role-reversal activities. *Helps individuals to gain insight and understanding of other person's feelings and point of view.*[3]
- Provide educational materials and information. *Enhances learning to assist in developing positive relationships among family members.*[4]
- Assist family members to identify situations that may create problems and lead to stress/anxiety. *Thinking ahead can help individuals anticipate helpful actions to handle or prevent conflict and untoward consequences.*[4]
- Refer to classes or community resources as appropriate. *Family Effectiveness, self-help, psychotherapy, religious affiliations can provide new information to assist family members to learn and apply to enhancing family interactions.*[4]
- Involve family members in setting goals and planning for the future. *When individuals are involved in the decision making, they are more committed to carrying through on plan to enhance family interactions as life goes on.*[2]

DOCUMENTATION FOCUS

Assessment/Reassessment
• Assessment findings, including family composition, developmental stage of family, and role expectations.
• Cultural or religious values and beliefs regarding family and family functioning.
• Family communication patterns.
• Motivation and expectations for change.

Planning
• Plan of care, specific interventions, and who is involved in planning.
• Educational plan.

Implementation/Evaluation
• Each individual's response to interventions, teaching, and actions performed.
• Attainment or progress toward desired outcome(s).
• Modifications to lifestyle and treatment plan.

Discharge Planning
• Long-term needs, noting who is responsible for actions to be taken.
• Specific referrals made.

References

1. Townsend, M. (2003). *Psychiatric Mental Health Nursing Concepts of Care*. 4th ed. Philadelphia: F. A. Davis.
2. Gordon, T. (2000). *Parent Effectiveness Training*. Updated ed. New York: Three Rivers Press.
3. Doenges, M. E., Townsend, M. C., Moorhouse, M. F. (1998). *Psychiatric Care Plans: Guidelines for Individualizing Care*. 3d ed. Philadelphia: F. A. Davis.
4. Doenges, M. E., Moorhouse, M. F., Geissler-Murr, A. C. (2004). *Nurse's Pocket Guide: Diagnoses, Interventions, and Rationales*. 9th ed. Philadelphia: F. A. Davis.
5. Schoenborn, C. Marital status and health: United States, 1999–2002. Advance Data from Vital and Health Statistics, volume 351. Retrieved March 2007 from www.cdc.gov/nchs/data/ad/ad351.pdf.
6. Marriage and family processes. Kearl's Guide to the Sociology of the Family. Retrieved July 2007 from www.trinity.edu/~mkearl/family.html.
7. Lipson, J. G., Dibble, S. L., Minarik, P. A. (1996). *Culture & Nursing Care: A Pocket Guide*. San Francisco: UCSF Nursing Press.

Fatigue

DEFINITION: An overwhelming sustained sense of exhaustion and decreased capacity for physical and mental work at usual level

RELATED FACTORS

Psychological
Stress; anxiety; boring lifestyle; depression

Environmental
Noise; lights; humidity; temperature

⊕ Cultural ⊗ Collaborative ▲ Community/Home Care ⟋ Diagnostic Studies ∞ Pediatric/Geriatric/Lifespan Medications

Situational
Occupation; negative life events

Physiological
Increased physical exertion; sleep deprivation
Pregnancy; disease states; malnutrition; anemia
Poor physical condition
[Altered body chemistry (e.g., medications, drug withdrawal, chemotherapy)]

DEFINING CHARACTERISTICS

Subjective
Verbalization of an unremitting or overwhelming lack of energy; inability to maintain usual routines or level of physical activity
Perceived need for additional energy to accomplish routine tasks; increase in rest requirements
Tired; inability to restore energy even after sleep
Feelings of guilt for not keeping up with responsibilities
Compromised libido
Increase in physical complaints

Objective
Lethargic; listless; drowsy; lack of energy
Compromised concentration
Disinterest in surroundings; introspection
Decreased performance, [accident-prone]

Sample Clinical Applications: Anemia, hypothyroidism, cancer, multiple sclerosis (MS), Lyme disease, postpolio syndrome, AIDS, chronic renal failure, chronic fatigue syndrome (CFS), depression

DESIRED OUTCOMES/EVALUATION CRITERIA

Sample NOC linkages:
Endurance: Capacity to sustain activity
Energy Conservation: Personal actions to manage energy for initiating and sustaining activity
Activity Tolerance: Physiological response to energy-consuming movements with daily activities

Client Will (Include Specific Time Frame)
• Report improved sense of energy.
• Identify basis of fatigue and individual areas of control.
• Perform activities of daily living (ADLs) and participate in desired activities at level of ability.
• Participate in recommended treatment program.

(continues on page 332)

Fatigue (continued)
ACTIONS/INTERVENTIONS

Sample (NIC) linkages:
Energy Management: Regulating energy use to treat or prevent fatigue and optimize function
Exercise Promotion: Facilitation of regular physical exercise to maintain or advance to a higher level of fitness and health
Nutrition Management: Assisting with or providing a balanced dietary intake of foods and fluids

NURSING PRIORITY NO. 1

To assess causative/contributing factors:

- Identify presence of physical and/or psychological conditions (e.g., pregnancy, infectious processes, blood loss, anemia, autoimmune disorders [e.g., MS, lupus, rheumatoid arthritis], trauma, chronic pain syndromes [e.g., arthritis], cardiopulmonary disorders, cancer or cancer treatments, hepatitis, AIDS, major depressive disorder, anxiety states, substance use or abuse). *Important information can be obtained from knowing if fatigue is a result of an underlying condition or disease process (acute or chronic); whether an exacerbating or remitting condition is in exacerbation; and/or whether fatigue has been present over a long time without any identifiable cause.*
- Note diagnosis of CFS. *This condition has been defined as a distinct disorder (affecting children and adults) characterized by chronic (often relapsing but always debilitating) fatigue, lasting for at least 6 months (often for much longer), causing impairments in overall physical and mental functioning and without an apparent etiology.[1]*
- Note client's age, gender, and developmental stage. *Some studies show a prevalence of fatigue in adolescent girls.[11]*
- Assess general well-being—cardiovascular and respiratory status, musculoskeletal strength, emotional health, and nutritional and fluid status. *Underlying conditions (e.g., anemia, heart failure, depression, or malnutrition) may be causing or exacerbating fatigue.*
- Note changes in life (e.g., relationship problems, family illness, injury or death; expanded responsibilities or demands of others, job-related conflicts) that can be causing or exacerbating level of fatigue. *Stress may be the result of dealing with disease or situational crises, dealing with the "unknowns" or trying to meet expectations of others.[2] Also, grief and depression can sap energy and cause avoidance of social and/or physical interactions that could stimulate the mind and body. Note: Persons with AIDS and the elderly are especially prone to this fatigue because they experience significant losses, often on a regular or recurring basis.[3,4]*
- Assess sleep pattern—hours and quality of sleep. *Sleep disturbance is both a contributor to and a manifestation of fatigue (e.g., a client with chronic pain or depression may be sleeping long periods but not experience refreshing sleep, or may not be able to fall or stay asleep).*
- Determine ability to participate in activities and level of mobility. *While many illness conditions negatively affect client's energy and activity tolerance, if the client is not engaged in light to moderate exercise, he or she may simply adjust to more sedentary activities, which can in turn exacerbate deconditioning and debilitation (CFS, cancer). However, there are certain conditions (e.g., MS and postpolio syndrome) where the client's ability to do things*

reduces as he or she does them (e.g., at the beginning of a walk the client feels okay, but fatigue sets in [out of proportion to the activity] and the client is exhausted as if running a marathon).[5,6]

- Review medication regimen and use. *Many medications have the potential side effect of causing/exacerbating fatigue (e.g., beta-blockers, chemotherapy agents, narcotics, sedatives, muscle relaxants, antiemetics, antidepressants, antiepileptics, diuretics, cholesterol-lowering drugs, HIV treatment agents, and combinations of drugs and/or substances).*
- Assess psychological and personality factors that may affect reports of fatigue level. *Client with severe or chronic fatigue may have issues affecting desire to be active (or work), resulting in secondary gain from exaggerating fatigue reports.*
- Evaluate aspect of "learned helplessness" that may be manifested by giving up. *Can perpetuate a cycle of fatigue, impaired functioning, increased anxiety and fatigue.*

NURSING PRIORITY NO. 2

To determine degree of fatigue/impact on life:

- Ask client to describe fatigue, noting particular phrases (e.g., drained, exhausted, lousy, weak, lazy, worn out, whole-body tiredness). *Helpful in clarifying client's expressions for symptoms, pattern and timing of fatigue, which varies over time and may also vary in duration, unpleasantness, and intensity from person to person.[7]*
- Have client rate fatigue (using 1–10 or similar scale) and describe its effects on ability to participate in desired activities. *Fatigue may vary in intensity, and is often accompanied by irritability, lack of concentration, difficulty making decisions, problems with leisure, relationship difficulties that can add to stress level and aggravate sleep problems.[12]*
- Assess severity of fatigue using a recognized scale (e.g., the Multidimensional Assessment of Fatigue [MAF], Piper Fatigue Self-Report Scale, Global Fatigue Index), as appropriate. *In initial evaluations, these scales can help determine manifestation, intensity, duration, and emotional meaning of fatigue. The scales can be used in ongoing evaluations to determine current status and estimate response to treatment strategies.[2,7–9,13,14]*
- Measure blood pressure and heart and respiratory rate before and after activity as indicated. *Physiological response to activity (e.g., changes in blood pressure or heart or respiratory rate) may indicate need for interventions to improve cardiovascular health, pulmonary status and conditioning.* (Refer to risk for Activity Intolerance for additional interventions.)
- Review availability and current use of assistance with daily activities, support systems, and resources.
- Evaluate need for individual assistance or assistive devices. *Certain conditions causing fatigue (e.g., postpolio syndrome) worsen with overuse of weakened muscles. Client benefits from protection provided by braces, canes, power chairs, and so forth.[6,7]*

NURSING PRIORITY NO. 3

To assist client to cope with fatigue and manage with individual limitations:

- Accept reality of client's fatigue and avoid underestimating effect on quality of life the client experiences. *Fatigue is subjective and often debilitating (e.g., clients with cancer, AIDS, or MS are prone to more frequent episodes of severe fatigue following minimal energy expenditure and require longer recovery period; postpolio clients often display a cumulative effect if they fail to pace themselves and rest when early signs of fatigue are encountered).[5,7,10]*
- Active-listen concerns, encourage expression of feelings. *Provides support to help client deal with very frustrating and taxing situation.*

Nursing Diagnoses in Alphabetical Order

- Treat underlying conditions where possible (e.g., manage pain, depression, or anemia; treat infections, reduce numbers of interacting medications) *to reduce fatigue caused by treatable conditions.*
- Involve client/SO/caregivers(s) in planning care *to incorporate their input, choices, and assistance.*
- Encourage client to do whatever activity possible (e.g., self-care, sit up in chair, walk for 5 minutes), pacing self, increasing activity level gradually. Schedule activities for periods when client has the most energy, *to maximize participation.*
- Structure daily routines and establish realistic activity goals with client, especially when depression is a factor in fatigue. *May enhance client's commitment to efforts and promote sense of self-esteem in accomplishing goals.*
- Instruct client/caregivers in alternate ways of doing familiar activities and methods to conserve energy, such as the following:[2,3,7–10,13]
  Sit instead of standing during daily care or other activities.
  Adjust the level or height of work surface for ergonomic benefit and to prevent bending over.
  Carry several small loads instead of one large load.
  Use assistive devices (e.g., wheeled walkers or chairs, electrically raised chairs, stair-climbers).
  Plan steps of activity before beginning so that all needed materials are at hand.
  Take frequent short rest breaks and return to activity.
  Delegate tasks or duties whenever possible.
  Combine and simplify activities.
  Ask for and accept assistance.
  Say "no" or "later."
- Provide environment conducive to relief of fatigue, avoid temperature and humidity extremes. *Temperature and level of humidity are known to affect exhaustion (especially in clients with MS).*[5]
- Encourage nutritional foods, refer to dietitian as indicated. *Nutritionally balanced diet with proteins, complex carbohydrates, vitamins, and minerals may boost energy. Frequent, small meals and simple-to-digest foods are beneficial when combating fatigue. Reduced amounts of caffeine and sugar can improve sleep and energy.*[3,7,10]
- Provide supplemental oxygen as needed. *If fatigue is related to oxygenation/perfusion problems, oxygen may improve energy level and ability to be active.* (Refer to ND Activity Intolerance for additional interventions.)
- Provide diversional activities (e.g., visiting with friends/family, TV/music, doing hobbies or schoolwork). *Participating in pleasurable activities can refocus energy and diminish feelings of unhappiness, sluggishness, worthlessness, which can accompany fatigue.* (Refer to deficient Diversional Activity for additional interventions.)
- Avoid over or understimulation (cognitive and sensory). *Impaired concentration can limit ability to block competing stimuli and distractions.*
- Recommend or implement routines that promote restful sleep, such as the following:
  Regular sleep hours at night with beneficial nighttime rituals
  Short naps during day hours
  Mild exercise, yoga, tai chi
  Quiet activities in the evening
  Meditation, visualization
  Warm baths
  Refer to NDs Insomnia, Sleep Deprivation for additional interventions.

* Instruct in or refer for stress-management skills of visualization, deep breathing, relaxation, and biofeedback *to deal with situation, aid in relaxation, and to reduce boredom, pain, and sense of fatigue.*

* Participate in comprehensive rehabilitation program with physical or occupational therapist, exercise or rehabilitation physiologist. *Collaborative program with short-term achievable goals enhances likelihood of success and may motivate client to adopt a lifestyle for enhancement of health.*[2,7,8]

* Discuss appropriateness of other therapies (e.g., massage, acupuncture, osteopathic or chiropractic manipulations). Complementary therapies may be helpful in reducing muscle tension and pain to promote relaxation and rest.

NURSING PRIORITY NO. 4

To promote wellness (Teaching/Discharge Considerations):

* Discuss therapy regimen relating to individual causative factors (e.g., physical and/or psychological illnesses) and help client/SO(s) to understand relationship of fatigue to illness. Promotes acceptance of situation, allowing client to focus attention on finding ways to live with fatigue.

* Assist client/SO(s) to develop plan for activity and exercise within individual ability. *Enhances sense of control and commitment to attaining goals.*

* Stress necessity of allowing sufficient time to finish activities. *Client is more likely to succeed when he or she does not feel rushed and is allowed to proceed at a measured pace.*

* Instruct client in ways to monitor response to activity and significant signs/symptoms to heed. *Changes in pulse or respiratory rate, or development of worsened or unrelenting fatigue is a signal to stop, rest, and to modify activity level.*

* Promote overall health measures (e.g., good nutrition, adequate fluid intake, appropriate vitamin and iron supplementation).

* Encourage client to develop assertiveness skills and prioritizing of goals and activities.

* Discuss burnout syndrome when appropriate and actions client can take to change individual situation.

* Assist client to identify appropriate coping behaviors. *Promotes sense of control and improves self-esteem.*

* Identify support groups and resources (e.g., condition-specific groups, reliable Web sites) *to provide information, share experiences, enhance problem-solving.*

* Refer to community resources for assistance with routine needs (e.g., Meals on Wheels, homemaker or housekeeper services, yard care, transportation options).

* Refer to counseling or psychotherapy as indicated *to deal with stressors and effects of condition.*

DOCUMENTATION FOCUS

Assessment/Reassessment
* Manifestations of fatigue and other assessment findings.
* Degree of impairment and effect on lifestyle.
* Expectations of client/SO relative to individual abilities and specific condition.

Planning
* Plan of care, specific interventions, and who is involved in the planning.
* Teaching plan.

Implementation/Evaluation
- Client's response to interventions, teaching, and actions performed.
- Attainment or progress toward desired outcome(s).
- Modifications to plan of care.

Discharge Planning
- Discharge needs and who is responsible actions to be taken.
- Specific referrals made.

References

1. Fukuda, K., et al. (1994). The chronic fatigue syndrome: A comprehensive approach to its definition and study. International Chronic Fatigue Syndrome Study Group. *Ann Intern Med*, 121(12), 953–959.
2. Vogin, G. (2001). Colorectal cancer: Coping with fatigue. Cleveland Clinic Condition Center. Retrieved July 2007 from www.webmd.com/colorectalcancer/colorectal_cancer_coping _with_fatigue?page=1.
3. Zimmerman, J. (2002). Nutrition for health and healing in HIV. ACRIA Update, 11(2). Retrieved July 2007 from www.thebody.com/content/art14418.html.
4. Ackley, B. J. (2002). Fatigue. In Ackley, B. J., Ladwig, G. B. (eds). *Nursing Diagnosis Handbook: A Guide to Planning Care*. 5th ed. St. Louis, MO: Mosby.
5. Understanding the unique role of fatigue in multiple sclerosis. Multiple Sclerosis Encyclopedia Web site. Retrieved July 2007 from www.mult-sclerosis.org/fatigue.html.
6. Perlman, S. (1999). Coping with fatigue of post-polio syndrome. *Rancho Los Amigos Post Polio Support Group Newsletter*.
7. Wells, J. N., Fedric, T. (2001). Helping patients manage cancer-related fatigue. *Home Healthcare Nurse*, 19(8), 486.
8. Veterans Health Administration, Department of Defense. (2001). Clinical practice guidelines for the management of medically unexplained symptoms: Chronic pain and fatigue. Retrieved July 2007 from www.oqp.med.va.gov/cpg/cpgn/mus/D/CFS_Summary.pdf. Washington, DC: Veterans Health Administration, Department of Defense.
9. Tolan, R. W., Stewart, J. M. (2001). Chronic fatigue syndrome. Retrieved July 2007 from www.emedicine.com/ped/topic2795.htm.
10. American Health Consultants. (1996). *Common Sense about AIDS: Fighting Fatigue Requires Battle on Many Fronts*. Atlanta: American Health Consultants.
11. ter Wolbeek, M., et al. (2006). Severe fatigue in adolescents: A common phenomenon? *Pediatrics* 117(6), e1078–e1086.
12. Barton-Burke, M. (2006). Cancer-related fatigue and sleep disturbances: Further research on the prevalence of these two symptoms in long-term cancer survivors can inform education, policy, and clinical practice. *Am J Nurs*, 106(3 suppl), 72–77.
13. Belza, B. (1994). The impact of fatigue on exercise performance. *Arthritis Care Res*, 7(4), 176–180.
14. Trendall, J. (2005). Concept analysis: Chronic fatigue. *J Adv Nurs*, 32(5), 1126–1131.

Fear [specify focus]

DEFINITION: Response to perceived threat [real or imagined] that is consciously recognized as a danger

RELATED FACTORS

Innate origin (e.g., sudden noise, height, pain, loss of physical support), innate releasers (neurotransmitters); phobic stimulus
Learned response (e.g., conditioning, modeling from or identification with others)
Unfamiliarity with environmental experience(s)
Separation from support system in potentially stressful situation (e.g., hospitalization, hospital procedures [or treatments])
Language barrier, sensory impairment

DEFINING CHARACTERISTICS

Subjective
Report of apprehension; excitement; being scared; alarm; panic; terror; dread; decreased self-assurance; increased tension; jitteriness
Cognitive: Identifies object of fear; stimulus believed to be a threat
Physiological: Anorexia, nausea, fatigue, dry mouth, [palpitations]

Objective
Cognitive: Diminished productivity, learning ability, or problem-solving
Behaviors: Increased alertness; avoidance [or flight]; attack behaviors; impulsiveness; narrowed focus on the source of the fear
Physiological: Increased pulse; vomiting; diarrhea; muscle tightness; increased respiratory rate; dyspnea; increased systolic blood pressure; pallor; increased perspiration; pupil dilation

Sample Clinical Applications: Phobias, hospitalization/diagnostic procedures, diagnosis of chronic or life-threatening condition

DESIRED OUTCOMES/EVALUATION CRITERIA

Sample NOC linkages:
Fear Self-Control: Personal actions to eliminate or reduce disabling feelings of apprehension, tension, or uneasiness from an identifiable source
Coping: Personal actions to manage stressors that tax an individual's resources
Fear Level: Severity of manifested apprehension, tension, or uneasiness arising from an identifiable source

Client Will (Include Specific Time Frame)
- Acknowledge and discuss fears, recognizing healthy versus unhealthy fears.
- Verbalize accurate knowledge of and sense of safety related to current situation.
- Demonstrate understanding through use of effective coping behaviors (e.g., problem-solving) and resources.
- Display lessened fear as evidenced by appropriate range of feelings and relief of signs/symptoms (specific to client).

(continues on page 338)

Fear (continued)
ACTIONS/INTERVENTIONS

Sample NIC linkages:
Anxiety Reduction: Minimizing apprehension, dread, foreboding, or uneasiness related to an unidentified source or anticipated danger
Security Enhancement: Intensifying a patient's sense of physical and psychological safety
Coping Enhancement: Assisting a patient to adapt to perceived stressors, changes, or threats that interfere with meeting life demands and roles

NURSING PRIORITY NO. 1

To assess degree of fear and reality of threat perceived by the client:

- Ascertain client's/SO('s) perception of what is occurring and how this affects life. *Fear is a natural reaction to frightening events and how client views the event will determine how he or she will react.*[1]
- Determine client's age and developmental level. *Helps in understanding usual or typical fears experienced by individuals (e.g., toddler has entirely different fears than adolescent or older person with dementia).*[3]
- Note ability to concentrate, level of attention, degree of incapacitation (e.g., "frozen with fear," inability to engage in necessary activities). *Indicative of extent of anxiety or fear related to what is happening and need for specific interventions to reduce physiological reactions. Presence of severe reaction (phobia), requires more intensive intervention.*[1,4]
- Compare verbal and nonverbal responses. *Noting congruencies or incongruencies can help to identify client's misperceptions of situation and what actions may be helpful.*[1]
- Be alert to signs of denial or depression. *Client may deny existence of problem until overwhelmed and unable to deal with situation. Depression may be associated with fear that interferes with productive life and daily activities.*[2]
- Identify sensory deficits that may be present, such as vision or hearing impairment. *Affects reception and interpretation. Inability to correctly sense and perceive stimuli leads to misunderstanding, increasing fear.*[4]
- Measure vital signs and physiological responses to situation. *Provides baseline information of extent of response for comparison as needed. Stabilization can indicate effectiveness of interventions by diminished response to identified fear.*[6]
- Investigate client's reports of subjective experiences (may reflect delusions or hallucinations). *It is important to understand how the client views the situation and identify need for reality orientation and further evaluation.*[4]
- Be alert to and evaluate potential for violence. *Client who is fearful may feel need to protect himself or herself and strike out at closest person. Proactive planning can avert or manage violent behaviors.*[5]
- Assess family dynamics. *Actions and responses of family members may exacerbate or soothe fears of client.*[1] (Refer to NDs Anxiety, readiness for enhanced family Coping, compromised/disabled family Coping, interrupted Family Processes for additional interventions.)

NURSING PRIORITY NO. 2

To assist client/SOs in dealing with fear/situation:

- Stay with the very fearful client or make arrangements to have someone else be there. *Provides nonthreatening environment in which the presence of a calm, caring person can provide reassurance that individual will be safe. Sense of abandonment can exacerbate fear.*[6]

- Active-listen client concerns. *Conveys message of belief in competence and ability of client. Promotes understanding of issues when client feels listened to, so problem-solving can begin.*[2]
- Acknowledge normalcy of fear, pain, despair, and give "permission" to express feelings appropriately and freely. *Feelings are real, and it is helpful to bring them out in the open so they can be discussed and dealt with.*[6]
- Present objective information when available and allow client to use it freely. Avoid arguing about client's perceptions of the situation. *Limits conflicts when fear response may impair rational thinking.*[6]
- Speak in simple sentences and concrete terms, include written materials as appropriate. *Intense state of fear interferes with reception and interpretation of verbal information; supplementing it with written information facilitates understanding and retention of information.*[4]
- Provide opportunity for questions, answering honestly. *Enhances sense of trust and promotes positive nurse-client relationship in which individual can verbalize fears and begin to problem-solve.*[1]
- ∞ Manage environmental factors, such as loud noises, harsh lighting, changing person's location without knowledge of family/SO, strangers in care area or unfamiliar people, high traffic flow, *which can cause or exacerbate stress, especially to very young or to older individuals.*
- ∞ Be truthful with client when painful procedures are anticipated; be present, provide physical contact (e.g., hugging, refocusing attention, rocking a child) as appropriate, *to soothe fears and provide assurance.*[9]
- Modify procedures as possible (e.g., substitute oral for intramuscular medications, combine blood draws or use fingerstick method) *to limit degree of stress, avoid overwhelming a fearful individual.*[3]
- Promote client control where possible and help client identify and accept those things over which control is not possible. *Life changes and stressful events are viewed differently by each individual. Providing the client with opportunity to make own decision when possible strengthens internal locus of control. Individual with external locus of control may attribute feelings of anxiety and fear to an external source and may perceive it as beyond his or her control.*[1]
- Provide touch, Therapeutic Touch, massage, and other adjunctive therapies as indicated. *Aids in meeting basic human need, decreasing sense of isolation, and assisting client to feel less anxious. Note: Therapeutic Touch requires the nurse to have specific knowledge and experience to use the hands to correct energy field disturbances by redirecting human energies to help or heal.* (Refer to ND disturbed Energy Field.)[2,7]
- Encourage contact with a peer who has successfully dealt with a similarly fearful situation. *Provides a role model, which can enhance sense of optimism. Client is more likely to believe others who have had similar experience(s).*[1]

NURSING PRIORITY NO. 3

To assist client in learning to use own responses for problem-solving:

- Acknowledge usefulness of fear for taking care of self. *Provides new idea that can be a motivator to focus on dealing appropriately with situation.*[1]
- Explain relationship between disease and symptoms if appropriate. *Providing accurate information promotes understanding of why the symptoms occur, allaying anxiety about them.*[1]
- Identify client's responsibility for the solutions while reinforcing that the nurse will be available for help if desired or needed. *Enhances sense of control, self-worth, and confidence in own ability, diminishing fear.*[8]

- Determine internal and external resources for assistance (e.g., awareness and use of effective coping skills in the past; SOs who are available for support). *Provides opportunity to recognize and build on resources client/SO may have used successfully in the past.*[1]
- Explain actions and procedures within level of client's ability to understand and handle being aware of how much information client wants *to prevent confusion or overload. Complex and/or anxiety-producing information can be given in manageable amounts over an extended period as opportunities arise and facts are given; individual will accept what he or she is ready for.*[8]
- Discuss use of antianxiety medications and reinforce use as prescribed. *Antianxiety agents may be useful for brief periods to assist client to reduce anxiety to manageable levels, providing opportunity for initiation of client's own coping skills.*[1]

NURSING PRIORITY NO. 4

To promote wellness (Teaching/Discharge Considerations):

- Support planning for dealing with reality. *Assists in identifying areas in which control can be exercised and those in which control is not possible, enabling client to handle fearful situation or feelings.*[1]
- Assist client to learn relaxation, visualization, or guided imagery skills (e.g., imagining a pleasant place, use of music or tapes, deep breathing, meditation, and mindfulness). *Promotes release of endorphins and aids in developing internal locus of control, reducing fear and anxiety. May enhance coping skills, allowing body to go about its work of healing. Note: Mindfulness is a method of being in the here and now, concentrating on what is happening in the moment.*[7,8]
- Encourage regular physical activity. Assist client or refer to physical therapist to develop exercise program within limits of ability. *Provides a healthy outlet for energy generated by feelings and promotes relaxation. Has been shown to raise endorphin levels to enhance sense of well-being.*[2]
- Provide for and deal with sensory deficits in appropriate manner (e.g., speak clearly and distinctly, use touch carefully as indicated by situation). *Hearing or visual impairments, other deficits can contribute to feelings of fear. Recognizing and providing for appropriate contact can enhance communication, promoting understanding.*[4]
- Refer to support groups, community agencies and organizations as indicated. *Provides information, ongoing assistance to meet individual needs, and opportunity for discussing concerns.*[2]

DOCUMENTATION FOCUS

Assessment/Reassessment
- Assessment findings, noting individual factors contributing to current situation, source of fear.
- Manifestations of fear.

Planning
- Plan of care and who is involved in the planning.
- Teaching plan.

Implementation/Evaluation
- Client's responses to treatment plan, interventions, and actions performed.
- Attainment or progress toward desired outcome(s).
- Modifications to plan of care.

Discharge Planning
* Long-term needs and who is responsible for actions to be taken.
* Specific referrals made.

References

1. Townsend, M. C. (2003). *Psychiatric Mental Health Nursing Concepts of Care*. 4th ed. Philadelphia: F. A. Davis.
2. Doenges, M. E., Moorhouse, M. F., Geissler-Murr, A. C. (2004). *Nurse's Pocket Guide: Diagnoses, Interventions, and Rationales*. 9th ed. Philadelphia: F. A. Davis.
3. Lawrence, S. (2005). When health fears are overblown. Retrieved February 2007 from www.webmd.com/balance/features.
4. Cox, H. C., et al. (2002). *Clinical Applications of Nursing Diagnosis: Adult, Child, Women's, Psychiatric, Gerontic, and Home Health Considerations*. 4th ed. Philadelphia: F. A. Davis.
5. Lewis, M. I., Dehn, D. S. (1999). Violence against nurses in outpatient mental health settings. *J Psychosoc Nurs*, 37(6), 28.
6. Bay, E. J., Algase, D. L. (1999). Fear and anxiety. A simultaneous concept analysis. *Nurs Diagn*, 10, 103.
7. Olson, M., Sneed, N. (1995). Anxiety and therapeutic touch. *Issues Ment Health Nurs*, 16(2), 97.
8. Kabat-Zinn, J. (1994). *Wherever You Go There You Are, Mindfulness Meditation in Everyday Life*. New York: Hyperion.

ineffective infant Feeding Pattern

DEFINITION: Impaired ability of an infant to suck or coordinate the suck/swallow response resulting in inadequate oral nutrition for metabolic needs

RELATED FACTORS

Prematurity
Neurological impairment or delay
Oral hypersensitivity
Prolonged NPO
Anatomic abnormality

DEFINING CHARACTERISTICS

Subjective
[Caregiver reports infant is unable to initiate or sustain an effective suck]

Objective
Inability to initiate or sustain an effective suck
Inability to coordinate sucking, swallowing, and breathing

Sample Clinical Applications: Prematurity, cleft lip/palate, thrush, hydrocephalus, cerebral palsy, fetal alcohol syndrome, respiratory distress, severe developmental delay

(continues on page 342)

ineffective infant Feeding Pattern (continued)
DESIRED OUTCOMES/EVALUATION CRITERIA

Sample (NOC) linkages:
Swallowing Status: Oral Phase: Preparation, containment, and posterior movement of fluids and/or solids in the mouth
Breastfeeding Establishment: Infant: Infant attachment to and sucking from the mother's breast for nourishment during the first 3 weeks of breastfeeding
Hydration: Adequate water in the intracellular and extracellular compartments of the body

Infant Will (Include Specific Time Frame)
• Display adequate output as measured by sufficient number of wet diapers daily.
• Demonstrate appropriate weight gain.
• Be free of aspiration.

ACTIONS/INTERVENTIONS

Sample (NIC) linkages:
Lactation Counseling: Use of an interactive helping process to assist in maintenance of successful breastfeeding
Bottle Feeding: Preparation and administration of fluids to an infant via a bottle
Nutrition Monitoring: Collection and analysis of patient data to prevent or minimize malnourishment

NURSING PRIORITY NO. 1

To identify contributing factors/degree of impaired function:

● Assess infant's suck, swallow, and gag reflexes. *Provides comparative baseline and useful in determining appropriate feeding method.*
● Note developmental age, structural abnormalities (e.g., cleft lip/palate), mechanical barriers (e.g., endotracheal [ET] tube, ventilator). *These factors (infant maturity and structural/mechanical barriers to infant feeding) help to determine plan of care.*[1,2,4]
● Determine level of consciousness, neurological impairment, seizure activity, presence of pain. *Provides baseline information and identifies areas of special need.*[1,2]
● Observe parent/infant interactions *to determine level of bonding and comfort that could impact stress level during feeding activity.*
● Note type and scheduling of medications. *May cause sedative effect, or otherwise impair feeding activity.*[2]
● Compare birth and current weight and length measurements. *Monitors effectiveness of infant feeding technique.*[1,2,4]
● Assess signs of stress when feeding (e.g., tachypnea, cyanosis, fatigue, lethargy). *Detects areas of increased need for alternate feeding methods and/or rest periods.*[1]
● Note presence of behaviors indicating continued hunger after feeding. *Determines if infant is receiving adequate amount during feeding.*[2,4]

NURSING PRIORITY NO. 2

To promote adequate infant intake:

- Determine appropriate method for feeding (e.g., special nipple or feeding device, gavage or enteral tube feeding) and choice of breast milk or formula to meet infant needs. *Individualizes care and maintains infant health status.*[1]
- Review early infant feeding cues (e.g., rooting, lip smacking, sucking fingers or hand) versus late cue of crying. *Early recognition of infant hunger promotes timely and more rewarding feeding experience for infant and mother*[5]
- Demonstrate techniques or procedures for feeding. Note proper positioning of infant, "latching-on" techniques, rate of delivery of feeding, frequency of burping. (Refer to ND ineffective Breastfeeding as appropriate.) *Models appropriate feeding methods, increases parental knowledge base and confidence.*[2-4]
- Limit duration of feeding to maximum of 30 minutes based on infant's response (e.g., signs of fatigue) *to balance energy expenditure with nutrient intake.*
- Monitor caregiver's efforts. Provide feedback and assistance as indicated. *Enhances learning, encourages continuation of efforts.*[2,3]
- Refer mother to lactation specialist for assistance and support in dealing with unresolved issues (e.g., teaching infant to suck). *Provides resource for future needs and problem-solving. Begins pattern of resource utilization.*[2-4]
- Emphasize importance of calm/relaxed environment during feeding *to reduce detrimental stimuli and enhance mother/infant's focus on feeding activity.*
- Adjust frequency and amount of feeding according to infant's response. *Prevents infant's frustration associated with under- or overfeeding.*
- Advance diet, adding solids or thickening agent as appropriate for age and infant needs. *Provides for infant's nutrition and health needs.*[2,4]
- Alternate feeding techniques (e.g., nipple and gavage) according to infant's ability and level of fatigue. *Individualizes plan of care to enhance successful feeding.*[1]
- Alter medication or feeding schedules as indicated to minimize sedative effects. *Altered states of function and consciousness interfere with feeding and may lead to choking or aspirating.*[1]

NURSING PRIORITY NO. 3

To promote wellness (Teaching/Discharge Considerations):

- Instruct caregiver in techniques to prevent or alleviate aspiration. *Helps parent/caregiver feel more confident, promotes infant safety.*[1,4]
- Discuss anticipated growth and development goals for infant, corresponding caloric needs. *Accommodating infant maturity and development help to individualize and update plan of care.*[1,2,5]
- Suggest recording infant's weight and nutrient intake periodically. *Monitors effectiveness of infant feeding technique by providing measurable data. Provides positive reinforcement to implementation of care plan.*[1,2,4]
- Recommend participation in classes as indicated (e.g., first aid, infant cardiopulmonary resuscitation [CPR]). *Increases knowledge base for infant safety and caregiver confidence.*[2-4]
- Refer to support groups (e.g., La Leche League, parenting support groups, stress reduction, or other community resources as indicated).
- Provide bibliotherapy including appropriate Web sites for further information.

Nursing Diagnoses in Alphabetical Order

DOCUMENTATION FOCUS

Assessment/Reassessment
- Type and route of feeding, interferences to feeding and reactions.
- Infant's measurements.

Planning
- Plan of care, specific interventions, and who is involved in planning.
- Teaching plan.

Implementation/Evaluation
- Infant's response to interventions (e.g., amount of intake, weight gain, response to feeding) and actions performed.
- Caregiver's involvement in infant care, participation in activities, response to teaching.
- Attainment or progress toward desired outcome(s).
- Modifications to plan of care.

Discharge Planning
- Long-term needs, referrals made, and who is responsible for follow-up actions.

References

1. Creasy, R., Resnik, R. (1999). *Maternal-Fetal Medicine*. 4th ed. Philadelphia: W. B. Saunders.
2. London, M., et al. (2003). *Maternal-Newborn & Child Nursing; Family-Centered Care*. Upper Saddle River, NJ: Prentice Hall.
3. Ladewig, P., et al. (2002). *Contemporary Maternal-Newborn Nursing Care*. 5th ed. Upper Saddle River, NJ: Prentice Hall.
4. Lowdermilk, D., Perry, S., Bobak, I. (2001). *Maternity & Women's Health Care*. 6th ed. St. Louis, MO: Mosby.
5. American Academy of Family Physicians. Breastfeeding (position paper). Retrieved February 2007 from www.aafp.org/online/en/home/policy/policies/b/breastfeedingpositionpaper.html.

readiness for enhanced Fluid Balance

DEFINITION: A pattern of equilibrium between fluid volume and chemical composition of body fluids that is sufficient for meeting physical needs and can be strengthened

RELATED FACTORS

To be developed by nurse researchers and submitted to NANDA

DEFINING CHARACTERISTICS

Subjective
Expresses willingness to enhance fluid balance
No excessive thirst

Objective
Stable weight; no evidence of edema
Moist mucous membranes
Intake adequate for daily needs

Cultural   Collaborative   Community/Home Care   Diagnostic Studies   Pediatric/Geriatric/Lifespan   Medications

Straw-colored urine; specific gravity within normal limits; urine output appropriate for intake

Good tissue turgor; [no signs of] dehydration

Sample Clinical Applications: Heart failure, irritable bowel syndrome, Addison's disease, enteral or parenteral feeding

DESIRED OUTCOME/EVALUATION CRITERIA

Sample (NOC) linkages:
Hydration: Adequate water in the intracellular and extracellular compartments of the body
Fluid Balance: Water balance in the intracellular compartments of the body
Risk Control: Personal actions to prevent, eliminate, or reduce actual, modifiable health threats

Client Will (Include Specific Time Frame)
• Maintain fluid volume at a functional level as indicated by adequate urinary output, stable vital signs, moist mucous membranes, good skin turgor.
• Demonstrate behaviors to monitor fluid balance.
• Be free of thirst.
• Be free of evidence of fluid deficit or fluid overload.

ACTIONS/INTERVENTIONS

Sample (NIC) linkages:
Fluid Management: Promotion of fluid balance and prevention of complications resulting from abnormal or undesired fluid levels
Fluid Monitoring: Collection and analysis of patient data to regulate fluid balance
Surveillance: Purposeful and ongoing acquisition, interpretation, and synthesis of patient data for clinical decision making

NURSING PRIORITY NO. 1

To assess potential for fluid imbalance, ways that client is managing:

● Note presence of factors with potential for fluid imbalance: (1) diagnoses or disease processes (e.g., hyperglycemia, ulcerative colitis, COPD, burns, cirrhosis of the liver, vomiting, diarrhea, hemorrhage) or situations (e.g., diuretic therapy; hot/humid climate, prolonged exercise, heat exhaustion; fever; diuretic effect of caffeine or alcohol) that may lead to deficits; or (2) conditions or situations potentiating fluid excess (e.g., renal failure, cardiac failure, stroke, cerebral lesions, renal or adrenal insufficiency, psychogenic polydipsia, acute stress, anesthesia, surgical procedures, excessive or rapid infusion of IV fluids). *Body fluid balance is regulated by intake (food and fluid), output (kidney, gastrointestinal [GI] tract, skin, and lungs), and regulatory hormonal mechanisms. Balance is maintained within a relatively narrow margin and can be easily disrupted by multiple factors.*[4]
∞ ● Determine potential effects of age and developmental stage. *Elderly individuals have less body water than younger adults, decreased thirst response, and reduced effectiveness of compensatory mechanisms (e.g., kidneys are less efficient in conserving sodium and water). Infants and children have a relatively higher percentage of total body water and metabolic rate, and are often less able than adults to control their fluid intake.*[1,2,5]

- Evaluate environmental factors that could impact fluid balance. *Persons with impaired mobility, diminished vision or confined to bed cannot as easily meet their own needs and may be reluctant to ask for assistance. Persons whose work environment is restrictive or outside may also have greater challenges in meeting fluid needs.*[3]
- Assess vital signs (e.g., temperature, blood pressure, heart rate), skin and mucous membrane moisture, and urine output. Weigh as indicated. *Predictors of fluid balance that should be in client's usual range in a healthy state.*[4]
- Ascertain motivation and expectations for change. *Motivation to improve and high expectations can encourage client to make changes that will improve his or her life. However, unrealistic expectations may hamper efforts.*

NURSING PRIORITY NO. 2

To prevent occurrence of imbalance:

- Monitor intake and output (I&O) (e.g., frequency of voids or diaper changes) as appropriate, being aware of insensible losses (e.g., diaphoresis in hot environment, use of oxygen or permanent tracheostomy) and "hidden sources" of intake (e.g., foods high in water content) *to ensure accurate picture of fluid status.*[4]
- Weigh client regularly and compare with recent weight history. *Useful in early recognition of water retention or unexplained losses.*[1,4]
- Establish or review individual fluid needs and replacement schedule with client. Distribute fluids over 24-hour period. *Enhances likelihood of cooperation with meeting therapeutic goals while avoiding periods of thirst if fluids are restricted.*[1]
- Encourage regular oral intake of fluids (e.g., between meals, additional fluids during hot weather or when exercising) interspersed with high-fluid-content foods of client's choice. *Adds variety to maximize intake while maintaining fluid balance.*[1]
- Provide adequate free water with enteral feedings.
- Administer or discuss judicious use of medications as indicated (e.g., antiemetics, antidiarrheals, antipyretics, and diuretics). *Medications may be indicated to prevent fluid imbalance if individual becomes ill.*[1]

NURSING PRIORITY NO. 3

To promote optimum wellness (Teaching/Discharge Considerations):

- Discuss client's individual conditions/factors that could cause occurrence of fluid imbalance as appropriate, paying special attention to environmental factors such as hot/humid climate, lack of air conditioning, outdoor work setting *so that client/SO can take corrective action and modify risks.*[1,3,6]
- Identify and instruct in ways to meet specific fluid needs (e.g., keep fluids near at hand, carry water bottle when leaving home, or measure specific 24-hour fluid portions if restrictions apply) *to manage fluid intake over time.*[1,3]
- Instruct client/SO(s) in how to measure and record I&O, including weighing diapers or continence pads when used, *if data needed for home management.*
- Establish regular schedule for weighing *to help monitor changes in fluid status.*
- Identify actions (if any) client may take to correct imbalance (e.g., limiting salt or caffeine intake, as needed use of diuretics, tight control of blood sugar).
- Review and instruct in medication regimen and administration and discuss potential for interactions or side effects that could disrupt fluid balance.[1,4,5]
- Instruct in signs and symptoms indicating need for immediate or further evaluation and follow-up to prevent complications and/or allow for timely intervention.[1,4,5]

DOCUMENTATION FOCUS

Assessment/Reassessment
• Individual findings, including factors affecting ability to manage (regulate) body fluids.
• I&O, fluid balance, changes in weight, and vital signs.
• Results of diagnostic studies and laboratory tests.
• Motivation and expectations for change.

Planning
• Plan of care and who is involved in the planning.
• Teaching plan.

Implementation/Evaluation
• Client's responses to treatment, teaching, and actions performed.
• Attainment or progress toward desired outcome(s).
• Modifications to plan of care.

Discharge Planning
• Long-term needs, noting who is responsible for actions to be taken.
• Specific referrals made.

References

1. Cox, H. C., et al. (2002). *Clinical Applications of Nursing Diagnosis: Adult, Child, Women's, Psychiatric, Gerontic, and Home Health Considerations.* 4th ed. Philadelphia: F. A. Davis.
2. Miller-Huey, R. Hydration in elders: More than just a glass of water. Today's Caregiver. Retrieved July 2007 from www.caregiver.com/articles/general/hydration_in_elders.htm.
3. Curtis, R. (1997). Heat-related illnesses & fluid balance: Outdoor action guide. *National Ag Safety Database (NASD)* (Available at www.nasdonline.org/document/1420/d001215/heat-related-illnesses-amp-fluid-balance-outdoor-action.html). Princeton, NJ: Princeton University.
4. Metheny, N. (2000). *Fluid and Electrolyte Balance: Nursing Considerations.* 4th ed. Philadelphia: J. B. Lippincott.
5. Engle, J. (2002). *Pocket Guide to Pediatric Assessment.* 4th ed. St. Louis, MO: Mosby.
6. Bennett, J. A. (2000). Dehydration: Hazards and benefits. *Geriatr Nurs, 21*(2), 84–88.

deficient Fluid Volume: hyper/hypotonic

DEFINITION: [Decreased intravascular, interstitial, and/or intracellular fluid. This refers to dehydration with changes in sodium.]

[**NOTE:** NANDA has restricted deficient Fluid Volume to address only isotonic dehydration. For client needs related to dehydration associated with alterations in sodium, the authors have provided this second diagnostic category.]

RELATED FACTORS

[Hypertonic dehydration: uncontrolled diabetes mellitus or insipidus, hyperosmolar hyperglycemic nonketotic syndrome (HHNS), increased intake of hypertonic fluids or IV therapy, inability to respond to thirst reflex, inadequate free water supplementation (high-osmolarity enteral feeding formulas), renal insufficiency or failure]

[Hypotonic dehydration: chronic illness, malnutrition, excessive use of hypotonic IV solutions (e.g., D5W), renal insufficiency]

(continues on page 348)

deficient Fluid Volume: hyper/hypotonic (continued)
DEFINING CHARACTERISTICS

Subjective
[Reports of fatigue, nervousness, exhaustion]
[Thirst]

Objective
[Increased urine output, dilute urine (initially), or decreased output, oliguria]
[Weight loss]
[Decreased venous filling; hypotension (postural)]
[Increased pulse rate; decreased pulse volume and pressure]
[Decreased skin turgor; dry skin and mucous membranes]
[Increased body temperature]
[Change in mental status (e.g., confusion)]
[Hemoconcentration; altered serum sodium]

Sample Clinical Applications: Diabetes mellitus, diabetic ketoacidosis, renal failure, conditions requiring IV therapy or enteral feeding, heat exhaustion or stroke, presence of draining wounds or fistulas

DESIRED OUTCOMES/EVALUATION CRITERIA

Sample NOC linkages:
Fluid Balance: Water balance in the intracellular and extracellular compartments of the body
Hydration: Adequate water in the intracellular and extracellular compartments of the body
Electrolyte and Acid/Base Balance: Balance of electrolytes and nonelectrolytes in the intracellular and extracellular compartments of the body

Client Will (Include Specific Time Frame)
• Maintain fluid volume at a functional level as evidenced by individually adequate urinary output, stable vital signs, moist mucous membranes, good skin turgor.
• Verbalize understanding of causative factors and purpose of individual therapeutic interventions and medications.
• Demonstrate behaviors to monitor and correct deficit as indicated when condition is chronic.

ACTIONS/INTERVENTIONS

Sample NIC linkages:
Fluid/Electrolyte Management: Regulation and prevention of complications from altered fluid and/or electrolyte levels
Hypovolemia Management: Expansion of intravascular fluid volume in a patient who is volume depleted
Shock Prevention: Detecting and treating a patient at risk for impending shock

NURSING PRIORITY NO. 1

To assess causative/precipitating factors:

● Note possible medical diagnoses or disease processes that may lead to fluid deficits:
   (1) fluid loss (e.g., diarrhea, vomiting; fever; excessive sweating; heat stroke; diabetic

Excess fluid intake
Excess sodium intake
[Drug therapies such as chlorpropamide, tolbutamide, vincristine, triptylines, carbamazepine]

DEFINING CHARACTERISTICS

Subjective[2,9]
Anxiety
[Difficulty breathing]

Objective
Edema; anasarca; weight gain over short period of time
Intake exceeds output; oliguria; specific gravity changes
Adventitious breath sounds [rales or crackles]; changes in respiratory pattern; dyspnea; orthopnea
Pulmonary congestion; pleural effusion; pulmonary artery pressure [PAP] changes; blood pressure changes[3]
Increased central venous pressure [CVP]; jugular vein distention; positive hepatojugular reflex
S_3 heart sound
Change in mental status, restlessness
Decreased Hb/Hct, azotemia, altered electrolytes

Sample Clinical Applications: Congestive heart failure, renal failure, cirrhosis of liver, cancer, toxemia of pregnancy, conditions associated with SIADH (e.g., meningitis, encephalitis, Guillain-Barré syndrome), schizophrenia (where polydipsia is a prominent feature)

DESIRED OUTCOMES/EVALUATION CRITERIA

Sample NOC linkages:
Fluid Balance: Water balance in the intracellular and extracellular compartments of the body
Electrolyte and Acid/Base Balance: Balance of electrolytes and non-electrolytes in the intracellular and extracellular compartments of the body
Cardiac Pump Effectiveness: Adequacy of blood volume ejected from the left ventricle to support systemic perfusion pressure

Client Will (Include Specific Time Frame)
• Stabilize fluid volume as evidenced by balanced intake and output (I&O), vital signs within client's normal limits, stable weight, and free of signs of edema.
• Verbalize understanding of individual dietary and fluid restrictions.
• Demonstrate behaviors to monitor fluid status and reduce recurrence of fluid excess.
• List signs that require further evaluation.

(continues on page 358)

---

ketoacidosis; burns, draining wounds; gastrointestinal [GI] obstruction; salt-wasting diuretics; rapid breathing or mechanical ventilation, surgical drains); (2) limited intake (e.g., sore throat or mouth; client dependent on others for eating and drinking; vomiting); (3) fluid shifts (e.g., ascites, effusions, burns, sepsis); and (4) environmental factors (e.g., isolation, restraints, malfunctioning air conditioning, exposure to extreme heat).

• Determine effects of age, gender. Obtain weight and measure subcutaneous fat and muscle mass (influences total body water [TBW], which is approximately 60% of an adult's weight and 75% of an infant's weight).[1] *In general, men have higher TBW than women, and the elderly's TBW is less than that of a youth. Elderly individuals are often at risk because of decreased thirst reflex, repeated infections, chronic conditions, and polypharmacy.[2,9] Infants/young children and other nonverbal persons cannot describe thirst. Worldwide, dehydration (secondary to diarrheal illness) is the leading cause of infant and child mortality.[3,9]*

• Evaluate nutritional status, noting current intake, weight changes, problems with oral intake, use of supplements/tube feedings.

• Collaborate with physician to identify or characterize the nature of fluid and electrolyte imbalance(s). *Dehydration is often categorized according to serum sodium concentration. Isonatremic (i.e., isotonic) dehydration is the most common type of dehydration. However, hypernatremic (also called "hypertonic dehydration" when relatively less sodium than water is lost) and hyponatremic (or hypotonic dehydration when relatively less water than sodium is lost) can both cause neurological complications, and thus may be more dangerous.[3] More than one cause may exist at a given time (e.g., increased loss of salt and water caused by diuretics that leads to decreased fluid intake as a result of lethargy and confusion).[5,10,11]*

NURSING PRIORITY NO. 2

To evaluate degree of fluid deficit:

• Obtain history of usual pattern of fluid intake and recent alterations. *Intake may be reduced because of current physical or environmental issues (e.g., swallowing problems, vomiting, severe heat wave with inadequate fluid replacement); or a behavior pattern (e.g., elderly person refuses to drink water trying to control incontinence).[8]*

• Assess vital signs, including temperature (often elevated), pulse (elevated), respirations, and blood pressure (may be low). Measure blood pressure (lying, sitting, standing) *to evaluate orthostatic blood pressure*, and monitor invasive hemodynamic parameters as indicated (e.g., central venous pressure [CVP]) *to determine degree of intravascular deficit and replacement needs.[7-9]*

• Note presence of dry mucous membranes, poor skin turgor, delayed capillary refill, flat neck veins, reports of thirst or weakness, child crying without tears, sunken eyeballs, fever, weight loss, little or no urine output. *Assessment signs of dehydration that client/SO may notice.[8,9]*

• Note change in usual mentation, behavior, and functional abilities (e.g., confusion, falling, loss of ability to carry out usual activities, lethargy, dizziness) *These signs indicate sufficient dehydration to cause poor cerebral perfusion and/or electrolyte imbalance.[10,11]*

• Observe and measure urinary output hourly or for 24 hours as indicated. Note color *(may be dark because of concentration)* and specific gravity *(high number associated with dehydration with usual range being 1.010–1.025).[4]*

• Estimate or measure other fluid losses, (e.g., gastric, respiratory, and wound losses) *to more accurately determine fluid replacement needs.[8]*

• Review laboratory data (e.g., hemoglobin/hematocrit [Hb/Hct]; electrolytes [sodium, potassium, chloride, bicarbonate]; blood urea nitrogen [BUN], creatinine [Cr]) *to evaluate body's response to fluid loss and to determine replacement needs.[4]*

DOCUMENTATION FOCUS

Assessment/Reassessment
• Assessment findings, including degree of deficit and current sources of fluid intake.
• I&O, fluid balance, changes in weight or edema, urine-specific gravity, and vital signs.
• Results of diagnostic studies.

Planning
• Plan of care and who is involved in planning.
• Teaching plan.

Implementation/Evaluation
• Client's responses to interventions, teaching, and actions performed.
• Attainment or progress toward desired outcome(s).
• Modifications to plan of care.

Discharge Planning
• Long-term needs, plan for correction, and who is responsible for actions to be taken.
• Specific referrals made.

References

1. Kolecki, P., Meckhoff, C. R. (2001). Shock, hypovolemic. Retrieved August 2003 from www.emedicine.com.
2. Cox, H. C., et al. (2002). *Clinical Applications of Nursing Diagnosis: Adult, Child, Women's, Psychiatric, Gerontic, and Home Health Considerations.* 4th ed. Philadelphia: F. A. Davis, 88.
3. Mentes, J. C. (1998). *Hydration Management. The Iowa Veterans Affairs Nursing Research Consortium.* Iowa City: University of Iowa Gerontological Nursing Interventions Research Center, Research Dissemination Core.
4. Ellsbury, D. L., George, C. S. (2006 update). Dehydration. Retrieved July 2007 from www.emedicine.com/ped/topic556.htm.
5. Welch, J. (1998). Isotonic dehydration. Retrieved August 2003 from http://gucfm.georgetown.edu/welchjj/netscut/fen/isotonic_dehydration.html.
6. Cavanaugh, B. M. (1999). *Nurse's Manual of Laboratory and Diagnostic Tests.* 3d ed. Philadelphia: F. A. Davis.
7. Koch, H., Graber, M. A. Pediatrics: Vomiting, diarrhea, and dehydration. *University of Iowa Family Practice Handbook.* Retrieved August 2003 from www.vh.org. 4th ed.
8. Fluid and Electrolyte imbalances. In Doenges, M. E., Moorhouse, M. F., Geissler-Murr, A. C. (eds). (2002). *Nursing Care Plans: Guidelines for Individualizing Patient Care* (CD-ROM). 6th ed. Philadelphia: F. A. Davis.
9. Mayo Clinic Staff. (2007). Dehydration. Retrieved February 2007 from www.mayoclinic.com/health/dehydration/DS00561/DSECTION=1.
10. Diel-Oplinger, L., Kaminski, M. F. (2004). Choosing the right fluid to counter hypovolemic shock. *Nursing,* 34(3), 52–54.

excess Fluid Volume

DEFINITION: Increased isotonic fluid retention

RELATED FACTORS

Compromised regulatory mechanism [e.g., syndrome of inappropriate antidiuretic hormone (SIADH), or decreased plasma proteins as found in conditions such as malnutrition, draining fistulas, burns, organ failure]

---

excess Fluid Volume (continued)
ACTIONS/INTERVENTIONS

Sample NIC linkages:
Hypervolemia Management: Reduction in extracellular or intracellular fluid volume and prevention of complications in a patient who is fluid overloaded
Electrolyte Management: Promotion of electrolyte balance and prevention of complications resulting from abnormal or undesired serum electrolyte levels
Peritoneal Dialysis [or] Hemodialysis Therapy: Administration and monitoring of dialysis solution into and out of the peritoneal cavity/or management of extracorporeal passage of the patient's blood through a dialyzer

NURSING PRIORITY NO. 1

To assess causative/precipitating factors:

● Note presence of medical conditions or situations (e.g., heart failure, chronic kidney disease, renal or adrenal insufficiency, excessive or rapid infusion of IV fluids, cerebral lesions, psychogenic polydipsia, acute stress, anesthesia, surgical procedures, decreased or loss of serum proteins) *that can contribute to excess fluid intake or retention.*[1]
● Determine or estimate amount of fluid intake from all sources: oral, intravenous, enteral feedings, ventilator, and so forth.
● Review nutritional issues (e.g., intake of sodium, potassium, and protein). *Imbalances in these areas are associated with fluid imbalances.*

NURSING PRIORITY NO. 2

To evaluate degree of excess:

● Compare current weight with admission or previously stated weight. Weigh daily or on a regular schedule, as indicated. *Provides a comparative baseline and evaluates the effectiveness of diuretic therapy when used (i.e., if I&O is 1 L negative, weight loss of 2.2 pounds should be noted).*[8] *Note: Volume overload can occur over weeks to months in clients with unrecognized renal failure where lean muscle mass is lost and fluid overload occurs with relatively little change in weight.*[4]
● Measure vital signs and invasive hemodynamic parameters (e.g., CVP, PAP/pulmonary capillary wedge pressure [PCWP]) if available. *Blood pressures may be high because of excess fluid volume, or be low if cardiac failure is occurring.*
● Note presence of tachycardia, irregular rhythms. Auscultate heart tones for S_3, ventricular gallop. *Signs suggestive of heart failure, which results in decreased cardiac output and tissue hypoxia.*[7]
● Auscultate breath sounds for presence of crackles or congestion. Record occurrence of exertional breathlessness, dyspnea at rest, or paroxysmal nocturnal dyspnea. *Indication of pulmonary congestion and potential of developing pulmonary edema that can interfere with oxygen—carbon dioxide exchange at the capillary level.*[3]
● Note presence and location of edema (e.g., puffy eyelids, dependent swelling ankles and feet if ambulatory or up in chair; sacrum and posterior thighs when recumbent). Determine whether lower extremity edema is new or increasing. *Heart failure and renal failure are associated with dependent edema because of hydrostatic pressures, with dependent edema being a defining characteristic for excess fluid. Generalized edema (e.g., upper extremities and eyelids) is associated with nephrotic syndrome.*[2]

- Assess for presence of neck vein distention/hepatojugular reflux with head of bed elevated 30 to 45 degrees. *Signs of increased intravascular volume.*[6]
- Measure abdominal girth *to evaluate changes that may indicate increasing fluid retention and edema.*[7]
- Measure and record I&O accurately. Include "hidden" fluids (e.g., IV antibiotic additives, liquid medications, ice chips). Calculate 24-hour fluid balance (plus or minus). Note patterns, times, and amount of urination (e.g., nocturia, oliguria).[6]
- Evaluate mentation for restlessness, anxiety, confusion, and personality changes. *Signs of decreased cerebral oxygenation (e.g., cerebral edema) or electrolyte imbalance (e.g., hyponatremia).*[1,9]
- Assess appetite; note presence of nausea/vomiting. Assess neuromuscular reflexes *to determine presence of problems associated with imbalance of electrolytes (e.g., glucose, sodium, potassium, calcium).*[9]
- Observe skin and mucous membranes. *Edematous tissues are prone to ischemia and breakdown or ulceration.*[5]
- Review laboratory data (e.g., blood urea nitrogen [BUN]/creatinine [Cr], hemoglobin [Hb]/hematocrit [Hct], serum albumin, proteins, and electrolytes; urine specific gravity, osmolality, and sodium excretion) and chest radiograph. *These tests may be repeated not only to ascertain baseline imbalances, but also to monitor response to therapy.*

NURSING PRIORITY NO. 3

To promote mobilization/elimination of excess fluid:

- Restrict fluid intake as indicated (especially when sodium retention is less than water retention or when fluid retention is related to renal failure).[6]
- Provide for sodium restrictions if needed (as might occur in sodium retention in excess of water retention). *Restricting sodium favors renal excretion of excess fluid and may be more useful than fluid restriction.*[1]
- Set an appropriate rate of fluid intake or infusion throughout 24-hour period. Maintain steady rate of all IV infusions *to prevent exacerbation of excess fluid volume and to prevent peaks and valleys in fluid level.*[6]
- Administer medications (e.g., diuretics, cardiotonics, plasma or albumin volume expanders) in order to improve cardiac output and kidney function, thereby *reducing congestion and edema.*
- Evaluate edematous extremities *to enhance venous return and prevent further edema formation.*[7]
- Encourage bedrest when ascites is present and place in semi-Fowler's position as appropriate. *May promote recumbency-induced diuresis and facilitate respiratory effort when movement of the diaphragm is limited/breathing is impaired because of lung congestion.*
- Prepare for and assist with procedures as indicated (e.g., peritoneal or hemodialysis, mechanical ventilation). *May be done to correct volume overload, electrolyte and acid-base imbalances, or to support individual during shock state.*[7]

NURSING PRIORITY NO. 4

To maintain integrity of skin and tissues:

- Promote early ambulation *to mobilize fluids and prevent or limit damage from venous stasis complications.*
- Change position frequently *to reduce tissue pressure and risk of skin breakdown.*[7]

Nursing Diagnoses in Alphabetical Order

- Offer frequent mouth care when fluids are restricted using nondrying mouthwash, hard candies, and so forth, *to promote comfort of dry mucous membranes and prevent oral complications.*[7]
- Avoid use of restraints, use safety precautions if client is confused or debilitated as may occur with cerebral edema, electrolyte imbalance, heart failure, and so forth. *There is an increased risk of skin and tissue trauma with the use of restraints as well as increased agitation that may lead to more serious injury or death.*[7]
- Refer to NDs impaired Oral Mucous Membrane, impaired or risk for impaired Skin/Tissue Integrity for additional interventions.

NURSING PRIORITY NO. 5

To promote wellness (Teaching/Discharge Considerations):

- Consult dietitian as needed *to develop dietary plan and identify foods to be limited or omitted*:
  Review dietary restrictions and safe substitutes for salt (e.g., lemon juice or spices such as oregano).
  Discuss fluid restrictions and "hidden sources" of fluids (e.g., foods high in water content such as fruits, ice cream, sauces, custard). Use small drinking cup or glass.
  Avoid salty or spicy foods, as they increase thirst or fluid retention. Suck ice chips, hard candy, or slices of lemon *to help allay thirst.*[7]
- Suggest chewing gum, use of lip balm *to reduce discomforts of fluid restrictions.*[7]
- Instruct client/family in ways to keep track of intake. For example, use a marked water bottle or container; refill as needed.[6]
- Measure output, encourage use of voiding record when it is appropriate, or weigh daily and report gain of more than 2 lb/day (or as indicated by individual situation). *If weight is higher than target weight, fluid is likely being retained.*[6,7]
- Review drug regimen and side effects of agents used to increase urine output or manage hypertension, kidney disease, or heart failure. *Many drugs have an impact on kidney function and fluid balance, especially in the elderly or those with cardiac and kidney impairments.*
- Stress need for mobility or frequent position changes *to prevent stasis and reduce risk of tissue injury.*[7]
- Identify "danger" signs requiring notification of healthcare provider *to ensure timely evaluation and intervention.*[6]

DOCUMENTATION FOCUS

Assessment/Reassessment
- Assessment findings, noting existing conditions contributing to and degree of fluid retention (vital signs; amount, presence and location of edema; and weight changes).
- I&O, fluid balance.
- Results of laboratory tests and diagnostic studies.

Planning
- Plan of care and who is involved in the planning.
- Teaching plan.

Implementation/Evaluation
- Response to interventions, teaching, and actions performed.
- Attainment or progress toward desired outcome(s).
- Modifications to plan of care.

Discharge Planning
• Long-term needs, noting who is responsible for actions to be taken.

References

1. Fauci, A. S., et al. (eds). (1998). *Harrison's Principles of Internal Medicine.* 14th ed. New York: McGraw-Hill, 268, 1292–1293.
2. Rios, H., et al. (1991). Validation of defining characteristics of four nursing diagnoses using a computerized database. *J Prof Nurs*, 7, 293–299.
3. Matheny, N. (2000). *Fluid and Electrolyte Balance: Nursing Considerations.* 4th ed. Philadelphia: J. B. Lippincott.
4. Veterans Health Administration, Department of Defense. VHA/DoD clinical practice guideline for the management of chronic kidney disease and pre-ERSD in the primary care setting. Retrieved August 2003 from www.guideline.gov.
5. Cullen, L. (1992). Interventions related to fluid and electrolyte imbalance. *Nurs Clin North Am*, 27, 569–597.
6. American Medical Directors Association (AMDA). (2004 update). Hydration management. Retrieved July 2007 from (www.guideline.gov). Columbia, MD: National Guideline Clearinghouse.
7. Doenges, M. E., Moorhouse, M. F., Geissler-Murr, A. C. (2002). Fluid and electrolyte imbalances. *Nursing Care Plans: Guidelines for Individualizing Patient Care* (CD-ROM). 6th ed. Philadelphia: F. A. Davis.
8. Riggs, J. M. (2006). Manage heart failure. *Nurs Crit Care*, 1(4), 18–28.
9. Astle, S. M. (2005). Restoring electrolyte balance. *RN*, 68(5), 31–34.

risk for deficient Fluid Volume

DEFINITION: At risk for experiencing vascular, cellular, or intracellular dehydration

RISK FACTORS

Extremes of age or weight
Loss of fluid through abnormal routes (e.g., indwelling tubes)
Knowledge deficiency
Factors influencing fluid needs (e.g., hypermetabolic states)
Medications (e.g., diuretics)
Excessive losses through normal routes (e.g., diarrhea)
Deviations affecting access, intake, or absorption of fluids (e.g., physical immobility)

NOTE: A risk diagnosis is not evidenced by signs and symptoms, as the problem has not occurred; rather, nursing interventions are directed at prevention.
Sample Clinical Applications: Conditions with fever, diarrhea, nausea, vomiting; irritable bowel syndrome, draining wounds, dementia, depression, eating disorders

DESIRED OUTCOMES/EVALUATION CRITERIA

Sample **NOC** linkages:
Fluid Balance: Water balance in the intracellular and extracellular compartments of the body

(continues on page 362)

risk for deficient Fluid Volume (continued)

Client Will (Include Specific Time Frame)
• Maintain fluid volume at a functional level as evidenced by individually adequate urinary output with normal specific gravity, stable vital signs, moist mucous membranes, good skin turgor, and prompt capillary refill.
Risk Control: Personal actions to prevent, eliminate, or reduce modifiable health threats
Knowledge: Disease Process: Extent of understanding conveyed about a specific disease process

Client/Caregiver Will (Include Specific Time Frame)
• Identify individual risk factors and appropriate interventions.
• Demonstrate behaviors or lifestyle changes to prevent development of fluid volume deficit.

ACTIONS/INTERVENTIONS

Sample NIC linkages:
Fluid Monitoring: Collection and analysis of patient data to regulate fluid balance
Hemodynamic Regulation: Optimization of heart rate, preload, afterload, and contractility
Teaching: Disease Process: Assisting the patient to understand information related to a specific disease process

NURSING PRIORITY NO. 1

To assess causative/contributing factors:

● Note possible conditions/processes *that may lead to fluid deficits*: (1) fluid loss (e.g., indwelling tubes, diarrhea, vomiting, fever, excessive sweating, diabetic ketoacidosis; burns, other draining wounds; gastrointestinal [GI] obstruction; use of diuretics); (2) limited intake (e.g., extremes of age, immobility, client dependent on others for eating and drinking; lack of knowledge related to fluid intake; heat exhaustion or stroke); (3) fluid shifts (e.g., ascites, effusions, burns, sepsis); or (4) environmental factors (e.g., isolation, restraints, very high ambient temperatures, malfunctioning air conditioning).[4,8]

∞ ● Determine effects of age, gender. Obtain weight and measure subcutaneous fat/muscle mass. These factors affect ratio of lean body mass to body fat, influencing total body water (TBW). *In general, men have higher TBW than women, and the elderly's TBW is less than that of a youth. Elderly individuals are often at risk for underhydration because of a decreased thirst reflex, repeated infections, and chronic conditions. They may not be aware of water or nutritional needs, may be depressed or cognitively impaired, incontinent, and taking many medications.*[2] *Infants, children, and developmentally delayed individual cannot verbalize or self-manage thirst. Worldwide, dehydration (secondary to diarrheal illness) is the leading cause of infant and child mortality.*[3]

● Evaluate nutritional status, noting current food intake, type of diet (e.g., client is NPO or is on a restricted or pureed diet). Note problems *that can negatively affect fluid intake (e.g., impaired mentation, nausea, wired jaws, immobility, insufficient time for meals, lack of finances restricting availability of food).*

● Refer to NDs deficient Fluid Volume: [hyper/hypotonic] or [isotonic] for additional interventions.

NURSING PRIORITY NO. 2

To prevent occurrence of deficit:

- Monitor intake and output (I&O) balance being aware of altered intake or output, as well as insensible losses *to ensure accurate picture of fluid status.*[4]
- Weigh client and compare with recent weight history. Perform serial weights to determine trends.[5]
- Monitor vital signs for changes (e.g., orthostatic hypotension, tachycardia, fever) *that may cause dehydration.*[4]
- Assess skin turgor and oral mucous membranes *for signs of dehydration.*
- Review laboratory data (e.g., hemoglobin [Hb]/hematocrit [Hct], electrolytes, blood urea nitrogen [BUN]/creatinine [Cr]) as indicated *to evaluate fluid and electrolyte status.*[4]
- Administer medications as appropriate (e.g., antiemetics, antidiarrheals, antipyretics) *to stop or limit fluid losses.*[4,5]
- Determine individual fluid needs and establish replacement schedule. Distribute fluids over 24 hours *to prevent periods of thirst.*[5]
- Provide supplemental fluids (tube feed, IV) as indicated. *Fluids may be given in this manner if client is unable to take oral fluid or is NPO for procedures.*
- Encourage oral intake:[4-6]
  Provide water and other fluids to a minimum amount daily (up to 2.5 L/day or amount determined by healthcare provider for client's age, weight, and condition).
  Offer fluids between meals and regularly throughout the day.
  Allow adequate time for eating and drinking at meals.
  Provide fluids in manageable cup, bottle, or with drinking straw.
  Ensure that immobile or restrained client is assisted.
  Encourage a variety of fluids in small frequent offerings, attempting to incorporate client's preferred beverage and temperature (e.g., iced or hot).
  Limit fluids that tend to exert a diuretic effect (e.g., caffeine, alcohol).
  Promote intake of high-water content foods (e.g., popsicles, gelatin, soup, eggnog, watermelon) or electrolyte replacement drinks (e.g., Smartwater, Gatorade, Pedialyte), as appropriate.
  Encourage client to increase fluids when engaged in exercise or physical exertion, or during hot weather.
- Review diet orders to remove any nonessential fluid and salt restrictions.
- Provide nutritionally balanced diet and/or enteral feedings, when indicated (avoiding use of hyperosmolar or excessively high-protein formulas) and provide adequate amount of free water with feedings.

NURSING PRIORITY NO. 3

To promote wellness (Teaching/Discharge Considerations):

- Discuss individual risk factors or potential problems and specific interventions *to reduce risk of heat injury and dehydration (e.g., proper clothing and bedding for infants and elderly during hot weather, use of room cooler or fan for comfortable ambient environment).*[7]
- Review appropriate use of medications and inform client of side effects of medications *that have potential for causing or exacerbating dehydration.*
- Encourage client/caregiver to maintain diary of food and fluid intake, number and amount of voidings, and estimate of other fluid losses (e.g., wounds, liquid stools) as necessary *to determine replacement needs.*

Nursing Diagnoses in Alphabetical Order

NURSING PRIORITY NO. 2

To evaluate degree of compromise:

- Evaluate respirations:

  Observe respiratory rate, depth. *Increasing both rate and depth of respirations increases alveolar ventilation and occurs normally in response to exercise and stressors. Tachypnea is usually present to some degree and can progress to hyperventilation with shallow respirations, dyspnea, and respiratory depression.*[1]

  Note client's reports/perceptions of breathing ease. *Client may report a range of symptoms (e.g., air hunger; shortness of breath with speaking, activity, or at rest).*

  Observe for dyspnea on exertion, gasping; changing positions frequently to ease breathing; tendency to assume three-point position (bending forward while supporting self by placing one hand on each knee) *to maximize respiratory effort.*

  Note use of accessory muscles (e.g., scalene muscles, pectoralis minor, sternocleidomastoids, and external intercostal muscles) *to assist diaphragm in increasing volume of thoracic cavity, which aids in inspiration.*[2]

  ∞ Observe infants/young children for nasal flaring and sternal retractions *indicating increased work of breathing or respiratory distress.*

  Note use of abdominal muscles during expiration (normally a passive process) *to reduce thoracic dimensions and overcome airway resistance to expiration.*[2]

- Evaluate lungs:

  Auscultate and percuss chest, describing presence or absence of breath sounds, note adventitious breath sounds. *Although air may be heard moving through the lung fields, breath sounds may be faint because of decreased airflow or areas of consolidation. In this nursing diagnosis, ventilatory effort is insufficient to deliver enough oxygen, or to get rid of sufficient amounts of carbon dioxide. Abnormal breath sounds are indicative of numerous problems (e.g., hypoventilation such as might occur with atelectasis or presence of secretions, improper endotracheal (ET) tube placement, collapsed lung) and must be evaluated for further intervention.*[3,4]

- Note character and effectiveness of cough mechanism. *Affects ability to clear airways of secretions.*

- Evaluate skin and mucous membrane color noting areas of pallor or cyanosis, for example, peripheral (nailbeds) versus central (around lips or earlobes) or general duskiness. *Duskiness and central cyanosis are indicative of advanced hypoxemia.*[4]

- Evaluate behavior:

  Assess level of consciousness and mentation changes. *Decreased level of consciousness impairs one's ability to protect the airway, potentially adversely affecting oxygenation that in turn further impairs mentation.*

  Note somnolence, restlessness, reports of headache on arising.

  Assess energy level and activity tolerance, noting reports or evidence of fatigue, weakness, problems with sleep *that are associated with decreased oxygenation.*

- Monitor vital signs:

  Measure temperature. *High fever greatly increases metabolic demands and oxygen consumption.*

  Monitor heart rate and rhythm. *Tachycardia and dysrhythmias may be noted as heart reacts to ischemia, especially during activity.*

  Monitor blood pressure. *BP can be variable, depending on underlying condition and cardiopulmonary response.*

  Note increased pulmonary artery or right ventricular wedge pressures in critically ill client with central lines. *Indicative of increased pulmonary vascular resistance.*

● Review pertinent diagnostic data (e.g., ABGs, hemoglobin [Hb], red blood cells [RBCs], electrolytes); chest radiography. Evaluate pulse oximetry (can be commomplace measurement along with vital signs in many facilities) and pulmonary function studies (e.g., lung volumes and capacities) *to determine presence and degree of lung function, and/or respiratory insufficiency and acid-base status; also used to monitor response to therapies. Client in respiratory failure typically shows hypoxemia and metabolic acidosis and is high risk for developing respiratory acidosis.*[5,8]

NURSING PRIORITY NO. 3

To correct/improve existing deficiencies:

● Elevate head of bed or position client appropriately. *Elevation or upright position facilitates respiratory function by gravity; however, client in severe distress will seek position of comfort. In ventilated client, prone position may be implemented in some clients to improve pulmonary perfusion and increase oxygen diffusion.*[4]

● Provide airway adjuncts and suction as indicated *to clear or maintain open airway, and when client is unable to clear secretions, or to improve gas diffusion when client is showing desaturation of oxygen by oximetry or ABGs.*[4,6,7]

● Encourage frequent position changes, deep-breathing exercises or directed coughing, use of incentive spirometer, and chest physiotherapy as indicated. *Promotes optimal chest expansion, mobilization of secretions, and oxygen diffusion.*[4]

● Provide supplemental oxygen (via cannula, mask) using lowest concentration possible *dictated by pulse oximetry, ABGs, and client symptoms/underlying condition.*

● Ensure availability of proper emergency equipment, including ET/tracheostomy set and suction catheters appropriate for age and size of infant/child/adult. Avoid use of face mask in elderly emaciated client.

● Prepare for and assist with intubation and mechanical ventilation. *The decision to intubate and ventilate is made on a clinical diagnosis of increased work of breathing, hypoventilation, impaired mental status, or presence of a moribund state.*[5]

● Monitor and adjust ventilator settings (e.g., FIo_2, tidal volume, inspiratory and expiratory ratio, sigh, positive end–expiratory pressure [PEEP]) as indicated when mechanical support is being used.

● Monitor for carbon dioxide narcosis (e.g., change in level of consciousness, changes in O_2 and CO_2 blood gas levels, flushing, decreased respiratory rate and headaches), *which may occur in clients receiving long-term oxygen therapy.*[8]

● Maintain adequate intake *for mobilization of secretions*, but avoid fluid overload *that may increase pulmonary congestion.*

● Provide psychological support. Active-listen questions and concerns. Address client's/SO's fears and anxiety that may be present. Maintain calm attitude while working with client/SOs. *Anxiety is contagious, and associated agitation can increase oxygen consumption and dyspnea.*

● Encourage adequate rest and limit activities to within client tolerance. Promote calm, restful environment. *Facilitates relaxation and helps limit oxygen needs and consumption.*[4]

● Administer medications as indicated (e.g., inhaled and systemic glucocorticosteroids, antibiotics, bronchodilators, methylxanthines, expectorants, heparin) to treat underlying conditions. Medications may be aerosolized or nebulized for enhanced response and limitation of side effects.[4]

● Monitor therapeutic and adverse effects or interactions of drug therapy *to determine efficacy and need for change.*

● Use sedation judiciously *to avoid depressant effects on respiratory functioning.*[4]

● Minimize blood loss from procedures (e.g., blood draws—especially in neonates/infants, hemodialysis) *to limit effects of anemia and related gas diffusion impairment.*

- Assist with procedures as individually indicated (e.g., transfusion, phlebotomy, bronchoscopy) *to improve respiratory function/oxygen-carrying capacity.*
- Keep environment allergen/pollutant-free *to reduce irritant effect of dust and chemicals on airways.*

NURSING PRIORITY NO. 4

To promote wellness (Teaching/Discharge Considerations):

- Review risk factors, particularly genetic, environmental, and employment-related conditions (e.g., sickle-cell anemia, altitude sickness, exposure to toxins) *to help client/SO prevent complications or manage risk factors.*
- Discuss implications of smoking related to the illness or condition. Encourage client and SO(s) to stop smoking, attend cessation programs as necessary *to reduce health risks and or prevent further decline in lung function.*[9]
- Review oxygen-conserving techniques (e.g., organizing tasks before beginning, sitting instead of standing to perform tasks, eating small meals, performing slower-purposeful movements) *to reduce oxygen demands.*[4]
- Reinforce need for adequate rest, while encouraging activity and exercise (e.g., upper and lower extremity endurance and strength training, and flexibility) *to decrease dyspnea and improve quality of life.*[10]
- Emphasize the importance of good general nutrition *for improving stamina and reducing the work of breathing.*[4,10]
- Refer to dietitian *for nutritional assessment and individual dietary plan as indicated.*[10]
- Instruct in the use of relaxation, stress-reduction techniques as appropriate.
- Review job description and work activities *to identify need for job modifications or vocational rehabilitation.*[4]
- Discuss home oxygen therapy use and instruct in safety concerns as indicated *to ensure client's safety, especially when used in the very young, fragile elderly, or when cognitive or neuromuscular impairment is present.*[4]
- Identify specific supplier for supplemental oxygen and necessary respiratory devices, as well as other individually appropriate resources, such as home-care agencies, Meals on Wheels, and so forth, to facilitate independence.[4]

DOCUMENTATION FOCUS

Assessment/Reassessment
- Assessment findings, including respiratory rate, character of breath sounds; frequency, amount, and appearance of secretions; presence of cyanosis; laboratory findings; and mentation level.
- Conditions that may interfere with oxygen delivery or exchange.

Planning
- Plan of care, specific interventions, and who is involved in the planning.
- Liters of supplemental oxygen, ventilator settings.
- Teaching plan.

Implementation/Evaluation
- Client's responses to treatment, teaching, and actions performed.
- Attainment or progress toward desired outcome(s).
- Modifications to plan of care.

Discharge Planning
- Long-term needs, identifying who is responsible for actions to be taken.
- Community resources for equipment and supplies postdischarge.
- Specific referrals made.

References

1. Seay, S. J., Gay, S. L., Strauss, M. (2002). Tracheostomy emergencies. *Am J Nurs*, 102(3), 59.
2. Waldorf, A. (2003). Pulmonary structure and function and gas exchange and transport. Online course: Physiology of Exercise and Health. Cal State San Marcos. iLearn (Internet Learning Environments and Resource Network). Retrieved from http://courses.csusm.edu/resources/indexarchive/spring03.html.
3. Cox, H. C., et al. (2002). *Clinical Applications of Nursing Diagnosis: Adult, Child, Women's, Psychiatric, Gerontic, and Home Health Considerations.* 4th ed. Philadelphia: F. A. Davis, 256–261.
4. Doenges, M. E., Moorhouse, M. F., Geissler-Murr, A. C. (2002). *Nursing Care Plans: Guidelines for Individualizing Patient Care.* 6th ed. Philadelphia: F. A. Davis.
5. Carcillo, J. A., Fields, A. I. (2002). Clinical practice parameters for hemodynamic support of pediatric and neonatal patients in septic shock. *Crit Care Med*, 30(6), 1365–1378.
6. Fink, J. B., Hess, D. R. (2002). Secretion clearance techniques. In Hess, D. R., et al. (eds). *Respiratory Care: Principles and Practices.* Philadelphia: W. B. Saunders.
7. Blair, K. A. (1999). The aging pulmonary system. In Stanley, M., Beare, P. G. (eds). *Gerontological Nursing: A Health Promotion/Protection Approach.* 2d ed. Philadelphia: F. A. Davis.
8. Argyle, B. (1996). Blood Gases Computer Program. Retrieved July 2007 from Mad Scientist Software's Blood Gas tutorialwww.madsci.com/manu/indexgas.htm.
9. Anderson, N. R. (2006). The role of the home healthcare nurse in smoking cessation: Guidelines for successful intervention. *Home Healthcare Nurse*, 24(7), 424–431.
10. McAllister, M. (2005). Promoting physiologic-physical adaptation in chronic obstructive pulmonary disease: Pharmacotherapeutic evidence-based research and guidelines. *Home Healthcare Nurse*, 23(8), 523–531.

risk for unstable blood Glucose Level

DEFINITION: Risk for variation of blood glucose/sugar levels from the normal range

RISK FACTORS

Lack of acceptance of diagnosis; deficient knowledge of diabetes management (e.g., action plan)

Lack of diabetes management or adherence to diabetes management (e.g., action plan); inadequate blood glucose monitoring; medication management

Dietary intake; weight gain or loss; rapid growth periods; pregnancy

Physical health status or activity level

Stress; mental health status

Developmental level

NOTE: A risk diagnosis is not evidenced by signs and symptoms, as the problem has not occurred, rather, nursing interventions are directed at prevention.

Sample Clinical Applications: Diabetes mellitus, diabetic ketoacidosis, hypoglycemia, gestational diabetes, corticosteroid use, total parenteral nutrition (TPN)

(continues on page 374)

Nursing Diagnoses in Alphabetical Order

risk for unstable blood Glucose Level (continued)
DESIRED OUTCOMES/EVALUATION CRITERIA

Sample **NOC** linkages:
Knowledge: Diabetes Management: Extent of understanding conveyed about diabetes mellitus, its treatment, and the prevention of complications
Diabetes Self-Management: Personal actions to manage diabetes mellitus, its treatment, and prevent disease progression
Blood Glucose Level: Extent to which glucose levels in plasma and urine are maintained in normal range

Client Will (Include Specific Time Frame)
• Acknowledge factors that may lead to unstable glucose.
• Verbalize understanding of body and energy needs.
• Verbalize plan for modifying factors to prevent or minimize shifts in glucose level.
• Maintain glucose in satisfactory range.

ACTIONS/INTERVENTIONS

Sample **NIC** linkages:
Hyperglycemia Management: Preventing and treating above-normal blood glucose levels
Teaching: Disease Process: Assisting the patient to understand information related to a specific disease process
Teaching: Prescribed Medication: Preparing a patient to safely take prescribed medications and monitor for their effects

NURSING PRIORITY NO. 1

To assess risk/contributing factors:

● Determine individual factors as listed in Risk Factors. *Client or family history of diabetes; known diabetic with poor glucose control; eating disorders (e.g., morbid obesity); poor exercise habits; failure to recognize changes in glucose needs or control due to adolescent growth spurts or pregnancy can result in problems with glucose stability.*
● Ascertain client's/SO's knowledge and understanding of condition and treatment needs.
● Identify individual perceptions and expectations of treatment regimen.
● Note influence of cultural or religious factors impacting dietary practices, taking responsibility for own care, expectations of outcomes. *These factors will influence client's ability to manage condition and must be considered when planning care.*
● Determine client's awareness and ability to be responsible for dealing with situation. *Age, developmental level, and current health status affect client's ability to provide for own safety.*
● Assess client family/SO(s) support of client. *Client may need assistance with lifestyle changes (e.g., food preparation, consumption, timing of intake and/or exercise, administration of medications).*
● Note availability and use of resources.

NURSING PRIORITY NO. 2

To assist client to develop preventative strategies to avoid glucose instability:

● Ascertain whether client/SOs are adept at operating client's home glucose-monitoring device. *All available machines will provide satisfactory readings if properly used, maintained, and routinely calibrated.*[1]

- Provide information on balancing food intake, antidiabetic agents, and energy expenditure.
- Review medical necessity for regularly scheduled lab screening tests for diabetes. *Tests including fasting and daily glucose levels, HgbA1c help identify acute and long-term glucose control.*[2,3]
- Discuss home glucose-monitoring according to individual parameters (e.g., six times per day for normal day and more frequently during times of stress) *to identify and manage glucose fluctuations.*[2]
- Identify common situations that contribute to client's glucose instability on daily, occasional, or crisis basis. *Multiple factors can be in play at any time, such as missing meals, an adolescent growth spurt, infection or other illness.*
- Review client's diet, especially carbohydrate intake. *Glucose balance is determined by the amount of carbohydrates consumed, which should be determined in needed grams/day.*[4]
- Encourage client to read labels and choose foods described as having a low glycemic index, higher fiber, and low-fat content. *These foods produce a slower rise in blood glucose and more stable release of insulin.*[5]
- Discuss how client's antidiabetic medication(s) work. *Drugs and combinations of drugs work in varying ways with different blood glucose control and side effects. Understanding drug actions can help client avoid or reduce risk of potential for hypoglycemic reactions.*[6]

For client receiving insulin:

- Emphasize importance of checking expiration dates of medication, inspecting insulin for cloudiness if it is normally clear, and monitoring proper storage and preparation (when mixing required). *Affects insulin absorbability and effectiveness.*[1]
- Review type(s) of insulin used (e.g., rapid, short, intermediate, long-acting, premixed) and delivery method (e.g., subcutaneous, intramuscular injection; inhaled; pump). Note time when short-acting and long-acting insulins are administered. Remind client that only short-acting insulin is used in pump. *Affects timing of effects and provides clues to potential timing of glucose instability.*[1,7]
- Check injection sites periodically. *Insulin absorption can vary from day to day in healthy sites and is less absorbable in lumpy sites.*[7]
- Ascertain that all injections are being given. *Children, teenagers, and elderly client may forget injections or be unable to self-inject, may need reminders and supervision.*[7]

NURSING PRIORITY NO. 3

To promote wellness (Teaching/Discharge Considerations):

- Review individual risk factors and provide information *to assist client in efforts to avoid complications, such as caused by chronic hyperglycemia and acute hypoglycemia. Note: Hyperglycemia is most commonly caused by alterations in nutrition needs, inactivity, or inadequate use of antidiabetic medications. Hypoglycemia is the most common complication of antidiabetic therapy, stress, and exercise.*[1,8-10]
- Emphasize consequences of actions and choices —both immediate and long term. *Close control of glucose levels over time has been shown to delay onset and reduce severity of complications enhancing quality of life.*
- Engage client/family/caregiver in formulating plan *to manage blood glucose level incorporating lifestyle, age, developmental level, physical and psychological ability to manage condition.*
- Consult with dietitian about specific dietary needs based on individual situation (e.g., growth spurt, pregnancy, change in activity level following injury).
- Encourage client to develop a system for self-monitoring *to provide a sense of control and enable client to follow own progress and assist with making choices.*

⊛ • Refer to appropriate community resources, diabetic educator, and/or support groups as needed *for lifestyle modification, medical management, referral for insulin pump or glucose monitor, financial assistance for supplies, and so forth.*

DOCUMENTATION FOCUS

Assessment/Reassessment
- Findings related to individual situation, risk factors, current caloric intake and dietary pattern; prescription medication use; monitoring of condition.
- Client's/caregiver's understanding of individual risks and potential complications.
- Results of laboratory tests and fingerstick testing.

Planning
- Plan of care and who is involved in planning.
- Teaching plan.

Implementation/Evaluation
- Individual responses to interventions, teaching, and actions performed.
- Specific actions and changes that are made.
- Attainment or progress toward desired outcomes.
- Modifications to plan of care.

Discharge Planning
- Long-term plans for ongoing needs, monitoring, and management of condition, and who is responsible for actions to be taken.
- Sources for equipment and supplies.
- Specific referrals made.

References

1. Monitoring diabetes control. Diabetes Manual. Royal Children's Hospital. Retrieved January 2009 from www.rch.org.au/diabetesmanual/manual.cfm?doc_id=2738.
2. Gardner, B. M. (2002). Current approaches to type 2 diabetes mellitus. Article for Medscape CME. American Academy of Family Physicians (AAFP) 2002 Annual Scientific Assembly Common Clinical Problem Update and Family Medicine research. Retrieved September 2009 from www.medscape.com/viewarticle/444348.
3. Buse, J. B. (2003). Normal A1c but unstable blood glucose. Retrieved January 2007 from www.medscape.com/viewarticle/46302.
4. Moshang, J. (2005). The growing problem of type 2 diabetes. *LPN*, 1(3), 26–34.
5. Diabetes and healthy eating. Better Health Channel Fact Sheet (2000–2004). Victoria, Australia. Retrieved January 2007 from www.betterhealth.vic.gov.au.
6. Davis, J. L. (2006). New type 2 diabetes treatment options. Retrieved January 2007 from www.webmd.com/content/Article/129/117304.htm.
7. Haines, C. (2006). Diabetes: Treating diabetes with insulin. Retrieved January 2007 from www.webmd.com/content/Article/46/1667_50931.htm.
8. Iscoe, K. E., et al. (2006). Efficacy of continuous real-time blood glucose monitoring during and after prolonged high-intensity cycling exercise: Spinning with a continuous glucose monitoring system. *Diabetes Technol Ther*, 8(6), 627–635.
9. McLeod, M. E. (2006). Interventions for clients with diabetes mellitus. In Ignativicius, D. D., Workman, M. L. (eds). *Medical-Surgical Nursing: Critical Thinking for Collaborative Care.* 5th ed. Philadelphia: Elsevier Saunders.
10. Asp, A. A. (2005). Diabetes mellitus. In Copstead, L. C., Banasik, J. L. (eds). *Pathophysiology.* 3d ed. Philadelphia: Elsevier Saunders.

Grieving

DEFINITION: A normal complex process that includes emotional, physical, spiritual, social, and intellectual responses and behaviors by which individuals, families, and communities incorporate an actual, anticipated, or perceived loss into their daily lives

RELATED FACTORS

Anticipatory loss/loss of significant object (e.g., possessions, job, status, home, parts and processes of body)
Anticipatory loss or death of a significant other

DEFINING CHARACTERISTICS

Subjective
Anger; pain; suffering; despair; blame
Alteration in activity level, sleep or dream patterns
Making meaning of the loss; personal growth
Experiencing relief

Objective
Detachment; disorganization; psychological distress; panic behavior
Maintaining the connection to the deceased
Alterations in immune or neuroendocrine function

Sample Clinical Applications: Cancer, traumatic injuries (e.g., brain or spinal cord), amputation, chronic or debilitating conditions (e.g., renal failure, chronic obstructive pulmonary disease [COPD], multiple sclerosis [MS], amyotrophic lateral sclerosis [ALS]), genetic or birth defects, community disaster

DESIRED OUTCOMES/EVALUATION CRITERIA

Sample NOC linkages:
Grief Resolution: Adjustment to actual or impending loss
Caregiver Emotional Health: Emotional well-being of a family care provider while caring for a family member

Client Will (Include Specific Time Frame)
• Identify and express feelings (e.g., sadness, guilt, fear) freely and effectively.
• Acknowledge impact or effect of the grieving process (e.g., physical problems of eating, sleeping) and seek appropriate help.
• Look toward and plan for future, one day at a time.

Sample NOC linkages:
Community Competence: Capacity of a community to collectively problem-solve to achieve community goals

Community Will (Include Specific Time Frame)
• Recognize needs of citizens, including underserved population.
• Activate or develop plan to address identified needs.

(continues on page 378)

Grieving (continued)
ACTIONS/INTERVENTIONS

Sample (NIC) linkages:
Grief Work Facilitation: Assistance with the resolution of a significant loss
Grief Work Facilitation: Perinatal Death: Assistance with the resolution of a perinatal loss
Dying Care: Promotion of physical comfort and psychological peace in the final phase of life

NURSING PRIORITY NO. 1

To assess causative/contributing factors:

● Determine circumstances of current situation (e.g., sudden death, prolonged fatal illness, loved one kept alive by extreme medical interventions). *Grief can be anticipatory (mourning the loss of loved one's former self before actual death) or actual. Both types of grief can provoke a wide range of intense and often conflicting feelings. Grief also follows losses other than death (e.g., traumatic loss of a limb, or loss of home by a tornado, loss of known self due to brain injury).*[11]
● Determine significance of loss to community (e.g., school bus accident with loss of life, major storm with damage to community infrastructure, financial failure of major employer).
● Determine client's perception of anticipated or actual loss and meaning to him or her. "What are your concerns?" "What are your fears? Your greatest fear?" "How do you see this affecting you and your lifestyle?" *Identifying the needs to be addressed and acknowledging the client's responses are integral to planning care.*[9] *Some individuals may use anticipatory grieving as a defense against the inevitable loss. While some people may find this helpful when the loss occurs, many people find that intense feelings occur regardless of the period of anticipation.*[2]
● Ascertain response of family/SO(s) to client's situation/concerns. *Family concerns affect client and need to be listened to and appropriate interventions taken. Problems may arise if family completes grieving prematurely and disengages from the dying member, who then feels abandoned at a time when the support is needed.*[2]

NURSING PRIORITY NO. 2

To determine current response:

● Note emotional responses, such as withdrawal, angry behavior, crying. Provide information about normal stages of grieving. *Awareness allows for appropriate choice of interventions because individuals handle grief in different ways. Knowledge promotes understanding of emotional responses.*[4]
● Observe client's body language and check out meaning with the client. Note congruency of body language with verbalizations. *Body language is open to interpretation and needs to be validated so misinterpretation does not occur. Client may be saying one thing, but often body language is saying something else; identifying incongruencies can provide opportunity for individual to understand self in relation to grieving process.*[2]
● Note cultural and religious factors and expectations that may impact client's responses to situation. *Beliefs vary with the individual/community and will affect responses to the situation (e.g., Arab Americans may want to pray in silence or private; African Americans may*

use faith and root healers in conjunction with biomedical resources; groups may congregate at site of disaster or at church to grieve together).[5,8]

- Determine impact on general well-being (e.g., increased frequency of minor illnesses, exacerbation of chronic condition, problems with eating, activity level, sexual desire, role performance [e.g., work, parenting]). *Indicators of severity of feelings client is experiencing and need for specific interventions to resolve these issues.*[5]
- Note family communication and interaction patterns. *Dysfunctional patterns of communication such as avoidance, preaching, giving advice can block effective communication and isolate family members.*[3]
- Discuss with client and family/SOs, and others as appropriate, plans that need to be made as well as anticipated adjustments and role changes related to the situation. Encourage and answer questions as needed. *This type of discussion will bring concerns out in the open and help with adaptation to the loss.*[5,11]
- Determine availability and use of community resources and support groups. *Appropriate use of support can help the individual feel less isolated and can promote feelings of inclusion and comfort.*[6]
- Note community plans in place to deal with major loss (e.g., team of crisis counselors stationed at a school to address the loss of classmates; vocational counselors or retraining programs, outreach of services from neighboring communities).

NURSING PRIORITY NO. 3

To assist client/community to deal with situation:

- Provide open environment and trusting relationship. *Promotes a free discussion of feelings and concerns in a safe environment where client can reveal innermost fears and beliefs about anticipated loss.*[2]
- Use therapeutic communication skills of Active-listening, silence, acknowledgment. Respect client desire or request not to talk. *These skills convey belief in ability of client to deal with situation and develop a sense of competence. Client may not be ready to discuss feelings and situation, and respecting client's own timeline conveys confidence.*[2,3]
- Inform children about the anticipated or actual death or loss in age-appropriate language. *Providing accurate information about loss or change in life situation will help the child begin the mourning process.*[10]
- Give permission to child to express feelings about situation and ask questions, being careful to provide honest answers within child's understanding. *Adults may be uncomfortable or upset talking about death or loss, and children may be excluded from adult conversation about what is happening.*[10]
- Provide puppets or play therapy for toddlers/young children. *Young children do not have the ability to express their feelings verbally; use of play may help them express grief and help deal with loss in ways that are appropriate to the age.*[2]
- Permit appropriate expressions of anger, fear. Note hostility toward spiritual power or feelings of abandonment. *Anger is a normal part of the grieving process, and talking about these feelings allows individual to think about them and move on, coming to some resolution regarding the anticipated loss.*[6] (Refer to ND Spiritual Distress for additional interventions.)
- Provide information about normalcy of individual grief reaction. *Many people are not familiar with grief and are concerned that what they are experiencing is not normal. Letting them know that grief takes many forms and what they are feeling is all right helps them deal with what is happening.*[9]

Nursing Diagnoses in Alphabetical Order

- Be honest when answering questions, providing information. *Enhances nurse-client relationship, promoting trust and confidence.*[2]
- Provide assurance to child that cause for situation is not his or her own doing, bearing in mind age and developmental level. *May lessen sense of guilt and affirm there is no need to assign blame to self or any family member.*[2]
- Provide hope within parameters of individual situation. *Assisting client to find the positives will help with management of current situation.* Do not give false reassurance. *Comments such as "Everything will be all right" or "Don't worry" are not helpful and convey lack of understanding to the client.*[2]
- Review past life experiences and previous loss(es), role changes, and coping skills used, noting strengths and successes. *Useful in dealing with current situation and problem-solving existing needs.*[4]
- Discuss control issues, such as what is in the power of the individual to change and what is beyond control. *Recognition of these factors helps client focus energy for maximal benefit and outcome on what can be done.*[4]
- Incorporate family/SO(s) in problem-solving. *Encourages family to support and assist client to deal with situation while meeting needs of family members.*[6]
- Determine client's status and role in family (e.g., parent, sibling, child), and address loss of family member role. *Client's illness affects usual activities in the role he or she has in the family, and inevitably affects all the other family members as responsibilities are taken over by them.*[6]
- Instruct in use of visualization and relaxation techniques. *These skills can be helpful to reduce anxiety and stress and help client and family members manage grief more effectively.*[7]
- Use sedatives or tranquilizers with caution. *While the use of these medications may be helpful in the short term, too much dependence on them may retard passage through the grief process.*[2]
- Mobilize resources when client is the community. *When anticipated loss affects community as a whole, such as closing of manufacturing plant, impending disaster (e.g., wildfire, terrorist concerns), multiple supports will be required to deal with size and complexity of situation. Indeed, when more people are directly or indirectly involved in the anticipated or actual loss, emotions and anxiety tend to be amplified and transmitted, thus complicating the situation.*[1]
- Encourage community members/groups to engage in talking about event or loss and verbalizing feelings. Seek out underserved populations to include in process. *Increases likelihood that the needs of the entire community are identified and addressed.*
- Encourage individuals to participate in activities to deal with loss and rebuild community. *Exercising control in a productive manner empowers individuals and promotes rebuilding of life and community.*

NURSING PRIORITY NO. 4

To promote wellness (Teaching/Discharge Considerations):

- Provide information that feelings are okay and are to be expressed appropriately. Set limits regarding destructive behavior. *Talking about feelings can facilitate the grieving process, but destructive behavior can be damaging to the self-esteem.*[2]
- Discuss recurring nature of grief reactions. *On birthdays, major holidays, at times of significant personal events, or anniversary of loss, intense grief reactions may occur for a long time after the loss. If these reactions start to disrupt day-to-day functioning, client may need to seek help.*[1] (Refer to NDs such as ineffective community Coping, complicated Grieving.)

🏠 ● Encourage continuation of usual activities and schedule, and involvement in appropriate exercise program, as appropriate and able. *Promotes sense of control and self-worth, enabling client to feel more positive about ability to handle situation.*[6]

🏠 ● Identify and promote involvement of family and social support systems. *A supportive environment enhances the effectiveness of interventions and promotes a successful grieving process.*[4]

🏠 ● Discuss and assist with planning for future or funeral, as appropriate. *Involving family members in this discussion assures that everyone knows what is desired and what is planned, thus avoiding unexpected disagreements.*[4]

☣ ● Refer to additional resources, such as pastoral care, counseling or psychotherapy, organized community support groups, as indicated, for both client and family/SO. *Useful for ongoing needs and facilitation of grieving process.*[6,8]

🏠 ● Identify resources and develop community plan to address anticipated large-scale losses. *Preparation for complex challenges facilitates prompt response as needs occur.*

🏠 ● Support community efforts to strengthen support and develop plan to foster recovery and growth.

DOCUMENTATION FOCUS

Assessment/reassessment
• Assessment findings, including client's perception of anticipated loss and signs/symptoms that are being exhibited.
• Responses of family/SO(s) or community members, as indicated.
• Availability and use of resources.

Planning
• Plan of care and who is involved in planning.
• Teaching plan.

Implementation/Evaluation
• Client's response to interventions, teaching, and actions performed.
• Attainment or progress toward desired outcome(s).
• Modifications to plan of care.

Discharge planning
• Long term needs and who is responsible for actions to be taken.
• Specific referrals made.

References

1. Sharma, V. P. (1996). Normal mourning and "complicated grief". Retrieved March 2007 from www.Mindpub.com/art045.htm.
2. Townsend, M. C. (2003). *Psychiatric Mental Health Nursing Concepts of Care.* 4th ed. Philadelphia: F. A. Davis.
3. Gordon, T. (2000). *Parent Effectiveness Training.* Updated ed. New York: Three Rivers Press.
4. Cox, H. C., et al. (2002). *Clinical Applications of Nursing Diagnosis: Adult, Child, Women's, Psychiatric, Gerontic, and Home Health Considerations.* 4th ed. Philadelphia: F. A. Davis.
5. Lipson, J. G., Dibble, S. L., Minarik, P. A. (1996). *Culture & Nursing Care: A Pocket Guide.* San Francisco: UCSF Nursing Press.
6. Doenges, M. E., Townsend, M. C., Moorhouse, M. F. (1998). *Psychiatric Care Plans: Guidelines for Individualizing Care.* 3d ed. Philadelphia: F. A. Davis.
7. Pearce, J. C. (2002). *The Biology of Transcendence: A Blueprint of the Human Spirit.* Rochester, VT: Park Street Press.

8. Matzo, M., et al. (2002). Teaching cultural consideration at the end of life. End of Life Nursing Education Consortium program recommendations. *J Contin Edu Nurs*, 33(6), 270–278.

9. Neeld, E. H. (2003). *Seven Choices*. 4th ed. Austin, TX: Centerpoint Press.

10. Riely, M. (2003). Facilitating Children's Grief. *J School Nurs*, 19(4), 212–218.

11. Anticipatory grief. Retrieved March 2007 from Featured Columns under Life Topics/Grief & Loss for Psychologist 4therapy Web site, www.4therapy.com.

complicated Grieving

DEFINITION: A disorder that occurs after the death of a significant other, in which the experience of distress accompanying bereavement fails to follow normative expectations and manifests in functional impairment

RELATED FACTORS

Death or sudden death of a significant other
Emotional instability
Lack of social support
[Loss of significant object (e.g., possessions, job, status, home, parts and processes of body)]

DEFINING CHARACTERISTICS

Subjective
Verbalizes anxiety; lack of acceptance of the death; persistent, painful memories; distressful feelings about the deceased; self-blame
Verbalizes feelings of anger; disbelief; detachment from others
Verbalizes feeling dazed; empty; stunned; in shock
Decreased sense of well-being; fatigue; low levels of intimacy; depression
Yearning

Objective
Decreased functioning in life roles
Persistent emotional distress; separation or traumatic distress
Preoccupation with thoughts of the deceased; longing for the deceased; searching for the deceased; self-blame
Experiencing somatic symptoms of the deceased
Rumination
Grief avoidance

Sample Clinical Applications: Death of significant other, traumatic loss, depression, attempted suicide

DESIRED OUTCOMES/EVALUATION CRITERIA

Sample NOC linkages:
Depression Level: Severity of melancholic mood and loss of interest in life events
Grief Resolution: Adjustment to actual or impending loss
Psychosocial Adjustment: Life Change: Adaptive psychosocial responses of an individual to a significant life change

Cultural　Collaborative　Community/Home Care　Diagnostic Studies　Pediatric/Geriatric/Lifespan　Medications

Client Will (Include Specific Time Frame)
• Acknowledge presence and impact of dysfunctional situation.
• Demonstrate progress in dealing with stages of grief at own pace.
• Participate in work and self-care and activities of daily living (ADLs), as able.
• Verbalize a sense of progress toward resolution of the grief and hope for the future.

ACTIONS/INTERVENTIONS

Sample NIC linkages:
Grief Work Facilitation: Assistance with the resolution of a significant loss
Grief Work Facilitation: Perinatal Death: Assistance with the resolution of a perinatal loss
Coping Enhancement: Assisting a patient to adapt to perceived stressors, changes, or threats that interfere with meeting life demands and roles

NURSING PRIORITY NO. 1

To determine causative/contributing factors:

• Identify loss that is present. Note circumstances of death such as sudden or traumatic (e.g., fatal accident, homicide), related to socially sensitive issue (e.g., AIDS, suicide), or associated with unfinished business (e.g., spouse died during time of crisis in marriage, son has not spoken to parent for years). *These situations can sometimes cause individual to become stuck in grief and unable to move forward with life.*[11–13]
• Determine significance of the loss to client (e.g., presence of chronic condition leading to divorce or disruption of family unit and change in lifestyle or financial security). *The more complicated or devastating the loss is to the individual, the more likely she or he will have difficulty reaching resolution.*
• Identify cultural or religious beliefs and expectations *that may impact or dictate client's response to loss.*
• Ascertain response of family/SO(s) to situation (e.g., sympathetic or urging client to "just get over it"). Assess needs of SO(s). *Response of family members will affect how client is dealing with situation—this information is important for planning care to enable all members to effectively cope with events.*[9]

NURSING PRIORITY NO. 2

To determine degree of impairment/dysfunction:

• Observe for cues of sadness (e.g., sighing, faraway look, unkempt appearance, inattention to conversation, somatic complaints such as exhaustion, headaches). *Indicators of the extent of grief and how individual is dealing with situation.*[6]
• Identify stage of grief being expressed: denial, isolation, anger, bargaining, depression, acceptance. *Helps to establish how client is dealing with grieving and degree of difficulty client is having adjusting to the death or loss.*[10]
• Listen to words and communications indicative of renewed or intense grief (e.g., constantly bringing up death or loss even in casual conversation long after event; outbursts of anger at relatively minor events; expressing desire to die), *indicating person is possibly unable to adjust/move on from feelings of intense grief.*[12]
• Determine level of functioning, ability to care for self, and use of support systems and community resources. *Individual may be incapacitated by depth of loss and be unable to manage day-to-day activities adequately, necessitating intervention and assistance.*[6]

- Be aware of avoidance behaviors (e.g., anger; withdrawal; long periods of sleeping or refusing to interact with family; sudden or radical changes in lifestyle; inability to handle everyday responsibilities at home, work, or school; conflict). *Additional indicators of depth of grieving being experienced and need for more intensive support and monitoring to help client deal effectively with death or loss.*[10,11]
- Determine if client is engaging in reckless or self-destructive behaviors (e.g., substance abuse, heavy drinking, promiscuity, or aggression) *to identify safety issues.*[1]
- Identify cultural factors and ways individual(s) has dealt with previous loss(es). *Way of expressing self may reflect cultural background and religious beliefs. Understanding cultural expectations will help put current behavior and responses in context and determine the nature and degree of dysfunction.*[8]
- Perform or refer for psychological testing, as indicated (e.g., Beck's Depression Scale). *Determines degree of depression and indication of need for medication.*[2]

NURSING PRIORITY NO. 3

To assist client/others to deal appropriately with loss:

- Encourage verbalization without confrontation about realities. *It is helpful to listen without correcting misperceptions in the beginning, allowing free flow of expression. Provides opportunity for reflection aiding resolution and acceptance.*[6]
- Encourage client to choose topics of conversation and refrain from forcing client to "face the facts." *Talking freely about concerns can help client identify what is important to deal with and how to cope with situation.*[9]
- Active-listen feelings and be available for support or assistance. Speak in soft, caring voice. *Communicates acceptance and caring, enabling client to seek own answers to current situation.*[3]
- Encourage expression of anger, fear and anxiety. (Refer to appropriate NDs.) *These feelings are part of the grieving process, and to accomplish the work of grieving, they need to be expressed and accepted.*[9]
- Permit verbalization of anger with acknowledgment of feelings and setting of limits regarding destructive behavior. *Enhances client safety, promotes resolution of grief process by encouraging expression of feelings that are not usually accepted, and supports self-esteem.*[2]
- Acknowledge reality of feelings of guilt or blame, including hostility toward spiritual power. Do not minimize loss; avoid clichés and easy answers. (Refer to ND Spiritual Distress.) *Reinforces that feelings are acceptable and allows client to become aware of own thoughts and begin to deal with feelings.*[1,7]
- Respect the client's needs and wishes for quiet, privacy, talking, or silence. *Individual may not be ready to talk about or share grief and needs to be allowed to make own timeline.*[6]
- Give "permission" to be at this point when the client is depressed. *Assures client that feelings are normal and can be a starting point to deal in a positive manner with loss/death that has occurred.*[9]
- Provide comfort and availability as well as caring for physical needs. *Client needs to know he or she will be supported and helped when not able to care for self.*[6]
- Reinforce use of previously effective coping skills. Instruct in and encourage use of visualization and relaxation techniques. *Identifying and discussing how client has dealt with loss in the past can provide opportunities in the current situation. Use of these techniques helps client to learn to relax and consider options for dealing with loss.*[2]
- Assist SOs to cope with client's response. Include age-specific interventions. *Family/SO(s) may not understand/be intolerant of client's distress and inadvertently hamper client's*

progress. Family members, including children, may express their feelings in anger, result-ing in punishment for behavior that is deemed unacceptable rather than recognized as the basis in grief.[10]

- Include family/SO(s) in setting realistic goals for meeting needs of client and family members. *Involving all members enhances the probability that each member will express their needs and hear what the needs of others are, ensuring a more effective outcome.*[2]
- Use sedatives or tranquilizers with caution. *While the use of these medications may be helpful in the short term, too much dependence on them may retard passage through the grief process.*[2]
- Refer to mental health provider for specific diagnostic studies and intervention in issues associated with complicated grief.[13]
- Refer to ND Grieving for additional interventions as appropriate.

NURSING PRIORITY NO. 4

To promote wellness (Teaching/Discharge Considerations):

- Discuss with client/SO healthy ways of dealing with difficult situations. *Identifying ways individual(s) has dealt with losses in the past will help identify strengths and successes and what might be useful in the current situation.*[2]
- Have individual(s) identify familial, religious, and cultural factors that have meaning. *One's family of origin has a major impact on what the individuals learn about these issues and how to deal with losses. Identifying and discussing how they affect the current situation may help bring loss into perspective and facilitate grief resolution.*[8]
- Encourage involvement in usual activities, exercise, and socialization within limits of physical ability and psychological state. *Keeping life to a somewhat normal routine can provide individual(s) with some sense of control over events that are not controllable.*[8]
- Suggest client keep a journal of experiences and feelings. *As client writes about what is happening, new insights may occur. Reading over what has been written can help individual see progress that has been made and begin to have hope for the future.*[9]
- Advocate planning for the future as appropriate to individual situation (e.g., staying in own home after death of spouse, returning to sporting activities following traumatic amputation, choice to have another child or to adopt, rebuilding home following a disaster). *Provides a sense of control and purpose and ensures that individual's wishes will be heard and respected.*[10]
- Identify volunteer opportunities (e.g., working with children at risk, raising funds for favorite charity, investigating new employment or relocation opportunities, participating in community reorganization or clean up). *Exercising control in a productive manner empowers individuals and promotes rebuilding of life and community.*
- Refer to other resources (e.g., pastoral care, family counseling, psychotherapy, organized support groups—widow's group) as indicated. *Provides additional support to resolve situation, continue grief work.*[8]

DOCUMENTATION FOCUS

Assessment/Reassessment
- Assessment findings, including meaning of loss to the client, current stage of the grieving process, and responses of family/SOs.
- Cultural or religious beliefs and expectations.
- Availability and use of resources.

Planning
• Plan of care and who is involved in the planning.
• Teaching plan.

Implementation/Evaluation
• Client's response to interventions, teaching, and actions performed.
• Attainment or progress toward desired outcome(s).
• Modifications to plan of care.

Discharge Planning
• Long-term needs and who is responsible for actions to be taken.
• Specific referrals made.

References

1. Lubit, R. (2005). Acute treatment of disaster survivors. Retrieved March 2007 from www.emedicine.com/med/topic3540.htm.
2. Townsend, M. C. (2003). *Psychiatric Mental Health Nursing Concepts of Care*. 4th ed. Philadelphia: F. A. Davis.
3. Gordon, T. (2000). *Parent Effectiveness Training*. Updated ed. New York: Three Rivers Press.
4. Cox, H. C., et al. (2002). *Clinical Applications of Nursing Diagnosis: Adult, Child, Women's, Psychiatric, Gerontic, and Home Health Considerations*. 4th ed. Philadelphia: F. A. Davis.
5. Lipson, J. G., Dibble, S. L., Minarik, P. A. (1996). *Culture & Nursing Care: A Pocket Guide*. San Francisco: UCSF Nursing Press.
6. Doenges, M. E., Townsend, M. C., Moorhouse, M. F. (1998). *Psychiatric Care Plans: Guidelines for Individualizing Care*. 3d ed. Philadelphia: F. A. Davis.
7. Pearce, J. C. (2002). *The Biology of Transcendence: A Blueprint of the Human Spirit*. Rochester, VT: Park Street Press.
8. Matzo, M., et al. (2002). Teaching cultural consideration at the end of life. End of Life Nursing Education Consortium program recommendations. *J Contin Edu Nurs*, 33(6), 270–278.
9. Neeld, E. H. (2003). *Seven Choices*. 4th ed. Austin, TX: Centerpoint Press.
10. Riely, M. (2003). Facilitating children's grief. *J School Nurs*, 19(4), 212–218.
11. Sharma, V. P. (1996). Normal mourning and "complicated grief." Retrieved March 2007 from www.Mindpub.com/art045.htm.
12. Sometimes grief becomes complicated, unresolved or stuck. Retrieved March 2007 from Featured Columns under Life Topics/Grief & Loss for Psychologist 4therapy Web site, www.4therapy.com.
13. Kersting, K. (2004). A new approach to complicated grief. *Monitor on Psychology*, 35(10), 51.

risk for complicated Grieving

DEFINITION: At risk for a disorder that occurs after the death of a significant other, in which the experience of distress accompanying bereavement fails to follow normative expectations and manifests in functional impairment

RISK FACTORS

Death of a significant other
Emotional instability
Lack of social support

Cultural Collaborative Community/Home Care Diagnostic Studies Pediatric/Geriatric/Lifespan Medications

[Loss of significant object (e.g., possessions, job, status, home, parts and processes of body)]

NOTE: A risk diagnosis is not evidenced by signs and symptoms, as the problem has not occurred; rather, nursing interventions are directed at prevention.

Sample Clinical Applications: Death of significant other, depression

DESIRED OUTCOMES/EVALUATION CRITERIA

Sample (NOC) linkages:
Personal Resiliency: Positive adaptation and function of an individual following significant adversity or crisis
Grief Resolution: Adjustment to actual or impending loss
Psychosocial Adjustment: Life Change: Psychosocial adaptation of an individual to a life change

Client Will (Include Specific Time Frame)
• Acknowledge awareness of individual factors affecting client in this situation. (See Risk Factors.)
• Identify emotional responses and behaviors occurring after the death or loss.
• Participate in therapy to learn new ways of dealing with anxiety and feelings of inadequacy.
• Discuss meaning of loss to individual or family.
• Verbalize a sense of beginning to deal with grief process.

ACTIONS/INTERVENTIONS

Sample (NIC) linkages:
Grief Work Facilitation: Assistance with the resolution of a significant loss
Grief Work Facilitation: Perinatal Death: Assistance with the resolution of a perinatal loss
Coping Enhancement: Assisting a patient to adapt to perceived stressors, changes, or threats that interfere with meeting life demands and roles

NURSING PRIORITY NO. 1

To identify risk/contributing factors:

• Determine loss that has occurred and meaning to client. Note if death was sudden or traumatic (e.g., fatal accident, homicide), related to socially sensitive issue (e.g., AIDS, suicide), or associated with unfinished business (e.g., spouse died during time of crisis in marriage, son has not spoken to parent for years). *These situations can sometimes cause individual to become stuck in grief and unable to move forward with life.*[1]

∞ • Ascertain circumstances surrounding loss of fetus/infant/child (e.g., gestational age of fetus, multiple miscarriages, death due to violence or fatal illness). *Repeated losses and/or violent death can increase client's/SO's sense of futility and compromise resolution of grieving process.*[2]

∞ • Meet with both parents following loss of child *to determine how they are dealing with the loss together and individually. Death of a child is often more difficult for parents/family, based on individual values and sense of life unlived.*[2]

• Note stage of grief client is experiencing (e.g., denial, anger, bargaining, depression). *Stages of grief may progress in a predictable manner or stages may be random or revisited.*[3]

🏠 ● Assess client's ability to manage activities of daily living and period of time since loss has occurred. *Periods of crying, feelings of overwhelming sadness, loss of appetite, and insomnia can occur with grieving; however, when they persist and interfere with normal activities, client may need additional assistance.*[3]

🏠 ● Note availability and use of support systems, community resources.

● Listen to words and communications indicative of renewed or intense grief (e.g., constantly bringing up death or loss even in casual conversation long after event; outbursts of anger at relatively minor events; expressing desire to die), *indicating person is possibly unable to adjust or move on from feelings of intense grief.*[4]

🌐 ● Identify cultural or religious beliefs and expectations that may impact or dictate client's response to loss. *These factors affect current situation and may help bring loss into perspective and promote grief resolution.*[5]

● Assess status of relationships or marital difficulties and adjustments to loss. *Responses of family/SOs affect how client deals with situation.*[6]

NURSING PRIORITY NO. 2

To assist client to deal appropriately with loss:

● Discuss meaning of loss to client, Active-listen to responses without judgment. *The more complicated or devastating the loss is to the individual, the more likely she or he will have difficulty reaching resolution.*

● Respect client's desire for quiet, privacy, talking, or silence. *Individual may not be ready to talk about or share grief and needs to be allowed to make own time line.*[3]

● Encourage expression of feelings, including anger, fear, and anxiety. Let client know that all feelings are okay, while setting limits on destructive behavior. *These feelings are part of the grieving process, and to accomplish the work of grieving, they need to be expressed and accepted.*[3,6]

● Acknowledge client's sense of relief when death follows a long and debilitating course. *Sadness and loss are still there, but the death may be a release, or client may feel guilty about having a sense of relief.*

● Assist SOs/family to understand and be tolerant of client's feelings and behavior. *Family/SO(s) may not understand or be intolerant of client's distress and inadvertently hamper client's progress. Family members, including children, may express their feelings in anger, resulting in punishment for behavior that is deemed unacceptable, rather than recognizing the basis in grief.*[8]

NURSING PRIORITY NO. 3

To promote wellness (Teaching/Discharge Considerations):

🏠 ● Assist client/SOs to identify successful coping skills they have used in the past. *These can be used in current situation to facilitate dealing with grief.*[3]

🏠 ● Support client and family in setting goals for meeting needs of members for moving on beyond the grieving process.

🏠 ● Encourage resuming involvement in usual activities, exercise, and socialization within physical and psychological abilities. *Keeping life to a somewhat normal routine can provide individual with some sense of control over events that are not controllable.*[5]

🏠 ● Advocate planning for the future as appropriate to individual situation (e.g., staying in own home after death of spouse, returning to sporting activities following traumatic amputation, choice to have another child or to adopt, rebuilding home following a disaster). *Provides a sense of control and purpose and ensures that individual's wishes will be heard and respected.*[8]

● Refer to other resources, as needed, such as psychotherapy, family counseling, religious references or pastor, grief support group. *Depending upon meaning of the loss, individual may require ongoing support to work through grief.*[5]

DOCUMENTATION FOCUS

Assessment/Reassessment
• Assessment findings, including meaning of loss to the client, current stage of the grieving process, psychological status, and responses of family/SOs.
• Cultural or religious beliefs, expectations, and rituals.
• Availability and use of resources.

Planning
• Plan of care and who is involved in the planning.
• Teaching plan.

Implementation/Evaluation
• Client's response to interventions, teaching, and actions performed.
• Attainment or progress toward desired outcome(s).
• Modifications to plan of care.

Discharge Planning
• Long-term needs and who is responsible for actions to be taken.
• Specific referrals made.

References

1. Sharma, V. P. (1996). Normal mourning and "complicated grief". Retrieved March 2007 from www.Mindpub.com/art045.htm.
2. Doenges, M. E., Moorhouse, M. F., Murr, A. C. (2006). Risk for dysfunctional grieving. *Nurse's Pocket Guide: Diagnoses, Prioritized Interventions, and Rationales*. 10th ed. Philadelphia: F. A. Davis.
3. Doenges, M. E., Townsend, M. C., Moorhouse, M. F. (1998). *Psychiatric Care Plans: Guidelines for Individualizing Care*. 3d ed. Philadelphia: F. A. Davis.
4. Sometimes grief becomes complicated, unresolved or stuck. Retrieved March 2007 from Featured Columns under Life Topics/Grief & Loss for Psychologist 4therapy Web site, www.4therapy.com.
5. Matzo, M., et al. (2002). Teaching cultural considerations at the end of life. End of Life Nursing Education Consortium program recommendations. *J Contin Edu Nurs*, 33(6), 212–218.
6. Neeld, E. H. (2003). *Seven Choices*. 4th ed. Austin, TX: Centerpoint Press.
7. Kersting, K. (2004). A new approach to complicated grief. *Monitor on Psychology*, 35(10), 51.
8. Riely, M. (2003). Facilitating children's grief. *J School Nurs*, 19(4), 212–218.

delayed Growth and Development

DEFINITION: Deviations from age-group norms

RELATED FACTORS

Inadequate caretaking, [physical or emotional neglect or abuse]
Indifference, inconsistent responsiveness, multiple caretakers
Separation from significant others
Environmental and stimulation deficiencies
Effects of physical disability [handicapping condition]
Prescribed dependence [insufficient expectations for self-care]
[Physical or emotional illness (chronic, traumatic), such as chronic inflammatory disease, pituitary tumors, impaired nutrition/metabolism, greater-than-normal energy requirements, prolonged/painful treatments, prolonged or repeated hospitalizations]
[Sexual abuse]
[Substance use or abuse]

DEFINING CHARACTERISTICS

Subjective
Inability to perform self-care or self-control activities appropriate for age

Objective
Delay or difficulty in performing skills typical of age group; [loss of previously acquired skills, precocious or accelerated skill attainment]
Altered physical growth
Flat affect, listlessness, decreased responses
[Sleep disturbances, negative mood or response]

Sample Clinical Applications: Congenital or genetic disorders, prematurity, infection, nutritional problems (malnutrition, anorexia, failure to thrive), toxic exposures (e.g., lead), substance abuse, endocrine disorders, abuse or neglect, Down syndrome or developmental delay

DESIRED OUTCOMES/EVALUATION CRITERIA

Sample NOC linkages:
Child Development: [specify age group]: Milestones of physical, cognitive, and psychosocial progression by [specify] months/years of age
Physical Maturation: Female [or] Male: Normal physical changes in the female/male that occur with the transition from childhood to adulthood
Growth: Normal increase in bone size and body weight during growth years

Client Will (Include Specific Time Frame)
• Perform motor, social, and expressive skills typical of age group within scope of present capabilities.
• Perform self-care and self-control activities appropriate for age.
• Demonstrate weight and growth stabilization or progress toward age-appropriate size.

Sample **NOC** linkages:
Knowledge: Parenting: Extent of understanding conveyed about provision of a nurturing and constructive environment for a child from 1 to 17 years of age

Parents/Caregivers Will (Include Specific Time Frame)
• Verbalize understanding of growth or developmental delay or deviation and plan(s) for intervention.

ACTIONS/INTERVENTIONS

Sample **NIC** linkages:
Developmental Enhancement: Child [or] Adolescent : Facilitating or teaching parents/caregivers to facilitate the optimal gross motor, fine motor, language, cognitive, social, and emotional growth of preschool and school-age children/of individuals during the transition from childhood to adulthood
Nutritional Monitoring: Collection and analysis of patient data to prevent or minimize malnourishment
Developmental Care: Structuring the environment and providing care in response to the behavioral cues and states of the preterm infant

NURSING PRIORITY NO. 1

To assess causative/contributing factors:

● Determine existing condition(s) (e.g., limited intellectual capacity, physical disabilities, accelerated physical growth, early or delayed puberty, chronic illness, tumors, genetic anomalies, substance use or abuse, violence, poverty, birth of multiples, minimal length of time between pregnancies). *These conditions contribute to growth or developmental deviation, necessitating specific evaluation and interventions depending on the situation.*[6]

● Determine developmental delays using standard screening tests assessing cognitive abilities, communication, and social interactions. *Developmental surveillance is a flexible, ongoing process that involves the use of both skilled observation of the child and concerns of parents, health professionals, teachers, and others to identify children with variations in normal growth and development.*[1,10,11]

● Review results of lab tests (e.g., pituitary hormones) and diagnostic studies (e.g., radiographs, bone scans assessing bone growth plates and age) *to evaluate problems with growth and assist in determining interventions and treatment needs.*

● Active-listen to client's/parents' concerns about body size and actual or perceived limitations, ability to perform competitively (e.g., ability to participate in desired activities and lifestyle, perform in sports, body building). *Helps in identifying actual needs and provides emotional support in situation that is often difficult to manage over the years.*

● Ascertain cultural beliefs, norms, and values. *What is considered normal or abnormal growth and development may be influenced by familial and cultural perceptions.*[5]

● Determine nature of parenting/caretaking activities. *Presence of conflict and negative interaction between parent/caregiver and child (e.g., inadequate, inconsistent parenting, unrealistic or insufficient expectations; lack of stimulation, limit-setting, and responsiveness) interferes with the development of age-appropriate skills and maturation.*[1,3,12]

● Assess occurrence and frequency of significant stressful events, losses, separation, and environmental changes (e.g., loss, separation, abandonment, divorce; death of parent/sibling;

aging; unemployment, new job; moves; new baby/sibling, marriage, new stepparent). *Lack of resolution or repetition of stressor can have a cumulative effect over time and result in regression in/or deterioration of functional level.*

🏠 • Determine presence of environmental risk factors (e.g., exposure to toxins; active substance abusers in home; or child of parent(s) who are abusive, neglectful, or mentally disabled).[13,14]

🏠 • Note severity and pervasiveness of situation (e.g., long-term physical or emotional abuse versus situational disruption or inadequate assistance during period of crisis or transition). *Problems existing over a long period may have more severe effects and require longer course of treatment to reverse.*

🔘 • Evaluate home, day-care, hospital, or institutional environment *to determine adequacy of care provided, including nourishing meals, healthy sleep and rest time, stimulation, diversional or play activities.*

NURSING PRIORITY NO. 2

To determine degree of deviation from growth/developmental norms:

● Measure present growth age and stage. Record height and weight over time. *Provides baseline for identification of needs and determines trends and effectiveness of therapy.*[2]

● Determine expectations for current height and weight percentiles. *Measurements are compared to "standard" or normal range for children of same gender and age to determine degree of deviation.*[2]

● Note chronological age, familial factors (e.g., body build and stature) *to help determine individual developmental expectations (e.g., when child should roll over, sit up alone, speak first words, attain a certain weight and height), and how the expectations may be altered by child's condition. Pediatrician may screen with a motor quotient (MQ), which is child's age calculated by milestones met divided by chronological age and multiplied by 100. MQ between 50 and 70 requires further evaluation.*[3,9]

● Identify present developmental age and stage. Note reported deficits in functional level or evidence of precocious development. *Provides comparative baseline.*

● Review expected skills and activities, using authoritative text (e.g., Gesell, Musen/Congor), reports of neurological examinations, or assessment tools (e.g., Draw-a-Person, Denver Developmental Screening Test, Bender's Visual Motor Gestalt test, Early Language Milestone [ELM] Scale 2, and developmental language disorders [DLD]). *Provides guide for evaluation of growth and development, and for comparative measurement of individual's progress.*[4]

● Note degree of individual deviation, multiple skills affected (e.g., speech, motor activity, socialization vs. one area of difficulty such as toileting) and whether difficulty is temporary or permanent (e.g., setback or delay vs. irreversible condition, such as brain damage, stroke).

● Note signs of sexual maturation in child (e.g., development of pubic or axillary hair, breast enlargement, presence of body odor, acne, rapid linear growth, and adolescent-type behavior, with or without maturation of gonads). *Precocious puberty in females before age 8 or males before age 10 may occur because of lesions of hypothalamus or intracranial tumors.*

● Evaluate sexual behavior, as indicated. Investigate sexual acting-out behaviors inappropriate for age. *May indicate sexual abuse.*

● Note findings of psychological evaluation of client and family *to determine factors that may impact growth or development of client, or impair the psychological health of the family.*

NURSING PRIORITY NO. 3

To correct/minimize growth deviations and associated complications:

- Assist in therapies to treat or correct underlying medical or psychological conditions (e.g., intestinal malabsorption, malnourishment; infant feeding problems; kidney failure, congenital heart disease; cystic fibrosis, inflammatory bowel disease; bone or cartilage conditions; endocrine disorders [e.g., hypothyroidism, diabetes, growth hormone abnormalities], adverse side effects of medications; mental illness, substance abuse) as appropriate.[10] *May result in restoration of more normal developmental levels or growth patterns.*

- Collaborate with physician, nutritionist, and other specialists (e.g., physical or occupational therapist) in developing plan of care. *Multidisciplinary team care increases likelihood of developing a well-rounded plan of care that meets client's/family's specialized and varied needs.*

- Recommend involvement in regular exercise and sports program *to enhance muscle tone and strength and appropriate body building.*

- Administer and monitor responses to medications. *May be given to stimulate growth as appropriate, or possibly to shrink tumor when present.* Stress necessity of not stopping medications without approval of healthcare provider *in order to maximize benefit and limit adverse side effects.*

- Discuss appropriateness and potential complications of surgical interventions or radiation therapy when indicated *(e.g., to treat pituitary tumor, bone-lengthening procedures).*

- Plan for and stress importance of periodic evaluations. *Growth rates are measured in terms of how much a child grows within a specified time. These rates vary dramatically as a child grows (normal growth is a discontinuous process) and must be evaluated periodically over time to ascertain that child has definite growth disturbance. Accelerated or slowed growth rates are rarely normal and warrant further evaluation.*[2]

NURSING PRIORITY NO. 4

To assist clients (and/or caregivers) to prevent, minimize, or overcome delay/regressed or precocious development:

- Assist with treatment of underlying condition (e.g., inborn errors of metabolism—galactosemia, phenylketonuria; attention deficit disorder, autism), correct environmental factors (e.g., removal of lead paint) as appropriate.

- Provide anticipatory guidance for parents/care providers regarding expectations for client's development *to clarify misconceptions and assist them in dealing with reality of situation. May help in providing nurturing care.*[7]

- Describe realistic, age-appropriate patterns of development to parent/caregiver, whether child's deviation is likely to be temporary or permanent (setback or delay vs. permanent brain injury); and promote activities and interactions that support developmental tasks where client is at this time. *Increases likelihood of commitment to interventions in keeping with the child's current status and potential. Each child will have own unique strengths and difficulties. Some children will catch up with other children in early childhood; some will have problems into adulthood.*[1,5,6]

- Encourage recognition that certain deviations/behaviors are appropriate for a specific developmental age level (e.g., 14-year-old child functioning at level of 6-year-old child is not able to anticipate the consequences of his or her actions) or chronological age (e.g., 9-year-old is displaying pubertal changes). *Promotes acceptance of client as presented and helps shape expectations reflecting actual situation.*

Nursing Diagnoses in Alphabetical Order

- Encourage participation in "early intervention services" for child birth to 3 years of age with developmental delays. *Federally funded entitlement program for qualified child (e.g., Down syndrome or cerebral palsy; prematurity; deprived physical or social environment) aimed at maximizing child's development. Services include nursing, occupational, physical, or speech therapy; service coordination, social work, and assistive technologies.*[12]
- Communicate with client at appropriate cognitive level of development. Give client tasks and responsibilities appropriate to age or functional level *to model age and cognitively appropriate caregiver skills.*[8]
- Encourage client to perform activities of daily living (ADLs) as able. Discuss appropriateness of appearance, grooming, touching, language, play, safety, and other associated developmental issues. *Promotes independence and helps client develop sense of what is appropriate for age.*
- Involve client in opportunities to practice progress in activities of life or to try new behaviors (e.g., role play, group activities). *Facilitates learning process/retention of new skills.*
- Encourage setting of short-term, realistic goals for achieving developmental potential. Evaluate progress on continual basis *to increase complexity of tasks/goals as indicated.*
- Collaborate with additional professional resources (e.g., occupational, rehabilitation, or speech therapists; special education teacher; job counselor) *to address specific individual needs.*
- Maintain positive, hopeful attitude. Support self-actualizing nature of the client and attempts to achieve or return to optimal level of self-control or self-care activities.
- Provide positive feedback for efforts, successes, and adaptation while minimizing failures. *Encourages continuation of efforts, improving outcome.*
- Identify equipment needs and refer to suppliers (e.g., adaptive or growth-stimulating computer programs, communication devices) *to provide client/caregivers access to assistive devices that could improve involvement in and quality of life.*
- Assist client/caregivers to accept and adjust to irreversible developmental deviations (e.g., Down syndrome is not currently correctable). *Helps refocus attention and energy to areas that can be changed or improved.*
- Assist client/family to identify lifestyle changes that may be required (e.g., care for handicaps [blindness, musculoskeletal or cognitive deficits], proper use of assistive devices, learning new skills, development of routines and support systems).
- Provide support for caregiver during transitional crises (e.g., residential schooling, institutionalization).
- Refer family/client for counseling or psychotherapy to deal with issues of grief and loss, time and stress management, lifestyle changes, abuse or neglect and other needs as indicated.

NURSING PRIORITY NO. 5

To promote wellness (Teaching/Discharge Considerations):

- Provide information regarding normal growth and development process as appropriate. *Individuals need to know about normal process so deviations can be recognized when necessary.*
- Avoid blame when discussing contributing factors. *Parent/caregivers usually feel inadequate and blame themselves for being "a poor parent/care provider." Adding blame further diverts the individual's focus from learning new behaviors or making changes to achieve the desired outcomes.*
- Review reasonable expectations for individual without restricting potential (i.e., set realistic goals that, if met, can be advanced). *Provides hope for achievement and promotes continued personal growth.*
- Recommend involvement in regular exercise and sports medicine program *to enhance muscle tone and strength, and appropriate body building.*

- Review use of medications (e.g., steroids, growth hormones), *which can affect body growth and development. Potential for good and for harm exists in the use of these agents.*
- Recommend wearing medical alert bracelet when taking replacement hormones. *Provides information in case of an emergency.*
- Discuss consequences of substance use or abuse. *May be involved in the problems of growth and development that individual is experiencing.*[14]
- Suggest genetic testing or counseling for family/client dependent on causative factors. *May be necessary for planning for future pregnancies.*
- Stress importance of periodic reassessment of growth and development (e.g., periodic laboratory studies *to monitor hormone levels and nutritional status*). *Aids in evaluating effectiveness of interventions over time, and promotes early identification of need for additional actions, avoid preventable complications.*
- Encourage attendance at appropriate educational programs (e.g., parenting and expectant parent classes, infant stimulation sessions, seminars on life stresses, aging process). *Can provide information for client/family to learn to manage current situation and adapt to future changes.*
- Provide pertinent reference materials including reliable Web sites regarding normal growth and development as appropriate. *Bibliotherapy provides opportunity to review data at own pace, enhancing likelihood of retention.*
- Discuss community responsibilities (e.g., services required to be provided to school-age child). Include social worker or special education team in planning process *to meet educational, physical, psychological, and monitoring needs of child.*
- Identify community resources: public health programs such as Women, Infants, and Children (WIC), well-baby care provider; nutritionist, substance abuse programs; early intervention programs, seniors' activity or support groups, gifted and talented programs, Sheltered Workshop, crippled children's services, medical equipment and supplier. *Provides additional assistance to support family efforts in treatment program.*
- Refer to social services as indicated *to determine and monitor safety of client and consideration of placement in foster care.*
- Refer to the NDs interrupted Family Processes, impaired Parenting for additional interventions.

DOCUMENTATION FOCUS

Assessment/Reassessment
- Assessment findings, individual needs, including current growth status and trends, or developmental level and evidence of regression.
- Caregiver's understanding of situation and individual role.
- Cultural beliefs or values and expectations.
- Drug use or substance abuse.
- Safety of individual and need for placement.

Planning
- Plan of care and who is involved in the planning.
- Teaching plan.

Implementation/Evaluation
- Client's responses to interventions, teaching, and actions performed.
- Caregiver response to teaching.
- Attainment or progress toward desired outcome(s).
- Modifications to plan of care.

Discharge Planning
• Identified long-term needs and who is responsible for actions to be taken.
• Specific referrals made; sources for assistive devices, educational tools.

References

1. Curry, D. M., Duby, J. C. (1994). Developmental surveillance by pediatric nurses. *Pediatr Nurs*, 20, 40–44.
2. Leglar, J. D., Rose, L. C. (1998). Assessment of abnormal growth curves. "Problem-Oriented Diagnoses" series for Department of Family Practice. University of Texas Health Science Center; American Academy of Family Physicians. Retrieved July 2007 from www.aafp.org/afp/980700ap/legler.html.
3. Developmental delays: A pediatrician's guide to your children's health and safety. Retrieved July 2007 from www.keepkidshealthy.com/welcome/conditions/developmentaldelays.html.
4. American Academy of Child and Adolescent Psychiatry. (1999). Practice parameters for the assessment and treatment of children, adolescents, and adults with mental retardation and co-morbid mental disorders. *J Am Acad Child Adolesc Psychiatry*, 38(12 suppl), 55S–76S.
5. Leininger, M. M. (1996). *Transcultural Nursing: Theories, Research and Practices*. 2d ed. Hilliard, OH: McGraw-Hill.
6. Engel, J. (2002). *Mosby's Pocket Guide to Pediatric Assessment*. St. Louis, MO: Mosby.
7. Denehy, J. A. (1990). Anticipatory guidance. In Craft, M. J., Denehy, J. A. (eds). *Nursing Interventions for Infants and Children*. Philadelphia: W. B. Saunders.
8. McCloskey, J. C., Bulechek, G. M. (eds). (1992). *Nursing Interventions Classification (NIC)*. St. Louis, MO: Mosby.
9. Educating parents of extra-special children: Developmental delays. Retrieved January 2004 from www.epeconline.com/DevelopmentalDelays.html.
10. Kemp, S., Gungor, N. (2005). Growth failure. Retrieved March 2007 from www.emedicine.com/ped/topic902.htm.
11. Owens, T. A. (2005). Medical encyclopedia: Delayed growth. Retrieved March 2007 from http://nim.nih.gov/medlineplus/ency/article/003021.htm.
12. Blann, L. E. (2005). Early intervention for children and families with special needs. *MCN, Am J Matern Child Nurs*, 30(4), 263–267.
13. Grenz, K., et al. (updated 2005). Preventive services for children and adolescents. Institute for Clinical Systems Improvement [ICSI]. Article for National Guideline Clearinghouse. Retrieved February 2007 from www.guideline.gov.
14. Schiffman, R. F. (2004). Drug and substance use in adolescents. *MCN, Am J Matern Child Nurs*, 29(1), 21–27.

risk for disproportionate Growth

DEFINITION: At risk for growth above the 97th percentile or below the third percentile for age, crossing two percentile channels; disproportionate growth

RISK FACTORS

Prenatal
Maternal nutrition or infection; multiple gestation
Substance use or abuse; teratogen exposure
Congenital or genetic disorders [e.g., dysfunction of endocrine gland, tumors]

🌐 Cultural   Collaborative   🏠 Community/Home Care   Diagnostic Studies   ∞ Pediatric/Geriatric/Lifespan   Medications

Individual
Prematurity
Malnutrition; caregiver/individual maladaptive feeding behaviors; insatiable appetite; anorexia; [impaired metabolism, greater-than-normal energy requirements]
Infection; chronic illness [e.g., chronic inflammatory diseases]
Substance [use]/abuse [including anabolic steroids]

Environmental
Deprivation, poverty
Violence, natural disasters
Teratogen, lead poisoning

Caregiver
Abuse
Mental illness or retardation, severe learning disability

NOTE: A risk diagnosis is not evidenced by signs and symptoms, as the problem has not occurred; rather, nursing interventions are directed at prevention.
Sample Clinical Applications: Congenital or genetic disorders, prematurity, infection, nutritional problems (malnutrition, anorexia, failure to thrive, excessive intake or obesity), toxic exposures (e.g., lead), abuse or neglect, endocrine disorders, pituitary tumor

DESIRED OUTCOMES/EVALUATION CRITERIA

Sample (NOC) linkages:
Growth: Normal increase in bone size and body weight during growth years
Weight: Body Mass: Extent to which body weight, muscle, and fat are congruent to height, frame, gender, and age

Client Will (Include Specific Time Frame)
• Receive appropriate nutrition as dictated by individual needs.
• Demonstrate weight and growth stabilizing or progress toward age-appropriate size.
• Participate in plan of care as appropriate for age and ability.
Sample (NOC) linkages:
Child Development: [specify age group]: Milestones of physical, cognitive, and psychosocial progression by [specify] months/years of age

Client/Caregiver Will (Include Specific Time Frame)
• Verbalize understanding of potential for growth delay or deviation and plan for prevention

ACTIONS/INTERVENTIONS

Sample (NIC) linkages:
Nutritional Monitoring: Collection and analysis of patient data to prevent or minimize malnourishment
Teaching: Infant [or] Toddler Nutrition [specify age]: Instruction on nutrition and feeding practices during the first, second, and third years of life
Weight Management: Facilitating maintenance of optimal body weight and percent body fat

NURSING PRIORITY NO. 1

To assess causative/contributing factors:

- Determine factors or condition(s) existing that could contribute to growth deviation as listed in Risk Factors, including familial history (e.g., pituitary tumors, Marfan's syndrome, genetic anomalies); prematurity with complications; use of certain drugs or substances during pregnancy; maternal diabetes or other chronic illness; poverty or inability to attend to nutritional issues; eating disorders and so forth. *Information essential to developing plan of care.*[1]
- Identify nature and effectiveness of parenting and caregiving activities. *Inadequate, inconsistent caregiving, unrealistic or insufficient expectations, lack of stimulation, inadequate limit-setting; lack of responsiveness indicates problems in parent-child relationship.*[4]
- Note severity and pervasiveness of situation (e.g., individual/SO showing effects of long-term physical or emotional abuse or neglect vs. individual experiencing recent-onset situational disruption or inadequate resources during period of crisis or transition).
- Evaluate nutritional status. *Overfeeding or malnutrition (protein and other basic nutrients) on a constant basis prevents individual from reaching healthy growth potential, even if no disorder or disease exists.*
- Review results of studies such as x-rays, bone scans, magnetic resonance imaging (MRI) *to determine bone age and extent of bone and soft-tissue overgrowth; presence of tumors*; note laboratory studies (e.g., growth hormone levels and other endocrine studies) *to identify pathology.*
- Determine cultural, familial, and societal values that may impact situation or parental expectations (e.g., some cultures equate a "plump" baby with a healthy baby; childhood obesity is now a risk for American children and parents are concerned about child's food intake; expectations for "normal growth").
- Assess significant stressful events, losses, separation, and environmental changes (e.g., abandonment, divorce, death of parent/sibling, aging, move).
- Assess cognition, awareness, orientation, behavior of the client/caregiver. *Actions such as withdrawal or aggression, reactions to environment and stimuli provide information for identifying needs and planning care.*[1]
- Active-listen concerns about body size, ability to perform competitively (e.g., sports, body building) *to ascertain the potential for inappropriate use of anabolic steroids or other drugs.*

NURSING PRIORITY NO. 2

To prevent/limit deviation from growth norms:

- Determine chronological age, familial factors (body build/stature) to clarify growth expectations. Note reported losses or alterations in functional level. *Provides comparative baseline.*
- Identify present growth age and stage. *Measurements are compared to "standard" or normal range for children of same gender and age.*
- Review expectations for current height and weight percentiles and degree of deviation. Plan for periodic evaluations. *Growth rates are measured in terms of how much a child grows within a specified time. These rates vary dramatically as a child grows (normal growth is a discontinuous process) and must be evaluated periodically over time to ascertain that child has definite growth disturbance. Accelerated or slowed growth rates are rarely normal and warrant further evaluation.*[1]
- Investigate deviations in height, weight, and head size. *Deviations may include weight only (increased or decreased) or height (increased or decreased) and head size (disproportionate to rest of body). These deviations may be seen alone or in combination, all requiring*

additional testing over time to determine cause and effect on child's growth and development. Some are more urgent than others (e.g., small head size is evaluated further/treated as soon as identified, whereas short stature may require a longer evaluation period to determine if developmental problem exists).[1]

- Determine if child's growth is above 97th percentile (very tall and large) for age. *Child should be further evaluated for endocrine disorders or pituitary tumor (could result in gigantism). Other disorders may be characterized by excessive weight for height (e.g., hypothyroidism, Cushing's syndrome), abnormal sexual maturation or abnormal body/limb proportions.*[2,8]

- Determine if child's growth is below third percentile (very short and small) for age. *Child should have further evaluations for failure to thrive related to intrauterine growth retardation, prematurity or very low birth weight, small parents, poor nutrition, stress or trauma, or medical condition (e.g., intestinal disorders with malabsorption, diseases of heart, kidneys, diabetes mellitus). Treatment of underlying condition may alter or improve child's growth pattern.*[3,9,10]

- Assist with therapies *to treat or correct underlying conditions (e.g., Crohn's disease, cardiac problems, or renal disease); endocrine problems (e.g., hyperpituitarism, hypothyroidism, type 1 diabetes mellitus, growth hormone abnormalities); genetic or intrauterine growth retardation; infant feeding problems, nutritional deficits.*

- Include nutritionist and other specialists as indicated (e.g., physical or occupational therapist) in developing plan of care. *Helpful in determining specific dietary needs for growth and weight issues, assistive devices, or appropriate exercise and rehabilitation programs.*[6]

- Note reports of changes in facial features, joint pain, lethargy, sexual dysfunction, or progressive increase in hat, glove, ring, or shoe size in adults, especially after age 40. *Individual should be referred for further evaluation for hyperpituitarism or growth hormone imbalance and acromegaly.*

NURSING PRIORITY NO. 3

To promote wellness (Teaching/Discharge Considerations):

- Provide information regarding growth issues, as appropriate, including pertinent reference materials, including books, audiovisual materials, credible Web sites and so forth. *Provides opportunity to review data at own pace, enhancing likelihood of retention, and opportunity to make informed decisions.*

- Discuss with pregnant women and adolescents consequences of substance use or abuse. *Prevention of growth disturbances depends on many factors but includes the cessation of smoking, alcohol, and many drugs that have the potential for causing central nervous system (CNS) or orthopedic disorders in the fetus.*[5,7]

- Refer for genetic screening as appropriate. *There are many reasons for referral, including (and not limited to) positive family history of a genetic disorder (e.g., fragile X syndrome, muscular dystrophy), woman with exposure to toxins or potential teratogenic agents, women older than 35 years at delivery, previous child born with congenital anomalies, history of intrauterine growth retardation, and so forth.*

- Address parent/caregiver issues (e.g., parental abuse, learning deficiencies, environment of poverty) *where they could impact client's ability to thrive.*

- Promote client lifestyle that prevents or limits complications (e.g., management of obesity, hypertension, sensory or perceptual impairments), regular medical follow-up, nutritionally balanced meals, socialization for age and development, and so forth, *to enhance functional independence and quality of life.*

- Recommend involvement in regular monitored exercise and sports program *to enhance muscle tone and strength, and appropriate body building.*

- Review medications being considered (e.g., appetite stimulant, growth hormone, thyroid replacement, antidepressant) noting potential side effects/adverse reactions *to promote adherence to regimen and reduce risk of untoward responses.*
- Identify available community resources as appropriate (e.g., public health programs such as Women, Infants, and Children [WIC] program, medical equipment suppliers, nutritionist, substance abuse programs, specialists in endocrine problems/genetics).
- Stress importance of regular follow-up with healthcare provider *to monitor progress of growth and weight changes.*

DOCUMENTATION FOCUS

Assessment/Reassessment
- Assessment findings, individual needs, current growth status and trends.
- Caregiver's understanding of situation and individual role.
- Cultural or familial values and expectations.

Planning
- Plan of care and who is involved in the planning.
- Teaching plan.

Implementation/Evaluation
- Client's responses to interventions, teaching, and actions performed.
- Caregiver response to teaching.
- Attainment or progress toward desired outcome(s).
- Modifications to plan of care.

Discharge Planning
- Identified long-term needs and who is responsible for actions to be taken.
- Specific referrals made, sources for assistive devices, educational tools.

References

1. Leglar, J. D., Rose, L. C. (1998). Assessment of abnormal growth curves. "Problem-Oriented Diagnoses" series for Department of Family Practice. University of Texas Health Science Center; American Academy of Family Physicians. Retrieved July 2007 from www.aafp.org/afp/980700ap/legler.html.
2. Gigantism. (2003). Fact sheet: University of Pennsylvania Health System. Retrieved July 2007 from http://pennhealth.com/ency/article/001174.htm.
3. Endocrinology and short stature. (2001). Patient fact sheets. Endocrine Society. Retrieved March 2007 from www.endosociety.org.
4. Gordon, T. (2000). *Parent Effectiveness Training*. Updated ed. New York: Three Rivers Press.
5. Maloni, J. A., et al. (2003). Implementing evidence-based practice: Reducing risk for low birth weight through pregnancy smoking cessation. *J Obstet Gynecol Neonat Nurs*, 32(5), 676–682.
6. American Dietetic Association. (1997). Nutrition in comprehensive program planning for persons with developmental disabilities. *J Am Diet Assoc*, 97(2), 189–193.
7. Schiffman, R. F. (2004). Drug and substance use in adolescents. *MCN Am J Matern Child Nurs*, 29(1), 21–27.
8. Ferry, R. J., Shim, M. (2006). Gigantism and acromegaly. Retrieved March 2007 from www.emedicine.com/ped/topic2634.htm.
9. Kemp, S., Gungor, N. (2005). Growth failure. Retrieved March 2007 from www.emedicine.com/ped/topic902.htm.
10. Owens, T. A. (2005). Medical encyclopedia: Delayed growth. Retrieved March 2007 from http://nim.nih.gov/medlineplus/ency/aritcle/003021.htm.

ineffective Health Maintenance

DEFINITION: Inability to identify, manage, and/or seek out help to maintain health [This diagnosis contains components of other NDs. We recommend subsuming health maintenance interventions under the "basic" nursing diagnosis when a single causative factor is identified (e.g., deficient Knowledge [specify], ineffective self Health Management, chronic Confusion, impaired verbal Communication, [disturbed Thought Process], ineffective Coping, compromised family Coping, delayed Growth and Development).]

RELATED FACTORS

Deficient communication skills [written, verbal, or gestural]
Unachieved developmental tasks
Inability to make appropriate judgments
Perceptual or cognitive impairment
Diminished or lack of gross motor skills; diminished or lack of fine motor skills
Ineffective individual/family coping; complicated grieving; spiritual distress
Insufficient resources (e.g., equipment, finances); [lack of psychosocial supports]

DEFINING CHARACTERISTICS

Subjective
Lack of expressed interest in improving health behaviors
[Reported compulsive behaviors]

Objective
Demonstrated lack of knowledge regarding basic health practices
Inability to take the responsibility for meeting basic health practices; history of lack of health-seeking behavior
Demonstrated lack of adaptive behaviors to environmental changes
Impairment of personal support system
[Observed compulsive behaviors]

Sample Clinical Applications: Chronic conditions (e.g., multiple sclerosis [MS], rheumatoid arthritis, chronic pain), brain injury or stroke, spinal cord injury or paralysis, laryngectomy, dementia, Alzheimer's disease, developmental delay

DESIRED OUTCOMES/EVALUATION CRITERIA

Sample **NOC** linkages:
Health Promoting Behavior: Personal actions to sustain or increase wellness
Knowledge: Health Behavior: Extent of understanding conveyed about the promotion and protection of health
Participation in Health Care Decisions: Personal involvement in selecting and evaluating healthcare options to achieve desired outcome

Client Will (Include Specific Time Frame)
• Identify necessary health maintenance activities.
• Verbalize understanding of factors contributing to current situation.
• Assume responsibility for own healthcare needs within level of ability.
• Adopt lifestyle changes supporting individual healthcare goals.

(continues on page 402)

ineffective Health Maintenance (continued)

Sample (NOC) linkages:
Risk Detection: Personal actions to identify personal health threats
Social Support: Reliable assistance from others

SO/Caregiver Will (Include Specific Time Frame)
• Verbalize ability to cope adequately with existing situation, provide support and monitoring as indicated.

ACTIONS/INTERVENTIONS

Sample (NIC) linkages:
Health System Guidance: Facilitating a patient's location and use of appropriate health services
Support System Enhancement: Facilitation of support to patient by family, friends, and community
Health Education: Developing and providing instruction and learning experiences to facilitate voluntary adaptation of behavior conducive to health in individuals, families, groups, or communities

NURSING PRIORITY NO. 1

To assess causative/contributing factors:

• Identify risk factors in client's personal and family history, including health values, religious or cultural beliefs, and expectations regarding healthcare. *May not view current situation as a problem or be unaware of routine health maintenance practices and needs.*[11]

• Note client's age (e.g., very young or elderly age); cognitive, emotional, physical, and developmental status; and level of dependence and independence. *Client's status may range from complete dependence (dysfunctional) to partial or relative independence and determines type of interventions/support needed.*[1]

• Note whether impairment is related to an acute or sudden onset situation, or a progressive illness or long-term health problem. *Determines type and intensity, and length of time support may be required.*[4]

• Ascertain client's ability and desire to learn. Determine barriers to learning (e.g., can't read, speaks or understands different language, is overcome with stress or grief). *May not be physically, emotionally, or mentally capable at present because of current situation or may need information in small, manageable increments.*[1]

• Assess communication skills and ability or need for interpreter. Identify support person requiring or willing to accept information. *Ability to understand is essential to identification of needs and planning care. May need to provide the information to another individual if client is unable to comprehend.*[9]

• Evaluate for substance use/abuse (e.g., alcohol/other drugs). *Affects client's desire and ability to accept responsibility for self.*[6]

• Note client's desire and level of ability to meet health maintenance needs as well as self-care activities of daily living (ADLs). *Care may begin with helping client make a decision to improve situation, as well as identifying factors that are currently interfering with meeting needs.*[3]

• Note setting where client lives (e.g., long-term care facility, homebound, or homeless). *May contribute to inability or desire to meet healthcare needs.*[10]

Cultural   Collaborative   Community/Home Care   Diagnostic Studies   Pediatric/Geriatric/Lifespan   Medications

- Ascertain recent changes in lifestyle. *For instance, a man whose spouse dies and who has no skills for taking care of his own/family's health needs may need assistance to learn how to manage new situation, or newly unemployed individual without healthcare benefits may require referral to public assistance agencies.*[8]
- Determine level of adaptive behavior, knowledge, and skills about health maintenance, environment, and safety. *Will determine beginning point for planning and intervening to help client learn necessary skills to maintain health in a positive manner.*[7]
- Evaluate environment *to note individual adaptation needs (e.g., supplemental humidity, air purifier, change in heating system).*[1]
- Note client's use of professional services and resources (i.e., appropriate or inappropriate, nonexistent).[9]

NURSING PRIORITY NO. 2

To assist client/caregiver(s) to maintain and manage desired health practices:

- Discuss with client/SO beliefs about health and reasons for not following prescribed plan of care. *Determines client's view about current situation and potential for change.*
- Identify realistic health goals and develop plan with client/SO(s) for self-care. *Allows for incorporating existing disabilities with client's/SO's desires, adapting and organizing care as necessary.*[1]
- Involve comprehensive specialty health teams when available or indicated (e.g., pulmonary, psychiatric, enterostomal, IV therapy, nutritional support, substance abuse counselors).[9]
- Provide time to Active-listen concerns of client/SO(s). *Provides opportunity to clarify expectations and misconceptions.*
- Provide anticipatory guidance *to maintain and manage effective health practices during periods of wellness and to identify ways client can adapt when progressive illness or long-term health problems occur.*[9,11]
- Encourage socialization, "buddy system," and personal involvement *to enhance support system, provide pleasant stimuli, and limit permanent regression.*[2]
- Provide for communication and coordination between healthcare facility teams and community healthcare providers *to promote continuation of care and maximize outcomes.*[2]
- Monitor adherence to prescribed medical regimen *to problem-solve difficulties in adherence and alter the plan of care as needed.*[1]

NURSING PRIORITY NO. 3

To promote wellness (Teaching/Discharge Considerations):

- Provide information about individual healthcare needs, using client's preferred learning style (e.g., pictures, words, video, Internet). *Can help client to understand own situation and enhance cooperation with the plan of care.*[8]
- Limit amount of information presented at one time, especially when dealing with elderly or cognitively impaired client. Present new material through self-paced instruction when possible. *Allows client time to process and store new information.*[8]
- Help client/SO(s) prioritize healthcare goals. Provide a written copy to those involved in planning process *for future reference/revision as appropriate. Promotes planning to enable the client to maintain a healthy and productive lifestyle.*[10]
- Assist client/SO(s) to develop stress-management skills. *Knowing ways to manage stress helps individual to develop and maintain a healthy lifestyle.*[3]
- Identify ways to make adaptations in exercise program *to meet client's changing needs and abilities, and environmental concerns.*[5]

- ⊕ • Identify signs and symptoms requiring further screening, evaluation, and follow-up. Essential to identify developing problems that could interfere with maintaining well-being.[10,11]
- ⊕ • Make referral as needed for community support services (e.g., homemaker or home attendant, Meals on Wheels, skilled nursing care, community or free clinic, Well-Baby Clinic, senior citizen healthcare activities). *May need additional assistance to maintain self-sufficiency.*[9]
- ⊕ • Refer to social services as indicated. *May need assistance with financial, housing, or legal concerns (e.g., conservatorship).*[2]
- ⊕ • Refer to support groups as appropriate (e.g., senior citizen groups, Alcoholics or Narcotics Anonymous, Red Cross, or Salvation Army). *Provides information and help for specific needs or at times of crisis.*[9]
- ⊕ • Arrange for hospice service for client with terminal illness. *Will help client and family deal with end-of-life issues in a positive manner.*[3,4]

DOCUMENTATION FOCUS

Assessment/Reassessment
- Assessment findings, including individual abilities, family involvement, and support factors.
- Cultural or religious beliefs, healthcare values, and expectations.
- Availability and use of resources.

Planning
- Plan of care and who is involved in planning.
- Teaching plan.

Implementation/Evaluation
- Responses of client/SO(s) to plan, interventions, teaching, and actions performed.
- Attainment or progress toward desired outcome(s).
- Modifications to plan of care.

Discharge Planning
- Long-term needs and who is responsible for actions to be taken.
- Specific referrals made.

References

1. Bohny, B. (1997). A time for self-care: Role of the home healthcare nurse. *Home Healthcare Nurs*, 15(4), 281–286.
2. Callaghan, P., Morrissey, G. (1993). Social support and health: A review. *J Adv Nurs*, 18(2), 203–210.
3. Dossey, B. M., Dossey, L. (1998). Body-mind-spirit: Attending to holistic care. *Am J Nurs*, 98(8), 35–38.
4. Gregory, C. M. (1997). Caring for caregivers: Proactive planning eases burden on caregivers. *AWHONN Lifelines*, 1(2), 51–53.
5. Lai, S. C., Cohen, M. N. (1999). Promoting lifestyle changes. *Am J Nurs*, 99(4), 63–67.
6. Larsen, L. S. (1998). Effectiveness of counseling intervention to assist family caregivers of chronically ill relatives. *J Psychosoc Nurs*, 36(8), 26–32.
7. MacNeill, D., Weis, T. (1998). Case study: Coordinating care. *Continuing Care*, 17(4), 78.
8. McCrory Pocinki, K. (1991). Writing for an older audience: Ways to maximize understanding and acceptance. *J Nutr Elder*, 11(1–2), 69–77.
9. Stuifbergen, A. (1997). Health promotion: An essential component of rehabilitation for persons with chronic disabling conditions. *Adv Nurs Sci*, 19(4), 138–147.

 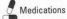

10. Public Health Foundation. *Healthy People 2010 Toolkit: A Field Guide for Health Planning* (Available at www.healthypeople.gov/state/toolkit/). Washington, DC: Author.
11. Health maintenance evaluation: Replacing the "annual physical". Fact sheet for Palo Alto Medical Foundation. Retrieved March 2007 from www.pamf.org/children/maintenance/healtheval.html.

ineffective self Health Management

DEFINITION: Pattern of regulating and integrating into daily living a therapeutic regimen for treatment of illness and its sequelae that is unsatisfactory for meeting specific health goals

RELATED FACTORS

Complexity of healthcare system or therapeutic regimen
Decisional conflicts
Economic difficulties
Excessive demands made (e.g., individual, family); family conflict
Family patterns of healthcare
Inadequate number of cues to action
Knowledge deficit; regimen
Mistrust of regimen or healthcare personnel
Perceived seriousness, susceptibility, barriers, or benefits
Powerlessness
Social support deficits

DEFINING CHARACTERISTICS

Subjective
Verbalizes desire to manage the illness
Verbalizes difficulty with prescribed regimen

Objective
Failure to include treatment regimens in daily living, or take action to reduce risk factors
Makes choices in daily living ineffective for meeting the health goals
[Unexpected acceleration of illness symptoms]

Sample Clinical Applications. Chronic conditions (e.g., chronic obstructive pulmonary disease [COPD], multiple sclerosis [MS], arthritis, chronic pain, end-stage liver or renal failure) or new diagnoses necessitating lifestyle changes

DESIRED OUTCOMES/EVALUATION CRITERIA

Sample NOC linkages:
Treatment Behavior: Illness or Injury: Personal actions to palliate or eliminate pathology
Health Beliefs: Personal convictions that influence health behaviors
Adherence Behavior: Self-initiated actions to promote wellness, recovery, and rehabilitation

(continues on page 406)

NURSING PRIORITY NO. 2

To help client/SO(s) to create/maintain a safe, growth-promoting environment:

- Coordinate planning with multidisciplinary team and client/SO as appropriate. *Coordination and cooperation of team improves motivation and maximizes outcomes.*
- Assist client/SO(s) to develop plan for maintaining a clean, healthful environment. *Activities such as sharing of household tasks or repairs between family members, contract services, exterminators, trash removal can promote ongoing maintenance.*
- Discuss home environment or perform home visit as indicated *to determine client's ability to care for self, to identify potential health and safety hazards, and to determine adaptations that may be needed (e.g., wheelchair-accessible doors and hallways, safety bars in bathroom, safe place for child play, clean water available, working cook stove or microwave, screens on windows).*[2]
- Assist client/SO(s) to identify and acquire necessary equipment and services (e.g., chair or stair lifts; commode chair; safety grab bar; structural adaptations; service animals; aids for hearing, seeing, mobility; trash removal; cleaning supplies) *to meet individual needs.*[3]
- Identify resources available for appropriate assistance (e.g., visiting nurse, budget counseling, homemaker, Meals on Wheels, physical or occupational therapy, social services).[2]
- Discuss options for financial assistance with housing needs. *Client may be able to stay in home with minimal assistance or may need significant assistance over a wide range of possibilities, including removal from the home.*[2]

NURSING PRIORITY NO. 3

To promote wellness (Teaching/Discharge Considerations):

- Evaluate client at each community contact or before facility discharge *to determine if home maintenance needs are ongoing in order to initiate appropriate referrals.*[3]
- Discuss environmental hazards *that may negatively affect health or ability to perform desired activities.*
- Discuss long-term plan *for taking care of environmental needs (e.g., assistive personnel, specialized controls for electrical equipment, trash removal and pest control services).*[4]
- Provide information necessary for the individual situation. *Helps client/family decide what can be done to improve situation.*[3]
- Identify ways to access/use community resources and support systems (e.g., extended family, neighbors, church group, seniors program).
- Refer to NDs Caregiver Role Strain, compromised family Coping, ineffective Coping, risk for Injury, deficient Knowledge [specify], Self-Care Deficit [specify] for additional interventions as appropriate.

DOCUMENTATION FOCUS

Assessment/Reassessment
- Assessment findings include individual (cognitive, emotional, and physical functioning) and environmental factors, specific safety concerns.
- Availability and use of support systems.

Planning
- Plan of care and who is involved in planning; support systems and community resources identified.
- Teaching plan.

Implementation/Evaluation
- Client's/SO's responses to interventions, teaching, and actions performed.
- Attainment or progress toward desired outcome(s).
- Modifications to plan of care.

Discharge Planning
- Long-term needs and who is responsible for actions to be taken.
- Specific referrals made, equipment needs/resources.

References

1. Townsend, M. C. (2003). *Psychiatric Mental Health Nursing Concepts of Care*. 4th ed. Philadelphia: F. A. Davis.
2. MSU Extension. (2003). Home maintenance and repair. Retrieved July 2007 from http://web1.msue.msu.edu/msue/imp/mod02/master02.html.
3. Fenn, M. (1998). Health promotion: Theoretical perspectives and clinical application. *Holis Nurs Pract*, 19(2), 1–7.
4. Schmelling, S. (2005). Home, adapted home. *Rehabil Manage*, 18(6), 12–19.
5. Gibbons, S., Lauder, W., Ludwick, R. (2006). Self-neglect: A proposed new NANDA diagnosis. *Int J Nurs Terminol Classif*, 17(1), 10–18.

readiness for enhanced Hope

DEFINITION: A pattern of expectations and desires that is sufficient for mobilizing energy on one's own behalf and can be strengthened

RELATED FACTORS

To be developed by nurse researchers and submitted to NANDA

DEFINING CHARACTERISTICS

Subjective

Expresses desire to enhance: hope; belief in possibilities; congruency of expectations with desires; ability to set achievable goals; problem-solving to meet goals
Expresses desire to enhance: sense of meaning to life; interconnectedness with others; spirituality

Sample Clinical Applications: Any acute or chronic condition, or healthy individual looking to improve well-being

DESIRED OUTCOMES/EVALUATION CRITERIA

Sample **NOC** linkages:
Hope: Optimism that is personally satisfying and life supporting
Quality of Life: Extent of positive perception of current life circumstances
Personal Well-Being: Extent of positive perception of one's health status

Client Will (Include Specific Time Frame)
- Identify and verbalize feelings related to expectations and desires.
- Verbalize belief in possibilities for the future.

(continues on page 416)

readiness for enhanced Hope (continued)

• Discuss current situation and desire to enhance hope.
• Set short-term goals that will lead to behavioral changes to meet desire for enhanced hope.

ACTIONS/INTERVENTIONS

Sample NIC linkages:
Hope Inspiration: Enhancing the belief in one's capacity to initiate and sustain actions
Self-Awareness Enhancement: Assisting a patient to explore and understand his or her thoughts, feelings, motivations, and behaviors
Spiritual Growth Facilitation: Facilitation of growth in patient's capacity to identify, connect with, and call upon the source of meaning, purpose, comfort, strength, and hope in his or her life

NURSING PRIORITY NO. 1

To determine needs and desire for improvement:

- Review familial and social history to identify past situations (e.g., illness, emotional conflicts, alcoholism) that have led to decision to improve life. *When trials of life have been resolved, individuals may look toward making life better.*[1]
- Determine current physical condition of client/SO. *Treatment regimen and indicators of healing can influence ability to promote positive feelings of hope.*[2]
- Ascertain client's perception of current state and expectations or goals for the future (e.g., general well-being, prosperity, independence). *Perception is more important than reality in individual's mind and can help to pursue realistic goals for self.*[3]
- Identify spiritual beliefs/cultural values that guide or influence client's spirituality and view of self. *Influences sense of hope and connectedness.*[4]
- Determine meaning of life or reasons for living, belief in God or higher power. *Helps client to clarify beliefs and how they relate to desire for improvement in life.*[6]
- Ascertain motivation and expectations for change. Note congruency of expectations with desires for change. *Motivation to improve and high expectations can encourage client to make changes that will improve his or her life. However, presence of unrealistic expectations may hamper efforts.*[3,4]
- Note degree of involvement in activities and relationships with others. *Interactions with others can promote a sense of connectedness and enjoyment of relationships.*[3]

NURSING PRIORITY NO. 2

To assist client to achieve goals and strengthen sense of hope:

- Establish a therapeutic relationship showing positive regard and hopefulness for the client. *Enhances feelings of worth and comfort, inspiring client to continue pursuit of goals.*[3]
- Help client recognize areas that are in his or her control versus those that are not. *To be most effective, client needs to expend energy in those areas where he or she has control and let the others go.*[2]
- Assist client to develop manageable short-term goals. *Success at short-term goals that are manageable will lead to attainment of long-term goals too.*[2]
- Identify activities to achieve goals, and facilitate contingency planning. *Promotes dealing with situation in manageable steps, enhancing chances for success and sense of control.*[5]

- Explore interrelatedness of relationship between unresolved emotions, anxieties, fears, and guilt. *Provides opportunity to address issues that may be limiting individual's ability to improve life situation.*[5]
- Assist client to acknowledge current coping behaviors and defense mechanisms that may hamper moving toward goals. *Allows client to focus on coping mechanisms that are more successful in problem-solving.*[3]
- Encourage client to concentrate on progress not perfection. *If client can accept that perfection is difficult or not always the desirable outcome, he or she may be able to view own accomplishments with pride.*[3]
- Involve client in care and explain all procedures thoroughly, answering questions truthfully. *Enhances trust and relationship, promoting hope for a positive outcome.*[2]
- Express hope to client and encourage SO(s) and other health team members to do so. *Enhances client's sense of hope and belief in possibilities of a positive outcome.*[1]
- Identify ways to strengthen sense of interconnectedness or harmony with others *to support sense of belonging and connection that promotes feelings of wholeness and hopefulness.*[1]

NURSING PRIORITY NO. 3

To promote optimum wellness:

- Demonstrate and encourage use of relaxation techniques, guided imagery, and meditation activities. *Learning to relax can help client decrease tension resulting in refreshment of body and mind, enabling individual to perform and think more successfully.*[3]
- Provide positive feedback for efforts taken to improve situation, growth in use of skills, and learning efforts. *Acknowledges client's efforts as individual is moving forward in learning new skills, and reinforces gains.*[3]
- Explore ways that beliefs give meaning and value to daily living. *As client's understanding of these issues improves, hope for the future is strengthened.*[1]
- Encourage life-review by client. *Acknowledges own successes, identifies opportunity for change, and clarifies meaning in life.*[5]
- Identify ways for spiritual expression, strengthening spirituality. *There are many options for enhancing spirituality through connectedness with self and others (e.g., volunteering, mentoring, involvement in religious activities). (Refer to ND: readiness for enhanced Spiritual Well-Being.)*[5]
- Encourage client to join groups with similar or new interests. *Expanding knowledge and making friendships with new people will widen horizons for the individual.*
- Refer to community resources and support groups, spiritual advisor as indicated.

DOCUMENTATION FOCUS

Assessment/Reassessment
- Assessment findings, including client's perceptions of current situation, relationships, sense of desire for enhancing life.
- Cultural or spiritual values and beliefs.
- Motivation and expectations for improvement.

Planning
- Plan of care and who is involved in planning.
- Teaching plan.

after cardiac arrest or brain injury) requiring interventions to protect client from adverse affects.[6,7]

🏠 • Identify factors that client can control (if any), such as protection from environment, adequate heat in home; layering clothing and blankets; minimize heat loss from head with hat or scarf; appropriate cold-weather clothing; avoidance of alcohol or other drugs if anticipating exposure to cold; potential risks for future hypersensitivity to cold, etc.

🏠 • Discuss signs/symptoms of early hypothermia (e.g., changes in mentation, somnolence, impaired coordination, slurred speech) *to facilitate recognition of problem and timely intervention. Information may be especially important if client works or plays outdoors (e.g., camping, skiing, hiking).*[1,2,5]

🌀 • Identify assistive community resources, as indicated (e.g., social services, emergency shelters, clothing suppliers, food bank, public service company, financial resources). *Individual/ SO may be in need of numerous resources if hypothermia was associated with inadequate housing, homelessness, malnutrition.*

DOCUMENTATION FOCUS

Assessment/Reassessment
• Findings, noting degree of system involvement, respiratory rate, electrocardiogram (ECG) pattern, capillary refill, and level of mentation.
• Graph temperature.

Planning
• Plan of care and who is involved in planning.
• Teaching plan.

Implementation/Evaluation
• Responses to interventions, teaching, and actions performed.
• Attainment or progress toward desired outcome(s).
• Modifications to plan of care.

Discharge Planning
• Long-term needs, identifying who is responsible for each action.

References

1. Curtis, R. (2002). Outdoor Action guide to hypothermia and cold weather injuries. Princeton University Outdoor Action. Retrieved July 2007 from www.princeton.edu/~oa/safety/hypocold.html.
2. Decker, W., et al. (2001, updated 2005). Hypothermia. Retrieved July 2007 from www.emedicine.com/emerg/topic279.htm.
3. Doenges, M. E., Moorhouse, M. F., Geissler-Murr, A. C. (2002). Surgical intervention. *Nursing Care Plans: Guidelines for Individualizing Patient Care.* 6th ed. Philadelphia: F. A. Davis, 771–772.
4. State of Alaska cold injuries and cold water near drowning guidelines. (2003). Retrieved July 2007 from www.chems.alaska.gov/EMS/documents/AKColdInj2005.pdf.
5. Li, J., Decker, W. (2005). Hypothermia. Retrieved March 2007 from www.emedicine.com/emerg/topic279.htm.
6. Good, K. K., et al. (2006). Postoperative hypothermia—The chilling consequences. *AORN J,* 83(5), 1055–1066.
7. Calver, P., et al. (2005). The big chill: Improving the odds after cardiac arrest. CE Home Study Program for RNweb. Retrieved March 2007 from www.rnweb.com.

disturbed personal Identity

DEFINITION: Inability to maintain an integrated and complete perception of self

RELATED FACTORS

Low self-esteem; dysfunctional family processes
Situational crises; stages of growth and development; social role change
Ingestion of or inhalation of toxic chemicals; use of psychoactive drugs
Cultural discontinuity; discrimination or prejudice
Manic states; multiple personality disorder; psychiatric disorders (e.g., psychoses, depression, dissociative disorder); organic brain syndromes
Cult indoctrination

DEFINING CHARACTERISTICS

Subjective
Disturbed body image or relationships; delusional description of self
Fluctuating feelings about self; feelings of strangeness or emptiness
Uncertainty about goals, or cultural or ideological values (e.g., beliefs, religion and moral questions)
Gender confusion
Unable to distinguish between inner and outer stimuli

Objective
Contradictory personal traits
Ineffective coping or role performance

Sample Clinical Applications: Schizophrenia, dissociative disorders, borderline personality disorder, developmental delay, autism, gender identity conflict, dementia, traumatic injury (e.g., amputation, spinal cord injury [SCI], brain injury)

DESIRED OUTCOMES/EVALUATION CRITERIA

Sample NOC linkages:
Identity: Distinguish between self and nonself and characterize one's essence
Distorted Thought Self-Control: Self-restraint of disruption in perception, thought processes, and thought content
Anxiety Self-Control: Personal actions to eliminate or reduce feelings of apprehension, tension, or uneasiness from an unidentifiable source

Client Will (Include Specific Time Frame)
• Acknowledge threat to personal identity.
• Integrate threat in a healthy, positive manner (e.g., state anxiety is reduced, make plans for the future).
• Verbalize acceptance of changes that have occurred.
• State ability to identify and accept self (long-term outcome).

(continues on page 434)

disturbed personal Identity (continued)
ACTIONS/INTERVENTIONS

Sample (NIC) linkages:
Self-Esteem Enhancement: Assisting a patient to increase his or her personal judgment of self-worth
Self-Awareness Enhancement: Assisting a patient to explore and understand his or her thoughts, feelings, motivations, and behaviors
Decision-Making Support: Providing information and support for a person who is making a decision regarding healthcare

NURSING PRIORITY NO. 1

To assess causative/contributing factors:

● Ascertain client's perception of the extent of the threat to self and how client is handling the situation. *Many factors can affect an individual's self-image: illness (chronic or terminal), injuries, changes in body structure (amputation, spinal cord damage, burns), and client's view of what has happened will affect development of plan of care and interventions to be used.*[1,6]

● Determine speed of occurrence of threat. *An event, such as an accident or sudden diagnosis of diabetes, cancer, that has happened quickly may be more threatening.*[7]

● Have client define own body image. *Body image is the basis of personal identity, and client's perception will affect how changes are viewed, may prevent achievement of ideals and expectations, and have a negative effect.*[1]

∞ ● Note age of client. *An adolescent may struggle with the developmental task of personal/ sexual identity, whereas an older person may have more difficulty accepting or dealing with a threat to identity, such as progressive loss of memory or aging body changes.*[3]

🏠 ● Assess availability and use of support systems. Note response of family/SO(s). *During stressful situations, support is essential for client to cope with changes that are occurring. Engaging family in choosing supportive interventions will help client and family members deal with situation or illness.*[3]

∞ ● Note withdrawn or automatic behavior, regression to earlier developmental stage, general behavioral disorganization, or display of self-mutilation behaviors in adolescent or adult; delayed development, preference for solitary play, unusual display of self-stimulation in child. *Indicators of poor coping skills and need for specific interventions to help client develop sense of self and identity. Inability to identify self interferes with interactions with others.*[3]

● Be aware of physical signs of panic state. *Presence of severe anxiety state may progress to panic when concerns seem overwhelming to client.* (Refer to ND Anxiety.)

● Determine presence of hallucinations or delusions, distortions of reality. *Indicators of presence of psychosis and need for immediate interventions to deal with inability to distinguish between self and nonself.*[1,3]

NURSING PRIORITY NO. 2

To assist client to manage/deal with threat:

● Make time to listen to, or Active-listen client, encouraging appropriate expression of feelings, including anger and hostility. *Conveys a sense of confidence in client's ability to identify extent of threat, how it is affecting sense of identity, and how to deal with feelings in acceptable ways.*[7,8]

- Note use of alcohol or other drugs. *Individual may turn to these substances to relieve painful feelings, especially in the presence of fearful diagnoses (e.g., cancer, multiple sclerosis [MS]).*[8]
- Provide calm environment. *Feelings of anxiety are contagious, and calm surroundings can help client to relax, maintain control, and be able to think more clearly about how illness or situation can be managed effectively.*[9]
- Use crisis-intervention principles when indicated. *May be necessary to help client restore equilibrium when situation escalates.*[1]
- Discuss client's commitment to an identity. *Those who have made a strong commitment to an identity tend to be more comfortable with self and happier than those who have not.*[3]
- Assist client to develop strategies to cope with threat to identity. *Reduces anxiety, promotes self-awareness, and enhances self-esteem, enabling client to deal with threat more realistically.*[10]
- Engage client in activities appropriate to individual situation. *Using activities such as a mirror for visual feedback, tactile stimulation to reconnect with parts of the body (amputation, unilateral neglect), can help to identify self as an individual.*[2]
- Provide for simple decisions, concrete tasks, calming activities. *Promotes sense of control and positive expectations to enable client to regain sense of self.*[3]
- Allow client to deal with situation in small steps. *May have difficulty coping with larger picture when in stress overload. Taking small steps promotes feelings of success and ability to manage illness or situation.*[9]
- Encourage client to develop and participate in an individualized exercise program. *While walking is an excellent beginning program, it is helpful to choose activities that client enjoys. Exercise releases endorphins, thereby reducing stress and anxiety, promoting a sense of well-being.*[1]
- Provide concrete assistance as needed. *Until basic-level needs, such as activities of daily living (ADLs) and food, are met, individual is unable to deal with higher-level needs. Once these needs are met, client can begin to deal with threat to identity.*[1]
- Take advantage of opportunities to promote growth. Realize that client will have difficulty learning while in a dissociative state. *Alterations in mental status can interfere with ability to process information, and new information can increase confusion and disorientation.*[3]
- Maintain reality orientation without confronting client's irrational beliefs. *Client may become defensive, blocking opportunity to look at other possibilities. Arguing does not change the perceptions and can interfere with or damage nurse-client relationship.*[1]
- Use humor judiciously when appropriate. *While humor can lift spirits and provide a moment of levity, it is important to note the mood or receptiveness of the client before using it.*[3]
- Discuss options for dealing with issues of gender identity. *Identification of client's concerns about role dysfunction or conflicting feelings about sexual identity will indicate need for therapy, possible gender-change surgery when client is a transsexual, or other available choices.*[2]
- Refer to NDs disturbed Body Image, Self-Esteem [specify], Spiritual Distress.

NURSING PRIORITY NO. 3

To promote wellness (Teaching/Discharge Considerations):

- Provide accurate information about threat to and potential consequences for individual in current situation. *Fear and anxiety regarding the threat represented by the illness or situation can be potentiated by lack of knowledge, unknown consequences, and inaccurate beliefs. Accurate information can help client incorporate new knowledge into changed self-concept.*[7]

- ● Assist client and SO(s) to acknowledge and integrate threat into future planning. *A diagnosis, accident, etc., can require major life changes, such as wearing identification bracelet when prone to mental confusion; a new lifestyle to accommodate change of gender for transsexual client; diet and medication routine with the diagnosis of diabetes mellitus. Planning can help the client to make the changes required to move forward with new life.*[4,5]
- ● Refer to appropriate support groups. *May need additional assistance, such as day-care program, counseling or psychotherapy, gender identity, family or marriage counseling, parenting classes.*[2]

DOCUMENTATION FOCUS

Assessment/Reassessment
- Findings, noting degree of impairment.
- Nature of and client's perception of the threat.

Planning
- Plan of care and who is involved in the planning.
- Teaching plan.

IMPLEMENTATION/EVALUATION

- Client's response to interventions, teaching, and actions performed.
- Attainment or progress toward desired outcome(s).
- Modifications to plan of care.

Discharge Planning
- Long-term needs and who is responsible for actions to be taken.
- Specific referrals made.

References

1. Townsend, M. (2006). *Psychiatric Mental Health Nursing: Concepts of Care.* 5th ed. Philadelphia: F. A. Davis.
2. Doenges, M., Moorhouse, M., Murr, A. (2006). *Nursing Care Plans: Guidelines for Individualizing Patient Care.* 7th ed. Philadelphia: F. A. Davis.
3. Doenges, M., Townsend, M., Moorhouse, M. (1998). *Psychiatric Care Plans: Guidelines for Individualizing Care.* 3d ed. Philadelphia: F. A. Davis.
4. Pinhas-Hamiel, O., et al. (1996). Increased incidence of non-insulin-dependent diabetes mellitus among adolescents. *J Pediatr*, 128(8), 608.
5. Deckelbaum, R. J., Williams, C. L. (2001). Childhood obesity: The health issue. *Obesity Res*, 9(5), 239s–243s.
6. Badger, J. M. (2001). Burns: The psychological aspect. *Am J Nurs*, 101(11), 38–41.
7. Bartol, T. (2002). Putting a patient with diabetes in the driver's seat. *Nursing*, 32(2), 53–55.
8. Bruera, E., et al. (1995). The frequency of alcoholism among patients with pain due to terminal cancer. *J Pain Symptom Manage*, 10(8), 599–603.
9. Paice, J. (2002). Managing psychological conditions in palliative care. *Am J Nurs*, 102(11), 36–43.
10. Cox, H., et al. (2002). *Clinical Applications of Nursing Diagnosis: Adult, Child, Women's, Psychiatric, Gerontic, and Home Health Considerations.* 4th ed. Philadelphia: F. A. Davis.

readiness for enhanced Immunization Status

DEFINITION: A pattern of conforming to local, national, or international standards of immunization to prevent infectious disease(s) that is sufficient to protect a person, family, or community and can be strengthened

RELATED FACTORS

To be developed by nurse researchers and submitted to NANDA

DEFINING CHARACTERISTICS

Subjective
Expresses desire to enhance:
Knowledge of immunization standards
Immunization status
Identification of providers of immunizations
Record-keeping of immunizations
Identification of possible problems associated with immunizations
Behavior to prevent infectious diseases

Sample Clinical Applications: Newborn, infant, school-age children, young adults, pregnancy, chronic health conditions, international travelers

DESIRED OUTCOMES/EVALUATION CRITERIA

Sample NOC linkages:
Immunization Behavior: Personal actions to obtain immunization to prevent a communicable disease

Client Will (Include Specific Time Frame)
• Express understanding of immunization recommendations.
• Develop plan to obtain appropriate immunizations.
• Identify and adopt behaviors to reduce risk of infectious disease.
• Maintain and update immunization records.
Community Health Status: Immunity: Resistance of community members to the invasion and spread of an infectious agent that could threaten public health

Community Will (Include Specific Time Frame)
• Provide information to community regarding immunization requirements or recommendations.
• Identify underserved populations requiring immunization support and ways to meet their needs.
• Develop a plan to provide mass immunizations in time of major threat or disease outbreak.

ACTIONS/INTERVENTIONS

Sample NIC linkages:
Immunization/Vaccination Management: Monitoring immunization status, facilitating access to immunizations, and providing immunizations to prevent communicable disease

NURSING PRIORITY NO. 1

To determine current immunization status:

- Assess client's history of immunizations. *Response may vary widely, depending on client's age (infant to adult), cultural influences, travel history, family beliefs about immunization, and medical conditions (e.g., some vaccines should not be given to children with certain cancers or persons taking immunosuppressant drugs or with serious allergies to eggs).*[1]
- Ascertain motivation and expectations for change. *Motivation to improve and high expectations can encourage client to make changes that will improve his or her life. However, unrealistic expectations may hamper efforts.*
- Determine if adult client works in or frequents high-risk areas (e.g., emergency first responder, hospital or long-term facility, doctor's office, home care, child-care provider, homeless or immigrant shelters or clinics, correctional facility, international travel) *to review potential exposures and determine new vaccines or boosters client may need.*
- Address client/SO concerns (e.g., client may wonder if annual flu shots are truly beneficial or whether adult boosters may be needed for particular immunizations received in childhood; parent is concerned about safety of vaccine supply). *Helps to clarify plans and deal with misconceptions or myths.*[2]
- Ascertain presence or discuss conditions that may preclude client receiving specific immunizations *(e.g., history of prior adverse reaction, current fever or illness, pregnancy, undergoing cancer or other immunosuppressant treatments).*
- Review community plan for dealing with immunizations and disease outbreak. *Identifies strengths to build on and limitations to be addressed.*

NURSING PRIORITY NO. 2

To assist client/SO/community to develop/strengthen plan to meet identified needs:

- Review parents' knowledge and information regarding immunizations recommended or required to enter school: (1) prior to kindergarten (e.g., hepatitis B, rotavirus, *Haemophilus influenzae*, mumps/measles/rubella [MMR], varicella, and hepatitis A); (2) by junior high or middle school age: diphtheria/pertussis/tetanus [DPT]; human papillomavirus; (3) for college freshmen planning to live in dorm: meningitis, *to document status, plan for boosters, and/or discuss appropriate intervals for follow-up.*[1-4]
- Discuss protective benefit of each vaccine, route of administration, expected side effects, and potential adverse reactions. *Information necessary for client/SO to make informed decisions.*
- Discuss appropriate time intervals for all recommended immunizations, as well as catch-up and booster options for children birth to 18 years.[4]
- Review travel requirements for client preparing for international travel *to ascertain potential for contracting vaccine-preventable disease in geographic area of client's travel so that vaccines can be provided if needed.*[3]
- Inform of exemptions when client/SO desires. *Some states permit medical, religious, personal, and philosophical exemptions when parent does not want child to participate in immunization programs.*[5] Refer to appropriate care providers for further discussion or intervention.
- Define and discuss current needs and anticipated or projected concerns of community health-promotion programs. *Agreement on scope and parameters of needs is essential for effective planning.*
- Prioritize goals *to facilitate accomplishment.*

- Identify available community resources (e.g., persons, groups, financial, governmental, as well as other communities). *Inclusion of all stakeholders enhances support for plan and increases likelihood of success.*
- Seek out and involve underserved and at-risk groups within the community. *Supports communication and commitment of community as a whole.*

NURSING PRIORITY NO. 3

To promote optimum wellness:

- Review reasons to continue immunization programs. *Viruses and bacteria that cause vaccine-preventable disease and death still exist and can be passed on to people who are not protected, increasing medical, social, and economic costs.*[6]
- Provide reliable vaccine information in written form or Web sites (e.g., brochures and fact sheets from the Centers for Disease Control and Prevention [CDC], American Academy of Pediatrics, National Network for Immunization Information). *Allows client/SO to review at own pace in order to make informed decisions.*[1-4]
- Identify community resources for obtaining immunizations such as Public Health Department/community clinic, family physician.
- Discuss management of common side effect symptoms (e.g., muscle pain, rash, fever, site swelling).
- Support development of community plans for maintaining or enhancing efforts *to increase immunization level of population.*
- Establish mechanism for self-monitoring of community needs and evaluation of efforts.
- Use multiple formats for client instruction (e.g., TV, radio, print media, billboards, and computer bulletin boards, speakers' bureau, reports to community leaders/groups on file and accessible to the public), *to keep community informed regarding immunization needs, disease prevention.*

DOCUMENTATION FOCUS

Assessment/Reassessment
- Assessment findings of immunization status, potential risks, disease exposure.
- Identified areas of concern, strengths and limitations.
- Understanding of immunization needs, safety, and disease prevention.
- Motivation and expectations for change.

Planning
- Action plan and who is involved in planning.
- Teaching plan.

Implementation/Evaluation
- Individual/family responses to interventions, teaching, and actions performed.
- Response of community entities to the actions performed.
- Attainment or progress toward desired outcome(s).
- Modifications to plan.

Discharge Planning
- Identified needs for follow-up care, support systems.
- Specific referrals made.
- Short- and long-term plans to deal with current, anticipated, and potential community needs and who is responsible for follow-through.
- Coalitions formed.

References

1. Mosocco, D. (2007). Clipboard: Childhood vaccines. *Home Healthcare Nurse*, 25(1), 7–8.
2. Engle, J. (2002). *Mosby's Pocket Guide to Pediatric Assessment*. 4th ed. St. Louis, MO: Mosby.
3. Centers for Disease Control and Prevention. (2007). Adult immunization schedule. Fact sheet for National Immunization Program. Retrieved March 2007 from www.cdc.gov/nip.
4. Centers for Disease Control and Prevention. (2006). Recommended immunization schedules for persons aged 0–18 years—United States. *Morbidity and Mortality Weekly Report*, 55(51–52), Q1–Q4.
5. Salmon, D. A., et al. (2005). Factors associated with refusal of childhood vaccines among parents of school-aged children: A case-control. *Arch Pediatr Adolesc Med*, 159(5), 470–476.
6. Centers for Disease Control and Prevention. (2003). What would happen if we stopped vaccinations? Fact sheet for National Immunization Program. Retrieved March 2007 from www.cdc.gov/nip.

disorganized Infant Behavior

DEFINITION: Disintegrated physiological and neurobehavioral responses of infant to the environment

RELATED FACTORS

Prenatal
Congenital or genetic disorders; teratogenic exposure; [exposure to drugs]

Postnatal
Prematurity; oral or motor problems; feeding intolerance; malnutrition
Invasive procedures; pain

Individual
Gestational or postconceptual age; immature neurological system
Illness; [infection]; [hypoxia or birth asphyxia]

Environmental
Physical environment inappropriateness
Sensory inappropriateness, overstimulation, or deprivation
Lack of containment within environment

Caregiver
Cue misreading; cue knowledge deficit
Environmental stimulation contribution

DEFINING CHARACTERISTICS

Objective
Regulatory problems: Inability to inhibit startle; irritability
State-organization system:
Active-awake (fussy, worried gaze); quiet-awake (staring, gaze aversion)
Diffuse sleep; state-oscillation

🌐 Cultural Collaborative 🏠 Community/Home Care Diagnostic Studies ∞ Pediatric/Geriatric/Lifespan Medications

Irritable crying

Attention-interaction system: Abnormal response to sensory stimuli (e.g., difficult to soothe, inability to sustain alert status)

Motor system:

Finger splay; fisting; hands to face; hyperextension of extremities

Tremors; startles; twitches; jittery; uncoordinated movement

Changes to motor tone; altered primitive reflexes

Physiological:

Bradycardia; tachycardia; arrhythmias

Skin color changes

"Time-out signals" (e.g., gaze, grasp, hiccough, cough, sneeze, sigh, slack jaw, open mouth, tongue thrust)

Feeding intolerances

Sample Clinical Applications: Prematurity, congenital or genetic disorders, meconium aspiration, respiratory distress syndrome, small for gestational age

DESIRED OUTCOMES/EVALUATION CRITERIA

Sample **NOC** linkage:

Neurological Status: Ability of the peripheral and central nervous system (CNS) to receive, process, and respond to internal and external stimuli

Infant Will (Include Specific Time Frame)

• Exhibit organized behaviors that allow the achievement of optimal potential for growth and development as evidenced by modulation of physiological, motor, state, and attentional-interactive functioning.

Sample **NOC** linkages:

Child Development [specify age 1, 2 month]: Milestones of physical, cognitive, and psychosocial progression by [specify] months of age

Growth: Normal increase in bone size and body weight during growth years

Parent/Caregiver Will (Include Specific Time Frame)

• Recognize individual infant cues.

• Identify appropriate responses (including environmental modifications) to infant's cues.

• Verbalize readiness to assume caregiving independently.

ACTIONS/INTERVENTIONS

Sample **NIC** linkages:

Environmental Management: Manipulation of the patient's surroundings for therapeutic benefit

Developmental Care: Structuring the environment and providing care in response to the behavioral cues and states of the preterm infant

Newborn Care: Management of neonate during the transition to extrauterine life and subsequent period of stabilization

NURSING PRIORITY NO. 1

To assess causative/contributing factors:

- Determine infant's chronological and developmental age; note length of gestation. *These factors (prematurity, infant maturity, and stages of development) help to determine plan of care.*[1,2,5]
- Observe for cues suggesting presence of situations that may result in pain or discomfort. *Some behavior that appears to be disorganized may be caused by a pain source that once identified may be alleviated.*[1]
- Determine adequacy of physiological support. *Identifies areas of additional need.*[1]
- Evaluate level and appropriateness of environmental stimuli. *Infant behavior is affected by a wide range of stimuli. Careful assessment narrows focus of concerns.*[2]
- Ascertain parents' understanding of infant's needs and abilities. *Identifies knowledge base and areas of learning needed.*[2–4]
- Listen to parents' concerns about their capabilities to meet infant's needs. *Active-listening can reassure parents, pinpoint areas to be addressed, as well as provide opportunity to correct misconceptions.*[2,3]

NURSING PRIORITY NO. 2

To assist parents in providing coregulation to the infant:

- Provide a calm, nurturant physical and emotional environment. *Provides optimal infant comfort. Models behavior for parent(s) and optimizes learning.*[2,3]
- Encourage parents to hold infant, including skin-to-skin contact as appropriate. Touch enhances parent-infant bonding, as well as provides means of calming.[3] Research suggests skin-to-skin contact or kangaroo care (KC) may have a positive effect on infant development by enhancing neurophysiological organization as well as an indirect effect by improving parental mood, perceptions, and interactive behavior.[6]
- Model gentle handling of baby and appropriate responses to infant behavior. *Provides cues to parent.*[3]
- Support and encourage parents to be with infant and participate actively in all aspects of care. *Situation may seem overwhelming to new parents. Emotional and physical support enhances coping. Parents who are able to help in the care of their infant express lower levels of helplessness and powerlessness.*[1,2]
- Provide positive feedback for progressive parental involvement in caregiving process. *Transfer of care from staff to parents progresses along a continuum as parents' confidence level increases, and they are able to take on more complex care activities.*[7]
- Discuss infant growth and development, pointing out current status and progressive expectations as appropriate. *Augments parent knowledge of coregulation.*[2]
- Incorporate the parents' observations and suggestions into plan of care. *Demonstrates valuing of parents' input and encourages continued involvement.*[2,4]

NURSING PRIORITY NO. 3

To deliver care within the infant's stress threshold:

- Provide a consistent caregiver. *Facilitates recognition of infant cues or changes in behavior. Communication is optimized if family is familiar with caregiver.*[2]
- Identify infant's individual self-regulatory behaviors (e.g., sucking, mouthing; grasp, hand-to-mouth, face behaviors; foot clasp, brace; limb flexion, trunk tuck; boundary seeking).

- Support hands to mouth and face; offer pacifier or nonnutritive sucking at the breast with gavage feedings. *Provides opportunities for infant to self-regulate.*[2]
- Avoid aversive oral stimulation, such as routine oral suctioning; suction ET tube only when clinically indicated. *Maximizes infant comfort, preventing undue/noxious stimulation.*[1,2]
- Use Oxyhood large enough to cover the infant's chest so arms will be inside the hood. *Allows for hand-to-mouth self-calming activities during this therapy.*[2]
- Provide opportunities for infant to grasp. *Helps with development of motor function skills.*[2]
- Provide boundaries or containment during all activities. Use swaddling, nesting, bunting, caregiver's hands as indicated. *Enhances infant's feelings of security and safeness. Avoids startle reflex and accompanying distress.*[2,3]
- Allow adequate time and opportunities to hold infant. Handle infant very gently, move infant smoothly, slowly, and contained, avoiding sudden or abrupt movements. *Provides comfort to infant and models behavior to parent(s).*[3]
- Maintain normal alignment, position infant with limbs softly flexed, shoulders and hips adducted slightly. Use appropriate-sized diapers. *Avoids unnecessary discomfort.*[2]
- Evaluate chest for adequate expansion, placing rolls under trunk if prone position indicated. *Provides for ease of respirations.*[2]
- Avoid restraints, including at IV sites. If IV board is necessary, secure to limb positioned in normal alignment. *Optimizes comfort and movement.*[1,2]
- Provide a sheepskin, egg-crate mattress, waterbed, or gel pillow or mattress for infant who does not tolerate frequent position changes. *Minimizes tissue pressure and risk of tissue injury.*[2]
- Visually assess color, respirations, activity, invasive lines without disturbing infant. Assess with "hands on" every 4 hours as indicated and prn. *Allows for undisturbed rest and quiet periods.*[2,3]
- Schedule daily activities, time for rest, and organization of sleep and wake states to maximize tolerance of infant. Defer routine care when infant in quiet sleep. *Gives infant a sense of routine and also provides for undisturbed rest and quiet periods.*[2,3]
- Provide care with baby in side-lying position. Begin by talking softly to the baby, then placing hands in containing hold on baby, allow baby to prepare. Proceed with least invasive manipulations first. *Gradual build from comforting touch, to nursing care, to invasive interventions decreases overall stress of infant. Shortens perception of "being bothered" time and facilitates more rapid calming phase.*[3]
- Respond promptly to infant's agitation or restlessness. Provide "time-out" when infant shows early cues of overstimulation. Comfort and support the infant after stressful interventions. *Decreases stress for both infant and family. Facilitates calming phase.*[3]
- Remain at infant's bedside for several minutes after procedures and caregiving to monitor infant's response and provide necessary support. *Allows for more rapid intervention(s) if infant becomes overstressed.*[3]
- Administer analgesics as individually appropriate. *Maintains optimal comfort.*[1-4]

NURSING PRIORITY NO. 4

To modify the environment to provide appropriate stimulation:

- Introduce stimulation as a single mode and assess individual tolerance.

LIGHT/VISION
- Reduce lighting perceived by infant, introduce diurnal lighting (and activity) when infant achieves physiological stability. (Daylight levels of 20–30 candles and nightlight levels of

less than 10 candles are suggested.) Change light levels gradually to allow infant time to adjust. *Lowering light levels reduces visual stimulation, provides comforting environment. Diurnal lighting allows the stable infant to begin perception of day and night cycles and to establish circadian rhythms.*[1]

- Protect the infant's eyes from bright illumination during examinations and procedures, as well as from indirect sources such as neighboring phototherapy treatments. *Prevents retinal damage and reduces visual stressors.*[2]

 ● Deliver phototherapy (when required) with Biliblanket devices if available. *Alleviates need for eye patches to protect vision.*[2]

- Provide caregiver face (preferably parent's) as visual stimulus when infant shows readiness (awake, attentive). *Begins process of visual recognition.*[1]

SOUND
- Identify sources of noise in environment and eliminate/reduce *to minimize auditory stimulus, reduces startle response in infant, provides comforting environment:*[2]
  Speak in a low voice.
  Reduce volume on alarms and telephones to safe but not excessive volume.
  Pad metal trash can lids.
  Open paper packages such as IV tubing and suction catheters slowly and at a distance from bedside.
  Conduct rounds or report away from bedside.
  Place soft, thick fabric such as blanket rolls and toys near infant's head *to absorb sound.*
  Keep all incubator portholes closed, closing with two hands *to avoid loud snap with closure and associated startle response.*
- Refrain from playing musical toys or tape players inside incubator. *Even very soft sounds echo in an enclosed space. What an adult may find soothing is likely to overstimulate an infant.*[2,3]
- Avoid placing items on top of incubator; if necessary to do so, pad surface well. *Contact with the external parts of the incubator causes reverberation inside the chamber.*
- Conduct regular decibel (dB) checks of interior noise level in incubator (recommended not to exceed 60 dB). *Verifies that decibel levels are within acceptable range.*[2]
- Provide auditory stimulation to console, support infant before and through handling or to reinforce restfulness. *Provides modeling of behavior for family and increased comfort for infant.*[3]

OLFACTORY
- Be cautious in exposing infant to strong odors (e.g., alcohol, Betadine, perfumes). *Olfactory capability of the infant is very sensitive.*[1]
- Place a cloth or gauze pad scented with milk near the infant's face during gavage feeding. *Enhances association of milk with act of feeding and gastric fullness.*[2]
- Invite parents to leave a handkerchief near infant that they have scented by wearing close to their body. *Strengthens infant recognition of parents.*[2]

VESTIBULAR
- Move and handle the infant slowly and gently. Do not restrict spontaneous movement. *Maintains comfort while at the same time encouraging motor function skill.*[2]
- Provide vestibular stimulation *to console, stabilize breathing/heart rate, or enhance growth.* Use a waterbed (with or without oscillation), a motorized, moving bed or cradle; or rocking in the arms of a caregiver.

GUSTATORY

● Dip pacifier in milk and offer to infant for sucking and tasting during gavage feeding. *Further enhances feeding recognition with touch and taste cues.*[2]

TACTILE

● Maintain skin integrity and monitor closely. Limit frequency of invasive procedures. *Decreases chance of infections. Decreases infant discomfort.*[1]
● Minimize use of chemicals on skin (e.g., alcohol, povidone-iodine, solvents) and remove afterward with warm water. *Chemical compounds remove the natural protective mechanisms of skin, and infants are often very sensitive to integumentary injury.*[1]
● Limit use of tape and adhesives directly on skin. Use DuoDerm under tape. *Helps prevent dermal injury and allergic reactions.*[1]
● Touch infant with a firm, containing touch, avoid light stroking. Provide a sheepskin, soft linen. *Note:* Tactile experience is the primary sensory mode of the infant. *Light stroking can cause tickle sensations that are irritating rather than pleasurable. Firm touch is reassuring.*[2]
● Encourage frequent parental holding of infant (including skin-to-skin). Supplement activity with extended family, staff, volunteers. *For family members, touch enhances bonding. If family is not readily available, infant needs regular skin-to-skin contact from caregivers for comfort and reassurance.*[3]

NURSING PRIORITY NO. 5

To promote wellness (Teaching/Discharge Considerations):

● Evaluate home environment to identify appropriate modifications. *Helps the family identify needs and begin to mentally prepare for infant homecoming.*[3]
● Identify community resources (e.g., early stimulation program, qualified childcare facilities or respite care, visiting nurse, home-care support, specialty organizations). *Begins process of resource utilization.*[2–4]
● Determine sources for equipment and therapy needs. *Facilitates transition to at-home care.*[3]
● Refer to support or therapy groups as indicated. *Provides role models, facilitates adjustment to new roles and responsibilities, and enhances coping.*[2,3]
● Provide contact number, as appropriate (e.g., primary nurse). *Supports adjustment to home setting, enhances problem-solving.*[3]
● Refer to additional NDs such as risk for impaired Attachment, risk for Caregiver Role Strain, compromised/disabled/readiness for enhanced family Coping, delayed Growth and Development.

DOCUMENTATION FOCUS

Assessment/Reassessment
• Findings, including infant's cues of stress, self-regulation, and readiness for stimulation; chronological and developmental age.
• Parent's concerns, level of knowledge.

Planning
• Plan of care and who is involved in the planning.
• Teaching plan.

Implementation/Evaluation
• Infant's responses to interventions and actions performed.
• Parents' participation and response to interactions and teaching.
• Attainment or progress toward desired outcome(s).
• Modifications of plan of care.

Discharge Planning
• Long-term needs and who is responsible for actions to be taken.
• Specific referrals made.

References

1. Creasy, R., Resnik, R. (1999). *Maternal-Fetal Medicine*. 4th ed. Philadelphia: W. B. Saunders.
2. London, M., et al. (2003). *Maternal-Newborn & Child Nursing; Family-Centered Care*. Upper Saddle River, NJ: Prentice Hall.
3. Ladewig, P., et al. (2002). *Contemporary Maternal-Newborn Nursing Care*. 5th ed. Upper Saddle River, NJ: Prentice Hall.
4. Lowdermilk, D., Perry, S., Bobak, I. (2001). *Maternity & Women's Health Care*. 6th ed. St. Louis, MO: Mosby.
5. Mandeville, L., Troiano, N. (1999). *High-Risk & Critical Care: Intrapartum Nursing*. 2d ed. Philadelphia: Lippincott.
6. Feldman, R., et al. (2002). Comparison of skin-to-skin (kangaroo) and traditional care: Parenting outcomes and preterm infant development. *Pediatrics*, 110(1), 16–26.
7. Scharer, K., Brooks, G. (1994). Mothers of chronically ill neonates and primary nurses in the NICU: Transfer of care. *Neonatal Network*, 13(5), 37–46.

readiness for enhanced organized Infant Behavior

DEFINITION: A pattern of modulation of the physiological and behavioral systems of functioning (i.e., autonomic, motor, state-organizational, self-regulators, and attentional-interactional systems) in an infant that is satisfactory but that can be improved

RELATED FACTORS

Prematurity
Pain

DEFINING CHARACTERISTICS

Objective
Stable physiological measures
Definite sleep-wake states
Use of some self-regulatory behaviors
Response to stimuli (e.g., visual, auditory)

Sample Clinical Applications: Prematurity, congenital or genetic disorders, meconium aspiration, respiratory distress syndrome, small for gestational age

⊕ Cultural Ⓐ Collaborative 🏠 Community/Home Care ⬗ Diagnostic Studies ∞ Pediatric/Geriatric/Lifespan   Medications

DESIRED OUTCOMES/EVALUATION CRITERIA

Sample (NOC) linkage:
Neurological Status: Ability of the peripheral and central nervous system (CNS) to receive, process, and respond to internal and external stimuli

Infant Will (Include Specific Time Frame)
- Continue to modulate physiological and behavioral systems of functioning.
- Achieve higher levels of integration in response to environmental stimuli.

Sample (NOC) linkages:
Child Development: [specify age group 1/2 months]: Milestones of physical, cognitive, and psychosocial progression by [specify] months of age
Knowledge: Infant Care: Extent of understanding conveyed about caring for a baby from birth to first birthday

Parent/Caregiver Will (Include Specific Time Frame)
- Identify cues reflecting infant's stress threshold and current status.
- Develop or modify responses (including environment) to promote infant adaptation and development.

ACTIONS/INTERVENTIONS

Sample (NIC) linkages:
Developmental Care: Structuring the environment and providing care in response to the behavioral cues and states of the preterm infant
Environmental Management: Manipulation of the patient's surroundings for therapeutic benefit

NURSING PRIORITY NO. 1

To assess infant status and parental skill level:

- Determine infant's chronological and developmental age; note length of gestation. *These factors (prematurity, infant maturity, and stages of development) help to determine plan of care.*[1,2,5]
- Identify infant's individual self-regulatory behaviors: suck, mouth; grasp, hand-to-mouth, face behaviors; foot clasp, brace; limb flexion, trunk tuck; boundary seeking. *Assessing the infant's own regulatory coping tools alerts family and caregiver when infant is entering a stress cycle and helps determine if the infant needs assistance coping. This knowledge also helps development of a care plan if situation warrants.*[1,2,4]
- Observe for cues suggesting presence of situations that may result in pain/discomfort. *Some behavior that appears to be disorganized may be caused by a pain source that once identified may be alleviated.*[1]
- Evaluate level and appropriateness of environmental stimuli. *Infant behavior is affected by a wide range of stimuli. Careful assessment narrows focus of concerns.*[2]
- Ascertain parents' understanding of infant's needs and abilities. *Identifies knowledge base and areas of additional learning need.*[2-4]
- Listen to, or Active-listen parents' perceptions of their capabilities to promote infant's development. *When parents feel their thoughts and concerns are heard, they will feel reassured that they will be able to handle situation.*[2,3]

NURSING PRIORITY NO. 2

To assist parents to enhance infant's integration:

- Provide positive feedback for parental involvement in caregiving process. *Transfer of care from staff to parents progresses along a continuum as parents' confidence level increases, and they are able to take on more responsibility.*[7]
- Discuss use of skin-to-skin contact (kangaroo care—KC) as appropriate. *Research suggests KC may have a positive effect on infant development by enhancing neurophysiological organization as well as an indirect effect by improving parental mood, perceptions, and interactive behavior.*[6]
- Review infant growth and development, pointing out current status and progressive expectations. *Increases parental knowledge base and level of confidence.*[2–4]
- Identify cues reflecting infant stress. *Attention to cues allow for early intervention in case of problem development.*[2–4]
- Discuss parents' perceptions of needs and provide recommendations for modifications of environmental stimuli, activity schedule, sleep, and pain control needs. *While care provided is satisfactory, some modifications may enhance infant's integration and development.*[1,4]
- Incorporate parents' observations and suggestions into plan of care. *Demonstrates value of and regard for parents' input and enhances sense of ability to deal with situation.*[2,4]

NURSING PRIORITY NO. 3

To promote wellness (Teaching/Learning Considerations):

- Identify community resources (e.g., visiting nurse, home-care support, childcare). *Begins process of resource utilization.*[2–4]
- Refer to support group or individual role model *to facilitate ongoing adjustment to new roles and responsibilities, and problem-solving.*[2,3]
- Refer to additional NDs, for example, readiness for enhanced family Coping.

DOCUMENTATION FOCUS

Assessment/Reassessment
- Findings, including infant's self-regulation and readiness for stimulation; chronological and developmental age.
- Parents' concerns, level of knowledge.

Planning
- Plan of care and who is involved in the planning.
- Teaching plan.

Implementation/Evaluation
- Infant's responses to interventions and actions performed.
- Parents' participation and response to interactions/teaching.
- Attainment or progress toward desired outcome(s).
- Modifications of plan of care.

Discharge Planning
- Long-term needs and who is responsible for actions to be taken.
- Specific referrals made.

References

1. Creasy, R., Resnik, R. (1999). *Maternal-Fetal Medicine*. 4th ed. Philadelphia: W. B. Saunders.
2. London, M., Ladewig, P., Ball, J., Bindler, R. (2003). *Maternal-Newborn & Child Nursing: Family-Centered Care*. Upper Saddle River, NJ: Prentice Hall.
3. Ladewig, P., et al. (2002). *Contemporary Maternal-Newborn Nursing Care*. 5th ed. Upper Saddle River, NJ: Prentice Hall.
4. Lowdermilk, D., Perry, S., Bobak, I. (2001). *Maternity & Women's Health Care*. 6th ed. St. Louis, MO: Mosby.
5. Mandeville, L., Troiano, N. (1999). *High-Risk & Critical Care: Intrapartum Nursing*. 2d ed. Philadelphia: Lippincott.
6. Feldman, R., et al. (2002). Comparison of skin-to-skin (kangaroo) and traditional care: Parenting outcomes and preterm infant development. *Pediatrics*, 110(1), 16–26.
7. Scharer, K., Brooks, G. (1994). Mothers of chronically ill neonates and primary nurses in the NICU: Transfer of care. *Neonatal Network*, 13(5), 37–46.

risk for disorganized Infant Behavior

DEFINITION: Risk for alteration in integration and modulation of the physiological and behavioral systems of functioning (i.e., autonomic, motor, state, organizational, self-regulatory, and attentional-interactional systems)

RISK FACTORS

Pain

Oral or motor problems

Environmental overstimulation

Lack of containment within environment

Invasive or painful procedures

Prematurity; [immaturity of the central nervous system; genetic problems that alter neurological and/or physiological functioning, conditions resulting in hypoxia and/or birth asphyxia]

[Malnutrition; infection; drug addiction]

[Environmental events or conditions such as separation from parents, exposure to loud noise, excessive handling, bright lights]

NOTE: A risk diagnosis is not evidenced by signs and symptoms, as the problem has not occurred; rather, nursing interventions are directed at prevention.

Sample Clinical Applications: Prematurity, congenital or genetic disorders, meconium aspiration, respiratory distress syndrome, small for gestational age

DESIRED OUTCOMES/EVALUATION CRITERIA

Sample **NOC** linkages:

Preterm Infant Organization: Extrauterine integration of physiological and behavioral function by the infant born 24 to 37 (term) weeks gestation

Neurological Status: Ability of the peripheral and central nervous system to receive, process, and respond to internal and external stimuli

(continues on page 450)

Nursing Diagnoses in Alphabetical Order

risk for disorganized Infant Behavior (continued)

Infant Will (Include Specific Time Frame)
• Exhibit organized behaviors that allow the achievement of optimal potential for growth and development as evidenced by modulation of physiological, motor, state, and attentional-interactive functioning.

Sample (NOC) linkages:
Child Development: [specify age group 1/2 months]: Milestones of physical, cognitive, and psychosocial progression by [specify] months of age
Knowledge: Infant Care: Extent of understanding conveyed about caring for a baby from birth to 1 year

Parent/Caregiver Will (Include Specific Time Frame)
• Identify cues reflecting infant's stress threshold and current status.
• Develop or modify responses (including environment) to promote infant adaptation and development.

ACTIONS/INTERVENTIONS AND DOCUMENTATION FOCUS

Refer to ND disorganized Infant Behavior for Actions/Interventions and Documentation Focus.

risk for Infection

DEFINITION: At increased risk for being invaded by pathogenic organisms

RISK FACTORS

Inadequate primary defenses (broken skin, traumatized tissue, decrease in ciliary action, stasis of body fluids, change in pH secretions, altered peristalsis)
Inadequate secondary defenses (e.g., decreased hemoglobin, leukopenia, suppressed inflammatory response)
Inadequate acquired immunity; immunosuppression
Tissue destruction; increased environmental exposure to pathogens; invasive procedures
Chronic disease, malnutrition, trauma
Pharmaceutical agents (e.g., immunosuppressants, [antibiotic therapy])
Rupture of amniotic membranes
Insufficient knowledge to avoid exposure to pathogens

NOTE: A risk diagnosis is not evidenced by signs and symptoms, as the problem has not occurred; rather, nursing interventions are directed at prevention.
Sample Clinical Applications: Immune suppressed conditions (e.g., HIV positive, AIDS, cancer), chronic obstructive pulmonary disease (COPD), long-term use of steroids (e.g., asthma, rheumatoid arthritis, systemic lupus erythematosus [SLE]), diabetes mellitus, malnutrition, surgical or invasive procedures, substance abuse, burns, pregnancy/preterm labor

DESIRED OUTCOMES/EVALUATION CRITERIA

Sample **NOC** linkages:
Immune Status: Natural and acquired appropriately targeted resistance to internal and external antigens
Knowledge: Infection Management: Extent of understanding conveyed about infection, its treatment, and the prevention of complications
Risk Control: Personal actions to prevent, eliminate, or reduce modifiable health threats

Client Will (Include Specific Time Frame)
• Verbalize understanding of individual causative or risk factor(s).
• Identify interventions to prevent or reduce risk of infection.
• Demonstrate techniques, lifestyle changes to promote safe environment.
• Achieve timely wound healing; be free of purulent drainage or erythema; be afebrile.

ACTIONS/INTERVENTIONS

Sample **NIC** linkages:
Infection Protection: Prevention and early detection of infection in a patient at risk
Infection Control: Minimizing the acquisition and transmission of infectious agents
Surveillance: Purposeful and ongoing acquisition, interpretation, and synthesis of patient data for clinical decision making

NURSING PRIORITY NO. 1

To determine risk/contributing factors:

• Assess for presence of host-specific factors that affect immunity:[1,12-14]
• **Extremes of age:** *Newborns and the elderly are more susceptible to disease and infection than general population.*
• **Presence of underlying disease:** *Client may have disease that directly impacts immune system (e.g., cancer, AIDS, autoimmune disorder) or may be weakened by prolonged disease condition or treatment.*
• **Lifestyle:** *Personal habits or living situations such as persons sharing close quarters and/or equipment (e.g., college dorm, group home, long-term care facility, day care, correctional facility); IV drug use and shared needles, unprotected sex can increase susceptibility to infections.*
• **Nutritional status:** *Malnutrition weakens the immune system; elevated serum glucose levels (e.g., administration of total parenteral nutrition [TPN] or poorly controlled diabetes mellitus) provides growth media for pathogens.*
• **Trauma:** Loss of skin or mucous membrane integrity, or invasive procedures (e.g., surgery or invasive procedures: urinary catheterizations, oral intubation, parenteral injection, sharps and needle sticks) *are common paths of pathogen entry.*
• **Certain medications:** *Steroids, chemotherapeutic agents directly affect immune system. Long-term or improper antibiotic treatment can disrupt body's normal flora and result in increased susceptibility to antibiotic-resistant organisms.*
• **Presence or absence of immunity:** *Natural immunity may be acquired as a result of development of antibodies to a specific agent following infection, preventing recurrence of specific disease (e.g., chicken pox). Active immunization (via vaccination, e.g., measles, polio) and passive immunization (e.g., antitoxin or immunoglobulin administration) can prevent certain communicable diseases.*

- **Environmental exposure:** *May be accidental or intentional (e.g., act of terrorism).*
- Observe skin/tissues surrounding injuries (e.g., knife cuts, toe injuries, insect or animal bites); also inspect insertion sites of invasive lines, sutures, surgical incisions, wounds. *Redness, warmth, swelling, pain, red streaks are signs of developing localized infection that may have systemic implications if treatment is delayed.*[9,10,14,17]
- Assess and document skin conditions around insertions of orthopedic pins, wires, and tongs. *Direct connection to bone increases the risk of infections in bone sites that can lead to osteomyelitis, bone loss, and long-term delays of healing.*[9,10,14,17]
- Review laboratory values (e.g., white blood cell [WBC] count and differential, blood, urine, sputum, or wound cultures) *to identify presence of pathogens and treatment options.*
- Note onset of fever, chills, diaphoresis, altered level of consciousness. *Signs and symptoms of sepsis (systemic infection), requiring intensive medical treatment and evaluation for source of infection and specific pathogen.*

NURSING PRIORITY NO. 2

To reduce/correct existing risk factors:

HEALTHCARE ENVIRONMENT

- Emphasize proper handwashing techniques (using antibacterial soap and running water) before and after all care contacts, and after contact with items likely to be contaminated. Wash hands after glove removal. Instruct client/SO/visitors to wash hands, as indicated. *A first-line defense against healthcare-associated infections (HAI).*[1,3,15]
- Provide clean, well-ventilated environment (may require turning off central air-conditioning and opening window for good ventilation; room with negative air pressure, etc.).[6]
- Post visual alerts in healthcare settings instructing clients/SO to inform healthcare providers if they have symptoms of respiratory infections or influenza-like symptoms. *Can limit or prevent transmission to and from client and may reveal additional cases.*[1,8,11,12,15]
- Monitor client's visitors/caregivers for respiratory illnesses. Offer masks and tissues to client/visitors who are coughing or sneezing *to limit exposures, reduce cross-contamination.*
- Encourage parents of sick children to keep them away from child care settings and school until afebrile for 24 hours.
- Provide for isolation as indicated (e.g., wound/skin, respiratory, reverse). Educate staff in infection-control procedures. *Reduces risk of cross-contamination.*[18]
- Stress proper use of personal protective equipment (PPE) by staff/visitors as dictated by agency policy *for particular exposure risk (e.g., airborne, droplet, splash risk), including mask or respiratory filter of appropriate particulate regulator, gowns, aprons, head covers, face shields, protective eyewear.*[1,4,6,8,11]
- Include information in preoperative teaching about ways *to reduce potential for postoperative infection (e.g., respiratory measures to prevent pneumonia, wound or dressing care, avoidance of others with infection).*[5,9]
- Encourage early ambulation, deep breathing, coughing, position changes, and early removal of endotracheal and/or nasal or oral feeding tubes *for mobilization of respiratory secretions and prevention of aspiration and respiratory infections.*[15,16]
- Monitor and assist with use of adjuncts (e.g., respiratory aids such as incentive spirometry) *to prevent pneumonia.*[15,16]
- Maintain adequate hydration and electrolyte balance *to prevent imbalances that would predispose to infection.*
- Provide or encourage balanced diet, emphasizing proteins to feed the immune system. Immune function is affected by protein intake, the balance between omega-6 and omega-3 fatty acid intake, and adequate amounts of vitamins A, C, and E and the minerals zinc and iron. A deficiency of these nutrients puts the client at an increased risk of infection.[2]

- Handle and properly package tissue and fluid specimens.[1,7]
- Administer prophylactic antibiotics and immunizations as indicated.
- Assist with medical procedures (e.g., wound or joint aspiration, incision and drainage of abscess, bronchoscopy) as indicated.
- Administer and monitor medication regimen (e.g., antimicrobials, drip infusion into osteomyelitis, subeschar clysis, topical antibiotics) and note client's response *to determine effectiveness of therapy and presence of side effects.*

MEDICAL DEVICES

- Maintain sterile technique for invasive procedures (e.g., IV, urinary catheter, tracheostomy care, pulmonary suctioning).[1]
- Use disposable equipment whenever possible. Sterilize reusable equipment and surfaces according to manufacturer recommendations.[1,8]
- Dispose of needles and sharps in approved containers *to reduce risk of needle stick or sharps injury.*[1,8]
- Choose proper vascular access device based on anticipated treatment duration and solution or medication to be infused and best available aseptic insertion techniques; cleanse incisions and insertion sites daily/per facility protocol with appropriate solution *to reduce potential for catheter-related bloodstream infections.*[17]
- Maintain appropriate hang times for parenteral solutions (IVs, additives, nutritional solutions) *to reduce opportunity for contamination and bacterial growth.*[2]
- Assist with weaning from mechanical ventilator as soon as possible *to reduce risk of ventilator-associated pneumonia (VAP).*[18]
- Fill bubbling humidifiers or nebulizers with sterile water—not distilled or tap water. Use heat and moisture exchangers (HME) instead of heated humidifier with mechanical ventilator.[16,18]

SKIN/TISSUES

- Change surgical or other wound dressings as needed or indicated, using proper technique for changing and disposing of contaminated materials.[8,9,19]
- Cleanse incisions and insertion sites daily and as needed with povidone-iodine or other appropriate solution *to prevent growth of bacteria.*[9]
- Separate touching surfaces of excoriated skin (e.g., in herpes zoster, burns, weeping dermatitis) and apply appropriate skin barriers. Use gloves when caring for open lesions *to minimize autoinoculation or transmission of viral diseases.*[9]
- Perform or instruct in daily mouth care. Include use of antiseptic mouthwash for individuals in acute or long-term care settings *at high-risk for nosocomial or healthcare associated infections.*[18]
- Provide regular urinary catheter or perineal care. *Reduces risk of ascending urinary tract infection.*
- Cover perineal and pelvic region dressings or casts with plastic when using bedpan *to prevent contamination when wound is in perineal or pelvic region.*
- Discuss routine or preoperative body shower or scrubs when indicated (e.g., orthopedic, plastic surgery) *to reduce bacterial colonization.*[15]

COMMUNITY

- Recommend individuals/staff isolate self at home when ill *to prevent spread of infection to others, including coworkers.*[11]
- Alert infection control officer/proper authorities to presence of specific infectious agents and number of cases as required. *Provides for case finding and helps curtail outbreak.*[11,21]

- Group/cohort individuals with same diagnosis or exposure as resources require. *Limited resources (as may occur with an outbreak or epidemic) may dictate a wardlike environment but need for regular precautions to control spread of infection still exists.*[11]
- Encourage contacting healthcare provider for prophylactic therapy as indicated following exposure to individuals with infectious disease (e.g., tuberculosis, hepatitis, influenza).

NURSING PRIORITY NO. 3

To promote wellness (Teaching/Discharge Considerations):

- Review individual nutritional needs, appropriate exercise program, and need for rest *to enhance immune system function and healing.*[2,10,11]
- Instruct client/SO(s) in techniques to protect the integrity of skin, care for lesions, temperature measurement, and prevention of spread of infection in the home setting. *Provides basic knowledge for self-help and self-protection.*[7,10]
- Emphasize necessity of taking antivirals or antibiotics as directed (e.g., dosage and length of therapy). *Premature discontinuation of treatment when client begins to feel well may result in return of infection and potentiate drug-resistant strains.*[20]
- Discuss importance of not taking antibiotics or using "leftover" drugs unless specifically instructed by healthcare provider. *Inappropriate use can lead to development of drug-resistant strains or secondary infections.*[10]
- Discuss the role of smoking and secondhand smoke in respiratory infections. Refer to smoking cessation programs as indicated.
- Promote safer-sex practices and reporting sexual contacts of infected individuals *to prevent the spread of HIV or other sexually transmitted diseases.*[1,10,20]
- Encourage high-risk persons, including healthcare workers, to have influenza and pneumonia vaccinations *to reduce individual risk as well as help prevent spread of flu and viral pneumonias to others.*[1,11,21]
- Promote childhood immunization program. Encourage adults to update immunizations as appropriate.[12]
- Discuss precautions with client engaged in international travel, and refer for immunizations *to reduce incidence and transmission of global infections.*[13]
- Review use of prophylactic antibiotics if appropriate *(e.g., before dental work for clients with history of rheumatic fever, heart valve replacements).*[10]
- Identify resources available to the individual (e.g., substance abuse or rehabilitation, or needle-exchange program as appropriate; available or free condoms).
- Provide information and involve in appropriate community and national education programs *to increase awareness of and prevention of communicable diseases.*[1,10,11]
- Refer to NDs risk for Disuse Syndrome; ineffective Health Maintenance; impaired Home Maintenance; readiness for enhanced Immunization Status for additional interventions as appropriate.

DOCUMENTATION FOCUS

Assessment/Reassessment
- Individual risk factors that are present, including recent and current antibiotic therapy.
- Wound and/or insertion sites, character of drainage or body secretions.
- Signs/symptoms of infectious process.

Planning
- Plan of care, specific interventions, and who is involved in planning.
- Teaching plan.

Implementation/Evaluation
- Responses to interventions, teaching, and actions performed.
- Attainment or progress toward desired outcome(s).
- Modifications to plan of care.

Discharge Planning
- Discharge needs and who is responsible for actions to be taken.
- Specific referrals made.

References

1. Mechanisms of transmission and pathogenic organisms in the health care setting and strategies for prevention and control. (2001). Elements One and Two of online course of Infection Control Learning Institute. Retrieved September 2003 from www.proceo.com.
2. Lehmann, S. (1991). Immune function and nutrition: The clinical role of the intravenous nurse. *J Intraven Nurs*, 14, 406–420.
3. Garner, J., Favero, M. (1986). CDC Guideline for handwashing and hospital environmental control. *Am J Infection Control*, 16, 28–40.
4. Borton, D. (1997). Isolation precautions: Clearing up the confusion. *Nursing*, 21(1), 49–51.
5. Emori, L., Culver, D., Horan, T. (1995). National Nosocomial Infections Surveillance System (NNIS): Description of surveillance methods. *Am J Infection Control*, 19, 259–267.
6. Garner, J. S. (1996). Guideline for isolation precautions in hospitals. *Infect Control Hosp Epidemiol*, 17(1), 53–80.
7. Friedman, M. M. (2002). Improving infection control in home care: From ritual to science-based practice. *Home Healthcare Nurse*, 18(2), 99–106.
8. World Health Organization (WHO). Hospital hygiene and infection control. Retrieved October 2009 from www.who.int/water_sanitation_health/medicalwaste/148to158.pdf.
9. Thompson, J. (2000). A practical guide to wound care. *RN*, 63(1), 48–52.
10. Androwich, I., Burkhart, L., Gettrust, K. V. (1996). *Community and Home Health Nursing*. Albany, NY: Delmar.
11. Doenges, M. E., Moorhouse, M. F., Geissler-Murr, A. C. (2002). Care plan: Disaster considerations; and ND infection, risk for, in numerous care plans. *Nursing Care Plans: Guidelines for Individualizing Patient Care*. 6th ed. Philadelphia: F. A. Davis.
12. Goldrick, B. A., Goetz, A. M. (2006). 'Tis the season for influenza. Nurse Pract, 31(12), 24–33.
13. Hunter, A., Denman-Vitale, S., Garzon, L. (2007). Global infections: Recognition, management, and prevention. *Nurse Pract*, 32(2), 34–41.
14. Romero, D. V., Treston, J., O'Sullivan, A. L. (2006). Hand-to-hand combat: Preventing MRSA infection. *Adv Wound Care*, 19(6), 328–333.
15. Houghton, D. (2006). HAI prevention: The power is in your hands. *Nurs Manage*, 37(5 suppl), 1–7.
16. Lorente, L., et al. (2006). Ventilator-associated pneumonia using a heated humidifier or a heat and moisture exchanger: A randomized controlled trial. *Crit Care*, 10, 4.
17. Rosenthal, K. (2006). Guarding against vascular site infection. *Nurs Manage*, 37(4), 54–66.
18. Tablan, O. C., et al. (2004) Guidelines for preventing health-care associated pneumonia, 2003—Recommendations of CDC and Healthcare Infection Control Practices Advisory Committee. *Morbidity and Mortality Weekly Report*, 53(RRO3), 1–36.
19. Odom-Forren, J. (2006). Preventing surgical site infections. *Nursing*, 36(6), 59–63.
20. Kirton, C. (2005). The HIV/AIDS epidemic: A case of good news/bad news. *Nursing Made Incredibly Easy!*, 3(2), 28–40.
21. Lashley, F. R. (2006). Emerging infectious diseases at the beginning of the 21st century. *Online J Issues Nurs*, 11(1). Retrieved March 2007 from www.nursingworld.org.ojin/topic29_1.htm.

risk for Injury

DEFINITION: At risk of injury as a result of environmental conditions interacting with the individual's adaptive and defensive resources

RISK FACTORS

Internal
Physical (e.g., broken skin, altered mobility); tissue hypoxia; malnutrition
Abnormal blood profile (e.g., leukocytosis/leukopenia, altered clotting factors, thrombocytopenia, sickle cell, thalassemia, decreased hemoglobin)
Biochemical dysfunction; sensory dysfunction
Integrative or effector dysfunction; immune-autoimmune dysfunction
Psychological (affective, orientation); developmental age (physiological, psychosocial)

External
Biological (e.g., immunization level of community, microorganism)
Chemical (e.g., pollutants, poisons, drugs, pharmaceutical agents, alcohol, nicotine, preservatives, cosmetics, dyes); nutritional (e.g., vitamins, food types)
Physical (e.g., design, structure, and arrangement of community, building, and/or equipment), mode of transport
Human (e.g., nosocomial agents, staffing patterns; cognitive, affective, psychomotor factors)

NOTE: A risk diagnosis is not evidenced by signs and symptoms, as the problem has not occurred; rather, nursing interventions are directed at prevention.
Sample Clinical Applications: Seizure disorder, dementia, AIDS, cataracts, glaucoma, Parkinson's disease, substance abuse, malnutrition, developmental delay/mental retardation. In reviewing this ND, it is apparent there is much overlap with other diagnoses. We have chosen to present generalized interventions. Although there are commonalities to injury situations, we suggest that the reader refer to other primary diagnoses as indicated, such as risk for acute/chronic Confusion; risk for Contamination; impaired Environmental Interpretation Syndrome; risk for Falls; ineffective Health Maintenance; impaired Home Maintenance; risk for Infection; impaired physical Mobility; impaired/risk for impaired Parenting; risk for Poisoning; impaired/risk for impaired Skin Integrity; disturbed Thought Processes; risk for Trauma; risk for other-directed Violence; Wandering for additional interventions.

DESIRED OUTCOMES/EVALUATION CRITERIA

Sample (NOC) linkage:
Physical Injury Severity: Severity of injuries from accidents and trauma

Client Will (Include Specific Time Frame)
• Be free of injury.

Sample (NOC) linkages:
Personal Safety Behavior: Personal actions that prevent physical injury to self
Risk Control [specify]: Personal actions to prevent, eliminate, or reduce modifiable health threats [e.g., alcohol/drug use, altered visual function]

Client/Caregivers Will (Include Specific Time Frame)
• Verbalize understanding of individual factors that contribute to possibility of injury.
• Demonstrate behaviors, lifestyle changes to reduce risk factors and protect self from injury.
• Modify environment as indicated to enhance safety.

ACTIONS/INTERVENTIONS

Sample **NIC** linkages:
Surveillance: Safety: Purposeful and ongoing collection and analysis of information about the patient and the environment for use in promoting and maintaining client safety
Risk Identification: Analysis of potential risk factors, determination of health risks, and prioritization of risk-reduction strategies for an individual or group
Environmental Management: Safety: Manipulation of the patient's surroundings for therapeutic benefit

NURSING PRIORITY NO. 1

To evaluate degree/source of risk inherent in the individual situation:

● Identify client at risk (e.g., acute illness, surgery, trauma; chronic illness conditions with weakness, immunosuppression, or prolonged immobility; acute or chronic confusion, dementia, head injury; use of multiple medications; use of alcohol or other drugs; mental illness, emotional liability; cultural, familial, and socioeconomic factors adversely affecting lifestyle and home; exposure to environmental chemicals or other hazards).
● Note age and gender. *Children, young adults, elderly persons, and men are at greater risk for injury reflecting client's ability or desire to protect self and influencing choice of interventions or teaching.*[15]
● Evaluate developmental level, decision-making ability, level of cognition, competence, and independence. *Determines client's/SO's ability to attend to safety issues.*
● Assess mood, coping abilities, personality styles (i.e., temperament, aggression, impulsive behavior, level of self-esteem). *May result in carelessness or increased risk-taking without consideration of consequences.*[1,2]
● Evaluate individual's emotional and behavioral response to violence in surroundings (e.g., neighborhood, television, peer group). *May affect client's view of and regard for own or others' safety.*[1,2,15]
● Assess muscle strength, gross and fine motor coordination *to identify risk for falls.*
● Observe client for signs of injury and age (e.g., old or new bruises, history of fractures, frequent absences from school or work). Determine potential for abusive behavior by family members/SO(s)/peers. *Client or care providers may require further evaluation or investigation for abuse.*[5]
● Perform thorough assessments regarding safety issues when planning for client care and discharge. *Failure to accurately assess and intervene or refer regarding these issues can place the client at needless risk and creates negligence issues for the healthcare practitioner.*[14]
● Ascertain knowledge of safety needs and injury prevention, and motivation to prevent injury in home, community, and work setting. *Information may reveal areas of misinformation, lack of knowledge, need for teaching.*[1]
● Note socioeconomic status and availability and use of resources.

NURSING PRIORITY NO. 2

To assist client/caregiver to reduce or correct individual risk factors:

- Provide healthcare within a culture of safety (e.g., adherence to nursing standards of care and facility safe-care policies) *to prevent errors resulting in client injury, promote client safety, and model safety behaviors for client/SO:*[14]

  Maintain bed or chair in lowest position with wheels locked.

  Provide seat raisers for chairs, use stand-assist, repositioning, or lifting devices as indicated.

  Ensure that pathway to bathroom is unobstructed and properly lighted.

  Place assistive devices (e.g., walker, cane, glasses, hearing aid) within reach.

  Instruct client/SO to request assistance, as needed; make sure call light is within reach and client knows how to operate.

  Monitor environment for potentially unsafe conditions or hazards, modify as needed.

- ∞ Place confused elderly client or young child near nurses' station *to provide for frequent observation.*[6]

  Orient or reorient client to environment, as needed.

  Safety lock exit and stairwell doors *when client can wander away.*

  Avoid use of restraints. *Restraints can increase client's agitation and risk of entrapment and death.*

- Administer medications and infusions using "6 rights" system (right client, right medication, right route, right dose, right time, right documentation).[8]

  Inform and educate client/SO regarding all treatments and medications.

- Provide client/SO information regarding client's specific disease or condition and consequences of continuing unhealthy behaviors (e.g., increase in oral cancer among teenagers using smokeless tobacco; fetal alcohol syndrome or neonatal addiction in prenatal women using tobacco, alcohol, or other drugs) *to enhance decision making, clarify expectations and individual needs.*

- Determine if risk-prone behavior is occurring or likely to occur *to initiate appropriate wellness counseling and referrals.*

- Review client's level of physical activity in his or her lifestyle *to determine changes or adaptations that may be required by current situation.*

- Refer to physical or occupational therapist as appropriate *to identify high-risk tasks, conduct site visits; select, create, modify equipment or assistive devices; and provide education about body mechanics and musculoskeletal injuries, in addition to providing therapies as indicated.*[6]

- Perform home assessment and identify safety issues such as:[1–13]

  locking up medications and poisonous substances;

  using window grates or locks *to prevent young children from falls*;

  installing handrails, ramps, bathtub safety tapes;

  using electrical outlet covers or lockouts;

  locking exterior doors *to prevent confused individual from wandering off while SO is engaged in other household activities*;

  removing matches, smoking materials, and knobs from the stove *so young children or confused individual do not turn on burner and leave it unattended*;

  properly placing alarms and fire extinguishers;

  discussing safe use of oxygen;

  obtaining medical alert device or home monitoring service.

- Review specific employment concerns or worksite issues and needs (e.g., ergonomic chairs and workstations; proper fitting safety equipment, footwear; regular use of safety glasses or goggles and ear protectors; safe storage of hazardous substances; number of hours worked per shift/week).

- Demonstrate and encourage use of techniques to reduce or manage stress and vent emotions such as anger, hostility. *Identifying and dealing with emotions appropriately enables individual to maintain control of behavior and avoid possibility of violent outbursts.*[2,5,7]
- Discuss importance of self-monitoring of factors that can contribute to occurrence of injury (e.g., fatigue, anger, irritability). *Client/SO may be able to modify risk through monitoring of actions, or postponement of certain actions, especially during times when client is likely to be highly stressed.*
- Encourage participation in self-help programs, such as assertiveness training, anger management, positive self-image *to enhance self-esteem.*
- Review expectations caregivers have of children, cognitively impaired, and/or elderly family members. Discuss concerns about discipline practices.[13]
- Discuss need for and sources of supervision (e.g., before- and after-school programs, elderly day care).

NURSING PRIORITY NO. 3

To promote wellness (Teaching/Discharge Considerations):

- Identify individual needs and resources for safety education (e.g., home hazard information; fall prevention; firearm safety; cardiopulmonary resuscitation [CPR]/first aid).[3,10,11]
- Stress importance of correct use of child safety seats, car seat belt restraints, bicycle or other helmets; regular use of sports safety equipment; etc.
- Provide instruction or refer to classes for back safety and proper use of injury-prevention devices. Recommend use of ergonomic bed and chair as appropriate.
- Provide telephone numbers and other contact numbers as individually indicated (e.g., doctor, 911, poison control, police, elder advocate).
- Provide bibliotherapy including written resource lists and reliable Web sites *for later review and self-paced learning.*
- Refer to other resources as indicated (e.g., counseling or psychotherapy, budget counseling, and parenting classes).
- Refer to or assist with community education programs *to increase awareness of safety measures and resources available to the individual.*[4]
- Promote community awareness about the problems of design of buildings, equipment, transportation, and workplace practices that contribute to accidents.[4]
- Identify community resources, neighbors, or friends to assist elderly or handicapped individuals in providing such things as structural maintenance, removal of snow and ice from walks and steps, and so forth.
- Identify emergency escape plans and routes for home and community *to be prepared in the event of natural or man-made disaster (e.g., fire, hurricane, earthquake, toxic chemical release).*[4]

DOCUMENTATION FOCUS

Assessment/Reassessment
- Individual risk factors, noting current physical findings (e.g., bruises, cuts).
- Client's/caregiver's understanding of individual risks and safety concerns.

Planning
- Plan of care and who is involved in planning.
- Teaching plan.

Implementation/Evaluation
• Individual responses to interventions, teaching, and actions performed.
• Specific actions and changes that are made.
• Attainment or progress toward desired outcome(s).
• Modifications to plan of care.

Discharge Planning
• Long-term plans for discharge needs, lifestyle and community changes, and who is responsible for actions to be taken.
• Specific referrals made.

References

1. Gorman-Smith, D., Tolan, P. (1998). The role of exposure to community violence and developmental problems among inner city youth. *Dev Psychopathol*, 10(1), 101–116.
2. National Center for Injury Prevention and Control. Youth violence in the United States. Retrieved July 2007 from www.cdc.gov/ncipc/factsheets/yvfacts.htm.
3. Gun safety. ENA Fact sheet. Retrieved July 2007 from www.ena.org/ipinstitute/fact/ENAIPFactSheet-GunSafety.pdf.
4. Doenges, M. E., Moorhouse, M. F., Geissler-Murr, A. C. (2002). Care plan: Disaster considerations; and ND infection, risk for, in numerous care plans. *Nursing Care Plans: Guidelines for Individualizing Patient Care*. 6th ed. Philadelphia: F. A. Davis.
5. National Center for Injury Prevention and Control. Intimate partner violence. Retrieved July 2007 from www.cdc.gov/ncipc/factsheets/ipvfacts.htm.
6. Nelson, A., (2003). Safe patient handling & movement. *Am J Nurs*, 103(3), 32–43.
7. National Center for Injury Prevention and Control. Sexual violence. Retrieved July 2007 from www.cdc.gov/ncipc/factsheets/svfacts.htm.
8. Gosdon, M. J. (2009). Using technology to reduce medication errors. *Nursing*, 39(6), 57–58.
9. Bicycle/Helmet Safety. Retrieved January 2004 from www.ena.org.
10. Emergency Nurses Association. Water safety. Retrieved January 2004 from www.ena.org.
11. National Center for Injury Prevention and Control. Drowning prevention. Retrieved July 2007 from www.cdc.gov/ncipc/factsheets/drown.htm.
12. National Center for Injury Prevention and Control. Suicide in the United States. Retrieved July 2007 from www.cdc.gov/ncipc/factsheets/suifacts.
13. Safety for older consumers' home safety checklist. Consumer Product Safety Commission (CPSC) document no. 701. Retrieved July 2007 from www.gardencitymi.org/departments/fire/seniorsafetychecklist.pdf.
14. Keepnews, D., Mitchell, P. H. (2003). Health systems' accountability for patient safety. *Online J Issues Nurs*, 8(2). Retrieved March 2007 from http://nursingworld.org/ojin/topic22/tpc22_2.htm.
15. Schwebel, D. C., Barton, B. K. (2005). Contributions of multiple risk factors to child injury. *J Pediatr Psychol*, 30(7), 553–61.

risk for perioperative positioning Injury

DEFINITION: At risk for injury as a result of the environmental conditions found in the perioperative setting

RISK FACTORS

Disorientation; sensory or perceptual disturbances due to anesthesia
Immobilization; muscle weakness; [preexisting musculoskeletal conditions]

Obesity; emaciation; edema
[Elderly]

NOTE: A risk diagnosis is not evidenced by signs and symptoms, as the problem has not occurred; rather, nursing interventions are directed at prevention.

Sample Clinical Applications: Operative procedures, arthritis, obesity, malnutrition, peripheral vascular disease

DESIRED OUTCOMES/EVALUATION CRITERIA

Sample NOC linkages:
Risk Detection: Personal actions to identify personal health threats
Risk Control: Personal actions to prevent, eliminate, or reduce modifiable health threats
Tissue Perfusion: Peripheral: Adequacy of blood flow through the small vessels of the extremities to maintain tissue function

Client Will (Include Specific Time Frame)
• Be free of injury related to perioperative disorientation.
• Be free of untoward skin and tissue injury or changes lasting beyond 24 to 48 hours post-procedure.
• Report resolution of localized numbness, tingling, or changes in sensation related to positioning within 24 to 48 hours as appropriate.

ACTIONS/INTERVENTIONS

Sample NIC linkages:
Positioning: Intraoperative: Moving the patient body part to promote surgical exposure while reducing the risk of discomfort and complications
Skin Surveillance: Collection and analysis of patient data to maintain skin and mucous membrane integrity
Circulatory Precautions: Protection of a localized area with limited perfusion

NURSING PRIORITY NO. 1

To identify individual risk factors/needs:

• Consider anticipated type and length of procedure, type of anesthesia to be used, and customary required position (e.g., supine, lithotomy, prone, lateral, sitting) *to increase awareness of potential postoperative complications (e.g., supine position may cause low back pain and skin pressure at heels, elbows, and sacrum; lateral chest position can cause shoulder and neck pain, or eye and ear injury on the client's downside. Also normal defense mechanisms are altered due to anesthetic agents and medications as well as forced prolonged immobility during the procedure).*[1,2,8]

∞ • Review client's history, noting age, weight, height, nutritional status, physical limitations (e.g., prostheses, implants, range-of-motion restrictions) and preexisting conditions (vascular, respiratory, circulatory, neurological, immunocompromise). *These factors affect choice of position for the procedure (e.g., elderly person with no subcutaneous padding or severe arthritis). Presence of certain conditions can cause the risk of skin and tissue integrity problems during surgery (e.g., diabetes mellitus, obesity, presence of peripheral vascular disease, level of hydration, temperature of extremities).*[1,2,10,11]

- Evaluate and document client's preoperative reports of neurological, sensory or motor deficits *for comparative baseline of perioperative and postoperative sensations.*
- Assess the individual's responses to preoperative sedation and medication, noting level of sedation or adverse effects (e.g., drop in blood pressure) and report to surgeon as indicated. *Hypotension is a common factor associated with nerve ischemia.*[3]
- Evaluate environmental conditions/safety issues surrounding the sedated client (e.g., client alone in holding area, side rails up on bed and cart, use of tourniquets and arm boards, need for local injections) *that predispose client to potential tissue injury.*[1,3,9,11]

NURSING PRIORITY NO. 2

To position client to provide protection for anatomical structures and to prevent injury:

- Stabilize and lock transport cart or bed when transferring client to and from operating room table. Provide body and limb support for client during transfers, using adequate numbers of personnel *to prevent client fall, shear and friction injuries, as well as to prevent injury to personnel.*[4,11]
- Position client, using appropriate positioning equipment or devices, *to provide protection for anatomic structures and to prevent injury:*[1,2]

  Keep head in neutral position (when client in supine position) and arm boards at less than 90-degree angle and level with floor *to prevent neural injuries.*

  Maintain cervical neck alignment and provide protection or padding for forehead, eyes, nose, chin, breasts, genitalia, knees, and feet *when client in prone position.*

  Protect bony prominences and pressure points on dependent side (e.g., axillary roll for dependent axilla, lower leg flexed at hip, upper leg straight padding between knees, ankles, and feet) *when client in lateral position.*

  Place legs in stirrups simultaneously, adjusting stirrup height to client's legs, maintaining symmetrical position, pad popliteal space as indicated *to reduce risk of peroneal and tibial nerve damage, prevent muscle strain, and reduce risk of hip dislocation when lithotomy position used.*

- Check that positioning equipment is correct size for client, is firm and stable, and is adjusted accordingly.[2,4]
- Use gel pads or similar devices over the operating room bed. *Decreases pressure at any given point by redistributing overall pressures across a larger surface area.*[2,8]
- Limit use of pillows, blankets, molded foam devices, towels, and sheet rolls, *which may produce only a minimum of pressure reduction or contribute to friction injuries.*[2]
- Place safety straps strategically *to secure client for specific procedure.* Avoid pressure on extremities when securing straps *to limit possibility of compromising circulation and pressure injuries.*[4]
- Realign or maintain body alignment during procedure as needed. *Changes in position may expose or damage otherwise protected body tissue. The position change may be planned, or imperceptible, and may result from adding or deleting positioning devices, adjusting the procedure bed in some manner, or moving the client on the procedure bed.*[2]
- Apply and periodically reposition padding of pressure points/bony prominences (e.g., arms, shoulders, ankles) and neurovascular pressure points (e.g., breasts, knees, ears) *to maintain position of safety and prevent injury from prolonged pressure.*
- Protect body from contact with metal parts of the operating table, *which could produce electrical injury or burns.*[1,5]
- Position extremities to facilitate periodic evaluation of hands, fingers, and toes. *Prevents accidental trauma from moving table attachments; allows for repositioning of extremities to*

prevent neurovascular injuries from prolonged pressure. Extremities should not extend beyond the end of operating table to reduce risk of compression or stretch injury.[6,10]

- Check peripheral pulses and skin color and temperature periodically *to monitor circulation.*
- Ascertain that eyelids are closed and secured *to prevent corneal abrasions.*[6]
- Prevent pooling of prep and irrigating solutions, and body fluids. *Pooling of liquids in areas of high pressure under client increases risk of pressure ulcer development and presents electrical hazard.*[7,8]
- Reposition slowly at transfer and in bed (especially halothane-anesthetized client) *to prevent severe drop in blood pressure, dizziness, or unsafe transfer.*
- Position client following extubation *to protect airway and facilitate respiratory effort.*
- Determine specific postoperative positioning guidelines (e.g., head of bed slightly elevated following spinal anesthesia *to prevent headache;* turn to unoperated side following pneumonectomy *to facilitate maximal respiratory effort).*[1]

NURSING PRIORITY NO. 3

To promote wellness (Teaching/Discharge Considerations):

- Maintain equipment in good working order *to identify potential hazards in the surgical suite and implement corrections as appropriate.*[8]
- Provide perioperative teaching relative to client safety issues (including not crossing legs during procedures performed under local or light anesthesia, postoperative needs or limitations, and signs/symptoms requiring medical evaluation) *to reduce incidence of preventable complications.*
- Inform client and postoperative caregivers of expected or transient reactions (e.g., low backache, localized numbness, and reddening or skin indentations, which should quickly resolve) *to help them identify problems or concerns that require follow-up.*
- Assist with therapies and perform nursing actions, including skin care measures, application of elastic stockings, early mobilization *to enhance circulation and venous return, and promote skin and tissue integrity.*
- Encourage and assist with frequent range-of-motion exercises *to prevent or reduce joint stiffness.*
- Refer to appropriate resources, as needed.

DOCUMENTATION FOCUS

Assessment/Reassessment
- Findings, including individual risk factors for problems in the perioperative setting and need to modify routine activities or positions.
- Periodic evaluation of monitoring activities.

Planning
- Plan of care and who is involved in planning.
- Teaching plan.

Implementation/Evaluation
- Response to interventions and actions performed.
- Attainment or progress toward desired outcome(s).
- Modifications to plan of care.

Discharge Planning
- Long-term needs and who is responsible for actions to be taken.

References

1. Doenges, M. E., Moorhouse, M. F., Geissler-Murr, A. C. (2002). Surgical intervention. *Nursing Care Plans: Guidelines for Individualizing Patient Care.* 6th ed. Philadelphia: F. A. Davis, 766–767.
2. Association of Perioperative Registered Nurses (AORN). (2001). *AORN Standards and Recommended Practices for Perioperative Nursing.* Denver, CO: Author.
3. Prevention of injuries in the anaesthetized patient. (1997–2004). Retrieved July 2007 from www.surgical-tutor.org.uk/default-home.htm?principles/perioperative/perioperative_injuries .htm~right.
4. Gruendemann, B. J., Fernsebner, B. (1995). *Comprehensive Perioperative Nursing,* vol. 1. Boston: Jones & Bartlett.
5. Rothrock, J. (1996). *Perioperative Nursing Care Planning.* St. Louis, MO: Mosby.
6. Spry, C. (1997). *Essentials of Perioperative Nursing.* Gaithersburg, MD: Aspen.
7. Meeker, M., Rothrock, J. (1999). *Alexander's Care of the Patient in Surgery.* 11th ed. St. Louis, MO: Mosby.
8. Lafreniere, R., Berguer, R., Seifert, P. C. (2005). Preparation of the operating room. Retrieved March 2007 www.medscape.com/viewarticle/503004.
9. Dunn, D. (2005). Preventing perioperative complications in special populations. *Nursing,* 35(11), 36–43.
10. Renter, T. A. Upper extremity positioning injuries during operative/other invasive procedures. Anesthesia Consulting. Retrieved March 2007 from www.anesthesia-consulting.com.
11. Dunn, D. (2006). Age-smart care: Preventing perioperative complications in older adults. *Nursing,* 4(3), 30–39.

Insomnia

DEFINITION: A sustained disruption in amount and quality of sleep that impairs functioning

RELATED FACTORS

Intake of stimulants or alcohol; medications; gender-related hormonal shifts

Stress (e.g., ruminative presleep pattern); depression, fear, anxiety, grief

Impairment of normal sleep pattern (e.g., travel, shift work, parental responsibilities, interruptions for interventions); inadequate sleep hygiene (current)

Activity pattern (e.g., timing, amount)

Physical discomfort (e.g., body temperature, pain, shortness of breath, cough, gastroesophageal reflux, nausea, incontinence/urgency)

Environmental factors (e.g., ambient noise, daylight/darkness exposure, ambient temperature/humidity, unfamiliar setting

DEFINING CHARACTERISTICS

Subjective
Patient reports:
Difficulty falling or staying asleep
Waking up too early
Dissatisfaction with sleep (current); nonrestorative sleep
Sleep disturbances that produce next-day consequences; lack of energy; difficulty concentrating; changes in mood

Decreased health status or quality of life
Increased accidents

Objective
Observed lack of energy
Observed changes in affect
Increased work or school absenteeism

Sample Clinical Applications: Chronic pain, substance use or abuse, hyperthyroidism, pulmonary diseases (e.g., COPD, asthma), sleep apnea, restless leg syndrome, depression, Alzheimer's disease, senile dementia, anxiety disorders, bipolar disorders, pregnancy—prenatal or postnatal period

DESIRED OUTCOMES/EVALUATION CRITERIA

Sample (NOC) linkages:
Sleep: Natural periodic suspension of consciousness during which the body is restored
Rest: Quality and pattern of diminished activity for mental and physical rejuvenation

Client Will (Include Specific Time Frame)
• Verbalize understanding of sleep impairment.
• Identify individually appropriate interventions to promote sleep.
• Adjust lifestyle to accommodate chronobiological rhythms.
• Report improvement in sleep or rest pattern.
• Report increased sense of well-being and feeling rested.

ACTIONS/INTERVENTIONS

Sample (NIC) linkages:
Sleep Enhancement: Facilitation of regular sleep/wake cycle
Relaxation Therapy: Use of techniques to encourage and elicit relaxation for the purpose of decreasing undesirable signs and symptoms such as pain, muscle tension, or anxiety
Environmental Management: Comfort: Manipulation of the patient's surroundings for promotion of optimal comfort

NURSING PRIORITY NO. 1

To identify causative/contributing factors:

● Identify presence of Related Factors that can contribute to insomnia (e.g., chronic pain, arthritis, dyspnea; movement disorders; dementia; obesity; pregnancy, menopause; psychiatric disorders); metabolic diseases (e.g., hyperthyroidism and diabetes); prescribed and over-the-counter (OTC) drugs; alcohol, stimulant or other recreational drug use; circadian rhythm disorders (e.g., shift work, jet lag); environmental factors (e.g., noise, no control over thermostat, uncomfortable bed); major life stressors (e.g., grief, loss, finances).[1–6,12,13]

∞ ● Note age. *Increased sleep latency (time required to fall asleep), decreased sleep efficiency, and increased awakenings are common in the elderly.*[2]

∞ ● Observe parent-infant interactions and provision of emotional support. Note mother's sleep-wake pattern. *Lack of knowledge of infant cues or problem relationships may create tension interfering with sleep. Structured sleep routines based on adult schedules may not meet child's needs.*[7]

- Ascertain presence and frequency of enuresis, incontinence, or need for frequent nighttime voidings, interrupting sleep.[2]
- Assist with or review psychological assessment, noting individual and personality characteristics *if anxiety disorders or depression could be affecting sleep.*
- Determine recent traumatic events in client's life (e.g., a death in family, loss of job). *Physical and emotional trauma often affects client's sleep patterns and quality for a short period of time. This disruption can become long term and require more intensive assessment and intervention.* [2,3]
- Review client's medication regimen, including prescription (e.g., beta-blockers, steroids, antihypertensives, bronchodilators, weight-loss drugs, thyroid preparations, sedatives); OTC products (e.g., decongestants); herbals. *Use or timing may be interfering with falling asleep or staying asleep requiring adjustments such as change in dose or time medication is taken, or choice of drug prescribed.* [8,13]
- Note caffeine and alcohol intake. *May interfere with falling asleep, or duration and quality of sleep.*
- Assist with diagnostic testing (e.g., EEG, full-night sleep studies) *to determine cause and type of sleep disturbance.*

NURSING PRIORITY NO. 2

To determine sleep pattern and dysfunction(s):

- Observe or obtain feedback from client/SO(s) regarding client's sleep problems, usual bedtime, rituals or routines, number of hours of sleep, time of arising, and environmental needs *to determine usual sleep pattern and provide comparative baseline.*
- Listen to subjective reports of sleep quality (e.g., client never feels rested or feels sleepy during day). *Provides opportunity to address misconceptions or unrealistic expectations and plan for interventions.* [9]
- Determine type of insomnia (e.g., transient, short term, chronic). *Transient episodes are occasional restless nights caused by such factors as jet lag, first night in a new bed, and so forth. Short-term insomnia lasts a few weeks and arises from temporary stressful experience, such as pressures at work, loss of job, death in family, and usually resolves over time as client adapts to stressor. Chronic insomnia lasts for more than 3 weeks and can be caused by many physical and psychological factors as well as use/misuse of medications and drugs.* [5]
- Investigate whether client snores and in what position(s) this occurs. Also determine if obese individual experiences loud periodic snoring, along with unusual nighttime activities (e.g., sitting upright, sleepwalking); morning headaches, sleepiness, depression. *Sleep studies may need to be done to rule out obstructive sleep disorder.* [2,4]
- Note alteration of habitual sleep time such as change of work pattern or rotating shifts, change in normal bedtime (hospitalization). *Helps identify circumstances that are known to interrupt sleep patterns resulting in mental and physical fatigue, affecting concentration, interest, energy, and appetite.* [6]
- Observe physical signs of fatigue (e.g., restlessness, hand tremors, thick speech).
- Graph "circadian" rhythms of individual's biological internal chemistry per protocol as indicated. *Note: Studies have shown sleep cycles are affected by body temperature at onset of sleep.*
- Assist with diagnostic testing (e.g., electroencephalogram [EEG], electrooculogram [EOG], and electromyogram [EMG]; psychological assessment/testing, chronological chart). *Polysomnography (the three electrical tests noted above) are performed in a sleep laboratory to*

measure several parameters of sleep, including brain wave activity, eye movement, and leg muscle tone. These tests may be performed after initial clinical evaluation or symptom management fails to discover or resolve a particular sleep disturbance or point to appropriate interventions and treatments.[1,2,4]

NURSING PRIORITY NO. 3

To assist client to establish optimal sleep/rest patterns:

- Collaborate in treatment of underlying medical problem (e.g., obstructive sleep apnea, pain, gastroesophageal reflux disease [GERD], lower urinary tract infection [UTI]/prostatic hypertropy; depression, complicated grief).
- Arrange care to provide for uninterrupted periods for rest. *Allows for longer periods of sleep, especially during night.*[9]
- Limit fluid intake in evening if nocturia is a problem to reduce need for nighttime elimination.[10]
- Provide quiet environment and comfort measures (e.g., back rub, washing hands and face, cleaning and straightening sheets). *Promotes relaxation and readiness for sleep.*[9]
- Administer pain medications (if required) 1 hour before sleep *to relieve discomfort and take maximum advantage of analgesic and sedative effect.*[5]
- Discuss and implement effective age-appropriate bedtime rituals (e.g., going to bed at same time each night, drinking warm milk, rocking, story reading, cuddling, favorite blanket or toy) *to enhance client's ability to fall asleep, reinforce that bed is a place to sleep, and promote sense of security for child or confused elder.*[7]
- Recommend limiting intake of chocolate and caffeinated or alcoholic beverages, especially prior to bedtime. *Substances known to impair falling asleep or staying asleep. Alcohol may help individual fall asleep, but ensuing sleep is fragmented.*[7]
- Explore other sleep aids (e.g., warm bath or milk, light protein snack before bedtime, soothing music, favorite TV show). *Nonpharmaceutical aids may enhance falling asleep free of concern of medication side effects such as morning hangover or drug dependence.*[5]
- Develop behavioral program for insomnia, such as:[1-6,13]
  - establishing routine at bedtime and arising;
  - thinking relaxing thoughts when in bed;
  - avoid napping in the daytime;
  - refrain from reading or watching TV in bed;
  - getting out of bed if not asleep in 15 minutes;
  - limiting sleep to 7 hours a night;
  - getting up the same time each day—even on weekends and days off;
  - getting adequate exposure to bright light during day;
  - individually tailoring stress-reduction program, music therapy, relaxation routine.
- Recommend and assist with implementing program to "reset" sleep clock (chronotherapy when client has delayed sleep onset insomnia). *These sleep-wake problems are common among shift workers and airplane travelers. Shift workers can benefit by adhering to a set routine and ensuring that noises and interruptions are kept to a minimum. Those who travel across time zones can benefit by adjusting their sleep time to match the time zone of their arrival and avoiding caffeine and alcohol.*[11]
- Use barbiturates or other sleeping medications sparingly. *Research indicates long-term use of these medications can actually induce sleep disturbances.*
- Encourage routine use of continuous positive airway pressure (CPAP) therapy when indicated to obtain optimal benefit of treatment for sleep apnea.

- Monitor effects of therapeutic use of amphetamines or stimulants (such as may be used for attention deficit disorder or narcolepsy). *Use of these medications can induce or potentiate sleep disturbances.*[8]

- Refer to sleep specialist as indicated or desired. *Follow-up evaluation and intervention may be needed when insomnia is having a serious impact on client's quality of life, productivity, and safety (e.g., on the job, at home, on the road).*[2,15]

NURSING PRIORITY NO. 4

To promote wellness (Teaching/Discharge Considerations):

- Assure client that occasional sleeplessness should not threaten health. *Knowledge that occasional insomnia is universal and usually not harmful may promote relaxation and relief from worry, which can perpetuate the problem.*[4]

- Assist client to develop individual program of relaxation. Demonstrate techniques (e.g., biofeedback, self-hypnosis, visualization, progressive muscle relaxation). *Methods that reduce sympathetic response and decrease stress can help induce sleep, particularly in persons suffering from chronic and long-term sleep disturbances.*[3]

- Encourage participation in regular exercise program during day *to aid in stress control and release of energy. Note: Exercise at bedtime may stimulate rather than relax client and actually interfere with sleep.*[2]

- Investigate use of aids (e.g., sleep mask, darkening shades or curtains, earplugs, monotonous sounds [white noise]) *to block out ambient light and noise.*

- Assist individuals with insomnia associated with shift work to develop individual schedule *to take advantage of peak performance times as identified in chronobiological chart.*

- Recommend midmorning nap if one is required. *Napping, especially in the afternoon, can disrupt normal sleep patterns.*

- Assist client to deal with grieving process if grief is causing or exacerbating insomnia. (Refer to ND Grieving.)

DOCUMENTATION FOCUS

Assessment/Reassessment
- Assessment findings, including specifics of sleep pattern (current and past) and effects on lifestyle and level of functioning.
- Medications, interventions, previous therapies tried.
- Results of testing.

Planning
- Plan of care and who is involved in planning.
- Teaching plan.

Implementation/Evaluation
- Client's response to interventions, teaching, and actions performed.
- Attainment or progress toward desired outcome(s).
- Modifications to plan of care.

Discharge Planning
- Long-term needs and who is responsible for actions to be taken.
- Specific referrals made.

References

1. National Sleep Foundation. When you can't sleep: ABCs of ZZZs. Retrieved July 2007 from www.sleepfoundation.org.
2. Grandjean, C. K., Gibbons, S. W. (2000). Assessing geriatric sleep complaints. *Nurse Pract: Am J Prim Health Care*, 25(9), 25.
3. Cox, H. C., et al. (2002). Sleep pattern, disturbed. *Clinical Applications of Nursing Diagnosis: Adult, Child, Women's, Psychiatric, Gerontic, and Home Health Considerations*. 4th ed. Philadelphia: F. A. Davis, 375–380.
4. National Institute of Neurological Disorders and Stroke (NINDS). Brain basics: Understanding sleep. Retrieved July 2007 from www.ninds.nih.gov/disorders/brain_basics/understanding _sleep.htm.
5. Bahr, R. T. (1999). Sleep disturbances. In Stanley, M., Beare, P. G. (eds). *Gerontological Nursing: A Health Promotion/Protection Approach*. 2d ed. Philadelphia: F. A. Davis, 335–341.
6. Pronitis-Ruotolo, D. (2001). Surviving the night shift: Making Zeitgerber work for you. *Am J Nurs*, 101(7), 63.
7. Olds, S., London, M., Ladwig, P. (1999). *Maternal-Newborn Nursing: A Family and Community-Based Approach*. 6th ed. Upper Saddle River, NJ: Prentice Hall.
8. Deglin, J. H., Vallerand, A. H. (2003). *Davis's Drug Guide for Nurses*. 8th ed. Philadelphia: F. A. Davis.
9. Doenges, M. E., Moorhouse, M. F., Geissler-Murr, A. C. (2004). *Nurse's Pocket Guide; Diagnoses, Interventions and Rationales.* 9th ed. Philadelphia: F. A. Davis.
10. Townsend, M. C. (2000). *Psychiatric Mental Health Nursing Concepts of Care*. 4th ed. Philadelphia: F. A. Davis.
11. Somer, E., Snyderman, N. L. (1999). *Food & Mood: The Complete Guide to Eating Well and Feeling Your Best*. 2d ed. New York: Owl Books.
12. Vij, S., Gentili, A. (2005). Sleep disorder, geriatric. Retrieved December 2006 from www.emedicine.com/med/topic3179.htm.
13. Hertz, G., Cataletto, M. E. (2006). Sleep dysfunction in women. Retrieved December 2006 from www.emedicine.com/med/topic656.htm.
14. Turkowski, B. B. (2006). Managing insomnia. *Orthop Nurs*, 25(5), 339–345.
15. Nadolski, M. (2005). Getting a good night's sleep: Diagnosing and treating insomnia. *Plast Surg Nurs*, 25(4), 167–173.

decreased Intracranial Adaptive Capacity

DEFINITION: Intracranial fluid dynamic mechanisms that normally compensate for increases in intracranial volume are compromised, resulting in repeated disproportionate increases in intracranial pressure (ICP) in response to a variety of noxious and nonnoxious stimuli

RELATED FACTORS

Brain injuries
Sustained increase in ICP = 10 to 15 mm Hg
Decreased cerebral perfusion pressure ≤50 to 60 mm Hg
Systemic hypotension with intracranial hypertension

(continues on page 470)

decreased Intracranial Adaptive Capacity (continued)
DEFINING CHARACTERISTICS

Objective

Repeated increases in ICP of > 10 mm Hg for more than 5 minutes following a variety of external stimuli

Disproportionate increase in ICP following stimulus

Elevated P_2 ICP waveform

Volume pressure response test variation (volume-pressure ratio 2, pressure-volume index <10)

Baseline ICP ≤10 mm Hg

Wide amplitude ICP waveform

[Altered level of consciousness—coma]

[Changes in vital signs, cardiac rhythm]

Sample Clinical Applications: Traumatic brain injury (TBI), cerebral edema, stroke, cranial tumors/hematomas, hydrocephalus

DESIRED OUTCOMES/EVALUATION CRITERIA

Sample NOC linkages:

Tissue Perfusion: Cerebral: Adequacy of blood flow through the cerebral vasculature to maintain brain function

Neurological Status: Ability of the peripheral and central nervous system to receive, process, and respond to internal and external stimuli

Client Will (Include Specific Time Frame)
- Demonstrate stable ICP as evidenced by normalization of pressure waveforms and response to stimuli.
- Display improved neurological signs.

ACTIONS/INTERVENTIONS

Sample NIC linkages:

Cerebral Edema Management: Limitation of secondary cerebral injury resulting from swelling of brain tissue

Cerebral Perfusion Promotion: Promotion of adequate perfusion and limitation of complications for a patient experiencing or at risk for inadequate cerebral perfusion

Intracranial Pressure (ICP) Monitoring: Measurement and interpretation of patient data to regulate intracranial pressure

NURSING PRIORITY NO. 1

To assess causative/contributing factors:

- Determine factors related to individual situation (e.g., TBI, infection such as meningitis or encephalitis; brain tumor) and potential for increased ICP. *Deterioration in neurological signs/symptoms or failure to improve after initial insult may reflect decreased adaptive capacity.*[1]
- Review results of diagnostic imaging (e.g., cerebral computed tomography [CT] scans) *to note location, type, and severity of tissue injury.*

- Monitor for change in intracranial pressure (e.g., worsening neurological signs or variations in ICP monitor waveform and pressure) and corresponding event (e.g., coughing, suctioning, position change, noise such as monitor alarms, family visit). *Elevated pressure can be caused by the injury, environmental stimuli, or treatment modalities.*[1,2]

NURSING PRIORITY NO. 2

To note degree of impairment:

- Evaluate level of consciousness using Glasgow Coma Scale (GCS). *GCS assesses eye opening (e.g., awake, opens only to painful movement, keeps eyes closed), position or movement (e.g., spontaneous, purposeful, posturing), pupils (size, shape, equality, light reactivity), and consciousness or mental status (e.g., comatose, responds to pain, awake or confused). Low numbers (e.g., <9) are typically seen in clients with severe head injury and impaired cerebral perfusion requiring critical care interventions.*[1-3,7]
- Note purposeful and nonpurposeful motor response (e.g., posturing), comparing right and left sides. *Posturing and abnormal flexion of extremities usually indicates diffuse cortical damage. Absence of spontaneous movement on one side indicates damage to the motor tracts in the opposite cerebral hemisphere.*[1]
- Test for presence or absence of reflexes (e.g., blink, cough, gag, Babinski's reflex), nuchal rigidity. *Helps identify location of injury (e.g., loss of blink reflex suggests damage to the pons and medulla, absence of cough and gag reflexes reflects damage to medulla, and presence of Babinski's reflex indicates injury along pyramidal pathways in the brain).*[1]
- Monitor vital signs and cardiac rhythm before, during, and after activity. *Helps determine parameters for "safe" activity. Mean arterial blood pressure should be maintained above 90 mm Hg to maintain cerebral perfusion pressure (CCP) greater than 70 mm Hg, which reflects adequate blood supply to the brain. Fever in brain injury can be associated with injury to the hypothalamus or bleeding, systemic infection (e.g., pneumonia), or drugs. Hyperthermia exacerbates cerebral ischemia. Irregular respiration patterns can suggest location of cerebral insult. Cardiac dysrhythmias can be due to brainstem injury and stimulation of the sympathetic nervous system. Bradycardia may occur with high ICP.*[1,3]
- Monitor pulse oximetry or arterial blood gases (ABGs), particularly pH, CO_2, and PaO_2. *$PaCO_2$ level of 28 to 30 mm Hg decreases cerebral blood flow while maintaining adequate cerebral oxygenation, while a PaO_2 of less than 65 mm Hg may cause cerebral vascular dilation.*[1-3]
- Monitor urine output and serum sodium (Na). *Posttraumatic neuroendocrine dysfunction can result in a hyponatremic or hypernatremic state. When hyponatremia exists, cerebral edema or syndrome of inappropriate antidiuretic hormone (SIADH) can occur requiring correction with fluid restriction and hypertonic IV solution. Hypernatremia can occur because of injury to the hypothalamus or pituitary stalk, causing diabetes insipidus (DI), resulting in huge urine losses, or can be the result of excessive diuresis due to use of mannitol or furosemide administered to reduce cerebral edema.*[3]

NURSING PRIORITY NO. 3

To minimize/correct causative factors/maximize perfusion:

- Elevate head of bed as individually appropriate. *Optimal head of bed position is determined by both ICP and coronary perfusion pressure (CPP) measurements—that is, which degree of elevation lowers ICP while maintaining adequate cerebral blood flow.*[4] *Studies show that in most cases, 30 degrees elevation significantly decreases ICP while maintaining cerebral blood flow.*[1,7,8]

- Maintain head and neck in neutral position, supporting with small towel rolls or pillows *to maximize venous return. Note: Lateral and rotational neck flexion has been shown to be the most consistent trigger of sustained increases in ICP.* [5]

- Avoid causing hip flexion of 90 degrees or more. *Hip flexion may trap venous blood in the intra-abdominal space, increasing abdominal and intrathoracic pressure, and reducing venous outflow from the head, increasing cerebral pressure.* [6]

- Limit or prevent activities such as coughing, vomiting, straining at stool and avoid or restrict use of restraints. *These factors often increase intrathoracic/abdominal pressures or agitation and markedly increasing ICP.* [1]

- Suction with caution and only when needed, limiting to two passes of 10 seconds each with negative pressure no more than 120 mm Hg. Pass catheter just beyond end of endotracheal (ET) tube without touching tracheal wall or carina. Administer lidocaine intratracheally if indicated, *to reduce cough reflex.* [3]

- Hyperoxygenate before suctioning as appropriate *to minimize hypoxia. Note: Routine hyperventilation is to be avoided; however, therapeutic hyperventilation (PaCO$_2$ of 30–35 mm) may be used for a short period of time in acute neurological deterioration to reduce intracranial hypertension, while other methods of ICP control are initiated.* [3,8,9]

- Investigate increased restlessness *to determine causative factors and initiate corrective measures as indicated:*

  Decrease extraneous stimuli and provide comfort measures (e.g., quiet environment, soft voice, tapes of familiar voices played through earphones, back massage, gentle touch as tolerated) *to reduce central nervous system (CNS) stimulation and promote relaxation.* [1,5]

  Limit painful procedures (e.g., venipunctures, redundant neurological evaluations) to those that are absolutely necessary *in order to minimize preventable elevations in ICP.* [1,3]

  Provide rest periods between care activities and limit duration of procedures. Lower lighting and noise levels, schedule and limit activities *to provide restful environment and limit spikes in ICP associated with noxious stimuli.* [1]

  Encourage family/SOs to talk to client. *Familiar voices appear to have a relaxing effect on many comatose individuals (thereby reducing ICP).* [1]

- Administer and restrict fluid intake as necessary, administer IV fluids via pump or control device *to maintain intravascular volume sufficient to maintain cerebral perfusion while preventing inadvertent vascular overload, cerebral edema, and increased ICP.* [1]

- Weigh as indicated. Calculate fluid balance every shift/daily *to determine fluid needs and maintain hydration, and prevent fluid overload.* [1]

- Monitor and manage body temperature. Regulate environmental temperature and bed linens, use cooling blanket as indicated *to decrease metabolic and oxygen needs when fever present or when therapeutic hypothermia therapy is used. Lowering the body temperature has been shown to lower ICP and improve outcomes for recovery.* [3]

- Provide appropriate safety measures/initiate treatment for seizures *to prevent injury and increase of ICP or hypoxia.*

- Administer medications (e.g., antihypertensives, diuretics, analgesics, sedatives, antipyretics, vasopressors, antiseizure drugs, neuromuscular blocking agents, and corticosteroids) as appropriate *to maintain cerebral homeostasis and manage symptoms associated with neurological injury.*

- Administer enteral or parenteral nutrition *to achieve positive nitrogen balance, reducing effects of post–brain injury metabolic and catabolic states, which can lead to complications such as immunosuppression, infection, poor wound healing, loss of body mass, and multiple organ dysfunction.* [3]

⊕ Cultural   Ⓐ Collaborative   🏠 Community/Home Care   ⟋ Diagnostic Studies   ∞ Pediatric/Geriatric/Lifespan   Ⴑ Medications

⊕ • Prepare client for surgery as indicated (e.g., evacuation of hematoma or space-occupying lesion) *to reduce ICP and enhance circulation.*

NURSING PRIORITY NO. 4

To promote wellness (Teaching/Discharge Considerations):

• Identify signs/symptoms suggesting increased ICP (in client at risk without an ICP monitor), for example, restlessness, deterioration in neurological responses. Review appropriate interventions.

DOCUMENTATION FOCUS

Assessment/Reassessment
• Neurological findings noting right and left sides separately (e.g., pupils, motor response, reflexes, restlessness, nuchal rigidity); GCS.
• Response to activities and events (e.g., changes in pressure waveforms or vital signs).
• Presence and characteristics of seizure activity.

Planning
• Plan of care and who is involved in planning.
• Teaching plan.

Implementation/Evaluation
• Response to interventions and actions performed.
• Attainment or progress toward desired outcome(s).
• Modifications to plan of care.

Discharge Planning
• Future needs, plan for meeting them, and determining who is responsible for actions.
• Referrals as identified.

References

1. Doenges, M. E., Moorhouse, M. F., Geissler-Murr, A. C. (2002). Craniocerebral trauma (acute rehabilitative phase). *Nursing Care Plans: Guidelines for Individualizing Patient Care.* 6th ed. Philadelphia: F. A. Davis.
2. Brain Trauma Foundation, American Association of Neurological Surgeons. (2000). Part 1: Guidelines for the management of severe traumatic brain injury. Retrieved July 2007 from www.guideline.gov/summary/summary.aspx?doc_id=3794.
3. Acute care management of severe traumatic brain injuries. (2001). *Crit Care Nurse Q*, 23(4), 1.
4. Simmons, B. J. (1997). Management of intracranial hemodynamics in the adult: A research analysis of head positioning and recommendations for clinical practice and future research. *J Neurosci Nurs*, 29, 44.
5. Mitchell, P. H., Habermann, B. (1999). Rethinking physiological stability: Touch and intracranial pressure. *Biol Res Nurs*, 1(1), 12–19.
6. Vos, H. R. (1993). Making headway with intracranial hypertension. *Am J Nurs*, 93, 28.
7. Salinas, P., Hanbali, F. (2006). Closed head trauma. Retrieved March 2007 from www.emedicine.com/med/topic3403.htm.
8. Reddy, L. (2006). Heads up on cerebral bleeds. *Nursing*, 3(5), 4–9. Suppl, ED Insider.
9. Zink, E. K., McQuillan, K. (2005). Managing traumatic brain injury. *Nursing*, 35(9), 36–43.

neonatal Jaundice

DEFINITION: The yellow-orange tint of the neonate's skin and mucous membranes that occurs after 24 hours of life as a result of unconjugated bilirubin in the circulation

RELATED FACTORS

Neonate age 1 to 7 days
Feeding pattern not well established
Abnormal weight loss (>7–8% in breastfeeding newborn; 15% in term infant)
Stool (meconium) passage delayed
Infant experiences difficulty making transition to extrauterine life

DEFINING CHARACTERISTICS

Objective
Yellow-orange skin; yellow sclera
Abnormal skin bruising
Abnormal blood profile (hemolysis; total serum bilirubin > 2 mg/dL; inherited disorder; total serum bilirubin in high risk range [for] age in hour-specific nomogram)

Sample Clinical Applications: Newborn, premature infant

DESIRED OUTCOMES/EVALUATION CRITERIA

Sample (NOC) linkages:
Newborn Adaptation: Adaptive response to the extrauterine environment by a physiologically mature newborn during the first 28 days

Infant Will (Include Specific Time Frame):
• Display decreasing bilirubin levels with resolution of jaundice.
• Be free of central nervous system (CNS) involvement or complications associated with therapeutic regimen.
Knowledge: Treatment Procedure: Extent of understanding conveyed about a procedure required as part of a treatment regimen

Parent/Caregiver Will (Include Specific Time Frame):
• Verbalize understanding of cause, treatment, and possible outcomes of hyperbilirubinemia.
• Demonstrate appropriate care of infant.

ACTIONS/INTERVENTIONS

Sample (NIC) linkages:
Phototherapy: Neonate: Use of light therapy to reduce bilirubin levels in newborn infants
Breastfeeding Assistance: Preparing a new mother to breastfeed her infant

NURSING PRIORITY NO. 1

To assess causative/contributing factors:

● Determine infant and maternal blood group and blood type. *ABO incompatibilities affect 20% of all pregnancies and most commonly occur in mothers with type O blood, whose*

⊕ Cultural   ⊗ Collaborative   🏠 Community/Home Care   ✏ Diagnostic Studies   ∞ Pediatric/Geriatric/Lifespan   💊 Medications

anti A and anti-D antibodies pass into fetal circulation, causing red blood cell (RBC) agglutination and hemolysis.[1]

- Note gender, race, and place of birth. *Risk of developing jaundice is higher in males, infants of East Asian or American Indian descent, and those living at high altitudes. Incidence is lower for African American infants.*[2]
- Review intrapartal record for specific risk factors, such as low birth weight (LBW) or intrauterine growth retardation (IUGR), prematurity, abnormal metabolic processes, vascular injuries, abnormal circulation, sepsis, or polycythemia. *The risk of significant neonatal jaundice is increased in LBW or premature infants, presence of congenital infection, or maternal diabetes.*[2] *Studies suggest neonates at 36 to 37 weeks gestation are four to five times more likely to develop hyperbilirubinemia than those born at 40 weeks.*[3] *Also, certain clinical conditions may cause a reversal of the blood-brain barrier, allowing bound bilirubin to separate either at the level of the cell membrane or within the cell itself, increasing the risk of CNS involvement.*
- Note use of instruments or vacuum extractor for delivery. Assess infant for presence of birth trauma, cephalhematoma, and excessive ecchymosis or petechiae. *Resorption of blood trapped in fetal scalp tissue and excessive hemolysis may increase the amount of bilirubin being released and cause jaundice.*[7]
- Review infant's condition at birth, noting need for resuscitation or evidence of excessive ecchymosis or petechiae, cold stress, asphyxia, or acidosis. *Asphyxia and acidosis reduce affinity of bilirubin to albumin increasing the amount of unbound circulating (indirect) bilirubin, which may cross the blood-brain barrier causing CNS toxicity.*[2]
- Evaluate maternal and prenatal nutritional levels; note possible neonatal hypoproteinemia, especially in preterm infant. *One gram of albumin carries 16 mg of unconjugated bilirubin; therefore, lack of sufficient albumin (hypoproteinemia) in the newborn increases risk of jaundice.*
- Assess infant for signs of hypoglycemia such as jitteriness, irritability, and lethargy. Obtain heelstick glucose levels as indicated. *Hypoglycemia necessitates use of fat stores for energy-releasing fatty acids, which compete with bilirubin for binding sites on albumin.*
- Determine successful initiation and adequacy of breastfeeding. *Poor caloric intake and dehydration associated with ineffective breastfeeding increases risk of developing hyperbilirubinemia.*[1]
- Evaluate infant for pallor, edema, or hepatosplenomegaly. *These signs may be associated with hydrops fetalis, Rh incompatibility, and in-utero hemolysis of fetal RBCs.*
- Evaluate for jaundice in natural light, noting sclera and oral mucosa, yellowing of skin immediately after blanching, and specific body parts involved. Assess oral mucosa, posterior portion of hard palate, and conjunctival sacs in dark-skinned newborns. *Detects evidence/degree of jaundice generally first noted on face and progressing to trunk and then extremities.*[1,6] *Clinical appearance of jaundice is evident at bilirubin levels > 5 mg/dL in full-term infant. Estimated degree of jaundice is as follows: face, 4 to 8 mg/dL; trunk, 10 to 12 mg/dL; groin, 8 to 16 mg/dL; arms/legs, 11 to 18 mg/dL, and hands/feet, 15 to 20 mg/dL. Note: Yellow underlying pigment may be normal in dark-skinned infants.*[1,6,7]
- Note infants age at onset of jaundice. *Aids in differentiating type of jaundice (i.e., physiological, breast milk induced, or pathological). Physiological jaundice usually appears between the second and third days of life, as excess RBCs needed to maintain adequate oxygenation for the fetus are no longer required in the newborn and are hemolyzed, thereby releasing bilirubin.*[2,6] *Breast milk jaundice usually appears between the fourth and the seventh days of life, affecting approximately 16% of breastfed infants.*[6] *Pathological jaundice occurs within the first 24 hours of life, or when the total serum bilirubin level rises by more than 5 mg/dL per day.*[2,7]

NURSING PRIORITY NO. 2

To evaluate degree of compromise:

- Review laboratory studies including total serum bilirubin and albumin levels, hemoglobin (Hb)/hematocrit (Hct), reticulocyte count *to monitor severity of problem and need for, or effectiveness, of therapy.*[2] *Note: Excessive unconjugated bilirubin has an affinity for extravascular tissue, including the basal ganglia of brain tissue.*[7]
- Calculate plasma bilirubin-albumin binding capacity. *Aids in determining risk of kernicterus and treatment needs.*[1] *When total bilirubin value divided by total serum protein level is <3.7, the danger of kernicterus is very low. However, the risk of injury is dependent on factors such as degree of prematurity, presence of hypoxia or acidosis, and drug regimen (e.g., sulfonamides, chloramphenicol).*[7]
- Assess infant for progression of signs and behavioral changes associated with bilirubin toxicity. *Early-stage toxicity involves neurodepression—lethargy, poor feeding, high-pitched cry, diminished or absent reflexes; late-stage hypotonia, neuro-hyperreflexia—twitching, convulsions, opisthotonos, fever. Behavior changes associated with kernicterus usually occur between the 3rd and 10th days of life and rarely occur prior to 36 hours of life.*
- Evaluate appearance of skin and urine, noting brownish-black color. *An uncommon side effect of phototherapy, particularly in presence of cholestatic jaundice, involves exaggerated pigment changes (bronze baby syndrome), which may occur if conjugated bilirubin levels rise. The changes in skin color may last for 2 to 4 months but are not associated with harmful sequelae.*

NURSING PRIORITY NO. 3

To correct hyperbilirubinemia and prevent associated complications:

- Keep infant warm and dry; monitor skin and core temperature frequently. *Prevents cold stress and the release of fatty acids that compete for binding sites on albumin thus increasing the level of freely circulating bilirubin.*
- Initiate early oral feedings within 4 to 6 hours following birth, especially if infant is to be breastfed. *Establishes proper intestinal flora necessary for reduction of bilirubin to urobilinogen and decreases reabsorption of bilirubin from bowel by promoting passage of meconium stool.*[7]
- Encourage frequent breastfeeding—8 to 12 times per day. Assist mother with pumping of breasts as needed to maintain milk production. *Interruption of breastfeeding is rarely necessary unless serum levels reach 20 mg/dL; however, breastfeeding support may increase frequency and efficacy of intake.*[2,5–7]
- Administer small amounts of breast milk substitute (L-aspartic acid or enzymatically hydrolyzed casein [EHC]) for 24 to 48 hr if indicated. *Use of feeding additives is under investigation with mixed results for inhibition of beta-glucuronidase leading to increased fecal excretion of bilirubin.*[4,5]
- Apply transcutaneous jaundice meter, as indicated. *Provides noninvasive screening of jaundice, quantifying skin color in relation to total serum bilirubin.*
- Initiate phototherapy per protocol, using fluorescent bulbs placed above the infant, or fiber-optic pad or blanket (except for newborn with Rh disease). *Primary therapy for neonates with unconjugated hyperbilirubinemia. Three separate processes work to convert bilirubin isomers to water-soluble isomers and the formation of lumirubin. The photoisomers are then excreted in urine, stool, and bile.*[2]
- Apply eye patches ensuring correct fit during periods of phototherapy *to prevent retinal injury.* Remove eye covering during feedings or other care activities as appropriate *to provide visual stimulation and interaction with caregivers/parents.*[8]

- Avoid application of lotion or oils to skin of infant receiving phototherapy *to prevent dermal irritation or injury.*[8]
- Reposition infant every 2 hours *to ensure all areas of skin are exposed to bililight when fiber-optic pad or blanket is not used.*[8]
- Cover male groin with small pad *to protect from heat-related injury to testes.*[8]
- Monitor infant's weight loss, urine output and specific gravity, and fecal water loss from loose stools associated with phototherapy *to determine adequacy of fluid intake.*[2] *Note: Infant may sleep for longer periods in conjunction with phototherapy, increasing risk of dehydration if frequent feeding schedule is not maintained.*
- Administer intravenous immunoglobulin (IVIG) to neonates with Rh or ABO isoimmunization. *Rate of hemolysis in Rh disease or other cases of immune hemolytic jaundice usually exceeds the rate of bilirubin reduction related to phototherapy. IVIG inhibits antibodies that cause red cell destruction helping to limit the rise in bilirubin levels.*[2-5]
- Administer enzyme induction agent (phenobarbital) as appropriate. *May be used on occasion to stimulate hepatic enzymes to enhance clearance of bilirubin.*[2]
- Assist with preparation and administration of exchange transfusion. *Exchange transfusions are occasionally required in cases of severe hemolytic anemia unresponsive to other treatment options, or in presence of acute bilirubin encephalopathy as evidenced by hypertonia, arching, retrocollis, opisthotonos, fever, high-pitched cry.*[1,2] *Procedure removes serum bilirubin, provides bilirubin-free albumin increasing binding sites for bilirubin; and treats anemia by providing RBCs that are not susceptible to maternal antibodies.*
- Document events during transfusion, carefully recording amount of blood withdrawn and injected (usually 7–20 mL at a time). *Helps prevent errors in fluid replacement. Amount of blood exchanged is approximately 170 mL/kg of body weight. A double-volume exchange ensures that between 75% and 90% of circulating RBCs are replaced.*

NURSING PRIORITY NO. 4

To promote wellness (Teaching/Discharge Considerations):

- Provide information about types of jaundice and pathophysiological factors and future implications of hyperbilirubinemia. *Promotes understanding, corrects misconceptions, and may reduce fear and feelings of guilt.*
- Review means of assessing infant status (feedings, intake/output, stools, temperature, and serial weights if scale available) and for monitoring increasing bilirubin levels (e.g., observing blanching of skin over bony prominence or behavior changes), especially if infant is to be discharged early. *Enables parents to monitor infant's progress, and to recognize signs of increasing bilirubin levels. Note: Persistence of jaundice beyond 2 weeks in formula-fed infant or 3 weeks in breastfed infant requires further evaluation.*[7]
- Provide parents with 24-hour emergency telephone number and name of contact person, stressing importance of reporting increased jaundice or changes in behavior. *Promotes independence and provides for timely evaluation and intervention. Refer to lactation specialist to enhance or reestablish breastfeeding process.*[6]
- Arrange appropriate referral for home phototherapy program if necessary. *Lack of available support systems may necessitate use of visiting nurse to monitor home phototherapy program.*
- Provide written explanation of home phototherapy, safety precautions, and potential problems. *Home phototherapy is recommended only for full-term infants after the first 48 hours of life, whose serum bilirubin levels are between 14 and 18 mg/dL, with no increase in direct reacting bilirubin concentration.*
- Make appropriate arrangements for follow-up testing of serum bilirubin at same laboratory facility. *Treatment is discontinued once serum bilirubin concentrations fall below 14 mg/dL.*

Nursing Diagnoses in Alphabetical Order

Untreated or chronic hyperbilirubinemia can lead to permanent damage such as high-pitch hearing loss, cerebral palsy, or mental retardation. [7]

● Discuss possible long-term effects of hyperbilirubinemia and the need for continued assessment and early intervention. *Neurologic damage associated with kernicterus includes cerebral palsy, mental retardation, sensory difficulties, delayed speech, learning difficulties, death.*

DOCUMENTATION FOCUS

Assessment/Reassessment
• Assessment findings, risk or related factors.
• Adequacy of intake—hydration level, character and number of stools.
• Laboratory results—bilirubin trends.

Planning
• Plan of care, specific interventions, and who is involved in the planning.
• Teaching plan and resources provided.

Implementation/Evaluation
• Client's responses to treatment and actions performed.
• Parents understanding of teaching.
• Attainment or progress toward desired outcome(s).
• Modifications to plan of care.

Discharge Planning
• Long-term needs, identifying who is responsible for actions to be taken.
• Community resources for equipment and supplies postdischarge.
• Specific referrals made.

References

1. American Academy of Pediatrics. (2004). Treatment of hyperbilirubinema in the newborn infant 35 or more weeks of gestation. *Pediatrics*, 114(1), 297–316.
2. Hansen, T. W. R. (2007). Neonatal Jaundice. Retrieved March 2009 from http://emedicine.medscape.com/article/974786-overview.
3. Sarici, S. U., et al. (2004). Incidence, course, and prediction of hyperbilirubinemia in near-term and term newborns. *Pediatrics*, 113(4), 775–780.
4. Gourley, G. R., et al. (2005). A controlled, randomized, double-blind trial of prophylaxis against jaundice among breastfed newborns. *Pediatrics*, 116(2), 385–391.
5. Canadian Paediatric Society Position Statement. (2007). Guidelines for detection, management and prevention of hyperbilirubinemia in term and late preterm newborn infants (35 or more weeks' gestation). *Paediatr Child Health*, 12(suppl B), 1B–12B.
6. Deshpande, P. G. (2008). Breast milk jaundice. Retrieved March 2009 from http://emedicine.medscape.com/article/973629-overview.
7. Porter, M. L., Dennis, B. L. (2002). Hyperbilirubinemia in the term newborn. *Am Fam Physician*, 65(4), 599–606.
8. Phototherapy. (2008). *Lippincott's Nursing Procedures*. 5th ed. Philadelphia: Lippincott Williams & Wilkins, 895–897.

deficient Knowledge [Learning Need] [specify]

DEFINITION: Absence or deficiency of cognitive information related to specific topic necessary for clients/SO(s) to make informed choices regarding condition, treatment, or lifestyle changes

RELATED FACTORS

Lack of exposure or recall
Information misinterpretation; [inaccurate or incomplete information presented]
Unfamiliarity with information resources
Cognitive limitation
Lack of interest in learning; [request for no information]

DEFINING CHARACTERISTICS

Subjective
Verbalization of the problem
[Request for information]
[Statements reflecting misconceptions]

Objective
Inaccurate follow-through of instruction or performance of test
Inappropriate or exaggerated behaviors (e.g., hysterical, hostile, agitated, apathetic)
[Development of preventable complication]

Sample Clinical Applications: Any newly diagnosed disease or traumatic injury, progression of or deterioration in a chronic condition

DESIRED OUTCOMES/EVALUATION CRITERIA

Sample **NOC** linkages:
Knowledge: [specify—42 choices]: Extent of understanding conveyed about a specific disease process, the promotion and protection of health, maintaining optimal health, etc.
Information Processing: Ability to acquire, organize, and use information

Client Will (Include Specific Time Frame)
• Participate in learning process.
• Identify interferences to learning and specific action(s) to deal with them.
• Exhibit increased interest and assume responsibility for own learning by beginning to look for information and ask questions.
• Verbalize understanding of condition or disease process and treatment.
• Identify relationship of signs/symptoms to the disease process and correlate symptoms with causative factors.
• Perform necessary procedures correctly and explain reasons for the actions.
• Initiate necessary lifestyle changes and participate in treatment regimen.

(continues on page 480)

deficient Knowledge (continued)
ACTIONS/INTERVENTIONS

Sample (NIC) linkages:
Teaching: Individual [or 29 other choices]: Planning, implementation, and evaluation of a teaching program designed to address a patient's particular needs
Learning Facilitation: Promoting the ability to process and comprehend information
Learning Readiness Enhancement: Improving the ability and willingness to receive information

NURSING PRIORITY NO. 1

To assess readiness to learn and individual learning needs:

- Ascertain level of knowledge, including anticipatory needs. *Learning needs can include many things (e.g., disease cause and process, factors contributing to symptoms, procedures for symptom control, needed alterations in lifestyle, ways to prevent complications). Client may or may not ask for information or may express inaccurate perceptions of health status and needed behaviors to manage self-care.*[1]
- Engage in Active-listening. *Conveys expectation of confidence in client's ability to determine learning needs and best ways of meeting them.*[5]
- Determine client's ability and readiness and barriers to learning. *Client may not be physically, emotionally, or mentally capable at this time and may need time to work through and express emotions before learning.*[1]
- Be alert to signs of avoidance. *May need to allow client to suffer the consequences of lack of knowledge before client is ready to accept information.*[1]
- Identify SO(s)/family members requiring information. Providing appropriate information to others can provide reinforcement for learning, as everyone will understand what is to be expected.[4]

NURSING PRIORITY NO. 2

To determine other factors pertinent to the learning process:

- Note personal factors (e.g., age, developmental level, gender, social and cultural influences, religion, life experiences, level of education, emotional stability) *that affect ability and desire to learn and assimilate new information, take control of situation, accept responsibility for change.*[2,11]
- Determine blocks to learning, including (1) language barriers (e.g., can't read or write, speaks or understands a different language than that spoken by teacher); (2) physical factors (e.g., cognitive impairment, sensory deficits [e.g., aphasia, dyslexia, hearing or vision impairment]); (3) physical constraints (e.g., acute illness, activity intolerance, impaired thought processes); (4) complexity of material to be learned (e.g., caring for colostomy, giving own insulin injections); (5) forced change in lifestyle (e.g., smoking cessation); or (6) have stated no need or desire to learn. *Many factors affect the client's ability and desire to learn, and his or her expectations of the learning process must be addressed if learning is to be successful.*[1,11]
- Assess the level of the client's capabilities and the possibilities of the situation. *May need to assist SO(s) or caregivers to learn by introducing one new idea, by building on previous information, or by finding pictures to demonstrate an idea, and so forth, to adapt teaching to client's specific needs.*[6]

NURSING PRIORITY NO. 3

To assess the client's/SO's motivation:

- Identify motivating factors for the individual (e.g., client needs to stop smoking because of advanced lung cancer, or client wants to lose weight because family member died of complications of obesity). *Motivation may be negative (e.g., smoking causes lung cancer) or positive (e.g., client wants to promote health/prevent disease). Provides information that can guide content specific to client's situation and motivations.*[3,12]
- Provide information relevant only to the situation. *Reducing the amount of information at any one given time helps to keep the client focused and prevents client from feeling overwhelmed.*[4]
- Provide positive reinforcement rather than negative reinforcers (e.g., criticism and threats). *Enhances cooperation and encourages continuation of efforts.*[5]

NURSING PRIORITY NO. 4

To establish priorities in conjunction with client:

- Determine client's most urgent need from both client's and nurse's viewpoint. *Identifies whether client and nurse are together in their thinking and provides a starting point for teaching and outcome planning for optimal success.*[6]
- Discuss client's perception of need. *Takes into account the client's personal desires/needs and values/beliefs, providing a basis for planning appropriate care.*[6]
- Differentiate "critical" content from "desirable" content. *Identifies information that must be learned now as well as content that could be addressed at a later time. Client's emotional state may preclude hearing much of what is presented, and by only providing what is essential, client may hear it.*[3]

NURSING PRIORITY NO. 5

To determine the content to be included:

- Identify information that needs to be remembered (cognitive) at client's level of development and education. *Enhances possibility that information will be heard and understood.*[6]
- Identify information having to do with emotions, attitudes, and values (affective). *The affective learning domain addresses a learner's emotions toward learning experiences, and attitudes, interest, attention, awareness, and values are demonstrated by affective behaviors. Knowing the client's affective state enhances learning possibilities.*[7,12]
- Identify psychomotor skills that are necessary for learning. *Psychomotor learning involves both cognitive learning and muscular movement. The phases for learning these skills are cognitive (what), associative (how), and autonomous (practice to automaticity). Learners need to know what, why, and how they will learn. For instance, papers need to be typed, so the psychomotor skill will be touch typing. The individual will learn touch typing finger placement and how to type smoothly and rhythmically.*[8]

NURSING PRIORITY NO. 6

To develop learner's objectives:

- State objectives clearly in learner's terms to meet learner's (not instructor's) needs. *Understanding why the material is important to the learner provides motivation to learn.*[8]
- Identify outcomes (results) to be achieved. *Understanding what the outcomes will be helps the client realize the importance of learning the material, providing the motivation necessary to learning.*[8]

- Recognize level of achievement, time factors, and short-term and long-term goals. *Learning progresses in stages. Stage 1: unconsciously unskilled where we don't know we don't know. Stage 2: consciously unskilled, we know we don't know and start to learn. Stage 3: consciously skilled, we know how to do it but need to think and work hard to do it. And stage 4: we become unconsciously skilled, where the new skills are easier and even seem natural.*[9]
- Include the affective goals (e.g., reduction of stress). *The learner's emotional behaviors affect the learning experience and need to be actively addressed for maximum effectiveness.*[7]

NURSING PRIORITY NO. 7

To identify teaching methods to be used:

- Determine client's/SO's method of accessing information and preferred learning mode (e.g., auditory, visual, kinesthetic; group classes, one-to-one instruction, online) and include in teaching plan. *Using multiple modes of instruction facilitates learning and enhances retention, especially when faced with a stressful situation, illness or new treatment regimen.*[3,10]
- Involve the client/SO(s) by using age-appropriate materials tailored to client's interest and literacy skills (e.g., interactive programmed books, questions, dialogue, and audio/visual materials). *Accesses familiar mental images at client's developmental level to help individual learn more effectively.*[3,12,13]
- Involve with others who have same problems, needs, or concerns. *Group presentations, support groups provide role models and opportunity for sharing of information to enhance learning.*
- Use team and group teaching as appropriate.

NURSING PRIORITY NO. 8

To facilitate learning:

- Provide mutual goal-setting and learning contracts. Clarifies expectations of teacher and learner.
- Provide written information/guidelines and self-learning modules for client to refer to as necessary. *Reinforces learning process.*
- Pace and time learning sessions and learning activities to individual's needs. Involve and evaluate effectiveness of learning activities with client. *Client statements, questions, comments provide feedback about ability to grasp information being presented.*
- Provide an environment that is conducive to learning *to limit distractions and allow client to focus on the material presented.*
- Be aware of factors related to teacher in the situation (e.g., vocabulary, dress, style, knowledge of the subject, and ability to impart information effectively) *that may affect client's reaction to teacher or ability to learn from this individual.*
- Begin with information the client already knows and move to what the client does not know, progressing from simple to complex. *Can arouse interest and limit sense of being overwhelmed.*[12]
- Deal with the client's anxiety or other strong emotions. Present information out of sequence, if necessary, dealing first with material that is most anxiety-producing *when the anxiety is interfering with the client's learning process.*
- Provide active role for client in learning process, including questions and discussion. *Promotes sense of control over situation.*
- Have client paraphrase content in own words, perform return demonstration, and explain how learning can be applied in own situation *to enhance internalization of material and to evaluate learning.*[3]

- Provide for feedback (positive reinforcement) and evaluation of learning and acquisition of skills. *Validates current level of understanding and identifies areas requiring follow-up.*[5]
- Be aware of informal teaching and role modeling that takes place on an ongoing basis. *Answering specific questions and reinforcing previous teaching during routine contacts or care enhances learning on a regular basis.*[1]
- Assist client to use information in all applicable areas (e.g., situational, environmental, personal). *Enhances learning to promote better understanding of situation or illness.*[1]

NURSING PRIORITY NO. 9

To promote wellness (Teaching/Discharge Considerations):

- Provide access information for contact person *to answer questions and validate information after discharge.*[1]
- Identify available community resources and support groups *to assist with problem-solving, provide role models, and support personal growth/change.*[4]
- Provide additional learning resources (e.g., bibliography, reliable Web sites, audio/visual media), as appropriate. *May assist with further learning and promote learning at own pace.*[7]

DOCUMENTATION FOCUS

Assessment/Reassessment
- Individual findings, learning style, and identified needs; presence of learning blocks (e.g., hostility, inappropriate behavior).

Planning
- Plan for learning, methods to be used, and who is involved in the planning.
- Teaching plan.

Implementation/Evaluation
- Responses of the client/SO(s) to the learning plan and actions performed.
- How the learning is demonstrated.
- Attainment or progress toward desired outcome(s).
- Modifications to plan of care.

Discharge Planning
- Additional learning and referral needs.

References

1. Bohny, B. A. (1997). A time for self-care: Role of the home healthcare nurse. *Home Healthcare Nurse*, 15(4), 281–286.
2. Purnell, L. D., Paulanka, B. J. (1998). Purnell's model for cultural competence. *Transcultural Health Care. A Culturally Competent Approach*. Philadelphia: F. A. Davis.
3. Duffy, B. (1997). Using a creative teaching process with adult patients. *Home Healthcare Nurse*, 15(2), 102–108.
4. Bartholomew, L. K. (2000). Watch, discover, think, and act: A model for patient education program development. *Patient Educ Couns*, 39(2–3), 269–280.
5. Gordon, T. (2000). *Parent Effectiveness Training*. Updated ed. New York: Three Rivers Press.
6. Townsend, M. C. (2003). *Psychiatric Mental Health Nursing Concepts of Care*. 4th ed. Philadelphia: F. A. Davis.
7. Bloom, B. Bloom's learning domains. Encyclopedia of Educational Technology. Retrieved March 2004 from http://coe.sdsu.edu/eet/Articles/BloomsLD/.

8. Cook, S. L. Strategies for psychomotor skills. Instructional Strategies. Retrieved March 2004 from www.signaleader.com/IDTPortfolio/IT800/psychomotor.html.

9. Adams, L. Learning a new skill is easier said than done. *Gordon Training International.* Retrieved July 2007 from www.gordontraining.com/article-learning-a-new-skill-is-easier-said -than-done.html.

10. Kolb, D. A. (1984). *Experiential Learning: Experience as the Source of Learning and Development.* Englewood Cliffs, NJ: Prentice Hall.

11. Understanding transcultural nursing. (2005). *Nursing*, 35(1), 14–23. Suppl: Career Directory.

12. Anderson, N. R. (2006). The role of the home healthcare nurse in smoking cessation: Guidelines for successful intervention. *Home Healthcare Nurse*, 24(7), 424–431.

13. Pieper, B., Sieggreen, M., Freeland, B. (2006). Discharge information needs of clients after surgery. *J Wound, Ostomy Continence Nurs*, 33(3), 281–290.

readiness for enhanced Knowledge [specify]

DEFINITION: The presence or acquisition of cognitive information related to a specific topic that is sufficient for meeting health-related goals and can be strengthened

RELATED FACTORS

To be developed by nurse researchers and submitted to NANDA

DEFINING CHARACTERISTICS

Subjective
Expresses an interest in learning
Explains knowledge of the topic; describes previous experiences pertaining to the topic

Objective
Behaviors congruent with expressed knowledge

Sample Clinical Applications: As a health-seeking behavior, the patient may be healthy or this diagnosis can occur in any clinical condition

DESIRED OUTCOMES/EVALUATION CRITERIA

Sample NOC linkages:
Knowledge: [specify—42 choices]: Extent of understanding conveyed about a specific disease process, the promotion and protection of health, maintaining optimal health, etc.
Information Processing: Ability to acquire, organize, and use information

Client Will (Include Specific Time Frame)
• Exhibit responsibility for own learning by seeking answers to questions.
• Verify accuracy of informational resources.
• Verbalize understanding of information gained.
• Use information to develop individual plan to meet healthcare needs/goals.

🌐 Cultural 😀 Collaborative 🏠 Community/Home Care ✏ Diagnostic Studies ∞ Pediatric/Geriatric/Lifespan 💊 Medications

ACTIONS/INTERVENTIONS

Sample (NIC) linkages:
Teaching: Individual: Planning, implementation, and evaluation of a teaching program designed to address a patient's particular needs
Learning Facilitation: Promoting the ability to process and comprehend information
Learning Readiness Enhancement: Improving the ability and willingness to receive information

NURSING PRIORITY NO. 1

To develop plan for learning:

- Verify client's level of knowledge about specific topic. *Provides opportunity to assure accuracy and completeness of knowledge base for future learning.*[4]
- Determine motivation and expectation for learning. *Provides insight useful in developing goals and identifying information needs.*[4]
- Assist client to identify learning goals and measurable outcomes. *Helps to frame or focus content to be learned. Provides motivation for learning and a measure to evaluate learning process.*[5,8]
- Ascertain preferred methods of learning (e.g., auditory, visual, interactive, or "hands-on"). *Identifies best approaches for the individual to facilitate learning process.*[5]
- Note personal factors (e.g., age and developmental level, gender, social and cultural influences, religion, life experiences, level of education) *that may impact learning style, choice of informational resources, willingness to take control of situation, accept responsibility for change.*[2]
- Determine challenges to learning: language barriers (e.g., client cannot read, speaks or understands language other than that of care provider, dyslexia), physical factors (e.g., sensory deficits such as vision or hearing impairments, aphasia), physical stability (e.g., acute illness, activity intolerance), difficulty of material to be learned. *Identifies special needs to be addressed if learning is to be successful.*[6]

NURSING PRIORITY NO. 2

To facilitate learning:

- Provide information in varied formats appropriate to client's learning style (e.g., audiotapes, print materials, videos, classes or seminars, online). *Use of multiple formats increases learning and retention of material.*[3]
- Provide information about additional or outside learning resources (e.g., bibliotherapy, pertinent Web sites). *Promotes ongoing learning at own pace.*[7]
- Discuss ways to verify accuracy of informational resources. *Encourages independent search for learning opportunities while reducing likelihood of acting on erroneous or unproven data that could be detrimental to client's well-being.*[4]
- Identify available community resources and support groups. *Provides additional opportunities for role modeling, skill training, anticipatory problem-solving, and so forth.*[1]
- Be aware of and discuss informal teaching and role modeling that takes place on an ongoing basis. *Incongruencies in community or peer role models, support group feedback, print advertisements, popular music and videos may exist, creating questions and potentially undermining learning process.*[4]

NURSING PRIORITY NO. 3

To enhance optimum wellness:

- Assist client to identify ways to integrate and use information in all applicable areas (e.g., situational, environmental, personal). *Ability to apply or use information increases desire to learn and retention of information.*[5]

- Encourage client to journal, keep a log, or graph as appropriate. *Provides opportunity for self-evaluation of effects of learning, such as better management of chronic condition, reduction of risk factors, acquisition of new skills.*[6,9]

DOCUMENTATION FOCUS

Assessment/Reassessment
- Individual findings, learning style and identified needs, presence of challenges to learning.
- Motivation and expectations for learning.

Planning
- Plan for learning, methods to be used, and who is involved in the planning.
- Educational plan.

Implementation/Evaluation
- Responses of the client/SO(s) to the educational plan and actions performed.
- How the learning is demonstrated.
- Attainment or progress toward desired outcome(s).
- Modifications to lifestyle or treatment plan.

Discharge Planning
- Additional learning and referral needs.

References

1. Bohny, B. A. (1997). A time for self-care: Role of the home healthcare nurse. *Home Healthcare Nurse*, 15(4), 281–286.
2. Purnell, L. D., Paulanka, B. J. (1998). Purnell's model for cultural competence. *Transcultural Health Care: A Culturally Competent Approach*. Philadelphia: F. A. Davis.
3. Duffy, B. (1997). Using a creative teaching process with adult patients. *Home Healthcare Nurse*, 15(2), 102–108.
4. Bartholomew, L. K. (2000). Watch, discover, think, and act: A model for patient education program development. *Patient Educ Couns*, 39(2–3), 269–280.
5. Clark, D. (1999). Learning styles, or how we go from the unknown to the known. Retrieved July 2007 from www.nwlink.com/~donclark/hrd/learning/styles.html.
6. Townsend, M. C. (2003). *Psychiatric Mental Health Nursing Concepts of Care*. 4th ed. Philadelphia: F. A. Davis.
7. Bloom, B. Bloom's learning domains. Encyclopedia of Educational Technology. Retrieved July 2007 from http://coe.sdsu.edu/eet/articles/BloomsLD/.
8. Cook, S. L. Strategies for psychomotor skills. Instructional Strategies. Retrieved March 2004 from www.signaleader.com/IDTPortfolio/IT800/psychomotor.html.
9. Adams, L. Learning a new skill is easier said than done. Gordon Training International. Retrieved July 2007 from www.gordontraining.com/article-learning-a-new-skill-is-easier-said-than-done.html.

sedentary Lifestyle

DEFINITION: Reports a habit of life that is characterized by a low physical activity level

RELATED FACTORS

Lack of interest, motivation, or resources (time, money, companionship, facilities)
Lack of training for accomplishment of physical exercise
Deficient knowledge of health benefits of physical exercise

DEFINING CHARACTERISTICS

Subjective
Verbalizes preference for activities low in physical activity

Objective
Chooses a daily routine lacking in physical exercise
Demonstrates physical deconditioning

Sample Clinical Applications: Chronic or debilitating conditions (e.g., arthritis, multiple sclerosis [MS], chronic obstructive pulmonary disease [COPD], heart failure, paralysis), chronic pain, obesity, depression

DESIRED OUTCOMES/EVALUATION CRITERIA

Sample NOC linkages:
Knowledge: Prescribed Activity: Extent of understanding conveyed about prescribed activity and exercise
Physical Fitness: Performance of physical activities with vigor
Endurance: Capacity to sustain activity

Client Will (Include Specific Time Frame)
• Verbalize understanding of importance of regular exercise to general well-being.
• Identify necessary precautions, safety concerns, and self-monitoring techniques.
• Formulate and implement realistic exercise program with gradual increase in activity.

ACTIONS/INTERVENTIONS

Sample NIC linkages:
Exercise Promotion: Facilitation of regular physical activity to maintain or advance to a higher level of fitness and health
Teaching: Prescribed Activity/Exercise: Preparing a patient to achieve or maintain a prescribed level of activity

NURSING PRIORITY NO. 1

To assess precipitating/etiological factors:

• Identify client's specific condition(s) (e.g., obesity, depression, MS, arthritis, Parkinson's disease, surgery, hemiplegia or paraplegia, chronic pain, brain injury) *that may contribute to immobility or the onset and continuation of inactivity or sedentary lifestyle.*

- Assess client's age, developmental level, motor skills, ease and capability of movement, posture and gait. *Determines type and intensity of needed interventions related to activity.*[1]
- Determine client's current weight and body mass index (BMI); note dietary habits. *If client is overweight and BMI is not in healthy range, weight-loss program will be needed.*[8]
- Assess physical capabilities to participate in exercise/activities, noting attention span, physical limitations and tolerance, level of interest or desire, and safety needs. *Identifies barriers that need to be addressed.*[1,6]
- Review usual activities, work requirements/environment. *Absence of regular exercise, stressful job with little physical exercise increases likelihood of deconditioning and affects choice of interventions and need for involvement of primary healthcare provider in determining safe program.*[8]
- Note emotional and behavioral responses to problems associated with self- or condition-imposed sedentary lifestyle. *Feelings of frustration and powerlessness may impede attainment of goals.*[2]
- Determine family dynamics and support provided by family/friends. *Major lifestyle change will require support of others to achieve and maintain goals or client is at increased risk of slipping back into "old" ways.*[8]
- Discuss availability of resources (e.g., financial for gym membership, transportation, exercise facility or gym at work site, proximity of bike path, safety of neighborhood for outdoor activity).

NURSING PRIORITY NO. 2

To motivate and stimulate client involvement:

- Establish therapeutic relationship, acknowledging reality of situation and client's feelings. *Changing a lifelong habit can be difficult, and client may feel discouraged with body and hopeless to turn situation around into a positive experience.*[2]
- Ascertain client's perception of current activity and exercise patterns, impact on life, and cultural expectations of client/others. *Helps to determine whether or not client perceives need for change, and potential limitations in choices for activities.*[8]
- Discuss client's stated motivation for change. *Concerns of client/SOs regarding threats to personal health/longevity, or acceptance by teen peers may be sufficient to cause client to initiate change; however, client must want to change for himself or herself in order to sustain change.*[4,8]
- Review necessity for and benefits of regular exercise. *Research confirms that exercise has benefits for the whole body (e.g., can boost energy, enhance coordination, reduce muscle deterioration, improve circulation, lower blood pressure, produce healthier skin and a toned body, prolong youthful appearance). Regular exercise has also been found to boost cardiac fitness in both conditioned and out-of-shape individuals.*[4]
- Counsel client regarding individual health risks. *Focuses attention on own situation and helps prioritize needs, making change more manageable.*[8]
- Involve client, SO/parent, or caregiver in developing exercise plan and goals *to meet individual needs, desires, and available resources.* Also increases commitment to program and successful attainment of goals.
- Introduce activities at client's current level of functioning, progressing to more complex activities, as tolerated. *Reduces likelihood of overwhelming client at the beginning and maintains interest over time.*
- Recommend mix of age and gender-appropriate activities or stimuli (e.g., movement classes, walking, hiking, jazzercise, swimming, biking, skating, bowling, golf, weight training).

Cultural Collaborative Community/Home Care Diagnostic Studies Pediatric/Geriatric/Lifespan Medications

Activities need to be personally meaningful for client to derive the most enjoyment and to sustain motivation to continue with program.[2,6]

- Encourage change of scenery (indoors and outdoors where possible) and periodic changes in the personal environment when client is confined inside.

NURSING PRIORITY NO. 3

To promote optimal level of function and prevent exercise failure:

- Assist with treatment of underlying condition impacting participation in activities *to maximize function within limitations of situation.* Refer to dietitian for weight-loss program, as indicated.
- Collaborate with physical medicine specialist or occupational or physical therapist in providing active or passive range-of-motion exercises, isotonic muscle contractions. *Techniques such as gait training, strength training, and exercise to improve balance and coordination can be helpful in rehabilitating client.*[1]
- Schedule ample time to perform exercise activities balanced with adequate rest periods.[1]
- Provide for safety measures as indicated by individual situation, including environmental management and fall prevention. (Refer to ND risk for Falls.)
- Reevaluate ability/commitment periodically. *Changes in strength or endurance signal readiness for progression of activities or possibly to decrease exercise if overly fatigued. Wavering commitment may require change in types of activities, addition of a workout buddy to reenergize involvement.*[2,5]
- Discuss discrepancies in planned and performed activities with client aware and unaware of observation. Suggest methods for dealing with identified problems. *May be necessary when client is using avoidance or controlling behavior or is not aware of own abilities due to anxiety or fear.*[2,5]

NURSING PRIORITY NO. 4

To promote wellness (Teaching/Discharge Considerations):

- Review components of physical fitness: (1) muscle strength and endurance, (2) flexibility, (3) body composition (muscle mass, percentage of body fat), and (4) cardiovascular health. *Fitness routines need to include all elements to attain maximized benefits and prevent deconditioning.*[4,5,7]
- Instruct in safety measures, as individually indicated (e.g., warm-up and cooldown activities; taking pulse before, during, and after activity; adequate intake of fluids, especially during hot weather or strenuous activity; wearing reflective clothing when jogging or reflectors on bicycle; locking wheelchair before transfers; judicious use of medications; supervision, as indicated).[1]
- Recommend keeping an activity or exercise log, including physical and psychological responses, changes in weight, endurance, body mass. *Provides visual evidence of progress or goal attainment and encouragement to continue with program.*[2,6]
- Encourage client to involve self in exercise *as part of wellness management for the whole person.*[3,6]
- Encourage parents to set a positive example for children *by participating in exercise and engaging in an active lifestyle.*[3,6]
- Identify community resources, charity activities, support groups. *Community walking/hiking trails, sports leagues, and so forth, provide free/low-cost options. Activities such as 5k walks for charity, participation in Special Olympics, or age-related competitive games*

provide goals to work toward. Note: Some individuals may prefer solitary activities; however, most individuals enjoy supportive companionship when exercising.[3,4]

🏠 ● Discuss alternatives for exercise program in changing circumstances (e.g., walking the mall during inclement weather, using exercise facilities at hotel when traveling, water aerobics at local swimming pool, joining a gym).

🏠 ● Promote individual participation in community awareness of problem and discussion of solutions. *Physical inactivity (and associated diseases) is a major public health problem that affects large numbers of people in all regions of the world. Recognizing the problem and future consequences may empower the global community to develop effective measures to promote physical activity and improve public health.*[7]

🏠 ● Promote community goals for increasing physical activity, such as school-based physical education; Sports, Play, and Active Recreation for Kids (SPARK); "buddy" system or contracting for specific physical activities; and Physician-Based Assessment and Counseling for Exercise (PACE) *to address national concerns about obesity and major barriers to physical activity, such as time constraints, lack of training in physical activity, or behavioral change methods, and lack of standard protocols.*[3,6,7,9]

DOCUMENTATION FOCUS

Assessment/Reassessment
• Individual findings, including level of function and ability to participate in specific or desired activities, motivation for change.

Planning
• Plan of care and who is involved in the planning.
• Teaching plan.

Implementation/Evaluation
• Responses to interventions, teaching, and actions performed.
• Attainment or progress toward desired outcome(s).
• Modifications to plan of care.

Discharge Planning
• Discharge and long-term needs, noting who is responsible for each action to be taken.
• Specific referrals made.
• Sources of and maintenance for assistive devices.

References

1. Boesch, C., Meyers, J., Habersaat, A. (2005). Maintenance of exercise capacity and physical activity patterns after cardiac rehabilitation. *Cardiopulm Rehabil*, 25(1), 14–21.
2. Sallis, J. F. (1996). The role of behavioral science in improving health through physical activity. *Summary of presentation. Science Writers Briefing, December 1996*: Sponsored by OBSSR and the American Psychological Association.
3. Wehling-Weepie, A. K., McCarthy, A. (2002). A healthy lifestyle program: Promoting child health in schools. *J School Nurs*, 18(6), 322.
4. McCormack, B. N., Yorkey, M. (2005). *Ten Great Things Exercise Can Do for You.* New York: Wiley Pub, American Media.
5. Lai, S. C., Cohen, M. N. (1999). Promoting lifestyle changes. *Am J Nurs*, 99(4), 63.
6. Fitness at any age. (2006). Retrieved March 2007 from www.medicinenet.com.
7. World Health Organization (WHO). (2007). Sedentary lifestyle: A global public health problem. "Move for health" information sheet. Retrieved March 2007 from www.who.int.

8. Morantz, C. (2004). Obesity and sedentary lifestyle guidelines. American Academy of Family Physicians. Retrieved July 2007 from http://findarticles.com/p/articles/mi_m3225/is_10_69/ai_n6048509.

9. Task Force on Community Preventive Services—Independent Expert Panel. (May 2002). Recommendations to increase physical activities in communities. *Am J Prev Med*, 22(2 suppl), 67–72.

risk for impaired Liver Function

DEFINITION: At risk for a decrease in liver function that may compromise health

RISK FACTORS

Viral infection (e.g., hepatitis A, hepatitis B, hepatitis C, Epstein-Barr); HIV co-infection
Hepatotoxic medications (e.g., acetaminophen, statins)
Substance abuse (e.g., alcohol, cocaine)

NOTE: A risk diagnosis is not evidenced by signs and symptoms, as the problem has not occurred; rather, nursing interventions are directed at prevention.
Sample Clinical Applications: Hepatitis, HIV, substance abuse, drug overdose (acetaminophen), Epstein-Barr infection

DESIRED OUTCOMES/EVALUATION CRITERIA

Sample **NOC** linkages:
Knowledge: Disease Process: Extent of understanding conveyed about a specific disease process
Treatment Behavior: Illness or Injury: Personal actions to palliate or eliminate pathology

Client Will (Include Specific Time Frame)
• Verbalize understanding of individual risk factors that contribute to possibility of liver damage/failure.
• Demonstrate behaviors, lifestyle changes to reduce risk factors and protect self from injury.
• Be free of signs of liver failure as evidenced by liver function studies within normal range, and absence of jaundice, hepatic enlargement, or altered mental status.

ACTIONS/INTERVENTIONS

Sample **NIC** linkages:
Risk Identification: Analysis of potential risk factors, determination of health risk, and prioritization of risk-reduction strategies for an individual or group
Infection Protection: Prevention and early detection of infection in a patient at risk
Substance Use Treatment: Supportive care of patient/family members with physical and psychosocial problems with the use of alcohol or drugs

NURSING PRIORITY NO. 1

To identify individual risk factors/needs:

- Determine presence of condition(s) as listed in Risk Factors, noting whether problem is acute (e.g., viral hepatitis, acetaminophen overdose) or chronic (e.g., alcoholic cirrhosis). *Influences choice of interventions.*[1]
- Note client history of known/possible exposure to virus, bacteria, or toxins *that can damage liver*:[2–8]

  Works in high-risk occupation (e.g., performs tasks that involve contact with blood, blood-contaminated body fluids, other body fluids, or sharps).

  Injects drugs, especially if client shared a needle; received tattoo or piercing with an unsterile needle.

  Received blood or blood products prior to 1992.

  Ingested contaminated food or water or experienced poor sanitation practices by food-service workers.

  Close contact (e.g., lives with or has sex with infected person or carrier).

  Regular exposure to toxic chemicals (e.g., carbon tetrachloride cleaning agents, bug spray, paint fumes, and tobacco smoke).

  Uses prescription drugs (e.g., sulfonamides, phenothiazines, isoniazid).

  Ingests certain herbal remedies or mega doses of vitamins.

  Uses alcohol with medications (including over-the-counter [OTC] medications).

  Consumes alcohol heavily and/or over long period of time.

  Ingested acetaminophen (accidentally, as may occur when client takes too large a dose, or has several medications containing acetaminophen over time; or intentionally, as may occur with suicide attempt).

  Travels internationally to or immigrates from countries such as China, Africa, Southeast Asia, Middle East *(where hepatitis is endemic)*.

- Review results of laboratory tests (e.g., liver function studies, such as alanine aminotransferase [ALT], alkaline phosphatase [ALP], bilirubin, gamma-glutamyl transferase [GGT], lactic acid dehydrogenase [LDH], albumin, total protein and prothrombin time (PT), drug levels, hepatitis titers) and diagnostic studies *that indicate presence of hepatotoxic condition and need for medical treatment.*[9]

NURSING PRIORITY NO. 2

To assist client to reduce or correct individual risk factors:

- Assist with medical treatment of underlying condition (e.g., hepatitis, alcoholism, drug overdose) *to support organ function and minimize liver damage.*
- Educate client/SO on way(s) to prevent exposure to or incidence of hepatitis infections and limit damage to liver:[7]

  Practice safer sex (e.g., avoid multiple-partner sex, wear condoms, avoid sex with partners known to be infected).

  Avoid injecting drugs or sharing needles.

  Use proper protective equipment when working in high-risk occupations, such as health-care, emergency services, chemical manufacturing.

  Avoid tap water and practice good hygiene and sanitation when traveling internationally.

  Use harsh cleansers and aerosol products in well-ventilated room; wear mask and gloves, cover skin, and wash well afterward. *Insecticides and other chemicals can reach the liver through skin and destroy liver cells.*

⊕ Cultural ⊗ Collaborative 🏠 Community/Home Care ▱ Diagnostic Studies ∞ Pediatric/Geriatric/Lifespan ⚱ Medications

- Discuss safe use and concerns about client's medication regimen (e.g., acetaminophen, NSAIDs, herbal or vitamin supplements, phenobarbital, cholesterol-lowering drugs such as statins, certain antibiotics [e.g., sulfonamides, isonicotinyl hydrazine (INH)]; certain cardiovascular drugs [e.g., amiodarone, hydralazine]; certain antidepressants [e.g., tricyclics]) known to cause hepatotoxicity, either alone or in combination, or in overdose situation. *Note:* Many OTC and prescription medicines, even "natural" or herbal remedies, contain chemicals that can harm the liver over time. Very high doses of certain pain relievers (e.g., acetaminophen) can cause liver failure.[9–12]

- Encourage client who is routinely taking acetaminophen for pain management to read labels, determine strength of medication, note safe number of doses over 24 hours, become familiar with "hidden" sources of acetaminophen (e.g., Nyquil, Vicodin), and limit alcohol intake *to avoid or limit risk of liver damage.*[8]

- Stress importance of responsible drinking (e.g., men should limit alcohol to no more than two drinks/day, and women, one drink/day); or avoid alcohol altogether when indicated (if client has any kind of liver disease) *to reduce incidence of cirrhosis and severity of liver damage or failure.*[7]

- Encourage smoking cessation. *The additives in cigarettes pose a challenge to the liver by reducing the liver's ability to eliminate toxins.*[7]

- Encourage client with liver dysfunction to avoid fatty foods. *Fat interferes with normal function of liver cells and can cause additional damage and permanent scarring to liver cells when they can no longer regenerate.*[11]

- Refer to nutritionist, as indicated, for dietary needs, including proteins, vitamins, *to promote healing.*

- Discuss signs/symptoms (e.g., increased abdominal girth; rapid weight loss or gain; increased peripheral edema; dyspnea, fever; blood in stool or urine; excess bleeding of any kind; jaundice) *that warrant prompt notification of healthcare provider for evaluation and treatment of severe liver dysfunction, possible organ failure.*[12]

- Refer to specialist or liver treatment center, as indicated. *May be beneficial for client with chronic liver disease when decompensating, for client with hepatitis and other coexisting disease condition (e.g., HIV), or for client with intolerance to treatment due to side effects.*

NURSING PRIORITY NO. 3

To promote wellness (Teaching/Discharge Considerations):

- Emphasize importance of hand hygiene, use of bottled water, and avoidance of fresh produce, raw meat, or seafood *if client is traveling to area where hepatitis A is endemic or food- or waterborne illness is a risk.*[13]

- Instruct in measures including protection from blood or other body fluids, sharps safety; safer sex practices; avoiding needle sharing; body tattoos and piercings *to prevent occupational and nonoccupational exposures to hepatitis.*

- Discuss need and refer for vaccination, as indicated (e.g., healthcare and public safety worker, children under 18, international traveler, recreational drug user, men who have sex with other men, client with clotting disorders or liver disease, anyone sharing household with an infected person) *to prevent exposure and transmission of blood or body fluid hepatitis and limit risk of liver injury.*[13]

- Discuss appropriateness of prophylaxis immunizations. *Although the best way to protect against hepatitis B and C infections is to prevent exposure to viruses, postexposure prophylaxis (PEP) should be initiated promptly to prevent or limit severity of infection, especially in persons with close contact with infected individual or in client with compromised immune system.*[14]

- Provide information regarding availability of gamma globulin, immune serum globulin (ISG), heptatitis B immune globulin (H-BIG), HB vaccine (Recombivax HB, Engerix-B), through health department or family physician.
- Stress necessity of follow-up care (in client with chronic liver disease) *to monitor liver function and effectiveness of interventions* and importance of adherence to therapeutic regimen *to prevent or minimize permanent liver damage.*
- Refer to community resources for immunizations/drug/alcohol treatment program, as indicated.

DOCUMENTATION FOCUS

Assessment/Reassessment
- Assessment findings, including individual risk factors.
- Results of laboratory tests and diagnostic studies.

Planning
- Plan of care and who is involved in planning.
- Teaching plan.

Implementation/Evaluation
- Response to interventions, teaching, and actions performed.
- Attainment or progress toward desired outcome(s).
- Modifications to plan of care.

Discharge Planning
- Long-term needs, plan for follow-up and who is responsible for actions to be taken.
- Specific referrals made.

References

1. Smith, D. H. (2007). Managing acute acetaminophen toxicity. *Nursing*, 37(1), 58–63.
2. Bockhold, K. M. (2000). Who's afraid of hepatitis C? *Am J Nurs*, 100(5), 26.
3. Lambright, J. A. (1999). Preventing hepatitis. *Nursing*, 29(8), 66.
4. Shovein, J. T., Camozo, R. J., Hyams, I. (2000). Hepatitis A: How benign is it? *Am J Nurs*, 100(3), 43.
5. Klainberg, M. (1999). Primary biliary cirrhosis. *Amer J Nurs*, 99(12), 38.
6. American Liver Society and National Institutes for Health. (2003). Viral hepatitis: A through E and beyond. NIH Publication No. 03-4762. Retrieved July 2007 from http://digestive.niddk.nih.gov/ddiseases/pubs/viralhepatitis/index.htm.
7. American Liver Society and National Institutes for Health. (2006). You are at risk for liver damage or disease if . . . . NIH Fact Sheet. Retrieved July 2007 from http://digestive.niddk.nih.gov/ddiseases/pubs/viralhepatitis/index.htm.
8. Fong, T. (2002). Acetaminophen (Tylenol) liver damage. MedicineNet. Retrieved December 2006 from www.medicinenet.com.
9. American Association for Clinical Chemistry. (2006). Liver panel. Lab Tests Online. Retrieved July 2007 from http://labtestsonline.org/understanding/analytes/liver_panel/glance.html.
10. Liver blood enzymes. (2005). MedicineNet. Retrieved December 2006 from www.medicinenet.com.
11. Cormier, M. (2005). The role of hepatitis C support groups. *Gastroenterol Nurs*, 28(3 suppl), S4–S9.
12. Whiteman, K., McCormick, C. (2005). When your patient is in liver failure. *Nursing*, 35(4), 58–63.
13. Durston, S. (2005). What you need to know about viral hepatitis. *Nursing*, 35(8), 36–41.
14. Kania, D. S., Scott, C. M. (2007). Postexposure prophylaxis considerations for occupational and nonoccupational exposures. *Adv Emerg Nurs J*, 29(1), 20–32.

Cultural ⊗ Collaborative ⌂ Community/Home Care ▱ Diagnostic Studies ∞ Pediatric/Geriatric/Lifespan Medications

risk for Loneliness

DEFINITION: At risk for experiencing discomfort associated with a desire or need for more contact with others

RISK FACTORS

Affectional deprivation
Physical or social isolation
Cathectic deprivation
[Problems of attachment for infants or adolescents]
[Chaotic family relationships]

NOTE: A risk diagnosis is not evidenced by signs and symptoms, as the problem has not occurred; rather, nursing interventions are directed at prevention.
Sample Clinical Applications: Debilitating conditions (e.g., multiple sclerosis [MS], chronic obstructive pulmonary disease [COPD], renal failure), cancer, AIDS, major depression

DESIRED OUTCOMES/EVALUATION CRITERIA

Sample NOC linkages:
Loneliness Severity: Severity of emotional, social, or existential isolation response
Social Involvement: Social interactions with persons, groups, or organizations

Client Will (Include Specific Time Frame)
• Identify individual difficulties and ways to address them.
• Engage in desired social activities.
• Report involvement in interactions or relationship client views as meaningful.

Sample NOC linkages:
Knowledge: Parenting: Extent of understanding conveyed about provision of a nurturing and constructive environment for a child from 1 year through 17 years of age

Parent Will (Include Specific Time Frame)
• Provide infant with consistent and loving caregiving.
• Participate in programs for adolescents and families.

ACTIONS/INTERVENTIONS

Sample NIC linkages:
Socialization Enhancement: Facilitation of another person's ability to interact with others
Hope Inspiration: Enhancing the belief in one's capacity to initiate and sustain actions
Emotional Support: Provision of reassurance, acceptance, and encouragement during times of stress

NURSING PRIORITY NO. 1

To identify causative/precipitating factors:

● Differentiate between ordinary loneliness and a state of constant sense of dysphoria. *Being alone is a different state than loneliness.*[3]

∞ • Note client's age and duration of problem—that is, situational (e.g., leaving home for college) or chronic. *Adolescents may experience lonely feelings related to the changes that are happening as they become adults. Elderly individuals incur multiple losses associated with aging, loss of spouse, decline in physical health, and changes in roles, thus intensifying feelings of loneliness.*[3,12]

• Determine degree of distress, tension, anxiety, restlessness present. Note history of frequent illnesses, accidents, crises. Identifies somatic complaints that can result from loneliness. *Individuals under stress tend to have more illnesses and accidents related to inattention and anxiety.*[6]

• Note presence and proximity of family/SO(s). *Loneliness may not be related to being alone, but knowing that family is available can help with planning care. Client may be estranged from other family members or they may not be willing to be involved with client.*[6]

• Discuss with client whether there is a person(s) in his or her life who is trustworthy and who will listen with empathy to the feelings that are expressed.

🏠 • Determine how individual perceives and deals with solitude. *Client may see being alone as positive, allowing time to pursue own interests, or may view solitude as sad and long for lost objects, such as spouse.*[6,13]

∞ • Review issues of separation from parents as a child, loss of SO(s)/spouse. *Early separation from parents often affects the individual as other losses occur throughout life, leading to feelings of inadequacy and inability to deal with current situation.*[6,13]

• Assess sleep and appetite disturbances, ability to concentrate. *Feelings of loneliness often accompany depression, and identifying whether client is adequately taking care of self is important to planning care.*[7]

• Note expressions of "yearning" for an emotional partnership. *Widows and widowers are particularly prone to feelings of loneliness. Going from being a "couple" to being alone is a difficult transition, and these feelings are indicative of a desire to return to the "couple" state.*[7]

• Assess feelings of loneliness in client who is receiving palliative care. *These individuals often feel alienated and lonely as they face the end of their life and may need additional socialization to help them feel valued.*[5]

NURSING PRIORITY NO. 2

To assist client to identify feelings and situations in which he or she experiences loneliness:

• Establish therapeutic nurse-client relationship. *Provides a sense of connection with someone, thereby enabling client to feel free to talk about feelings of loneliness and current situation that is related to these feelings.*[1,10]

• Discuss individual concerns about feelings of loneliness and relationship between loneliness and lack of SOs. Note desire and willingness to change situation. *Motivation or lack thereof can facilitate or impede achieving desired outcomes. Often feelings of loneliness arise from underlying depression related to loss, thus affecting individual's coping abilities.*[7]

• Support expression of negative perceptions of others and whether client believes they are true. *Provides opportunity for client to clarify reality of situation, recognize own denial. Individual's view of the world is colored by feelings of loneliness and depression.*[1]

• Accept client's expressions of loneliness as a primary condition and not necessarily as a symptom of some underlying condition. *Provides a beginning point, which will allow the client to look at what loneliness means in life without having to search for deeper meaning.*[1,2]

NURSING PRIORITY NO. 3

To assist client to become involved:

- Discuss reality versus perception of situation. Have client identify people with whom he or she interacts on a regular basis. *Provides opportunity for reality check and beginning to understand own feelings of loneliness related to what is happening in own life.*[2,13]
- Discuss importance of emotional bonding (attachment) between infants/young children, parents/caregivers, as appropriate. *Understanding the importance of attachment provides parents with information that will help them take measures to ensure that this bonding occurs.*[2]
- Involve in classes such as assertiveness, language and communication, social skills. *Addressing individual needs will enhance socialization and provide client with the skills to become involved in social activities, thus promoting self-confidence and alleviating feelings of loneliness.*[3,8,11]
- Role-play situations that are new or are anxiety-provoking for client. *Practicing new situations helps develop self-confidence and provides client with information about what to expect and how to deal with the unexpected in a positive manner.*[2]
- Discuss positive health habits, including personal hygiene, exercise activity of client's choosing. *Improves feelings of self-esteem, thus enabling client to feel more confident in social situations.*[7]
- Identify individual strengths and areas of interest that client identifies and is willing to pursue. *Provides opportunities for involvement with others to develop new social skills.*[7,11]
- Encourage attendance at support groups (e.g., therapy, separation or grief, religious). *Participating in these activities can meet individual needs and help client begin to deal with feelings of loneliness.*[7]
- Help client establish plan for progressive involvement, beginning with a simple activity, such as calling an old friend, speaking to a neighbor, and then leading to more complicated interactions and activities. *Taking small steps promotes success, and confidence is gained as each step is taken, thus helping the client to be more involved and to resolve feelings of loneliness.*[7]
- Provide opportunities for interactions in a supportive environment (e.g., have client accompanied as in a "buddy system") during initial attempts to socialize. *Helps reduce stress, provides positive reinforcement, and facilitates successful outcome.*[7]

NURSING PRIORITY NO. 4

To promote wellness (Teaching/Discharge Considerations):

- Let client know that loneliness can be overcome. *It is up to the individual to build self-esteem and learn to feel good about self.*[4,13]
- Encourage involvement in special-interest groups (e.g., computers, bird watchers) or charitable services (e.g., serving in a soup kitchen, youth groups, animal shelter). *Becoming involved with others takes focus off of self and own concerns, promotes feelings of self-worth, and encourages client to again be an active part of society.*[7]
- Suggest volunteering for church committee or choir; attending community events with friends and family; becoming involved in political issues or campaigns; or enrolling in classes at local college or continuing education programs, as able. *When client is willing to become involved in these kinds of activities, perception of loneliness fades into the background, and even though individual may still be lonely, the sense of loneliness is not so pervasive.*[7]
- Refer to appropriate counselors for help with relationships, social skills, or other identified needs. *May provide additional assistance to help client deal with feelings of loneliness and isolation.*[9,10]

• Refer to NDs Anxiety, Hopelessness, and Social Isolation, for additional interventions, as appropriate.

DOCUMENTATION FOCUS

Assessment/Reassessment
• Assessment findings, including client's perception of problem, availability of resources or support systems.
• Client's desire and commitment to change.

Planning
• Plan of care and who is involved in planning.
• Teaching plan.

Implementation/Evaluation
• Response to interventions, teaching, and actions performed.
• Attainment or progress toward desired outcome(s).
• Modifications to plan of care.

Discharge Planning
• Long-term needs, plan for follow-up, and who is responsible for actions to be taken.
• Specific referrals made.

References

1. Doenges, M. E., Townsend, M., Moorhouse, M. F. (1998). *Psychiatric Care Plans: Guidelines for Individualizing Care.* 3d ed. Philadelphia: F. A. Davis.
2. Townsend, M. (2006). *Psychiatric Mental Health Nursing: Concepts of Care.* 5th ed. Philadelphia: F. A. Davis.
3. Lipson, J. G., Dibble, S. L., Minarik, P. A. (1999). *Culture & Nursing Care: A Pocket Guide.* San Francisco: UCSF Nursing Press.
4. Doenges, M. E., Moorhouse, M. F., Geissler-Murr, A. C. (2006). *Nurse's Pocket Guide: Diagnoses, Interventions, and Rationales.* 11th ed. Philadelphia: F. A. Davis.
5. Paice, J. (2002). Managing psychological conditions in palliative care. *Am J Nurs,* 102(11), 36–43.
6. Killeen, C. (1998). Loneliness, an epidemic in modern society. *J Adv Nurs,* 28(4), 762–770.
7. McAuley, E., et al. (2000). Social relations, physical activity, and well-being in older adults. *Prev Med,* 31(5), 608–617.
8. Acorn, S., Bampton, E. (1992). Patient's loneliness: A challenge for rehabilitation nurses. *Rehabil Nurs,* 17(1), 22–25.
9. Davidson, L., Stayner, D. (1997). Loss, loneliness, and the desire for love: Perspectives on the social lives of people with schizophrenia. *Psychiatr Rehabil J,* 20(3), 3–12.
10. Robinson, K. (2007). Loneliness. University of New York at Buffalo. Retrieved March 2007 from http://ub-counseling.buffalo.edu/loneliness.shtml.
11. Finch, A. (2007). Fed up with feeling alone? Retrieved February 2007 from www.selfesteem4women.com/_lib/eZine/articles/cc_0408.php.
12. Evans, M. Loneliness. Self-Help Information Counseling and Testing Center. Retrieved March 2007 from http://darkwing.uoregon.edu/~counsel/loneliness.htm.
13. Seepersad, S. (2007). Loneliness in attachment and family. Retrieved March 2007 from www.webofloneliness.com/publications/critical/pubintro.htm.

risk for disturbed Maternal/Fetal Dyad

DEFINITION: At risk for disruption of the symbiotic maternal/fetal dyad as a result of co-morbid or pregnancy-related complications

RELATED FACTORS

Complications of pregnancy (e.g., premature rupture of membranes [PROM], placenta previa or abruption, late prenatal care, multiple gestation)
Compromised O_2 transport (e.g., anemia, asthma, hypertension, seizures, premature labor, hemorrhage; [sickle cell anemia])
Impaired glucose metabolism (e.g., diabetes, steroid use)
Physical abuse
Substance abuse (e.g., tobacco, alcohol, drugs)
Treatment related side effects (e.g., medications, surgery, chemotherapy)

NOTE: A risk diagnosis is not evidenced by signs and symptoms, as the problem has not occurred; rather, nursing interventions are directed at prevention.
Sample Clinical Applications: High-risk pregnancy, prenatal substance abuse, pregnancy-induced hypertension (PIH), maternal diabetes mellitus, prenatal hemorrhage, prenatal infection, premature dilatation of cervix, abdominal trauma, domestic violence

DESIRED OUTCOMES/EVALUATION CRITERIA

Sample **NOC** linkages:
Maternal Status Antepartum: Extent to which maternal well-being is within normal limits from conception to the onset of labor
Fetal Status Antepartum: Extent to which fetal signs are within normal limits from conception to the onset of labor
Prenatal Health Behavior: Personal action to promote a healthy pregnancy and a healthy newborn

Client Will: (Include Specific Time Frame)
• Verbalize understanding of individual risk factors or condition(s) that may impact pregnancy.
• Engage in necessary alterations in lifestyle and daily activities to manage risks.
• Participate in screening procedures as indicated.
• Identify signs/symptoms requiring medical evaluation or intervention.
• Display fetal growth within normal limits (WNL) and carry pregnancy to term.

ACTIONS/INTERVENTIONS

Sample **NIC** linkages:
High-Risk Pregnancy Care: Identification and management of a high risk pregnancy to promote healthy outcomes for mother and baby
Surveillance: Late Pregnancy: Purposeful and ongoing acquisition, interpretation, and synthesis of maternal-fetal data for treatment, observation, or admission

---

Nursing Diagnoses in Alphabetical Order

NURSING PRIORITY NO. 1

To identify individual risk/contributing factors:

- Review history of previous pregnancies for presence of complications, such as PROM, placenta previa, miscarriage or pregnancy losses due to premature dilation of the cervix, preterm labor and deliveries, previous birth defects, hyperemesis gravidarum, or repeated urinary tract or vaginal infections.[22,23]
- Obtain history about prenatal screening and amount and timing of care. *Prenatal screening can detect inherited and congenital abnormalities long before birth providing opportunities for informed parental decisions, such as repair of abnormality in utero or helping mother understand a procedure. Lack of prenatal care or late prenatal care may be result of ignorance of or fear about pregnancy, or be the result of inadequate finances or other support, and can place both mother and fetus at risk.[9,23]*
- Note conditions potentiating vascular changes and reduced placental circulation (e.g., diabetes, PIH, cardiac problems, smoking) or those that alter oxygen-carrying capacity (e.g., asthma, anemia, Rh incompatibility, hemorrhage). *Extent of maternal vascular involvement and reduction of oxygen-carrying capacity have a direct influence on uteroplacental circulation and gas exchange.[10,18]*
- Note maternal age. *Maternal age above 35 years is associated with increased risk of placental separation or abruptio placentae, spontaneous abortions, preterm delivery or stillbirths, fetal chromosomal abnormalities and malformations; and intrauterine growth retardation (IUGR). The most common maternal complications in this age group are PIH and gestational diabetes. In pregnant adolescents (younger than 15) the most common high-risk conditions include PIH, anemia, labor dysfunction, cephalopelvic disproportion and low-birth-weight, and preterm delivery.[2,5,11,14,23]*
- Ascertain current and past dietary patterns and practices. *Client may be malnourished, underweight or obese (weight <100 lb or > 200 lb), may reveal preconception eating disorders that can have a negative impact on fetal organ development—especially brain tissue in the early weeks of pregnancy.[1,3,15,23]*
- Assess for severe, unremitting nausea and vomiting, especially when it persists after the first trimester. *Hyperemesis gravidarum places mother at risk for substantial weight loss and fluid and electrolyte imbalances, and exposes the developing fetus to acidotic state and malnutrition. Development of hyperemesis gravidarum may require hospitalization.[14,19,23]*
- Note history of exposure to teratogenic agents, infectious diseases (e.g., tuberculosis, influenza, measles); high-risk occupations; exposure to toxic substances such as lead, organic solvents, carbon monoxide; use of certain over-the-counter (OTC) or prescription medications; substance use or abuse (including illicit drugs and alcohol).[4,6,7,14,18]
- Identify family or cultural influences in pregnancy. *Family history may include multiple births or congenital diseases, or generational abuse, or lack of support or finances. Cultural background may identify health risks associated with nationality (e.g., sickle cell in people of African descent or Tay-Sachs disease in people of Eastern European Jewish ancestry); or religious practices (e.g., exclusion of dairy products, no maternal immunizations for rubella), which can impact health of mother or fetal development.[11,14]*
- Review laboratory studies. *Low hemoglobin suggests anemia, which is associated with hypoxia. Blood type and Rh group may reveal incompatibility risks; elevated serum glucose seen in gestational diabetes mellitus (GDM), elevated liver function studies suggest hypertensive liver involvement; drop in platelet count may be associated with PIH and HELLP (hemolysis, elevated liver enzymes, and low platelet) syndrome. Nutritional studies may*

reveal decreased levels of serum proteins, electrolytes, minerals, and vitamins essential to maternal health and fetal development.[9,15,23]

- Review vaginal, cervical, or rectal cultures and serology results. *May reveal presence of sexually transmitted diseases (STDs), a virus of the TORCH (toxoplasmosis, other, rubella, cytomegalovirus, herpes simplex) group, or Listeria; or identify active/carrier state of hepatitis, HIV, AIDS.*[12,13,22]
- Assist in screening for and identifying genetic or chromosomal disorders. *Disorders such as phenylketonuria (PKU) or sickle cell anemia necessitate special treatment to prevent negative effects on fetal growth.*[11]
- Investigate current home situation. *May have history of unstable relationship, or inadequate/lack of housing which affects safety as well as general well-being.*[20]

NURSING PRIORITY NO. 2

To monitor maternal/fetal status:

- Weigh client and compare current weight with pregravid weight. Have client record weight between visits. *Underweight clients are at risk for anemia, inadequate protein/calorie intake, vitamin or mineral deficiencies, and PIH. Overweight women are at risk for possible changes in the cardiovascular system that create risks for development of PIH, GDM, and hyperinsulinemia of the fetus, resulting in macrosomia. Research indicates increased risk of fetal distress and cesarean delivery. Sudden weight gain of 2 or more pounds in a week may indicate PIH.*[3,15,23]
- Assess fetal heart rate (FHR), noting rate and regularity. Have client monitor fetal movement daily as indicated. *Tachycardia in a term infant may indicate a compensatory mechanism to reduced oxygen levels and/or presence of sepsis. A reduction in fetal activity occurs before bradycardia.*[23]
- Test urine for presence of ketones. *Indicates inadequate glucose utilization and breakdown of fats for metabolic processes.*[10,23]
- Provide information and assist with procedures as indicated, for example:[9,14,23]
  Amniocentesis: *May be performed for genetic purposes or to assess fetal lung maturity. Spectrophotometric analysis of the fluid may be done to detect bilirubin after 26 weeks gestation.*
  Ultrasonography: *Assesses gestational age of fetus, detects presence of multiples, or fetal abnormalities. Locates placenta (and amniotic fluid pockets before amniocentesis, if performed), monitors clients at risk for reduced/inadequate placental perfusion (such as adolescents; clients older than 35 years; and clients with diabetes, PIH, cardiac/kidney disease, anemia, or respiratory disorders).*
  Biophysical profile (BPP): *Assesses fetal well-being through ultrasound evaluation to measure amniotic fluid index (AFI), FHR and nonstress test (NST) reactivity, fetal breathing movement, body movement (large limbs), and muscle tone (flexion and extension).*
  Contraction stress test (CST): *A positive CST with late decelerations indicates a high-risk client/fetus with possible reduced uteroplacental reserves.*
- Screen for abuse during pregnancy. *Prenatal abuse is correlated with a low maternal weight gain, infections, anemia, delay in seeking prenatal care until the third trimester, and preterm delivery.*[20]
- Screen for preterm uterine contractions, which may or may not be accompanied by cervical dilatation. *Occurs in 6% to 7% of all pregnancies and may result in delivery of a preterm infant if tocolytic management is not successful in reducing uterine contractility and irritability.*[21]

NURSING PRIORITY NO. 3

To maintain or improve maternal and fetal well-being:

- Instruct client in reportable symptoms, and monitor for unusual symptoms at each prenatal visit (e.g., vaginal bleeding, headache along with blurred vision and ankle swelling, faintness, persistent vomiting). *Provides opportunity for early intervention in event of developing complications.*[15,23]
- Assist in treatment of underlying medical condition(s) that have potential for causing maternal or fetal harm.[10]
- Assess perceived impact of complication on client and family members. Encourage verbalization of concerns. *Family stress often occurs in an uncomplicated pregnancy, and it is amplified in a high-risk pregnancy, where concerns focus on the health of both the client and the fetus. Family is strengthened if all members have a chance to express fears openly and work cooperatively.*[23]
- Facilitate positive adaptation to situation, through Active-listening, acceptance, and problem-solving. *Helps in successful accomplishment of the psychological tasks of pregnancy, although the high-risk couple may remain ambivalent as a self-protective mechanism against possible loss of the pregnancy or fetal death.*[23]
- Develop dietary plan with client that provides necessary nutrients (calories, protein, vitamins and minerals) *to create new tissue and to meet increased maternal metabolic needs.*[16,18]
- Promote fluid intake of at least two quarts of noncaffeinated fluid per day. *Prevents dehydration, which may compromise optimal uterine and placental functioning and increase uterine irritability, which could potentiate premature labor.*
- Encourage client to participate in individually appropriate adaptations and self-care techniques, such as scheduling rest periods two to three times a day, avoiding overexertion or heavy lifting, or maintaining contact with family and daily life if bedrest is required. *Medical problems necessitating special therapy or restrictions at home or hospitalization significantly disrupt normal routines and cause stress. Preventive problem-solving promotes participation in own care and enhances self-confidence, sense of control, and client/couple satisfaction.*[23]
- Review medication regimen. *Prepregnancy treatment for chronic conditions may require alteration for maternal/fetal safety.*
- Review availability and use of resources. *Presence or absence of supportive resources can make the difference for the client and family in being able to manage the situation.*
- Administer Rh immune globulin (RhIgG) to client at 28 weeks gestation in Rh-negative clients with Rh-positive partners, or following amniocentesis, if indicated. *RhIgG helps reduce incidence of maternal isoimmunization in nonsensitized mothers and helps prevent erythroblastosis fetalis and fetal red blood cell (RBC) hemolysis.*[23,24]
- Encourage modified or complete bedrest as indicated. *Activity level may need modification, depending on symptoms of uterine activity, cervical changes, or bleeding. Side-lying position increases renal and placental perfusion, which is effective in preventing supine hypotensive syndrome.*[23] *Note: Bedrest may result in generalized weakness, raising safety concerns when client is out of bed.*
- Provide supplemental oxygen as appropriate. *Increases the oxygen available for fetal uptake, especially in presence of severe anemia or sickle cell crisis or when maternal/fetal circulation is compromised.*
- Prepare for and assist with intrauterine fetal exchange transfusion as indicated by titers (Kleihauer-Betke test). *If excess fetal RBC hemolysis occurs, transfusion into fetal*

🌐 Cultural   Collaborative   🏠 Community/Home Care   Diagnostic Studies   ∞ Pediatric/Geriatric/Lifespan   Medications

peritoneal cavity with RhO-negative blood replaces hemolyzed RBC's when fetus is determined at risk of dying before 32 weeks' gestation.[24]

NURSING PRIORITY NO. 4

To promote wellness (Teaching/Discharge Considerations):

- Emphasize the normalcy of pregnancy, focus on pregnancy milestones, "countdown to birth." *Avoids or limits perception of "sick role," promotes sense of hope that modifications or restrictions serve a worthwhile purpose.*[23]

- Discuss implications of preexisting condition and possible impact on pregnancy. *Pregnancy may have no effect, or may reduce or exacerbate severity of symptoms of chronic conditions. Repeat sickle cell crises predispose client and fetus to increased mortality and morbidity rates. Client with MS or spinal cord injury (SCI) may have decreased ability to sense uterine contractions or presence of labor necessitating closer monitoring.*[10]

- Provide information about risks of weight reduction during pregnancy and about nourishment needs of client and fetus. *Prenatal calorie restriction and resultant weight loss may result in nutrient deficiency or ketonemia, with negative effects on fetal central nervous system (CNS) and possible IUGR.*[18]

- Encourage smoking cessation, refer to community program or support group as indicated. *Severe adverse effects of smoking on the fetus may be reduced if mother quits smoking early in pregnancy, and pregnancy outcomes can still be improved if mother stops smoking as late as 32 weeks gestation.*[17]

- Help client/couple plan restructuring of roles or activities necessitated by complication of pregnancy. *Education, support, and assistance in maintenance of family integrity help foster growth of its individual members and reduce stress that the client may feel from her dependent role.*[23]

- Have client demonstrate new behaviors or therapeutic techniques. *During pregnancy, control of condition may require specific modified or new behaviors. Demonstration allows accurate assessment of learning.*

- Recommend client assess uterine tone and presence of contractions for one hour, once or twice a day as indicated *to monitor uterine irritability or early indication of premature labor.*[21]

- Encourage close monitoring of blood glucose levels, as appropriate. *Type 1 or insulin-dependent diabetes mellitus (IDDM) clients generally need to check blood glucose levels 4 to 12 times/day because insulin needs may increase two to three times above pregravid baseline.*[10]

- Demonstrate technique and specific equipment used when FHR monitoring is done in the home setting. *Provides opportunity for more detailed information regarding fetal well-being in a less stressful environment. Enhances sense of active involvement.*

- Identify danger signals requiring immediate notification of healthcare provider (e.g., PROM, preterm labor, vaginal drainage or bleeding). *Recognizing risk situations encourages prompt evaluation and intervention, which may prevent or limit untoward outcomes.*[21,22]

- Review availability and use of resources. *Presence or absence of supportive resources can make the difference for the client and family in being able to manage the situation.*[22]

- Refer to community service agencies (e.g., visiting nurse, social service) or resources, such as Sidelines. *Community supports may be needed for ongoing assessment of medical problem, family status, coping behaviors, and financial stressors. Note: Sidelines is a national telephone support group for pregnant women on bedrest.*

- Refer for counseling if family does not sustain positive coping and growth. *May be necessary to promote growth and to prevent family disintegration.*

DOCUMENTATION FOCUS

Assessment/Reassessment
- Assessment findings, weight, signs of pregnancy, safety concerns.
- Specific risk factors, comorbidities, and treatment regimen.
- Results of screening laboratory tests and diagnostic studies.
- Participation in prenatal care.
- Cultural beliefs and practices.

Planning
- Plan of care, specific interventions, and who is involved in the planning.
- Community resources for equipment or supplies.
- Specific referrals made.
- Teaching plan.

Implementation/Evaluation
- Client/fetal response to treatment and actions performed.
- Client's response to teaching provided.
- Attainment or progress toward desired outcome(s).
- Modifications to plan of care.

References

1. National Institute of Child Health and Human Development. (2006). High-risk pregnancy. Retrieved March 2009 from www.nichd.nih.gov/health/topics/high_risk_pregnancy.cfm.
2. Cleary-Goldman, J., et al. (2005). Impact of maternal age on obstetric outcome. *Obstet Gynecol*, 105(5), 983–990.
3. Ehrenberg, H. M., et al. (2009). Maternal obesity, uterine activity, and the risk of spontaneous preterm birth. *Obstet Gynecol*, 113(1), 48–52.
4. Surgeon General. (2005, rev. 2007). Surgeon General's advisory on alcohol use in pregnancy. Retrieved March 2009 from www.surgeongeneral.gov/pressreleases/sg02222005.html.
5. Miller, D. A. (2005). Is advanced maternal age an independent risk factor for uteroplacental insufficiency? *Am J Obstet Gynecol*, 192(6), 1974–1982.
6. March of Dimes. (2006). Fact sheets: Illicit drug use during pregnancy. Retrieved March 2009 from www.marchofdimes.com/professionals/14332_1169.asp.
7. Dharan, V. B., Parvianen, E. L. K. (2009). Psychosocial and environmental pregnancy risks. Retrieved March 2009 from http://emedicine.medscape.com/article/259346-overview.
8. Gibson, P., Carson, M. P. (2007). Hypertension and pregnancy. Retrieved March 2009 from http://emedicine.medscape.com/article/261435-overview.
9. Yale Medical Group. High-risk pregnancy: Maternal and fetal testing. Retrieved March 2009 from http://ymghealthinfo.org/content.asp?pageid=P02469.
10. Yale Medical Group. High-risk pregnancy: Pregnancy and medical conditions. Retrieved March 2009 from http://ymghealthinfo.org/content.asp?pageid=P02483.
11. Yale Medical Group. High-risk pregnancy: Prenatal counseling. Retrieved March 2009 from http://ymghealthinfo.org/content.asp?pageid=P02493.
12. Centers for Disease Control and Prevention. (2008). STDs and pregnancy. CDC fact sheet. Retrieved March 2009 from www.cdc.gov/std/STDFact-STDs&Pregnancy.htm.
13. U.S. Department of Health and Human Services. (2008). HIV during pregnancy, labor and delivery, and after birth. Retrieved March 2009 from http://aidsinfo.nih.gov/ContentFiles/Perinatal_FS_en.pdf.
14. Complications and high-risk conditions of the prenatal period. (2008). *Straight A's in Maternal-Neonatal Nursing*. 2d ed. Philadelphia: Lippincott Williams & Wilkins.
15. Holloway, B., Moredich, C., Aduddell, K. (2006). *OB Peds Women's Health Notes: Nurse's Clinical Pocket Guide*. Philadelphia: F. A. Davis.

16. RDAs for Pregnant Women. (2007). *Lippincott Manual of Nursing Practice Pocket Guides: Maternal-Neonatal Nursing.* Philadelphia: Lippincott Williams & Wilkins.
17. Barclay, L., Vega, C. (2009). Severe adverse effects of smoking may be reversible if mothers quit early in pregnancy. Retrieved April 2009 from http://cme.medscape.com/viewarticle/590543?src=cmemp.
18. National Institute of Child Health and Human Development. (2009). Care before and during pregnancy—Prenatal care. Retrieved March 2009 from www.nichd.nih.gov/womenshealth/research/pregbirth/prenatal_care.cfm.
19. Yale Medical Group. High-risk pregnancy: Hyperemesis gravidarum. Retrieved March 2009 from http://ymghealthinfo.org/content.asp?pageid=P02457.
20. Centers for Disease Control and Prevention. Violence and reproductive health. Retrieved April 2009 from www.cdc.gov/reproductivehealth/violence/index.htm.
21. Institute of Medicine. (2006). Preterm birth: Causes, consequences, and prevention. Retrieved April 2009 from http://books.nap.edu/openbook.php?record_id=11622&page=R1.
22. Ross, M. G., Eden, R. D. (2009). Preterm labor. Retrieved April 2009 from http://emedicine.medscape.com/article/260998-overview.
23. Ricci, S. S., Kyle, T. (2008). *Maternity and Pediatric Nursing.* Philadelphia: Lippincott Williams & Wilkins.
24. National Heart, Lung, and Blood Institute. (2008). Rh incompatibility. Retrieved April 2009 from www.nhlbi.nih.gov/health/dci/Diseases/rh/rh_what.html.
25. Maloni, J. A., et al. (2002). Dysphoria among high-risk pregnant hospitalized women on bed rest: A longitudinal study. *Nurs Res*, 51(2), 92–99.

impaired Memory

DEFINITION: Inability to remember or recall bits of information or behavioral skills [Impaired memory may be attributed to physiopathological or situational causes that are either temporary or permanent]

RELATED FACTORS

Hypoxia; anemia
Fluid and electrolyte imbalance; decreased cardiac output
Neurological disturbances [e.g., brain injury, concussion]
Excessive environmental disturbances; [manic state, fugue, traumatic event]
[Substance use or abuse; effects of medications]
[Age]

DEFINING CHARACTERISTICS

Subjective
[Reported] experiences of forgetting
Inability to recall recent or past events or factual information [or familiar persons, places, items]

Objective
[Observed] experiences of forgetting
Inability to determine if a behavior was performed
Inability to learn, retain new skills, or information
Inability to perform a previously learned skill

(continues on page 506)

impaired Memory (continued)

Forgets to perform a behavior at a scheduled time

Sample Clinical Applications: Brain injury, stroke, dementia, Alzheimer's disease, hypoxia (e.g., chronic obstructive pulmonary disease [COPD], anemia, altitude sickness), alcohol intoxication or substance abuse

DESIRED OUTCOMES/EVALUATION CRITERIA

Sample **NOC** linkages:

Memory: Ability to cognitively retrieve and report previously stored information
Cognition: Ability to execute complex mental processes

Client Will (Include Specific Time Frame)
• Verbalize awareness of memory problems.
• Establish methods to help in remembering essential things when possible.
• Accept limitations of condition and use resources effectively.

ACTIONS/INTERVENTIONS

Sample **NIC** linkages:
Memory Training: Facilitation of memory
Surveillance: Safety: Purposeful and ongoing collection and analysis of information about the patient and the environment for use in promoting and maintaining patient safety

NURSING PRIORITY NO. 1

To assess causative factor(s)/degree of impairment:

• Determine physical and biochemical factors (e.g., recent surgery, infections, brain injury, use of multiple medications, exposure to toxic substances, use or abuse of alcohol or other drugs, pain, depression) *that may be related to changes in memory.*

∞ • Note client's age and potential for depression symptoms in elderly. *Depressive disorders are particularly prevalent in older adults (approximately 15%) who report inability to concentrate and poor memory. Kuljis calls it a prevalent myth that substantial memory loss is a normal aspect of aging, barring effects of illness or injury. However, it is known that memory is somehow altered in the aging process and that generally, memory for past occurrences is superior to the retention and recall of more recent information.*[1,2,5,6]

• Note presence and degree of anxiety. *Can increase the client's confusion and disorganization and further interfere with attempts at recall.* (Refer to ND Anxiety for additional interventions as indicated.)

• Collaborate with medical and psychiatric providers *to evaluate extent of impairment to orientation, attention span, ability to follow directions, send/receive communication, and appropriateness of response.*

• Assist with or review results of cognitive testing (e.g., Blessed Information-Memory-Concentration [BIMC] test, Clinical Dementia Rating [CDR] Scale, Mini-Mental State Examination [MMSE]). *Although the etiology for some memory impairments may be obvious or established by client/SO/caregiver report, a combination of tests may be needed to complete picture of the client's overall condition and prognosis.*[3,6]

- Evaluate skill proficiency levels. *Evaluation may include many self-care activities (e.g., daily grooming, steps in preparing a meal, participating in a lifelong hobby, balancing a checkbook, and driving ability) to determine level of independence or needed assistance.*
- Ascertain how client/family view the problem (e.g., practical problems of forgetting to turn off the stove, client gets lost when driving, or role and responsibility impairments related to loss of memory and concentration) *to determine significance and impact of problem and suggest direction of interventions, especially as relates to basic safety issues.*[1]

NURSING PRIORITY NO. 2

To maximize level of function:

- Assist with treatment of underlying conditions (e.g., electrolyte imbalance, anemia, drug interactions/reaction to medications, alcohol or other drug intoxication, malnutrition, vitamin deficiencies, pain) *where treatment can improve memory processes.*
- Orient and reorient client, as needed, to environment. Introduce self with each client contact *to meet client's safety and comfort needs.* (Refer to NDs acute/chronic Confusion for additional interventions as appropriate.)
- Implement appropriate memory-retraining techniques (e.g., keeping calendars, writing lists, memory cue games, mnemonic devices, using computers) *to provide restorative or compensatory training for cognitive function.*[4]
- Assist in and instruct client and family in associate-learning tasks (e.g., practice sessions recalling personal information, reminiscing, locating a geographic location [Stimulation Therapy]). *Practice may improve performance and integrate new behaviors into the client's coping strategies.*
- Support and reinforce client's efforts to remember information or behavioral skills. *Can decrease anxiety levels and perhaps help with further memory recovery.*
- Encourage ventilation of feelings of frustration, helplessness, and so forth. Refocus attention to areas of control and progress *to diminish feelings of powerlessness or hopelessness.*
- Provide for and emphasize importance of pacing learning activities and getting sufficient rest *to avoid fatigue that may further impair cognitive abilities.*
- Monitor client's behavior and assist in use of stress-management techniques (e.g., music therapy, reading, television, games, socialization) *to reduce frustration and enhance enjoyment of life.*
- Structure teaching methods and interventions *to client's level of functioning or potential for improvement.*[5]
- Determine client's response to and effects of medications prescribed to improve attention, concentration, memory processes, and to lift spirits or modify emotional responses. *Medications used for cognitive enhancement can be effective, but benefits need to be weighed against whether quality of life is improved when considering side effects and cost of drugs.*[3]

NURSING PRIORITY NO. 3

To promote wellness (Teaching/Discharge Considerations):

- Assist client/SO(s) to establish compensation strategies *to improve functional lifestyle and safety, such as menu planning with a shopping list; timely completion of tasks on a daily planner; and checklists at the front door to ascertain that lights and stove are off before leaving.*[6]
- Teach client and family/care providers memory involvement tasks, such as reminiscence and memory practice exercises *geared toward improving client's functional ability.*[6]

Nursing Diagnoses in Alphabetical Order

- Refer to or encourage follow-up with counselors, rehabilitation programs, job coaches, social or financial support systems *to help deal with persistent or difficult problems.*
- Refer to rehabilitation services *that are matched to the needs, strengths, and capacities of individual and modified as needs change over time.*[4]
- Discuss and encourage safety interventions, as indicated (e.g., assistance with meal preparation, evaluation of driving abilities, cessation of tobacco use or its use only under supervision, removal of guns and other weapons) *to prevent injury to client/others.*[1]
- Identify resources to meet individual needs (e.g., home-care assistant, companion, Meals on Wheels), *thereby maximizing independence and general well-being.*

DOCUMENTATION FOCUS

Assessment/Reassessment
- Individual findings, testing results, and perceptions of significance of problem.
- Actual impact on lifestyle and independence.

Planning
- Plan of care and who is involved in planning process.
- Teaching plan.

Implementation/Evaluation
- Responses to interventions, teaching, and actions performed.
- Attainment or progress toward desired outcome(s).
- Modifications to plan of care.

Discharge Planning
- Long-term needs and who is responsible for actions to be taken.
- Specific referrals made.

References

1. Anderson, H. S., Kuljis, R. O. (2003, update 2008). Minimal cognitive impairment: Treatment & medication. Retrieved October 2009 from http://emedicine.medscape.com/article/1136393 -treatment.
2. Roussel, L. A. (1999). The aging neurological system. In Stanley, M., Beare, P. G. (eds). *Gerontological Nursing: A Health Promotion/Protection Approach.* 2d ed. Philadelphia: F. A. Davis.
3. About Alzheimer's. (2003). Physicians and care professionals educational materials. Alzheimer's Disease and Related Disorders Association (AARDA) Web site, www.alz.org.
4. NIH Consensus Panel. (1999). Rehabilitation of persons with traumatic brain injury. *JAMA,* 8(10), 974–983.
5. Mayo Clinic. (2006). Mild cognitive impairment prevalent in elderly population; Risk increases as age goes up and education goes down. Ascribe Health News Service. Retrieved January 2007 from www.mayoclinic.org/news2006-rst/3306.html.
6. Jacobs, D. H. (2006). Confusional states and acute memory disorders. Retrieved January 2007 from www.emedicine.com/neuro/topic435.htm.

impaired bed Mobility

DEFINITION: Limitation of independent movement from one bed position to another

RELATED FACTORS

Neuromuscular or musculoskeletal impairment
Insufficient muscle strength; deconditioning; obesity
Environmental constraints (i.e., bed size/type, treatment equipment, restraints)
Pain; sedating medications
Deficient knowledge
Cognitive impairment

DEFINING CHARACTERISTICS

Subjective
[Reported difficulty performing activities]

Objective
Impaired ability to turn side to side, move from supine to sitting or sitting to supine, "scoot," or reposition self in bed, move from supine to prone or prone to supine, from supine to long-sitting or long-sitting to supine

Sample Clinical Applications: Paralysis (e.g., spinal cord injury [SCI], stroke), traumatic brain injury, neuromuscular disorders (e.g., amyotrophic lateral sclerosis [ALS]), major chest or back surgery, severe depression, dementia, catatonic schizophrenia

DESIRED OUTCOMES/EVALUATION CRITERIA

Sample NOC linkages:
Body Positioning: Self-Initiated: Ability to change own body position independently with or without assistive device
Coordinated Movement: Adequacy of muscles to work together voluntarily for purposeful movement
Immobility Consequences: Physiological: Severity of compromise to physiological functioning due to impaired physical mobility

Client/Caregiver Will (Include Specific Time Frame)
• Verbalize willingness to and participates in repositioning program.
• Verbalize understanding of situation or risk factors, individual therapeutic regimen, and safety measures.
• Demonstrate techniques or behaviors that enable safe repositioning.
• Maintain position of function and skin integrity as evidenced by absence of contractures, foot drop, decubitus, and other skin disorders.
• Maintain or increase strength and function of affected and/or compensatory body part.

(continues on page 510)

impaired bed Mobility (continued)
ACTIONS/INTERVENTIONS

Sample NIC linkages:

Bed Rest Care: Promotion of comfort and safety and prevention of complications for a patient unable to get out of bed

Positioning: Deliberative placement of the client or a body part to promote physiological and/or psychological well-being

Teaching: Prescribed Activity/Exercise: Preparing a patient to achieve or maintain a prescribed level of activity

NURSING PRIORITY NO. 1

To identify causative/contributing factors:

- Determine diagnoses that contribute to current immobility (e.g., multiple sclerosis [MS], arthritis, Parkinson's disease, hemi-/para- or tetraplegia, fractures, multiple trauma, head injury, burns) *to identify interventions specific to client's mobility impairment and needs.*
- Note individual factors (e.g., surgery, casts, amputation, traction, pain, advanced age, general weakness or debilitation, severe depression, dementia) *that can contribute to problems related to bedrest and potential complications.*
- Determine degree of perceptual or cognitive impairment or ability to follow directions. *Impairments related to age, acute or chronic conditions (including severe depression, dementia), trauma, surgery, or medications require alternative interventions or changes in plan of care.*[1,3]

NURSING PRIORITY NO. 2

To assess functional ability:

- Determine functional level classification 1 to 4 *(level 1 requires use of equipment or device; level 2 requires help from another person for assistance; level 3 requires help from another person and equipment device; level 4 is totally dependent, does not participate in activity).*
- Note emotional and behavioral responses to problems of immobility. *Can negatively affect self-concept and self-esteem, autonomy, and independence. Feelings of frustration and powerlessness may impede attainment of goals. Social, occupational, and relationship roles can change, leading to isolation, depression, and economic consequences.*[4,5]
- Note presence of complications related to immobility. *Studies have shown that as much as 5.5% of muscle strength can be lost each day of rest and immobility.*[1] *Other complications include changes in circulation and impairments of organ function affecting the whole person (e.g., cognition, immune system function, emotional state).* (Refer to ND risk for Disuse Syndrome for additional interventions.)

NURSING PRIORITY NO. 3

To promote optimal level of function and prevent complications:

- Ascertain that dependent client is placed in best bed for situation (e.g., properly functioning equipment, correct size and support surface) *to promote environmental, client, and care provider safety.*[6]

 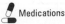

- Instruct client/care providers in bed capabilities (e.g., mobility functions and set positions) encouraging client to participate as much as possible, even if only to move head or run bed controls. *Promotes independence and purposeful movement.*
- Change client's position frequently, moving individual parts of the body (e.g., legs, arms, head) using appropriate support and proper body alignment. Encourage periodic changes in head of bed (if not contraindicated by conditions such as acute SCI), with client in supine and prone positions at intervals *to improve circulation, reduce tightening of muscles and joints, normalizing body tone, and more closely simulating body positions individual would normally use.*[2]
- Instruct caregivers in methods of moving client relative to specific situations (e.g., turning side to side, or prone or sitting) *to provide support for the client's body and to prevent injury to the lifter. Note: Positioning instructions and detailed sketches are available (e.g., Ossman)[7] on proper positions for certain conditions (e.g., paralyzed client) as well as the safe movement and positioning of body parts (e.g., rolling, bridging, scooting, sitting), which should become well known to caregivers in order to prevent injury to both the client and the caregivers.*
- Place client in upright position at intervals, or out of bed into upright chair, if condition allows. *Being vertical has been shown to reduce the work of heart, improve circulation and lung ventilation, and may improve cognition and awareness.*[3]
- Use egg-crate, alternating air-pressure, or water mattress; padding and positioning devices (e.g., foam wedge, pillows, hand rolls, etc., for bony prominences, feet, hands, elbows, head) *to prevent dermal injury or stress on tissues and reduce potential for disuse complications.*[3,6] Refer to ND risk for Peripheral Neurovascular Dysfunction for additional interventions.
- Perform and encourage regular skin examination for reddened or excoriated areas. Provide frequent skin care (e.g., cleansing, moisturizing, gentle massage) *to reduce pressure on sensitive areas and prevent development of problems with skin or tissue integrity.* Refer to NDs impaired Skin Integrity; impaired Tissue Integrity.
- Provide or assist with daily range-of-motion interventions (active and passive) *to maintain joint mobility, improve circulation, and prevent contractures.*
- Collaborate with rehabilitation team, physical or occupational therapists to create exercise and adaptive program designed specifically for client, identifying assistive devices (e.g., splints, braces, boots) and equipment (e.g., transfer board, sling, trapeze, hydraulic lift, specialty beds).
- Assist with activities of hygiene, feeding, and toileting, as indicated. Assist on and off bedpan and into sitting position (or use cardioposition bed or foot-egress bed) to facilitate elimination.
- Note change in strength to do more or less self-care (e.g., hygiene, feeding, toileting) *to promote psychological and physical benefits of self-care and to adjust level of assistance as indicated.*
- Administer medication before activity as needed for pain relief *to permit maximal effort and involvement in activity.*
- Provide diversional activities (e.g., television, books, music, games, visiting) as appropriate *to decrease boredom and potential for depression.*
- Ensure telephone or call bell is within reach, client is able to activate surveillance alarm if provided. *Provides individually appropriate methods for client to communicate needs for assistance.*
- Refer to NDs, Activity Intolerance, impaired physical Mobility, impaired wheelchair Mobility, risk for Disuse Syndrome, impaired Transfer Ability, impaired Walking for additional interventions.

Nursing Diagnoses in Alphabetical Order

NURSING PRIORITY NO. 4

To promote wellness (Teaching/Discharge Considerations):

 • Involve client/SO in determining activity schedule. *Promotes commitment to plan, maximizing outcomes.*

• Instruct all caregivers in safety concerns regarding body mechanics, as well as client's required positions and exercises *to prevent injury to both and to minimize potential for preventable complications.*

• Encourage continuation of regular exercise program *to maintain or enhance gains in strength and muscle control.*

• Obtain or identify sources for assistive devices. Demonstrate safe use and proper maintenance. *Promotes independence and enhances safety.*

DOCUMENTATION FOCUS

Assessment/Reassessment
• Individual findings, including level of function and ability to participate in specific or desired activities.

Planning
• Plan of care and who is involved in the planning.

Implementation/Evaluation
• Responses to interventions, teaching, and actions performed.
• Attainment or progress toward desired outcome(s).
• Modification to plan of care.

Discharge Planning
• Discharge and long-range needs, noting who is responsible for each action to be taken.
• Specific referrals made.
• Sources of and maintenance for assistive devices.

References

1. Pattillo, M. A., Stanley, M. (1999). The aging musculoskeletal system. In Stanley, M., Beare, P. G. (eds). *Gerontological Nursing: A Health Promotion/Protection Approach.* 2d ed. Philadelphia: F. A. Davis.
2. Kumagai, K. A. S. (1998). Physical management of the neurologically involved client: Techniques for bed mobility and transfers. In Chin, P. A., Finocchiaro, D., Rosebrough, A. (eds). *Rehabilitation Nursing Practice.* New York: McGraw-Hill.
3. Palmer, M., Wyness, M. A. (1988). Positioning and handling: Important considerations in the care of the severely head-injured patient. *J Neurosurg Nurs,* 20(1), 42–49.
4. Mass, M. L. (1989). *Impaired physical mobility.* Unpublished manuscript. Cited in research article for National Institutes for Health.
5. Hogue, C. C. (1984). Falls and mobility late in life: An ecological model. *J Am Geriatr Soc,* 32, 858–861.
6. Dionne, M. (2005). This bed is just right. *Rehabil Manage,* 18(1), 32–39.
7. Ossman, N. (1990). *Adult Positions, Transitions, and Transfers.* Psychological Corporation.

impaired physical Mobility

DEFINITION: Limitation in independent, purposeful physical movement of the body or of one or more extremities

RELATED FACTORS

Sedentary lifestyle; activity intolerance; disuse; deconditioning; decreased endurance; limited cardiovascular endurance

Decreased muscle strength or control mass; joint stiffness; contractures; loss of integrity of bone structures

Pain, discomfort

Neuromuscular or musculoskeletal impairment

Sensoriperceptual or cognitive impairment; developmental delay

Depressive mood state; anxiety

Malnutrition; altered cellular metabolism; body mass index (BMI) above 75th age-appropriate percentile

Deficient knowledge regarding value of physical activity; cultural beliefs regarding age-appropriate activity; lack of environmental supports (e.g., physical or social)

Prescribed movement restrictions; medications

Reluctance to initiate movement

DEFINING CHARACTERISTICS

Subjective

[Report of pain or discomfort on movement; unwillingness to move]

Objective

Limited range of motion; limited ability to perform gross fine or motor skills; difficulty turning

Slowed movement; uncoordinated or jerky movements, movement-induced tremor; decreased [slower] reaction time

Postural instability; gait changes

Engages in substitutions for movement (e.g., increased attention to other's activity, controlling behavior, focus on pre-illness disability/activity)

Sample Clinical Applications: Neuromuscular disorders (e.g., multiple sclerosis [MS], amyotrophic lateral sclerosis [ALS]), Parkinson's disease, traumatic injuries (e.g., fractures, spinal cord or brain injuries), rheumatoid arthritis, severe depression

SUGGESTED FUNCTIONAL LEVEL CLASSIFICATION

0—Completely independent
1—Requires use of equipment or device
2—Requires help from another person for assistance, supervision, or teaching
3—Requires help from another person and equipment device
4—Dependent, does not participate in activity

(continues on page 514)

impaired physical Mobility (continued)
DESIRED OUTCOMES/EVALUATION CRITERIA

Sample NOC linkages:
Mobility: Ability to move purposefully in own environment independently with or without assistive device
Immobility Consequences: Physiological: Severity of compromise in physiological functioning due to impaired physical mobility
Knowledge: Prescribed Activity: Extent of understanding conveyed about prescribed activity and exercise

Client Will (Include Specific Time Frame)
• Verbalize understanding of situation and individual treatment regimen and safety measures.
• Demonstrate techniques or behaviors that enable resumption of activities.
• Participate in activities of daily living (ADLs) and desired activities.
• Maintain position of function and skin integrity as evidenced by absence of contractures, footdrop, decubitus, and so forth.
• Maintain or increase strength and function of affected or compensatory body part.

ACTIONS/INTERVENTIONS

Sample NIC linkages:
Exercise Therapy [specify]: Use of active or passive body movement to maintain or restore flexibility; use of specific activity or exercise protocols to enhance or restore controlled body movement, and so forth
Pain Management: Alleviation of pain or a reduction in pain to a level of comfort acceptable to the patient
Traction/Immobilization Care: Management of a patient who has traction or a stabilizing device to immobilize and stabilize a body part

NURSING PRIORITY NO. 1

To identify causative/contributing factors:

● Determine diagnosis that contributes to immobility (e.g., MS, arthritis, Parkinson's disease, hemi-/paraplegia, depression, developmental delays). *These conditions can cause physiological and psychological problems that can seriously impact physical, social, and economic well-being.*[1]

● Note factors affecting current situation (e.g., surgery, fractures, amputation, tubings (chest tube, Foley catheter, IVs, pumps) and potential time involved (e.g., few hours in bed after surgery versus serious trauma requiring long-term bedrest or debilitating disease limiting movement). *Identifies potential impairments and determines type of interventions needed to provide for client's safety.*

● Assess client's developmental level, motor skills, ease and capability of movement, posture and gait *to determine presence of characteristics of client's unique impairment and to guide choice of interventions.*[8]

∞ ● Note older client's general health status. *Hogue identified mobility as the most important functional ability that determines the degree of independence and healthcare needs among older persons.*[2] *While aging per se does not cause impaired mobility, several predisposing factors in addition to age-related changes can lead to immobility (e.g., diminished body*

reserves of musculoskeletal system, chronic diseases, sedentary lifestyle, decreased ability to quickly and adequately correct movements affecting center of gravity). Thus, falls are a major source of morbidity and mortality for older persons.[3,6,8]

- Evaluate for presence and degree of pain, listening to client's description about manner in which pain limits mobility *to determine needed interventions for pain management.*[4]
- Ascertain client's perception of activity and exercise needs and impact of current situation. Identify cultural beliefs and expectations affecting recovery or response to long-term limitations. *Helps to determine client's expectations and beliefs related to activity and potential long-term effect of current immobility. Also identifies barriers that may be addressed (e.g., lack of safe place to exercise, focus on pre-illness or disability activity, controlling behavior, depression, cultural expectations, distorted body image).*[5]
- Assess nutritional status and client's report of energy level. *Deficiencies in nutrients and water, electrolytes and minerals can negatively affect energy and activity tolerance.*
- Determine history of falls and relatedness to current situation. *Client may be restricting activity because of weakness or debilitation, actual injury during a fall, or from psychological distress (i.e., fear and anxiety) that can persist after a fall.*[6-8] (Refer to ND risk for Falls for additional interventions.)

NURSING PRIORITY NO. 2

To assess functional ability:

- Determine degree of immobility in relation to 0–4 scale, noting muscle strength and tone, joint mobility, cardiovascular status, balance, and endurance. *Identifies strengths and deficits (e.g., ability to ambulate with or without assistive devices, or inability to transfer safely from bed to wheelchair) and may provide information regarding potential for recovery (e.g., client with severe brain injury may have permanent limitations because of impaired cognition affecting memory, judgment, problem-solving, and motor planning, requiring more intensive inpatient and long-term care).*[1,6]
- Determine degree of perceptual or cognitive impairment and ability to follow directions. *Impairments related to age, chronic or acute disease condition, trauma, surgery, or medications require alternative interventions or changes in plan of care.*[3]
- Observe movement when client is unaware of observation *to note any incongruency with reports of abilities.*
- Note emotional or behavioral responses to problems of immobility. *Can negatively affect self-concept and self-esteem, autonomy, and independence. Feelings of frustration and powerlessness may impede attainment of goals. Social, occupational, and relationship roles can change, leading to isolation, depression, and economic consequences.*[1,2]
- Determine presence of complications related to immobility (e.g., pneumonia, elimination problems, contractures, decubitus, anxiety). *Studies have shown that as much as 5.5% of muscle strength can be lost each day of rest and immobility.*[5] *Other complications include changes in circulation and impairments of organ function affecting the whole person (e.g., cognition, bone demineralization, venous pooling, and thromboembolic pneumonia, weakened immune system function, muscle contractures).* (Refer to ND risk for Disuse Syndrome.)

NURSING PRIORITY NO. 3

To promote optimal level of function and prevent complications:

- Assist with treatment of underlying condition(s) *to maximize potential for mobility and optimal function.*

- Discuss discrepancies in movement with client aware and unaware of observation and methods for dealing with identified problems. *May be necessary when client is using avoidance or controlling behavior or is not aware of own abilities due to anxiety or fear.*[7]
- Assist with or encourage client to reposition self on a regular schedule as dictated by individual situation (including frequent shifting of weight when client is wheelchair-bound) *to enhance circulation to tissues, reduce risk of tissue ischemia.*
- Review and encourage use of proper body mechanics *to prevent injury to client and caregiver.*
- Demonstrate and assist with use of side rails, overhead trapeze, roller pads, hydraulic lifts or chairs *for position changes and transfers.* Instruct in safe use of walker or cane *for ambulation.*
- Support affected body parts and joints using pillows or rolls, foot supports, shoes, gel pads, and so forth, *to maintain position of function and reduce risk of pressure ulcers.*
- Provide or recommend pressure-reducing mattress, such as egg-crate, or pressure-relieving mattress, such as alternating air-pressure or water. *Reduces tissue pressure and aids in maximizing cellular perfusion to prevent dermal injury.*
- Use padding and positioning devices (e.g., foam wedge, pillows, hand rolls) for bony prominences, feet, hands, elbows, head) *to prevent stress on tissues and reduce potential for disuse complications.*
- Collaborate with physical medicine specialist and occupational or physical therapists in providing range-of-motion exercise (active or passive), isotonic muscle contractions (e.g., flexion of ankles, push and pull exercises), assistive devices, and activities (e.g., early ambulation, transfers, stairs) *to limit or reduce effects and complications of immobility (e.g., contracture deformities, deep vein thromboses). Techniques such as gait training, strength training, and exercise to improve balance and coordination can be helpful in rehabilitating client.*[7]
- Encourage client's participation in self-care activities, physical or occupational therapies as well as diversional and recreational activities. *Reduces sensory deprivation, enhances self-concept and sense of independence, and improves body strength and function.*
- Provide client with ample time to perform mobility-related tasks. Schedule activities with adequate rest periods during the day *to reduce fatigue.*
- Avoid routinely assisting or doing for client those activities that client can do for self. *Caregivers can contribute to impaired mobility by being overprotective or helping too much.*
- Identify and encourage energy-conserving techniques for ADLs. *Limits fatigue, maximizing participation.*
- Provide for safety measures as indicated by individual situation, including environmental management and fall prevention. (Refer to ND risk for Falls.)
- Note change in strength to do more or less self-care (e.g., hygiene, feeding, toileting, therapies) *to promote psychological and physical benefits of self-care and to adjust level of assistance as indicated.*
- Administer medications before activity as needed for pain relief *to permit maximal effort and involvement in activity.*
- Perform and encourage regular skin examination and care *to reduce pressure on sensitive areas and to prevent development of problems with skin integrity.* (Refer to NDs risk for impaired Skin Integrity; risk for impaired Tissue Integrity for additional interventions.)
- Encourage adequate intake of fluids and nutritious foods. *Promotes well-being and maximizes energy production.*
- Refer to NDs Activity Intolerance, impaired bed Mobility, impaired wheelchair Mobility, impaired Transfer Ability, and impaired Walking for additional interventions.

NURSING PRIORITY NO. 4

To promote wellness (Teaching/Discharge Considerations):

🏠 ● Encourage client's/SO's involvement in decision making as much as possible. *Enhances commitment to plan, optimizing outcomes.*

🏠 ● Review importance and purpose of exercise *(e.g., increased cardiovascular and respiratory tolerance, improved flexibility, balance, and muscle strength and tone, enhanced sense of well-being).*

🏠 ● Discuss safe ways that client can exercise. *Multiple options provide client choices and variety (e.g., walking around the block with companion or in a mall during bad air days, participating in a water aerobics class, attending regular rehab sessions).*

🏠 ● Assist client/SO to learn safety measures as individually indicated. *May need instruction and to give return demonstration (e.g., use of heating pads, locking wheelchair before transfers, removal or securing of scatter or area rugs, judicious and accurate use of medications, supervised exercise).*[7]

🏠 ● Involve client and SO(s) in care, assisting them to learn ways of managing problems of immobility, especially when impairment is expected to be long term. *May need referral for support and community services to provide care, supervision, companionship, respite services, nutritional and ADL assistance, adaptive devices or changes to living environment, financial assistance and so forth.*[7,8]

🏠 ● Demonstrate use of standing aids and mobility devices (e.g., walkers, strollers, scooters, braces, prosthetics) and have client/care provider demonstrate knowledge about and safe use of device. Identify appropriate resources for obtaining and maintaining appliances or equipment. *Safe use of mobility aids promotes client's independence and enhances quality of life and safety for client and caregiver.*[9,10]

DOCUMENTATION FOCUS

Assessment/Reassessment
• Individual findings, including level of function and ability to participate in specific or desired activities.

Planning
• Plan of care and who is involved in the planning.
• Teaching plan.

Implementation/Evaluation
• Responses to interventions, teaching, and actions performed.
• Attainment or progress toward desired outcome(s).
• Modifications to plan of care.

Discharge Planning
• Discharge and long-term needs, noting who is responsible for each action to be taken.
• Specific referrals made.
• Sources of and maintenance for assistive devices.

References

1. Mass, M. L. (1989). *Impaired physical mobility.* Unpublished manuscript. Cited in research article for National Institutes for Health.
2. Hogue, C. C. (1984). Falls and mobility late in life: An ecological model. *J Am Geriatr Soc,* 32, 858–861.

dysfunctional gastrointestinal Motility (continued)

Pharmaceutical agents (e.g., narcotics/opiates, laxatives, antibiotics, anesthesia)
Food intolerance (e.g., gluten, lactose); ingestion of contaminants (e.g., food, water)
Sedentary lifestyle; immobility
Anxiety

DEFINING CHARACTERISTICS

Subjective
Absence of flatus
Abdominal cramping, pain
Diarrhea
Difficulty passing stool
Nausea; regurgitation

Objective
Change in bowel sounds (e.g., absent, hypoactive, hyperactive)
Abdominal distortion
Accelerated gastric emptying; diarrhea
Increased gastric residual; bile-colored gastric residual
Dry stool
Vomiting

Sample Clinical Applications: Abdominal or intestinal surgery, eating disorders, malnutrition, celiac disease, anemia, anxiety disorders, biliary cancer, cholecystectomy, Crohn's disease, irritable bowel syndrome, gastroesophageal reflux disease (GERD), gastritis, pancreatitis, quadriplegia, peritoneal dialysis, botulism, sepsis, multiple organ dysfunction syndrome, radiation therapy

DESIRED OUTCOMES/EVALUATION CRITERIA

Sample NOC linkages:
Gastrointestinal Function: Extent to which foods (ingested or tube-fed) are moved from ingestion to excretion
Knowledge: Treatment Regimen: Extent of understanding conveyed about a specific treatment regimen

Client Will (Include Specific Time Frame)
• Reestablish and maintain normal pattern of bowel functioning.
• Verbalize understanding of causative factors and rationale for treatment regimen.
• Demonstrate appropriate behaviors to assist with resolution of causative factors.

ACTIONS/INTERVENTIONS

Sample NIC linkages:
Bowel Management: Establishment and management of a regular pattern of bowel elimination
Tube Care: Gastrointestinal: Management of a patient with a gastrointestinal (GI) tube
Nutrition Therapy: Administration of food and fluids to support metabolic processes of a patient who is malnourished or at high risk for being malnourished

NURSING PRIORITY NO. 1

To assess causative/contributing factors:

- Note presence of conditions (e.g., congestive heart failure [CHF], major trauma, sepsis) affecting systemic circulation and perfusion. *Blood loss or shock can result in GI hypoperfusion and short-term and/or long-term GI dysfunction.*
- Determine presence of disorders causing localized or diffuse reduction in GI blood flow, such as esophageal varices, GI hemorrhage, pancreatitis, intraperitoneal hemorrhage *to identify client at higher risk for ineffective tissue perfusion.*
- Note presence of chronic or long-term disorders, such as GERD, hiatal hernia, inflammatory bowel (e.g., ulcerative colitis, Crohn's disease), malabsorption (e.g., dumping syndrome, celiac disease); short-bowel syndrome, as may occur after surgical removal of portions of the small intestine. *These conditions are associated with increased, decreased, or ineffective peristaltic activity.*
- Note client's age and developmental concerns. *Children are prone to infections causing gastroenteritis manifested by vomiting and diarrhea.[1] The elderly have problems associated with decreased motility (e.g., constipation is often a concern related to slower peristalsis, lack of sufficient fiber and fluid intake, chronic use of laxatives). Premature or low-birth-weight neonates are at risk for developing necrotizing enterocolitis (NEC).[18]*
- Note life style issues *that can affect GI circulation (e.g., people who regularly engage in competitive sports such as long-distance running, cycling); anorexia and bulimia.[4]*
- Review client's drug regimen. *Medications such as laxatives, antibiotics, anticholesterol agents, opiates, sedatives, iron preparations, NSAIDs may cause or exacerbate intestinal issues. In addition, likelihood of bleeding increases from use of medications such as anti-inflammatories, Coumadin, Plavix.[2,3]*
- Ascertain whether client is experiencing anxiety, stress, or other psychogenic factors *that can affect GI function.[5]*
- Review laboratory and other diagnostic studies. *Complete blood count (CBC) may be done to evaluate for bleeding, inflammation, toxicity, and infection. Metabolic panel may reveal hepatic dysfunction, electrolyte imbalances, or low albumin levels. Computed tomography (CT) or other scans, abdominal ultrasound can help identify conditions like kidney or gallstones. X-rays may show bowel dilation or obstruction, stool and gas patterns.[1,9,11,12] Changes in white blood cell (WBC) count with x-ray evidence of pneumoperitoneum (air in the abdominal cavity) in preterm neonate suggests NEC.[19]*

NURSING PRIORITY NO. 2

To note degree of dysfunction/organ involvement:

- Assess vital signs, noting presence of low blood pressure, elevated heart rate, fever. *May suggest hypoperfusion or developing sepsis. Fever in presence of bright red blood in stool may indicate ischemic colitis.*
- Ascertain presence and characteristics of abdominal pain. *Pain is a common symptom of GI disorders.[6] Diffuse pain may reflect hypoperfusion of the gastrointestinal tract, which is particularly vulnerable to even small decreases in circulating volume.[7] Midepigastric pain following meals and lasting several hours suggests abdominal angina due to atherosclerotic occlusive disease.[19] Tension pain caused by organ distention may develop in presence of bowel obstruction, constipation, or accumulation of pus or fluid. Inflammatory pain is deep and initially poorly localized, caused by irritation of either the visceral or the parietal peritoneum, as in acute appendicitis. Ischemic pain, most serious type of visceral pain, has*

sudden onset, is intense, progressive in severity, and not relieved by analgesics. Most common cause is strangulated bowel.[8]

- Investigate reports of pain out of proportion to degree of traumatic injury. *May reflect developing abdominal compartment syndrome.*[12]
- Inspect abdomen, noting contour. *Generalized distention may indicate presence of gas or fluid; local bulge could indicate hernia.*[7] Distention of the bowel results in accumulation of fluids (salivary, gastric, pancreatic, biliary, and intestinal) and gases formed from bacteria, swallowed air, or any food or fluid the client has consumed.[9]
- Auscultate abdomen. *Hypoactive bowel sounds may indicate ileus. Hyperactive bowels sounds may indicate early intestinal obstruction or irritable bowel or GI bleeding. Presence of bruit may indicated blood traveling through narrowed arteries such as aorta.*[9,11]
- Palpate abdomen, noting masses, enlarged organs (e.g., spleen, liver, or portions of colon), elicitation of pain with touch, pulsation of aorta.[9–11]
- Measure abdominal girth and compare with client's customary waist size/belt length *to monitor development or progression of distention possibly reflecting intra-abdominal bleeding, infection, or edema associated with toxins.*[10,12]
- Note frequency and characteristics of bowel movements. *Bowel movements by themselves are not necessarily diagnostic but need to be considered in total assessment because many different manifestations can occur. For example, diarrhea is the cardinal symptom of gastroenteritis, with severity depending on the causative organism. Both diarrhea and constipation can result from medications. Bloody diarrhea may indicate presence of ulcerative colitis, obstruction, or upper or lower gastrointestinal bleeding.*[1,9,14]
- Note presence of nausea, with or without vomiting, and relationship to food intake or other events, if indicated. *History of nausea and vomiting can provide important information about cause. For example, systemic conditions such as pregnancy, gastroenteritis, cancers, myocardial infarction, hepatitis, systemic infections, drug toxicity are often accompanied by nausea and vomiting. Timing of vomiting may be important too. For example, vomiting of large amounts several hours after eating can indicate delayed gastric emptying.*[5]
- Evaluate client's current nutritional status, noting ability to ingest and digest food. Inquire about food intolerances. Observe client's reactions to food, such as reluctance or refusal to eat, anorexia; anxiety—wants to eat but cannot retain food. *Health depends on the intake, digestion, and absorption of nutrients, which both affects and is affected by GI function.*
- Measure intra-abdominal pressure as indicated. *Tissue edema or free fluid collecting in the abdominal cavity leads to intra-abdominal hypertension, which, if untreated, can cause abdominal compartment syndrome with end-stage organ failure.*[20]

NURSING PRIORITY NO. 3

To correct/improve existing dysfunction:

- Collaborate in treatment of underlying conditions *to correct or treat disorders associated with clients current GI dysfunction.*
- Maintain GI rest when indicated—nothing by mouth, fluids only, gastric or intestinal decompression *to reduce intestinal bloating and risk of vomiting.*
- Measure GI output periodically, and note characteristics of drainage *to manage fluid losses and replacement needs and electrolyte balance.*
- Administer fluids and electrolytes as indicated *to replace losses and to improve GI circulation and function.*
- Encourage ambulation if able. *Promotes general circulation, stimulates peristalsis and intestinal function.*

- Collaborate with dietician or nutritionist *to provide diet sufficient in nutrients by best possible route—oral, enteral, parenteral.*
- Provide small, easily digested food and fluids when oral intake tolerated.
- Encourage rest after meals *to maximize blood flow to digestive system.*
- Manage pain with medications as ordered and nonpharmacologic interventions such as positioning, back rub, heating pad (unless contraindicated) *to enhance muscle relaxation and reduce discomfort.*[7]
- Report changes in nature or intensity of pain to physician, *as this may indicate worsening of condition, requiring more intensive interventions.*[13]
- Collaborate with physician in medication management. *Oral medications can be absorbed erratically and can change the therapeutic effect or lead to increased side effects of a particular drug.*[15] *Dose modification, discontinuation of certain drugs (e.g., laxatives, opioids, antidepressants, iron supplements), or alternative route of administration may be required over a long period of time to improve client's GI function.*[5,14,17]
- Prepare client for procedures and surgery as indicated. *May require a variety of interventions, including endoscopic procedures, appendectomy, bowel resection with/without ostomy, percutaneous transluminal angioplasty, abdominal-aortic bypass graft, mesenteric revascularization, or endarterectomy, and so forth, to treat problem causing or contributing to severe GI dysfunction.*

NURSING PRIORITY NO. 4

To promote wellness (Teaching/Discharge Considerations):

- Provide information regarding cause of GI dysfunction and treatment plans, utilizing best learning methods for client and including written information and bibliography of other resources for postdischarge learning. *May help client/SO to manage symptoms in a manner more acceptable to them if this is a long-term issue.*
- Discuss normal variations in bowel patterns *to help alleviate unnecessary concern, initiate planned interventions, or seek timely medical care. This may prevent overuse of laxatives or help client understand when food, fluid, or drug modifications are needed to prevent constipation.*[14]
- Encourage discussion of feelings regarding prognosis and long-term effects of condition. *Major or unplanned life changes can strain coping abilities, impairing functioning and jeopardizing relationships, and may even result in depression.*
- Discuss value of relaxation and distraction techniques *if anxiety is suspected to play a role in GI dysfunction.*[5]
- Identify necessary changes in lifestyle and assist client to incorporate disease management into activities of daily living (ADLs). *Promotes independence, enhances self-concept regarding ability to deal with change and manage own needs.*
- Review specific dietary changes or restrictions with client. *The client with GI disturbances may need to make various adaptations in food choices and eating habits (e.g., may need to avoid overeating in general, schedule mealtime in relation to activities and bedtime, avoid certain foods and/or alcohol)*
- Instruct in healthier variations in preparation of foods, as indicated—broiled instead of fried, spices added to foods instead of salt, addition of higher fiber foods, use of lactose-free dairy products—*when these factors are affecting GI health.*[11]
- Review use of dietary fiber as a means of managing constipation and incontinence. *Studies have shown that supplementation with dietary fiber from psyllium or gum arabic was associated with a decrease in incontinence and improved stool consistency.*[16]

- Discuss fluid intake appropriate to individual situation. *Water is necessary to general health and GI function. The individual may need encouragement and instruction about how to take in enough fluids or may need fluid restrictions for certain medical conditions.*

- Recommend maintenance of normal weight, or weight loss if client is obese, *to decrease risk associated with GI disorders such as GERD or gallbladder disease.*

- Recommend smoking cessation. *Risk for acquiring or exacerbating certain GI disorders (e.g., Crohn's disease) may be increased with smoking. It is theorized that smoking may decrease blood flow to the intestines or trigger a response in the immune system.*[13]

- Discuss medication regimen, including reasons for/consequences of failure to take prescribed long-term maintenance therapy (e.g., client with ulcerative colitis requires continuous treatment with 5-aminosalicylates to maintain remission). *Although many reasons are given for failing to take medications as prescribed, including denial of illness, forgetfulness, and costs of prescriptions, nonadherance negatively affects treatment efficacy and clients quality of life.*[17]

- Emphasize importance of avoiding use of NSAIDs (including aspirin), corticosteroids, some over-the-counter (OTC) drugs, vitamins containing potassium, mineral oil, or alcohol when taking anticoagulants. *These medications can be harmful to GI mucosa and increase risk of bleeding.*[9]

- Refer to NDs Constipation, Diarrhea, Bowel Incontinence for additional interventions.

DOCUMENTATION FOCUS

Assessment/Reassessment
- Individual findings, noting nature, extent and duration of problem; effect on independence and lifestyle.
- Dietary pattern, recent intake, food intolerances.
- Frequency and characteristics of stools.
- Characteristics of abdominal tenderness or pain, precipitators, and what relieves pain.

Planning
- Plan of care and who is involved in planning.
- Teaching plan.

Implementation/Evaluation
- Response to interventions, teaching, and actions performed.
- Attainment or progress toward desired outcome(s).
- Modifications to plan of care.

Discharge Planning
- Long-term needs and who is responsible for actions to be taken.
- Available resources, specific referrals made.

References

1. Sommers, M. S., Johnson, S. A., Beery, T. A. (2007). *Diseases and Disorders: A Nursing Therapeutics Manual*, 3d ed. Philadelphia: F. A. Davis.
2. Neal-Boylan, L. (2007). Health assessment of the very old person at home. *Home Healthcare Nurse*, 25(6), 388–398.
3. Tabloski, P. A. (ed). (2006). *Gerontological Nursing*. Upper Saddle River, NJ: Pearson Prentice-Hall.

4. Pasley, J. (2004). Introduction to gastrointestinal physiology, University of Arkansas Medical School Lecture. Retrieved October 2009 from www.uams.edu/m2008/notes/phys/pdf/April%2016%20Intro%20to%20GI%20Phys.pdf.

5. de Graef, A., Kyper, M. B., Hesselmann, G. M. (2006). Nausea and vomiting. National Guideline Clearinghouse. Retrieved January 2009 from www.guideline.gov.

6. Holcomb, S. S. (2008). Acute abdomen: What a pain! *Nursing*, 38(9), 34–40.

7. Sartin, J. S. (2005). Gastrointestinal disorders. In Copstead, L. E. C., Banasik, J. L. (eds). *Pathophysiology*, 3d ed. St. Louis, MO: Elsevier Saunders.

8. Schulman, C. (2002). End points of resuscitation: Choosing the right parameters to monitor. *Dimens Crit Care Nurs*, 21(1), 2–10.

9. Miller, S. K., Alpert, P. T. (2006). Assessment and differential diagnosis of abdominal pain. *Nurs Pract*, 31(7), 39–47.

10. Held-Warmkessel, J., Schiech, L. (2008). Responding to 4 gastrointestinal complications in cancer patients. *Nursing*, 38(7), 32–38.

11. Hogstel, M. O., Curry, L. C. (2005). *Health Assessment Through the Life Span*, 4th ed. Philadelphia: F. A. Davis.

12. Paula, R. (2006). Compartment syndrome, abdominal. Retrieved February 2009 from www.emedicine.medscape.com/article/829008-overview.

13. Day, M. W. (2008). Fight back against inflammatory bowel disease. *Nursing*, 38(11), 34–40.

14. Hill, R. (2007). Don't let constipation stop you up. *Nursing Made Incredibly Easy!* 5(5), 40–47.

15. Feigenbaum, K. (2006). Update on gastroparesis. *Gastroenterol Nurs*, 29(3), 239–244.

16. Zimmario, D., et al. (2001). Supplementation with dietary fiber improves fecal incontinence. *Nurs Res*, 50(4), 203–213.

17. Turnbough, L., Wilson, L. (2007). Take your medicine: Nonadherence issues in patients with ulcerative colitis. *Gastroenterol Nurs*, 30(3), 212–217.

18. American Pediatric Surgical Association. (2003). Necrotizing enterocolitis (NEC). Adapted from O'Neill, J. A., Grasfeld, J., Fonkalsrud, E. (eds). *Principles of Pediatric Surgery*, 2d ed. St. Louis, MO: Mosby. Retrieved February 2009 from www.eapsa.org/parents/resources/NEC.cfm.

19. Scott Conner, C. E. H., Ballinger, B. (2005). Abdominal angina. Retrieved February 2009 from www.emedicine.medscape.com/article/188618-overview.

20. Overview: Intra-abdominal hypertension and abdominal compartment syndrome. Retrieved February 2009 from www.abdominalcompartmentsyndrome.org.

risk for dysfunctional gastrointestinal Motility

DEFINITION: Risk for increased, decreased, ineffective, or lack of peristaltic activity within the gastrointestinal system

RISK FACTORS

Aging

Abdominal surgery; decreased gastrointestinal (GI) circulation

Food intolerance (e.g., gluten, lactose); change in food or water; unsanitary food preparation

Pharmaceutical agents (e.g., antibiotics, laxatives, narcotics/opiates, proton-pump inhibitors)

Gastroesophageal reflux disease (GERD)

Diabetes mellitus

Infection (e.g., bacterial, parasitic, viral)

(continues on page 528)

risk for dysfunctional gastrointestinal Motility (continued)

Sedentary lifestyle; immobility

Stress; anxiety

NOTE: A risk diagnosis is not evidenced by signs and symptoms, as the problem has not occurred; rather, nursing interventions are directed at prevention.

Sample Clinical Applications: Abdominal or intestinal surgery, eating disorders, malnutrition, celiac disease, anemia, anxiety disorders, biliary cancer, cholecystectomy, Crohn's disease, irritable bowel syndrome, GERD, gastritis, pancreatitis, quadriplegia, peritoneal dialysis, botulism, sepsis, multiple organ dysfunction syndrome, radiation therapy

DESIRED OUTCOMES/EVALUATION CRITERIA

Sample **NOC** linkages:

Gastrointestinal Function: Extent to which foods (ingested or tube-fed) are moved from ingestion to excretion

Knowledge: Treatment Regimen: Extent of understanding conveyed about a specific treatment regimen

Client Will (Include Specific Time Frame)
- Maintain normal pattern of bowel functioning.
- Verbalize understanding of individual risk factors and benefits of managing condition.
- Identify preventive interventions to reduce risk and promote normal bowel pattern.

ACTIONS/INTERVENTIONS

Sample **NIC** linkages:

Bowel Management: Establishment and management of a regular pattern of bowel elimination

Tube Care: Gastrointestinal: Management of a patient with a GI tube

Nutrition Therapy: Administration of food and fluids to support metabolic processes of a patient who is malnourished or at high risk for being malnourished

NURSING PRIORITY NO. 1

To identify individual risk factors/needs:

- Note presence of conditions affecting systemic circulation and perfusion such as congestive heart failure (CHF), major trauma, sepsis, and so forth. *Blood loss or shock can result in GI hypoperfusion, and short-term and/or long-term GI dysfunction.*[1]
- Determine presence of disorders that could cause reduction in GI blood flow, such as esophageal varices, pancreatitis; foreign body ingestion; increase of intra-abdominal pressure or abdominal hypertension; prior history of bowel obstruction or strangulated hernia; or prior abdominal surgery with adhesions, *to identify client at higher risk for changes in peristaltic activity.*[2,15]
- Assess client's current situation in conjunction with prior GI history. *Client may have an isolated incident putting him or her at risk (e.g., blunt force trauma to abdomen) or be at higher risk for recurrent GI dysfunction associated with history of a prior GI bleed or chronic condition such as Crohn's disease, long-term or severe alcoholism, ulcers, or diverticulitis.*

- Auscultate abdomen to evaluate peristaltic activity. *Hypoactive or hyperactive bowel sounds may indicate developing bowel disorders, such as chronic constipation, early intestinal obstruction, or acute viral gastroenteritis.*[9,10]
- Palpate abdomen for masses, enlarged organs (e.g., spleen, liver, or portions of colon); elicitation of pain with touch; pulsation of aorta *that could identify problem in GI system.*[9-11]
- Note frequency and characteristics of bowel movements. *Bowel movements by themselves are not necessarily diagnostic but need to be considered in total assessment because many different manifestations can occur.*[1,9,12]
- Ascertain presence and characteristics of abdominal pain. *Pain is a common symptom of GI disorders with location and type aiding in identifying underlying problems;*[8] *for example, diffuse pain may reflect hypoperfusion of the GI tract,*[13] *midepigastric pain following meals and lasting several hours suggests abdominal angina due to atherosclerotic occlusive disease,*[14] *or tension pain caused by organ distention may develop in presence of constipation or bowel obstruction.*
- Assess vital signs, noting presence of low blood pressure, elevated heart rate, fever. *May suggest hypoperfusion or developing sepsis.*
- Evaluate client's current nutritional status, noting ability to ingest and digest food. *Health depends on the intake, digestion, and absorption of nutrients, which both affects and is affected by gastrointestinal function.*
- Note client's age and developmental concerns. *Children are prone to infections causing gastroenteritis manifested by vomiting and diarrhea.*[1] *The elderly have problems associated with decreased motility (e.g., constipation is often a concern related to slower peristalsis, lack of sufficient fiber and fluid intake, chronic use of laxatives).*[3,4] *Premature or low-birth-weight neonates are at risk for developing necrotizing enterocolitis (NEC).*[5]
- Note life style issues *that can affect GI function (e.g., people who regularly engage in competitive sports such as long-distance running, cycling); anorexia and bulimia.*[6]
- Ascertain whether client is experiencing anxiety, stress, or other psychogenic factors *that can affect GI function.*[7]
- Review client's drug regimen. *Medications such as laxatives, antibiotics, anticholesterol agents, opiates, sedatives, iron preparations, NSAIDs may cause or exacerbate intestinal issues. In addition, likelihood of bleeding increases from use of medications such as anti-inflammatories, Coumadin, Plavix.*[3,4]
- Review laboratory and other diagnostic studies *to identify if conditions or disorders are present that may affect GI system or GI function.*

NURSING PRIORITY NO. 2

To reduce or correct individual risk factors:

- Discuss normal variations in bowel patterns *so client can initiate planned interventions or seek timely medical care. This may prevent overuse of laxatives or help client understand when food, fluid, or drug modifications are needed to prevent constipation.*[14]
- Collaborate in treatment of underlying conditions *to correct or treat disorders that could impact GI function.*
- Practice and promote hand hygiene and other infection precautions *to prevent transmission of infections that may cause/spread GI illnesses.*
- Maintain GI rest when indicated (e.g., nothing by mouth, fluids only, gastric or intestinal decompression after abdominal surgery) *to reduce intestinal bloating and reduce risk of vomiting.*
- Administer fluids and electrolytes as indicated *to replace losses and to maintain GI circulation and function.*

- Administer prescribed prophylactic medications (e.g., antiemetics, proton-pump inhibitors, antihistamines, anticholinergics, antibiotics) *to reduce potential for GI complications such as bleeding, ulceration of stomach mucosa, viral diarrheas, and so forth.*
- Collaborate with dietician or nutritionist *to provide diet sufficient in nutrients and provided by best possible route (e.g., oral, enteral, parenteral).*[2,16]
- Provide and encourage early ambulation following surgery or other procedures. Assist client with mobility issues to be as active as possible. Refer to physical therapy as indicated. *These measures can help reduce constipation or other GI complications associated with immobility.*
- Encourage relaxation and distraction techniques if anxiety is suspected to play a role in GI dysfunction.[5]

NURSING PRIORITY NO. 3

To promote wellness (Teaching/Discharge Considerations):

- Review measures to maintain bowel health:
  Use of dietary fiber and/or stool softeners. *Studies have shown that supplementation with dietary fiber from psyllium or gum arabic was associated with a decreased in incontinence and improved stool consistency.*[12,17]
  Fluid intake appropriate to individual. *Water is necessary to general health and GI function. The individual may need encouragement and instruction about how to take in enough fluids or may need fluid restrictions for certain medical conditions.*
  Establish or maintain regular bowel evacuation habits, incorporating privacy needs, assistance to bathroom on regular schedule, and so forth, as indicated.
  Emphasize benefits of regular exercise in promoting normal GI function.
- Discuss dietary recommendations with client/SO. *The client with potential for GI disturbances may elect to make adaptations in food choices and eating habits (e.g., to avoid overeating in general, schedule mealtime in relation to activities and bedtime, avoid certain foods and/or alcohol).*
- Instruct in healthier variations in preparation of foods as indicated (e.g., broiled instead of fried, spices added to foods instead of salt, addition of higher fiber foods, lactose-free dairy products) *when these factors may affect GI health.*
- Recommend maintenance of normal weight, or weight loss if client is obese, *to decrease risk associated with GI disorders such as GERD or gallbladder disease.*
- Collaborate with physician in medication management. *Oral medications can be absorbed erratically and can change the therapeutic effect or lead to increased side effects of a particular drug.*[18] *Dose modification, discontinuation of certain drugs (e.g., laxatives, opioids, antidepressants, iron supplements), or alternative route of administration may be required over a long period of time to improve client's GI function.*[12,19]
- Emphasize importance of discussing with physician current and new prescribed medications, and/or planned use of certain medications (e.g., NSAIDs [including aspirin], corticosteroids, some over-the-counter [OTC] drugs, herbals supplements), *which can be harmful to GI mucosa.*[20]
- Recommend smoking cessation. *Risk for acquiring or exacerbating certain GI disorders (e.g., Crohn's disease) may be increased with smoking.*[18]
- Review food- and waterborne illnesses, contamination and hygiene issues, as indicated, and make needed follow-up referrals. *Many different types of viruses, bacteria, and parasites can cause GI illnesses. This can affect a household, a day-care center, a college dorm, international travelers, or a whole segment of population. Information may be given to individuals, groups, and/or public in general.*

- Refer to appropriate resources (e.g., social services, public health services) for follow-up if client is at risk for ingestion of contaminated water or food sources or would benefit from teaching concerning food preparation and storage.
- Recommend and/or refer to physician for vaccines as indicated. The Centers for Disease Control and Prevention (CDC) makes recommendations for travelers and/or persons in high-risk areas or situations to receive certain vaccinations. *Typhoid vaccine, for example, is indicated for travel to areas where a person might be exposed to contaminated food or water. For young children susceptible to severe gastroenteritis, oral rotavirus vaccine can prevent about 75% of rotavirus gastroenteritis.*[21]

DOCUMENTATION FOCUS

Assessment/Reassessment
- Individual findings, noting specific risk factors.
- Dietary pattern, recent intake, food intolerances.
- Frequency and characteristics of stools.

Planning
- Plan of care and who is involved in planning.
- Teaching plan.

Implementation/Evaluation
- Response to interventions, teaching, and actions performed.
- Attainment or progress toward desired outcome(s).
- Modifications to plan of care.

Discharge Planning
- Long-term needs and who is responsible for actions to be taken.
- Available resources and specific referrals made.

References

1. Sommers, M. S., Johnson, S. A., Beery, T. A. (2007). *Diseases and Disorders: A Nursing Therapeutics Manual*, 3d ed. Philadelphia: F. A. Davis.
2. Goldberg, S. M. (2008). Identifying intestinal obstruction: Better safe than sorry. *Nurs Crit Care*, 3(5), 18–23.
3. Neal-Boylan, L. (2007). Health assessment of the very old person at home. *Home Healthcare Nurs*, 25(6), 388–398.
4. Tabloski, P. A. (ed). (2006). *Gerontological Nursing*. Upper Saddle River, NJ: Pearson Prentice-Hall.
5. American Pediatric Surgical Association. (2003). Necrotizing enterocolitis (NEC). Adapted from O'Neill, J. A., Grasfeld, J., Fonkalsrud, E. (eds). *Principles of Pediatric Surgery*, 2d ed. St. Louis, MO: Mosby. Retrieved February 2009 from www.eapsa.org/parents/resources/NEC.cfm.
6. Pasley, J. (2004). Introduction to gastrointestinal physiology. University of Arkansas Medical School Lecture. Retrieved February 2009 from www.uams.edu/m2008/notes/phys/pdf/April%2016%20Intro%20to%20GI%20Phys.pdf.
7. de Graef, A., Kyper, M. B., Hesselmann, G. M. (2006). Nausea and vomiting. National Guideline Clearinghouse. Retrieved January 2009 from www.guideline.gov.
8. Holcomb, S. S. (2008). Acute abdomen: What a pain! *Nursing*, 38(9), 34–40.
9. Miller, S. K., Alpert, P. T. (2006). Assessment and differential diagnosis of abdominal pain. *Nurse Pract*, 31(7), 39–47.
10. Hogstel, M. O., Curry, L. C. (2005). *Health Assessment Through the Life Span*, 4th ed. Philadelphia: F. A. Davis.

11. Held-Warmkessel, J., Schiech, L. (2008). Responding to 4 gastrointestinal complications in cancer patients. *Nursing*, 38(7), 32–38.
12. Hill, R. (2007). Don't let constipation stop you up. *Nursing Made Incredibly Easy!*, 5(5), 40–47.
13. Sartin, J. S. Gastrointestinal disorders. (2005). In Copstead, L. E. C., Banasik, J. L. (eds). *Pathophysiology*, 3d ed. St. Louis, MO: Elsevier Saunders.
14. Scott-Conner, C. E. H., Ballinger, B. (2005). Abdominal angina. Retrieved February 2009 from www.emedicine.medscape.com/article/188618-overview.
15. Overview: Intra-abdominal hypertension and abdominal compartment syndrome. Retrieved February 2009 from www.abdominalcompartmentsyndrome.org.
16. Glare, P. A., et al. (2008). Treatment of nausea and vomiting in terminally ill cancer patients. *Drugs*, 68(18), 2575–2590.
17. Zimmario, D., et al. (2001). Supplementation with dietary fiber improves fecal incontinence. *Nurs Res*, 50(4), 203–213.
18. Feigenbaum, K. (2006). Update on gastroparesis. *Gastroenterol Nurs*, 29(3), 239–244.
19. Day, M. W. (2008). Fight back against inflammatory bowel disease. *Nursing*, 38(11), 34–40.
20. Turnbough, L., Wilson, L. (2007). Take your medicine: Nonadherence issues in patients with ulcerative colitis. *Gastroenterol Nurs*, 30(3), 212–217.
21. Centers for Disease Control and Prevention (CDC). (2007 update). Vaccines and immunizations. Retrieved February 2009 from www.cdc.gov/vaccines/vpd-vac/child-vpd.htm.

Nausea

DEFINITION: A subjective unpleasant, wavelike sensation in the back of the throat, epigastrium, or abdomen that may lead to the urge or need to vomit

RELATED FACTORS

Treatment
Gastric irritation [e.g., alcohol, blood]
Gastric distention
Pharmaceuticals [e.g., analgesics—aspirin, nonsteroidal anti-inflammatory drugs, opioids, anesthesia, antiviral for HIV, steroids, antibiotics, chemotherapeutic agents]
[Radiation therapy or exposure]

Biophysical
Biochemical disorders (e.g., uremia, diabetic ketoacidosis, pregnancy)
Localized tumors (e.g., acoustic neuroma, primary or secondary brain tumors, bone metastases at base of skull); intra-abdominal tumors
Toxins (e.g., tumor-produced peptides, abdominal metabolites due to cancer)
Esophageal or pancreatic disease; liver or splenetic capsule stretch
Gastric distention [e.g., delayed gastric emptying, pyloric intestinal obstruction, external compression of the stomach, other organ enlargement that slows stomach functioning (squashed stomach syndrome)]
Gastric irritation [e.g., pharyngeal and/or peritoneal inflammation]
Motion sickness; Ménière's disease; labyrinthitis
Increased intracranial pressure; meningitis

Situational
Noxious odors or taste; unpleasant visual stimulation
Pain
Psychological factors; anxiety; fear

DEFINING CHARACTERISTICS

Subjective
Report of nausea ["sick to my stomach"]

Objective
Aversion toward food
Increased salivation; sour taste in mouth
Increased swallowing; gagging sensation

Sample Clinical Applications: Surgery, anesthesia, cancer, pregnancy, AIDS, gastritis, peptic ulcer disease, renal failure, brain injury, meningitis, panic disorders, phobias

DESIRED OUTCOMES/EVALUATION CRITERIA

Sample (NOC) linkages:
Nausea & Vomiting Severity: Severity of nausea, retching, and vomiting symptoms
Nausea & Vomiting Control: Personal actions to control nausea, retching, and vomiting symptoms
Appetite: Desire to eat when ill or receiving treatment

Client Will (Include Specific Time Frame)
• Be free of nausea.
• Manage chronic nausea, as evidenced by acceptable level of dietary intake.
• Maintain or regain weight, as appropriate.

ACTIONS/INTERVENTIONS

Sample (NIC) linkages:
Nausea Management: Prevention and alleviation of nausea
Vomiting Management: Prevention and alleviation of vomiting
Fluid Management: Promotion of fluid balance and prevention of complications resulting from abnormal or undesired fluid levels

NURSING PRIORITY NO. 1

To determine causative/contributing factors:

• Assess for presence of conditions of the gastrointestinal (GI) tract (e.g., peptic ulcer disease, cholecystitis, appendicitis, gastritis, intestinal blockage, ingestion of "problem" foods). *Dietary changes may be sufficient to decrease frequency of nausea in some situations.*
• Note systemic conditions that may result in nausea (e.g., pregnancy, cancer treatment, myocardial infarction, hepatitis, acid-base and metabolic disturbances, systemic infections, drug toxicity, migraine headache, presence of neurogenic causes—stimulation of the vestibular system, concussion, central nervous system [CNS] trauma/tumor). *Helpful in determining appropriate interventions/need for treatment of underlying conditions.*[4]

- Identify situations that client perceives as anxiety-inducing, threatening, or distasteful (e.g., "this is nauseating") such as might occur if client is having multiple diagnostic studies, facing surgery. *May be able to limit or control exposure to situations or take medication prophylactically.*
- Note psychological factors, including those that are culturally determined (e.g., eating certain foods considered repulsive in one's culture).[4]
- Determine if nausea is potentially self-limiting and/or mild (e.g., first trimester of pregnancy, 24-hour GI tract viral infection) or is severe and prolonged (e.g., cancer treatment, hyperemesis gravidarum). *Indicates potential degree of effect on fluid/electrolyte balance and nutritional status, and determines type and intensity of interventions.*[4]
- Record food intake and changes in symptoms *to help identify food intolerances when nausea is chronic.*
- Assess vital signs, especially for children and older clients, and note signs of dehydration. *Nausea may occur in the presence of postural hypotension or fluid volume deficit, or in severe hypertension.*
- Review medication regimen, especially in elderly client on multiple drugs. *Polypharmacy with drug interactions and side effects may cause or exacerbate nausea.*

NURSING PRIORITY NO. 2

To promote comfort and enhance intake:

- Collaborate with physician to treat underlying medical condition *when cause of nausea is known (e.g., infection, adverse side effect of medications, food allergies, GI reflux).*
- Administer and monitor response to medications used to treat underlying cause of nausea (e.g., vestibular, bowel obstruction, dysmotility of upper gut, infection or inflammation, toxins). *Note: Older individuals are more prone to side effects of antiemetic and anti-anxiety or antipsychotic medications (e.g., excessive sedation, extrapyramidal movements), and there is increased risk of aspiration in the sedated client.*[5,8]
- Select route of medication administration best suited to client's needs (i.e., oral, sublingual, injectable, rectal, transdermal).[7]
- Administer antiemetic on regular schedule before, during, and after administration of antineoplastic agents or radiation therapy as indicated. *Antiemetic agents may be administered prophylactically to prevent or limit severity of nausea and vomiting.*[1]
- Administer analgesics *when postoperative pain is a factor in nausea and vomiting.*[2]
- Review pain control regimen for client experiencing nausea. *Converting to long-acting opioids or combination drugs may decrease stimulation of the chemotactic trigger zone (CTZ), reducing the occurrence of narcotic-related nausea.*[5,8]
- Manage food and fluids.
  Have client try dry foods such as toast, crackers, or dry cereal before arising *when nausea occurs in the morning or throughout the day.*[8]
  Encourage client to begin with ice chips or sips/small amounts of fluids—4 to 8 ounces for adult, 1 ounce or less for child.[6]
  Advise client to drink liquids 30 minutes before or after meals instead of with meals.[8] Suggest sipping fluids slowly and using cool, clear liquids (e.g., water, ginger ale or lemon-lime soda, and electrolyte drinks).
  Recommend avoiding milk and other dairy products (especially during acute episodes), overly sweet, fried, or fatty foods, gas-forming vegetables (e.g., broccoli, cauliflower, cucumbers) *that may increase nausea and be more difficult to digest.*[4,6,8]
  Provide bland diet and snacks high in carbohydrates with substitutions of preferred foods (including bland, caffeine-free nondiet carbonated beverages; clear soup broth, nonacidic

fruit juice, gelatin, sherbet or ices, skinless chicken) *to reduce gastric acidity and improve nutrient intake.*[4,6,8]

Instruct client to eat small meals spaced throughout the day rather than large meals *so stomach does not feel too full.*[4,8]

Instruct client to eat and drink slowly, chewing food well *for easier digestion.*[8]

Advise client to suck on ice cubes or tart or hard candies, or to chew gum. *Keeps mucous membranes moist and can provide some fluid and nutrient intake.*

Provide frequent oral care (especially after vomiting) *to cleanse mouth and minimize "bad tastes."*

Time chemotherapy doses *for least interference with food intake.*

Monitor infusion rate of tube feeding, if present, *to prevent rapid administration that can cause gastric distention and produce nausea.*

- Manage environment.

Elevate head of bed or have client sit upright after meals *to promote digestion by gravity and eliminate feeling of fullness when that is causing nausea.*[8]

Avoid sudden changes in position.

Apply cool cloth to face and neck.

Provide clean, pleasant-smelling, quiet environment and fresh air with fan or open window.

Avoid offending odors (e.g., cooking smells, smoke, perfumes, mechanical emissions).[7,8]

- Discuss nonpharmacological measures.

Encourage slow, deep breathing *to promote relaxation.*

Use such distraction techniques as guided imagery, music therapy, chatting with family/friends, watching television *to refocus attention away from unpleasant sensations.*

Provide frequent oral care *to cleanse mouth and minimize "bad tastes."*

- Investigate use of electrical nerve stimulation, or acupressure point therapy (e.g., elastic band worn around wrist with small, hard bump that presses against acupressure point). *Some individuals with chronic nausea or history of motion sickness report this to be helpful and without the sedative effect of medication.*[3]

NURSING PRIORITY NO. 3

To promote wellness (Teaching/Discharge Considerations):

- Review individual factors or triggers causing nausea and ways to avoid problem (e.g., identifying offending medications or foods). *Provides necessary information for client to manage own care. Note: Some individuals develop anticipatory nausea (a conditioned reflex) that recurs each time he or she encounters the situation that triggers the reflex.*[8]

- Instruct in proper use, side effects, and adverse reactions of antiemetic medications. *Enhances client safety and effective management of condition.*

- Discuss appropriate use of over-the-counter (OTC) medications and herbal products (e.g., Dramamine, antacids, antiflatulents, ginger) or in the use of THC (Marinol).[6,8]

- Encourage use of nonpharmacological interventions. *Activities such as self-hypnosis, progressive muscle relaxation, biofeedback, guided imagery, and systemic desensitization promote relaxation, refocus client's attention, increase sense of control, and decrease feelings of helplessness.*[7]

- Advise client/SO to prepare and freeze meals in advance, have someone else cook, or use microwave or oven instead of stovetop cooking for days when nausea is severe or cooking is impossible, as with chemotherapy/radiation therapy.[8]

- Suggest wearing loose-fitting clothing *to reduce pressure on abdomen, if that is causing or exacerbating nausea.*[8]

- Recommend recording weight weekly, if appropriate, *to help monitor fluid and nutritional status.*

Nursing Diagnoses in Alphabetical Order

- Identify signs requiring immediate notification of healthcare provider (e.g., emesis appears bloody, black, or like coffee grounds; feeling faint) *to facilitate timely evaluation and intervention.*[8]
- Discuss potential complications and possible need for medical follow-up or alternative therapies. *Timely recognition and intervention may limit severity of complications (e.g., dehydration).*
- Review signs of dehydration and stress importance of replacing fluids and/or electrolytes (with products such as Gatorade for adults or Pedialyte for children) if vomiting occurs, especially in young children or frail elderly. *Increases likelihood of preventing potentially serious complications.*[6]

DOCUMENTATION FOCUS

Assessment/Reassessment
- Individual findings, including individual factors causing nausea.
- Baseline periodic weight, vital signs.
- Specific client preferences for nutritional intake.

Planning
- Plan of care and who is involved in planning.
- Teaching plan.

Implementation/Evaluation
- Response to interventions, teaching, and actions performed.
- Response to medication.
- Attainment or progress toward desired outcome(s).
- Modifications to plan of care.

Discharge Planning
- Individual long-term needs, noting who is responsible for actions to be taken.
- Specific referrals made.

References

1. American Society of Health System Pharmacists (ASHP). (1999). Therapeutic guidelines on the pharmacologic management of nausea and vomiting in adult and pediatric patients receiving chemotherapy or radiation therapy or undergoing surgery. *Am J Health Syst Pharm*, 56(8), 729.
2. Thompson, H. J. (1999). The management of post-operative nausea and vomiting. *J Adv Nurs*, 29(5), 1130–1136.
3. Mann, E. (1999). Using acupuncture and acupressure to treat postoperative emesis. *Prof Nurs*, 14(10), 691–694.
4. The American Gastroenterological Association Medical Position Statement: Nausea and Vomiting. (2001). *Gastroenterology*, 120(1), 261–262. Retrieved January 2004 from www .guideline.gov.
5. Hallenbeck, J., Weissman, D. (2007). Treatment of nausea and vomiting. Retrieved August 2007 from www.jasonprogram.org/nausea_treatment.htm.
6. Keim, S. M., Kent, M. (2005). Nausea and vomiting. Retrieved August 2007 from www .emedicinehealth.com/vomiting_and_nausea/article_em.htm.
7. National Comprehensive Cancer Network clinical practice guidelines: Nausea and vomiting: Treatment guidelines for patients with cancer. (2005). Retrieved August 2007 from www.cancer .org/downloads/CRI/NCCN_Nasuea.pdf.
8. Palliative care & symptom management: nausea & vomiting. Retrieved August 2007 from www.canceradvocacy.org/resources/essential/effects/nausea.aspx.

self Neglect

DEFINITION: A constellation of culturally framed behaviors involving one or more self-care activities in which there is a failure to maintain a socially accepted standard of health and well-being

RELATED FACTORS

Major life stressor; depression
Obsessive-compulsive disorder; schizotypal or paranoid personality disorders
Frontal lobe dysfunction and executive processing ability; cognitive impairment (e.g. dementia); Capgras syndrome
Functional impairment; learning disability
Lifestyle/choice; substance abuse; malingering
Maintaining control; fear of institutionalization

DEFINING CHARACTERISTICS

Objective
Inadequate personal or environmental hygiene
Nonadherence to health activities

Sample Clinical Applications: Mental illness (as in related factors); terminal illness—cancer, amyotrophic lateral sclerosis (ALS); debilitating conditions—multiple sclerosis (MS), Parkinson's disease; alcohol/drug abuse

DESIRED OUTCOMES/EVALUATION CRITERIA

Sample NOC linkages:
Self-Care Status: Ability to perform basic personal care activities and instrumental activities of daily living (IADLs)
Health Promoting Behaviors: Personal actions to sustain or increase wellness

Client Will (Include Specific Time Frame)
• Acknowledge difficulty maintaining hygiene practices.
• Demonstrate ability to manage lifestyle changes and medication regimen.
• Perform activities of daily living within level of own ability.

Caregiver Will (Include Specific Time Frame):
• Assist individual with personal and environmental hygiene as needed.
• Identify and assist client with medical, dental, and other healthcare appointments as indicated.

ACTIONS/INTERVENTIONS

Sample NIC linkages:
Self-Responsibility Facilitation: Encouraging a patient to assume more responsibility for own behavior
Self-Care Assistance: Assisting another to perform activities of daily living

NURSING PRIORITY NO. 1

To identify causative or precipitating factors:

- Determine existing health problems, age, developmental level, and cognitive psychological factors, including presence of delusions affecting ability to care for own needs. Use an appropriate screening instrument, such as the Elder Assessment Instrument (EAI). *A wide variety of impairments can cause a person to neglect hygiene needs, particularly aging, homelessness and dementia. Neglect and elder abuse is underreported, and the use of a good tool can help identify presence.*[2,3]
- Identify other problems which may interfere with ability to care for self. *Visual or hearing impairment, language barrier, emotional instability or lability can create difficulties for individual to manage daily tasks.*[2,4]
- Note recent life events or changes in circumstances. *Losses (e.g., loved one, financial security, physical independence) can trigger or exacerbate self-neglect behaviors.*[4]
- Review circumstances of client illness, possible monetary rewards, sympathy or attention from family. *On occasion self-neglect may be malingering as an attempt to gain something from others or relinquish unwanted responsibilities.*
- Perform mental status examination. *Mental illness (e.g., psychosis, depression, dementia) can affect individual's ability or desire to maintain self-care activities or care for home surroundings.*[5]
- Review studies evaluating frontal lobe dysfunction and possibility of Diogenes syndrome. *These clients present with severe self-neglect and may have coexisting medical and psychiatric conditions.*[10]
- Assess economic situation and living arrangements. *May live alone or with family members who are not helpful, or may be homeless; and may have little or no financial resources resulting in inability or lack of concern about personal well-being.*[4]
- Determine availability and use of resources. *Depending on disability of client, agencies can work together to develop a plan to meet needs, noting whether individual is availing self of help.*[6]
- Interview SO/family members to determine level of involvement and support. *Client may be exhibiting acting-out or paranoid behaviors, stressing caregivers who may not realize individual is unable to control self because of cognitive impairment.*

NURSING PRIORITY NO. 2

To determine degree of impairment:

- Perform head-to-toe assessment, inspecting scalp and skin; noting personal hygiene, body odor, rashes, bruising, skin tears, lesions, burns, presence of vermin; oral cavity for gum disease, inflammation, lesions, loose or broken teeth, fit of dentures. *Identifies specific needs and may reveal signs of trauma or abuse.*
- Obtain weight. Perform nutritional assessment as indicated. *Neglecting oneself often includes not eating meals regularly or failing to eat nutritionally balanced foods. When alcoholism or drug abuse is a part of neglect, individual may be severely malnourished.*[1,3]
- Review medication regimen. *In addition to neglecting self-care activities, client will likely not pay attention to taking prescriptions as ordered resulting in exacerbation of medical problem. Note: Some psychotropic medication may cause individual to "feel different" or not in control of self, resulting in reluctance to take drug.*[3]
- Determine willingness to change situation. *Depending on individual's situation (living alone, homeless, mental status), client may have difficulty committing to or be unwilling to change. May see change as a loss of independence.*[3]

NURSING PRIORITY NO. 3

To assist in correcting/dealing with situation:

- Develop multidisciplinary team specific to individual needs, such as case manager, physician, dietitian, physical or occupational therapist, rehabilitation specialist *to review assessment data and develop a plan appropriate to the individual situation, making use of client's capabilities and maximizing potential.*[6]
- Establish therapeutic relationship with client, family if available and willing to be involved. *Promotes trust and encourages input into planning process.*[7]
- Identify specific priorities and goals of client/SOs. *Helps client to look at possibilities for dealing with difficult situation of no longer being able to maintain lifestyle and moving on to a new way of managing.*[6]
- Promote client/SOs participation in problem identification and decision making. *Enhances commitment to plan when individual has input, and encourages participation, enhancing outcomes.*[7]
- Evaluate need for safety, balancing client's need for autonomy. *The ethical challenge of providing individual safety within the current laws for client's right to refuse care in face of self-neglect and self-destructive behaviors that can impact others as well as the client is difficult to manage.*[4,9]
- Perform home assessment. *Determines safety issues, cleanliness, compulsive hoarding, neglected property concerns, so plans can be made to take care of these matters if client is to remain in the home.*[7]
- Instruct in or review skills necessary for caring for self, using terms appropriate to client's level of understanding. *When individual is cognitively impaired or otherwise has difficulty processing information, instructions need to be simplified.*[5]
- Plan time for listening to client/SOs concerns. *Provides opportunity to determine whether plan is being followed and what the barriers to participation may be.*[7]
- Refer to NDs Self-Care Deficit, ineffective Health Maintenance, impaired Home Maintenance, and disturbed Sensory Perception for additional interventions as appropriate.

NURSING PRIORITY NO. 4

To promote wellness (Discharge/Evaluation Criteria):

- Establish remotivation or resocialization program when indicated. *Depending on where the client is residing, isolation may become a problem as individual withdraws from contact with others, and these programs may be helpful.*[2]
- Assist with setting up medication regimen. *Client may need help with arranging medications in specific ways to assure correct administration, especially in the presence of cognitive impairment.*[8]
- Discuss dietary needs and client's ability to provide nutritious meals. *May require support such as food stamps, community pantry, elder meal program, Meals on Wheels.*[1]
- Provide for ongoing evaluation of self-care program. *Helps to identify whether client is managing effectively or whether cognitive functioning is deteriorating and a new plan needs to be developed.*[1]
- Evaluate for appropriateness of providing a companion animal. *Taking responsibility for another life and sharing unconditional love can provide purpose and motivation for client to take more interest in own situation.*[4]
- Refer to support services such as home care, day care program, social services, food stamps, community clinic, physical or occupational therapy, senior services as indicated. *Provides for long-term support to facilitate client's independence and general well-being.*[8]

Nursing Diagnoses in Alphabetical Order

- Investigate alternative placements as indicated. *Client may require group home, assisted living, or long-term care, and it is best to place in least restrictive environment capable of meeting client's needs.*[9]
- Discuss need for respite for family members. *Care of cognitively impaired member can be wearing, and time away allows for renewing oneself and enhancing ability to cope with continued care responsibilities.*[5]
- Refer for counseling as indicated. Accurate mental health diagnoses indicates the need for appropriate services, psychiatric, social services, home care.[6]

DOCUMENTATION FOCUS

Assessment/Reassessment
- Individual findings, functional level and limitations, mental status.
- Personal safety issues.
- Needed resources, possible need for placement.

Planning
- Plan of care and who is involved in planning.
- Teaching plan.

Implementation/Evaluation
- Response to interventions, teaching, and actions performed.
- Attainment or progress toward desired outcomes.
- Modifications of plan of care.

Discharge Planning
- Long-term needs and who is responsible for actions to be taken.
- Type of assistance and resources needed.
- Specific referrals made.

References

1. Smith, S. M., et al. (2006). Nutritional status is altered in the self-neglecting elderly. *J Nutr Online*, 136(10), 2534–2541.
2. Abrams, R. C., et al. (2002). Predictors of self-neglect in community-dwelling elders. *Am J of Psychiatry*, 159(10), 1724–1730.
3. Fulmer, T. (2003). Elder abuse and neglect assessment. *Gerontal Nurs*, 29(1), 8–9.
4. National Center on Elder Abuse. Self-neglect: An update of the literature 2000–2005. Retrieved March 2009 from www.ncea.aoa.gov/NCEAroot/Main_Site/Library/CANE/CANE_Series/CANE_Selfneglectupdate.aspx.
5. Townsend, M. (2006). *Psychiatric Mental Health Nursing Concept of Care in Evidence-Based Practice.* 5th ed. Philadelphia: F. A. Davis.
6. Lauder, W., Anderson, I., Barclay, A. (2005). A framework for good practice in interagency interventions with cases of self-neglect. *J Psychiatr Ment Health Nurs*, 12(2), 192–198.
7. Lauder, E., Anderson, A., Barclay, A. (2005). Housing and self-neglect: The responses of health, social care and environmental health agencies. *J Interprof Care*, 19(4), 317–325.
8. Tierney, M., et al. (2004). Risk factors for harm in cognitively impaired seniors who live alone: A prospective study. *J Am Geriatr Soc*, 52(9), 1435–1441.
9. Nusbaum, N. (2004). Safety versus autonomy: Dilemmas and strategies in protection of vulnerable community-dwelling elderly. *Ann Long-Term Care*, 12(5), 50–53.
10. Campbell, H., et al. (2005). Diogenes syndrome: Frontal lobe dysfunction or multi-factorial disorder. *Geriatr Med*, 35(3), 77–79.

unilateral Neglect

DEFINITION: Impairment in sensory and motor response, mental representation, and spatial attention to body and the corresponding environment characterized by inattention to one side and overattention to the opposite side; left-side neglect is more severe and persistent than right-side neglect

RELATED FACTORS

Brain injury from cerebrovascular problems; neurological illness; trauma; tumor
Left hemiplegia from cerebrovascular accident (CVA) of the right hemisphere
Hemianopsia

DEFINING CHARACTERISTICS

Subjective
[Reports feeling that body part does not belong to own self]

Objective
Marked deviation of the eyes, head, or trunk (as if drawn magnetically) to the nonneglected side to stimuli and activities on that side
Failure to move eyes, head, limbs, or trunk in the neglected hemisphere despite being aware of a stimulus in that space; failure to notice people approaching from the neglected side
Displacement of sounds to the nonneglected side
Appears unaware of positioning of neglected limb
Lack of safety precautions with regard to the neglected side
Failure to eat food from portion of the plate on the neglected side; dress or groom neglected side
Difficulty remembering details of internally represented familiar scenes that are on the neglected side
Use of only vertical half of page when writing; failure to cancel lines on the half of the page on the neglected side; substitution of letters to form alternative words that are similar to the original in length when reading
Distortion or omission of drawing on the half of the page on the neglected side
Perseveration of visual motor tasks on nonneglected side
Transfer of pain sensation to the nonneglected side

Sample Clinical Applications: Traumatic brain injury, CVA/ruptured cerebral aneurysm, brain tumor, glaucoma

DESIRED OUTCOMES/EVALUATION CRITERIA

Sample NOC linkages:
Adaption to Physical Disability: Adaptive response to a significant functional challenge due to a physical disability
Self-Care: Activities of Daily Living (ADL): Ability to perform the most basic physical tasks and personal care activities independently with or without assistive device
Personal Safety Behavior: Personal actions that prevent physical injury to self

(continues on page 542)

unilateral Neglect (continued)

Client/Caregiver Will (Include Specific Time Frame)
• Acknowledge presence of sensory-perceptual impairment.
• Identify adaptive and protective measures for individual situation.
• Demonstrate behaviors, lifestyle changes necessary to promote physical safety.

Client Will (Include Specific Time Frame)
• Verbalize positive realistic perception of self, incorporating the current dysfunction.
• Perform self-care within level of ability.

ACTIONS/INTERVENTIONS

Sample (NIC) linkages:
Unilateral Neglect Management: Protecting and safely reintegrating the affected part of the body while helping the patient adapt to disturbed perceptual abilities
Positioning: Deliberative placement of the patient or a body part to promote physiological and/or psychological well-being
Environmental Management: Safety: Manipulation of the patient's surroundings for therapeutic benefit

NURSING PRIORITY NO. 1

To assess the extent of altered perception and the related degree of disability:

• Identify underlying condition or reason for alterations in sensory/motor/behavioral perceptions as noted in Related Factors.
• Observe client's behaviors (as noted in Defining Characteristics) *to determine the extent of impairment (e.g., failure to respond to stimuli, objects, or people on the contralesional side).*
• Ascertain client's/SO's perception of problem and changes and impact on life and future, noting differences in perceptions. *Client may or may not be aware of or able to express spatial perception problems or understand potential effect on future expectations.*
• Measure visual acuity and field of vision *to determine presence and degree of interference if problem is due to actual loss of visual field as can occur with some types of stroke, causing failure to (1) recognize an object or (2) define where an object is located. However, the client can have intact visual fields and still experience spatial neglect.*[1]
• Assess ability to distinguish between right and left. *Unilateral spatial neglect is observed in stroke, brain tumor, or accident victims with damage to the right parietal or parietal-occipital lobe, resulting in misperceptions of space opposite to brain damage. The individual with this condition has information from the left hemispace but no conscious awareness of the information; thus they will pay no attention to the left space.*[1–4]
• Assess sensory awareness (e.g., response to stimulus of hot and cold, dull or sharp); note problems with awareness of motion and proprioception. *Disturbances in these areas may be result of spinal cord injury (where loss of sensation affects body awareness) or brain lesion (where sensation may be intact but awareness is impaired).*
• Note physical signs of neglect (e.g., disregard for position of affected limb[s], bumping into walls when ambulating, shaving only right side of face, skin irritation or injury).
• Observe ability to function within limits of impairment. Compare with client's perception of own abilities. *Client may or may not be able to learn from mistakes or from observing others, depending on the location and severity of the brain lesion.*[5]

- Explore and encourage verbalization of feelings *to identify meaning of loss, dysfunction, or change to the client and impact it may have on assuming ADLs.*
- Review results of testing done to determine cause or type of neglect syndrome (e.g., sensory, motor, representational, personal, spatial, behavioral inattention). *Aids in distinguishing neglect from visual field cuts, impaired attention, and planning or visuospatial abilities.*[6][8]

NURSING PRIORITY NO. 2

To promote optimal comfort and safety for the client in the environment:

- Engage in treatment strategies *focused on training of attention to the neglected hemispace:*[1][5,8,9]

  Encourage use of vision and hearing aids if condition requires or client usually wears them *to improve sensory input and interpretation.*

  Remove excess stimuli from the environment *to decrease confusion and reactive stress.*

  Orient or reorient to physical environment and persons interacting with client. *Client with unilateral neglect can also have numerous other cognitive defects affecting ability to think, remember, speak or understand language, and/or interpret environment.*[5]

  Approach client, and instruct others to approach client from the unaffected side (e.g., right side, or side where vision is not impaired) *to enhance client's awareness and potential for communication.*

  Encourage client to turn head and eyes in full rotation and "scan" the environment *to compensate for visual field loss or if neglect therapies include scanning.*

  Position bedside table and objects (e.g., telephone/call bell, tissues) *within functional field of vision or awareness to facilitate self-care.*

  Place nonessential items (e.g., television, pictures, hairbrush) on affected side during postacute phase once client begins to cross midline *to encourage continuation of retraining behaviors.*

  Discuss affected side while touching, manipulating, and stroking affected side *to focus client's attention on area* and provide objects of various weight, texture, and size for the client to handle *to provide tactile stimuli.*

  Describe where affected areas of body are *when moving or repositioning client.*

  Use descriptive terms to identify body parts rather than "left" and "right"; for example, "Lift this leg" (point to leg) or "Lift your affected leg."

  Encourage client to accept affected limb or side as part of self even when it no longer feels like it belongs. Have client look at and handle affected side *to stimulate awareness* and bring the affected limb across the midline *for client to visualize during care.*

  Provide visual cues and assist client to position the affected extremity carefully and teach to routinely visualize placement of the extremity.

  Use a mirror to help client adjust position *by visualizing both sides of the body.*

- Provide assistance with ADLs (e.g., feeding, bathing, dressing, grooming, toileting), *which helps client tend to affected side or compensate for client's impairments.*

- Monitor neglected body part(s) for positioning and anatomic alignment, pressure points, skin irritation or injury, and dependent edema. *Increased risk of injury and pressure ulcer formation necessitates close observation and timely intervention.* (Refer to NDs risk for Peripheral Neurovascular Dysfunction, impaired Tissue Integrity.)

- Assist with ambulation or movement, using appropriate mobility and assistive devices *to promote safety of client and caregiver.*

- Protect from falls and/or collision with objects:

  Position furniture and equipment *so travel path is unobstructed.*

Remove articles that may create a safety hazard (e.g., footstool, throw rug).
Ensure adequate lighting in the environment.
Keep doors wide open or completely closed.
- Refer to NDs impaired Environmental Interpretation Syndrome, risk for Falls/Injury, and Self-Care Deficit (specify) for additional interventions regarding comfort and safety.

NURSING PRIORITY NO. 3

To promote wellness (Teaching/Discharge Considerations):

- Collaborate with rehabilitation team in strategies (e.g., sensory stimulation techniques such as tapping or stroking, active and passive range-of-motion exercises, and temporary restraint of healthy limb while practicing motor skills) *to assist client to compensate for deficits.*[5]
- Refer for or participate in neuropsychological therapies, as indicated. *Rehabilitation may address (1) visual attention deficits (e.g., scanning, training) or (2) spatial representation deficits (e.g., mental imagery training, eye patching, stimulation therapy).*[3]
- Acknowledge and accept feelings of despondency, grief, and anger. *When feelings are openly expressed, client can deal with them and move forward.* (Refer to ND Grieving as appropriate.)
- Encourage family members/SO(s) to treat client normally, to urge client to perform own care as able, and to include client in family activities and outings. *Promotes sense of self-worth and encourages participation in life activities to limit withdrawal and depression.*
- Reinforce to client the reality of the dysfunction and need to compensate. Avoid participating in the client's use of denial. *Delays dealing with reality of situation and limits progress toward goals.*
- Encourage client to continue rehabilitative services *to maximize recovery and enhance independence. Note: Research indicates that most clients with neglect show early recovery, particularly within the first month and marked improvement within 3 months. In approximately 10% of clients, classic (more severe) symptoms of spatial neglect persist after 6 months or longer. In these individuals, the deficit may be regarded as chronic neglect.*[9]
- Discuss and prepare for ongoing safety issues. *Client may continue to have some functional problems after apparent recovery of spatial neglect, including difficulty with navigating in familiar and unfamiliar environments and safe driving.*[9]
- Identify additional resources to meet individual needs (e.g., Meals on Wheels, home-care rehabilitation services) *to maximize independence, allow client to return to and succeed in community setting.*

DOCUMENTATION FOCUS

Assessment/Reassessment
- Individual findings, including extent of altered perception, degree of disability, effect on independence and participation in ADLs.

Planning
- Plan of care and who is involved in the planning.
- Teaching plan.

Implementation/Evaluation
- Responses to intervention, teaching, and actions performed.
- Attainment or progress toward desired outcome(s).
- Modifications to plan of care.

 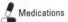

Discharge Planning

• Long-term needs and who is responsible for actions to be taken.

• Available resources, specific referrals made.

References

1. Walker, R., et al. (1994). Unilateral neglect: Clinical and experimental studies. *Review for Psyche: An Interdisciplinary Journal of Research on Consciousness.* Retrieved July 2007 from http://psyche.cs.monash.edu.au/v1/psyche-1-08-walker.html.
2. Mansoori, L. Hemispatial neglect syndrome. Student lecture for Brain, Thought and Action (MCDB 3650). University of Colorado. Boulder.
3. Ricci, R., Calhoun, J., Chatterjee, A. (2000). *Orientation bias in unilateral neglect: Representational contributions* (Research article). Philadelphia: Department of Neurology and the Center for Cognitive Neuroscience, University of Pennsylvania.
4. Sinclair, C. (2001). Brain organization as seen in unilateral spatial neglect. Retrieved July 2007 from http://serendip.brynmawr.edu/bb/neuro/neuro01/web2/Sinclair.html.
5. National Institute for Neurological Disorders and Stroke (NINDS). Post-stroke rehabilitation fact sheet. Retrieved July 2007 from www.ninds.nih.gov/disorders/stroke/poststrokerehab.htm.
6. Bates, B., Choi, J. Y., Duncan, P. W. (2005). Veterans Affairs/Department of Defense clinical practice guidelines for the management of adult stroke rehabilitation care: An executive summary. *Stroke*, 36(9), 2049–2056.
7. Plummer, P., Morris, M. E., Dunai, J. (2003). Assessment of unilateral neglect. *Phys Ther*, 83(8), 732–740.
8. Swan, L. (2001). Unilateral spatial neglect. *Phys Ther*, 81(9), 1572–1580.
9. Barrett, A. M., John, S. T. (2007). Spatial neglect. Retrieved July 2007 from www.emedicine.com/neuro/topic719.htm.

Noncompliance [ineffective Adherence] [specify]

DEFINITION: Behavior of person and/or caregiver that fails to coincide with a health-promoting or therapeutic plan agreed on by the person (or family or community) and healthcare professional; in the presence of an agreed-on health-promoting or therapeutic plan, person's or caregiver's behavior is fully or partially nonadherent and may lead to clinically ineffective or partially ineffective outcomes

[Author Note: When the plan of care is reviewed with client/SO, use of the term *noncompliance* may create a negative response and sense of conflict between healthcare providers and client. Labeling the client noncompliant may also lead to problems with third-party reimbursement. Where possible, use of the ND ineffective self Health Management is recommended.]

RELATED FACTORS

Healthcare plan

Duration

Cost; intensity; complexity

Financial flexibility of plan

Individual factors

Personal or developmental abilities; knowledge or skill relevant to the regimen behavior; motivational forces

(continues on page 546)

Noncompliance (continued)

Individual's value system; health beliefs, cultural influences, spiritual values, significant others

[Altered thought processes such as depression, paranoia]

[Difficulty changing behavior, as in addictions]

[Denial; issues of secondary gain]

Health system

Individual health coverage

Credibility of provider; client-provider relationships; provider continuity or regular follow-up; provider reimbursement; communication or teaching skills of the provider

Access or convenience of care; satisfaction with care

Network

Involvement of members in health plan; social value regarding plan

Perceived beliefs of significant others [SOs]

DEFINING CHARACTERISTICS

Subjective

Statements by client or SO(s) of failure to adhere; [does not perceive illness or risk to be serious, does not believe in efficacy of therapy, unwilling to follow treatment regimen or accept side effects or limitations]

Objective

Behavior indicative of failure to adhere

Objective tests (e.g., physiological measures, detection of physiological markers)

Failure to progress; evidence of development of complications or exacerbation of symptoms

Failure to keep appointments

Sample Clinical Applications: Any new diagnosis, chronic conditions, or situations requiring undesired or major lifestyle changes

DESIRED OUTCOMES/EVALUATION CRITERIA

Sample **NOC** linkages:

Compliance Behavior: Personal actions to promote wellness, recovery, and rehabilitation recommended by a health professional

Health Beliefs: [specify]: Personal convictions that influence health behaviors

Participation in Healthcare Decisions: Involvement in selecting and evaluating healthcare options to achieve desired outcomes

Client Will (Include Specific Time Frame)
• Verbalize accurate knowledge of condition and understanding of treatment regimen.
• Make choices at level of readiness based on accurate information.
• Verbalize commitment to mutually agreed-upon goals and treatment plan.
• Access resources appropriately.
• Demonstrate progress toward desired outcomes or goals.

ACTIONS/INTERVENTIONS

Sample NIC linkages:
Mutual Goal-Setting: Collaborating with patient to identify and prioritize care goals, then developing a plan for achieving those goals
Self-Modification Assistance: Reinforcement of self-directed change initiated by the patient to achieve personally important goals
Values Clarification: Assisting another to clarify her/his own values in order to facilitate effective decision making

NURSING PRIORITY NO. 1

To determine reason for alteration/disregard of therapeutic regimen/instructions:

- Determine client/SO(s) perception and understanding of the situation (illness, treatment). *Basic information needed to understand client's/SO's position and possible conflicts in order to develop plan of care.*[2]
- Listen to/Active-listen client's complaints, comments. *Conveys confidence in individual's ability to understand and manage own care.*[1] *Helps to identify client's thinking about the treatment regimen (e.g., may be concerned about side effects of medications or success of procedures or transplantation).*[11]
- Note language spoken, read, and understood. *Lack of understanding of words that are used in explanations may result in client lack of cooperation with therapeutic regimen.*[2,10]
- Identify developmental level as well as chronological age of client. *Determines how to interact with client on appropriate level to enhance relationship and ability to discuss lack of cooperation with medical regimen.*[2]
- Assess level of anxiety, locus of control, sense of powerlessness, and so forth. *Presence of these factors will affect how client is managing illness or situation and therapeutic regimen.*[1,11]
- Note length of illness. *People tend to become passive and dependent in long-term, debilitating illnesses and find it difficult to expend energy to follow through with therapeutic regimen.*[6]
- Clarify value system: cultural or religious values, health and illness beliefs and practices of the client/SO(s). *These factors will influence individual's view of the therapeutic regimen and willingness to follow through on some interventions; for instance, Mexican Americans may believe the future is in God's hands; women may delay Pap smears and mammograms because of modesty.*[10]
- Determine social characteristics, demographic and educational factors, as well as personality of the client. *Educated individuals may be more oriented to health promotion and disease prevention, while lower-socioeconomic individuals may be focused on the basics of living and may not pay attention to or follow healthcare recommendations. Personality characteristics such as suspiciousness, obsessive features may affect how client views medical regimen.*[9]
- Verify psychological meaning of the behavior (e.g., may be denial). Note issues of secondary gain. *Family dynamics, school or workplace issues, involvement in legal system may unconsciously affect client's decision regarding care and necessary follow-through.*[3]
- Assess availability and use of support systems and resources. *Failure to follow through with recommended therapies may be due to lack of or incorrect usage of support that is available.*[9]
- Be aware of nurses'/healthcare providers' attitudes and behaviors toward the client. Do they have an investment in the client's compliance or recovery? What is the behavior of the

client and healthcare provider when client is labeled "noncompliant"? *Some care providers may be enabling client whereas others' judgmental attitudes may impede treatment progress.*[1]

 ● Determine who (e.g., client, SO, other) manages the medication regime and whether individual knows what the medications are and why they are prescribed.

 ● Ascertain how client remembers to take medications and how many doses have been missed in the last 72 hours, last week, last 2 weeks, and last month. *While clients claiming to take their medication often do not, self-reported nonadherence is likely to be accurate and should be taken seriously.*[13]

● Identify factors that interfere with taking medications or lead to lack of adherence (e.g., depression, active alcohol or other drug use, low literacy, lack of support, lack of belief in treatment efficacy). *Forgetfulness is the most common reason given for not complying with the treatment plan.*[12]

NURSING PRIORITY NO. 2

To assist client/SO(s) to develop strategies for dealing effectively with the situation:

● Develop therapeutic nurse-client relationship. *Promotes trust, provides atmosphere in which client/SO(s) can freely express views or concerns and explore reasons for lack of compliance with therapeutic regimen. Adherence assessment is most successful when conducted in a positive, nonjudgmental atmosphere.*[1]

● Explore client involvement in or lack of mutual goal-setting. *Client will be more likely to follow through on goals he or she participated in developing.*[5,8]

● Review treatment strategies. Identify which interventions in the plan of care are most important in meeting therapeutic goals and which are least amenable to cooperation. *Sets priorities and encourages problem-solving areas of conflict, enabling client to make decisions related to choices of care.*[7]

● Contract with the client for participation in care. *Enhances commitment to follow-through.*[3]

 ● Encourage client to maintain self-care, providing for assistance when necessary. Accept client's evaluation of own strengths and limitations while working with client to improve abilities. *Promotes self-esteem, enabling client to have a sense of control over illness and treatment regimen.*[7]

 ● Provide for continuity of care in and out of the hospital or care setting, including long-range plans. *Supports trust, facilitates progress toward goals as client illness is dealt with over time.*[6,14]

 ● Provide information and help client to know where and how to find it on own. *Promotes independence and encourages informed decision making and control over illness, enhancing compliance with therapeutic regimen.*[4]

● Present information in manageable amounts, using verbal, written, and audiovisual modes at level of client's ability. *Individuals learn in many ways, and using different modes at client's own pace facilitates learning and enhances assimilation of the information.*[3]

 ● Have client/SO paraphrase instructions and information heard. *Validates understanding and reveals misconceptions so that corrections can be made and appropriate questions can be asked and answered.*[4]

● Accept the client's choice or point of view, even if it appears to be self-destructive. Avoid confrontation regarding beliefs. *Maintaining open communication is important to continuing to provide correct information and therapeutic relationship with the client/SO(s). If illness is terminal, accept client's wishes regarding continued care or treatments, providing what is accepted.*[1]

● Establish graduated goals or modified regimen as necessary. *Client with chronic obstructive pulmonary disease (COPD) who smokes a pack of cigarettes a day may be willing to reduce that amount but not give up smoking altogether. This choice may improve quality of life, and success with this goal may encourage progression to more advanced goals.*[3]

NURSING PRIORITY NO. 3

To promote wellness (Teaching/Discharge Considerations):

● Stress importance of the client's knowledge and understanding of the need for treatment or medication, as well as consequences of actions and choices. *Client who is not adhering to the treatment regimen may not have full information or may not understand the reasons for the recommendations. With full understanding, client can make a more informed decision about care.*[1,11,14]

● Develop a system for self-monitoring. *Provides a sense of control and enables the client to follow own progress, seek timely evaluation/intervention by healthcare provider, and assist with making choices.*[7]

● Suggest using a medication reminder system. *These have been shown to improve client adherence by a significant percentage.*

● Provide support systems to reinforce negotiated behaviors. Encourage client to continue positive behaviors, especially if client is beginning to see benefit. *Individuals who feel alone and do not hear any positive reinforcement for changes that have been made will have difficulty maintaining the changes. When clients do hear positive comments and see the results for themselves, they are more apt to be willing to continue treatment regimen.*[7,8]

● Refer to counseling or therapy or other appropriate resources. *May need additional assistance to resolve situation and enable client to progress as desired.*[1]

● Refer to NDs Anxiety; compromised family Coping; ineffective Coping; deficient Knowledge (specify); ineffective self Health Management.

DOCUMENTATION FOCUS

Assessment/Reassessment
• Individual findings, deviation from prescribed treatment plan, and client's reasons in own words.
• Cultural or religious values, beliefs, and expectations.
• Availability and use of resources.
• Involvement of SO/family.
• Consequences of actions to date.

Planning
• Plan of care and who is involved in planning.
• Teaching plan.

Implementation/Evaluation
• Response to interventions, teaching, and actions performed.
• Attainment or progress toward desired outcome(s).
• Modifications to plan of care.

Discharge Planning
• Long-term needs and who is responsible for actions to be taken.
• Specific referrals made.

References

1. Doenges, M., Townsend, M., Moorhouse, M. (1998). *Psychiatric Care Plans: Guidelines for Individualizing Care*. 3d ed. Philadelphia: F. A. Davis.
2. Locher, J., et al. (2002). Effects of age and casual attribution to aging on health-related behaviors associated with urinary incontinence in older women. *Gerontologist*, 42(4), 515–521.
3. Cox, H., et al. (2002). *Clinical Applications of Nursing Diagnoses: Adult, Child, Women's, Psychiatric, Gerontic, and Home Health Considerations*. 4th ed. Philadelphia: F. A. Davis.
4. Pinhas-Hamiel, O., et al. (1996). Increased incidence of non-insulin-dependent diabetes mellitus among adolescents. *J Pediatr*, 128(8), 608–615.
5. Deckelbaum, R. J., Williams, C. L. (2001). Childhood obesity: The health issue. *Obes Res*, 9(5), 239s–243s.
6. Badger, J. M. (2001). Burns: The psychological aspect. *Am J Nurs*, 101(11), 38–41.
7. Bartol, T. (2002). Putting a patient with diabetes in the driver's seat. *Nursing*, 32(2), 53–55.
8. Doughty, D. B. (2001). The state of ostomy care, tremendous progress, continued challenges. *J Wound Ostomy Continence Nurs*, 28(1), 1–2.
9. American Society of Pain Management Nurses. (2002). Position paper on pain management in patients with addictive disease. Pensacola, FL.
10. Lipson, J. G., Dibble, S. L., Minarik, P. A. (1999). *Culture & Nursing Care: A Pocket Guide*. San Francisco: UCSF Nursing Press.
11. Morrissey, P. (2005). Noncompliance after transplantation. Retrieved August 2007 from www.lifespan.org/rih/services/transplant/news/02-07.htm.
12. Human medication noncompliance. Retrieved August 2007 from www.alrt.com/humnonc.html.
13. Zuger, A. (2001). Adherence by any measure still matters. Retrieved August 2007 from http://aids-clinical-care.jwatch.org/cgi/content/full/2001/701/1.
14. Section 3: Antiretroviral therapy adherence. (2006). *Clinical Manual for Management of the HIV-Infected Adult*. AIDS Education and Training Centers. Retrieved April 2007 from at www.aidsetc.org/aetc/pdf/AETC-CM_092206.pdf, 3–11.

imbalanced Nutrition: less than body requirements

DEFINITION: Intake of nutrients insufficient to meet metabolic needs

RELATED FACTORS

Inability to ingest or digest food; inability to absorb nutrients
Biological, psychological, or economic factors
[Increased metabolic demands, such as with burns]
[Lack of information, misinformation, or misconceptions]

DEFINING CHARACTERISTICS

Subjective
Reported food intake less than RDAs (recommended daily allowances); lack of food
Lack of interest in food; aversion to eating; reported altered taste sensation; perceived inability to digest food
Satiety immediately after ingesting food
Abdominal pain or cramping
Lack of information, misinformation, or misconceptions [NOTE: The authors view these as related factors rather than defining characteristics.]

imbalanced Nutrition: less than body requirements (continued)

Objective

Body weight 20% or more under ideal [for height and frame]; [decreased subcutaneous fat or muscle mass]

Loss of weight with adequate food intake

Hyperactive bowel sounds; diarrhea; steatorrhea

Weakness of muscles required for swallowing or mastication; poor muscle tone

Sore buccal cavity, pale mucous membranes; capillary fragility

Excessive loss of hair [or increased growth of hair on body (lanugo)]; [cessation of menses]

[Abnormal laboratory studies (e.g., decreased albumin, total proteins; iron deficiency; electrolyte imbalances)]

Sample Clinical Applications: Cancer, AIDS, anorexia or bulimia nervosa, burns, facial trauma, brain injury, coma, stroke, Parkinson's disease, cleft lip/palate, anemia, dementia, Alzheimer's disease, major depression, schizophrenia

DESIRED OUTCOMES/EVALUATION CRITERIA

Sample (NOC) linkages:
Nutritional Status: Extent to which nutrients are available to meet metabolic needs
Knowledge: Diet: Extent of understanding conveyed about recommended diet
Weight Gain Behavior: Personal actions gain weight following voluntary or involuntary significant weight loss

Client Will (Include Specific Time Frame)
• Demonstrate progressive weight gain toward goal.
• Display normalization of laboratory values and be free of signs of malnutrition as reflected in Defining Characteristics.
• Verbalize understanding of causative factors when known and necessary interventions.
• Demonstrate behaviors, lifestyle changes to regain or maintain appropriate weight.

ACTIONS/INTERVENTIONS

Sample (NIC) linkages:
Nutrition Management: Assisting with or providing a balanced dietary intake of foods and fluids
Weight-Gain Assistance: Facilitating gain of body weight
Eating Disorders Management: Prevention and treatment of severe diet restrictions and overexercising or binging and purging of foods and fluids

NURSING PRIORITY NO. 1

To assess causative/contributing factors:

∞ • Identify client at risk for malnutrition (e.g., institutionalized elderly; client with chronic illness; child or adult living in poverty/low-income area; client with facial injuries or deformities; restrictive weight-loss program or surgical intervention; prolonged time of restricted intake, prior nutritional deficiencies; hypermetabolic states [e.g., hyperthyroidism]; malabsorption syndromes).[2,11,12]

- Obtain dietary history *to determine chronic problems and ongoing needs*:
  Increased caloric requirements with difficulty ingesting sufficient calories (e.g., cancer, burns)
- Maturational or developmental issues (e.g., premature baby with sucking difficulties, child with lack of emotional stimulation, frail elderly living alone)
  Swallowing problems (e.g., stroke, Parkinson's disease, cerebral palsy, other neuromuscular disorders)[2]
  Poor dentition: damaged or missing teeth, ill-fitting dentures, gum disease
  Decreased absorption (e.g., lactose intolerance, Crohn's disease)
  Diminished desire or refusal to eat (e.g., anorexia nervosa, cirrhosis, pancreatitis, alcoholism, bipolar disorder, chronic fatigue)[2,8]
  Treatment-related issues (e.g., chemotherapy, radiation, stomatitis, facial surgery, wired jaw)
  Personal or situational factors (e.g., inability to procure or prepare food, social isolation, grief, loss)[10]
- Assess pediatric concerns (e.g., changes in nutritional needs related to growth phase; congenital anomalies, including tracheoesophageal fistula, cleft lip/palate; metabolic or malabsorption problems, such as diabetes, phenylketonuria, cerebral palsy; chronic infections).[5]
- Determine lifestyle factors that may affect weight. *Socioeconomic resources, amount of money available for purchasing food, proximity of grocery store, and available storage space for food are all factors that may impact food choices and intake.*
- Evaluate impact of cultural, ethnic, and religious influences. *The nutritional balance of a diet is recognized by most cultures, with distinct theories of nutritional practices for health promotion and disease prevention. Foods are used for prevention or treatment of disease (e.g., client may believe in use of "hot" or "cold" foods to treat certain conditions; or use low-fat, low-sodium foods to prevent heart disease). Certain foods may be thought to cause a disease condition (e.g., upset stomach caused from eating too many cold foods). Special diets or food preparation may be cultural or religious based (e.g., kosher preparation for Jewish client or eating no meat or meat by-products for vegetarian).*[1]
- Explore specific eating habits, the meaning of food to client (e.g., never eats breakfast, snacks throughout entire day, fasts for weight control, no time to eat properly), and individual food preferences and intolerances/aversions. *Identifies poor eating practices to be corrected and provides insight into dietary interventions that may appeal to client.*
- Obtain history or review diary of daily portion (or calorie) intake, patterns and times of eating *to reveal recent changes in client's weight or appetite and identify strengths and weaknesses in client's dietary habits.*[2]
- Assess client's knowledge of nutritional needs and ways client is meeting these needs. *Identifies teaching needs and/or helps guide choice of interventions.*[2]
- Note availability and use of financial resources and support systems. *These factors affect or determine ability to acquire, prepare, and store food. Lack of support or socialization may impact client's desire to eat.*
- Assess medication regimen, noting possible drug side effects or interactions, allergies, use of laxatives, diuretics. *These factors may be affecting appetite, food intake, or absorption.*[2,10]
- Note client's ability to feed self or presence of interfering factors. *Difficulties such as paralysis, tremor, or injury to hands or arms with inability to grasp or lift utensils to mouth; cognitive impairments affecting coordination or remembering to eat, age and/or developmental issues may require input of multiple providers and therapists to develop individualized plan of care.*[2]

- Auscultate for presence and character of bowel sounds *to determine ability and readiness of intestinal tract to handle digestive processes (e.g., hypermotility accompanies vomiting or diarrhea, while absence of bowel sounds may indicate bowel obstruction).*
- Determine psychological factors that may affect food choices. Perform psychological assessment as indicated, *to assess body image and congruency with reality, or to identify factors (e.g., dementia, severe depression) that may be interfering with client's appetite and food intake.*[2]
- Note occurrence of amenorrhea, tooth decay, swollen salivary glands, or report of constant sore throat. *May be signs of eating disorder, such as bulimia, affecting eating patterns and requiring additional evaluation.*[7,8]
- Review usual activities and exercise program noting repetitive activities (e.g., constant pacing) or inappropriate exercise (e.g., prolonged jogging). *Individuals with dementia may pace or be in constant motion increasing energy needs. Clients who have eating disorders, such as anorexia or bulimia, may use obsessive activities as weight-control measures.*[8]

NURSING PRIORITY NO. 2

To evaluate degree of deficit:

- Assess current weight, compared to usual weight, and norms for age and body size *to identify changes (e.g., sudden loss related to medical illness vs. ongoing chronic depression with anorexia and weight loss; or toddler with failure to meet growth expectations) that affect choice of intervention and helps clarify expectations.*
- Obtain weights using same scale, same time of day, and same clothing, as much as possible *to provide for accurate comparison to evaluate effectiveness of therapeutic regimen.*[2]
- Calculate growth percentiles in infants/children using growth chart *to identify deviations from the norm.*[5]
- Measure or calculate body fat, body water, and muscle mass (via triceps skinfold or other anthropometric measurements), or calculate body mass index (BMI) *to establish baseline parameters and assist in determining therapeutic goals. Note: BMI = weight (lb)/height (inches squared) × 704. Desirable BMI is 23 to 25, with <19 being severely underweight.*[2,10]
- Observe for absence of subcutaneous fat or muscle wasting, loss of hair, fissuring of nails, delayed healing, gum bleeding, swollen abdomen, and so forth, that indicate protein-energy malnutrition.[11]
- Perform or review results of nutritional assessment using screening tools such as Mini Nutritional Assessment (MNA).[8,13]
- Review laboratory studies (e.g., serum albumin, prealbumin, transferrin, aminoacid profile, iron, blood urea nitrogen [BUN], nitrogen balance studies, glucose, liver function, electrolytes, total lymphocyte count, indirect calorimetry) *to determine degree of nutritional deficits and effect on body function dictating specific dietary needs. Note: Baseline screening may be done (e.g., albumin, cholesterol, and complete blood count [CBC]) to determine whether more in-depth evaluation is needed.*[2,6]
- Assist with or review results of diagnostic procedures (e.g., Schilling's test, D-xylose test, 72-hour stool fat, gastrointestinal [GI] endoscopy, gastric reflux scanning).[2]

NURSING PRIORITY NO. 3

To establish a nutritional plan that meets individual needs:

- Collaborate with interdisciplinary team *to set nutritional goals when client has specific dietary needs, malnutrition is profound, or long-term feeding problems exist.*[2,9,11]

- Calculate basal energy expenditure (BEE) using Harris-Benedict (or similar) formula and estimate energy and protein requirements.
- Establish ongoing method of evaluating intake (e.g., calories/day, percent of food consumed at each feeding) *to assist in determining both amount of food taken and what food groups are consumed or left uneaten, to identify nutritional deficits.*[2]
- Discuss with client/SO aspects of diet that can remain unchanged *to preserve those that are valuable or meaningful to individual, and enhance sense of control.* Negotiate with client aspects of diet that need to be changed, especially if eating or psychiatric disorder is limiting food intake.

NURSING PRIORITY NO. 4

To address specific underlying condition/treatment needs:

- Assist in treatments to correct or control underlying causative factors *to improve intake and utilization of nutrients:*[2,9]

Administer oral antifungal agent *to treat cutaneous lesions of the mouth (e.g., candidiasis) that limit client's ability or desire for food.*

Medicate for pain or nausea, and manage drug side effects *to increase physical comfort and appetite.*

Provide pureed foods, formula tube feedings, or parenteral nutrition infusions when indicated by client's condition (e.g., wired jaws or paralysis following stroke) and degree of malnutrition. *Enteral route is preferred when oral feeding is not appropriate; however, parenteral nutrition is recommended if client is not able to tolerate at least 50% of the goal rate of enteral feedings.*[9]

Consult occupational therapist *to identify appropriate assistive devices to facilitate independence in feeding and self-esteem.*

Consult speech therapist *to develop specific exercises or activities to address swallowing difficulties related to neurological problems (e.g., stroke, amyotrophic lateral sclerosis [ALS]).* (Refer to ND impaired Swallowing for additional interventions.)

Refer for dental care *to correct missing teeth or poorly fitting dentures that affect client's ability to chew food or enjoy process of eating.*

Develop or refer client to structured (behavioral modification) program of nutrition therapy, which may include documenting time/length of eating period, putting food in a blender, and tube-feeding food not eaten. *These programs are used to change the maladaptive eating behaviors of clients with anorexia and bulimia and ensure adequate caloric intake. Because "control" is central to the etiology of these disorders, it is important to ensure that the client is perceived to be "in control."*[8]

Recommend or support hospitalization for controlled environment, as indicated, in severe malnutrition or life-threatening situations.

NURSING PRIORITY NO. 5

To enhance dietary intake:

- Avoid or limit withholding of food (e.g., prolonged NPO for surgery) as much as possible and reinstitute oral feedings as early as possible *to reduce adverse effects of malnutrition.*
- Increase specific nutrients (e.g., protein, carbohydrates, fats, and calories), as needed, providing client with preferred food and seasoning choices where possible *to enhance intake.*[11]
- Determine when client prefers or tolerates largest meal of the day. Maintain flexibility in timing of food intake *to promote sense of control and give client opportunity to eat when feeling more rested, less pain or nausea, or family coming at mealtime, and so forth.*[2]

- Provide numerous small feedings as indicated; supplement with easily digested snacks *to reduce feeling of fullness that can accompany larger meals and to improve chances of increasing the amount of nutrients taken over 24-hour period.*[3]
- Promote adequate and timely fluid intake. *Fluid is essential to the digestive process and is often taken with meals. Fluids may need to be withheld before meals or with meals if interfering with food intake.*
- Encourage variety in food choices, varying textures and taste sensations (e.g., sweet, salty, fresh, methods of cooking) *to enhance food satisfaction and stimulate appetite.*[2]
- Offer and keep available to client finger foods and snacks *that are easy to self-feed.*
- Provide oral care before and after meals. *Reduces discomfort associated with nausea, vomiting, oral lesions, mucosal dryness and halitosis, making eating easier or food more palatable.*
- Encourage use of lozenges, gum, hard candy, beverages, and so forth, *to stimulate salivation when dryness is a factor.*
- Use alternative flavoring agents (e.g., lemon and herbs) *to enhance taste of foods, especially if salt is restricted.*
- Add nonfat milk powder to foods with a high liquid content (e.g., gravy, puddings, cooked cereal) and sugar or honey in beverages if carbohydrates are tolerated *to increase caloric value.*[2]
- Avoid foods that cause intolerances or increase gastric motility (e.g., gas-forming foods, hot or cold, spicy, caffeinated beverages, milk products, and the like) *to reduce postprandial discomfort that may discourage client from eating.*[4]
- Limit high-fat foods or fiber and bulk if indicated, *because they may lead to early satiety.*
- Offer supplement drinks (or dispense in 2- to 4-oz portions several times/day). *Client may view this as a "medication" and thus will drink it, improving intake and energy level.*[2]
- Promote pleasant, relaxing environment, including socialization when possible. *Promotes focus on activity of eating, enhancing intake.*[2]
- Prevent or minimize unpleasant odors and sights, or cooking odors. *Often have a negative effect on appetite or activate gag reflex.*
- Administer pharmaceutical agents as indicated. *Appetite stimulants, dietary supplements; digestive drugs or enzymes, vitamins and minerals (e.g., iron), antacids, anticholinergics, antiemetics, or antidiarrheals, and so forth, may be used to enhance intake, improve digestion, and correct nutritional deficiencies.*[?]

NURSING PRIORITY NO. 6

To promote wellness (Teaching/Discharge Considerations):

- Discuss myths client/SO(s) may have about weight and weight gain *to address misconceptions and perhaps improve motivation for needed behavior changes.*
- Emphasize importance of well-balanced, nutritious intake. Provide nutritional information as indicated, taking into account client's age and developmental stage (e.g., toddler, teenager, pregnant woman, elderly person with chronic disease), physical health and activity tolerance, financial and socioeconomic factors, and client/SOs potential for management of underlying conditions. *For example, older adults need same nutrients as younger adults, but in smaller amounts and with attention to certain components, such as calcium, fiber, vitamins, protein, and water.*[4] *Infants/children require small meals and constant attention to needed nutrients for proper growth and development while dealing with child's food preferences and eating habits.*[5]
- Address financial issues and identify ways to meet dietary needs using nutrient-dense, low-budget foods.

- Involve SO(s) in treatment plan as much as possible *to provide ongoing support and increase likelihood of accomplishing dietary goals.*
- Consult with dietitian/nutritional support team as necessary *for long-term needs.*[2,9]
- Involve client in developing behavior modification program appropriate to specific needs based on consistent, realistic weight gain goal. *Enhances commitment to change and likelihood of accomplishing desired outcomes.*[8]
- Provide positive regard, love, and acknowledgment of "voice within" guiding client with eating disorder. *These efforts encourage the client to recognize maladaptive eating patterns as defense mechanisms to ease the emotional pain and begin to resolve underlying issues and develop more adaptive coping strategies for dealing with stressful situations.*[8]
- Weigh weekly and document results *to monitor effectiveness of dietary plan.*
- Develop regular exercise/stress-reduction program. *Enhances general well-being, improves organ function/muscle tone, and increases appetite.*[2]
- Review medical regimen and provide information or assistance as necessary. Discuss drug side effects and potential interactions with other medications and over-the-counter drugs.
- Assist client to identify and access community resources such as food stamps, budget counseling, Meals on Wheels, community food banks, or other appropriate assistance programs.
- Refer for dental hygiene and professional care, counseling or psychiatric care, family therapy as indicated.
- Provide and reinforce client teaching regarding preoperative and postoperative dietary needs when surgery is planned.
- Assist client/SO(s) to learn how to blenderize food or perform tube feeding when indicated. *Promotes independence in self-care and sense of some degree of control in a difficult situation.*
- Refer to home health resources *for initiation and supervision of home nutrition therapy when used.*

DOCUMENTATION FOCUS

Assessment/Reassessment
- Baseline and subsequent assessment findings to include signs/symptoms and laboratory diagnostic findings.
- Caloric and nutrient intake.
- Individual cultural or religious restrictions, personal preferences.
- Availability and use of resources.
- Personal understanding and perception of problem.

Planning
- Plan of care and who is involved in planning.
- Teaching plan.

Implementation/Evaluation
- Client's responses to interventions, teaching, and actions performed.
- Results of periodic weigh-in.
- Attainment or progress toward desired outcome(s).
- Modifications to plan of care.

Discharge Planning
- Long-term needs and who is responsible for actions to be taken.
- Specific referrals made.

References

1. Purnell, L. D., Paulanka, B. J. (1998). *Transcultural Health Care: A Culturally Competent Approach*. Philadelphia: F. A. Davis, 33–35.
2. Lawhorne, L. S. (2001). Altered nutritional status: Guideline. American Medical Directors Association (AMDA). Columbia, MD. Retrieved July 2007 from www.guideline.gov.
3. Love, C. C., Seaton, H. (1991). Eating disorders: Highlights of nursing assessment and therapeutics. *Nurs Clin North Am*, 26, 667–697.
4. American Dietetic Association. (2005). Nutrition across the spectrum of aging. *J Am Diet Assoc*, 105(4), 616–633.
5. Engel, J. (2002). *Pocket Guide to Pediatric Assessment*. 4th ed. St. Louis, MO: Mosby.
6. Vogelzang, J. L. (2003). Making nutrition sense from OASIS. *Home Healthcare Nurse*, 21(9), 592–600.
7. Could you or someone you care about have an eating disorder? Retrieved July 2007 from www.eating-disorder.com.
8. Townsend, M. C. (2003). *Psychiatric Mental Health Nursing Concepts of Care*. 4th ed. Philadelphia: F. A. Davis.
9. Jacobs, D. G., Jacobs, D. O., Kudsk, K. A. (2004). Practice management guidelines for nutritional support of the trauma patient. *J Trauma*, 57(3), 660–678.
10. John A. Hartford Foundation Institute for Geriatric Nursing. (2003). Mealtime difficulties for older persons: Assessment and management. Retrieved July 2007 from www.guideline.gov.
11. Scheinfeld, N. S., Mokashi, A. (2007). Protein-energy malnutrition. Retrieved April 2007 from www.emedicine.com/derm/topic797.htm.
12. Sullivan, C. S., Logan, J., Kolasa, K. M. (2006). Medical nutrition therapy for the bariatric patient. *Nutr Today*, 41(5), 207–212.
13. DiMaria, R. A., Amelia, E. (2005). Nutrition in older adults: Intervention and assessment can curb the growing threat of malnutrition. *Am J Nurs*, 105(3), 40–50.

imbalanced Nutrition: more than body requirements

DEFINITION: Intake of nutrients that exceeds metabolic needs

RELATED FACTORS

Excessive intake in relationship to metabolic need

DEFINING CHARACTERISTICS

Subjective
Dysfunctional eating patterns (e.g., pairing food with other activities)
Eating in response to external cues (e.g., time of day, social situation)
Concentrating food intake at end of day
Eating in response to internal cues other than hunger (e.g., anxiety)
Sedentary activity level

Objective
Weight 20% over ideal for height and frame [obese]
Triceps skinfold >15 mm in men, >25 mm in women
[Percentage of body fat greater than 22% for trim women and 15% for trim men]

(continues on page 558)

imbalanced Nutrition: more than body requirements (continued)

Sample Clinical Applications: Bulimia nervosa, morbid obesity, diseases requiring long-term steroid use (e.g., chronic obstructive pulmonary disease [COPD]), conditions associated with immobility (e.g., stroke/paralysis, multiple sclerosis [MS], amputation), Alzheimer's disease, depression, developmental delay

DESIRED OUTCOMES/EVALUATION CRITERIA

Sample (NOC) linkages:
Weight Loss Behavior: Personal actions to lose weight through diet, exercise, and behavior modification
Knowledge: Diet: Extent of understanding conveyed about recommended diet
Nutritional Status: Extent to which nutrients are available to meet metabolic needs

Client Will (Include Specific Time Frame)
• Verbalize a more realistic self-concept or body image (congruent mental and physical picture of self).
• Demonstrate appropriate changes in lifestyle and behaviors, including eating patterns, food quantity/quality, and exercise program.
• Attain desirable body weight with optimal maintenance of health.

ACTIONS/INTERVENTIONS

Sample (NIC) linkages:
Weight-Reduction Assistance: Facilitating loss of weight or body fat
Nutrition Management: Assisting with or providing a balanced dietary intake of foods and fluids
Eating Disorders Management: Prevention and treatment of severe diet restrictions and overexercising or binging and purging of foods and fluids

NURSING PRIORITY NO. 1

To identify causative/contributing factors:

• Obtain weight history, noting if client has weight gain out of character for self or family, is or was obese child, or used to be much more physically active than is now *to identify trends. Note: Obesity is now the most prevalent nutritional disorder among children and adolescents in the United States.*[1]
• Assess risk and presence of factors or conditions associated with obesity (e.g., familial pattern of obesity; decreased basal metabolic rate or hypothyroidism; type 2 diabetes; pregnancy; menopause; chronic disorders, such as heart, kidney disease, chronic pain; food or other substance addictions; stressful or sedentary lifestyle; depression; use of certain medications such as steroids, birth control pills; physical disabilities or limitations; lack of socioeconomic resources for obtaining or preparing healthy foods) *to determine treatments and interventions that may be indicated in addition to weight management.*[1,13]
• Assess client's knowledge of own body weight and nutritional needs, and determine cultural expectations regarding size. Although nutritional needs are not always understood, being overweight or having large body size may not be viewed negatively by individual, since it is considered within relationship to family eating patterns, peer and cultural influences.[1] African American women's frame of reference for "normal body weight" is higher than

standard indicators.[2] Some cultures place importance on large body size (e.g., Samoan people or Cuban children).[3] *Life goals may dictate body size (e.g., wrestler, football lineman).*

- Identify familial and cultural influences regarding food. *People of many cultures place high importance on food and food-related events, while some cultures routinely observe fasting days (e.g., Arab, Greek, Irish, Jewish) that may be done for health or religious purposes.*[3]

- Ascertain how client perceives food and the act of eating. *Individual beliefs, values, and types of foods available influence what people eat, avoid, or alter. Client may be eating to satisfy an emotional need rather than physiological hunger, not only because food plays a significant role in socialization but also because food can offer comfort, sense of security, and acceptance.*[3,4]

- Assess dietary practices by means of diary covering several days, asking for recall of foods and fluids ingested; times, patterns, and place of eating; activities; whether alone or with other(s); and feelings before, during, and after eating. *Provides opportunity for individual to focus on and internalize realistic picture of the amount of food ingested and corresponding eating habits and feelings. Identifies patterns requiring change or a base on which to tailor dietary program.*[5]

- Calculate total calorie intake, using client's 24-hour recall or weekly food diary. Evaluate usual intake of different food groups. *Helps identify strengths and weaknesses. For example, client may report normal or excessive intake of food, but calories and intake of certain food groups (e.g., sweets and fats) are often underestimated.*[12–14]

- Ascertain previous dieting history. *Client may report experimentation with numerous types of diets, repeated dieting efforts ("yo-yo" dieting) with varying results, or may never have attempted a weight-management program.*

- Obtain comparative body drawing having client draw self on wall with chalk, then standing against it and having actual body outline drawn to note difference between the two. *Determines whether client's view of self-body image is congruent with reality.*[14]

- Ascertain occurrence of negative feedback from SO(s). *May reveal control issues, impact motivation for change.*

- Identify unhelpful eating behaviors (e.g., eating over sink, "gobbling, nibbling, or grazing") and address kinds of activities associated with eating (e.g., watching television or reading, being unmindful of eating or food) *that result in taking in too many calories as well as eliminating the joy of food because of failure to notice flavors or sensation of fullness or satiety.*[1,13,15]

- Review daily activity and exercise program *for comparative baseline and to identify areas for modification.*

- Review laboratory test results (e.g., total cholesterol and triglycerides, fasting glucose and insulin levels; thyroid and other hormones) *that may reveal medical conditions associated with obesity, and identify problems that may be treated with alterations in diet or medications.*[11,17]

NURSING PRIORITY NO. 2

To establish weight reduction program:

- Determine client's motivation for weight loss (e.g., for own satisfaction or self-esteem, to improve health status, or to gain approval from another person). *Client is more likely to succeed and maintain desired weight when change is for self (e.g., acceptance of self "as is," general well-being) rather than to please others.*

- Discuss myths client/SO may have about weight and weight loss *to address misconceptions and possibly enhance motivation for needed behavior changes.*

- Obtain commitment or contract for weight loss. *Verbal agreement to goals or written contract formalizes the plan and may enhance efforts and maximize outcomes.*

- Involve SO(s) in treatment plan as much as possible *to provide ongoing support and increase likelihood of success.*
- Obtain anthropometric measurements *to determine presence and severity of obesity*:
  Evaluate body fat, body water, and muscle mass via scale skin caliper measurements and scale weight (*direct* measurement), bioelectric impedance analysis (BIA), dual-energy x-ray absorptiometry (DEXA), and hydrostatic weighing (*indirect* measurement).[13]
  Calculate body mass index (BMI) *to estimate percentage of body fat. Note: Desirable BMI is 23 to 25, with >30 being obese and >40 being morbidly obese.*[6] *Children who are 120% or more of ideal body weight for height and age are considered obese.*[7]
  Determine waist-to-hip ratio (WHR). *A WHR >8.2 in women and >1.0 in men (apple-shaped fat distribution in abdomen or around torso) is associated with increased risk of complications of obesity (e.g., diabetes and cardiovascular disease).*[8–10,16]
- Set realistic goals (short- and long-term) for weight loss. *Reasonable weight loss (1 to 2 lb/week) has been shown to have more lasting effects than rapid weight loss, although sustaining motivation for small losses often makes it difficult for client to stick with a program. Note: A loss of 5% to 20% of total body weight can reduce many of the health risks associated with obesity in adults.*[1,19]
- Collaborate with physician, nutritionist *to develop and implement comprehensive weight-loss program that includes food, activity, behavior alteration, and support.*
- Calculate calorie requirements based on physical factors and activity. *While many weight-reduction programs focus on portion size and food components (e.g., low-fat, high-protein, low-glycemic foods), reducing calorie intake is essential for weight loss.*[14] *Calories are usually counted according to three substances—carbohydrates = 4 calories/g, protein = 4 calories/g, fats = 9 calories/g. Note: Alcohol (a fourth separate group) = 7 calories/g. Decreasing calories by 500/day or expending 500 calories/day through exercise results in a weight loss of about 1 pound/week.*[9]
- Provide information regarding specific nutritional needs. *Individual may be deficient in needed nutrients (e.g., proteins, vitamins, or minerals) or may eat too much of one food group (e.g., fats or carbohydrates). Depending on client's desires and needs, many weight-management programs are available that focus on particular factors (e.g., low carbohydrates, low fat, low calories). Reducing portion size and following a balanced diet along with increasing exercise is often what is needed to improve health.*[12,18,19]
- Discuss modifications to achieve healthy body weight:[14,15,19,20]
  Eat from each food group (fruits, vegetables, whole grains, lean meats, low-fat dairy, and oils).
  Start with small changes, such as adding one more vegetable/day, introducing healthier versions of favorite foods.
  Choose "nutrient-dense" forms of foods that provide substantial amounts of fiber, vitamins, electrolytes, and minerals.
  Avoid saturated fats, trans fats, cholesterol, salt (sodium), and added sugars.
  Focus on portion sizes: calorie-dense foods (high in fat and/or sugar) should be eaten in smaller quantities, whereas high-fiber foods can be eaten in larger quantities.
  Discuss smart snacks (e.g., low-fat yogurt with fruit, nuts, apple slices with peanut butter, low-fat string cheese) *to assist client in finding healthy options.*
- Stress need for adequate fluid intake and taking fluids between meals rather than with meals to provide fluid while leaving more room for food intake at meals *to assist in digestive process and to quench thirst, which is often mistakenly identified as hunger.*
- Encourage involvement in planned activity program of client's choice and within physical abilities. Refer to formal exercise program, if desired. *Moderately increased physical*

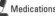

activity for 30 to 45 minutes 5 days/week can expend an additional 1500 to 2000 calories/ week, supporting both loss of pounds and maintenance of lower weight.[13,20,21]

- Recommend weighing only once/week, same time and clothes, and graph on chart. Measure and monitor body fat when possible *to track progress while focusing more on the idea of being health-conscious and responsible than what scale may reveal.*[13]
- Provide positive reinforcement and encouragement for efforts as well as actual weight loss. *Enhances commitment to program and enhances person's sense of self-worth.*
- Refer to bariatric physician/surgeon when indicated. *Evaluation for special measures may be needed (e.g., supervised fasting or bariatric surgery) for morbidly obese persons with BMI >40.*[9,22]

NURSING PRIORITY NO. 3

To promote wellness (Teaching/Discharge Considerations):

- Assist in and encourage periodic evaluation of nutritional status and alteration of dietary plan. *May be desired or needed for addressing special needs (e.g., diabetes mellitus, age considerations, very low calorie or fasting) and monitoring health status.*[21]
- Emphasize importance of avoiding fad diets *that may be harmful to health and often do not produce long-term positive results.*
- Identify and encourage finding ways to reduce tension when eating. *Promotes relaxation to permit focus on act of eating and awareness of satiety.*
- Review and discuss strategies to deal appropriately with stressful events *to avoid overeating as a means of coping.*
- Discuss importance of an occasional treat by planning for inclusion in diet *to avoid feelings of deprivation arising from self-denial.*
- Advise planning for special occasions (birthday or holidays) by reducing intake before event and/or eating "smart" *to redistribute or reduce calories and allow for participation in food events.*
- Discuss normalcy of ups and downs of weight loss; plateau, set point (at which weight is not being lost), hormonal influences, and so forth. *Prevents discouragement when progress stalls.*
- Encourage buying personal items and clothing *as a reward for weight loss or other accomplishments.* Suggest disposing of "fat clothes" *to encourage positive attitude of permanent change and remove "safety valve" of having wardrobe available "just in case" weight is regained.*
- Review prescribed drug regimen (e.g., appetite suppressants, hormone therapy, vitamin and mineral supplements) *for benefits or adverse side effects and drug interactions.*
- Recommend reading labels of nonprescription diet aids if used. *Herbals containing diuretics or ma huang (product similar to ephedrine) may cause adverse side effects in vulnerable persons.*
- Encourage parents and school dieticians to model and offer good nutritional choices (e.g., offer vegetables, fruits, and lower-fat foods in daily meals and snacks) *to assist child in accepting healthy foodstyles.*[23]
- Refer to community support groups or psychotherapy, as indicated, *to provide role models, address issues of body image or self-worth.*
- Provide contact number for dietitian/nutritionist and/or audiovisual materials, bibliography, reliable Internet sites for resources *to address ongoing nutrition needs and dietary changes.*
- Refer to NDs disturbed Body Image and ineffective Coping for additional interventions, as appropriate.

DOCUMENTATION FOCUS

Assessment/Reassessment
- Individual findings, including current weight, dietary pattern; perceptions of self, food, and eating; motivation for loss, support or feedback from SO(s).
- Results of laboratory and diagnostic testing.
- Results of weekly weigh-in.

Planning
- Plan of care, specific interventions, and who is involved in planning.
- Teaching plan.

Implementation/Evaluation
- Responses to interventions, weekly weight, and actions performed.
- Attainment or progress toward desired outcome(s).
- Modifications to plan of care.

Discharge Planning
- Long-term needs and who is responsible for actions to be taken.
- Specific referrals made.

References

1. Freemark, M. (2002, update 2006). Obesity. Retrieved July 2007 from www.emedicine.com/ped/topic1699.htm.
2. Gore, S. V. (1999). African-American women's perceptions of weight: Paradigm shift for advanced practice. *Holist Nurs Pract*, 13(4), 71–79.
3. Purnell, L. D., Paulanka, B. J. (1998). *Transcultural Health Care: A Culturally Competent Approach*. Philadelphia: F. A. Davis, 22.
4. Leininger, M. E. (1988). Transcultural eating patterns and nutrition: Transcultural nursing and anthropological perspectives. *Holist Nurs Pract*, 3(1), 16–25.
5. Fleury, J. (1991). Empowering potential: A theory of wellness motivation. *Nurs Res*, 40, 288.
6. Lawhorne, L. S. (2001). Altered nutritional status: Guideline. American Medical Directors Association (AMDA). Columbia, MD. Retrieved July 2007 from www.guideline.gov.
7. Engel, J. (2002). Dimensions of Nutritional Assessment. *Pocket Guide to Pediatric Assessment*. 4th ed. St. Louis, MO: Mosby, 58.
8. Stanley, M. (1999). The aging gastrointestinal system, with nutritional considerations. In Stanley, M., Beare, P. G. (eds). *Gerontological Nursing: A Health Promotion/Protection Approach*. 2d ed. Philadelphia: F. A. Davis.
9. Galletta, G. M. (2003). Obesity and weight control. Retrieved November 2003 from www.emedicine.com.
10. Lutz, C. A., Przytulski, K. R. (2001). *Nutrition and Diet Therapy*. 3d ed. Philadelphia: F. A. Davis.
11. Woods, A. (2003). X marks the spot: Understanding metabolic syndrome. *Nursing Made Incredibly Easy!*, 1(1), 19–26.
12. Nonas, C. A. (1998). A model for chronic obesity through dietary treatment. *J Am Diet Assoc* (suppl 2), S16.
13. Mathur, R. (2007). Obesity. Retrieved April 2007 from www.medicinet.com.
14. Anne Collins Weight Management Program. (2000–2007). Food portion size and calorie intake. Retrieved July 2007 from www.annecollins.com/food-portion-size-weight-management.htm.
15. U.S. Department of Health and Human Services, Department of Agriculture. The Dietary Guidelines for Americans, 2005. Retrieved July 2007 from www.heatlhierus.gov/dietaryguidelines.

  Cultural   Collaborative   Community/Home Care   Diagnostic Studies   Pediatric/Geriatric/Lifespan   Medications

16. U.S. Department of Health and Human Services, National Institutes of Heath. (2004). Weight and waist measurement. Fact sheet. Weight-control Information Network (WIN). Retrieved July 2007 from http://win.niddk.nih.gov/statistics/index.htm.

17. Lab test: Insulin. Retrieved July 2007 from www.labtestsonline.org/understanding/analytes/insulin/test.html.

18. Rippe, J. M., Hess, S. (1998). The role of physical activity in the prevention and management of obesity. *J Am Diet Assoc* (suppl 2), S9.

19. Miller, C. K., et al. (2007). A reduced-carbohydrate diet improves outcomes in patients with metabolic syndrome: A transitional study. *Top Clin Nutr*, 22(1), 82–91.

20. Wing, R., Phelan, S. (2005). Long-term weight loss maintenance. *Am J Clin Nutr*, 82(1 suppl), 222S–225S.

21. Meadows, M. (2006). Nutrition: Healthy eating. Retrieved April 2007 from www.medicinet.com.

22. Beauchamp-Johnson, B. M. (2006). Scale down bariatric surgery risks. *Nurs Manage*, 37(9), 27–32.

23. Doheny, K. (2006). Adults with children at home consume more fat, study shows. Retrieved January 2007 from www.webmd.com/content/Article/131/117923.htm.

readiness for enhanced Nutrition

DEFINITION: A pattern of nutrient intake that is sufficient for meeting metabolic needs and can be strengthened

RELATED FACTORS

To be developed by nurse researchers and submitted to NANDA

DEFINING CHARACTERISTICS

Subjective
Expresses knowledge of healthy food and fluid choices or willingness to enhance nutrition
Eats regularly
Attitude toward eating or drinking is congruent with health goals

Objective
Consumes adequate food or fluid
Follows an appropriate standard for intake (e.g., the food pyramid or American Diabetic Association Guidelines)
Safe preparation or storage for food or fluids

Sample Clinical Applications: As a health-seeking behavior the client may be healthy or this diagnosis can occur in any clinical condition

DESIRED OUTCOMES/EVALUATION CRITERIA

Sample NOC linkages:
Nutritional Status: Extent to which nutrients are available to meet metabolic needs
Knowledge: Diet: Extent of understanding conveyed about recommended diet
Weight Maintenance Behavior: Personal actions to maintain optimum body weight

(continues on page 564)

readiness for enhanced Nutrition (continued)

Client Will (Include Specific Time Frame)
• Demonstrate behaviors to attain or maintain appropriate weight.
• Be free of signs of malnutrition.
• Be able to safely prepare and store foods.

ACTIONS/INTERVENTIONS

Sample NIC linkages:
Nutritional Counseling: Use of an interactive helping process focusing on the need for diet modification
Teaching: Prescribed Diet: Preparing a patient to correctly follow a prescribed diet
Weight Management: Facilitating maintenance of optimal body weight and percent body fat

NURSING PRIORITY NO. 1

To determine current nutritional status and eating patterns:

- Assess client's knowledge of current nutritional needs and ways client is meeting these needs. *Provides baseline for further teaching or interventions.*
- Assess eating patterns and food and fluid choices in relation to any health-risk factors and health goals. *Helps to identify specific strengths and weaknesses that can be addressed.*
- Determine that age-related and developmental needs are met. *These factors are constantly present throughout the life span, although differing for each age group. For example, older adults need same nutrients as younger adults, but in smaller amounts and with attention to certain components, such as calcium, fiber, vitamins, protein, and water.[1] Infants/children require small meals and constant attention to needed nutrients for proper growth and development while dealing with child's food preferences and eating habits.[2]*
- Evaluate influence of cultural and religious factors *to determine what client considers to be normal dietary practice as well as to identify food preferences and restrictions, and eating patterns that can be strengthened or altered if indicated.[3]*
- Assess how client perceives food, food preparation, and the act of eating *to determine client's feeling and emotions regarding food (including the use of food for celebrations or as a reward) and self-image.*
- Ascertain occurrence of or potential for negative feedback from SO(s). *May reveal control issues that could impact client's motivation for and commitment to change.*
- Determine patterns of hunger and satiety. *Helps identify strengths and weaknesses in eating patterns and potential for change (e.g., person predisposed to weight gain may need a different time for a big meal than evening or may need teaching as to what foods reinforce feelings of satisfaction).*
- Assess client's ability to shop for, safely store, and prepare foods *to determine if health information or financial resources might be needed.*

NURSING PRIORITY NO. 2

To assist client/SO(s) to develop plan to meet individual needs:

- Determine motivation and expectation for change. *Motivation to improve and high expectations can encourage client to make changes that will improve his or her life. However, presence of unrealistic expectations may hamper efforts. Client may actually be satisfied with current nutritional state and eating behaviors or may be changing some aspect of food intake or preparation in response to new dietary information or change in health status.*

- Assist in obtaining or review results of individual testing, such as weight and height, body fat percent, lipids, glucose, complete blood count (CBC), total protein, and so forth, *to determine that client is healthy and/or identify dietary changes that may be helpful in attaining health goals.*[5]

- Encourage client's beneficial eating patterns and habits (e.g., controlling portion size, eating regular meals, reducing high-fat, high-sugar, or fast-food intake; following specific dietary program and drinking water and healthy beverages). *Provides reinforcement and supports client's efforts to incorporate changes into lifestyle habits and continue with new behaviors.*[6,7]

- Provide instruction and reinforce information regarding special needs. *Client/SO may benefit from or desire assistance in learning new eating habits or following medically prescribed diets (e.g., very low-calorie diet, tube-feedings, diabetic or renal dialysis diet).*[4]

- Encourage the client to carefully read food labels, instructing in meaning of labeling, as indicated, *to assist client/SO in making healthful choices.*[7]

- Review safe preparation and storage of food *to maintain maximal nutrient value and avoid foodborne illnesses.*

- Consult with or refer to nutritionist/physician, as indicated. *Client/SO may benefit from advice regarding specific nutrition or dietary issues or may require regular follow-up to determine that needs are being met when following a medically prescribed program.*

- Develop a system for self-monitoring *to provide a sense of control and enable the client to track own progress as well as to assist in making informed choices.*[6]

NURSING PRIORITY NO. 3

To promote optimum wellness (Teaching/Discharge Considerations):

- Review individual risk factors and provide additional information or response to concerns. *Assists the client with motivation and decision making.*

- Provide bibliotherapy and help client/SO(s) identify and evaluate resources they can access on their own. *Reinforces learning, allows client to progress at own pace, and encourages client to be responsible for own learning. When referencing the Internet and nontraditional or unproven resources, the individual must exercise some restraint and determine the reliability of the source and information before acting on it.*

- Encourage variety and moderation in dietary plan *to decrease boredom and encourage client in efforts to make healthy choices about eating and food.*

- Discuss use of nutritional supplements, over-the-counter (OTC) and herbal products. *Confusion may exist regarding the need for and use of these products in a balanced dietary regimen.*

- Assist client to identify and access community resources, when indicated. *May benefit from assistance, such as food stamps, budget counseling, Meals on Wheels, community food banks, and other assistance programs.*

DOCUMENTATION FOCUS

Assessment/Reassessment
- Baseline information, client's perception of need.
- Nutritional intake and metabolic needs.
- Motivation and expectations for change.

Planning
• Plan of care, specific interventions, and who is involved in planning.
• Teaching plan.

Implementation/Evaluation
• Client's responses to interventions, teaching, and actions performed.
• Attainment or progress toward desired outcome(s).
• Modifications to plan of care.

Discharge Planning
• Long-term needs and actions to be taken.
• Support systems available, specific referrals made, and who is responsible for actions to be taken.

References

1. American Dietetic Association. (2005). Nutrition across the spectrum of aging. *J Am Diet Assoc*, 105(4), 616–633.
2. Engel, J. (2002). *Pocket Guide to Pediatric Assessment.* 4th ed. St. Louis, MO: Mosby.
3. Purnell, L. D., Paulanka, B. J. (1998). *Transcultural Health Care: A Culturally Competent Approach.* Philadelphia: F. A. Davis.
4. Pignone, M. P. (2003). Counseling to promote a healthy diet in adults: A summary of the evidence for the U.S. Preventive Services Task Force. *Am J Prev Med*, 24(1), 75–92.
5. Vogelzang, J. L. (2003). Making nutrition sense from OASIS. *Home Healthcare Nurse*, 21(9), 592–600.
6. Anne Collins Weight Management Program. (2000–2007). Food portion size and calorie intake. Retrieved July 2007 from www.annecollins.com/food-portion-size-weight-management.htm.
7. U.S. Department of Health and Human Services, Department of Agriculture. *Dietary Guidelines for Americans,* 2005. Retrieved July 2007 from www.healthierus.gov/dietaryguidelines.

risk for imbalanced Nutrition: more than body requirements

DEFINITION: At risk for an intake of nutrients that exceeds metabolic needs

RISK FACTORS

Dysfunctional eating patterns; pairing food with other activities; eating in response to external cues (e.g., time of day, social situation) or internal cues other than hunger (e.g., anxiety); concentrating food intake at end of day

Parental obesity

Rapid transition across growth percentiles in children; reported use of solid food as major food source before 5 months of age

Higher baseline weight at beginning of each pregnancy

Observed use of food as reward or comfort measure

[Frequent, repeated dieting]

[Alteration in usual activity patterns; sedentary lifestyle]

[Majority of foods consumed are concentrated, high-calorie or fat sources]

[Lower socioeconomic status]

NOTE: A risk diagnosis is not evidenced by signs and symptoms, as the problem has not occurred; rather, nursing interventions are directed at prevention.

Sample Clinical Applications: Bulimia nervosa, diseases requiring long-term steroid use (e.g., chronic obstructive pulmonary disease [COPD]), conditions associated with immobility (e.g., stroke, paralysis, multiple sclerosis [MS], amputation), Alzheimer's disease, depression, developmental delay

DESIRED OUTCOMES/EVALUATION CRITERIA

Sample NOC linkages:
Weight Maintenance Behavior: Personal actions to maintain optimum body weight
Knowledge: Diet: Extent of understanding conveyed about recommended diet
Nutritional Status: Nutrient Intake: Adequacy of usual pattern of nutrient intake

Client/Caregiver Will (Include Specific Time Frame)
• Verbalize understanding of body and energy needs.
• Identify lifestyle and cultural factors that predispose to obesity.
• Demonstrate behaviors, lifestyle changes to reduce risk factors.
• Acknowledge responsibility for own actions and need to "act, not react" to stressful situations.

Sample NOC linkages:
Weight: Body Mass: Extent to which body weight, muscle, and fat are congruent to height, frame, gender, and age

Client Will (Include Specific Time Frame)
• Maintain weight at a satisfactory level for height, body build, age, and gender.

ACTIONS/INTERVENTIONS

Sample NIC linkages:
Weight Management: Facilitating maintenance of optimal body weight and percent body fat
Nutritional Counseling: Use of an interactive helping process focusing on the need for diet modification
Nutrition Management: Assisting with or providing a balanced dietary intake of foods and fluids

NURSING PRIORITY NO. 1

To assess potential factors for undesired weight gain:

• Note presence of factors or conditions that can contribute to weight gain or obesity (e.g., familial pattern of obesity; decreased basal metabolic rate or hypothyroidism; type 2 diabetes; pregnancy; menopause; chronic disorders such as heart, kidney disease, chronic pain; food or other substance addictions; stressful and/or sedentary lifestyle; depression; use of certain medications such as steroids, birth control pills; physical disabilities or limitations; lack of socioeconomic resources for obtaining or preparing healthy foods) *to determine treatment needs and possible behavioral changes for weight management.*[7]

∞ • Note client's particular situation and number of risk factors *to help determine level of concern. For example, a high correlation exists between obesity in parents and children, which may reflect (in part) family patterns of food intake, exercise, selection of leisure activity (e.g., amount of television watching), family and cultural patterns of food selection. Also family studies (e.g., twin and adoption) suggest genetic factors.*[1,2]

⊕ • Evaluate familial and cultural influences *that often place high importance on food and food-related events, or groups that place importance on large body size or frame of reference for "normal body weight" is higher than standard indicators (e.g., athletes such as football players or wrestlers; African American women, Samoan people, or Cuban children).*[2]

∞ • Note client's age and activity level and exercise patterns *to identify areas where changes might be useful to prevent obesity and promote health. For example, older adults need same nutrients as younger adults but in smaller amounts and with attention to certain components, such as calcium, fiber, vitamins, protein, and water.*[4] *Infants/children require small meals and constant attention to needed nutrients for proper growth and development while dealing with child's food preferences and eating habits.*[5]

∞ • Calculate growth percentiles in infants/children using growth chart *to identify deviations from the norm.*

⊘ • Review laboratory data (e.g., growth hormones, thyroid, glucose and insulin levels, lipids, total protein) *to determine health status and presence of endocrine or metabolic disorders, thus dictating specific dietary needs.*[6]

• Assess eating patterns in relation to risk for obesity and disease conditions. *Food choices and amounts of certain food groups are known to impact health (in both children and adults) and cause or exacerbate disease conditions (e.g., heart disease, diabetes, hypertension, gallstones, colon cancer).*[3,8]

• Determine patterns of hunger and satiety. *Eating patterns often differ in those who are predisposed to weight gain and may include such factors as skipping meals (decreases the metabolic rate), fasting and binging (causes wide fluctuations in glucose and insulin), eating or overeating in response to emotions (e.g., loneliness, anger, happiness).*

• Note history of dieting and kinds of diets used. *Client may have tried multiple diets with varying degrees of success in the past, but often has history of regaining weight ("yo-yo" dieting) or finding that diets are not desirable.*

🏠 • Determine whether binging or purging (bulimia) is a factor *to identify potential for eating disorder requiring in-depth intervention.*

• Identify personality characteristics (e.g., rigid thinking patterns, external locus of control, negative body image or self-concept, negative monologues [self-talk], and dissatisfaction with life) *that are often associated with obesity.*

• Determine psychological significance of food to the client (e.g., derives love and comfort from food, uses food to escape deep unhappiness, eats when stressed or anxious).

• Listen to concerns and assess motivation to prevent weight gain. *If client's concern regarding weight control are motivated for reasons other than personal well-being (e.g., partner's expectations or demands), the likelihood of success is decreased.*

NURSING PRIORITY NO. 2

To assist client to develop preventive program to avoid weight gain:

• Assess client's knowledge of nutritional needs and ways client is meeting these needs. *Provides baseline for further teaching and/or interventions.*

- Provide information, as indicated, on nutrition, taking into account client's age and developmental stage (e.g., toddler, teenager, pregnant woman, elderly person with chronic disease), physical health and activity tolerance, financial and socioeconomic factors, and client's/SO's potential for management of risk factors.
- Review guidelines for achieving and maintaining healthy body weight:[9,10]
  Eat from each food group (fruits, vegetables, whole grains, lean meats, low-fat dairy and oils).
  Start with small changes, such as adding one more vegetable/day, introducing healthier versions of favorite foods.
  Choose "nutrient-dense" forms of foods that provide substantial amounts of fiber, vitamins, electrolytes, and minerals.
  Avoid saturated fats, trans fats, cholesterol, salt (sodium), and added sugars.
  Focus on portion sizes: calorie-dense foods (high in fat and/or sugar) should be eaten in smaller quantities, whereas high-fiber foods can be eaten in larger quantities.
  Discuss smart snacks (e.g., low-fat yogurt with fruit, nuts, apple slices with peanut butter, low-fat string cheese) *to assist client in finding healthy options.*
- Review healthy eating patterns or habits (e.g., eating slowly and only when hungry; stopping when full; avoiding skipping meals; eating foods from every food group; using smaller plates; chewing food thoroughly; making healthy food choices even when eating fast food). *Most fast foods and packaged foods are highly processed or are high in sugar, fat, and calories.*
- Encourage involvement in planned exercises of client's choice and within physical abilities. Refer to formal exercise program, if desired. *Promotes incorporation of active lifestyle.*[11]
- Assist client to develop strategies for reducing stressful thinking or actions. *Promotes relaxation, reduces likelihood of stress or comfort eating.*

NURSING PRIORITY NO. 3

To promote wellness (Teaching/Discharge Considerations):

- Provide information about individual risk factors *to enhance decision making and support motivation.*
- Consult with nutritionist *to address client-specific issues (e.g., food groups, dietary restrictions that might be needed for certain chronic diseases such as kidney disease or diabetes).*
- Provide information to new mothers about nutrition for developing babies *to reduce potential for childhood obesity related to lack of knowledge.*
- Encourage parents and school dietitians to model and offer good nutritional choices (e.g., offer vegetables, fruits, and lower-fat foods in daily meals and snacks) *to assist child in accepting healthy foodstyles.*[2,3]
- Encourage the client to make a commitment to lead an active life, to manage food habits, and to develop a system for self-monitoring *to provide a sense of control and assist with making choices.*
- Provide bibliography including reliable Internet sites for resources *to reinforce learning, address ongoing nutrition needs, support informed decision making.*
- Refer to support groups and appropriate community resources for behavior modification, as indicated. *Provides role models and assistance for making lifestyle changes.*

DOCUMENTATION FOCUS

Assessment/Reassessment

- Findings related to individual situation, risk factors, current caloric intake and dietary pattern; activity level.
- Baseline height and weight, growth percentile.
- Results of laboratory tests.
- Motivation to reduce risks or prevent weight problems.

Planning

- Plan of care and who is involved in the planning.
- Teaching plan.

Implementation/Evaluation

- Response to interventions, teaching, and actions performed.
- Attainment or progress toward desired outcome(s).
- Modifications to plan of care.

Discharge Planning

- Long-term needs, noting who is responsible for actions to be taken.
- Specific referrals made.

References

1. Freemark, M. (2002, update 2006). Obesity. Retrieved July 2007 from www.emedicine.com/ped/topic1699.htm.
2. Purnell, L. D., Paulanka, B. J. (1998). *Transcultural Health Care: A Culturally Competent Approach*. Philadelphia: F. A. Davis.
3. Galletta, G. M., Khandwala, H. M. (2005). Obesity. Retrieved October 2009 from www.emedicine.com.
4. American Dietetic Association. (2005). Nutrition across the spectrum of aging. *J Am Diet Assoc*, 105(4), 616s–633s.
5. Engel, J. (2002). *Pocket Guide to Pediatric Assessment*. 4th ed. St. Louis, MO: Mosby.
6. Vogelzang, J. L. (2003). Making nutrition sense from OASIS. *Home Healthcare Nurse*, 21(9), 592–600.
7. Mathur, R. (2007). Obesity. Retrieved April 2007 from www.medicinet.com.
8. Doheny, K. (2006). Adults with children at home consume more fat, study shows. Retrieved January 2007 from www.webmd.com/content/Article/131/117923.htm.
9. Anne Collins Weight Management Program. (2000–2007). Food portion size and calorie intake. Retrieved July 2007 from www.annecollins.com/food-portion-size-weight-management.htm.
10. U.S. Department of Health and Human Services, Department of Agriculture. *Dietary Guidelines for Americans,* 2005. Retrieved July 2007 from www.healthierus.gov/dietaryguidelines.
11. Rippe, J. M., Hess, S. (1998). The role of physical activity in the prevention and management of obesity. *J Am Diet Assoc*, 98(2 suppl), S31–S38.

impaired Oral Mucous Membrane

DEFINITION: Disruption of the lips and/or soft tissue of the oral cavity

RELATED FACTORS

Dehydration; NPO for more than 24 hours; malnutrition

Decreased salivation; medication side effects; diminished hormone levels (women); mouth breathing

Deficient knowledge of appropriate oral hygiene

Ineffective oral hygiene; barriers to oral self-care/professional care

Mechanical factors (e.g., ill-fitting dentures; braces; tubes [endotracheal/nasogastric], surgery in oral cavity); loss of supportive structures; trauma; cleft lip/palate

Chemical irritants (e.g., alcohol, tobacco, acidic foods, regular use of inhalers or other noxious agents)

Chemotherapy; immunosuppression; immunocompromised; decreased platelets; infection; radiation therapy

Stress; depression

DEFINING CHARACTERISTICS

Subjective
Xerostomia [dry mouth]
Oral pain or discomfort
Reports bad taste in mouth; diminished taste; difficulty eating or swallowing

Objective
Coated tongue; smooth atrophic; geographic tongue
Gingival or mucosal pallor
Stomatitis; hyperemia; gingival hyperplasia; macroplasia; vesicles; nodules; papules
White patches or plaques, spongy patches; white curdlike exudate
Oral lesions or ulcers; fissures; bleeding; cheilitis; desquamation; mucosal denudation
Purulent drainage or exudates; presence of pathogens; enlarged tonsils
Edema
Halitosis
Gingival recession, pocketing deeper than 4 mm; [carious teeth]
Red or bluish masses (e.g., hemangiomas)
Difficult speech

Sample Clinical Applications: Oral trauma, cancer, chemo-/radiation therapy, malnutrition, infection, oral surgery, cleft lip/palate, conditions requiring endotracheal (ET) intubation (e.g., brain injury, stroke, spinal cord injury [SCI], chronic obstructive pulmonary disease [COPD], acute respiratory distress syndrome, amyotrophic lateral sclerosis [ALS])

(continues on page 572)

impaired Oral Mucous Membrane (continued)
DESIRED OUTCOMES/EVALUATION CRITERIA

Sample **NOC** linkages:
Self-Care: Oral Hygiene: Ability to care for own mouth and teeth independently with or without assistive device
Tissue Integrity: Skin & Mucous Membranes: Structural intactness and normal physiological function of skin and mucous membranes

Client/Caregiver Will (Include Specific Time Frame)
• Verbalize understanding of causative factors.
• Identify specific interventions to promote healthy oral mucosa.
• Demonstrate techniques to restore and maintain integrity of oral mucosa.

Sample **NOC** linkages:
Oral Hygiene: Condition of the mouth, teeth, gums, and tongue

Client Will (Include Specific Time Frame)
• Report or demonstrate a decrease in signs/symptoms as noted in Defining Characteristics.

ACTIONS/INTERVENTIONS

Sample **NIC** linkages:
Oral Health Restoration: Promotion of healing for a patient who has an oral mucosa or dental lesion
Oral Health Maintenance: Maintenance and promotion of oral hygiene and dental health for the patient at risk for developing oral or dental lesions
Oral Health Promotion: Promotion of oral hygiene and dental care for a patient with normal oral and dental health

NURSING PRIORITY NO. 1

To identify causative/contributing factors affecting oral health:

• Note presence of conditions (e.g., oral infections; facial fractures, head or neck cancer radiation; or systemic diseases such as Sjögren syndrome, systemic lupus erythematosus [SLE], rheumatoid arthritis, scleroderma, sarcoidosis, amyloidosis, hypothyroidism, diabetes) *that can affect health of oral tissues.*[10-12]

• Determine type of oral mucous membrane problem (e.g., severe or chronic dry mouth [xerostomia] associated with lack of saliva; abnormal tongue surfaces; gingivitis or periodontal disease; ulcerations or other lesions) *that may cause inflammation affecting ability to eat or more serious complications.*[1]

• Investigate reports of oral pain to determine possible source (e.g., oral lesion, gum disease, tooth abscess) *to identify needed interventions and reduce risk of complications such as systemic infection.*[1]

• Collaborate in evaluating abnormal lesions of mouth, tongue, and cheeks (e.g., white or red patches, ulcers). *White ulcerated spots may be canker sores, especially in children; white curd patches (thrush) are common in infants. Reddened, swollen bleeding gums may indicate infection, poor nutrition, or poor oral hygiene. A red tongue may be related to vitamin deficiencies.*[2] *Malignant lesions are more common in elderly than younger persons (especially if there is a history of smoking or alcohol use), and many elderly persons rarely visit a dentist.*[3]

- Note use of tobacco (including smokeless) and alcohol, *which may predispose mucosa to effects of nutritional deficiencies, infection, cell damage, and cancer.*[10,12]
- Observe for chipped or sharp-edged teeth. Note fit of dentures or other prosthetic devices when used. *Factors that increase the risk of injury to delicate tissues.*
- Review client's medications and evaluate possibility of side effects. *Many drugs (e.g., anticholinergics, antidepressants, anti-Parkinson's drugs, antihistamines or decongestants, urinary antispastics, antipsychotics, diuretics, hypnotics, systemic bronchodilators, muscle relaxants, reserpine, laxatives, beta-blockers, narcotics) can impair salivary function and promote xerostomia.*[8,10]
- Determine nutrition and fluid intake and reported changes (e.g., avoiding eating, reports change in taste, chews painstakingly, swallows numerous times for even small bites, unexplained weight loss). *Malnutrition and dehydration are associated with problems with oral mucous membranes.*[6,10]
- Determine allergies to foods, drugs, or other substances *that may result in irritation of oral mucosa.*
- Review oral hygiene practices, noting frequency and type (e.g., brushing, flossing, water appliances). Inquire about client's professional dental care, regularity and date of last dental examination.
- Evaluate client's ability to provide self-care and availability of necessary equipment and assistance. *Client's age (very young or elderly) impacts ability to provide self-care, as well as current health issues (e.g., disease condition or treatment, weakness), and client's habits and lifestyle.*[4]

NURSING PRIORITY NO. 2

To correct identified/developing problems:

- Collaborate in treatment of underlying conditions (e.g., structural defects, infections) *that may correct or limit problem with oral tissues.*
- Routinely inspect oral cavity and recommend client establish regular schedule of self-inspection, such as when performing oral care activities. *Can help with early identification and management of mucous membrane concerns.*
- Adjust medication regimen *to reduce use of drugs with potential for causing or exacerbating painful dry mouth.*
- Administer medications, as ordered, (e.g., NSAIDs, antibiotics, antifungal agents, including antimicrobial mouth rinse or spray) *to treat oral infections or reduce potential for bacterial overgrowth.*[8–10]
- Provide anesthetic lozenges or analgesics such as Stanford solution, viscous lidocaine (Xylocaine), sulfacrate slurry, as indicated *to provide protection and reduce oral discomfort or pain.*[10]
- Discuss safe use of products used to treat xerostomia (e.g., artificial salivas mimic natural saliva to relieve soft tissue discomfort, are more effective and longer lasting than simple rinses but do not stimulate natural salivary gland production; cholinergic agonist preparations [e.g., pilocarpine, cevimeline] do stimulate saliva production).[13]
- Encourage use of tart, sour foods and drinks; chewing sugar-free gum or sucking hard candy to *stimulate saliva.*[11] Use citrus foods and liquids with caution *because may irritate mucosa and increase pain.*[13]
- Provide or encourage regular oral care (including after meals and at bedtime, and frequently to critically ill client):
  Use water, or rinses of normal saline or sodium bicarbonate solutions. *Note: Other rinses, including those containing chlorhexidine or sucralfate, available by prescription, and*

---

glutamine, an over-the-counter (OTC) amino acid typically sold in powder form, can be costly, and studies have not demonstrated healing with their use.[10]

Avoid mouthwashes containing alcohol *(drying effect)* or hydrogen peroxide *(drying and foul tasting).*[5,13]

Use soft-bristle brush or sponge/cotton-tip applicators to cleanse teeth and tongue. *Brushing the teeth is the most effective way of reducing plaque and manage periodontal disease.*[6]

Floss gently or use Waterpik *to remove food particles that promote bacterial growth and gum disease.*

Use foam sticks *to swab mouth, tongue, and gums when client has no teeth.*

Use lemon/glycerin swabs with caution. *Glycerin absorbs water and actually dries the oral cavity; can result in decreased salivary amylase, as well as erosion of tooth enamel.*[6,13]

Provide or assist with denture care, as needed. *Evidence-based protocol for denture care states that dentures are to be removed and scrubbed at least once daily, removed and rinsed after every meal, and kept in an appropriate solution at night.*[7]

- Change position of ET tube or airway every 8 hours and as needed when client is on ventilator *to minimize pressure on fragile tissues and improve access to all areas of oral cavity.*

- Suction oral cavity *if client cannot swallow secretions. Saliva contains digestive enzymes that may be erosive to exposed tissues (such as might occur because of heavy drooling following radical neck surgery).*

- Use gentle low-intensity suctioning *to reduce risk of aspiration in intubated clients or those with decreased gag or swallow reflexes.*[8]

- Lubricate lips and provide commercially prepared oral lubricant solution, when indicated. Encourage use of chewing gum, hard candy, and so forth, *to stimulate flow of saliva to neutralize acids and limit bacterial growth.*[10]

- Encourage adequate fluids *to prevent dehydration and oral dryness, and limit bacterial overgrowth.*[8]

- Suggest use of vaporizer or room humidifier *to increase humidity if client is mouth breather or ambient humidity is low.*[13]

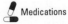 - Implement diet modifications, as indicated:[10]

Offer foods with adequate nutrients and vitamins to promote healing *when deficits are impairing health of oral tissues.*

Avoid sharp, hard, coarse, spicy, salty, and acidic foods *that can irritate or damage fragile mucosa and existing ulcers.*

Include bland, low-acid, high-protein foods (e.g., milk shakes, bananas, applesauce, mashed potatoes, cooked cereals, soft-boiled or scrambled eggs, cottage cheese, macaroni and cheese, pudding, custard, and gelatin) *that are nutrient-dense and easy to eat.*

Provide moderate temperature foods and fluids, soft or pureed foods, popsicles, frozen yogurt or ice cream *that may be soothing to sensitive mucosa.*

Drink liquids with meals and use gravies and sauces *to make food easier to swallow.*[13]

Avoid dry foods, such as crackers, cookies, and toast, or soften them with liquids before eating.[13]

NURSING PRIORITY NO. 3

To promote wellness (Teaching/Discharge Considerations):

- Recommend regular dental checkups and care, and episodic evaluation of oral health prior to certain medical treatments (e.g., chemotherapy, radiation) *to maintain oral health and reduce risks associated with impaired tissues.*[8]

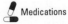 - Review current oral hygiene concerns and provide informational resources including reliable Web sites about oral health *to reinforce learning, encourage proper care.*

- Promote general health and mental health habits *to prevent negative effects that altered immune response can exert on oral mucosa.*
- Provide nutritional information *to correct deficiencies, reduce mucosal inflammation or gum disease, and prevent dental caries.*
- Instruct parents in oral hygiene techniques and proper dental care for infants/children (e.g., safe use of pacifier, brushing of teeth and gums, avoidance of sweet drinks and candy, recognition and treatment of thrush). *Encourages early initiation of good oral health practices and timely intervention for treatable problems.*
- Emphasize importance of limiting nighttime regimen of bottle of milk for infant in bed. Suggest pacifier or use of water during night *to prevent bottle syndrome with decaying of teeth.*
- Discuss special mouth care required during and after illness or trauma, or following surgical repair (e.g., cleft lip/palate, facial fractures, jaw surgery) *to facilitate healing.*
- Recommend avoiding alcohol, smoking or chewing tobacco, *which can contribute to mucosal inflammation.*
- Identify need for and demonstrate use of special appliances (e.g., power toothbrushes, dental water jets, flossing instruments, applicators). *Enhances independence in self-care.*
- Identify community resources (e.g., low-cost dental clinics, smoking cessation resources, cancer information services or support group, Meals on Wheels, food stamps, home-care aide) *to meet individual needs.*

DOCUMENTATION FOCUS

Assessment/Reassessment
- Condition of oral mucous membranes, routine oral care habits and interferences.
- Availability of oral care equipment and products.
- Knowledge of proper oral hygiene and care.
- Availability and use of resources.

Planning
- Plan of care and who is involved in planning.
- Teaching plan.

Implementation/Evaluation
- Responses to interventions, teaching, and actions performed.
- Attainment or progress toward desired outcome(s).
- Modifications to plan of care.

Discharge Planning
- Long-term needs and who is responsible for actions to be taken.
- Specific referrals made, resources for special appliances.

References

1. Carl, W., Havens, J. (2000). The cancer patient with severe mucositis. *Cur Rev Pain*, 4(3), 197–202.
2. Engel, J. (2002). *Pocket Guide to Pediatric Assessment.* 4th ed. St. Louis, MO: Mosby, 155–156.
3. Aubertin, M. A. (1997). Oral cancer screening in the elderly: The home healthcare nurse's role. *Home Healthcare Nurse*, 15(9), 594–604.
4. White, R. (2000). Nurse assessment of oral health: A review of practice and education. *Br J Nurs*, 9(5), 260–266.
5. Winslow, E. H. (1994). Don't use H_2O_2 for oral care. *Am J Nurse*, 94(3), 19.

6. Stiefel, K. A. (2000). Improving oral hygiene for the seriously ill patient: Implementing research-based practice. *Medsurg Nurs*, 9(1), 40–43, 46.
7. Curzio, J., McCowan, M. (2000). Getting research into practice: Developing oral hygiene standards. *Br J Nurs*, 9(7), 434–438.
8. Trieger, N. (2004). Oral care in the intensive care unit. *Am J Crit Care*, 13(1), 24.
9. Munro, C., Grap, M. J. (2004). Oral health and care in the intensive care unit: State of science. *Am J Crit Care*, 13(1), 25–33.
10. Dahlin, C. (2004). Oral complications at the end of life. *Am J Nurs*, 104(7), 40–47.
11. Stegeman, C. A. (2005). Oral manifestations of diabetes. *Home Healthcare Nurse*, 23(4), 233–240.
12. Oral cancer. (2006). Retrieved April 2007 from www.medicinenet.com.
13. McKee, C. D. (1999). Xerostomia. Retrieved August 2007 from http://findarticles.com/p/articles/mi_m3374/is_7_21/ai_54563620/pg_1.

acute Pain

DEFINITION: Unpleasant sensory and emotional experience arising from actual or potential tissue damage or described in terms of such damage (International Association for the Study of Pain); sudden or slow onset of any intensity, from mild to severe, with an anticipated or predictable end and a duration of less than 6 months

RELATED FACTORS

Injuring agents (biological, chemical, physical, psychological)

DEFINING CHARACTERISTICS

Subjective
Verbal report of pain; coded report [may be less from clients younger than age 40, men, and some cultural groups]
Changes in appetite

Objective
Observed evidence of pain
Guarding behavior; protective gestures; positioning to avoid pain
Facial mask; sleep disturbance (eyes lack luster, beaten look, fixed or scattered movement, grimace)
Expressive behavior (e.g., restlessness, moaning, crying, vigilance, irritability, sighing)
Distraction behavior (e.g., pacing, seeking out other people and/or activities, repetitive activities)
Change in muscle tone (may span from listless [flaccid] to rigid)
Diaphoresis; change in blood pressure, heart rate, or respiratory rate; pupillary dilation
Self-focusing; narrowed focus (altered time perception, impaired thought process, reduced interaction with people and environment)

Sample Clinical Applications: Traumatic injuries, surgical procedures, infections, cancer, burns, skin lesions, gangrene, thrombophlebitis, pulmonary embolus, neuralgia

DESIRED OUTCOMES/EVALUATION CRITERIA

Sample (NOC) linkages:
Pain Level: Severity of observed or reported pain
Pain Control: Personal actions to control pain
Pain: Adverse Psychological Response: Severity of observed or reported adverse cognitive and emotional responses to physical pain

Client Will (Include Specific Time Frame)
• Report pain is relieved or controlled.
• Follow prescribed pharmacological regimen.
• Verbalize methods that provide relief.
• Demonstrate use of relaxation skills and diversional activities as indicated for individual situation.

ACTIONS/INTERVENTIONS

Sample (NIC) linkages:
Pain Management: Alleviation of pain or a reduction in pain to a level of comfort that is acceptable to the patient
Analgesic Administration: Use of pharmacological agents to reduce or eliminate pain
Environmental Management: Comfort: Manipulation of the patient's surroundings for promotion of optimal comfort

NURSING PRIORITY NO. 1

To assess etiology/precipitating contributory factors:

● Note client's age, developmental level, and current condition (e.g., infant/child, critically ill, ventilated, sedated, or cognitively impaired client) *affecting ability to report pain parameters.*[13,14]
● Obtain client's assessment of pain to include location, characteristics, onset, duration, frequency, quality, intensity. Identify precipitating or aggravating and relieving factors.
● Use pain rating scale appropriate for age and cognition (e.g., 0 to 10 scale, facial expression or Wong-Baker faces pain scale [pediatric, nonverbal], adolescent pediatric pain tool [APPT], pain assessment scale for seniors with limited ability to communicate [PACSLAC]; behavioral pain scale [BPS]).[1,2,17]
● Note possible pathophysiological and psychological causes of pain (e.g., inflammation, tissue trauma, burns, fractures, surgery; infections, heart attack, angina; abdominal conditions [e.g. appendicitis, cholecystitis] grief, fear, anxiety, depression, personality disorders). *Acute pain is that which follows an injury, trauma, or procedure such as surgery, or occurs suddenly with the onset of a painful condition (e.g., herniated disk, migraine headache, pancreatitis).*[3,15]
● Note anatomical location of surgical incisions or procedures. *This can influence the amount of postoperative pain experienced; for example, vertical or diagonal incisions are more painful than transverse or S-shaped. Presence of known and unknown complication(s) may make the pain more severe than anticipated.*[4,5,10]
● Determine history or presence of chronic conditions (e.g., multiple sclerosis [MS], stroke, diabetes, depression) *that may also cause pain, or be associated with an exacerbation of pain symptoms, or interfere with accurate assessment of acute pain.*[2]

- Assess client's perceptions of pain, along with behaviors and cultural expectations regarding pain. *Client's perception of and expression of pain is influenced by age, developmental stage, underlying problem causing pain, cognitive, behavioral and sociocultural factors.*[2]
- Note client's attitude toward pain and use of specific pain medications, including any history of substance abuse. *Client may have beliefs restricting use of medications, or may have a high tolerance for drugs because of recent or current use, or may not be able to take pain medications at all if participating in a substance abuse recovery program.*
- Note client's locus of control (internal or external). *Individuals with external locus of control may take little or no responsibility for pain management.*
- Determine medications (e.g., skeletal muscle relaxants, antibiotics, antidepressants, anticoagulants), alcohol or other drugs currently being used, and any medication allergies *that affect choice of analgesics.*[4,5]
- Collaborate with other medical providers in pain assessment, including neurological and psychological factors (pain inventory, psychological interview) as appropriate when pain persists.
- Assist with and review results of laboratory tests and diagnostic studies depending on results of history and physical examination.

NURSING PRIORITY NO. 2

To evaluate client's response to pain:

- Perform pain assessment each time pain occurs. Document and investigate changes from previous reports and evaluate results of pain interventions *to demonstrate improvement in status or to identify worsening of underlying condition/developing complications.*[6,16]
- Accept client's description of pain. Be aware of the terminology client uses for pain experience (e.g., young child may say "owie"; elderly may say "it aches so bad"). *Pain is a subjective experience and cannot be felt by others.*[2] *Note: Some elderly clients experience a reduction in perception of pain or have difficulty localizing or describing pain, and pain may be manifested as a change in behavior (e.g., restlessness, increased confusion or wandering, acting out).*
- Note cultural influences affecting pain response. *Verbal or behavioral cues may have no direct relationship to the degree of pain perceived (e.g., client may deny pain even when feeling uncomfortable, or reactions can be stoic or exaggerated, reflecting cultural and familial norms). These factors affect client's and caregiver's attitudes and beliefs regarding the pain experience, expressions of pain, and expectations regarding pain management.*[2,9,14]
- Observe nonverbal cues (e.g., how client walks, holds body, guarding behaviors; sleeplessness; grimacing facial expressions; distraction behaviors, narrowed focus; crying, poor feeding, lethargy in infants). Ask others who know client well (e.g., spouse, parent) to identify behaviors that may indicate pain in persons who cannot communicate verbally. *Helpful in recognizing presence of pain; however, cues not congruent with verbal reports indicate need for further evaluation.*[1–6,9]
- Assess for referred pain, as appropriate, *to help determine possibility of underlying condition or organ dysfunction causing pain to be perceived in area other than site of the problem.*
- Monitor vital signs during episodes of pain. *Blood pressure, respiratory and heart rate are usually altered in acute pain.*[1,2,4,5]
- Ascertain client's knowledge of and expectations about pain management. *Provides baseline for interventions and teaching, provides opportunity to allay common fears and misconceptions (e.g., fears about addiction to opiates, belief that complete pain relief is possible in every situation) or to address expected side effects of analgesics (e.g., constipation).*[2]

- Review client's previous experiences with pain and methods found either helpful or unhelpful for pain control in the past. *Useful in determining appropriate interventions.*
- Be aware of client's "Right to Treatment" *that includes prevention of or adequate relief from pain*[7] *and that failure to meet the standard of assessing for pain can be considered negligence.*[8]

NURSING PRIORITY NO. 3

To assist client to explore methods for alleviation/control of pain:

- Determine client's acceptable level of pain and pain control goal. *Client may not be 100% pain free but may feel that a "3" is a manageable level of discomfort, while another may require medication for pain at the same level, because the experience is subjective.*[1,2,4–6,9]
- Determine factors in client's lifestyle (e.g., alcohol or other drug use or abuse) that can affect responses to analgesics and/or choice of interventions for pain management.[14]
- Note when pain occurs (e.g., only with ambulation, every evening) *to medicate prophylactically as appropriate.*
- Collaborate in treatment of underlying condition or disease processes causing pain and proactive management of pain (e.g., epidural analgesia, nerve blockade for postoperative pain, surgical plication of a nerve, implantation of nerve stimulator).
- Work with client *to prevent rather than "chase" pain.* Use flow sheet to document pain, therapeutic interventions, response, and length of time before pain recurs. Instruct client to report pain as soon as it begins, *because timely intervention is more likely to be successful in alleviating pain.*[2,11]
- Encourage verbalization of feelings about the pain *to evaluate coping abilities and to identify areas of additional concern.*[1,11]
- Review procedures and expectations, and inform client when treatments will hurt. Discuss pain management methods that will be used *to reduce concerns of the unknown and muscle tension associated with anxiety or fear.*
- Use puppets or dolls for explanations and teaching, when indicated, *to demonstrate procedures for child and enhance understanding to reduce level of anxiety or fear.*
- Provide or promote nonpharmacological pain management:
  Quiet environment, calm activities
  Comfort measures (e.g., back rub, change of position, use of heat or cold compresses)
  Use of relaxation exercises (e.g., focused breathing, visualization, guided imagery)
  Diversional or distraction activities, such as television and radio, socialization with others, commercial or individualized tapes (e.g., "white" noise, music, instructional)
  Presence of parent during painful procedures *to comfort child*
  Identification of ways to avoid or minimize pain; *splinting incision during cough, keeping body in good alignment and using proper body mechanics, and resting between activities can reduce occurrence of muscle tension or spasms, or undue stress on incision*
- Establish collaborative approach for pain management based on client's understanding about and acceptance of available treatment options. *Pharmacological management is based on client's symptomatology and mechanism of pain as well as tolerance for pain and for the various analgesics. Pain medications may include pills, injections, intravenous dosing or patient-controlled analgesia (PCA), or regional analgesia (e.g., epidural and spinal blocking).*[2–5,11,14,16]
- Administer analgesics to maximal dosage as needed *to maintain "acceptable" level of pain. The type of medication(s) ordered depends on the type and severity of pain (e.g., acetaminophen and NSAIDs are commonly used to treat mild to moderate pain, while opiates [e.g., morphine, oxycodone and fentanyl] are used to treat moderate to severe pain). Note: Combinations of medications may be used on prescribed intervals.*[5,12]

Nursing Diagnoses in Alphabetical Order

- Notify physician/healthcare provider if regimen is inadequate to meet pain control goal. Assist client to prevent (rather than treat pain) and alter drug regimen based on individual needs. *Once established, pain is more difficult to suppress. Increasing dosage, changing medication, or using a stepped program (e.g., switching from injection to oral route, or lengthening time interval between doses) helps in self-management of pain.*[4,7]
- Evaluate and document client's response to analgesics and assist in transitioning or altering drug regimen based on individual needs and planned interventions *to limit adverse effects and barriers to adequate use of analgesics.*[2]
- Evaluate for adverse medication effects (e.g., decrease in mental acuity, change in thought processes, confusion or delirium, urinary retention, severe nausea, vomiting, pruritus). *Intolerable symptoms that usually require change of medication(s).*[2,3,5,11,12]
- Demonstrate and monitor use of self-administration/PCA that involves client in plan *to administer own IV pain medication or bolus additional dose when on continual basis drip.*[2–5,11,12]
- Provide information and monitor use of site-specific medications (e.g., spinal, epidural, regional anesthesia) *that might be used for certain procedures such as back surgery or amputation, labor and delivery).*[3,4,11,12]
- Instruct client in use of transcutaneous electrical stimulation (TENS) unit when ordered.

NURSING PRIORITY NO. 4

To promote wellness (Teaching/Discharge Considerations):

- Acknowledge the pain experience and convey acceptance of client's response to pain. *Reduces defensive responses, promotes trust, and enhances cooperation with regimen.*
- Involve client and SO/family in pain management program. *Provides additional support for the client and increases the likelihood of attaining goals when involved parties understand the process and feel a part of the solution.*
- Encourage adequate rest periods *to prevent fatigue that can impair ability to manage or cope with pain.*
- Review nonpharmacological measures for lessening pain. *Relaxation skills and techniques such as self-hypnosis, biofeedback, and Therapeutic Touch (TT) have no detrimental side effects.*
- Provide information and discuss pain management before planned procedures. *The primary concern of most clients/families is pain and discomfort following surgery or invasive procedure.*
- Address impact of pain on lifestyle and independence. *Understanding that pain can be manageable and that there are ways to maximize level of functioning promotes hope and cooperation with regimen.*
- Encourage performance of individualized physical therapy/exercise program. *Promotes active role in preventing muscle spasms or contractures, enhances sense of control.*
- Discuss ways SO(s) can assist client with pain management. *Helping to reduce precipitating factors that may cause or exacerbate pain (e.g., need to walk distances or climb stairs; strenuous activity, including household chores and yard work; noisy environment), supporting timely pain control, encouraging eating nutritious meals to enhance wellness, and providing gentle massage to reduce muscle tension facilitate recovery and pain control.*
- Identify specific signs/symptoms and changes in pain requiring evaluation by healthcare provider. *Provides opportunity to modify pain management regimen and allows for timely intervention for developing complications.*

DOCUMENTATION FOCUS

Assessment/Reassessment
- Individual assessment findings, including client's description of response to pain, specifics of pain inventory, expectations of pain management, and acceptable level of pain.

- Locus of control and cultural beliefs affecting response to pain.
- Prior medication use; substance abuse.

Planning
- Plan of care and who is involved in planning.
- Teaching plan.

Implementation/Evaluation
- Response to interventions, teaching, and actions performed.
- Attainment or progress toward desired outcome(s).
- Modifications to plan of care.

Discharge Planning
- Long-term needs, noting who is responsible for actions to be taken.
- Specific referrals made.

References

1. Engel, J. (2002). *Pocket Guide to Pediatric Assessment*. 4th ed. St. Louis, MO: Mosby, 249–259.
2. Young, D. (1999). *Acute pain management* (Research Dissemination Core). Iowa City: University of Iowa Gerontological Nursing Interventions Research Center.
3. Information about pain management options. Retrieved July 2007 from www.seanesthesiology.com/handler.cfm?categoryID=35&ParentID=23.
4. Clinical practice guideline for the management of postoperative pain (version 1.2). (2002). Department of Defense, Veterans Health Administration. Washington, DC. Retrieved July 2007 from www.guidelines.gov.
5. Ameres, M. J., Yeh, B. (2001, update 2005). Pain after surgery. Retrieved July 2007 from www.emedicine.com.
6. Smith, R., Curci, M., Silverman, A. (2002). Pain management: The global connection. *Nurs Manage*, 33(6), 26–29.
7. Acute pain management: Operative or medical procedures and trauma. (1992). (Clinical Practice Guideline) Publication No. AHCPR 92-0019. Rockville, MD: Agency for Health Care Policy and Research, Public Health Service, U.S. Dept of Health and Human Services.
8. Porter, S. (2001). Pain, pain go away. American Academy of Family Physicians: FP Report (excerpt JCAHO 2001 Pain Standards). Retrieved October 2009 from www.aafp.org/fpr/20010300/05.
9. Purnell, L. D., Paulanka, B. J. (1998). *Transcultural Health Care: A Culturally Competent Approach*. Philadelphia: F. A. Davis.
10. Doenges, M. E., Moorhouse, M. F., Geissler-Murr, A. C. (2002). ND Pain, acute. *Nurse's Pocket Guide: Diagnoses, Interventions and Rationales*. 8th ed. Philadelphia: F. A. Davis.
11. Assessment and management of acute pain. (2002, update 2006). Institute for Clinical Systems Improvement (ICSI). Bloomington, MN. Available at www.guideline.gov.
12. Michael, J. A. (2002). Pain medicine, types. Retrieved December 2003 from www.eirmc.org.
13. Pasero, C., McCaffrey, M. (2005). No self-report means no pain-intensity rating. *Am J Nurs*, 105(10), 50–53.
14. Mann, A. R. (2006). Manage the power of pain. *Men in Nursing*, 1(4), 20–28.
15. D'Arcy, Y. (2007). Managing pain in a patient who's drug-dependent. *Nursing*, 37(3), 36–40.
16. Wheeler, M. S. (2006). Pain assessment and management in the patient with mild to moderate cognitive impairment. *Home Healthcare Nurse*, 24(6), 354–359.
17. Zwakhalen, S., et al. (2006). Pain in elderly people with severe dementia: A systematic review of behavioural pain assessment tools. *BMC Geriatrics*, 6(3). Retrieved August 2007 from www.biomedcentral.com/1471-2318/6/3.

NURSING PRIORITY NO. 3

To promote wellness (Teaching/Discharge Considerations):

🏠 ● Involve all available members of the family in learning. *Promotes understanding and effective communication when each individual has the same information and is able to ask questions and clarify what has been heard.*[2,5]

🏠 ● Provide information appropriate to the situation, including time management, limit setting, and stress-reduction techniques. *Facilitates satisfactory implementation of plan and new behaviors.*[5]

🏠 ● Discuss parental beliefs about childrearing, punishment and rewards. *Identifying these beliefs allows opportunity to provide new information regarding effective alternatives to spanking and/or yelling.*

🔄 ● Develop support systems appropriate to the situation. *Extended family, friends, social worker, home-care services may be needed to help parents cope positively with what is happening.*[3]

🏠 ● Assist parent to plan time and conserve energy in positive ways. *Enables individual to cope more effectively with difficulties as they arise.*[3]

🏠 ● Encourage parents to identify positive outlets for meeting their own needs. *Going out for dinner or dating, making time for their own interests and each other promotes general well-being, helps reduce burnout.*[3,9]

🔄 ● Refer to appropriate support or therapy groups as indicated. *Underlying issues may interfere with adaptation to situation and additional support may help individuals to deal more effectively with them.*[5]

🔄 ● Identify community resources (e.g., childcare services). *Will assist with individual needs to provide respite and support.*[3]

🔄 ● Report and take necessary actions, as legally and professionally indicated, if child's safety is a concern. *Parents may believe corporal punishment is the best way to have children behave but may lead to abuse.*

● Refer to NDs ineffective Coping, compromised family Coping, risk for Violence [specify], Self-Esteem [specify], interrupted Family Processes as appropriate.

DOCUMENTATION FOCUS

Assessment/Reassessment
- Individual findings, including parenting skill level, deviations from normal parenting expectations.
- Family makeup and developmental stages.
- Interactions between parent and child.
- Availability and use of support systems and community resources.

Planning
- Plan of care and who is involved in planning.
- Teaching plan.

Implementation/Evaluation
- Parent(s')/child's responses to interventions, teaching, and actions performed.
- Attainment or progress toward desired outcome(s).
- Modification to plan of care.

Discharge Planning
- Long-term needs and who is responsible for actions to be taken.
- Specific referrals made.

References

1. Townsend, M. C. (2006). *Psychiatric Mental Health Nursing Concepts of Care.* 5th ed. Philadelphia: F. A. Davis.
2. Gordon, T. (2000). *Parent Effectiveness Training.* Updated ed. New York: Three Rivers Press.
3. Cox, H. C., et al. (2002). *Clinical Applications of Nursing Diagnosis: Adult, Child, Women's, Psychiatric, Gerontic, and Home Health Considerations.* 4th ed. Philadelphia: F. A. Davis.
4. Lipson, J. G., Dibble, S. L., Minarik, P. A. (1996). *Culture & Nursing Care: A Pocket Guide.* San Francisco: UCSF Nursing Press.
5. Doenges, M. E., Townsend, M. C., Moorhouse, M. F. (1998). *Psychiatric Care Plans. Guidelines for Individualizing Care.* 3d ed. Philadelphia: F. A. Davis.
6. Gordon, T. (1989). *Teaching Children Self-Discipline: At Home and at School.* New York: Random House.
7. Gordon, T. (2000). *Family Effectiveness Training Video.* Solana Beach, CA: Gordon Training International.
8. Neeld, E. H. (1997). *Seven Choices.* 3d ed. Austin, TX: Centerpoint Press.
9. Adams, L. *The language of love.* Retrieved April 2007 from www.gordontraining.com/The_Language_of_Love.html.

readiness for enhanced Parenting

DEFINITION: A pattern of providing an environment for children or other dependent person(s) that is sufficient to nurture growth and development and can be strengthened

RELATED FACTORS

To be developed by nurse researchers and submitted to NANDA

DEFINING CHARACTERISTICS

Subjective
Expresses willingness to enhance parenting
Children or other dependent person(s) express(es) satisfaction with home environment

Objective
Emotional support of children [or dependent person(s)]; evidence of attachment
Needs of children [or dependent person(s)] are met (e.g., physical and emotional)
Exhibits realistic expectations of children [or dependent person(s)]

Sample Clinical Applications: As a health-seeking behavior, the client/family may be healthy or this diagnosis can be associated with any clinical condition

DESIRED OUTCOMES/EVALUATION CRITERIA

Sample (NOC) linkages:
Parenting Performance: Parental actions to provide a child with a nurturing and constructive physical, emotional, and social environment
Knowledge: Parenting: Extent of understanding conveyed about provision of a nurturing and constructive environment for a child from 1 year through 17 years of age
Parenting: Psychosocial Safety: Parental actions to protect a child from social contacts that might cause harm or injury

(continues on page 594)

readiness for enhanced Parenting (continued)

Client Will (Include Specific Time Frame)
• Verbalize realistic information and expectations of parenting role.
• Identify own strengths, individual needs, and methods or resources to meet them.
• Participate in activities to enhance parenting skills.
• Demonstrate improved parenting behaviors.

ACTIONS/INTERVENTIONS

Sample (NIC) linkages:
Parent Education: Childrearing Family: Assisting parents to understand and promote the physical, psychological, and social growth and development of their toddler, preschool, or school-age child/children
Parent Education: Adolescent: Assisting parents to understand and help their adolescent children
Parenting Promotion: Providing parenting information, support, and coordination of comprehensive services to high-risk families

NURSING PRIORITY NO. 1

To determine need/motivation for improvement:

● Ascertain motivation and expectations for change. *Motivation to improve and high expectations can encourage client to make changes that will improve skills. However, unrealistic expectations may hamper efforts.*
● Note family constellation: two-parent, single, extended family, or child living with other relative, such as grandparent/sibling; or relationship of dependent person (e.g., foster family). *Understanding makeup of the family provides information about needs to assist them in improving their family connections.*[1]
● Determine developmental stage of the family (e.g., new child, adolescent, child leaving or returning home, retirement). *These maturational crises bring changes in the family that can provide opportunity for enhancing parenting skills and improving family interactions.*[1]
● Assess family relationships and identify needs of individual members, noting any special concerns that exist, such as birth defects, illness, hyperactivity. *The family is a system, and when members make decisions to improve parenting skills, the changes affect all parts of the system. Identifying needs, special situations, and relationships can help to develop plans to bring about effective change.*[1]
● Assess parenting skill level, taking into account the individual's intellectual, emotional, and physical strengths and weaknesses. *Identifies areas of need for education, skill training, and information on which to base plan for enhancing parenting skills.*[2,4]
● Observe attachment behaviors among parent(s) and child(ren), recognizing cultural background, which may influence expected behaviors. *Behaviors such as eye-to-eye contact, use of en face position, talking to infant in high-pitched voice are indicative of attachment behaviors in American culture but may not be appropriate in another culture. Failure to bond is thought to affect subsequent parent-child interactions.*[3,4]
● Determine presence and effectiveness of support systems, role models, extended family, and community resources available to the parent(s). *Parents desiring to enhance abilities and improve family life can benefit by role models that help them strengthen own style of parenting.*[2,3]
● Note cultural or religious influences on parenting, expectations of self/child, sense of success or failure. *Expectations may vary with different cultures; for example, Arab Americans*

hold children to be sacred, but childrearing is based on negative rather than positive rein-forcements and parents are stricter with girls than boys. These beliefs may interfere with ability to improve parenting skills when there is conflict between the two.[3,4]

NURSING PRIORITY NO. 2

To foster development of parenting skills:

- Create an environment in which relationships can be strengthened and needs of each individual family member can be met. *A safe environment in which individuals can freely express their thoughts and feelings optimizes learning and positive interactions among family members enhancing relationships.[2,5]*
- Make time for listening to concerns of the parent(s). *Promotes sense of importance and of being heard and identifies accurate information regarding needs of the family for enhancing relationships.[2]*
- Encourage expression of feelings, such as frustration, anger while setting limits on unacceptable behaviors. *Identification of feelings promotes understanding of self and enhances connections with others in the family. Unacceptable behaviors result in feelings of anger and diminished self-esteem and can lead to problems in the family relationships.[3]*
- Emphasize parenting functions rather than mothering/fathering skills. *By virtue of gender, each person brings something to the parenting role; however, nurturing tasks can be done by both parents, enhancing family relationships.[5]*
- Encourage attendance at skill classes, such as Parent Effectiveness Training. *Assists in developing communication skills of Active-listening, I-messages, and problem-solving techniques to improve family relationships and promote a win-win environment.[2]*

NURSING PRIORITY NO. 3

To promote optimum parenting skills/wellness:

- Involve all members of the family in learning. *The family system benefits from all members participating in learning new skills to enhance family relationships.[1]*
- Encourage parents to identify positive outlets for meeting their own needs. *Activities such as going out for dinner/dating, making time for their own interests and each other promotes general well-being, enhances family relationships, and improves family functioning.[2]*
- Provide information as indicated, including time management, stress-reduction techniques. *Learning about positive parenting skills, understanding growth and developmental expectations, and ways to reduce stress and anxiety promotes individual's ability to deal with problems that may arise in the course of family relationships.[1,6]*
- Discuss current "family rules," identifying areas of needed change. *Rules may be imposed by adults, rather than through a democratic process, involving all family members, leading to conflict and angry confrontations. Setting positive family rules with all family members participating can promote an effective, functional family.[2,6]*
- Discuss need for long-term planning and ways in which family can maintain desired positive relationships. *Each stage of life brings its own challenges, and understanding and preparing for each stage enables family members to move through them in positive ways, promoting family unity and resolving inevitable conflicts with win-win solutions.[6]*

DOCUMENTATION FOCUS

Assessment/Reassessment

- Individual findings, including parenting skill level, parenting expectations, family makeup, and developmental stages.

- Availability and use of support systems and community resources.
- Motivation and expectations for change.

Planning
- Plan for enhancement, who is involved in planning.

Implementation/Evaluation
- Family members' responses to interventions, teaching, and actions performed.
- Attainment or progress toward desired outcome(s).
- Modifications to plan.

Discharge Planning
- Long-term needs and who is responsible for actions to be taken.
- Modification to plan.

References

1. Townsend, M. C. (2006). *Psychiatric Mental Health Nursing Concepts of Care*. 5th ed. Philadelphia: F. A. Davis.
2. Gordon, T. (2000). *Parent Effectiveness Training*. Updated ed. New York: Three Rivers Press.
3. Doenges, M. E., Townsend, M. C., Moorhouse, M. F. (1998). *Psychiatric Care Plans: Guidelines for Individualizing Care*. 3d ed. Philadelphia: F. A. Davis.
4. Lipson, J. G., Dibble, S. L., Minarik, P. A. (1999). *Culture & Nursing Care: A Pocket Guide*. San Francisco: UCSF Nursing Press.
5. Doenges, M. E., Moorhouse, M. F., Geissler-Murr, A. C. (2007). *Nurses' Pocket Guide: Diagnoses, Interventions, and Rationales*. 11th ed. Philadelphia: F. A. Davis.
6. Gordon, T. (1989). *Teaching Children Self-Discipline: At Home and at School*. New York: Random House.

risk for impaired Parenting

DEFINITION: Risk for inability of the primary caretaker to create, maintain, or regain an environment that promotes the optimum growth and development of the child

Note: It is important to reaffirm that adjustment to parenting in general is a normal maturational process that elicits nursing behaviors to prevent potential problems and to promote health.

RISK FACTORS

Infant or child
Altered perceptual abilities; attention deficit-hyperactivity disorder
Difficult temperament; temperamental conflicts with parental expectation
Premature birth; multiple births; not gender desired
Handicapping condition; developmental delay
Illness; prolonged separation from parent

Knowledge
Unrealistic expectations of child; deficient knowledge about child development or health maintenance, parenting skills

Low educational level or attainment; lack of cognitive readiness for parenthood; low cognitive functioning
Poor communication skills
Inability to respond to infant cues
Preference for physical punishment

Physiological
Physical illness

Psychological
Young parental age
Closely spaced pregnancies; high number of pregnancies; difficult birthing process
Sleep disruption or deprivation
Depression; history of mental illness or substance abuse
Disability

Social
Stress; job problems; unemployment; financial difficulties; poor home environment; relocation
Situational or chronic low self-esteem
Lack of family cohesiveness; marital conflict; change in family unit; inadequate child care arrangements
Role strain; single parent; father/mother of child not involved; parent-child separation
Poor or lack of parental rode model; lack of valuing of parenthood
Unplanned or unwanted pregnancy; late or lack of prenatal care
Low socioeconomic class; poverty; lack of resources or access to resources; lack of transportation
Poor problem-solving skills; maladaptive coping strategies
Lack of social support network; social isolation
History of being abused or being abusive; legal difficulties

NOTE: A risk diagnosis is not evidenced by signs and symptoms, as the problem has not occurred; rather, nursing interventions are directed at prevention.
Sample Clinical Applications: Prematurity, multiple births, genetic or congenital defects, chronic illness (parent/child), substance abuse, physical or psychological abuse, major depression, developmental delay, schizophrenia

DESIRED OUTCOMES/EVALUATION CRITERIA

Sample NOC linkages:
Parenting Performance: Parental actions to provide a child a nurturing and constructive physical, emotional, and social environment
Knowledge: Parenting: Extent of understanding conveyed about provision of a nurturing and constructive environment for a child from 1 year to 17 years of age
Social Support: Reliable assistance from other persons

Client Will (Include Specific Time Frame)
• Verbalize awareness of individual risk factors.
• Identify own strengths, individual needs, and methods or resources to meet them.

(continues on page 598)

risk for impaired Parenting (continued)

• Demonstrate behavior or lifestyle changes to reduce potential for development of problem or reduce or eliminate effects of risk factors.
• Participate in activities, classes to promote growth.

ACTIONS/INTERVENTIONS

Sample (NIC) linkages:
Parenting Promotion: Providing parenting information, support, and coordination of comprehensive services to high-risk families
Parent Education: Childbearing Family: Assisting parents to understand and promote the physical, psychological, and social growth and development of their toddler, preschool, or school-aged child/children
Family Integrity Promotion: Promotion of family cohesion and unity
• **Refer to impaired Parenting for Actions/Interventions and Documentation Focus.**

ineffective peripheral tissue Perfusion

DEFINITION: Decrease in blood circulation to the periphery that may compromise health

RELATED FACTORS

Deficient knowledge of aggravating factors (e.g., smoking, sedentary lifestyle, trauma, obesity, salt intake, immobility)
Deficient knowledge of disease process (e.g., diabetes, hyperlipidemia; [peripheral artery disease, chronic venous insufficiency])
Hypertension
Sedentary lifestyle
Smoking

DEFINING CHARACTERISTICS

Subjective
Extremity pain; claudication
Paresthesia; [altered sensations]

Objective
Diminished or absent pulses; [diminished arterial pulsations; bruits; blood pressure changes in extremities]
Altered skin characteristics (color, elasticity, hair, moisture, nails, sensation, temperature)
Skin color pale on elevation; color does not return to leg on lowering it; [skin erythema or dependent rubor with chronic dryness, scaling, flaking]
Varicosities; [spider veins]
Edema
Altered motor function
Delayed peripheral wound healing; [ulcerations]

Sample Clinical Applications: Atherosclerosis, coronary artery disease, Raynaud's disease, peripheral vascular disease, Buerger's disease, thrombophlebitis, diabetes mellitus, sickle cell anemia

DESIRED OUTCOMES/EVALUATION CRITERIA

Sample (NOC) linkages:
Tissue Perfusion: Peripheral: Adequacy of blood flow through the small vessels of the extremities to maintain tissue function
Knowledge: Disease Process: Extent of understanding conveyed about a specific disease process and prevention of complications

Client Will (Include Specific Time Frame)
• Demonstrate increased perfusion as individually appropriate (e.g., skin warm and dry, peripheral pulses present and strong, absence of edema, free of pain or discomfort).
• Verbalize understanding of condition, therapy regimen, side effects of medications, and when to contact healthcare provider.
• Demonstrate behaviors or lifestyle changes to improve circulation (e.g., engage in regular exercise, cessation of smoking, weight reduction, disease management).

ACTIONS/INTERVENTIONS

Sample (NIC) linkages:
Circulatory Care: Arterial Insufficiency: Promotion of arterial circulation
Circulatory Care: Venous Insufficiency: Promotion of venous circulation

NURSING PRIORITY NO. 1

To assess causative/contributing factors:

• Note current situation or presence of conditions that can affect perfusion to all body systems (e.g., congestive heart failure, lung disorders, major trauma, septic or hypovolemic shock, coagulopathies, sickle cell anemia) *affecting systemic circulation and perfusion.*
• Determine history of conditions associated with thrombus or emboli (e.g., problems with coronary or cerebral circulation, stroke; high-velocity trauma with fractures, abdominal or orthopedic surgery, long periods of immobility; inflammatory diseases; chronic lung disease; diabetes with coexisting peripheral vascular disease; estrogen therapy; cancer and cancer therapies; presence of central venous catheters *to identify client at higher risk for venous stasis, vessel wall injury, and hypercoagulability.*[1,2,14,15]
• Identify presence of high-risk factors or conditions (e.g., smoking, uncontrolled hypertension, obesity, pregnancy, pelvic tumor, paralysis, hypercholesterolemia, varicose veins, arthritis, sepsis). *Places client at greater risk for developing peripheral vascular disease (PVD) (including arterial blockage and chronic venous insufficiency) with associated complications.*[3,4,14]
• Note location of restrictive clothing, pressure dressings, circular wraps, cast or traction device *that may restrict circulation to limb.*
• Review results of diagnostic studies (e.g., x-rays, Doppler ultrasound, angiography/other imaging scans, arterial and/or venous pressure measurements; treadmill exercise test; endoscopy, biopsy of ulcerations) *to determine location and severity of condition.*[5]

- Ascertain impact on functioning and lifestyle. *For example, leg pain may restrict ambulation, or person may develop skin ulceration and healing problems that seriously impact quality of life.*

NURSING PRIORITY NO. 2

To evaluate degree of impairment:

- Assess skin color, temperature, moisture, and whether changes are widespread or localized. *Helps in determining location and type of perfusion problem.*
- Compare skin temperature and color with other limb when assessing extremity circulation. *Helps differentiate type of problem (e.g., deep redness in both hands triggered by vibrating machinery is associated with functional PVD, such as Raynaud's disease; edema, redness, swelling in calf of one leg is associated with localized thrombophlebitis).*[1,5,14-16]
- Assess presence, location, and degree of swelling or edema formation. Measure circumference of extremities, noting differences in size. *Useful in identifying or quantifying edema in involved extremity.*
- Measure capillary refill *to determine adequacy of systemic circulation.*
- Note client's nutritional and fluid status. *Protein-energy malnutrition and weight loss make ischemic tissues more prone to breakdown. Dehydration reduces blood volume and compromises peripheral circulation.*[14]
- Inspect lower extremities for skin texture (e.g., atrophic; shiny appearance; lack of hair; dry, scaly, reddened skin) and skin breaks or ulcerations *that often accompany diminished peripheral circulation.*[2,3,6,14]
- Palpate arterial pulses (bilateral femoral, popliteal, dorsalis pedis, and postero-tibial), using handheld Doppler if indicated *to determine level of circulatory problem (e.g., client with intermittent claudication may have palpable pulses which disappear after ambulation).*[2,5]
- Determine pulse equality as well as intensity (e.g., bounding, normal, diminished, or absent) and compare with unaffected extremity *to evaluate distribution and quality of blood flow, and success or failure of therapy.*[2]
- Evaluate extremity pain reports, noting associated symptoms (e.g., cramping or heaviness, discomfort with walking, progressive temperature or color changes, paresthesia). Determine time (day or night) that symptoms are worse, precipitating or aggravating events (e.g., walking), and relieving factors (e.g., rest, sitting down with legs in dependent position, oral analgesics) *to help isolate and differentiate problems such as intermittent chronic claudication versus loss of function and pain due to acute sustained ischemia related to loss of arterial blood flow.*[2,3]
- Assess motor and sensory function. *Problems with ambulation, hypersensitivity or loss of sensation, numbness and tingling are changes that can indicate neurovascular dysfunction or limb ischemia, requiring more evaluation for differentiation of problem.*[2,6]
- Check for calf tenderness or pain on dorsiflexion of foot (Homans' sign), swelling and redness. *Indicators of deep vein thrombosis (DVT), although DVT is often present without a positive Homans' sign.*[1,15]
- Review laboratory studies such as clotting times, hemoglobin/hematocrit (Hb/Hct), renal/cardiac function tests; and diagnostic studies (e.g., Doppler ultrasound, magnetic resonance angiography [MRA], venogram, contrast angiography, resting ankle-brachial index [ABI], leg segmental arterial pressure measurements) *to determine location and degree of impairment.*[1-3,6]

NURSING PRIORITY NO. 3

To maximize tissue perfusion:

- Collaborate in treatment of underlying conditions, such as diabetes, hypertension, cardiopulmonary conditions, blood disorders, traumatic injury, hypovolemia, hypoxemia *to maximize systemic circulation and organ perfusion.*
- Administer medications such as antiplatelet agents, thrombolytics, antibiotics *to improve tissue perfusion and organ function.*[1,2,4,6,15,16]
- Administer fluids, electrolytes, nutrients, and oxygen as indicated *to promote optimal blood flow, organ perfusion and function.*
- Assist with or prepare for medical procedures such as endovascular stent placement, surgical revascularization procedures, thrombectomy, sympathectomy *to improve peripheral circulation.*
- Assist with application of elasticized tubular support bandages, adhesive elastic or Velcro wraps (e.g., Circ-Aid), paste bandage (Unna boot), multilayer bandage regimens, sequential pneumatic compression devices, and custom-fitted compression stockings as indicated *to provide graduated compression of lower extremity in presence of venous stasis ulcer.*[13,15]
- Collaborate with wound care specialist if arterial or venous ulcerations are present. *In-depth wound care may include debridement and various specialized dressings that provide optimal moisture for healing, prevention of infection and further injury.*[14,15]
- Provide interventions to promote peripheral circulation and limit complications:[1–3,7]
  Encourage early ambulation when possible, and recommend regular exercise. *Enhances venous return. Studies indicate exercise training may be an effective early treatment for intermittent claudication.*[8]
  Recommend or provide foot and ankle exercises when client unable to ambulate freely *to reduce venous pooling and increase venous return.*[15]
  Provide pressure-relieving devices for immobilized client (e.g., air mattress, foam or sheepskin padding, bed or foot cradle) *to reduce excessive tissue pressure that could lead to skin breakdown.*
  Apply intermittent compression devices and/or elastic compression stockings to lower extremities *to limit venous stasis, improve venous return and reduce risk of DVT or tissue ulceration in client who is limited in activity, or otherwise at risk.*[9,14–16]
  Assist with or cue client to change position at timed intervals rather than using presence of pain as signal to change positions, *because sensation may be impaired.*[6]
  Elevate the legs when sitting, but avoid sharp angulation of the hips or knees *to enhance venous return and minimize edema formation.*
  Avoid massaging the leg in presence of thrombosis *to reduce risk for embolus.*
  Avoid, or carefully monitor, use of heat or cold, such as hot water bottle, heating pad, or icepack. *Tissues may have decreased sensitivity due to ischemia, increasing risk of dermal injury.*
- Refer to ND risk for Peripheral Neurovascular Dysfunction, risk for impaired Skin Integrity, impaired Tissue Integrity, and disturbed Sensory Perception for additional interventions as appropriate.

NURSING PRIORITY NO. 4

To promote wellness (Teaching/Discharge Considerations):

- Discuss relevant risk factors (e.g., family history, obesity, age, smoking, hypertension, diabetes, clotting disorders) and potential outcomes of atherosclerosis (e.g., systemic and

---

peripheral vascular disease conditions). *Information necessary for client to make informed choices about remedial risk factors and commit to lifestyle changes as appropriate to prevent onset of complications or manage symptoms when condition present.*[10,11]

- ● Identify necessary changes in lifestyle and assist client to incorporate disease management into activities of daily living (ADLs). *Promotes independence, enhances self-concept regarding ability to deal with change and manage own needs.*

- ● Emphasize need for regular exercise program *to enhance circulation and promote general well-being.*[12]

- ● Refer to dietitian for well-balanced, low-saturated-fat, low-cholesterol diet, or other modifications as indicated *to promote weight loss and/or lower cholesterol levels.*

- ● Discuss care of dependent limbs, foot care as appropriate. *When circulation is impaired, changes in sensation place client at risk for development of lesions or ulcerations that are often slow to heal.*

- ● Discourage sitting or standing for long periods, wearing constrictive clothing, crossing legs, *which can restrict circulation and lead to edema.*

- ● Provide education about relationship between smoking and peripheral vascular circulation, as indicated. *Smoking contributes to development and progression of peripheral vascular disease and is associated with higher rate of amputation in presence of Buerger's disease.*[10,17]

- ● Educate client/SO in reportable symptoms, including any changes in pain level, difficulty walking, nonhealing wounds *to provide opportunity for timely evaluation and intervention.*

- ● Stress need for regular medical and laboratory follow-up *to evaluate disease progression and response to therapies, including medications for desired and untoward effects.*

- ● Review medication regimen with client/SO. *Client may be on various drugs (e.g., antiplatelet agents, blood viscosity–reducing agents, vasodilators, anticoagulants, or cholesterol-lowering agents) for treatment of the particular vascular disorder. Any of these medications have harmful side effects and require client teaching and medical monitoring.*[5,14–16]

- ● Emphasize importance of avoiding use of aspirin, some over-the-counter (OTC) drugs and supplements, and alcohol when taking anticoagulants.

- ● Refer to community resources such as smoking cessation assistance, weight control program, exercise group *to provide support for lifestyle changes.*

DOCUMENTATION FOCUS

Assessment/Reassessment
- Individual findings, noting nature, extent, and duration of problem, effect on independence and lifestyle.
- Characteristics of pain, precipitators, and what relieves pain.
- Pulses and blood pressure, including above and below suspected lesion as appropriate.

Planning
- Plan of care and who is involved in planning.
- Teaching plan.

Implementation/Evaluation
- Response to interventions/teaching, actions performed.
- Attainment or progress toward desired outcome(s).
- Modifications to plan of care.

Discharge Planning
- Long-term needs and who is responsible for actions to be taken.
- Available resources, specific referrals made.

References

1. Stockman, J. (2008) In too deep: Understanding deep vein thrombosis. *Nursing Made Incredibly Easy!*, 6(2), 29–38.
2. Sieggreen, M. (2008). Understanding critical limb ischemia. *Nursing*, 38(10), 50–55.
3. Stephens, E. (updated 2009). Peripheral vascular disease. Retrieved March 2009 from www.emedicine.com/emerg/topic862.htm.
4. Nieves, J., Capone-Swearer, D. (2006). The clot that changes lives. *Nursing 2006 Critical Care*, 1(3), 18–28.
5. American Heart Association (AHA). (2009). What is peripheral vascular disease? Retrieved March 2009 from www.americanheart.org/presenter.jhtml?identifier=4692.
6. Blach, D. A., Ignatavicius, D. D. (2006). Interventions for clients with vascular problems. In Ignatavicius, D. D., Workman, M. L. (eds). *Medical–Surgical Nursing: Critical Thinking for Collaborative Care*. 5 ed. St. Louis, MO: Elsevier Saunders.
7. Bartley, M. K. (2006). Keep venous thromboembolism at bay. *Nursing*, 36(10), 36–41.
8. Barclay, L. (2009). Hospital-supervised exercise may prevent need for surgery in patients with claudication. Retrieved March 2009 from http://cme.medscape.com/viewarticle/587997.
9. Amaragiri, S. V., Lees, T. A. (2000). Elastic compression stockings for prevention of deep vein thrombosis. Cochrane Database Syst Rev CD001484. Retrieved March 2009 from www.mrw.interscience.wiley.com/cochrane/clsysrev/articles/CD001484/frame.html.
10. Sieggreen, M. Y. (2006). Getting a leg up on managing venous ulcers. *Nursing Made Incredibly Easy!*, 4(6), 52–60.
11. Baldwin, K. M. (2006). Stroke: It's a knock-out punch. *Nursing Made Incredibly Easy!*, 4(2), 10–23.
12. Frost, K. L., Topp, R. (2006). A physical activity Rx for the hypertensive patient. *Nurse Pract*, 31(4), 29–37.
13. Moses, S. (2008). Unnas boot. Family practice notebook. Retrieved March 2009 from www.fpnotebook.com/Surgery/Pharm/UnsBt.htm.
14. Calianno, C., Holton, S. J. (2007). Fighting the triple threat of lower extremity ulcers. *Nursing*, 37(3), 57–63.
15. Kehl-Pruett, W. (2006). Deep vein thrombosis in hospitalized patients: A review of evidence-based guidelines for prevention. *Dimens Crit Care Nurs*, 25(2), 53–59.
16. Wipke-Tevis, D. D., Sae-Sia, W. (2004). Caring for vascular leg ulcers. *Home Healthcare Nurse*, 22(4), 237–247.
17. Johns Hopkins Vasculitis Center. Buerger's disease. Retrieved March 2009 from http://vasculitis.med.jhu.edu/typesof/buergers.html.

risk for decreased cardiac tissue Perfusion

DEFINITION: Risk for a decrease in cardiac (coronary) perfusion

RISK FACTORS

Coronary artery spasm; cardiac surgery; cardiac tamponade
Lack of knowledge of modifiable risk factors (e.g., smoking, sedentary lifestyle, obesity); hypertension; hyperlipidemia
Birth control pills
Drug abuse
Elevated C-reactive protein; hypoxemia; hypoxia
Family history of coronary artery disease

NOTE: A risk diagnosis is not evidenced by signs and symptoms, as the problem has not occurred; rather, nursing interventions are directed at prevention.

Sample Clinical Applications: Angina, coronary artery disease, hypertension, congestive heart failure, diabetes, cardiac surgery, pericarditis, sepsis, anemia, hemorrhagic shock, cocaine use

DESIRED OUTCOMES/EVALUATION CRITERIA

Sample NOC linkages:
Tissue Perfusion: Cardiac: Adequacy of blood volume through the coronary vasculature to maintain heart function
Cardiac Disease Self-Management: Personal actions to manage heart disease, its treatment, and prevent disease progression

Client Will (Include Specific Time Frame)
• Demonstrate adequate coronary perfusion as individually appropriate (e.g., vital signs within clients normal range, free of chest pain or discomfort).
• Identify individual risk factors.
• Verbalize understanding of treatment regimen.
• Demonstrate behaviors or lifestyle changes to maintain or maximize circulation (e.g., cessation of smoking, relaxation techniques, exercise program, dietary plan).

ACTIONS/INTERVENTIONS

Sample NIC linkages:
Cardiac Precautions: Prevention of an acute episode of impaired cardiac function by minimizing myocardial oxygen consumption or increasing myocardial oxygen supply
Hemodynamic Regulation: Optimization of heart rate, preload, afterload, and contractility

NURSING PRIORITY NO. 1

To identify individual risk factors:

• Note presence of conditions such as congestive heart failure, major trauma with blood loss, recent coronary artery bypass graft (CABG) surgery, use of intra-aortic balloon pump, chronic anemia, sepsis, etc. *Conditions such as these can affect systemic circulation, tissue oxygenation, and organ function.*[1]
• Note client's age and gender when assessing risk for coronary artery spasm or myocardial infarction. *Risk for heart disorders increases with age, and men are still considered at higher risk for myocardial infarction and experience them earlier in life.*[2] *Although studies show that men have experienced a decline in coronary heart disease mortality in the last two decades, due in part to national awareness campaigns, women have not experienced the same recognition and treatment or similar decline in coronary heart disease mortality.*[3]
• Identify life style issues such as obesity, smoking, high cholesterol, excessive alcohol intake, use of drugs such as cocaine, and physical inactivity *that can raise client's risk for coronary artery disease and impaired cardiac tissue perfusion.*[2]
• Determine presence of breathing problems, such as obstructive sleep apnea with oxygen desaturation. *Can produce alveolar hypoventilation, respiratory acidosis, and hypoxia, which can result in cardiac dysrhythmias and cardiac dysfunction.*[8]
• Determine if client is experiencing usual degree/long-term stress or may have underlying psychiatric disorder (e.g., anxiety or panic) *that may cause or exacerbate coronary artery disease and affect cardiac function.*[5]

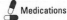

- Review client's medications, noting current use of any vasoactive drugs (e.g., dopamine, dobutamine, nitroglycerin, calcium channel blockers, beta blockers). *These medications may be used in emergent situations or to manage blood pressure over time and can exert undesirable and potentially dangerous secondary effects in addition to their intended primary effects. For example, dobutamine given to increase myocardial contractility can also cause tachycardia and hypotension, which increases myocardial workload and oxygen consumption.*[9]
- Review diagnostic studies and laboratory tests (e.g., electrocardiogram [ECG], echocardiogram, angiography, Doppler ultrasound, chest radiography; pulse oximetry, oxygen saturation, capnometry, or arterial blood gases [ABGs]; electrolytes, blood urea nitrogen/Creatinine (BUN/Cr), cardiac enzymes) *to identify conditions requiring treatment, and response to therapies.*[7,10,11]

NURSING PRIORITY NO. 2

To determine changes in cardiac status:

- Investigate reports of chest pain, noting changes in characteristics of pain *to evaluate for potential myocardial ischemia or inadequate systemic oxygenation or perfusion of organs. Note:* chest pain is often difficult to diagnose due to variability in symptoms. Leading causes of chest pain (other than heart) include musculoskeletal, gastrointestinal, and pulmonary systems, as well as psychiatric disorders such as panic disorders.[4-6]
- Monitor vital signs, especially noting blood pressure changes, including hypertension or hypotension *reflecting systemic vascular resistance problems that alter oxygen consumption and cardiac perfusion.*[1]
- Assess heart sounds and pulses for dysrhythmias. *Can be caused by inadequate myocardial or systemic tissue perfusion, electrolyte or acid-base imbalances.*
- Assess for restlessness, fatigue, changes in level of consciousness, decreased capillary refill time, diminished peripheral pulses, and pale, cool skin. *Signs and symptoms of inadequate systemic perfusion, which can cause or affect cardiac function.*[1]
- Inspect for pallor, mottling, cool and clammy skin, and diminished pulses. *Systemic vasoconstriction resulting from reduced cardiac output may be evidenced by poor skin or tissue perfusion and diminished pulses.*
- Investigate reports of difficulty breathing; note respiratory rate outside of acceptable parameters, which can be *indicative of oxygen exchange problems with potential for cardiac dysfunction.*[7]

NURSING PRIORITY NO. 3

To maintain/maximize cardiac perfusion:

- Collaborate in treatment of underlying conditions such as hypovolemia, chronic obstructive pulmonary disease (COPD), diabetes, chronic atrial fibrillation, *to correct or treat disorders that could influence cardiac perfusion or organ function.*
- Maintain hemodynamic stability when client is in postoperative phase of coronary artery bypass-graft (CABG) surgery *to keep vital organs adequately perfused. Risk factors in this time frame include dysrhythmias, hypotension or hypertension, cardiac tamponade, and pulmonary dysfunction.*[12]
- Provide supplemental oxygen as indicated *to improve or maintain cardiac and systemic tissue perfusion.*
- Administer fluids and electrolytes as indicated *to maintain systemic circulation and optimal cardiac function.*

- Administer medications (e.g., antihypertensive agents, analgesics, antidysrhythmics, bronchodilators, fibrinolytic agents) *to treat underlying conditions, to prevent thromboembolic phenomena, and to maintain cardiac tissue perfusion and organ function.*[12]
- Collaborate with dietician or nutritionist to provide easily digestible diet sufficient in nutrients, low in cholesterol and fat and high in complex carbohydrates *to provide energy and reduce substances harmful to coronary arteries.*[2,16]
- Provide periods of undisturbed rest and calming environment *to reduce myocardial workload.*

NURSING PRIORITY NO. 4

To promote wellness (Teaching/Discharge Considerations):

- Discuss the risk factors (e.g., family history, obesity, age, smoking, hypertension, diabetes, clotting disorders) and potential outcomes of atherosclerosis (e.g., systemic and cardiac disease conditions). *Information necessary for client to make informed choices about remedial risk factors and commit to lifestyle changes as appropriate to prevent onset of complications or manage symptoms when condition present.*[2]
- Review difference between modifiable and nonmodifiable risk factors *to assist client/SO in understanding those areas in which he/she can take action or make healthy choices.*

    Recommend maintenance of normal weight or weight loss if client is obese *to decrease risk associated with overweight and obesity.*[2]

    Review specific dietary concerns with client, e.g., reducing animal and dairy fats, increasing plant foods—fruits, vegetables, olive oil and nuts.[16]

    Encourage smoking cessation, when indicated, offering information about stop-smoking aids and programs. *Smoking causes vasoconstriction compromising perfusion. Smoking cessation is important in the medical management of many contributors to heart attack. These include atherosclerosis (fatty buildups in arteries), thrombosis (blood clots), coronary artery spasm, and cardiac dysrhythmia (heart rhythm problems).*[17]

    Encourage client to engage in regular exercise *to enhance circulation and promote general well-being.*[18]

    Discuss drug use where indicated (including cocaine, methamphetamines, alcohol) *to educate client regarding effect of drug on heart.*[19,20]

    Discuss coping and stress tolerance. Demonstrate and encourage use of relaxation or stress management techniques *to decrease tension level, thereby improving heart health.*[21]

- Encourage client in high-risk categories (e.g., strong family history, diabetic, prior history of cardiac event) to have regular medical examinations *to provide timely intervention, when needed.*
- Discuss and review medications on regular basis *to manage those which affect cardiac function or those given to prevent blood pressure or thromboembolic problems.*
- Refer to educational or community resources, as indicated. *Client/SO may benefit from instruction and support provided by agencies to engage in healthier heart activities (e.g., weight loss, smoking cessation, exercise).*
- Instruct in blood pressure monitoring at home if indicated; advise purchase of home monitoring equipment; refer to community resources as indicated. *Facilitates management of hypertension which is a major risk factor for damage to blood vessels or organ function.*[21]

DOCUMENTATION FOCUS

Assessment/Reassessment
- Individual findings, noting specific risk factors.
- Vital signs, cardiac rhythm, presence of dysrhythmias.

Planning
- Plan of care and who is involved in planning.
- Teaching plan.

Implementation/Evaluation
- Response to interventions, teaching, and actions performed.
- Attainment or progress toward desired outcome(s).
- Modifications to plan of care.

Discharge Planning
- Long-term needs and who is responsible for actions to be taken.
- Available resources, specific referrals made.

References

1. Breitenbach, J. E. (2007). Putting an end to perfusion confusion. *Nursing Made Incredibly Easy!*, 5(3), 50–60.
2. American Heart Association (AHA). AHA scientific position: Risk factors and coronary heart disease. Retrieved February 2009 from www.americanheart.org/presenter.jhtml?identifier=4726.
3. Yawn, B., et al. (2004). Identification of women's coronary heart disease risk factors prior to first myocardial infarction. *J Womens Health*, 13(10), 1087–1096.
4. Fagring, A. J., Gaston-Johansson, F., Danielson, E. (2005). Description of unexplained chest pain and its influence on daily life in men and women. *Eur J Cardiovasc Nurs*, 4, 337–344.
5. Katerndahl, D. (2004) Panic and plaques: Panic disorder and coronary artery disease in patients with chest pain. *J Am Board Fam Pract*, 17(2), 114–126.
6. Cayley, W. E. (2005). Diagnosing the cause of chest pain. *Am Fam Physician*, 72(10), 2012–2012.
7. Schulman, C. (2002). End points of resuscitation: Choosing the right parameters to monitor. *Dimens Crit Care Nurs*, 21(1), 2–10.
8. De Olazabal, J. R., et.al. (1982). Disordered breathing and hypoxia during sleep in coronary artery disease. *Chest*, 1378(5), 548–552.
9. Miller, J. (2007). Keeping your patient hemodynamically stable. *Nursing*, 37(5), 36–41.
10. Task Force on Pulmonary Embolism, European Society of Cardiology. (2000). Guidelines on diagnosis and management of acute pulmonary embolism. Retrieved July 2007 from www.idealibrary.com.
11. Goldrich, G. (2006). Understanding the 12-lead ECG, part I. *Nursing*, 36(11), 36–41.
12. Mullen-Fortino, M., O'Brien, N. (2008). Caring for the patient after coronary artery bypass graft. *Nursing*, 38(3), 46–52.
13. Bartley, M. K. (2006). Keep venous thromboembolism at bay. *Nursing*, 36(10), 36–41.
14. Sieggreen, M. Y. (2006). Getting a leg up on managing venous ulcers. *Nursing Made Incredibly Easy!*, 4(6), 52–60.
15. Baldwin, K. M. (2006). Stroke: It's a knock-out punch. *Nursing Made Incredibly Easy!*, 4(2), 10–23.
16. Sacks, F. M., Katan, M. (2002). Randomized clinical trials on the effects of dietary fat and carbohydrate on plasma proteins and cardiovascular disease. *Am J Med*, 113(suppl 9B), 13–24.
17. Smoking cessation: AHA scientific position [citing 2004 Surgeon General's Report: The health consequences of smoking]. Retrieved February 2009 from www.americanheart.org/presenter.jhtml?identifier=4731.
18. Frost, K. L., Topp, R. (2006). A physical activity Rx for the hypertensive patient. *Nurse Pract*, 31(4), 29–37.
19. American Heart Association. (1998). American Heart Association journal report: Researchers discover how cocaine use may cause heart attacks. Retrieved February 2009 from www.sciencedaily.com/releases/1998/08/980807104412.htm.
20. Wright, N. M. J., et al. (2007). Cocaine and thrombosis: A narrative systematic review of clinical and in-vivo studies. *Subst Abuse Treat Prevent Policy*, 2, 27.

21. Blach, D. A. (2006). Assessment of the cardiovascular system. In Ignatavicius, D. D., Workman, M. L. (eds.). *Medical-Surgical Nursing: Critical Thinking for Collaborative Care* 5th ed. St. Louis, MO: Elsevier Saunders.

risk for ineffective cerebral tissue Perfusion

DEFINITION: At risk for a decrease in cerebral tissue circulation

RISK FACTORS

Head trauma; cerebral aneurysm; brain tumor; neoplasm of the brain
Carotid stenosis; aortic atherosclerosis; arterial dissection
Atrial fibrillation; sick sinus syndrome; atrial myxoma; left atrial appendage thrombosis
Recent myocardial infarction; akinetic left ventricular segment; dilated cardiomyopathy; mitral stenosis; mechanical prosthetic valve; infective endocarditis; embolism
Coagulopathy (e.g., sickle cell anemia, disseminated intravascular coagulation); abnormal partial thromboplastin time; abnormal prothrombin time
Hypertension; hypercholesterolemia
Substance abuse
Treatment-related side effects (cardiopulmonary bypass, medications); thrombolytic therapy

NOTE: A risk diagnosis is not evidenced by signs and symptoms, as the problem has not occurred; rather, nursing interventions are directed at prevention.
Sample Clinical Applications: Traumatic brain injury, atherosclerosis, hypertension, atrial fibrillation, mitral valve stenosis or replacement, transient ischemic attack, sickle cell anemia, cocaine use

DESIRED OUTCOMES/EVALUATION CRITERIA

Sample NOC linkages:
Tissue Perfusion: Cerebral: Adequacy of blood flow through the cerebral vasculature to maintain brain function
Risk Control: Personal actions to prevent, eliminate, or reduce modifiable health threats

Client Will (Include Specific Time Frame)
- Display neurological signs within clients normal range.
- Verbalize understanding of condition, therapy regimen, side effects of medications, and when to contact healthcare provider.
- Demonstrate behaviors or lifestyle changes to improve circulation (e.g., cessation of smoking, relaxation techniques, exercise program, dietary plan).

ACTIONS/INTERVENTIONS

Sample NIC linkages:
Cerebral Perfusion Promotion: Promotion of adequate perfusion and limitation of complications for a patient experiencing or at risk for inadequate cerebral perfusion

Surveillance: Purposeful and ongoing acquisition, interpretation, and synthesis of patient data for clinical decision making
Cerebral Edema Management: Limitation of secondary injury resulting from swelling of brain tissue

NURSING PRIORITY NO. 1

To assess causative/contributing factors:

- Determine history of conditions associated with thrombus or emboli such as stroke, complicated pregnancy, sickle cell disease, fractures (especially long bones or pelvis) *to identify client at higher risk for decreased cerebral perfusion related to bleeding and/or coagulation problems.*
- Note current situation or presence of conditions (e.g., congestive heart failure, major trauma, sepsis, hypertension) *that can affect all body systems and systemic circulation and perfusion.*
- Ascertain potential for presence of acute neurologic conditions, such as traumatic brain injury, tumors, hemorrhage, anoxic brain injury associated with cardiac arrest, and toxic or viral encephalopathies. *These conditions alter the relationship between intracranial volume and pressure, potentially increasing intracranial pressure and decreasing cerebral perfusion.*[1]
- Investigate client reports of headache, particularly when accompanied by loss of coordination, confusion, visual disturbances, difficulty understanding or using language, or a range of progressive neurological deficits. *These symptoms may accompany cerebral perfusion deficits associated with conditions such as stroke, transient ischemic attack (TIA), brain trauma, or cerebral arteriovenous malformations.*[2,5]
- Ascertain if client has history of cardiac problems (e.g., recent myocardial infarction, heart failure, heart valve dysfunction or replacement, chronic atrial fibrillation), *which can impair systemic and cerebral blood flow or cause thromboembolic events to brain.*[3]
- Determine presence of cardiac dysrhythmias. *Can be caused by inadequate myocardial perfusion, electrolyte imbalances, or be associated with brain injury (e.g., bradycardia can accompany traumatic injury; or stroke can be precipitated by dysrhythmias).*[3]
- Evaluate blood pressure. *Chronic or severe acute hypertension can precipitate cerebrovascular spasm and stroke. Low blood pressure or severe hypotension causes inadequate perfusion of brain, with adverse changes in consciousness/mentation.*[4]
- Verify proper use of antihypertensive medications. *Individuals may stop medication because of lack of symptoms, presence of undesired side effects, and/or cost of drug, potentiating risk of stroke.*
- Review medication regimen noting use of anticoagulants or antiplatelet agents and other drugs *that could cause intracranial bleeding.*
- Review pulse oximetry or arterial blood gases (ABGs), noting oxygenation level and saturation. *Hypoxia (PaO_2 level <60 mg Hg), or O_2 saturation level < 90%, is associated with reduced cerebral perfusion and increased morbidity and mortality from severe brain injury.*[3]
- Review laboratory studies (e.g., coagulation profiles, complete blood count, electrolytes, lipids, B-type natriuretic peptide [BNP]) *to identify disorders that increase risk of clotting or bleeding, or other conditions contributing to causing decreased cerebral perfusion.*
- Review results of diagnostic studies (e.g., x-rays, cardiac output; ultrasound or other imaging scans such as echocardiography, computed tomography [CT], or angiography) *to determine location and severity of disorder that can cause or exacerbate cerebral perfusion problems.*

NURSING PRIORITY NO. 2

To maximize tissue perfusion:

- Collaborate in treatment of underlying conditions (e.g., carotid stent placement, surgical reperfusion procedures, treatment of infections) as indicated *to improve systemic perfusion and organ function.*
- Restore or maintain fluid balance *to maximize cardiac output and prevent decreased cerebral perfusion associated with hypovolemia.*[1,2]
- Manage cardiac dysrhythmias—medication administration, assist with pacemaker insertion. *Reduces risk of diminished cerebral perfusion due to blood clots or low cardiac output.*[1,2]
- Restrict fluids, administer diuretics as indicated *to prevent diminished cerebral perfusion associated with hypertension and cerebral edema.*[1,2]
- Keep head in midline position *to promote venous drainage, preventing elevated intracranial pressure.*[1,2]
- Maintain optimal head of bed (HOB) placement (e.g., 0, 15, 30 degrees). *Various studies demonstrate different perfusion responses to HOB placement but indicate that cerebral perfusion is reduced when HOB elevated greater than 30 degrees.*[6]
- Control fever, monitor hypothermia therapy, and provide supplemental oxygen *as indicated to decrease cerebral metabolism and cerebral edema.*[1,2]
- Administer vasoactive medications, as indicated, *to increase cardiac output and/or adequate mean arterial pressure (MAP) to maintain cerebral perfusion.*[1,2]
- Administer other medications as indicated. *Steroids may be used to decrease edema, antihypertensives to manage high blood pressure, anticoagulants to prevent cerebral embolus.*[1,2]
- Prepare client for surgery as indicated (e.g., carotid endarterectomy, evacuation of hematoma or space-occupying lesion) *to improve cerebral perfusion.*
- Refer to NDs decreased Cardiac Output, decreased Intracranial Adaptive Capacity for additional interventions.

NURSING PRIORITY NO. 3

To promote wellness (Teaching/Discharge Considerations):

- Review modifiable risk factors, as indicated (e.g., obesity, diet, smoking, activity level, hypertension, diabetes, clotting disorders). *Information necessary for client to make informed choices about remedial actions to reduce risk factors, and to commit to lifestyle changes as appropriate.*[2,7]
  Uncontrolled hypertension: *Incidence of stroke increases with systolic blood pressure >140/90 mm Hg. Client at risk can learn to self-monitor blood pressure, take prescribed antihypertensive agents consistently, and identify symptoms to report to physician.*
  Smoking: *Causes vasoconstriction and increased arterial wall stiffness, increasing fibrinogen levels and platelet aggregation, and abnormal blood lipids. Smoking cessation immediately lowers risk of stroke.*
  Obesity and unhealthy diet: *Abdominal obesity has been associated with increased risk for ischemic stroke.[8] Diet high in cholesterol contributes to development of cerebral atherosclerosis. High intake of sodium can contribute to hypertension.*
  Physical inactivity: *Contributes to obesity and hypertension.*
  Excessive alcohol intake: *Linked to higher risk of stroke because it can cause hypertension, which is a major risk factor*[7]
  Illicit drug use—especially cocaine and methamphetamines: *Can significantly boost the risk of a deadly or debilitating stroke.*[9]

- Discuss impact of unmodifiable risk factors such as family history, age, race. *Understanding effects and interrelationship of all risk factors may encourage client to address what can be changed to improve general well-being and reduce individual risk.*

- Assist client to incorporate disease management into activities of daily living (ADLs), including regular exercise. *Promotes independence, enhances self-concept regarding ability to deal with change and manage own needs.*

- Emphasize necessity of routine follow-up and laboratory monitoring as indicated. *Important for effective disease management and possible changes in therapeutic regimen.*

- Refer to educational or community resources as indicated. *Client/SO may benefit from instruction and support provided by agencies to engage in healthy activities (e.g., weight loss, smoking cessation, exercise).*

DOCUMENTATION FOCUS

Assessment/Reassessment
- Individual findings, noting specific risk factors.
- Vital signs, blood pressure, cardiac rhythm.
- Medication regimen.
- Diagnostic studies, laboratory results.

Planning
- Plan of care and who is involved in planning.
- Teaching plan.

Implementation/Evaluation
- Response to interventions, teaching, and actions performed.
- Attainment or progress toward desired outcome(s).
- Modifications to plan of care.

Discharge Planning
- Long-term needs and who is responsible for actions to be taken.
- Available resources, specific referrals made.

References

1. Editorial Staff. (2007). Patho puzzler: Don't let your head explode over increased ICP. *Nursing Made Incredibly Easy!*, 5(2), 21–25.
2. Nieves, J., Capone-Swearer, D. (2006). The clot that changes lives. *Nursing*, 1(3), 18–28.
3. Agency for Healthcare Research and Quality (AHRQ). (2003). Pharmacologic management of heart failure and left ventricular systolic dysfunction: Effect in female, black, and diabetic patients, and cost-effectiveness. Summary, Evidence Report/Technology Association. AHRQ Publication No. 03-E044. Rockville, MD. Retrieved March 2009 from www.ahrq.gov/clinic/epcsums/hrtfailsum.htm.
4. Brain Trauma Foundation, American Association of Neurological Surgeons. (2007). Guidelines for the management of severe traumatic brain injury: Blood pressure and oxygenation. Retrieved March 2009 from www.guideline.gov.
5. Vacca, V. M., Vilolett, S. (2008). Teamwork integral to treating cerebral arteriovenous malformation. *Nursing*, 3(3), 20–27.
6. McIlvoy, L. H., Meyer, K. (2008). Cerebral perfusion promotion. In Ackley, B. J., et al. (eds). *Evidence-Based Nursing Care Guidelines: Medical-Surgical Interventions*. St. Louis, MO: Mosby Elsevier.
7. National Stroke Association (NSA). (2009 update) Various public information monographs regarding stroke risk reduction. Retrieved March 2009 from www.stroke.org/site/PageServer?pagename=RISKRED.

8. Thom, T., et al. (2006). Heart disease and stroke statistics—2006 update: A report from the American Heart Association Committee and Stroke Statistics Subcommittee. *Circulation*, 113(6), e85–e151.

9. Nauert, R. (2007). Coke and speed increase risk of stroke. Article reporting result of study at UT Southwestern. Retrieved March 2009 from http://psychcentral.com/news/2007/04/05/coke -and-speed-increase-stroke-risk.

risk for ineffective gastrointestinal Perfusion

DEFINITION: At risk for change in gastrointestinal circulation that may compromise health

RISK FACTORS

Acute gastrointestinal bleed or hemorrhage; [hypovolemia]

Trauma; abdominal compartment syndrome

Vascular disease (e.g., peripheral vascular disease, aortoiliac occlusive disease); abdominal aortic aneurysm

Poor left ventricular performance; hemodynamic instability

Coagulopathy (e.g.. sickle cell anemia, disseminated intravascular coagulation), abnormal partial thromboplastin time, abnormal prothrombin time; [emboli]

Gastrointestinal disease (e.g., duodenal or gastric ulcer, ischemic colitis, ischemic pancreatitis); gastric paresis; gastroesophageal varices

Liver dysfunction; renal failure; diabetes mellitus; stroke

Treatment-related side effects (e.g., cardiopulmonary bypass, medication, anesthesia, gastric surgery)

Smoking

Age >60 years; female gender

NOTE: A risk diagnosis is not evidenced by signs and symptoms, as the problem has not occurred; rather, nursing interventions are directed at prevention.

Sample Clinical Applications: Gastrointestinal (GI) bleed, atherosclerosis, sickle cell anemia, diabetes, pancreatitis, congestive heart failure (CHF), cirrhosis, hemorrhage shock

DESIRED OUTCOMES/EVALUATION CRITERIA

Sample **NOC** linkages:

Tissue Perfusion: Abdominal Organs: Adequacy of blood flow through the small vessels of the abdominal viscera to maintain organ function

Gastrointestinal Function: Extent to which foods (ingested or tube-fed) are moved from ingestion to evacuation

Client Will (Include Specific Time Frame)

• Demonstrate adequate tissue perfusion as evidenced by active bowel sounds; absence of abdominal pain, nausea, and vomiting.

• Verbalize understanding of condition, therapy regimen, side effects of medication, and when to contact healthcare provider.

• Engage in behaviors or lifestyle changes to improve circulation (e.g., smoking cessation, diabetic glucose control, medication management).

⊕ Cultural   🐛 Collaborative   🏠 Community/Home Care   🖊 Diagnostic Studies   ∞ Pediatric/Geriatric/Lifespan   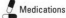 Medications

ACTIONS/INTERVENTIONS

Sample **NIC** linkages:

Surveillance: Purposeful and ongoing acquisition, interpretation, and synthesis of patient data for clinical decision making

Circulatory Care: Arterial Insufficiency: Promotion of arterial circulation

Gastrointestinal Intubation: Insertion of a tube into the GI tract

NURSING PRIORITY NO. 1

To assess causative/contributing factors:

- Note presence of conditions affecting systemic circulation/perfusion such as heart failure with left ventricular dysfunction, major trauma with hypotension, surgery with major blood loss, septic shock, and so forth. *Blood loss and hypovolemic or hypotensive shock can result in GI hypoperfusion and bowel ischemia.*[1]

- Determine presence of disorders such as esophageal varices, pancreatitis, abdominal or chest trauma, increase of intra-abdominal pressure or abdominal hypertension, prior history of bowel obstruction or strangulated hernia, or prior abdominal surgery with adhesions *that could cause local or regional reduction in GI blood flow.*[2–5,22]

- Identify client with history of bleeding or coagulation disorders, such as prior GI bleed, sickle cell anemia or other coagulopathies; cancer *to identify risk for potential bleeding problems complicating current situation (e.g., client having elective surgical procedure) or exacerbation of comorbidities.*

- Note client's age and gender. *Studies indicate that risk increases with age in both sexes and that risk is higher in men than women when assessing risk for GI bleed and abdominal aortic aneurysm.*[1,6] *Premature or low-birth-weight neonates are at risk for developing necrotizing enterocolitis (NEC).*[21]

- Investigate reports of abdominal pain, noting location, intensity, duration, and relationship to activities (e.g., eating, lifting heavy objects), trauma, surgery, or acute or chronic conditions causing displacement of abdominal organs accompanied by abdominal distention (e.g., peritonitis, cirrhosis, ascites), and so forth. *Many disorders can result in abdominal pain, some of which can include conditions affecting gastrointestinal perfusion such as postprandial abdominal angina due to occlusive mesenteric vascular disease, abdominal compartment syndrome, or other potential perforating disorders such as duodenal or gastric ulcer, or ischemic pancreatitis.*[4,7,8]

- Review routine medication regimen (e.g., NSAIDs, Coumadin, low-dose aspirin such as used for prophylaxis in certain cardiovascular conditions, corticosteroids). *Likelihood of bleeding increases from use of such medications.*[9–11]

- Note history of smoking, *which can potentiate vasoconstriction, or* excessive alcohol use or abuse, *which can cause general inflammation of the stomach mucosa and potentiate risk of GI bleeding, or liver involvement and esophageal varices.*

- Auscultate abdomen to evaluate peristaltic activity. *Hypoactive or absent bowels sounds may indicate intraperitoneal injury, bowel perforation and bleeding. Abdominal bruit can indicate abdominal aortic injury or aneurysm.*[5]

- Palpate abdomen for distension, masses, enlarged organs (e.g., spleen, liver, or portions of colon), elicitation of pain with touch, pulsation of aorta *that could identify problem in GI organs or circulation system.*[12–14]

- Percuss abdomen for fixed or shifting dullness over regions that normally contain air. *Can indicate accumulated blood or fluid.*[15]

- Measure and monitor progression of abdominal girth as indicated. *Abdominal distention can reflect bowel problems such as ileus or other bowel obstruction. It may also be indicative of organ failure (e.g., heart, liver, or kidney) or organ injury or enlargement/displacement with intra-abdominal fluid and gas accumulation. These condition can cause or exacerbate GI perfusion problems.*[8]
- Note reports of nausea or vomiting along with problems with elimination. *May reflect hypoperfusion of the GI tract, which is particularly vulnerable to even small decreases in circulating volume.*[16]
- Assess client with severe or prolonged vomiting, forceful coughing, lifting and straining activities, or childbirth, *which can result in a tear in the esophageal or stomach wall resulting in hemorrhage.*
- Evaluate stools for color and consistency. Test for occult blood, as indicated. *If bleeding is present, stools may be black or "tarry," currant-colored, or bright red. Consistency can range from normal with occult blood to thick liquid stools.*[1]
- Test gastric suction contents for blood when tube is used to decompress stomach and/or manage vomiting. *Can help in early identification of bleeding complications.*
- Assess vital signs noting sustained hypotension, *which can result in hypoperfusion of abdominal organs.*
- Review laboratory tests and other diagnostic studies (e.g., complete blood count [CBC], bilirubin, liver enzymes, electrolytes, stool guaiac; endoscopy, abdominal ultrasound or computed tomography [CT], aortic angiography, paracentesis) *to identify if conditions or disorders are present that may affect GI perfusion and function.*[8,13]
- Measure intra-abdominal pressure as indicated. *Tissue edema or free fluid collecting in the abdominal cavity leads to intra-abdominal hypertension, which if untreated can cause abdominal compartment syndrome with end-stage organ failure.*[23]

NURSING PRIORITY NO. 2

To reduce or correct individual risk factors:

- Collaborate in treatment of underlying conditions *to correct or treat disorders that could affect GI perfusion.*
- Administer fluids and electrolytes as indicated *to replace losses and to maintain GI circulation and function.*
- Administer prescribed prophylactic medications in at-risk clients during illness and hospitalization (e.g., antiemetics, proton-pump inhibitors, antihistamines, anticholinergics, antibiotics) *to reduce potential for stress-related GI complications such as bleeding, ulceration of stomach mucosa.*[17,18]
- Maintain gastric or intestinal decompression; when indicated, measure output periodically and note characteristics of drainage.
- Provide small and easily digested food and fluids when oral intake tolerated.
- Encourage rest after meals *to maximize blood flow to digestive system.*
- Prepare client for surgery as indicated. *May be a surgical emergency, for example, gastric resection, bypass graft, mesenteric endarterectomy.*
- Refer to NDs dysfunctional gastrointestinal Motility, Nausea, imbalanced Nutrition: Less than body requirements for additional interventions.

NURSING PRIORITY NO. 3

To promote wellness (Teaching/Discharge Considerations):

- Discuss individual risk factors (e.g., family history, obesity, age, smoking, hypertension, diabetes, clotting disorders) and potential outcomes of atherosclerosis (e.g., systemic and

peripheral vascular disease conditions). *Information necessary for client to make informed choices about remedial risk factors and commit to lifestyle changes as appropriate to prevent onset of complications or manage symptoms when condition present.*

- Identify necessary changes in lifestyle and assist client to incorporate disease management into activities of daily living (ADLs). *Promotes independence, enhances self-concept regarding ability to deal with change and manage own needs.*
- Encourage client to quit smoking, join Smoke-out, other smoking-cessation programs *to reduce risk of vasoconstriction compromising GI perfusion.*
- Establish regular exercise program *to enhance circulation and promote general well-being.*[19]
- Stress necessity of routine follow-up and laboratory monitoring as indicated. *Important for effective disease management and possible changes in therapeutic regimen.*
- Emphasize importance of discussing with primary care provider current and new prescribed medications, and/or planned use of certain medications (e.g., anticoagulants, NSAIDs including aspirin; corticosteroids, some over-the-counter [OTC] drugs, herbals supplements), *which can be harmful to GI mucosa, or cause bleeding.*[20]

DOCUMENTATION FOCUS

Assessment/Reassessment
- Individual findings, noting specific risk factors.
- Vital signs, adequacy of circulation.
- Abdominal assessment, characteristics of emesis/gastric drainage and stools.

Planning
- Plan of care and who is involved in planning.
- Teaching plan.

Implementation/Evaluation
- Response to interventions, teaching, and actions performed.
- Attainment or progress toward desired outcome(s).
- Modifications to plan of care.

Discharge Planning
- Long-term needs and who is responsible for actions to be taken.
- Available resources, specific referrals made.

References

1. Sommers, M. S., Johnson, S. A., Beery, T. A. (2007). *Diseases and Disorders: A Nursing Therapeutics Manual*, 3d ed. Philadelphia: F. A. Davis.
2. Goldberg, S. M. (2008). Identifying intestinal obstruction: Better safe than sorry. *Nurs Crit Care*, 3(5), 18–23.
3. Feigenbaum, K. (2006). Update on gastroparesis. *Gastroenterol Nurs*, 29(3), 239–244.
4. Kelso, L. A. (2008). Cirrhosis: Caring for patients with end-stage liver failure. *Nurse Pract*, 33(7), 24–30.
5. Blank-Reid, C. (2007). Abdominal trauma: Dealing with the damage. *Nursing*, 37(4 suppl: ED), 4–11.
6. Tan, W. A., Makaroun, M. S. (2007). Abdominal aortic aneurysm, rupture. Retrieved March 2009 from http://emedicine.medscape.com/article/416397.
7. Scott-Conner, C. E. H., Ballinger, B. (2007). Abdominal angina. Retrieved March 2009 from http://emedicine.medscape.com/article/188618.

8. Paula, R. (2009). Compartment syndrome, abdominal. Retrieved March 2009 from http://emedicine.medscape.com/article/829008.

9. Neal-Boylan, L. (2007). Health assessment of the very old person at home. *Home Healthcare Nurse*, 25(6), 388–398.

10. Tabloski, P. A. (ed.). (2006). *Gerontological Nursing*. Upper Saddle River, NJ: Pearson Prentice-Hall.

11. Estes, K., Thomure, J. (2008). Aspirin for the primary prevention of adverse cardiovascular events. *Crit Care Nurs Q*, 31(4), 324–339.

12. Miller, S. K., Alpert, P. T. (2006). Assessment and differential diagnosis of abdominal pain. *Nurse Pract*, 31(7), 39–47.

13. Hogstel, M. O., Curry, L. C. (2005). *Health Assessment Through the Life Span*, 4th ed. Philadelphia: F. A. Davis.

14. Held-Warmkessel, J., Schiech, L. (2008). Responding to 4 gastrointestinal complications in cancer patients. *Nursing*, 38(7), 32–38.

15. Dietzen, K. K. (2006). Assessment of the gastrointestinal system. In Ignatavicius, D. D., Workman, M. L. (eds.). *Medical-Surgical Nursing: Critical Thinking for Collaborative Care*, 5th ed. St. Louis, MO: Elsevier Saunders.

16. Schulman, C. (2002). End points of resuscitation: Choosing the right parameters to monitor. *Dimens Crit Care Nurs*, 21(1), 2–10.

17. Singh, H., et al. (2008). Gastrointestinal prophylaxis in critically ill patients. *Crit Care Nurs Q*, 31(4), 291–301.

18. Gisbert, J. P. (2004). *H. pylori* eradication therapy vs. antisecretory non-eradication therapy (with or without long-term maintenance antisecretory therapy) for the prevention of recurrent bleeding from peptic ulcer. Cochrane Collaboration. Cochrane Database Syst Rev, 2: CD004062.

19. Frost, K. L., Topp, R. (2006). A physical activity Rx for the hypertensive patient. *Nurse Pract*, 31(4), 29–37.

20. Turnbough, L., Wilson, L. (2007). Take your medicine: Nonadherence issues in patients with ulcerative colitis. *Gastroenterol Nurs*, 30(3), 212–217.

21. The American Pediatric Surgical Association. (2003). Necrotizing enterocolitis (NEC). Adapted from O'Neill, J. A., Grasfeld, J., Fonkalsrud, E. *Principles of Pediatric Surgery*, 2d ed. St. Louis, MO: Mosby. Retrieved February 2009 from www.eapsa.org/parents/resources/NEC.cfm.

22. Wolfe, T. R., Gallagher, J. (2006). Intra-abdominal hypertension: Pitfalls, prevalence and treatment options. *AACN News*. Retrieved March 2009 from www.wolfetory.com/pdf/Pocketalgorithm.pdf.

23. Overview: Intra-abdominal hypertension and abdominal compartment syndrome. Retrieved February 2009 from www.abdominalcompartmentsyndrome.org/acs/overview.html.

risk for ineffective renal Perfusion

DEFINITION: At risk for a decrease in blood circulation to the kidney that may compromise health

RISK FACTORS

Hypovolemia; [interruption of blood flow]; vascular embolism vasculitis

Hypertension; malignant hypertension; hyperlipidemia

Renal disease (polycystic kidney); polynephritis; exposure to toxins; bilateral cortical necrosis

Diabetes mellitus; malignancy

Cardiac surgery; cardiopulmonary bypass

Hypoxemia, hypoxia; metabolic acidosis

Cultural Collaborative Community/Home Care Diagnostic Studies Pediatric/Geriatric/Lifespan Medications

Multitrauma; abdominal compartment syndrome; burns; Infection (e.g, sepsis, localized infection); systemic inflammatory response syndrome

Treatment-related side effects (e.g., medications)

Advanced age

NOTE: A risk diagnosis is not evidenced by signs and symptoms, as the problem has not occurred; rather, nursing interventions are directed at prevention.

Sample Clinical Applications: Diabetes mellitus, hypertension, atherosclerosis, atrial fibrillation, sickle cell anemia, heat stroke, aortic aneurysm, shock states

DESIRED OUTCOMES/EVALUATION CRITERIA

Sample **NOC** linkages:

Kidney Function: Filtration of blood and elimination of metabolic waste products through the formation of urine

Knowledge: Disease Process: Extent of understanding conveyed about a specific disease process and prevention of complications

Client Will (Include Specific Time Frame)

- Demonstrate adequate renal perfusion as evidenced by urine output appropriate for individual, balanced intake and output, absence of edema formation or inappropriate weight gain.
- Verbalize understanding of condition, therapy regimen, side effects of medication, and when to contact healthcare provider.
- Engage in behaviors or lifestyle changes to improve circulation (e.g., smoking cessation, diabetic glucose control, medication management)

ACTIONS/INTERVENTIONS

Sample **NIC** linkages:

Fluid/Electrolyte Management: Regulation and prevention of complications from altered fluid and/or electrolyte levels

NURSING PRIORITY NO. 1

To assess causative/contributing factors:

- Determine history or presence of severe hypotension and hypoxemia; cardiogenic, hypovolemia, obstructive or septic shock, blunt or penetrating trauma with internal hemorrhage; surgery with excess bleeding or fluid loss, prolonged dehydration, poorly controlled dehydration, and so forth. *Conditions associated with decreased circulation and kidney ischemia.*[1,2]
- Note history or presence of abrupt onset or severe hypertension; persistent hypertension (160/100 mm Hg) over time; or hypertension resistent to appropriately dosed multidrug antihypertensive therapy, *which places client at high risk for kidney damage associated with renovascular hypertension.*[3,4]
- Assess hydration status. *Dehydration reduces glomerular filtration rate (GFR).*[5]
- Auscultate for bruit over each renal artery in abdomen at midclavicular line. *Bruit suggests renal artery stenosis, which is associated with renal insufficiency.*[3,5]
- Determine usual voiding pattern, and investigate reported deviations, such as low output or need for diuretics, *which may indicate problems with kidney perfusion associated with conditions such as hypovolemia, obstructive problem in urinary tract, shock states, heart failure, requiring further evaluation.*

Nursing Diagnoses in Alphabetical Order

risk for Poisoning (continued)
ACTIONS/INTERVENTIONS

Sample NIC linkages:
Medication Management: Facilitation of safe and effective use of prescription and over-the-counter (OTC) drugs
Environmental Management: Safety: Manipulation of the patient's surroundings for therapeutic benefit
Surveillance: Safety: Purposeful and ongoing collection and analysis of information about the patient and the environment for use in promoting and maintaining patient safety

NURSING PRIORITY NO. 1

To assess causative/contributing factors:

- Identify internal and external risk factors in client's environment (e.g., including infants/young children or frail elderly; confused or chronically ill person on multiple medications; person with suicidal ideation; illicit drug use/dealing [e.g., marijuana, cocaine, heroin]; drug manufacture in home [e.g., methamphetamines]; access or exposure to dangerous chemicals).
- Note age and cognitive status of client and care providers *to identify individuals who could be at higher risk for accidental poisoning. Babies, toddlers, and preschoolers are at risk because they are curious, like to put things into their mouths, and aren't aware of what's safe to eat. While school-age child can recognize danger and is at lower risk of unintentional poisoning, child is at risk for inadvertent overdose when taking medications without adequate supervision. The adolescent is at higher risk for experimentation due to natural inclination to take risks, peer pressure, and easy access to drugs and suicide attempts (with overdose of medications, and/or from illicit drug overdose or adverse reactions, or alcohol toxicity).*[2,3,12,13] *Elderly persons are at risk because of the higher number of prescription and OTC medications they consume (polypharmacy) and because of visual and cognitive impairments, which can cause them to forget what medications have been consumed and in what amounts they were taken. Elderly persons are also likely to share medications. In addition, the presence of nutritional deficits and renal or hepatic degeneration can reduce ability to detoxify drugs.*[4,5]
- Assess mood, coping abilities, personality styles (e.g., temperament, impulsive behavior, level of self-esteem) *that may result in carelessness and increased risk-taking without consideration of consequences, or suicidal actions.* (Refer to ND risk for Suicide.)
- Determine client's allergies to medications and foods *in order to avoid exposure to substances causing potentially lethal reaction.*
- Ascertain client's knowledge and use of medications. *Some individuals (especially elderly) believe that medication offers the solution to every health problem, a belief bolstered by frequent television, radio, and written advertising promising relief from a multitude of conditions from colds to sexual vitality. This often leads to multiple drug use (polypharmacy) and contributes to potential for overdose, adverse reactions (e.g., digoxin toxicity), and drug interactions.*[6,12]
- Determine specific drug hazards:
  Use of prescription, OTC medications, and culturally based home remedies. *These have potential for intentional and accidental overdose, as well as dangerous interactions. Drugs that are therapeutic in small doses may be deadly when taken in excess (e.g., beta-blockers, warfarin, digoxin). One of the most common problems is inadvertent overdosage of*

acetaminophen (Tylenol), either by increased dosing or by taking It with a combination product also containing acetaminophen. In children, the most serious accidental poisonings occur with iron, methadone, and tricyclic antidepressants.[1,5,7,14]

Availability or regular use of vitamins and mineral and herbal supplements. *Vitamins (especially A and D) are toxic in large doses, and iron is especially harmful to children.*[8,14] *Herbal drugs can be a source of poisoning (usually when taken chronically), due to toxicity of individual ingredients or from contaminants (e.g., mercury, lead, and arsenic).*[1]

Abuse of alcohol or other drugs (e.g., cocaine, methamphetamine, lysergic acid diethylamide [LSD], methadone). *These substances have potential for adverse reactions, cumulative affects with other substances, and risk for intentional and accidental overdose. Note: As little as 1 ounce of alcohol or a single dose of many drugs of abuse can cause serious injury/death in a small child.*[8,14]

- Identify environmental hazards:
  Storage of household chemicals (e.g., oven, toilet bowl, or drain cleaners; dishwasher products; bleach; hydrogen peroxide; fluoride preparations; essential oils; furniture polish; lighter fluid; lamp oil; kerosene; paints; turpentine; rust remover; lubricant oils; bug sprays or powders; fertilizers) *are readily available toxins in various forms that are often improperly stored.*[1,7,8]
  Review employment or work site safety *for exposure to chemicals, including vapors and fumes.*
  Refer to ND risk for Contamination for environmental issues.

- Review results of laboratory tests and toxicology screening, as indicated. *Guides treatment when overdose or accidental poisoning is known or suspected.*

NURSING PRIORITY NO. 2

To assist in correcting factors that can lead to accidental poisoning:

- Discuss medication safety with client/SO according to individual needs:
  Prevent accidental ingestion:[4–10,14,18]
  Stress importance of supervising infant/child, frail elderly, or individuals with cognitive limitations.
  Keep medicines and vitamins out of sight and reach of children or cognitively impaired persons
  Use child-resistant or tamper-resistant caps and locked medication cabinets.
  Recap medication containers immediately after obtaining current dosage. *Note: Many accidental poisonings occur when parent/caregiver steps away for a moment and child gets into product that was left out.*
  Code medicines for the visually impaired.
  Tell client to turn on light if the room is dark, and to put on glasses (if visually impaired) before taking or giving medications.
  Administer children's medications as drugs, not candy, *to prevent confusion.*
  Emphasize environmental safety regarding medications for all situations in which young child may be exposed (e.g., grandparents' home, day care, preschool).[11]
  Discuss vitamin use (especially those containing iron) *that can be poisonous to children if taken in large doses.*[11–13]
  Prevent duplication/possible overdose:[4–10]
  Review analgesic safety (e.g., acetaminophen is an ingredient in many OTC medications, and unintentional overdose can occur).[15,17]

Keep updated list of all medications (prescription, OTC, herbals, supplements) and review with healthcare providers when medications are changed, new ones added, or new healthcare providers are consulted.

Keep prescription medication in original bottle with label. Do not mix with other medication or place in unmarked containers.

Have responsible SO(s)/home health nurse supervise medication regimen/prepare medications for the cognitively or visually impaired, or obtain prefilled medicine boxes from pharmacy.

Take prescription medications and OTC drugs as prescribed on label.

Do not adjust medication dosage.

Retain and read safety information that accompanies prescriptions about expected effects, nuisance side effects, reportable and adverse affects, and how to manage forgotten dose.

Prevent taking medications that interact with one another or OTC/herbals/other supplements in an undesired or dangerous manner:[4–10]

Keep list of and reveal medication allergies, including type of reaction, to healthcare providers/pharmacist.

Wear medical alert bracelet or necklace, as appropriate.

Do not take outdated or expired medications. Do not save partial prescriptions to use another time.

Encourage discarding outdated or unused drug safely (disposing in hazardous waste collection areas, not down drain or toilet).

Do not take medications prescribed for another person.

Avoid mixing alcohol with medications (*potentiates effects of many drugs*).

Coordinate care when multiple healthcare providers are involved *to limit number of prescriptions and dosage levels.*

NURSING PRIORITY NO. 3

To promote wellness (Teaching/Discharge Considerations):

- Discuss general poison-prevention measures:[4–10]
- Encourage parent/caregiver to place safety stickers on dangerous products (drugs and chemicals) *to warn children of harmful contents.*
- Teach children about hazards of poisonous substances and to "ask first" before eating or drinking anything.
- Review drug side effects, potential interactions, and possibilities of misuse or overdosing (as with vitamin megadosing, etc.).[12]
- Discuss issues regarding drug use in home (e.g., alcohol, marijuana, heroin) *to provide opportunity to address potential for client's/SO's accidental overdose or accidental ingestion by children when drugs or drug paraphernalia are in the home.*[13]
- Provide list of emergency numbers (i.e., local or national poison control numbers, physician's office) to be placed by telephone *for use if poisoning occurs.*
- Instruct caregiver in event of poisoning, have product container on hand when contacting emergency provider.
- Discuss use of ipecac syrup in home. *The use of ipecac is controversial, as it may delay appropriate medical treatment (e.g., reduce the effectiveness of activated charcoal or oral antidotes) or be used inappropriately with adverse effects. Therefore, use in the home without direct advisement from poison control professionals is not recommended.*[16,17]
- Encourage client to obtain regular screening tests at prescribed intervals (e.g., prothrombin time/international normalized ratio [INR] for Coumadin; drug levels for Dilantin, digoxin; liver function studies when lipid-lowering agents [statins] are prescribed; or renal and

thyroid function and serum glucose levels for antimanics [lithium] use) to ascertain that circulating blood levels are within therapeutic range and absence of adverse effects.

- Ask healthcare provider/pharmacist about any considered medications if pregnant, nursing, or planning to become pregnant, *as some drugs are dangerous to fetus or nursing infant.*
- Refer substance abuser to detoxification programs, inpatient/outpatient rehabilitation, counseling, support groups, and psychotherapy.
- Encourage participation in community awareness and education programs (e.g., cardiopulmonary resuscitation [CPR] and first-aid class, home and workplace safety, hazardous materials disposal, access emergency medical personnel) *to assist individuals to identify and correct risk factors in environment, be prepared for emergency situation.*

DOCUMENTATION FOCUS

Assessment/Reassessment
- Identified risk factors noting internal and external concerns.

Planning
- Plan of care and who is involved in the planning.
- Teaching plan.

Implementation/Evaluation
- Response to interventions, teaching, and actions performed.
- Attainment or progress toward desired outcome(s).
- Modification to plan of care.

Discharge Planning
- Long-term needs and who is responsible for actions to be taken.
- Specific referrals made.

References

1. Bates, N. (2000). What's your poison? Retrieved July 2007 from www.dotpharmacy.com/uppoison.html.
2. Poisoning risk factors. (1997). *Information Sheet from Centers for Disease Control and Prevention* ("What Affects a Child's Risk of Poisoning?" Adapted from recommendations in Injury Prevention and Injury Control for Children and Youth). Atlanta, GA: Committee on Injury and Poison Prevention of the American Academy of Pediatrics.
3. Barela, T. (2001). What affects a child's risk of poisoning? TORCH magazine. Retrieved September 2003 from www.randolph.af.mil/se2/torch.
4. Stoehr, G. P. (1999). Pharmacology and older adults: The problem of polypharmacy. In Stanley, M., Beare, P. G. (eds). *Gerontological Nursing: A Health Promotion/Protection Approach.* 2d ed. Philadelphia: F. A. Davis, 66–73.
5. Older adults are at risk for poisoning exposures. (2002). News release from Illinois Poison Control Center. Retrieved September 2003 from www.mchc.org.
6. Nathan, M. S. (2001, update 2005). Poison proofing your home. Retrieved July 2007 from www.emedicinehealth.com.
7. Cohen, J. S. (2001, update 2005). Poisoning. Retrieved July 2007 from www.emedicinehealth.com.
8. Is my child at risk for poisoning during the holidays? (2003). Information Sheet. Retrieved September 2003 from www.phoenixchildrens.com.
9. Keep your children safe: Prevent accidental poisoning. Retrieved July 2007 from www.cnn.com/HEALTH/library/HQ/01263.html.
10. American Society of Health-System Pharmacists. Medications and you. Fact sheet. Retrieved July 2007 from www.safemedication.com.

11. Children's Hospital Boston. Poisons. Fact sheet. Retrieved July 2007 from www .childrenshospital.org/az/Site868.
12. Hingley, A. T. (2007). Preventing childhood poisoning. Retrieved April 2007 from www .kidsource.com/kidsource/content4/child.poison.fda.html.
13. Morris-Kukoski, C. L., Egland, A. G. (2006). Toxicity, deadly in a single dose. Retrieved July 2007 from www.emedicine.com/ped/topic2726.htm.
14. National Women's Health Resource Center Fact Sheet (2005). Medication safety. Retrieved July 2007 from www.healthywomen.org.
15. Smith, D. H. (2007). Managing acute acetaminophen toxicity. *Nursing*, 37(1), 58–63.
16. Manoguerra, A. S., Cobaugh, D. J. (2005). Guideline on the use of ipecac syrup in the out-of-hospital management of ingested poisons. *Clin Toxicol*, 43(1), 1–10.
17. American Academy of Clinical Toxicology. Position statement—Ipecac syrup. Retrieved April 2007 from www.clintox.org/Pos_Statements/Ipecac.html.
18. Doenges, M. E., Moorhouse, M. F., Geissler-Murr, A. C. (2004). ND: Poisoning, risk for. *Nurse's Pocket Guide: Diagnoses, Interventions, and Rationales.* 9th ed. Philadelphia: F. A. Davis.

Post-Trauma Syndrome [specify stage]

DEFINITION: Sustained maladaptive response to a traumatic, overwhelming event

RELATED FACTORS

Events outside the range of usual human experience
Serious threat to self or loved ones
Serious injury to self or loved ones; serious accidents (e.g., industrial, motor vehicle)
Abuse (physical and psychosocial); criminal victimization; rape
Witnessing mutilation or violent death; tragic occurrence involving multiple deaths
Disasters; sudden destruction of one's home or community; epidemics
Wars; being held prisoner of war; torture

DEFINING CHARACTERISTICS

Subjective
Intrusive thoughts or dreams; nightmares; flashbacks; [excessive verbalization of the traumatic event]
Palpitations; headaches [loss of interest in usual activities, loss of feeling of intimacy or sexuality]
Hopelessness; shame; guilt; [verbalization of survival guilt or guilt about behavior required for survival]
Anxiety; fear; grieving; depression
Reports of feeling numb
Gastric irritability; [change in appetite; sleep disturbance; chronic fatigue or easy fatigability]
Difficulty in concentrating

Objective
Hypervigilance; exaggerated startle response; irritability; neurosensory irritability
Anger; rage; aggression

Avoidance; repression; alienation; denial; detachment; psychogenic amnesia
Altered mood states; [poor impulse control or explosiveness]; panic attacks; horror
Substance abuse; compulsive behavior
Enuresis (in children)
[Difficulty with interpersonal relationships; dependence on others; work or school failure]
[Stages:
Acute Subtype: Begins within 6 months and does not last longer than 6 months.
Chronic Subtype: Lasts more than 6 months.
Delayed Subtype: Period of latency of 6 months or more before onset of symptoms.]

Sample Clinical Applications: Traumatic injuries, physical/psychological abuse, dissociative disorder

DESIRED OUTCOMES/EVALUATION CRITERIA

Sample NOC linkages:
Comfort Status: Psychospiritual: Psychospiritual ease related to self-concept, emotional well-being, source of inspiration, and meaning and purpose in one's life
Fear Self-Control: Personal actions to eliminate or reduce disabling feelings of apprehension or uneasiness from an identifiable source
Abuse Recovery: Emotional [or] Physical: Extent of healing of psychological/physical injuries due to abuse

Client Will (Include Specific Time Frame)
• Express own feelings and reactions, avoiding projection.
• Verbalize a positive self-image.
• Report reduced anxiety or fear when memories occur.
• Demonstrate ability to deal with emotional reactions in an individually appropriate manner.
• Demonstrate appropriate changes in behavior or lifestyle (e.g., share experiences with others, seek and get support from SO[s] as needed, change in job or residence).
• Report absence of physical manifestations (e.g., pain, chronic fatigue).
Refer to ND Rape-Trauma Syndrome for additional outcomes when trauma is the result of rape.

ACTIONS/INTERVENTIONS

Sample NIC linkages:
Support System Enhancement: Facilitation of support to patient by family, friends, and community
Counseling: Use of an interactive helping process focusing on the needs, problems, or feelings of the patient and significant others to enhance or support coping, problem-solving, and interpersonal relationships
Anxiety Reduction: Minimizing apprehension, dread, foreboding, or uneasiness related to an unidentified source or anticipated danger

NURSING PRIORITY NO. 1

To assess causative factor(s) and individual reaction:

ACUTE

- Observe for and elicit information about physical or psychological injury and note associated stress-related symptoms (e.g., numbness, headache, tightness in chest, nausea, pounding heart). *Anxiety is viewed as a normal reaction to a realistic danger or threat, and noting these factors can identify the severity of the anxiety the client is experiencing in the circumstances.*[4]
- Identify such psychological responses as anger, shock, acute anxiety, confusion, denial. Note laughter, crying, calm or agitated, excited (hysterical) behavior; expressions of disbelief, guilt and/or self-blame, labile emotions. *Indicators of severe response to trauma that client has experienced and need for specific interventions.*[9]
- Assess client's knowledge of and anxiety related to the situation. Note ongoing threat to self (e.g., contact with perpetrator and/or associates) or perception of others as threatening. *Client may be aware but speak as though the incident is related to someone else. Flashbacks may occur with the individual reliving the incident/event.*[9]
- Note occupation (e.g., police, fire, rescue, emergency department staff, corrections officer, mental health worker, disaster responders, soldier or support personnel in combat zone, as well as family members). *These occupations carry a high risk for constantly being involved in traumatic events and the potential for exacerbation of stress response and block to recovery.*[1] *In addition, family members are also subjected to the same trauma, because they see the same events repeated on TV news channels and hear stories repeated by their loved one(s) who were directly involved.*
- Identify social aspects of trauma or incident (e.g., disfigurement, chronic conditions or permanent disabilities, loss of home or community) *that affect ability to return to normal involvement in activities and work.*[9]
- Ascertain ethnic background, cultural and religious perceptions and beliefs about the occurrence. *Client may believe occurrence is retribution from God or result of some indiscretion on his or her part; client may in some way also blame themselves for the incident or occurrence. Individual's view of how he or she is coping may be influenced by cultural background, religious beliefs, and family influence.*[5,9]
- Determine degree of disorganization (e.g., task-oriented activity is not goal-directed, organized, or effective; individual is overwhelmed by emotion much of the time). *Presence of persistent frightening thoughts and memories, reliving the event, feeling emotionally numb and unable to be close to friends and family members, suffering from sleep and eating problems all interfere with ability to manage daily living, work, and relationships with others.*[9,14]
- Identify whether incident has reactivated preexisting or coexisting situations (physical or psychological). *Traumas or difficulties in client's life and how they were dealt with will affect how the client views the current trauma.*[7]
- Determine disruptions in relationships (e.g., family, friends, coworkers, SOs). *Support persons may not know how to deal with client/situation and may be oversolicitous or withdraw; either of these actions will be counterproductive to client's ability to cope with situation.*[9]
- Note withdrawn behavior, use of denial, and use of chemical substances or impulsive behaviors (e.g., chain-smoking, overeating). *Indicators of severity of anxiety and client's difficulty dealing with posttraumatic stress disorder (PTSD) and need for interventions to address these behaviors.*[9]
- Be aware of signs of increasing anxiety (e.g., silence, stuttering, inability to sit still). *Increasing anxiety may indicate risk for violence or need for medication or other measures to decrease anxiety and help client manage feelings.*[9]

- Note verbal and nonverbal expressions of guilt or self-blame when client has survived trauma in which others died. Validate congruency of observations with verbalizations. *Sense of own responsibility (blame) and guilt about not having done something to prevent incident or not having been "good enough" to deserve survival are strong beliefs, especially in individuals who are influenced by background, religious, and cultural factors.*[2]
- Assess signs and stage of grieving for self and others. *Identification and understanding of stages of grief assist with choice of interventions, planning of care, and movement toward resolution.*[2]
- Identify development of phobic reactions to ordinary articles (e.g., knives) and situations (e.g., walking in groups of people, strangers ringing doorbell). *These may trigger feelings from original trauma and need to be dealt with sensitively, accepting reality of feelings and stressing ability of client to deal with them.*[2]

CHRONIC (in addition to previous assessment)
- Evaluate continued somatic complaints. Investigate reports of new or changes in symptoms. *Reports of physical symptoms, such as gastric irritation, anorexia, insomnia, muscle tension, headache may accompany disorganization and need further evaluation and interventions.*[2]
- Note manifestations of chronic pain or pain symptoms in excess of degree of physical injury. *Psychological responses may magnify or exacerbate physical symptoms, indicating need for interventions to help client deal with pain.*[7]
- Be aware of signs of severe or prolonged depression; note presence of flashbacks, intrusive memories, nightmares, panic attacks, poor impulse control; and problems with memory or concentration; thoughts and perceptions; and conflict, aggression, or rage. *Symptoms are not uncommon following a trauma of such magnitude, although client may feel that he or she is "going crazy."*[4,13]
- Assess degree of dysfunctional coping (including substance use or abuse, suicidal ideation) and consequences. *Identifies needs and depth of interventions required. Individuals display different levels of dysfunctional behavior in response to stress, and often the choice of chemical substances or substance abuse is a way of deadening the psychic pain.*[2]

NURSING PRIORITY NO. 2

To assist client to deal with situation that exists:

ACUTE
- Allow the client to work through own kind of adjustment. If the client is withdrawn or unwilling to talk, do not force the issue. *Each person is an individual and has own ways of coping. Being there and allowing client to choose own path conveys sense of confidence in ability to deal with situation.*[10]
- Listen for expressions of fear of crowds or people. *May indicate continuing anxiety and difficulty reentering normal activities.*[9]
- Ascertain or monitor sleep pattern of children as well as adults. *Sleep disturbances or nightmares may develop, delaying resolution, impairing coping abilities, and interfering with return to desired lifestyle.*[7]
- Be aware of and assist client to use ego strengths in a positive way by acknowledging ability to handle what is happening. *Enhances self-concept and reduces sense of helplessness and powerlessness, thus enabling client to move on with life.*[3]
- Encourage client to learn stress-management techniques, such as deep breathing, meditation, relaxation, and exercise. *Reduces stress, enhancing coping skills and helping to resolve situation.*[11]

Nursing Diagnoses in Alphabetical Order

- Assist in dealing with practical concerns and effects of the incident, such as court appearances, altered relationships with SO(s), employment problems. *In the period immediately following the traumatic incident, individual is in a state of numbness and shock. Thinking becomes difficult, and assistance with practical matters will help manage necessary activities for the person to move through this time.*[10]
- Identify employment, community resource groups. *Provides opportunity for ongoing support to deal with recurrent stressors as individual regroups and moves forward.*[12]
- Administer anti-anxiety or sedative and hypnotic medications with caution.

CHRONIC

- Continue listening to expressions of concern. *May have recurring symptoms, thus necessitating the need to continue talking about the incident.*[9]
- Permit free expression of feelings (may continue from the crisis phase). Do not rush client through expressions of feelings too quickly, and refrain from providing false reassurances. *Client may believe pain or anguish is misunderstood and may be depressed. Statements such as "You don't understand" or "You weren't there" are a defense—a way of pushing others away—and need to be responded to with empathy and concern.*[10]
- Encourage client to talk out experience when ready, expressing feelings of fear, anger, loss or grief. (Refer to NDs Grieving, complicated Grieving.) *Client may need to repeat story over and over and needs to be accepted and assured that feelings are normal for the unusual event that has been experienced.*[9]
- Note whether feelings expressed appear congruent with events the client experienced. *Expressing feelings helps client recognize and identify them to enhance coping. Incongruency may indicate deeper conflict that can impede resolution.*[11]
- Encourage client to become aware and accepting of own feelings and reactions as being normal reactions in an abnormal situation. *There are no "bad" feelings, and awareness and acceptance enables client to deal with feelings once identified and move forward in recovery from traumatic event.*[6,14]
- Acknowledge reality of loss of self that existed before the incident. Assist client to move toward an acceptance of the potential for growth that exists within client. *Recognition that individual can never go back to being the person he or she was before the incident allows progress toward life as a different person.*[11]
- Continue to allow client to progress at own pace. *Taking own time to talk about what has happened, allowing feelings to be fully expressed, aids in the healing process. If rushed, client may believe he or she is not accepted or understood.*[2]
- Give "permission" to express and deal with anger at the assailant or situation in acceptable ways. *Being free to express anger appropriately allows it to be dissipated so underlying feelings can be identified and dealt with, thus strengthening coping skills.*[2]
- Avoid prompting discussion of issues that cannot be resolved. Keep discussion on practical and emotional level rather than intellectualizing the experience. *When feelings (the experience) are intellectualized, uncomfortable insights and/or awareness are avoided by the use of rationalization, blocking resolution of feelings and impairing coping abilities.*[2]
- Provide for sensitive, trained counselors/therapists and engage in therapies, such as psychotherapy in conjunction with medications, Implosive Therapy (flooding), hypnosis, relaxation, Rolfing, memory work, cognitive restructuring, Eye Movement Desensitization and Reprocessing (EMDR), physical and occupational therapies. *Although it is not necessary for the helping person to have experienced the same kind of trauma as the client, sensitivity and listening skills are important to helping the client confront fears and learn new ways to cope with what has happened. Therapeutic use of desensitization techniques (flooding, implosive therapy) provides for extinction through exposure to the fear. Body work can*

alleviate muscle tension. Some techniques (Rolfing) help to bring blocked emotions to awareness as sensations of the traumatic event are reexperienced.[9]

- Discuss use of psychotropic medication. *May be used to decrease anxiety, lift mood, aid in management of behavior, and ensure rest until client regains control of own self. Lithium may be used to reduce explosiveness; low-dose psychotropics may be used when loss of contact with reality is a problem.*[8]

NURSING PRIORITY NO. 3

To promote wellness (Teaching/Discharge Considerations):

- Assist client to identify and monitor feelings while therapy is occurring. *Promotes awareness and helps client know that control of feelings as they arise will help move beyond traumatic episode.*[9]
- Provide information about what reactions client may expect during each phase. Let client know these are common reactions and phrase in neutral terms of "You may or you may not. . . ." *Knowledge of what may be experienced helps reduce fear of the unknown, thereby enabling client to manage reactions if they occur. Use of neutral terms lets client understand that not all reactions may occur in own situation.*[3]
- Assist client to identify factors that may have created a vulnerable situation and that he or she may have power to change to protect self in the future. *While client is not responsible for event, may have unknowingly contributed to occurrence by their actions. Identifying those actions that are within their power to change provides sense of control over seemingly uncontrollable situations.*[9]
- Avoid making value judgments. *Client may be judging self and caregiver needs to convey nonjudgmental stance to allow individual to deal with feelings of guilt and recrimination, accepting fact that he or she did the best they were capable of in the circumstances.*[3]
- Discuss lifestyle changes client is contemplating and how they may contribute to recovery. *Client needs to evaluate appropriateness of plans and look at long-range consequences (e.g., moving away from effective support group) to make the best choice for the future.*[4]
- Assist with learning stress-management techniques. *Deep breathing, counting to 10, reviewing the situation, reframing skills assist client in developing constructive ways to cope with feelings of powerlessness and to regain control of self. Reframing stressors or situation in other words or positive ideas can help client recognize and consider alternatives.*[4]
- Discuss drug regimen, potential side effects of prescribed medications and necessity of prompt reporting of untoward effects.
- Discuss recognition of and ways to manage "anniversary reactions," reinforcing normalcy of recurrence of thoughts and feelings at this time. *Understanding that these feelings are to be expected and planning for them helps client get through the anniversary of the event with the least difficulty.*[10]
- Suggest support group for SO(s). *Family members may not understand client's reactions and need help with understanding them and learning how to deal with client in the most helpful manner.*[2]
- Encourage psychiatric consultation. *May need additional therapy if client is unable to maintain control, is violent or inconsolable, or does not seem to be making an adjustment. Participation in a group may be helpful.*[2]
- Refer for long-term family/marital counseling, if indicated. *Additional and ongoing support or therapy may be needed to help family resolve crisis and look at potential for growth. Client problems affect family members and other relationships, and further counseling may help resolve issues of enabling behavior and communication problems.*[12]
- Refer to NDs ineffective Coping, Grieving; complicated Grieving; Powerlessness.

DOCUMENTATION FOCUS

Assessment/Reassessment
• Individual findings, noting current dysfunction and behavioral or emotional responses to the incident.
• Specifics of traumatic event.
• Reactions of family/SO(s).
• Cultural or religious beliefs and expectations.
• Availability and use of resources.

Planning
• Plan of care and who is involved in the planning.
• Teaching plan.

Implementation/Evaluation
• Responses to interventions, teaching, and actions performed.
• Emotional changes.
• Attainment or progress toward desired outcome(s).
• Modifications to plan of care.

Discharge Planning
• Long-term needs and who is responsible for actions to be taken.
• Specific referrals made.

References

1. Doenges, M., Moorhouse, M., Geissler-Murr, A. (2002). *Nursing Care Plans: Guidelines for Individualizing Patient Care.* 6th ed. Philadelphia: F. A. Davis.
2. Doenges, M., Townsend, M., Moorhouse, M. (1998). *Psychiatric Care Plans: Guidelines for Individualizing Care.* 3d ed. Philadelphia: F. A. Davis.
3. Cox, H., et al. (2002). *Clinical Applications of Nursing Diagnoses: Adult, Child, Women's, Psychiatric, Gerontic, and Home Health Considerations.* 4th ed. Philadelphia: F. A. Davis.
4. Townsend, M. (2003). *Psychiatric Mental Health Nursing: Concepts of Care.* 4th ed. Philadelphia: F. A. Davis.
5. Lipson, J. G., Dibble, S. L., Minarik, P. A. (1996). *Culture & Nursing Care: A Pocket Guide.* San Francisco: UCSF Nursing Press.
6. Stuart, G. W. (2001). Anxiety responses and anxiety disorders. In Stuart, G. W., Laraia, M. T. (eds). *Principles and Practice of Psychiatric Nursing.* 7th ed. St. Louis, MO: Mosby.
7. Porth, C. M., Kunert, P. K. (2002). *Pathophysiology: Concepts of Altered Health States.* Philadelphia: J. B. Lippincott.
8. Townsend, M. (2001). *Nursing Diagnoses in Psychiatric Nursing: Care Plans and Psychotropic Medications.* 5th ed. Philadelphia: F. A. Davis.
9. National Institute of Mental Health. (2000). Anxiety disorders. NIH Publication No. 00-3879. Retrieved December 2003 from www.nimh.nih.gov.anxiety/anxiety.cfm.
10. Harper, N. E. (1997). *Seven Choices.* Austin, TX: Centerpoint Press.
11. Posttraumatic stress disorder—Part I. (June 1996). *Harvard Mental Health Letter.*
12. Posttraumatic stress disorder—Part II. (July 1996). *Harvard Mental Health Letter.*
13. Gore, T. A., Richards-Reid, G. M. (2006). Posttraumatic stress disorder. Retrieved April 2007 from www.emedicine.com/med/topic1900.htm.
14. Lubit, R. (2005). Acute treatment of disaster survivors. Retrieved April 2007 from www.emedicine.com/med/topic3540.htm.

risk for Post-Trauma Syndrome

DEFINITION: At risk for sustained maladaptive response to a traumatic, overwhelming event

RISK FACTORS

Occupation (e.g., police, fire, rescue, corrections, emergency room staff, mental health worker, [and their family members])
Perception of event; exaggerated sense of responsibility; diminished ego strength
Survivor's role in the event
Inadequate social support; nonsupportive environment; displacement from home
Duration of the event

NOTE: A risk diagnosis is not evidenced by signs and symptoms, as the problem has not occurred; rather, nursing interventions are directed at prevention.
Sample Clinical Applications: Traumatic injuries, physical/psychological abuse, dissociative disorder

DESIRED OUTCOMES/EVALUATION CRITERIA

Sample (NOC) linkages:
Fear Level: Severity of manifested apprehension, tension, or uneasiness arising from an identifiable source
Fear Self-Control: Personal actions to eliminate or reduce disabling feelings of apprehension and tension from an identifiable source
Grief Resolution: Adjustment to actual or impending loss

Client Will (Include Specific Time Frame)
• Verbalizes absence of disabling apprehension.
• Demonstrate ability to deal with emotional reactions in an individually appropriate manner.
• Deal with practical aspects of situation (e.g., court appearances, temporary housing, funeral services, rebuilding life).
• Report relief or absence of physical manifestations (pain, nightmares, flashbacks, fatigue) associated with event.

ACTIONS/INTERVENTIONS

Sample (NIC) linkages:
Crisis Intervention: Use of short-term counseling to help the patient cope with a crisis and resume a state of functioning comparable to or better than the precrisis state
Coping Enhancement: Assisting a patient to adapt to perceived stressors, changes, or threats that interfere with meeting life demands and roles
Support System Enhancement: Facilitation of support to patient by family, friends, and community

NURSING PRIORITY NO. 1

To assess contributing factors and individual reaction:

- Identify client who survived or witnessed traumatic event (e.g., airplane or motor vehicle crash, mass shooting, fire destroying home and lands, robbery at gunpoint, other violent act) *to recognize individual at high risk for post-trauma syndrome.*
- Note occupation (e.g., police, fire, emergency services personnel, rescue workers, disaster responders, soldiers and support personnel in combat areas, and family members). *Studies reveal a moderate to high percentage of posttraumatic stress disorders (PTSDs) develop in these populations when they have been exposed to one or more traumatic incidents.*[1,12] *In addition, family members are also at risk because they are subjected to the same trauma, as they see the events repeated on TV news channels/hear stories repeated by their loved one(s) who were directly involved.*
- Assess client's knowledge of and anxiety related to potential for work-related trauma incident (e.g., shooting in line of duty or viewing body of murdered child); and number, duration, and intensity of recurring situations (e.g., emergency medical technician [EMT] exposed to numerous on-the-job traumatic incidents; rescuers searching for victims of natural or man-made disasters). *Having information about these situations enables individuals to think about and plan for eventualities so anxiety can be dealt with in a positive manner.*[7]
- Ascertain ethnic background and cultural or religious perceptions and beliefs about the occurrence. *Client may believe occurrence is retribution from God, or result of some indiscretion on his or her part, or in some way blame themselves for the incident or occurrence. Individual's view of how he or she is coping may be influenced by cultural background, religious beliefs, and family influence.*[7]
- Identify how client's experiences may affect current situation. *Individual who has had previous experiences with traumatic events (e.g., firefighter who deals with trauma on a regular basis or person who has been involved in a trauma herself or himself) may be more susceptible to PTSD and ineffective coping abilities.*[2]
- Listen for comments of guilt, humiliation, shame, or taking on responsibility (e.g., "I should have been more careful/gone back to get her"; "Don't call me a hero; I couldn't save my partner"; "My kids are the same age as the ones who died"). *Expressing guilt for actions that individual might have taken can lead to ruminations about lack of responsible behavior, leading to anxiety and PTSD.*[9,12,13]
- Note verbal and nonverbal expressions of guilt or self-blame when client has survived trauma in which others died. *Sense of own responsibility (blame) and guilt about not having done something to prevent incident or not having been "good enough" to deserve surviving are strong beliefs, especially in individuals who are influenced by family background, religious, and cultural factors.*[2]
- Evaluate for life factors and stressors currently or recently occurring, such as displacement from home due to catastrophic event (e.g., illness or injury, fire, flood, violent storm, or earthquake) happening to individual whose child is dying of cancer or who suffered abuse as a child. *Cumulative effects of multiple events can put the individual at higher risk for developing PTSD (acute added to delayed onset reactions) and indicates need for preventive measures to be taken.*[4,12]
- Identify client's coping mechanisms. *Resolution of the posttrauma response is largely dependent on the coping skills the client has developed throughout own life and is able to bring to bear on current situation.*[4]

- Determine availability and usefulness of client's support systems, family, social, community, and so forth, being aware that family members themselves or community in general may also be at risk. *Having an effective available support system and talking with them about what is happening can help client and family members resolve feelings and move on with life in a positive manner.*[10]

NURSING PRIORITY NO. 2

To assist client to deal with situation that exists:

IMMEDIATE POSTINCIDENT

- Provide a calm, safe environment. *Client can deal with disruption of life more effectively when surrounded by quiet and by knowing he or she is safe.*[11]
- Assist with documentation for police report, as indicated, and stay with the client. *Developing accurate chain of evidence (maintaining sequencing and collection of evidence) and labeling each specimen and storing and packaging it properly provides important evidence for possibility of future prosecution.*[2]
- Listen to and investigate physical complaints. *Physical injuries may have occurred during incident, which may be masked by emotional reactions and limit client's ability to recognize them. These need to be identified and differentiated from anxiety symptoms so appropriate treatment may be instituted.*[2]
- Identify supportive persons (e.g., loved ones, spiritual advisor or pastor). *Having unconditional support from loving and caring others can help the client cope with the situation and move on to live more fully.*[2]
- Remain with client, listen as client recounts incident and concerns—possibly repeatedly. If client does not want to talk, accept silence. *Establishes trust, thus providing psychological support and allowing client opportunity to vent emotions.*[4]
- Encourage expression of feelings and reinforce that feelings and reactions to trauma are common and not indicators of weakness or failure. Note whether feelings expressed appear congruent with events the client experienced. *Expressing feelings helps client recognize and identify them to enhance coping. Incongruency may indicate deeper conflict that can impede resolution.*[7]
- Help child to express feelings about event using techniques appropriate to developmental level (e.g., play for young child, stories or puppets for preschooler, peer group for adolescent). *Children are more likely to express in play what they may not be able to verbalize directly. Adolescents may benefit from groups, gaining knowledge, support, decreased sense of isolation and improved coping skills.*[3]
- Assist with practical realities (e.g., temporary housing, money, notifications of family members, or other needs). *Dealing with these issues is necessary and helps client remain connected to reality and maintain sense of control over daily living concerns.*[2]

NURSING PRIORITY NO. 3

To assist client to deal with situation that exists:

- Evaluate client's perceptions of events and personal significance (e.g., police officer who is also a parent and is investigating death of a child). *Individuals perceive events depending on their previous experiences, cultural and religious background, and family of origin and will respond to any given trauma based on these factors. Incidents that touch a person's own life will be more difficult to deal with and may have a deeper effect.*[3]
- Provide emotional and physical presence *to strengthen client's coping abilities. Spending time with the client promotes trust and provides an opportunity for client to think about what will help in the current situation.*[4]

- Observe for signs and symptoms of stress responses, such as nightmares, reliving an incident, poor appetite, irritability, numbness and crying, family and relationship disruption. *These responses are normal in the early postincident time frame. If prolonged and persistent, the client may be experiencing PTSD.*[9]
- Identify and discuss client's strengths (e.g., very supportive family, usually copes well with stress) as well as vulnerabilities (e.g., client tends toward alcohol or other drugs for coping, client has witnessed a murder). *Knowing one's strengths and weaknesses helps client know what actions to take to cope with and prevent anxiety from becoming overwhelming.*[9]
- Discuss how individual coping mechanisms have worked in past traumatic events. *Awareness of previous successful experiences can help client remember coping skills that can be used to deal with current situation in a positive manner.*[4]

NURSING PRIORITY NO. 4

To promote wellness (Teaching/Discharge Considerations):

- 🏠 Educate high-risk persons and families about signs/symptoms of posttrauma response, especially if it is likely to occur in their occupation or life. *Awareness allows individual to be proactive and seek support and timely intervention as needed.*
- 🏠 Encourage client to identify and monitor feelings on an ongoing basis. *Promotes awareness of changes in ability to deal with stressors, allowing prompt intervention when necessary.*[5]
- 🏠 Encourage learning stress-management techniques, such as deep breathing, meditation, relaxation, exercise. *Reduces stress, enhancing coping skills and helping to resolve situation.*[6]
- 🏠 Recommend participation in debriefing sessions that may be provided following major events. *Dealing with the stressor promptly may facilitate recovery from event and prevent exacerbation. Debriefing is being used by many organizations who regularly deal with traumatic events to prevent the development of PTSD, although issues about best timing of debriefing continue to be debated.*[4]
- 🏠 Explain that posttraumatic symptoms can emerge months or sometimes years after a traumatic experience and that help or support can be obtained when needed or desired if client begins to experience intrusive memories or other symptoms.
- 🏠 Encourage individual to develop a survivor mentality. *People often have it within their means to head off life-threatening situations and even survive the worst when they plan for emergencies and think ahead about ways to survive, such as taking food, water, and protective gear on a day hike in case you get lost, fall and break a bone, or in other ways have to spend more time than anticipated.*[11]
- ⊗ Identify employment, community resource groups (e.g., Assistance Support and Self Help in Surviving Trauma [ASSIST], employee peer assistance programs, Red Cross or other survivor support services, Compassionate Friends). *Provides opportunity for ongoing support to deal with recurrent stressors as individual moves on with life.*[8,13]
- ⊗ Refer for individual or family counseling, as indicated. *May need additional assistance to prevent continuation of anxiety and the onset of PTSD.*[7]

DOCUMENTATION FOCUS

Assessment/Reassessment
- Identified risk factors noting internal and external concerns.
- Client's perception of event and personal significance.
- Cultural or religious beliefs and expectations.

Planning
- Plan of care and who is involved in the planning.
- Teaching plan.

Implementation/Evaluation
- Response to interventions, teaching, and actions performed.
- Attainment or progress toward desired outcome(s).

Discharge Planning
- Long-term needs and who is responsible for actions to be taken.
- Specific referrals made.

References

1. Doenges, M. E., Moorhouse, M. F., Geissler-Murr, A. C. (2002). *Nursing Care Plans: Guidelines for Individualizing Patient Care*. 6th ed. Philadelphia: F. A. Davis.
2. Doenges, M., Townsend, M., Moorhouse, M. (1998). *Psychiatric Care Plans: Guidelines for Individualizing Care*. 3d ed. Philadelphia: F. A. Davis.
3. Cox, H., et al. (2002). *Clinical Applications of Nursing Diagnoses: Child, Adult, Women's, Psychiatric, Gerontic, and Home Health Considerations*. 4th ed. Philadelphia: F. A. Davis.
4. Townsend, M. (2003). *Psychiatric Mental Health Nursing: Concepts of Care*. 4th ed. Philadelphia: F. A. Davis.
5. Stuart, G. W. (2001). Anxiety responses and anxiety disorders. In Stuart, G. W., Laraia, M. T. (eds). *Principles and Practice of Psychiatric Nursing*. 7th ed. St. Louis, MO: Mosby.
6. Porth, C. M., Kunert, P. K. (2002). *Pathophysiology: Concepts of Altered Health States*. Philadelphia: J. B. Lippincott.
7. National Institute of Mental Health. (2000). Anxiety disorders. NIH Publication No. 02-3879. Retrieved July 2007 from www.nimh.nih.gov.anxiety/anxiety.cfm.
8. Harper, N. E. (1997). *Seven Choices*. 5th ed. Austin, TX: Centerpoint Press.
9. Posttraumatic stress disorder—Part I. (June 1996). *Harvard Mental Health Letter*.
10. Posttraumatic stress disorder—Part II. (July 1996). *Harvard Mental Health Letter*.
11. Kamler, K. (2004). *Surviving the Extremes: A Doctor's Journey to the Limits of Human Endurance*. Boston: St. Martin's.
12. Davis, N. (2003). [Brief summaries from] Multi-Sensory Trauma Processing, A Manual for Understanding and Treating PTSD and Job-Related Trauma. Retrieved April 2007 from www.rescue-workers.com/1.htm.
13. Galea, S., Nandi, A., Vlahov, D. (2005). The epidemiology of post-traumatic stress disorders after disasters. *Epidemiol Rev*, 27(1), 78–91.

readiness for enhanced Power

DEFINITION: A pattern of participating knowingly in change that is sufficient for well-being and can be strengthened

RELATED FACTORS

To be developed by nurse researchers and submitted to NANDA

(continues on page 642)

readiness for enhanced Power (continued)
DEFINING CHARACTERISTICS

Subjective
Expresses readiness to enhance power; knowledge for participation in change; awareness of possible changes to be made; identification of choices that can be made for change
Expresses readiness to enhance freedom to perform actions for change; involvement in creating change; participation in choices for daily living and health

NOTE: Even though power (a response) and empowerment (an intervention approach) are different concepts, the literature related to both concepts supports the defining characteristics of this diagnosis.
Sample Clinical Applications: Any acute or chronic condition, or healthy individual looking to change life/improve well-being

DESIRED OUTCOMES/EVALUATION CRITERIA

Sample (NOC) linkages:
Personal Autonomy: Personal actions of a competent individual to exercise governance in life decisions
Decision-Making: Ability to make judgments and choose between two or more alternatives
Health Beliefs: Perceived Control: Personal conviction that one can influence a health outcome

Client Will (Include Specific Time Frame)
• Verbalize knowledge of what changes he or she want to make.
• Express awareness of own ability to be in charge of changes to be made.
• Participate in classes or group activities to learn new skills.
• State readiness to take power over own life.

ACTIONS/INTERVENTIONS

Sample (NIC) linkages:
Self-Responsibility Facilitation: Encouraging a patient to assume more responsibility for own behavior
Decision-Making Support: Providing information and support for a person who is making a decision regarding healthcare
Health System Guidance: Facilitating a patient's location and use of appropriate health services

NURSING PRIORITY NO. 1

To determine need/motivation for improvement:

● Determine current situation and circumstances that client is experiencing leading to desire to improve life. *Provides information to help client with planning for enhancing life.*[8]
● Ascertain motivation and expectations for change. *Motivation to improve and high expectations can encourage client to make changes that will improve his or her life. However, unrealistic expectations or motivation to please someone else may hamper efforts.*
● Identify emotional climate in which client and relationships live and work. *The emotional climate has a great impact between people. When a power differential exists in relationships, the atmosphere is largely determined by the person or people who have the power.*[4]

- Identify client locus of control: internal (expressions of responsibility for self and ability to control outcomes) or external (expressions of lack of control over self and environment). *Understanding locus of control can help client to work toward positive, internal control as he or she develops sense of ability to freely choose own actions.*[9]

 - Determine cultural factors or religious beliefs influencing client's self-view. *These factors can be strong determinants in individual's ability to change and view self as powerful and may complicate growth process.*[9]

- Assess degree of mastery client has exhibited in his or her life. *Helps client to understand how he or she has functioned in the past, how that applies to current situation, and what is needed to improve.*

- Note presence of family/SOs that can or do act as support systems for client. *When family understands and supports client's desires and efforts, he or she is more likely to be successful.*[6]

- Determine whether client knows or uses assertiveness skills. *Learning and enhancing these skills will help client to improve ability to take personal responsibility for own self and relationships with others.*[1,3,5,7]

NURSING PRIORITY NO. 2

To assist client to clarify needs relative to ability to improve feelings of power:

- Discuss how client is currently involved in creating change in life. *Provides a baseline to measure growth and suggests possibilities for change.*[8]

- Listen to and Active-listen client's perceptions and beliefs about the concept of power. *Enables client to identify underlying feelings and thoughts about this issue and how power can be gained in his or her life.*[8]

- Identify strengths, assets, and past coping strategies that were successful. *These strategies can be built on to enhance feelings of control.*[6]

- Discuss the importance of assuming personal responsibility for life and relationships. *This requires one to be open to new ideas and experiences, different values, and beliefs and to be inquisitive.*

- Identify things client can and or cannot control. *Avoids wasting time on things that are not in the control of the client.*

- Treat expressed desires and decisions with respect. Avoid critical parenting expressions. *Individual may express thoughts and opinions that are creative and out of the ordinary, and critical parenting responses such as "That's a dumb idea" can crush person's brainstorming.*[9]

NURSING PRIORITY NO. 3

To promote optimum wellness, enhancing power (Teaching/Discharge Considerations):

- Assist client to set realistic goals for the future. *Even though client is thinking creatively and brainstorming ideas, goals need to be planned step by step to reach the desired outcome.*[6]

- Provide accurate verbal and written information about client's concerns and life situation. *Reinforces learning and promotes self-paced review.*[8]

- Assist client to learn/use assertive communication skills. *These techniques require practice, but as the client becomes more proficient, they will help to develop relationships that are more effective.*[2,3]

- Use I-messages instead of You-messages. *I-messages acknowledge ownership of what is said, whereas You-messages suggest the other person is wrong or bad, fostering resentment and resistance instead of understanding and cooperation.*[8]

- Discuss importance of client paying attention to nonverbal communication. *Messages are often confusing or misinterpreted when verbal and nonverbal communications are not congruent.*[9]
- Help client learn to problem-solve differences. *Problem-solving process allows for each person involved to have input and promotes win-win solutions.*[8]
- Instruct and encourage use of stress-reduction techniques. *Relaxation helps individual to function more effectively, thus enhancing feelings of power.*[9]
- Refer to support groups or classes, as indicated, assertiveness training, effectiveness for women to "be your best." *Provides role models and allows individuals to learn from one another, thereby promoting problem-solving and enhancing learning.*[7]

DOCUMENTATION FOCUS

Assessment/Reassessment
- Individual findings, noting determination to improve sense of power, locus of control.
- Motivation and expectations for change.
- Cultural or religious beliefs affecting self-view.
- Locus of control.

Planning
- Plan of care, specific interventions, and who is involved in planning.
- Teaching plan.

Implementation/Evaluation
- Client's responses to interventions, teaching, and actions performed.
- Attainment or progress toward desired outcome(s).
- Modifications to plan of care.

Discharge Planning
- Long-term needs and who is responsible for actions to be taken.
- Specific referrals made.

References

1. Self-help brochures: Assertiveness. Retrieved April 2007 from www.couns.uiuc.edu/Brochures/assertiv.htm.
2. Organizational development & training tip sheet. (2002). Retrieved March 2007 from www.tufts.edu/hr/tips/assert.html.
3. Assertiveness training. Retrieved April 2007 from www.csusm.edu/caps/Assertiveness.html.
4. Adams, L. (2006). Working together: Climate—The emotional one that is. Retrieved March 2007 from www.gordontraining.com/pdf/wt-200612-climate-the-emotional-one-that-is.pdf.
5. Adams, L. (2007). Taking personal responsibility. Retrieved October 2009 from www.gordontraining.com/Taking_Personal_Responsibility.html.
6. Adams, L. (1989). *Be Your Best: Personal Effectiveness in Your Life and Your Relationships.* Rev. ed. New York: Penguin Group.
7. Alberte, R., Emmons, M. (1970). *Your Perfect Right.* San Luis Obispo, CA: Impact.
8. Family Effectiveness Training Program. (1997). Solana Beach, CA: Gordon Training International.
9. Townsend, M. (2006). *Psychiatric Mental Health Nursing Concepts of Care.* 5th ed. Philadelphia: F. A. Davis.

Cultural · Collaborative · Community/Home Care · Diagnostic Studies · Pediatric/Geriatric/Lifespan · Medications

Powerlessness [specify level]

DEFINITION: Perception that one's own action will not significantly affect an outcome; a perceived lack of control over a current situation or immediate happening

RELATED FACTORS

Healthcare environment [e.g., loss of privacy, personal possessions, control over therapies]
Interpersonal interaction [e.g., misuse of power, force; abusive relationships]
Illness-related regimen [e.g., chronic or debilitating conditions]
Lifestyle of helplessness [e.g., repeated failures, dependency]

DEFINING CHARACTERISTICS

Subjective
Low: Expressions of uncertainty about fluctuating energy levels
Moderate
Expressions of dissatisfaction or frustration over inability to perform previous tasks or activities
Expressions of doubt regarding role performance
Fear of alienation from caregivers
Reluctance to express true feelings; resentment; anger; guilt
Severe
Verbal expressions of having no control (e.g., over self-care, situation, outcome)
Depression over physical deterioration

Objective
Low: Passivity
Moderate
Dependence on others that may result in irritability
Inability to seek information regarding care
Passivity
Nonparticipation in care or decision making when opportunities are provided; does not monitor progress
Does not defend self-care practices when challenged
Severe
Apathy [withdrawal, resignation, crying]

Sample Clinical Applications: Chronic or debilitating conditions (e.g., chronic obstructive pulmonary disease [COPD], multiple sclerosis [MS]), cancer, spinal cord injury [SCI], major depressive disorder, somatization disorders

DESIRED OUTCOMES/EVALUATION CRITERIA

Sample (NOC) linkages:
Personal Autonomy: Personal actions of a competent individual to exercise governance in life decisions
Health Beliefs: Perceived Control: Personal conviction that one can influence a health outcome
Participation in Health Care Decisions: Personal involvement in selecting and evaluating healthcare options to achieve desired outcomes

(continues on page 646)

Powerlessness (continued)

Client Will (Include Specific Time Frame)
- Express sense of control over the present situation and future outcome.
- Make choices related to and be involved in care.
- Identify areas over which individual has control.
- Acknowledge reality that some areas are beyond individual's control.

ACTIONS/INTERVENTIONS

Sample (NIC) linkages:
Self-Responsibility Facilitation: Encouraging a patient to assume more responsibility for own behavior
Health System Guidance: Facilitating a patient's location and use of appropriate health services
Decision-Making Support: Providing information and support for a person who is making a decision regarding healthcare

NURSING PRIORITY NO. 1

To assess causative/contributing factors:

- Identify situational circumstances (e.g., strange environment, immobility, diagnosis of terminal or chronic illness, lack of support system(s), lack of knowledge about situation) affecting the client at this time. *Knowing the specific situation of the client is essential to planning care and empowering the individual.*[4]
- Determine client's perception and knowledge of condition and treatment plan. *Identifying how client views and understands what is happening and what the plan of care entails is essential to begin to help client feel empowered.*[2]
- Ascertain client response to treatment regimen. Does client see reason(s) for and understand it is in the client's interest, or is client compliant and helpless? *The manner in which the individual responds to the treatment indicates the depth of feelings of powerlessness and may interfere with progress.*[4]
- Identify client locus of control—internal (expressions of responsibility for self and ability to control outcomes—"I didn't quit smoking") or external (expressions of lack of control over self and environment—"Nothing ever works out"; "What bad luck to get lung cancer"). *Locus of control is a term used in reference to an individual's sense of mastery or control over events. Individuals view life change and stressful events differently. Those with internal locus of control tend to be more optimistic about their ability to deal with adversity even in the face of current difficulties. Individuals with external locus of control may attribute feelings of powerlessness to an external source perceiving it as beyond his or her control and will look to others to solve problems and take care of them.*[4,9]
- Note cultural or religious factors that may contribute to how client views self and is handling current situation. *One's values and beliefs may dictate gender roles and the individual's expectations of control, influencing the client's belief in ability to manage situation, participate in decision making, and direct own life.*[9,11]
- Assess degree of mastery client has exhibited in life. *How this individual has dealt with problems throughout life will help to understand feelings of powerlessness client is feeling during this crisis.*[4,5]
- Determine if there has been a change in relationships with SO(s). *Conflict in relationships may be contributing to sense of powerlessness. Domestic violence situations often leave the individuals involved feeling powerless to change what is happening.*[4]

- Note availability/use of resources. *Client who has few options for assistance or who is not knowledgeable about how to use resources needs to be given information and assistance to know how and where to seek help.*[3]
- Investigate healthcare providers and personal caregiver practices to determine if they support client control and responsibility. *Caregivers who do for the client what he or she is able to do for own self diminish client's sense of control. When client is given as much control over self as possible, sense of power is regained.*[3]

NURSING PRIORITY NO. 2

To assess degree of powerlessness experienced by the client:

- Listen to statements client makes: "They don't care"; "It won't make any difference"; "Are you kidding?" *Indicators of sense of powerlessness and hopelessness and need for specific interventions to provide sense of control over what is happening.*[2]
- Note expressions that indicate "giving up," such as "It won't do any good." *May indicate suicidal intent, indicating need for immediate evaluation and intervention.*[6]
- Note behavioral responses (verbal and nonverbal), including expressions of fear, interest or apathy, agitation, withdrawal. *These responses can show depth of anxiety, feelings of powerlessness over what is happening and indicate need for intervention to help client begin to look at situation with some sense of hope.*[6]
- Note lack of communication, flat affect, and lack of eye contact. *May indicate more severe state of mind, such as psychotic episode and need for immediate evaluation and treatment.*[4]
- Identify the use of manipulative behavior and reactions of client and caregivers. *Manipulation is used for management of powerlessness because of distrust of others, fear of intimacy, search for approval, and validation of sexuality.*[1,9]

NURSING PRIORITY NO. 3

To assist client to clarify needs relative to ability to meet them:

- Show concern for client as a person. *Communicates value of the individual, enhancing self-esteem.*[8]
- Make time to listen to or Active-listen client's perceptions and concerns and encourage questions. *Provides time for client to explore views and understand what is happening in order to come to some decisions about situation, enhancing sense of control.*[8,10]
- Accept expressions of feelings, including anger and hopelessness. *Communicates empathy and understanding of reality of those feelings and provides a point of discussion to move toward sense of control.*[4]
- Avoid arguing or using logic with hopeless client. *Client will not accept that anything can make a difference. Arguing denies client's reality and may impede client-nurse relationship.*[2]
- Deal with manipulative behavior by being straightforward and honest with your communication and letting client know that this is a better way to get needs met. *When client makes a commitment to stop using manipulation in life, steps can be taken to recognize the behaviors and feelings and begin to change them. Keeping a journal can help to identify these issues.*[9]
- Express hope for the client. *Although client may not accept expressions of hope, there is always hope of something, and when options are explored, client may begin to see there is hope.*[8]
- Identify strengths, assets, and past coping strategies that were successful. *Helps client to recognize own ability to deal with difficult situation, providing sense of power.*[5]

● Assist client to identify what he or she can do for self. Identify things the client can and cannot control. *Accomplishing something can provide a sense of control and helps client understand that there are things he or she can manage. Accepting that some things cannot be controlled helps client to stop wasting efforts and refocus energy.*[1]

● Encourage client to maintain a sense of perspective about the situation. *Discussing ways client can look at options and make decisions based on which ones will be best leads to the most effective solutions for situation.*[6]

NURSING PRIORITY NO. 4

To promote independence:

🏠 ● Use client's locus of control to develop individual plan of care. *Tailoring care to the individual's ability will maximize effectiveness. For instance, client with internal control can take control of own care, and those with external control may need to begin with small tasks and add as tolerated, moving toward learning to take more control of care.*[6]

🏠 ● Develop contract with client specifying goals agreed on. *When client is involved in planning, commitment to plan is enhanced, optimizing outcomes.*[2]

🏠 ● Treat expressed decisions and desires with respect. Avoid critical parenting behaviors. *Listening to client and accepting what is said, no matter what the content, helps client hear own words and begin to process information and feelings. Comments that are heard as critical or condescending will block communication and growth.*[1,10]

🏠 ● Provide client opportunities to control as many events as energy and restrictions of care permit. *Promotes sense of control over situation and helps client begin to feel more confident about own ability to manage what is happening.*[6,7]

🏠 ● Discuss needs openly with client and set up agreed-on routines for meeting identified needs. *Minimizes use of manipulation. Manipulative behavior is often used to influence others to do what the person thinks he or she should do. Usually this results in defensiveness or outright rebellion against what is suggested, resulting in lack of trust and withdrawal on the part of the person being manipulated.*[9]

● Minimize rules and limit continuous observation to the degree that safety permits. *Provides sense of control for the client while maintaining a safe environment for the client.*[6]

🏠 ● Support client efforts to develop realistic steps to put plan into action, reach goals, and maintain expectations. *Noting progress that is being made can provide a sense of control and diminish sense of powerlessness.*[6]

● Provide positive reinforcement for desired behaviors. *In behavioral therapy, the belief that when a behavior reinforces another behavior, the second behavior will recur is called a "positive reinforcer," and the function is called "positive reinforcement." By providing this reinforcement, the desired behaviors are more likely to continue.*[4]

● Direct client's thoughts beyond present state to future when appropriate. *Focusing on possibilities in small steps can help the client see that there can be hope in small things each day.*[1,8]

● Schedule frequent and regular contacts to check on client, deal with client needs, and let client know someone is available. *Communicates caring and concern for client and needs, reinforcing sense of worthiness.*[1]

● Involve SO(s) in client care as desired or appropriate. *Personal involvement by supportive family members can help client see the possibilities for resolving problems related to feelings of powerlessness.*[6]

NURSING PRIORITY NO. 5

To promote wellness (Teaching/Discharge Considerations):

🏠 • Instruct in and encourage use of anxiety- and stress-reduction techniques. *Most individuals react to stress in predictable physiological and psychological ways. Feelings of powerlessness related to client's situation can be relieved by use of these techniques.*[5]

🏠 • Provide accurate verbal and written information about what is happening and discuss with client/SO(s). Repeat as often as necessary. *Providing information in different modalities allows better access and opportunity for increased understanding. People do not always hear every piece of information the first time it is presented because of anxiety and inattention, so repetition helps to fill in the missed information.*[6]

🏠 • Assist client to set realistic goals for the future. *Provides opportunity for client to decide what direction is desired and to gain confidence from completion of each goal.*[10]

🏠 • Assist client to learn and use assertive communication skills. *Practicing a new way of expressing thoughts and requests provides the client with a skill to achieve desires and improve relationships.*[10]

🔄 • Facilitate return to a productive role in whatever capacity possible for the individual. Refer to occupational therapist or vocational counselor as indicated. *Feelings of powerlessness may result from inability to engage in or resume previous activities, and learning new ways to be productive enhances self-esteem and reduces feelings of powerlessness.*[6]

🏠 • Encourage client to think productively and positively and take responsibility for choosing own thoughts. *Negative thinking can result in feelings of powerlessness, and learning to use positive thinking can reverse this pattern, promoting feelings of control and self-worth.*[6]

🏠 • Model problem-solving process with client/SO(s). *Learning a problem-solving method that results in a win-win solution improves family relationships and promotes feelings of self-worth in those involved.*[10]

🏠 • Suggest client periodically review own needs and goals. *It is easy to become discouraged as time goes on, and reviewing, thinking about needs, and how previously set goals are relevant in the present helps to either renew those goals or develop new goals to meet current situation.*[6,8]

🔄 • Refer to support groups, counseling or therapy, and so forth, as indicated. *May need additional assistance to resolve current problems, long-standing issues, or troubled relationships.*[4]

DOCUMENTATION FOCUS

Assessment/Reassessment
• Individual findings, noting degree of powerlessness, locus of control, individual's perception of the situation.
• Specific cultural or religious factors.
• Availability and use of support system and resources.

Planning
• Plan of care and who is involved in the planning.
• Teaching plan.

Implementation/Evaluation
• Responses to interventions, teaching, and actions performed.
• Specific goals and expectations.
• Attainment or progress toward desired outcome(s).
• Modifications to plan of care.

Discharge Planning
• Long-term needs and who is responsible for actions to be taken.
• Specific referrals made.

References

1. Doenges, M., Moorhouse, M., Geissler-Murr, A. (2002). *Nursing Care Plans: Guidelines for Individualizing Patient Care*. 6th ed. Philadelphia: F. A. Davis.
2. Doenges, M., Townsend, M., Moorhouse, M. (1998). *Psychiatric Care Plans: Guidelines for Individualizing Care*. 3d ed. Philadelphia: F. A. Davis.
3. Cox, H., et al. (2002). *Clinical Applications of Nursing Diagnoses: Adult, Child, Women's, Psychiatric, Gerontic, and Home Health Considerations*. 4th ed. Philadelphia: F. A. Davis.
4. Townsend, M. (2006). *Psychiatric Mental Health Nursing: Concepts of Care*. 5th ed. Philadelphia: F. A. Davis.
5. Stuart, G. W. (2001). Anxiety responses and anxiety disorders. In Stuart, G. W., Laraia, M. T. (eds). *Principles and Practice of Psychiatric Nursing*. 7th ed. St. Louis, MO: Mosby.
6. Porth, C. M., Kunert, P. K. (2002). *Pathophysiology: Concepts of Altered Health States*. Philadelphia: J. B. Lippincott.
7. National Institute of Mental Health. (2000). Anxiety disorders. NIH Publication No. 00–3879. Retrieved December 2003 from www.nimh.nih.gov.anxiety/anxiety.cfm.
8. Neeld, E. H. (1997). *Seven Choices*. Austin, TX: Centerpoint Press.
9. Messina, J., Messina, C. Tools for handling control issues: Eliminating manipulation. Retrieved April 2007 from www.coping.org/control/manipul.htm.
10. Gordon, T. (2000). *Parent Effectiveness Training*. Updated ed. New York: Three Rivers Press.
11. Lipson, J. G., Dibble, S. L., Minarik, P. A. (1999). *Culture & Nursing Care: A Pocket Guide*. San Francisco: UCSF Nursing Press.

risk for Powerlessness

DEFINITION: At risk for perceived lack of control over a situation and/or one's ability to significantly affect an outcome

RISK FACTORS

Physiological
Illness [hospitalization, intubation, ventilator, suctioning]; dying
Acute injury; progressive debilitating disease process (e.g., spinal cord injury [SCI], multiple sclerosis [MS])
Aging [e.g., decreased physical strength, decreased mobility]

Psychosocial
Deficient knowledge (e.g., of illness or healthcare system)
Lifestyle of dependency
Inadequate coping patterns
Absence of integrality (e.g., essence of power)
Situational/chronic low self-esteem; disturbed body image

NOTE: A risk diagnosis is not evidenced by signs and symptoms, as the problem has not occurred; rather, nursing interventions are directed at prevention.
Sample Clinical Applications: New or unexpected diagnoses, chronic or debilitating conditions (e.g., chronic obstructive pulmonary disease [COPD], MS), cancer, SCI, major depressive disorder, somatization disorders

DESIRED OUTCOMES/EVALUATION CRITERIA

Sample (NOC) linkages:
Personal Autonomy: Personal actions of a competent individual to exercise governance in life decisions
Health Beliefs: Perceived Control: Personal conviction that one can influence a health outcome
Participation in Healthcare Decisions: Personal involvement in selecting and evaluating healthcare options to achieve desired outcomes

Client Will (Include Specific Time Frame)
• Express sense of control over the present situation and hopefulness about future outcomes.
• Verbalize positive self-appraisal in current situation.
• Make choices related to and be involved in care.
• Identify areas over which individual has control.
• Acknowledge reality that some areas are beyond individual's control.

ACTIONS/INTERVENTIONS

Sample (NIC) linkages:
Self-Responsibility Facilitation: Encouraging a patient to assume more responsibility for own behavior
Health System Guidance: Facilitating a patient's location and use of appropriate health services
Decision-Making Support: Providing information and support for a person who is making a decision regarding healthcare

NURSING PRIORITY NO. 1

To assess causative/contributing factors:

• Identify situational circumstances (e.g., acute illness, sudden hospitalization, diagnosis of terminal or debilitating or chronic illness, very young or aging with decreased physical strength and mobility, lack of knowledge about illness, healthcare system). *Necessary information to develop individualized plan of care for client.*[1]
• Determine client's perception and knowledge of condition and proposed treatment plan. *Identifying how client views and understands what is happening and what the plan of care entails is essential to help client feel empowered.*[7]
• Identify client locus of control—internal (expressions of responsibility for self and ability to control outcomes—"I didn't quit smoking") or external (expressions of lack of control over self and environment—"Nothing ever works out"; "What bad luck to get lung cancer"). *Locus of control is a term used in reference to an individual's sense of mastery or control over events. Individuals view life change and stressful events differently. Those with internal locus of control tend to be more optimistic about their ability to deal with adversity even in the face of current difficulties. Individuals with external locus of control may attribute feelings of powerlessness to an external source, perceiving it as beyond his or her control and will look to others to solve problems and take care of them.*[4,10]
• Note cultural or religious factors that may contribute to how client views self and is handling current situation. *One's values and beliefs may dictate gender roles and the individual's expectations of control, influencing the client's belief in ability to manage situation, participate in decision making, and direct own life.*[9,10]

- Assess client's self-esteem and degree of mastery client has exhibited in life situations. *Provides clues to client's ability to see self as in control and deal with current situation.*[7]

 - Note availability and use of resources, relationship with SO/family and degree of support provided to client. *Presence of support system and ability to use resources appropriately facilitates problem-solving, enhancing sense of control. Client who has few options for assistance or who is not knowledgeable about how to use resources needs to be given information and assistance to know how and where to seek help.*[3]

- Listen to statements client makes that might indicate feelings of possibility of loss of control (e.g., "They don't care"; "It won't make a difference"; "It won't do any good"). *Indicators of sense of powerlessness and hopelessness and need for specific interventions to provide sense of control over what is happening.*[4]

- Determine congruency of responses (verbal and nonverbal) and note expressions of fear, disinterest or apathy, or withdrawal. *These responses can show depth of anxiety over what is happening and indicate need for intervention to help client begin to look at situation with sense of hope.*[5]

- Be alert for signs of manipulative behavior and note reactions of client and caregivers. *Manipulation may be used for management of powerlessness because of fear and distrust.*[4,10]

NURSING PRIORITY NO. 2

To assist client to clarify needs and ability to meet them:

- Show concern for client as a person. Encourage questions. *Communicates value of the individual, enhancing self-esteem. Questions may reveal lack of information or concerns client may have.*[8]

- Make time to listen to client's perceptions of the situation as well as concerns. *Provides time for client to explore views and understand what is happening to come to some decisions about situation, enhancing sense of control.*[5]

- Accept expressions of feelings, including anger and reluctance to try to work things out. *Communicates unconditional regard for the client and encourages individual to think about options even though situation may be difficult.*[5]

- Express hope for client and encourage review of past experiences with successful strategies. *Provides an opportunity for person to remember and accept that he or she has managed difficult situations before and can apply these strategies in current situation.*[4]

- Assist client to identify what he or she can do to help self and what situations cannot be controlled. *Accomplishing something can provide a sense of control and helps client understand that there are things he or she can manage. Accepting that some things cannot be controlled helps client to stop wasting efforts and refocus energy.*[1,2]

NURSING PRIORITY NO. 3

To promote wellness (Teaching/Discharge Considerations):

 - Encourage client to be active in own healthcare management and to take responsibility for choosing own actions and reactions. *Discussing ways client can look at options and make decisions based on which ones will be best leads to the most effective solutions for situation.*[6,7]

 - Involve client/SO(s) in planning process, using client's locus of control. *Tailoring care to the individual's ability will maximize effectiveness. For instance, client with internal control can take control of own care, and those with external control may need to begin with small tasks and add as tolerated, moving toward learning to take more control of care.*[6]

Cultural   Collaborative   Community/Home Care   Diagnostic Studies   Pediatric/Geriatric/Lifespan   Medications

🏠 • Model problem-solving process with client and SOs. *Learning a problem-solving method that results in a win-win solution improves family relationships and promotes feelings of self-worth in those involved.*[8]

🏠 • Support client efforts to develop realistic steps to put plan into action, reach goals, and maintain expectations. *Noting progress that is being made can enhance sense of control.*[6]

🏠 • Provide accurate instructions in various modalities (e.g., verbal, written, audiovisual, Web sites) about what is happening and what realistically might happen. *Providing information in different formats allows better access and opportunity for increased understanding to support decision-making process.*[6]

🏠 • Identify resource books or classes for assertiveness training and stress-reduction, as appropriate. *Reinforces learning and promotes self-paced review.*[8]

🏠 • Suggest client periodically review own needs and goals. *Reviewing needs and how previously set goals are relevant in the present helps to either renew those goals or develop new goals to meet current situation.*[5]

⚕ • Refer to support groups for chronic conditions or disability (e.g., MS Society, Easter Seals, Alzheimer's, Al-Anon) or counseling or therapy, as appropriate. *May need additional assistance to manage difficulties of current situation.*[4]

DOCUMENTATION FOCUS

Assessment/Reassessment
• Individual findings, noting potential for powerlessness, locus of control, individual's perception of the situation.
• Cultural values or religious beliefs.
• Locus of control.
• SO/family involvement and support.
• Availability and use of resources.

Planning
• Plan of care and who is involved in the planning.
• Teaching plan.

Implementation/Evaluation
• Responses to interventions, teaching, and actions performed.
• Specific goals and expectations.
• Attainment or progress toward desired outcomes.
• Modifications to plan of care.

Discharge Planning
• Long-term needs and who is responsible for actions to be taken.
• Specific referrals made.

References

1. Doenges, M. E., Moorhouse, M. F., Geissler-Murr, A. C. (2002). *Nursing Care Plans: Guidelines for Individualizing Patient Care.* 6th ed. Philadelphia: F. A. Davis.
2. Doenges, M., Townsend, M., Moorhouse, M. (1998). *Psychiatric Care Plans: Guidelines for Individualizing Care.* 3d ed. Philadelphia: F. A. Davis.
3. Cox, H., et al. (2002). *Clinical Applications of Nursing Diagnoses: Adult, Child, Women's, Psychiatric, Gerontic, and Home Health Considerations.* 4th ed. Philadelphia: F. A. Davis.

4. Townsend, M. (2006). *Psychiatric Mental Health Nursing: Concepts of Care*. 5th ed. Philadelphia: F. A. Davis.
5. Stuart, G. W. (2001). Anxiety responses and anxiety disorders. In Stuart, G. W., Laraia, M. T. (eds). *Principles and Practice of Psychiatric Nursing*. 7th ed. St. Louis, MO: Mosby.
6. Porth, C. M., Kunert, P. K. (2002). *Pathophysiology: Concepts of Altered Health States*. Philadelphia: J. B. Lippincott.
7. National Institute of Mental Health. (2000). Anxiety disorders. NIH Publication No. 00-3879. Retrieved January 2004 from www.nimh.nih.gov.anxiety/anxiety.cfm.
8. Gordon, T. (2000). *Parent Effectiveness Training*. Updated ed. New York: Three Rivers Press.
9. Lipson, J. G., Dibble, S. L., Minarik, P. A. (1996). *Culture & Nursing Care: A Pocket Guide*. San Francisco: UCSF Nursing Press.
10. Messina, J., Messina, C. Tools for handling control issues: Eliminating manipulation. Retrieved April 2007 from www.coping.org/control/manipul.htm.

ineffective Protection

DEFINITION: Decrease in the ability to guard self from internal or external threats such as illness or injury

RELATED FACTORS

Extremes of age
Inadequate nutrition
Alcohol abuse
Abnormal blood profiles (e.g., leukopenia, thrombocytopenia, anemia, coagulation)
Drug therapies (e.g., antineoplastic, corticosteroid, immune, anticoagulant, thrombolytic)
Treatments (e.g., surgery, radiation)
Cancer; immune disorders

DEFINING CHARACTERISTICS

Subjective
Neurosensory alterations
Chilling
Itching
Insomnia; fatigue; weakness
Anorexia

Objective
Deficient immunity
Impaired healing; altered clotting
Maladaptive stress response
Perspiring [inappropriately]
Dyspnea; cough
Restlessness; immobility
Disorientation
Pressure sores

Sample Clinical Applications: Cancer, AIDS, systemic lupus, substance abuse, tuberculosis, dementia, Alzheimer's disease, anorexia or bulimia nervosa, diabetes mellitus, thrombophlebitis, conditions requiring long-term steroid use (e.g., chronic obstructive pulmonary disease [COPD], asthma, renal failure), major surgery

Authors' note: The purpose of this diagnosis seems to combine multiple NDs under a single heading for ease of planning care when a number of variables may be present. It is suggested that the user refer to specific NDs based on identified related factors and individual concerns for this client to find appropriate outcomes and interventions that are specifically tied to individual related factors that are present, such as:

Extremes of age: Includes concerns regarding body temperature or thermoregulation; memory or thought process, sensory-perceptual alterations; impaired mobility, risk for falls, sedentary lifestyle, self-care deficits; risk for trauma, suffocation, or poisoning; risk for skin or tissue integrity and fluid volume imbalances.

Inadequate nutrition: Brings up issues of nutrition (less or more than body requirements), risk for unstable blood glucose; risk for infection, delayed surgical recovery; impaired swallowing; disturbed thought processes, impaired skin or tissue integrity; trauma, ineffective coping, and interrupted family processes.

Alcohol [other drug] abuse: May be situational or chronic with problems ranging from ineffective breathing patterns, decreased cardiac output, impaired liver function, and fluid volume deficit to nutritional problems, infection, trauma, disturbed thought processes, and coping or family process difficulties.

Abnormal blood profile: Suggests possibility of fluid volume deficit, decreased tissue perfusion, impaired gas exchange, activity intolerance, or risk for infection or injury.

Drug therapies, treatments, and disease concerns: Includes ineffective tissue perfusion, activity intolerance; cardiovascular, respiratory, and elimination concerns; risk for infection, fluid volume imbalances, impaired skin or tissue integrity, impaired liver function; pain, nutritional problems, fatigue, sleep deprivation, ineffective therapeutic regimen management; and emotional responses (e.g., anxiety, sorrow, grief, coping).

Sample (NOC) linkages:

Cognition: Ability to execute complex mental processes

Blood coagulation: Extent to which blood clots within normal period of time

Immune Status: Natural and acquired appropriately targeted resistance to internal and external antigens

---

Sample (NIC) linkages:

Postanesthesia Care: Monitoring and management of the patient who has recently undergone general or regional anesthesia

Infection Protection: Minimizing the acquisition and transmission of infectious agents

Surveillance: Safety: Purposeful and ongoing collection and analysis of information about the patient and the environment for use in promoting and maintaining patient safety

Rape-Trauma Syndrome [specify]

DEFINITION: Sustained maladaptive response to a forced, violent sexual penetration against the victim's will and consent [Rape is not a sexual crime but a crime of violence and identified as sexual assault. Although attacks are most often directed toward women, men also may be victims.]

Note: This syndrome includes the following three subcomponents: [A] Rape-Trauma; [B] Compound Reaction; and [C] Silent Reaction. [All three are presented here.]

RELATED FACTORS

Rape [actual/attempted forced sexual penetration]

DEFINING CHARACTERISTICS

[A] Rape-Trauma
Acute phase

Subjective
Embarrassment; humiliation; shame; guilt; self-blame
Loss of self-esteem; helplessness; powerlessness
Shock; fear; anxiety; anger; revenge
Nightmare and sleep disturbances
Change in relationships; sexual dysfunction

Objective
Physical trauma [e.g., bruising, tissue irritation]; muscle tension/spasms
Confusion; disorganization; impaired ability to make decisions
Agitation; hyperalertness; aggression
Mood swings; vulnerability; dependence; depression
Substance abuse; suicide attempts
Denial; phobias; paranoia; dissociative disorders

[B Compound Reaction]—Retired from Taxonomy 2009
DEFINITION: Forced violent sexual penetration against the victim's will and consent; trauma syndrome that develops from this attack or attempted attack includes an acute phase of disorganization of the victim's lifestyle and a long-term process of reorganization of lifestyle

RELATED FACTORS

To be developed by nurse researchers and submitted to NANDA

DEFINING CHARACTERISTICS

Subjective
Acute phase
Emotional reactions (e.g., anger, embarrassment, fear of physical violence and death, humiliation, self-blame, revenge)

Multiple physical symptoms (e.g., gastrointestinal [GI] irritability, genitourinary discomfort, muscle tension, sleep pattern disturbance)
Reactivated symptoms of previous conditions (e.g., physical or psychiatric illness); substance abuse

Long-term phase
Changes in lifestyle (e.g., changes in residence, dealing with repetitive nightmares and phobias, seeking family or social network support)

[C Silent Reaction]—Retired from Taxonomy 2009
DEFINITION: Forced violent sexual penetration against the victim's will and consent; trauma syndrome that develops from this attack or attempted attack includes an acute phase of disorganization of the victim's lifestyle and a long-term process of reorganization of lifestyle

RELATED FACTORS

To be developed by nurse researchers and submitted to NANDA

DEFINING CHARACTERISTICS

Subjective
Increase in nightmares
Abrupt changes in relationships with men
Pronounced changes in sexual behavior

Objective
Increasing anxiety during interview (e.g., blocking of associations, long periods of silence; minor stuttering, physical distress)
No verbalization of the occurrence of rape
Sudden onset of phobic reactions

Sample Clinical Applications: Sexual assault, abuse

DESIRED OUTCOMES/EVALUATION CRITERIA

Sample **NOC** linkages:
Abuse Recovery: Physical: Extent of healing of physical injuries due to sexual abuse
Abuse Recovery: Emotional: Extent of healing of psychological injuries due to abuse
Coping: Personal actions to manage stressors that tax an individual's resources

---

Client Will (Include Specific Time Frame)
- Report absence of physical complications, pain, and discomfort.
- Deal appropriately with emotional reactions as evidenced by behavior and expression of feelings.
- Verbalize a positive self-image.
- Verbalize recognition that incident was not of own doing.
- Identify behaviors or situations within own control that may reduce risk of recurrence.
- Deal with practical aspects (e.g., court appearances).
- Demonstrate appropriate changes in lifestyle (e.g., change in job, residence) that contribute to recovery or seek and obtain support from SO(s), as needed.
- Interact with individuals or groups in desired and acceptable manner.

(continues on page 658)

Rape-Trauma Syndrome (continued)
ACTIONS/INTERVENTIONS

Sample **NIC** linkages:
Rape-Trauma Treatment: Provision of emotional and physical support immediately following a reported rape
Crisis Intervention: Use of short-term counseling to help the patient cope with a crisis and resume a state of functioning comparable to or better than the precrisis state
Counseling: Use of an interactive helping process focusing on the needs, problems, or feelings of the patient and significant others to enhance or support coping, problem-solving, and interpersonal relationships

NURSING PRIORITY NO. 1

To assess trauma and individual reaction, noting length of time since occurrence of event:

- Observe for and elicit information about physical injury and assess stress-related symptoms such as numbness, headache, tightness in chest, nausea, pounding heart, and so forth. *Indicators of degree of and reaction to trauma experienced by the client, which may occur immediately and in the days or weeks following the attack.*[3,4]
- Identify psychological responses: anger, shock, acute anxiety, confusion, denial. Note laughter, crying, calm or agitated, excited (hysterical) behavior, expressions of disbelief or self-blame. *Victim may exhibit expressed response pattern (compound reaction), displaying these feelings openly and freely as manifestations of experiencing the trauma of rape/sexual assault, and the accompanying feelings of fear of death, violation, powerlessness and helplessness. On the other hand, client may exhibit controlled (silent) response pattern with little or no emotion expressed. Any emotion is appropriate, as each person responds in own individual way; however, inappropriate behaviors or acting out may require intervention.*[1,4] Refer to NDs risk for self-/other-directed Violence.
- Note silence, stuttering, inability to sit still. *May be signs of increasing anxiety, thus indicating need for further evaluation and intervention. Anxiety is suppressed and client does not talk about the trauma, resulting in an overwhelming emotional burden.*[1]
- Determine degree of disorganization. *Initially, the individual may be in shock and disbelief, which is a normal response to the incident. The person may respond by withdrawing and be unable to manage activities of daily living, especially when the incident was particularly brutal, requiring assistance and treatment to enable her or him to recover and move on.*[4]
- Identify whether incident has reactivated preexisting or coexisting situations (physical or psychological). *The presence of these factors can affect how the client views the current trauma. Previous traumatic incidents that have not been effectively resolved may compound the current incident.*[1]
- Ascertain cultural values or religious beliefs that may affect how client views incident, self, and expectations of SO/family reaction. *Client may believe incident will bring shame on the family, blame self, or believe that family will blame client, thus affecting client's ability to reach out to others for support.*[6]
- Determine disruptions in relationships with men and with others (e.g., family, friends, co-workers, SO[s]). *Many women find that they react to men in general in a different way, seeing them as reminders of the assault.*[1]
- Identify development of phobic reactions to ordinary articles (e.g., knives) and situations (e.g., walking in groups of people, strangers ringing doorbell). *These are manifestations of*

extreme anxiety, and client will need to continue treatment to learn how to manage feelings.[4]

- Note degree of intrusive repetitive thoughts, sleep disturbances. *Survivor may notice disruptions in activities of daily living, reliving the attack, thoughts of recrimination, self-blame ("Why didn't I . . . ?"), nightmares. Although these factors are distressing and upsetting, they are part of the normal healing process.*[4]
- Assess degree of dysfunctional coping. *Client may turn to use of alcohol or other drugs, have suicidal or homicidal ideation, or display marked change in sexual behavior in an attempt to cope with traumatic event.*[4]

NURSING PRIORITY NO. 2

To assist client to deal with situation that exists:

- Explore own feelings (nurse/caregiver) regarding rape/incest issue prior to interacting with the client. *Since the feelings related to these incidents are so pervasive, the individual involved in caregiving needs to recognize own biases to prevent imposing them on the client.*[1]

ACUTE PHASE/IMMEDIATE CARE

- Stay with the client—do not leave child unattended. Listen but do not probe. Tell client you are sorry this has happened and that she or he is safe now. *During this phase, the client experiences a complete disruption of life as she or he has known it, and presence of caregiver may provide reassurance and sense of safety.*[2,4]
- Involve rape or sexual assault response team (SART), or sexual assault nurse examiner (SANE) when available. Provide same-sex examiner when appropriate. *Presence of the response team trained to collect evidence appropriately and sensitively provides assurance to the survivor that she or he is being taken care of. Client may react to someone who is the sex of the attacker and use of a same-sex examiner communicates sensitivity to her or his feelings at this difficult time.*[4,7]
- Be sensitive to cultural factors that may affect specifics of examination process. *For example, in some cultures, women cannot be examined without a male family member present. These issues need to be considered when treating the survivor.*[6]
- Evaluate client as dictated by age, gender, and developmental level. *Age of the survivor is an important consideration in deciding plan of care and appropriate interventions.*[4,8]
- Assist with documentation of incident for police and child-protective services reports, explaining each step of the procedure. Maintain sequencing and collection of evidence (chain of evidence), label each specimen, and store and package properly. Be careful to use nonjudgmental language. *It is crucial to provide accurate information to law enforcement for potential legal proceedings when perpetrator is charged.* Words can carry legal implications that may affect subsequent proceedings.[1]
- Provide environment in which client can talk freely about feelings and fears. *Client needs to talk about the incident and concerns, such as issues of relationship with or response of SO(s), pregnancy, sexually transmitted diseases (STDs) so they may be dealt with in a positive manner.*[4]
- Provide information about emergency birth control and prophylactic treatment for STDs and assist with finding resources for follow-through. *Promotes client's peace of mind and opportunity to prevent these conditions.*[4,8]
- Provide psychological support by listening and remaining with client. If client does not want to talk, accept silence. *May indicate Silent Reaction to the occurrence in which the individual contains their emotions, using all their energy to maintain composure.*[4]

Nursing Diagnoses in Alphabetical Order

- Listen to and investigate physical complaints. Assist with medical treatments, as indicated. *Emotional reactions may limit client's ability to recognize physical injury.*[4]
- Assist with practical realities. *Client may be so emotionally distraught that she or he may not be able to attend to needs for such things as safe temporary housing, money, or other issues that may need to be addressed. Assistance helps individual maintain contact with reality.*[4,5]
- Determine client's ego strengths and help him or her use them in a positive way by acknowledging client's ability to handle what is happening. *Validation of belief that person can deal with what has happened and move forward with life promotes self-acceptance and helps client begin this process.*[4,9]
- Identify supportive persons for this individual. *Client needs to know she or he can go to a strong system of friends, family, or advocate who will respond with empathy.*[4]

POSTACUTE PHASE

- Allow the client to work through own kind of adjustment. If client is withdrawn or unwilling to talk (Silent Reaction), do not force the issue. *Individuals react in many ways to the traumatic event of rape, and no response is abnormal. Factors that influence how the survivor deals with the situation are personality, support system, existing life problems and prior sexual victimization, relationship with the offender, degree of violence used, social and cultural influences, and ability to cope with stress.*[2,4]
- Listen for expressions of fear of crowds, men, and so forth. *May reveal developing phobias needing evaluation and appropriate interventions, ongoing therapy.*[2,4]
- Discuss specific concerns and fears. Identify appropriate actions and provide information as indicated. *May need diagnostic testing for pregnancy, sexually transmitted diseases, or other resources. Meeting these needs and providing information will help client begin the process of recovery.*[4]
- Include written instructions that are concise and clear regarding medical treatments, crisis support services, and so on. Encourage return for follow-up. *Reinforces teaching, provides opportunity to deal with information at own pace. Follow-up appointment provides opportunity for determining how client is managing feelings and what needs may not have been met.*[4]

LONG-TERM PHASE

- Continue listening to expressions of concern. Note persistence of somatic complaints (e.g., nausea, anorexia, insomnia, muscle tension, headache). *May need to continue to talk about the assault. Repeating the story helps client to move on, but continued somatic concerns may indicate developing posttraumatic stress disorder (PTSD).*[4,8]
- Permit free expression of feelings (may continue from the crisis phase). Refrain from rushing client through expressions of feelings too quickly and avoid reassuring inappropriately. *Client may believe pain and/or anguish is misunderstood and depression may limit responses.*[1]
- Acknowledge reality of loss of self that existed before the incident. Assist client to move toward an acceptance of the potential for growth that exists within individual. *Following this traumatic event, the individual will not be able to go back to the person they were before. Life will always have the memory of what happened, and client needs to accept that reality and move on in the best way possible.*[2]
- Continue to allow client to progress at own pace. *The process of grieving is a very individual one, and each person needs to know that she or he can take whatever time needed to resolve feelings and move on with life.*[4] (Refer to ND Grieving for additional interventions.)

- Give "permission" to express and deal with anger at the perpetrator and situation in acceptable ways. Set limits on destructive behaviors. *Facilitates resolution of feelings without diminishing self-concept.*[5]
- Keep discussion on practical and emotional level rather than intellectualizing the experience. *When the person talks about the incident intellectually, instead of identifying and talking about feelings, client avoids dealing with the feelings, thus inhibiting recovery.*[1]
- Assist in dealing with ongoing concerns about and effects of the incident, such as court appearance, STD, relationship with SO(s), and so forth. *Depending on degree of disorganization, client will need help to deal with these practical and emotional issues.*[4]
- Provide for sensitive, trained counselors, considering individual needs. *Male/female counselors may be best determined on an individual basis, as counselor's gender may be an issue for some clients, affecting ability to disclose and deal with feelings.*[1]

NURSING PRIORITY NO. 3

To promote wellness (Teaching/Discharge Considerations):

- Provide information about what reactions client may expect during each phase. Let client know these are common reactions and phrase in neutral terms of "You may or may not. . . ." *Such information helps client anticipate and deal with reactions if they are experienced. Note: Be aware that, although male rape perpetrators are usually heterosexual, the male victim may be concerned about his own sexuality and may exhibit a homophobic response.*[1]
- Assist client to identify factors that may have created a vulnerable situation and that she or he may have power to change to protect self in the future. *While client needs to be assured that she or he is not to blame for incident, the circumstances of the incident need to be assessed to identify factors that are within the individual's control to avoid a similar incident occurring.*[4]
- Avoid making value judgments. *The survivor often blames self about the incident and agonizes over the circumstances; therefore, nonjudgmental language is very important to help the person accept that the fault is not hers or his.*[1]
- Discuss lifestyle changes client is contemplating and how they will contribute to recovery. *Helps client evaluate appropriateness of plans. In the anxiety of the moment, the individual may believe that changing residence, job, or other aspects of her or his environment will be healing. In reality, these changes may not help and may make matters worse.*[4]
- Encourage psychiatric consultation if client is violent, inconsolable, or does not seem to be making an adjustment. Participation in a group may be helpful. *May need intensive professional help to come to terms with the assault.*[1]
- Refer to family or marital counseling, as indicated. *When relationships with family members are affected by the incident, counseling may be needed to resolve the issues.*[1,9]
- Refer to NDs Anxiety, ineffective Coping, Fear, complicated Grieving, and Powerlessness, as appropriate.

DOCUMENTATION FOCUS

Assessment/Reassessment
- Individual findings, including nature of incident, individual reactions and fears, degree of trauma (physical and emotional), effects on lifestyle.
- Cultural or religious factors.
- Reactions of family/SO(s).
- Samples gathered for evidence and disposition or storage (chain of evidence).

Planning
• Plan of action and who is involved in planning.
• Teaching plan.

Implementation/Evaluation
• Responses to interventions, teaching, and actions performed.
• Attainment or progress toward desired outcome(s).
• Modifications to plan of care.

Discharge Planning
• Long-term needs and who is responsible for actions to be taken.
• Specific referrals made.

References

1. Townsend, M. C. (2003). *Psychiatric Mental Health Nursing Concepts of Care.* 4th ed. Philadelphia: F. A. Davis.
2. Dealing with rape—Rape trauma syndrome. Retrieved January 2004 from www.rapecrisis.org.za/dealing/trauma.htm.
3. Cox, H. C., et al. (2002). *Clinical Applications of Nursing Diagnosis: Adult, Child, Women's, Psychiatric, Gerontic, and Home Health Considerations.* 4th ed. Philadelphia: F. A. Davis.
4. Rape trauma syndrome. Retrieved August 2007 from www.rapevictimadvocates.org/trauma.html.
5. Doenges, M. E., Moorhouse, M. F., Geissler-Murr, A. C. (2004). *Nurses' Pocket Guide: Diagnoses, Interventions, and Rationales.* 9th ed. Philadelphia: F. A. Davis.
6. Lipson, J., Dibble, S., Minarik, P. (1996). *Culture & Nursing Care: A Pocket Guide.* San Francisco: UCSF Nursing Press.
7. Menna, A. Rape trauma syndrome: The journey to healing belongs to everyone. Retrieved August 2007 from www.giftfromwithin.org/html/journey.html.
8. The Rape, Abuse, & Incest National Network (RAINN). Retrieved August 2007 from www.rainn.org/get-information/index.html.
9. Lauer, T. Rape trauma. *American Association for Marriage and Family Therapy.* Retrieved August 2007 from www.aamft.org/families/Consumer_Updates/RapeTrauma.asp.

readiness for enhanced Relationship

DEFINITION: A pattern of mutual partnership that is sufficient to provide each other's needs and can be strengthened

DEFINING CHARACTERISTICS

Subjective
Expresses:
Desire to enhance communication between partners
Satisfaction with sharing of information and ideas between partners
Satisfaction with fulfilling physical and emotional needs by one's partner
Satisfaction with complementary relation between partners
Identifies each other as a key person

Objective
Demonstrates:
Mutual respect between partners
Well-balanced autonomy and collaboration between partners
Mutual support in daily activities between partners
Understanding of partners insufficient (physical, social, psychological) function
Meets developmental goals appropriate for family life cycle stage

Sample Clinical Applications: Applicable in any setting, not dependent on presence of pathology although may be useful in chronic physical conditions or mental health challenges

DESIRED OUTCOMES/EVALUATION CRITERIA

Sample (NOC) linkages:
Social Interaction Skills: Personal behaviors that promote effective relationships
Role Performance: Congruence of an individual's role behavior with role expectations
Social Involvement: Social interactions with persons, groups, or communities

Client Will (Include Specific Time Frames)
• Verbalize a desire to learn more effective communication skills.
• Verbalizes understanding of current relationship with partner.
• Seek information to improve emotional and physical needs of both partners.
• Talk with partner about circumstances that can be improved.
• Develop realistic plans to strengthen relationship.

ACTIONS/INTERVENTIONS

Sample (NIC) linkages:
Role Enhancement: Assisting a patient, significant other, and/or family to improve relationships by clarifying and supplementing specific role behaviors
Socialization Enhancement: Facilitation of another person's ability to interact with others

NURSING PRIORITY NO. 1

To assess current situation and determine needs:

● Determine makeup of family: parents/children, older/younger. *Life changes, such as developmental, situational, health-illness can affect relationship between partners and require readjustment and thinking of ways to enhance situation.*[1]
● Discuss clients perception of needs and how partner sees desire to improve relationship. *Identifies thinking and whether both partners see the situation in the same way and individual expectations for change.*
● Identify use of effective communication skills. *May need to improve understanding of words partners use in discussion of sensitive subjects.*[4]
● Help client to identify thoughts and feelings when starting a discussion with partner. *A system of thinking (referred to as a paradigm) forms the basis for how we look at and experience life and determines how we perceive our world, forms the basis for our reality, and exists below our level of conscience.*[4]
● Ask partners how they deal with conflict. *Since conflict is a normal, natural, and inevitable part of life, this needs to be acknowledged, and individuals need to learn how to deal with it effectively.*[4]

Nursing Diagnoses in Alphabetical Order

- Ascertain client's view of sexual aspects of relationship. *Changes that occur with aging or medical conditions, such as hysterectomy, erectile dysfunction, can affect the relationship and need specific interventions to resolve.*[2]
- Identify cultural factors relating to individual's view of role in relationship. *Although changing, in America, men typically take care of financial affairs, car and house repairs, and women manage household and caregiving roles.*[1]
- Discuss how family as a whole functions. *Interrelationships with members of the family, personal and family history, and situational dynamics can improve the functioning of the whole family.*[2]

NURSING PRIORITY NO. 2

To assist the client to enhance existing situation:

- Maintain positive attitude toward client. *Promotes safe relationship in which client can feel free to speak openly and plan for a positive future.*[1]
- Have couple discuss paradigms that they have become aware of in own thinking that interfere with relationship. *These beliefs exist below our conscious mind, influencing our behavior, and whether we see the world in negative or positive ways.*[4]
- Determine how each person views themselves as a positive or negative person. *One's self-image influences behavior and how he or she relates to others. When emotional needs are met, individuals relate to others in positive ways, while unmet needs result in low self-image and insecurity.*[5]
- Discuss the skills of emotional intelligence, which are important for maintaining positive relationships. *This is the ability to recognize and effectively control our own emotions and to recognize the emotions of others.*[6]
- Help couple to recognize that surface symptoms of dysfunctional relationships are not the problems that need to be dealt with. *Underlying emotions influence our behaviors and individuals often are not aware of them and continue to deal with the superficial conflicts.*[6]
- Explore individual's emotional needs. *Relationships are often motivated by unconscious desires to gain acceptance, recognition, sense of being cared about or valued.*[5]
- Note client's awareness of nonverbal communications. *Body language, tone of voice, a roll of the eyes, or subtle movements convey strong messages, positive or negative, that need to be discussed and clarified.*[6]
- Discuss effective conflict resolution skills. *People tend to be afraid of conflict because effective ways to deal with it have not been learned and it often ends in a lose-lose situation.*[4]
- Encourage client to remain calm and focused regardless of circumstances. *Maintaining a calm demeanor helps individual to be able to think more clearly and be more rational in dealing with situation.*[6]
- Recommend cross-checking or verifying what listener believes speaker said. *Clarifies communication and allows speaker to respond or correct perception of listener as needed.*[5]
- Help partners to learn win-win method of conflict resolution. *Although conflict can damage a relationship, learning to listen to each other's needs can assist partners to arrive at mutually acceptable solutions.*[4]
- Role play ways to defuse arguments and repair injured feelings. *Provides a realistic situation wherein each person can identify own and partner's view and practice new ways of interacting.*[6]
- Provide open environment for partners to discuss sexual concerns and questions. *Problems may arise out of lack of information about these issues, and when individuals are comfortable with this knowledge, the relationship can be improved.*[2]

- Discuss nonblameful self-disclosure when having a dialogue. *Partners take turns talking about own needs and feelings without blaming the other, resulting in being able to find a solution in a climate of mutual consideration and respect.*[4]

NURSING PRIORITY NO. 3

To promote optimal functioning (Teaching/Discharge Considerations):

- Provide information for partners, using bibliotherapy, appropriate Web sites. *Promotes continuation of learning about how to enhance relationship.*[3]
- Encourage couple to use humor and playfulness in their relationship. *Sharing laughter and enjoying life helps to weather difficult times that may occur.*[6]
- Discuss the importance of being an empathic, understanding, and nonjudgmental listener when either partner has a problem. *The expectation that the partner will be willing to help by listening eases the anxiety of talking about major problems.*[5]
- Help individuals to learn to use Active-listening technique. *This avoids giving advice and helps other person to find own solution, enhancing self-esteem.*[4]
- Refer to support groups, classes on assertiveness, parenting, as indicated by individual needs.[3]
- Include family members in discussions as needed. *Knowing how the family relates as a whole will help improve relationships of partners as well as the other family members.*[3]
- Refer for care as indicated by psychological, physical problems of either individual. *May need further treatment and explanation to help partner understand these situations.*[1]

DOCUMENTATION FOCUS

Assessment/Reassessment
- Baseline information, individual's perception of situation and self.
- Reasons for desire to improve relationship and expectations for change.

Planning
- Plan of care and who is involved in planning.
- Teaching plan.

Implementation/Evaluation
- Response of partners to plan, interventions, and actions performed.
- Attainment or progress toward desired outcomes(s).

Discharge Planning
- Long-term plan and who is responsible for actions to be taken.

References

1. Doenges, M., Townsend, M., Moorhouse, M. (1998). *Psychiatric Care Plans: Guidelines for Individualizing Care.* 3d ed. Philadelphia: F. A. Davis.
2. Kuriansky, J. (2002). *The Complete Idiot's Guide to Healthy Relationships.* Indianapolis, IN: Alpha Books.
3. Branden, N. (1994). *Healthy Relationships.* New York: Bantam Books.
4. Gordon, T. (2000). *Parent Effectiveness Training.* Updated ed. New York: Three Rivers Press.
5. Hollister, W. G., Edgerton, J. W. (1974). Teaching relationship building skills. *Am J Public Health,* 64(1), 41–46.
6. Segal, J., Segal, R., Smith, M. Relationship help: Building great relationships using emotional intelligence. Retrieved March 2009 from www.helpguide.org/mental/improve_relationships.htm.

impaired Religiosity

DEFINITION: Impaired ability to exercise reliance on beliefs or participate in rituals of a particular faith tradition

RELATED FACTORS

Developmental and Situational
Life transitions; aging; end-stage life crises

Physical
Illness; pain

Psychological Factors
Ineffective support or coping
Anxiety; fear of death
Personal crisis; lack of security
Use of religion to manipulate

Sociocultural
Cultural or environmental barriers to practicing religion
Lack of social integration or sociocultural interaction

Spiritual
Spiritual crises; suffering

DEFINING CHARACTERISTICS

Subjective
Expresses emotional distress because of separation from faith community
Expresses a need to reconnect with previous belief patterns or customs
Questions religious belief patterns or customs
Difficulty adhering to prescribed religious beliefs and rituals (e.g., religious ceremonies, dietary regulations, clothing, prayer, worship/religious services, private religious behaviors/reading religious materials/media, holiday observances, meetings with religious leaders)

Sample Clinical Applications: Any acute or chronic condition, palliative care, end-of-life situation

DESIRED OUTCOMES/EVALUATION CRITERIA

Sample NOC linkages:
Spiritual Health: Connectedness with self, others, higher power, all life, nature, and the universe that transcends and empowers the self

Client Will (Include Specific Time Frame)
• Express ability to once again participate in beliefs and rituals of desired religion.
• Discuss beliefs and values about spiritual or religious issues.
• Attend religious or worship services of choice, as desired.
• Verbalize concerns about end-of-life issues and fear of death.

ACTIONS/INTERVENTIONS

Sample (NIC) linkages:

Spiritual Growth Facilitation: Facilitation of growth in patient's capacity to identify, connect with, and call upon the source of meaning, purpose, comfort, and hope in his or her life

Spiritual Support: Assisting the patient feel balance and connection with a greater power

NURSING PRIORITY NO. 1

To assess causative/contributing factors:

- Determine client's usual religious and spiritual beliefs, values and past spiritual commitment. *Provides a baseline for understanding current problem.*[5]
- Note client's/SO's reports and expressions of anger/concern, alienation from God, sense of guilt or retribution. *Perception of guilt may cause spiritual crisis and suffering resulting in rejection of religious beliefs or anger toward God.*[6]
- Determine sense of futility, feelings of hopelessness, lack of motivation to help self. *Indicators that client may see no, or only limited, options or personal choices, and treatment needs to be directed at finding what happened in client's life to bring about these feelings.*[5]
- Assess extent of depression client may be experiencing. *Some studies suggest that a focus on religion may protect against depression.*[7]
- Note recent changes in negative behaviors (e.g., withdrawal from others or religious activities, dependence on alcohol or medications). *Lack of connectedness with self and others impairs ability to trust others or feel worthy of trust from others or God.*[6,7]
- Identify cultural values and expectations regarding religious beliefs or practices. *Individuals grow up in a family that instills a value system within them. As the person grows up, ideas, values, and expectations may change or be strengthened by new information, different questioning, and alternative viewpoints, which may affect current situation.*[3]
- Note socioeconomic status of individual/family. *Women who are poor may have high levels of personal religiosity yet participate less in organized religion because they may feel stigmatized by their situation (e.g., single mothers, those receiving public assistance, or those engaging in a lifestyle that conflicts with church norms).*[2]

NURSING PRIORITY NO. 2

To assist client/SOs to deal with feelings/situation:

- Use therapeutic communication skills of reflection and Active-listening. *Communicates acceptance and enables client to find own solutions to concerns as situation is discussed and deeper meanings are discovered.*[4]
- Encourage expression of feelings about illness or condition, death. *As people age, they become more concerned about their own mortality, and others often see them as in poor health and as spiritual and religious. If they have been diagnosed with a terminal illness, they may be feeling more angry and rejecting of God than seeking his help.*[5,8]
- Discuss personal beliefs that may hinder participation in religious activities. *Provides opportunity for self reflection, such as own worthiness and ability to forgive self for past decisions/life choices.*
- Discuss differences between grief and guilt and help client to identify and deal with each. Point out consequences of actions based on guilt. *Individuals often feel guilty about the "what if's" of life. "If only I had done this!" "If only I had paid more attention!" "If only*

I had made him go to the doctor!" Most of these guilty feelings are not based on reality and, when they are acted on, the individual does not get the release he or she seeks.[5]

● Suggest use of journaling, reminiscence. *Promotes life review and can assist in clarifying values and ideas, recognizing and resolving feelings and situation.*[4]

 ● Encourage client to identify individuals who can provide needed support (e.g., spiritual advisor, parish nurse). *When client is seeking to restore reliance on religious beliefs, these providers can often be helpful.*[6]

● Review client's religious affiliation, associated rituals, and beliefs. *Helps client examine what was important in the past, and may trigger some desire to reconnect with these previous beliefs.*[6]

● Provide opportunity for nonjudgmental discussion of philosophical issues related to religious belief patterns and customs. *Open communication can assist client to check reality of perceptions and identify personal options and willingness to resume desired activities.*[1]

● Discuss desire to continue or reconnect with previous belief patterns and customs and perceived barriers. *As client begins to think about current feelings of alienation from previous religious connections, these discussions can help to clarify and allow client to think about how these beliefs can be regained.*[5]

● Identify ways to strengthen spiritual or religious expression. *There are multiple options for enhancing participation in faith community (e.g., joining women's/men's prayer or study group, volunteering time to community projects, singing in the choir, reading spiritual writings).*

● Involve client in refining healthcare goals and therapeutic regimen as appropriate. *Identifies role illness or condition is playing in current concerns about ability to and appropriateness of participating in desired religious activities.*[7]

NURSING PRIORITY NO. 3

To promote wellness (Teaching/Discharge Considerations):

● Help client identify spiritual counselor who could be helpful (e.g., minister, priest, spiritual advisor who has qualifications or experience) in dealing with specific concerns of client. *Provides answers to spiritual questions, assists in the journey of self-discovery, and can help client learn to accept and forgive self.*[6]

● Provide privacy for meditation or prayer, performance of rituals, as appropriate. *Many individuals prefer to pray or meditate in private so they can concentrate without interruption or questions from others.*

● Explore alternatives or modifications of ritual based on setting and individual needs and limitations. *Individual may not be able to go to a church or temple, so providing another setting—chapel in the hospital or quiet room with appropriate religious artifacts or material—can provide the setting desired.*[6]

● Provide bibliotherapy, including list of relevant resources and Web sites *for later reference promoting self-paced learning and ongoing support.*[4]

DOCUMENTATION FOCUS

Assessment/Reassessment
• Individual findings, including nature of spiritual conflict, effects of participation in treatment regimen.
• Physical and emotional responses to conflict.

Planning
- Plan of care and who is involved in planning.
- Teaching plan.

Implementation/Evaluation
- Responses to interventions, teaching, and actions performed.
- Attainment or progress toward desired outcomes(s).
- Modifications to plan of care.

Discharge Planning
- Long-term needs and who is responsible for actions to be taken.
- Available resources, specific referrals made.

References

1. Burkhardt, L. (2005). A click away: Documenting spiritual care. *J Cardiovasc Nurs*, 22(1), 6–12.
2. Sullivan, S. (2006). Faith and poverty: Personal religiosity and organized religion in the lives of low-income urban mothers. Retrieved August 2007 from www.bc.edu/bc_org/research/rapl/events/abstract_sullivan.html.
3. Lipson, J. G., Dibble, S. L., Minarik, P. A. (1999). *Culture & Nursing Care: A Pocket Guide.* San Francisco: UCSF Nursing Press.
4. Townsend, M. (2006). *Psychiatric Mental Health Nursing Concepts of Care.* 5th ed. Philadelphia: F. A. Davis.
5. Doenges, M., Moorhouse, M., Murr, A. (2006). *Nursing Care Plans: Guidelines for Individualizing Patient Care.* 7th ed. Philadelphia: F. A. Davis.
6. Doenges, M., Moorhouse, M., Murr, A. (2008). *Nurse's Pocket Guide: Diagnoses, Prioritized Interventions, and Rationales.* 11th ed. Philadelphia: F. A. Davis.
7. Murray-Swank, A., et al. (2006). *Religiosity, Psychosocial Adjustment, and Subjective Burden of Persons Who Care for Those with Mental Illness.* Arlington, VA: Psychiatric Services, American Psychiatric Association.
8. Mills, J. (2006). The ontology of religiosity: The oceanic feeling and the value of the lived experience. Huumanists. Retrieved April 2007 from www.huumanists.org/rh/mills.html.

readiness for enhanced Religiosity

DEFINITION: Ability to increase reliance on religious beliefs or participate in rituals of a particular faith tradition

RELATED FACTORS

To be developed by nurse researchers and submitted to NANDA

DEFINING CHARACTERISTICS

Subjective
Expresses desire to strengthen religious belief patterns or customs that had provided comfort or religion in the past

(continues on page 670)

readiness for enhanced Religiosity (continued)

Requests assistance to increase participation in prescribed religious beliefs (e.g., religious ceremonies, dietary regulations/rituals, clothing, prayer, worship/religious services, private religious behaviors, reading religious materials/media, holiday observances)

Requests assistance to expand religious options, religious materials, or experiences

Requests meeting with religious leaders or facilitators

Requests forgiveness or reconciliation

Questions or rejects belief patterns or customs that are harmful

Sample Clinical Applications: As a health-seeking behavior, the client/family may be healthy, or this diagnosis can be associated with any clinical condition or life process

DESIRED OUTCOMES/EVALUATION CRITERIA

Sample NOC linkages:
Spiritual Health: Connectedness with self, others, higher power, all life, nature, and the universe that transcends and empowers the self

Client Will (Include Specific Time Frame)
• Acknowledge need to strengthen religious affiliations and continue or resume previously comforting rituals.
• Verbalize willingness to seek help to enhance desired religious beliefs.
• Become involved in spiritually based programs of own choice.
• Recognize the difference between belief patterns and customs that are helpful and those that may be harmful.

ACTIONS/INTERVENTIONS

Sample NIC linkages:
Spiritual Growth Facilitation: Facilitation of growth in patient's capacity to identify, connect with, and call upon the source of meaning, purpose, comfort, and hope in his or her life
Spiritual Support: Assisting the patient to feel balance and connection with a greater power

NURSING PRIORITY NO. 1

To determine spiritual state/motivation for growth:

• Determine client's current thinking about desire to learn more about religious beliefs and actions.
• Ascertain religious beliefs or cultural values of family of origin and climate in which client grew up. *Early religious training deeply affects children and is carried on into adulthood. Conflict between family's beliefs and client's current learning may need to be addressed.*[7]
• Identify cultural values and expectations regarding religious beliefs and/or practices. *Individuals grow up in a family that instills a value system within them. As the person grows up, ideas, values, and expectations may change or be strengthened by new information, different questioning, and alternative viewpoints.*[3]
• Note socioeconomic status of individual/family. *Women who are poor may have high levels of personal religiosity, yet participate less in organized religion because they feel*

stigmatized by their situation (e.g., single mothers, those receiving public assistance, or those engaging in a lifestyle that conflicts with church norms).[2]

- Discuss client's spiritual commitment, beliefs, and values. *Enables examination of these issues and helps client learn more about self and what he or she desires/believes.*[7]
- Explore how spirituality and religious practices have affected client's life. *Some philosophers believe that the value of religiosity is the deepened sense of quality of life associated with practicing one's beliefs or tenets.*[8]
- Ascertain motivation and expectations for change. *The client's motivation needs to be for self and not for others, and client needs to understand own expectations to move forward with desire to improve status.*[4]

NURSING PRIORITY NO. 2

To assist client to integrate values and beliefs to strengthen sense of wholeness and achieve optimum balance in daily living:

- Establish nurse-client relationship in which dialogue can occur. *Client can feel safe in this relationship to say anything and know it will be accepted.*[5]
- Identify barriers and beliefs that may hinder growth or self-discovery. *Provides opportunity for self-reflection such as own worthiness and ability to forgive self for past decisions or life choices. Previous practices and beliefs may need to be considered and accepted or discarded in new search for religious beliefs.*[8]
- Discuss cultural beliefs of family of origin and how they have influenced client's religious practices. *As client expands options for learning new or other religious beliefs and practices, these influences will provide information for comparing and contrasting new information.*[7]
- Explore connection of desire to strengthen belief patterns and customs to daily life. *Becoming aware of how these issues affect the individual's daily life can enhance ability to incorporate them into everything he or she does.*[1]
- Identify ways in which individual can develop a sense of harmony with self and others. *Client may have some new beliefs that may or may not be shared with others, and discussing these can clarify understanding by each individual.*[1]

NURSING PRIORITY NO. 3

To enhance optimum wellness (Teaching/Discharge Considerations):

- Encourage client to seek out and experience different religious beliefs, services, and ceremonies, as desired. *Trying out different religions will give client more information to contrast and compare what will fit his or her belief system.*[6]
- Provide bibliotherapy or reading materials pertaining to spiritual issues. *Client may be interested in learning about new spiritual ideas, and finding resources that clarify thinking will help to develop own beliefs.*[4]
- Encourage client to engage in stress-reducing activities, such as meditation, relaxation exercises, or Mindfulness (method of being in the moment). *Promotes general well-being and sense of control over self and ability to choose desired religious activities.*[5]
- Encourage participation in religious activities, worship or religious services, prayer or study groups; volunteering in church choir or other needed duties; reading religious materials, viewing religious media. *Enhances client's knowledge and promotes connectedness with self, others, and/or higher power.*[4]
- Refer to community resources (e.g., parish nurse, religion classes, other support groups).

DOCUMENTATION FOCUS

Assessment/Reassessment
• Assessment findings, including client perception of needs and desire for growth.
• Motivation and expectations for change.

Planning
• Plan for growth and who is involved in planning.

Implementation/Evaluation
• Response to activities, learning, and actions performed.
• Attainment or progress toward desired outcome(s).
• Modifications to plan.

Discharge Planning
• Long-term needs, expectations, and plan of action.
• Specific referrals made.

References

1. Burkhardt, L. (2005). A click away: Documenting spiritual care. *J Cardiovasc Nurs*, 22(1), 6–12.
2. Sullivan, S. (2006). Faith and poverty: Personal religiosity and organized religion in the lives of low-income urban mothers. Retrieved August 2007 from www.bc.edu/bc_org/research/rapl/events/abstract_sullivan.html.
3. Lipson, J. G., Dibble, S. L., Minarik, P. A. (1999). *Culture & Nursing Care: A Pocket Guide*. San Francisco: UCSF Nursing Press.
4. Townsend, M. (2006). *Psychiatric Mental Health Nursing Concepts of Care*. 5th ed. Philadelphia: F. A. Davis.
5. Doenges, M., Moorhouse, M., Murr, A. (2006). *Nursing Care Plans: Guidelines for Individualizing Patient Care*. 7th ed. Philadelphia: F. A. Davis.
6. Doenges, M., Moorhouse, M., Murr, A. (2008). *Nurse's Pocket Guide: Diagnoses, Prioritized Interventions, and Rationales*. 11th ed. Philadelphia: F. A. Davis.
7. Murray-Swank, A., et al. (2006). *Religiosity, Psychosocial Adjustment, and Subjective Burden of Persons Who Care for Those with Mental Illness*. Arlington, VA: Psychiatric Services, American Psychiatric Association.
8. Mills, J. (2006). The ontology of religiosity: The oceanic feeling and the value of the lived experience. Huumanists. Retrieved April 2007 from www.huumanists.org/rh/mills.html.

risk for impaired Religiosity

DEFINITION: At risk for an impaired ability to exercise reliance on religious beliefs and/or participate in rituals of a particular faith tradition

RISK FACTORS

Developmental
Life transitions

Environmental
Lack of transportation
Barriers to practicing religion

⊕ Cultural ⊗ Collaborative 🏠 Community/Home Care ✏ Diagnostic Studies ∞ Pediatric/Geriatric/Lifespan Medications

Physical
Illness; hospitalization; pain

Psychological
Ineffective support, coping, or caregiving
Depression
Lack of security

Sociocultural
Lack of social interaction; social isolation
Cultural barrier to practicing religion

Spiritual
Suffering

NOTE: A risk diagnosis is not evidenced by signs and symptoms, as the problem has not occurred; rather, nursing interventions are directed at prevention.
Sample Clinical Applications: Any acute or chronic condition, palliative care, end-of-life situation

DESIRED OUTCOMES/EVALUATION CRITERIA

Sample **NOC** linkages:
Spiritual Health: Connectedness with self, others, higher power, all life, nature, and the universe that transcends and empowers the self

Client Will (Include Specific Time Frame)
• Express understanding of relation of situation or health status to thoughts and feelings of concern about ability to participate in desired religious activities.
• Seek solutions to individual factors that may interfere with reliance on religious beliefs or participation in religious rituals.
• Identify and use resources appropriately.

ACTIONS/INTERVENTIONS

Sample **NIC** linkages:
Religious Ritual Enhancement: Facilitating participation in religious practices
Spiritual Growth Facilitation: Facilitation of growth in patient's capacity to identify, connect with, and call upon the source of meaning, purpose, comfort, and hope in his or her life
Spiritual Support: Assisting the patient to feel balance and connection with a greater power

NURSING PRIORITY NO. 1

To assess causative/contributing factor:

● Ascertain current situation (e.g., illness, hospitalization, prognosis of death, depression, lack of support systems, financial concerns). *Identifies problems client is dealing with in the moment that may be affecting desire to be involved with religious activities.*[1]

- Note client's concerns, expressions of anger, belief that illness or condition is result of lack of faith. *Individual may blame own self for what has happened and could reject religious beliefs and/or God.*[6]
- Determine client's usual religious or spiritual beliefs, past or current involvement in specific church activities. *Provides an understanding of how client saw religion in own life before current disruption.*[1]
- Identify cultural values and expectations regarding religious beliefs and/or practices. *Individuals grow up in a family that instills a value system within them. As the person grows up, ideas, values, and expectations may change or be strengthened by new information, different questioning, and alternative viewpoints, which may affect current situation.*[3]
- Note quality of relationships with significant others and friends. *Individual may withdraw from others in relation to the stress of illness, pain, and suffering. Others may be encouraging client to rely on religious beliefs at a time when individual is questioning own beliefs in the current situation.*[1]
- Note socioeconomic status of individual/family. *Women who are poor may have high levels of personal religiosity, yet participate less in organized religion because they feel stigmatized by their situation (e.g., single mothers, those receiving public assistance, or those engaging in a lifestyle that conflicts with church norms).*[2]
- Assess lack of transportation or environmental barriers to participation in desired religious activities. *These barriers can be realistic in the face of such issues as poor bus systems, inability of individual to get to bus stop (physical problems of walking or distance to the bus stop), or inability to drive a car.*[2]
- Ascertain substance use or abuse. *Individuals often turn to use of various substances in distress, and this can affect the ability to deal with problems in a positive manner.*[7]

NURSING PRIORITY NO. 2

To assist client to deal with feelings/situation:

- Develop nurse-client relationship. *Individual can express feelings and concerns freely when he or she feels safe to do so.*[5]
- Discuss personal beliefs that may hinder participation in religious activities. *Provides opportunity for self-reflection such as own worthiness and ability to forgive self for past decisions or life choices.*
- Use therapeutic communication skills of Active-listening, reflection, and I-messages. *Helps client to find own solutions to problems/concerns and promotes sense of control.*[4]
- Have client identify and prioritize current and immediate needs. *Dealing with current needs is easier than trying to predict the future. Also, it is important to take care of basic needs before moving on to higher needs.*[4]
- Provide time for nonjudgmental discussion of individual's spiritual beliefs and fears about impact of current illness and/or treatment regimen. *Helps to clarify thoughts and promote ability to deal with stresses of what is happening.*[6]
- Review with client past difficulties in life and coping skills that were used at that time. *Recalling problems with family, peers and colleagues, or individuals in position of authority can help client to remember how those were handled and how those skills could be used in current situation.*
- Encourage client to discuss feelings about death and end-of-life issues when illness or prognosis is grave. *People are often afraid to talk about the possibility of their own death for fear it will bring reality to self and upset family.*[1]

NURSING PRIORITY NO. 3

To promote wellness (Teaching/Discharge Considerations):

- Have client identify support systems available. *Individual will usually know who can provide the best support for him or her in present situation. Family may not be the most supportive if they don't want to accept the reality of client's illness or situation.*[5]
- Help client learn relaxation techniques, meditation, guided imagery, and Mindfulness (living in the moment and enjoying it). *Learning to relax can help client to process information and make decisions in a more positive manner.*[4]
- Take the lead from the client in initiating participation in religious activities, prayer, other activities. *Client may be vulnerable in current situation and needs to be allowed to decide own participation in these actions. Living and participating in desired religious activities will help client to understand the tenets of his or her choice.*[8]
- Refer to appropriate resources such as crisis counselor, governmental agencies, spiritual advisor (who has qualifications or experience dealing with specific problems such as death or dying process, relationship problems, substance abuse, suicide), hospice, psychotherapy, Alcoholics or Narcotics Anonymous. *May require additional help to deal with current situation.*[4,6,7]

DOCUMENTATION FOCUS

Assessment/Reassessment
- Individual findings, including risk factors, nature of current distress.
- Physical and emotional response to distress.
- Access to and use of resources.

Planning
- Plan of care and who is involved in planning.
- Teaching plan.

Implementation/Evaluation
- Responses to interventions, teaching, and actions performed.
- Attainment or progress toward desired outcome(s).
- Modifications to plan of care.

Discharge Planning
- Long-term needs and who is responsible for actions to be taken.
- Available resources and specific referrals made.

References

1. Burkhardt, L. (2005). A click away: Documenting spiritual care. *J Cardiovasc Nurs*, 22(1), 6–12.
2. Sullivan, S. Faith and poverty: Personal religiosity and organized religion in the lives of low-income urban mothers. Retrieved August 2007 from www.bc.edu/bc_org/research/rapl/events/abstract_sullivan.html.
3. Lipson, J. G., Dibble, S. L., Minarik, P. A. (1999). *Culture & Nursing Care: A Pocket Guide.* San Francisco: UCSF Nursing Press.
4. Townsend, M. (2006) *Psychiatric Mental Health Nursing Concepts of Care.* 5th ed. Philadelphia: F. A. Davis.

5. Doenges, M., Moorhouse, M., Murr, A. (2006). *Nursing Care Plans: Guidelines for Individualizing Patient Care.* 7th ed. Philadelphia: F. A. Davis.
6. Doenges, M., Moorhouse, M., Murr, A. (2008). *Nurse's Pocket Guide: Diagnoses, Prioritized Interventions, and Rationales.* 11th ed. Philadelphia: F. A. Davis.
7. Murray-Swank, A., et al. (2006). *Religiosity, Psychosocial Adjustment, and Subjective Burden of Persons Who Care for Those with Mental Illness.* Arlington, VA: Psychiatric Services, American Psychiatric Association.
8. Mills, J. (2006). The ontology of religiosity: The oceanic feeling and the value of the lived experience. Huumanists. Retrieved April 2007 from www.huumanists.org/rh/mills.html.

Relocation Stress Syndrome

DEFINITION: Physiological and/or psychosocial disturbance following transfer from one environment to another

RELATED FACTORS

Losses; feeling of powerlessness
Lack of adequate support system; lack of predeparture counseling; unpredictability of experience
Isolation; language barrier
Impaired psychosocial health; passive coping
Decreased health status

DEFINING CHARACTERISTICS

Subjective
Anxiety (e.g., separation); anger
Insecurity; worry; fear
Loneliness; depression
Unwillingness to move; concern over relocation
Sleep disturbance

Objective
Move from one environment to another
Increased [frequency of] verbalization of needs
Pessimism; frustration
Increased physical symptoms or illness
Withdrawal; aloneness; alienation; [hostile behavior or outbursts]
Loss of identity, self-worth, or self-esteem; dependency
[Increased confusion, cognitive impairment]

Sample Clinical Applications: Chronic conditions (e.g., multiple sclerosis [MS], asthma, cystic fibrosis), brain injury, stroke, dementia, schizophrenia, developmental delay, end-of-life/hospice care

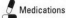

DESIRED OUTCOMES/EVALUATION CRITERIA

Sample (NOC) linkages:
Psychosocial Adjustment: Life Change: Adaptation psychosocial response of an individual to a significant life change
Quality of Life: Extent of positive perception of current life circumstances
Coping: Personal actions to manage stressors that tax an individual's resources

Client Will (Include Specific Time Frame)
• Verbalize understanding of reason(s) for change.
• Demonstrate appropriate range of feelings and lessened fear.
• Participate in routine and special or social events, as able.
• Verbalize acceptance of situation.
• Experience no catastrophic event.

ACTIONS/INTERVENTIONS

Sample (NIC) linkages:
Relocation Stress Reduction: Assisting the individual to prepare for and cope with movement from one environment to another
Hope Inspiration: Enhancing the belief in one's capacity to initiate and sustain actions
Family Involvement Promotion: Facilitating family participation in the emotional and physical care of the patient

NURSING PRIORITY NO. 1

To assess degree of stress as perceived/experienced by client and determine issues of safety:

• Determine situation or cause for relocation (e.g., planned move for new job, change in marital status, loss of home or community due to natural or man-made disaster, deterioration in health status or ability to care for self, caregiver burnout, elderly parent being requested to move closer to adult child). *Although nursing research has not currently validated the defining characteristics of relocation stress syndrome as a nursing diagnosis,[1,11] the belief that stress associated with relocation can be extreme is widely accepted in society. The effects of relocation can be minimal and transient, or very troubling and persistent.[2]*

∞ • Note client's age, developmental level, role in family. *Age and position in life cycle makes a difference in the impact of issues involved in relocating. For example, children can be traumatized by transfer to new school, loss of friends and familiar surroundings,[3] elderly persons may be affected by loss of their long-term home with its memories, neighborhood setting, and support persons.[12,13]*

⊕ • Identify cultural or religious concerns that may affect client's coping or impact social interactions and expectations. *Cultural norm may be that elders are cared for by family—not placed in a facility—causing client to feel abandoned; or individual may be required to defer to family decision maker and feel powerless in determining own destiny.[2,12,13]*

⊕ • Note ethnic ties and primary language spoken and read. *During times of stress, individuals may lapse into language of childhood. This affects healthcare providers who must try to reduce the client's feelings of alienation or confusion while communicating with client of another primary language, or client who is displaced from cultural attachments.[6]*

• Ascertain if client participated in the decision to relocate and perceptions about change(s), expectations for the future. *A forced relocation is much more stressful than one that is desired.[4] Client may be concerned that temporary placement will deplete savings or be fearful of being a burden on family members.*

🏠 • Determine involvement of family/SO(s). Note availability and use of support systems and resources. Ascertain presence or absence of comprehensive information and planning (e.g., when and how move took place, if the environment for the client is similar or greatly changed). *These factors can greatly affect client's ability to adjust to change.[4]*

• Note signs of increased stress in recently relocated client. *Client may report or demonstrate irritability, withdrawal, crying, moodiness, problems sleeping, or fatigue; "new" physical discomfort or pain (e.g., stomachaches, headaches, back pain); change in appetite; increased use of alcohol or other drugs; or greater susceptibility to colds.[2,5,12,13]*

• Observe behavior, noting presence of increasing anxiety, suspiciousness or paranoia, defensiveness. Compare with SO's/staff's description of customary responses. *Relocation may temporarily exacerbate mental deterioration (cognitive inaccessibility) and impair communication (social inaccessibility).*

• Identify issues of safety that may be involved, such as difficulty adjusting to new environment (e.g., navigating streets or choosing correct bus; locating dining hall or bathroom in facility), concerns of elopement or running away.

NURSING PRIORITY NO. 2

To assist client to deal with situation/changes:

🔵 • Collaborate in treatment of underlying conditions (e.g., chronic confusional states, brain injury, posttrauma rehabilitation) and physical stress symptoms *that are potentially exacerbating relocation stress or that may affect the length of time that relocation is required.*

• Encourage free expression of feelings about reason for relocation, including venting of anger; grief; loss of personal space, belongings, and friends; financial strains; powerlessness; and so forth. Acknowledge reality of situation and maintain hopeful attitude regarding move or change. *Bringing feelings out into the open helps clarify emotions and make feelings easier to deal with.[10,14]* Refer to NDs relating to client's particular situation (e.g., impaired Adjustment, ineffective Coping, Grieving) for additional interventions.

• Anticipate variety of emotions and reactions. *May vary from insomnia and loss of appetite to becoming involved with alcohol or other drugs, or exacerbation of health problems, onset of serious illness, or behavioral problems.[8]*

• Identify strengths and successful coping behaviors the individual has used previously. *Incorporating these into problem-solving builds on past successes.*

🏠 • Encourage client to maintain contact with friends (e.g., telephone, letters, e-mail, video or audio tapes, arranged visits) *to reduce sense of isolation.[9]*

🏠 • Provide client with information, list of organizations or community services (e.g., Welcome Wagon, senior citizens or teen clubs, churches, singles' groups, sports leagues) *to provide contacts for client to develop new relationships and learn more about the new setting.[10]*

🌐 • Obtain interpreter (where language differences exist) *to exchange information with the client/SO regarding residence or relocation wishes and to make helpful referrals.[6]*

🔵 • Refer to professionals (e.g., social worker, financial resources, mental healthcare provider, minister or spiritual advisor) if serious difficulties develop (e.g., depression, alcohol or other drug abuse, deteriorating behavior of child) *to assist client with special needs and/or persistent problems with adaptation.[5,15]*

🏠 • Take practical steps to alleviate stress for child. Encourage parents to walk with child to school or rehearse boarding the school bus, visit new classroom, contact friends child left behind, drive past places of interest to child, find a safe play place, unpack child's favorite toys, invite neighborhood children to a get-acquainted party, and so forth. *Helps child to maintain ties and develop new ones, thus reducing sense of loss and shifting focus to the future.*[3]

- Facilitate client's adjustment to new environment or facility:[4,7,9,13,16]

Determine client's usual schedule of activities and incorporate into facility routine, as possible. *Reinforces sense of importance of individual.*

Orient to surroundings and schedules, repeat directions, as needed.

Introduce to new staff members, roommate, other residents.

Provide clear, honest information about actions and events.

Provide consistency in daily routine; maintain same staff with client in new facility, as possible, during adjustment phase.

Address ways to preserve lifestyle (e.g., usual bath and bedtimes in new facility, involvement in church activities). *Helps reduce the sense of loss associated with move.*

Encourage individual/family to personalize area with pictures, own belongings, and the like as soon as possible. *Enhances sense of belonging, self-expression, and creation of personal space.*

Introduce socialization and diversional activities, such as meals with new acquaintances, art therapy, music, movies, etc. *Involvement increases opportunity to interact with others and form new friendships, thus decreasing isolation and stress reactions.*

Encourage hugging and use of touch unless client is paranoid or agitated at the moment. *Human connection reaffirms acceptance of individual.*

Place in private room, if appropriate, and include SO(s)/family in care activities, mealtime, and so forth. *Keeping client secluded may be needed under some circumstances (e.g., advanced Alzheimer's disease with fear or aggressive reactions) to decrease the client's stress reactions to new environment.*

Deal with aggressive behavior by imposing calm, firm limits. Control environment and protect others from client's disruptive behavior. *Promotes safety for client/others.*

Remain calm, place in a quiet environment, provide time-out, *to prevent escalation of disruptive behaviors (e.g., panic state, violence).*

- Anticipate and address feelings of distress in family/caregivers when placing loved one in a different environment (e.g., nursing home, foster care). *Support and referrals may be needed to help SOs in practical issues and adjustment.*

NURSING PRIORITY NO. 3

To promote wellness (Teaching/Discharge Considerations):

- Involve client in formulating goals and plan of care when possible. *Supports independence and commitment to achieving outcomes.*
- Encourage communication between client/family/SO *to provide mutual support and problem-solving opportunities.*[5]
- Discuss benefits of adequate nutrition, rest, and exercise *to maintain physical well-being and reduce adverse effects of stressful situation.*
- Instruct in anxiety and stress-reduction activities (e.g., meditation, other relaxation techniques, exercise program, group socialization), as able, *to enhance psychological well-being and coping abilities.*
- Encourage participation in activities, hobbies, or personal interactions, as appropriate. *Promotes creative endeavors, stimulating the mind.*
- Identify community support, or cultural or ethnic groups client can access.
- Support self-responsibility and coping strategies *to foster sense of control and self-worth.*

DOCUMENTATION FOCUS

Assessment/Reassessment
- Assessment findings, individual's perception of the situation and changes, specific behaviors.
- Cultural or religious concerns.
- Safety issues.

Planning
- Note plan of care, who is involved in planning, and who is responsible for proposed actions.
- Teaching plan.

Implementation/Evaluation
- Response to interventions (especially time-out or seclusion), teaching, and actions performed.
- Sentinel events.
- Attainment or progress toward desired outcome(s).
- Modifications to plan of care.

Discharge Planning
- Long-term needs and who is responsible for actions to be taken.
- Specific referrals made.

References

1. Mallick, M. J., Whipple, T. W. (2000). Validity of the nursing diagnosis of relocation stress syndrome. *Nurs Res*, 49(2), 97–100.
2. Conquering relocation stress. (2001). Public information article by the U.S. Army for military families. Retrieved September 2003 from www.usarec.army.
3. Chiaro, C. (2003). Preventing relocation stress, easing children's transition. Special report. *Colorado Springs Business Journal*.
4. Health impacts of relocation. Summary evidence review series: No. 11. Health impact assessment. (2002). Retrieved September 2003 from http://online.northumbria.ac.uk/faculties/hswe/hia/evidence/eleven.htm.
5. Solomon, A. (2000). Relocation stress: The warning signs. Retrieved July 2007 from www.therapyinla.com/psych/psych0100.html.
6. Purnell, L. D., Paulanka, B. J. (1998). Purnell's model for cultural competence. *Transcultural Health Care: A Culturally Competent Approach*. Philadelphia: F. A. Davis, 11–14.
7. Nypaver, J. M., Titus, M., Brugler, C. J. (1996). Patient transfer to rehabilitation: Just another move? Relocation stress syndrome. *Rehabil Nurs*, 21(2), 94–97.
8. Stress. Youth Center, Army Community Services. Retrieved January 2004 from www.armycommunityservices.org.
9. Cox, H. C., et al. (2002). ND Relocation Stress Syndrome, risk for. *Clinical Applications of Nursing Diagnosis: Adult, Child, Women's, Psychiatric, Gerontic, and Home Health Considerations*. 4th ed. Philadelphia: F. A. Davis.
10. Puskar, K. R., Dvorsak, K. G. (1991). Relocation stress in adolescents: Helping teenagers cope with a moving dilemma. *Pediatr Nurs*, 17(3), 298–297.
11. Walker, C. A., Curry, L. C., Hogstel, M. O. (2007). Relocation stress syndrome in older adults transitioning from home to long term care facility: Myth or reality? *J Psychosoc Nurs Ment Health Serv*, 45(1), 38–45.
12. Helpful moving tips: Family relocation checklist. (2004). Retrieved July 2007 from www.myarmylifetoo.com/.
13. Mintz, T. G. (2005). Relocation stress syndrome in older adults. *Social Work Today*, 5(6), 38–45.
14. Dion, R. (2005). Overcoming relocation stress. Military OneSource, PTSD Support Services. Retrieved July 2007 from www.ptsdsupport.net/relocation_stress.html.

15. Murphy, K. (2005). Anxiety: When is it too much? *Nursing Made Incredibly Easy!*, 3(5), 22–31.
16. Munche, J. A., McCarty, S. (2006). Geriatric rehabilitation. Retrieved April 2007 from www.emedicine.com/pmr/topic164.htm.

risk for Relocation Stress Syndrome

DEFINITION: At risk for physiological and/or psychosocial disturbance following transfer from one environment to another

RISK FACTORS

Move from one environment to another
Moderate to high degree of environmental change [e.g., physical, ethnic, cultural]
Lack of adequate support system or group; lack of predeparture counseling
Passive coping; feelings of powerlessness; losses
Moderate mental competence
Unpredictability of experiences

NOTE: A risk diagnosis is not evidenced by signs and symptoms, as the problem has not occurred; rather, nursing interventions are directed at prevention.
Sample Clinical Applications: Chronic conditions (e.g., multiple sclerosis [MS], asthma, cystic fibrosis), brain injury, stroke, dementia, schizophrenia, developmental delay

DESIRED OUTCOMES/EVALUATION CRITERIA

Sample **NOC** linkages:
Psychosocial Adjustment: Life Change: Psychosocial adaptation of an individual to a life change
Quality of Life: An individual's expressed satisfaction with current life circumstances
Grief Resolution: Adjustment to actual or impending loss

Client Will (Include Specific Time Frame)
• Verbalize understanding of reason(s) for change.
• Express feelings and concerns openly and appropriately.
• Experience no catastrophic event.

ACTIONS/INTERVENTIONS

Sample **NIC** linkages:
Discharge Planning: Preparation for moving a patient from one level of care to another within or outside the current healthcare agency
Relocation Stress Reduction: Assisting the individual to prepare for and cope with movement from one environment to another
Emotional Support: Provision of reassurance, acceptance, and encouragement during times of stress

NURSING PRIORITY NO. 1

To identify risk/contributing factors:

- Determine situation or cause for relocation (e.g., planned move for new job, change in marital status, loss of home or community due to natural or man-made disaster, deterioration in health status or ability to care for self, caregiver burnout, elderly parent being requested to move closer to adult child). *Although nursing research has not currently validated the defining characteristics of relocation stress syndrome as a nursing diagnosis,[1,5] the belief that stress associated with relocation can be extreme is widely accepted in society. The effects of relocation can be minimal and transient, or very troubling and persistent.[2]*

- Note client's age, developmental level, role in family. *Age and position in life cycle makes a difference in the impact of issues involved in relocating. For example, children can be traumatized by transfer to new school, loss of friends and familiar surroundings;[3] elderly persons may be affected by loss of their long-term home with its memories, neighborhood setting, and support persons.[4,6,7]*

- Identify cultural and/or religious concerns that may affect client's coping or impact social interactions, expectations. *Cultural norm may be that elders are cared for by family—not placed in a facility—causing client to feel abandoned; or individual may be required to defer to family decision maker and feel powerless in determining own destiny.[2,6,7]*

- Note ethnic ties and primary language spoken and read. *During times of stress, individuals may lapse into language of childhood. This affects healthcare providers who must try to reduce client's feelings of alienation while communicating, with client of another primary language, or client who is displaced from cultural, familial attachments.[2,8]*

- Ascertain if client has participated in the decision to relocate, perceptions about change(s), and expectations for the future. *Decision may have been made without client's input or understanding of event or consequences, which can impact adjustment. A forced relocation is much more stressful than one that is desired.[4,7] Client may be concerned that temporary placement will deplete savings or fearful of being a burden on family members and felt pressured to move.*

- Note whether relocation will be temporary (e.g., extended care for rehabilitation therapies, moving in with family while house being repaired after fire) or long term or permanent (e.g., move from home of many years, placement in long-term care facility). *To some degree, a temporary relocation is usually easier to cope with than a permanent relocation. However, any anticipated disruption of the client's usual way of living is upsetting, and emotional responses aren't always congruent with the magnitude of the event.*

- Determine involvement of family/SO(s). Note availability and use of support systems and resources. Ascertain presence or absence of comprehensive information and planning (e.g., when and how move will take place, if the environment for the client will be similar or greatly changed). *These factors can greatly affect client's ability to cope with change.[4]*

NURSING PRIORITY NO. 2

To prevent/minimize adverse response to change:

- Collaborate in treatment of underlying conditions (e.g., chronic confusional states, brain injury, posttrauma rehabilitation) and physical stress symptoms *that could exacerbate relocation stress or that affects length of time that relocation may be needed.*

- Provide information to client/SO as early in process as possible *to eliminate misconceptions and facilitate decision-making process. This can include obtaining audiovisual materials or Web sites about the new home, city, region, or country.[8,9]*

∞ • Discuss relocation or move with child. *Information for child must be aimed at level of understanding and interest.[3] Child lacks ability to put problem into perspective, so minor mishap may seem catastrophic. Also, child is more vulnerable to stress because he or she has less control over environment than most adults.[2,9]*

∞ • Avoid moving adolescent in middle of school year when possible. *Adolescent is vulnerable to emotional, social, and cognitive dysfunction because of the great importance of peer group and loss of friends and social standing caused by relocation.[9]*

🏠 • Involve client in placement choices when possible (e.g., move to nursing home or adult foster care) *to provide client with some control over the situation.*

🏠 • Encourage visit to new community, surroundings, or school before transfer when possible. *Provides opportunity to "get acquainted" with new situation, reducing fear of unknown.*

🏠 • Suggest contact with someone (friend, family, business associate) who has been to or lived in new area where move is being planned *to absorb some of their experience and knowledge.[8,9]*

🏠 • Take practical steps to alleviate stress for child. Encourage parents to walk with child to school or rehearse boarding the school bus, visit new classroom, contact friends child left behind, drive past places of interest to child, find a safe play place, unpack child's favorite toys, invite neighborhood children to a get-acquainted party, and so forth; *helps child to maintain ties and develop new ones, reducing sense of loss and shifting focus to the future.[3]*

• Encourage free expression of feelings about reason for relocation. Acknowledge reality of situation and maintain hopeful attitude regarding move or change. *Bringing feelings out into the open helps clarify emotion and make feelings easier to deal with.[9,10]*

NURSING PRIORITY NO. 3

To promote wellness (Teaching/Discharge Considerations):

🏠 • Involve client in formulating goals and plan of care when possible. *Fosters sense of control and self-worth, supports independence and commitment to achieving outcomes.*

🏠 • Encourage client/SO to accept that relocation is an adjustment and that it takes time to adapt to new circumstances or environment.

🏠 • Instruct in anxiety- and stress-reduction activities (e.g., meditation, other relaxation techniques, exercise program, group socialization) as able *to enhance psychological well-being and coping abilities.*

🏠 • Provide client with information and list of organizations or community services (e.g., Welcome Wagon, senior citizens or teen clubs, churches, singles' groups, sports leagues) *to provide contacts for client to develop new relationships and learn more about the new setting.[10]*

🏠 • Discuss safety issues regarding new environment (*e.g., how to navigate streets or choose correct bus; locate dining hall or bathroom in facility*), concerns of elopement or running away.

🏠 • Anticipate variety of emotions and reactions. *May vary from insomnia and loss of appetite to becoming involved with alcohol or other drugs, or exacerbation of health problems, onset of serious illness, or behavioral problems. Awareness provides opportunity for timely intervention.[6,9]*

• Refer to ND Relocation Stress Syndrome for additional interventions.

DOCUMENTATION FOCUS

Assessment/Reassessment
• Assessment findings, individual's perception of the situation/changes, specific behaviors.
• Cultural or religious concerns.
• Safety issues.

Planning
• Note plan of care, who is involved in planning, and who is responsible for proposed actions.
• Teaching plan.

Implementation/Evaluation
• Response to interventions (especially time-out/seclusion), teaching, and actions performed.
• Sentinel events.
• Attainment or progress toward desired outcome(s).
• Modifications to plan of care.

Discharge Planning
• Long-term needs and who is responsible for actions to be taken.
• Specific referrals made.

References

1. Mallick, M. J., Whipple, T. W. (2000). Validity of the nursing diagnosis of relocation stress syndrome. *Nurs Res*, 49(2), 97–100.
2. Conquering relocation stress. (2001). Public information article by the U.S. Army for military families. Retrieved September 2003 from www.usarec.army.
3. Chiaro, C. (2003). Preventing relocation stress, easing children's transition. Special report. *Colorado Springs Business Journal*.
4. Health impacts of relocation. Summary evidence review series: No. 11. Health impact assessment. (2002). Retrieved September 2003 from http://online.northumbria.ac.uk/faculties/hswe/hia/evidence/eleven.htm.
5. Walker, C. A., Curry, L. C., Hogstel, M. O. (2007). Relocation stress syndrome in older adults transitioning from home to long term care facility: Myth or reality? *J Psychosoc Nurs Ment Health Serv*, 45(1), 38–45.
6. Helpful moving tips: Family relocation checklist. (2004). Retrieved July 2007 from www.myarmylifetoo.com.
7. Mintz, T. G. (2005). Relocation stress syndrome in older adults. *Social Work Today*, 5(6), 38.
8. Solomon, A. (2000). Relocation stress: The warning signs. Psych Bytes. Retrieved July 2007 from www.therapyinla.com/psych/psych0100.html.
9. Dion, R. (2005). Overcoming relocation stress. Military OneSource, PTSD Support Services. Retrieved July 2007 from www.ptsdsupport.net/relocation_stress.html.10.
10. Cox, H. C., et al. (2002). ND Relocation Stress Syndrome, risk for. *Clinical Applications of Nursing Diagnosis: Adult, Child, Women's, Psychiatric, Gerontic, and Home Health Considerations*. 4th ed. Philadelphia: F. A. Davis.

(impaired individual Resilience)

DEFINITION: Decreased ability to sustain a pattern of positive responses to an adverse situation or crisis

RELATED FACTORS

Demographics that increase chance of maladjustment; large family size; minority status; poverty; gender
Vulnerability factors which encompass indices that exacerbate the negative effects of the risk condition; drug use; poor impulse control; violence in neighborhood

Low intelligence; low maternal education
Inconsistent parenting; parental mental illness
Psychological disorders; violence

DEFINING CHARACTERISTICS

Subjective
Depression; guilt; isolation; social isolation; low self-esteem; shame
Lower perceived health status
Renewed elevation of distress
Decreased interest in academic activities; vocational activities

Objective
Using maladaptive coping skills (i.e., drug use, violence, etc.)

Sample Clinical Applications: Substance abuse, mental health issues—depression, phobia, bipolar disorder, schizophrenia; chronic illness—renal failure, heart failure, cancer; debilitating conditions—multiple sclerosis (MS), Parkinson's disease, obesity; domestic abuse or violence

DESIRED OUTCOMES/EVALUATION CRITERIA

Sample **NOC** linkages:
Personal Resiliency: Positive adaptation and function of an individual following significant adversity or crisis
Hope: Optimism that is personally satisfying and life-supporting
Family Resiliency: Positive adaptation and function of the family system following significant adversity or crisis

Client Will (Include Specific Time Frame)
Acknowledge reality of current situation or crisis.
Express positive feelings about self and situation.
Seek appropriate resources to change circumstances that affect adaptation and resilience.
Be involved in programs to address problems presenting in life (e.g., substance abuse, low self-esteem, poverty).

ACTIONS/INTERVENTIONS

Sample **NIC** linkages:
Resiliency Promotion: Assisting individuals, families, and communities in development, use, and strengthening of factors to be used in coping with environmental and societal stressors
Hope Inspiration: Enhancing the belief in one's capacity to initiate and sustain actions
Family Mobilization: Utilization of family strengths to influence patient's health in a positive direction

frustration (and sometimes easier for the caregivers in terms of their time), it is important for client to do as much as possible for self to regain or maintain self-esteem, reduce helplessness, and promote optimal recovery.[2]

- Review coping skills (e.g., assertiveness, interpersonal relations, decision making, problem-solving, stigma management, and time management) *that are useful in managing a wide range of stressful conditions.* Encourage client to ask for assistance as needed or desired.[2,11]
- Schedule activities *to conform to client's normal schedule as much as possible (e.g., bathing at a relaxing time for client, rather than on a set routine).*[1]
- Plan activities to prevent or accommodate fatigue and/or exacerbation of pain *to conserve energy and promote maximum participation in self-care.*[2]
- Identify energy-saving behaviors *(e.g., sitting instead of standing when possible, organizing needs before beginning tasks).* Refer to NDs Activity Intolerance; Fatigue for additional interventions.
- Review medication needs (e.g., vitamins, nutritional supplements, pain reliever, antidepressants) *that may improve general well-being and ability to participate in self-care.*[1]
- Arrange for home visit, as indicated, *to assess environmental concerns that can impact client's abilities to care for self in home. If necessary modifications are not feasible or cannot be made, client may require temporary or long-term relocation or regular home-care assistance.*[2]
- Consult with rehabilitation professionals to identify and obtain assistive devices (e.g., modified eating utensils, modified clothing), mobility aids (e.g., rolling commode, shower chair), and home modification as necessary (e.g., adequate lighting; cutout under kitchen and bathroom sink; lowering cabinets and closet rods; handheld shower, raised toilet seat, grab bars for bathroom) *to optimize self-care efforts.*[1,3,10,12]
- Note availability and use of resources, supportive person(s) *to ascertain that client has means for sharing common concerns, needs, and wishes, as well as access to social support and approval (e.g., support group participants, family members, professionals).*[11]

NURSING PRIORITY NO. 4

To meet specific self-care needs:

FEEDING DEFICIT

- Assess client's need and ability to prepare food as indicated (including shopping, cooking, cutting food, opening containers, etc.). *Identifies specific assistance required.*
- Encourage food and fluid choices reflecting individual likes and abilities and that meet nutritional needs *to maximize food intake.*[4]
- Ascertain that client can swallow safely, checking gag and swallow reflexes, as indicated. Refer to ND impaired Swallowing for related interventions.
- Provide food and fluid of appropriate consistency *to facilitate swallowing.* Cut food into bite-size pieces *to prevent overfilling mouth and reduce risk of choking.*
- Assist client to handle utensils or in guiding utensils to mouth. *May require specialized equipment (e.g., rocker knife, plate guard, built-up handles) to increase independence, or assistance with movement of arms and hands.*[3]
- Assist client with cup, glass, or bottle for liquids, using straw or adaptive lids as indicated *to enhance fluid intake while reducing spills.*
- Allow client time for intake of sufficient food *for feeling satisfied or completing a meal.*[1]
- Assist client with social graces when eating with others; provide privacy *when manners might be offensive to others or client could be embarrassed.*
- Collaborate with nutritionist or physician *for special diets or feeding methods necessary to provide adequate nutrition.*[2]

● Feed client allowing adequate time for chewing and swallowing, *when client is not able to obtain nutrition by self-feeding.* Avoid providing fluids until client has swallowed food and mouth is clear. *Prevents "washing down" foods, reducing risk of choking.*[1]

BATHING DEFICIT

● Ask client/SO for input on bathing habits or cultural bathing preferences. *Creates opportunities for client to (1) keep long-standing routines (e.g., bathing at bedtime to improve sleep) and (2) exercise control over situation. This enhances self-esteem, while respecting personal and cultural preferences.*[5]

● Bathe or assist client in bathing, providing for any or all hygiene needs as indicated. *Type (e.g., bed bath, towel bath, tub bath, shower) and purpose (e.g., cleansing, removing odor, or simply soothing agitation) of bath is determined by individual need.*[1]

● Obtain hygiene supplies (e.g., soap, toothpaste, toothbrush, mouthwash, lotion, shampoo, razor, towels) for specific activity to be performed and place in client's easy reach *to provide visual cues and facilitate completion of activity.*

● Ascertain that all safety equipment is in place and properly installed (e.g., grab bars, antislip strips, shower chair, hydraulic lift) and that client/caregiver(s) can safely operate equipment *to prevent injury to client and caregivers.*[6]

● Instruct client to request assistance when needed and place call device within easy reach, *so client can summon help if bathing alone;* or stay with client *as dictated by safety needs.*

● Provide for adequate warmth (e.g., covering client during bed bath or warming bathroom). *Certain individuals (especially infants, the elderly, and very thin or debilitated persons) are prone to hypothermia and can experience evaporative cooling during and after bathing.*[7]

● Determine that client can perceive water temperature, adjust water temperature safely, or that water is correct temperature for client's bath or shower *to prevent chilling or burns. This step requires that client is cognitively and physically able to perceive hot and cold and to adjust faucets safely; otherwise, adequate supervision must be provided at all times.*[7]

● Assist client in and out of shower or tub as indicated. *Needs are variable (e.g., client may need to get into tub before running water; may require a shower chair, may be independent with one fixture and not another), requiring assessment of individual situations.*[1]

● Assist with or encourage client to complete hygiene steps (e.g., oral care, lotion application, applying deodorant, washing and styling hair). *These steps may be completed at same or different time as bathing, but are usually part of a daily routine that is necessary for client's physical well-being and emotional or social comfort.*[1]

DRESSING DEFICIT

● Ascertain that appropriate clothing is available. *Client may not have sufficient clothing, clothing may be inadequate for situation or weather conditions, or clothing may need to be modified for client's particular medical condition or physical limitations.*[2]

● Assist client in choosing clothing, or lay out clothing as indicated. *May be needed when client has cognitive, physical, or psychiatric conditions affecting ability to choose appropriate pieces of clothing or to maintain a satisfactory appearance.*[3]

● Dress client or assist with dressing, as indicated. *Client may need assistance in putting on or taking off items of clothing (e.g., shoes and socks, or over-the-head shirt), or may require partial or complete assistance with fasteners (e.g., buttons, snaps, zippers, shoelaces).*[1,2]

● Allow sufficient time for dressing and undressing *because tasks may be tiring, painful, and difficult to complete.*

● Use adaptive clothing as indicated (e.g., clothing with front closure, wide sleeves and pant legs, Velcro or zipper closures).

- Teach client to dress affected side first, then unaffected side (when client has paralysis or injury to one side of body) *to allow for easier manipulation of clothing.*[2]
- Provide for or assist with grooming activities (e.g., shaving, hair care, cleaning and clipping nails, makeup) on a routine, consistent basis. Encourage participation, guiding client's hand through tasks, as indicated. *Experiencing the normal process of a task through established routine and guided practice facilitates optimal relearning.*[8]

TOILETING DEFICIT

- Provide mobility assistance to bathroom or commode; or place on bedpan or offer urinal, as indicated. *Client might be impaired because of age, cognitive problems, weakness, acute injury or illness, requiring a range of interventions from complete care to help with walking.*[1,2]
- Direct cognitively impaired client to bathroom, if needed. *May need directions to the facilities or reminders to use the bathroom, and so forth.*[8]
- Observe for behaviors such as pacing, fidgeting, holding crotch *that may be indicative of need for prompt toileting.*[8]
- Provide privacy *to enhance self-esteem and improve ability to urinate or defecate.*[3]
- Assist with manipulation of clothing if needed, *to decrease incidence of functional incontinence caused by difficulty removing clothing/underwear.*[9]
- Observe need for and assist in obtaining modified clothing or fasteners *to assist client in manipulation of clothing, fostering independence in self-toileting.*
- Provide or assist with use of assistive equipment (e.g., raised toilet seat, support rails, spill-proof urinals, fracture pans, bedside commode) *to promote independence and safety in sitting down or arising from toilet, or for aiding elimination when client unable to go to bathroom.*[1,2]
- Keep toilet paper or wipes and hand-washing items within client's easy reach *to enhance self-cleansing efforts.*
- Implement bowel or bladder training/retraining programs as indicated. *This may include developing a schedule for toileting and other interventions as seen in NDs Bowel Incontinence, Constipation, impaired Urinary Elimination, Urinary Incontinence, [specify].*[1,2]

NURSING PRIORITY NO. 5

To promote wellness (Teaching/Discharge Considerations):

- Assist the client to become aware of rights and responsibilities in health and healthcare and to assess own health strengths—physical, emotional, and intellectual.
- Support client *in making health-related decisions and assist in developing self-care practices and goals that promote health.*
- Instruct in relaxation techniques (e.g., deep breathing, meditation, music, yoga) *to reduce frustration and enhance coping.*
- Provide for ongoing evaluation of self-care program *to note progress, identify changes in needs.*
- Modify program periodically *to accommodate changes in client's abilities. Assists client to adhere to plan of care to fullest extent.*
- Encourage keeping a journal *to note progress and identify factors affecting ability to perform self-care activities and to foster self-care and self-determination.*[1,3,11]
- Review safety concerns. Modify activities and environment *to reduce risk of injury and promote successful community functioning.*
- Refer to home-care provider, social services, physical or occupational therapy, rehabilitation and counseling resources as indicated.

- Arrange consult with community resources (e.g., Meals on Wheels, home care or visiting nurse service, senior services, nutritionist) *to provide long-term support and additional forms of assistance that may improve client's independence and self-care.*[2,3]
- Review instructions from other members of the healthcare team and provide written copy. *Provides clarification, reinforcement, and for periodic review by client/caregivers.*[1]
- Discuss respite or other care options with family. *Allows them free time away from the care situation to renew themselves, enhances coping abilities.* (Refer to ND Caregiver Role Strain for related interventions.)
- Assist or support family with alternative placements as necessary. *Enhances likelihood of finding individually appropriate situation to meet client's needs.*
- Be available for discussion of feelings (e.g., grieving, anger, frustration). *Provides opportunity for client/family to get feelings out in the open, realize the feelings are normal, and begin to problem-solve solutions as indicated.*
- Refer to NDs ineffective Coping; compromised family Coping; risk for Disuse Syndrome; risk for Falls/Injury/Trauma; impaired physical Mobility; Powerlessness; situational low Self-Esteem, as appropriate.

DOCUMENTATION FOCUS

Assessment/Reassessment
- Individual findings, functional level, and specifics of limitation(s).
- Needed resources and adaptive devices.
- Availability and use of community resources.
- Who is involved in care and provides assistance.

Planning
- Plan of care and who is involved in planning.
- Teaching plan.

Implementation/Evaluation
- Response to interventions, teaching, and actions performed.
- Attainment or progress toward desired outcome(s).
- Modifications of plan of care.

Discharge Planning
- Long-term needs and who is responsible for actions to be taken.
- Type of and source for assistive devices.
- Specific referrals made.

References

1. Doenges, M. E., Moorhouse, M. F., Geissler-Murr, A. C. (2004). ND: Self-Care Deficit: Bathing/hygiene, dressing/grooming, feeding, toileting. *Nurse's Pocket Guide: Diagnoses, Interventions, and Rationales.* 9th ed. Philadelphia: F. A. Davis.
2. Doenges, M. E., Moorhouse, M. F., Geissler-Murr, A. C. (2002). ND: Self-Care Deficit (specify). *Nursing Care Plans: Guidelines for Individualizing Patient Care.* 6th ed. Philadelphia: F. A. Davis, 238, 291, 545, 729.
3. Cox, H. C., et al. (2002). ND: Self Care Deficit (feeding, bathing-hygiene, dressing-grooming, toileting). *Clinical Applications of Nursing Diagnosis: Adult, Child, Women's, Psychiatric, Gerontic, and Home Health Considerations.* 4th ed. Philadelphia: F. A. Davis, 331–335.
4. Kayser-Jones, J., Schell, E. (1997). The mealtime experience of a cognitively impaired elder: Ineffective and effective strategies. *J Gerontol Nurs*, 23(7), 33.
5. Freeman, E. (1997). International perspectives on bathing. *J Gerontol Nurs*, 22(1), 40–44.

6. Schemm, R. L., Gitlin, L. N. (1998). How occupational therapists teach older patients to use bathing and dressing devices in rehabilitation. *Am J Occup Ther*, 52(4), 276–282.
7. Miller, M. (1997). Physically aggressive resident behavior during hygienic care. *J Gerontol Nurs*, 23(5), 24–39.
8. Sloane, P. (1995). Bathing the Alzheimer's patient in long term care: Results and recommendation from three studies. *Am J Alzheimer's Dis*, 10(4), 3–11.
9. Penn, C. (1996). Assessment of urinary incontinence. *J Gerontol Nurs*, 22, 8–19.
10. Baldwin, K. M. (2006). Stroke: It's a knock-out punch. *Nursing Made Incredibly Easy!*, 4(2), 10–23.
11. Livneh, H., Antonak, R. F. (2005). Psychosocial adaptation to chronic illness and disability: A primer for counselors (practice & theory). *J Couns Dev*. Excerpt retrieved July 2007 from www.accessmylibrary.com/coms2/summary_0286-19174530_ITM.
12. Singleton, J. K. Nurses' perspectives of encouraging client's care-of-self in a short-term rehabilitation unit within a long-term care facility. Retrieved July 2007 from www.rehabnurse.org/ce/010200/010200_a.htm.

readiness for enhanced Self-Care

DEFINITION: A pattern of performing activities for oneself that helps to meet health-related goals and can be strengthened

RELATED FACTORS

To be developed by nurse researchers and submitted to NANDA

DEFINING CHARACTERISTICS

Subjective
Expresses desire to enhance independence in maintaining life, health, personal development or well-being
Expresses desire to enhance knowledge for strategies for self-care
Expresses desire to enhance self-care or responsibility for self-care
[Note: Based on the definition and defining characteristics of this ND, the focus appears to be broader than simply meeting routine basic activities of daily living (ADLs) and addresses independence in maintaining overall health, personal development, and general well-being.]

Sample Clinical Applications: Presence of chronic physical or psychological conditions, or any individual seeking improved well-being or independence in meeting own needs

DESIRED OUTCOMES/EVALUATION CRITERIA

Sample **NOC** linkages:
Self-Care Status: Ability to perform basic personal care activities and household tasks
Self-Care: Instrumental Activities of Daily Living (IADL): Ability to perform activities to function in the home or community independently with or without assistive device
Self-Direction of Care: Care recipient actions taken to direct others who assist with or perform physical tasks and personal care

Client Will (Include Specific Time Frame)
- Maintain responsibility for planning and achieving self-care goals and general well-being.
- Demonstrate proactive management of chronic conditions, potential complications, or changes in capabilities.
- Identify and use resources appropriately.
- Remain free of preventable complications.

ACTIONS/INTERVENTIONS

Sample NIC linkages:
Self-Care Assistance: IADL: Assisting and instructing a person to perform instrumental activities of daily living needed to function in the home or community
Self-Modification Assistance: Reinforcement of self-directed change initiated by the patient to achieve personally important goals

NURSING PRIORITY NO. 1

To determine current self-care status and motivation for growth:

- Determine individual strengths and skills of the client *to incorporate into plan of care, enhancing likelihood of achieving outcomes.*[1]
- Ascertain motivation and expectations for change. *Motivation to improve and high expectations can encourage client to make changes that will improve his or her life. However, unrealistic expectations may hamper efforts.*
- Note availability and use of resources, and supportive person(s)*to ascertain that client has means for sharing common concerns, needs, and wishes as well as has access to social support and approval (e.g., support group participants, family members, professionals).*[2]
- Determine age, developmental issues, and presence of medical conditions resulting in very specific deficits (e.g., loss of visual or spatial orientation affecting driving, muscular weakness affecting fine motor coordination, peripheral neuropathy impairing sensory interpretation) *that could impact potential for growth or interrupt client's ability to meet own needs.*[1,3]
- Assess for potential challenges to enhanced participation in self-care (e.g., language barrier with healthcare providers, lack of information, insufficient time for discussion; sudden or progressive change in health status, catastrophic events).

NURSING PRIORITY NO. 2

To assist client/SO plan to meet individual needs:

- Discuss client's understanding of situation *to determine areas that can be clarified or strengthened.*
- Provide accurate and relevant information regarding current and future needs *so that client can incorporate into self-care plans while minimizing problems (e.g., stress, resistance) often associated with change.*[2]
- Promote client/SO participation in problem identification and decision making. *Optimizes outcomes and supports health promotion.*[4]
- Review coping skills (e.g., assertiveness, interpersonal relations, decision making, problem-solving, stigma management, and time management) *that are useful in managing a wide range of stressful conditions.* Encourage client to ask for assistance, as needed or desired.[2]

Nursing Diagnoses in Alphabetical Order

● Active-listen to client's/SO's concerns. *Exhibits regard for client's values and beliefs and provides opportunity to support positive responses and address questions or concerns.*[3]

 ● Encourage communication among those who are involved in the client's health promotion. *Periodic review provides clarification of issues, reinforcement of successful interventions, and possibility for early intervention, where needed, to manage chronic conditions.*

NURSING PRIORITY NO. 3

To promote optimum functioning (Teaching/Discharge considerations):

● Assist client to set realistic goals for the future. *Enhances likelihood of success and commitment to behavioral changes.*

● Support client in making health-related decisions and pursuit of self-care practices that promote health *to foster self-esteem and support positive self-concept.*

● Identify reliable reference sources (including Web sites) regarding individual needs and strategies for self-care. *Reinforces learning and promotes self-paced review.*

● Provide for ongoing evaluation of self-care program *to identify progress and needed changes for continuation of health, adaptation in management of limiting conditions.*

● Review safety concerns and modification of medical therapies or activities and environment, as needed, *to prevent injury and enhance successful functioning.*

● Refer to home-care provider, social services, physical or occupational therapy, rehabilitation, and counseling resources, as indicated or requested, *for education, assistance, and adaptive devices and modifications that may be desired.*[1]

● Identify additional community resources (e.g., senior services, handicap transportation van for appointments, accessible and safe locations for social or sports activities, Meals on Wheels) *to obtain additional forms of assistance that may improve client's independence and self-care.*[1]

DOCUMENTATION FOCUS

Assessment/Reassessment
• Individual findings, including strengths, health status, and any limitation(s).
• Availability and use of resources, support person(s), assistive devices.
• Motivation and expectations for change.

Planning
• Plan of care, specific interventions, and who is involved in planning.
• Teaching plan.

Implementation/Evaluation
• Client's responses to interventions, teaching, and actions performed.
• Attainment or progress toward desired outcome(s).
• Modifications to plan.

Discharge Planning
• Long-term needs and who is responsible for actions to be taken.
• Type of and source for assistive devices.
• Specific referrals made.

References:

1. Doenges, M. E., Moorhouse, M. F., Geissler-Murr, A. C. (2005). ND: Self-Care Deficit: Bathing/hygiene, dressing/grooming, feeding, toileting. *Nursing Diagnosis Manual: Planning, Individualizing, and Documenting Client Care.* Philadelphia: F. A. Davis.

2. Livneh, H., Antonak, R. F. (2005). Psychosocial adaptation to chronic illness and disability: A primer for counselors (practice & theory). *J Couns Dev*. Excerpt retrieved July 2007 from www.accessmylibrary.com/coms2/summary_0286-19174530_ITM.
3. Baldwin, K. M. (2006). Stroke: It's a knock-out punch. *Nursing Made Incredibly Easy!*, 4(2), 10–23.
4. Singleton, J. K. Nurses' perspectives of encouraging client's care-of-self in a short-term rehabilitation unit within a long-term care facility. Retrieved August 2007 from www.rehabnurse.org/ce/010200/010200_a.htm.

readiness for enhanced Self-Concept

DEFINITION: A pattern of perceptions or ideas about the self that is sufficient for well-being and can be strengthened

RELATED FACTORS

To be developed by nurse researchers and submitted to NANDA

DEFINING CHARACTERISTICS

Subjective
Expresses willingness to enhance self-concept
Accepts strengths or limitations
Expresses confidence in abilities
Expresses satisfaction with thoughts about self or sense of worthiness
Expresses satisfaction with body image, personal identity, or role performance

Objective
Actions are congruent with expressed feelings and thoughts

Sample Clinical Applications: As a health-seeking behavior, the client may be healthy or this diagnosis can occur in any clinical condition or life process

DESIRED OUTCOMES/EVALUATION CRITERIA

Sample **NOC** linkages:
Self-Esteem: Personal judgment of self-worth
Hope: Optimism that is personally satisfying and life-supporting
Personal Autonomy: Personal actions of a competent individual to exercise governance in life decisions

Client Will (Include Specific Time Frame)
- Verbalize understanding of own sense of self-worth.
- Participate in programs and activities to enhance self-esteem.
- Demonstrate behaviors or lifestyle changes to promote positive self-esteem.
- Participate in family, group, or community activities to enhance self-concept.

(continues on page 712)

readiness for enhanced Self-Concept (continued)
ACTIONS/INTERVENTIONS

Sample (NIC) linkages:
Self-Modification Assistance: Reinforcement of self-directed change initiated by the patient to achieve personally important goals
Self-Esteem Enhancement: Assisting a patient to increase his or her personal judgment of self-worth
Hope Instillation: Facilitation of the development of a positive outlook in a given situation

NURSING PRIORITY NO. 1

To assess current situation and desire to enhance self-concept:

- Determine current status of individual's belief about self. *Self-concept consists of the physical self (body image), personal self (identity), and self-esteem, and information about client's current thinking about self provides a beginning for making changes to improve self.*[1,2]
- Determine availability and quality of family/SO(s) support. *Presence of supportive people who reflect positive attitudes regarding the individual promotes a positive sense of self.*[1]
- Identify family dynamics, present and past. *Self-esteem begins in early childhood and is influenced by the perceptions of how the individual is viewed by significant others. Provides information about family functioning that will help to develop plan of care for enhancing client's self-concept.*[1,2]
- Note willingness to seek assistance, motivation for change. *Individuals who have a sense of their own self-image and are willing to look at themselves realistically will be better able to achieve desired growth.*[1]
- Determine client's concept of self in relation to cultural or religious ideals and beliefs. *Culture and religion play a major role in view individual has of self in relation to self-worth.*[3]
- Observe nonverbal behaviors and note congruence with verbal expressions. Discuss cultural meanings of nonverbal communication. *Incongruence between verbal and nonverbal communication requires clarification. Interpretation of nonverbal expressions is culturally determined and needs to be identified to avoid misinterpretation.*[1,3]

NURSING PRIORITY NO. 2

To promote client sense of self-esteem:

- Develop therapeutic relationship. Be attentive, validate client's communication, maintain open communication, use skills of Active-listening and I-messages. *Promotes trusting situation in which client is free to be open and honest with self and others.*[2–4]
- Accept client's perceptions and view of current status. *Avoids threatening existing self-esteem and provides opportunity for client to develop realistic plan for improving self-concept.*[3]
- Be aware that people are not programmed to be rational. *Individuals must seek information—choosing to learn, to think, rather than merely accepting/reacting—in order to have respect for self, facts, honesty, and to develop positive self-regard.*[3,7]
- Discuss client perception of self, confronting misconceptions and identifying negative self-talk. Address distortions in thinking, such as self-referencing (beliefs that others are focusing on individuals' weaknesses or limitations); filtering (focusing on negative and ignoring positive); catastrophizing (expecting the worst outcomes). *Addressing these issues openly allows client to identify things that may negatively affect self-concept and provides an opportunity for change.*[3,7,8]

- Have client list current and past successes and strengths. *Emphasizes fact that client is and has been successful in many actions taken.*[1,8]
- Use positive I-messages rather than praise. *Praise is a form of external control, coming from outside sources, whereas I-messages allow the client to develop internal sense of self-worth.*[4,5]
- Discuss what behavior does for client (positive intention). Ask what options are available to the client/SO(s). *Encourages thinking about what inner motivations are and what actions can be taken to enhance self-esteem.*[3]
- Provide reinforcement for progress noted. *Positive words of encouragement support development of effective coping behaviors, promotes continuation of efforts and personal growth.*[3,6]
- Allow client to progress at own rate. *Adaptation to a change in self-concept depends on its significance to the individual and disruption to lifestyle.*[3]
- Involve in activities or exercise program of choice, promote socialization. *Enhances sense of well-being and can help to energize client.*[3,6,8]

NURSING PRIORITY NO. 3

To promote enhanced sense of personal worth and happiness:

- Assist client to identify personally achievable goals. Provide positive feedback for verbal and behavioral indications of improved self-view. *Increases likelihood of success and commitment to change.*[3,6]
- Refer to vocational or employment counselor, educational resources, as appropriate. *Assists with improving development of social or vocational skills.*[3]
- Encourage participation in classes, activities, or hobbies that client enjoys or would like to experience. *Provides opportunity for learning new information or skills that can enhance feelings of success, improving self-concept.*[3,5]
- Reinforce that current decision to improve self-concept is ongoing. *Continued work and support are necessary to sustain behavior changes and personal growth.*[3,5]
- Discuss ways to develop optimism. *Optimism is a key ingredient in happiness and can be learned.*[7]
- Suggest enrolling in assertiveness training classes. *Promotes learning to assist with developing new skills of voice control, posture, eye contact, or expression of feelings in an assertive, rather than aggressive or passive manner to promote self-esteem.*[3]
- Emphasize importance of grooming and personal hygiene and assist in developing skills to improve appearance and dress for success. *Looking your best improves sense of self-worth, and presenting a positive appearance enhances how others see you. While these things are important, having an adequate foundation for the experience of competence and worth is essential to maintaining one's self-concept.*[1,6]

DOCUMENTATION FOCUS

Assessment/Reassessment
- Individual findings, including evaluations of self and others, current and past successes.
- Interactions with others, family dynamics, lifestyle.
- Cultural or religious influences.
- Motivation for and willingness to change.

Planning
- Plan of care and who is involved in planning.
- Educational plan.

Implementation/Evaluation

• Responses to interventions, teaching, and actions performed.
• Attainment or progress toward desired outcome(s).
• Modifications to plan of care.

Discharge Planning

• Long-term needs and who is responsible for actions to be taken.
• Specific referrals made.

References

1. Townsend, M. C. (2003). *Psychiatric Mental Health Nursing Concepts of Care.* 4th ed. Philadelphia: F. A. Davis.
2. Doenges, M. E., Townsend, M. C., Moorhouse, M. F. (1998). *Psychiatric Care Plans: Guidelines for Individualizing Patient Care.* 3d ed. Philadelphia: F. A. Davis.
3. Doenges, M. E., Moorhouse, M. F., Geissler-Murr, A. C. (2004). *Nurse's Pocket Guide: Diagnoses, Interventions, and Rationales.* 9th ed. Philadelphia: F. A. Davis.
4. Gordon, T., Adams, L. *Family Effectiveness Training, Video Home Program.* Available at www.gordontraining.com.
5. Gordon, T. (2000). *Parent Effectiveness Training.* Updated ed. New York: Three River Press.
6. FAQs about self-esteem. *National Association of Self-Esteem.* Retrieved October 2009 from www.self-esteem-nase.org/faq.php.
7. Schuman, W. Keeping your sunny side up. Retrieved April 2007 from www.beliefnet.com/story/147/story_14745_1.html.
8. Beland, N. (April–May 2005, updated November 2007). Special report: The pursuit of happiness. *Women's Health.* Retrieved December 2009 from http://womenshealthmag.com/health/how-to-be-happier.

chronic low Self-Esteem

DEFINITION: Long-standing negative self-evaluation/feelings about self or self-capabilities

RELATED FACTORS

Repeated negative reinforcement or failures
Lack of affection, approval, or membership in group
Perceived lack of belonging or respect from others
Perceived discrepancy between self and cultural or spiritual norms
Traumatic event or situation
Ineffective adaptation to loss
Psychiatric disorders
[Fixation in earlier level of development]
[Personal vulnerability]

DEFINING CHARACTERISTICS

Subjective
Self-negating verbalization
Expressions of shame or guilt
Evaluates self as unable to deal with events
Rejects positive or exaggerates negative feedback about self

🌐 Cultural 🅰 Collaborative 🏠 Community/Home Care ✏ Diagnostic Studies ∞ Pediatric/Geriatric/Lifespan 💊 Medications

Objective
Hesitant to try new things or situations
Frequent lack of success in work or life events
Overly conforming; dependent on others' opinions
Lack of eye contact
Nonassertive; passive; indecisive
Excessively seeks reassurance

Sample Clinical Applications: Chronic health conditions, degenerative diseases, eating disorders, substance abuse, depressive disorders, personality disorders, pervasive developmental disorders

DESIRED OUTCOMES/EVALUATION CRITERIA

Sample NOC linkages:
Self-Esteem: Personal judgment of self-worth
Personal Autonomy: Personal actions of a competent individual to exercise governance in life decisions
Hope: Optimism that is personally satisfying and life-supporting

Client Will (Include Specific Time Frame)
• Verbalize understanding of negative evaluation of self and reasons for this problem.
• Participate in treatment program to promote change in self-evaluation.
• Demonstrate behaviors or lifestyle changes to promote positive self-image.
• Verbalize increased sense of self-worth in relation to current situation.
• Participate in family, group, or community activities to enhance change.

ACTIONS/INTERVENTIONS

Sample NIC linkages:
Self-Esteem Enhancement: Assisting a patient to increase his or her personal judgment of self-worth
Emotional Support: Provision of reassurance, acceptance, and encouragement during times of stress
Body Image Enhancement: Improving a patient's conscious and unconscious perceptions and attitudes toward his or her body

NURSING PRIORITY NO. 1

To assess causative/contributing factors:

● Determine factors in current situation that can exacerbate low self-esteem, noting age and developmental level of individual. *Identifying potentially aggravating occurrences (e.g., family crises, physical disfigurement from an accident or illness, feelings of abandonment by SO resulting in social isolation) are important for developing plan of care and choosing appropriate interventions that help client develop a sense of self-worth.*[1]
● Assess content of negative self talk. Note client's perceptions of how others view him or her. *Constant repetition of negative words and thoughts reinforce idea that individual is worthless and belief that others view him or her in a negative manner. Identifying these negative ruminations and bringing them to the client's awareness enables person to begin to replace them with positive thoughts.*[1]

- Note nonverbal behavior (e.g., nervous movements, lack of eye contact). *Incongruencies between verbal and nonverbal communication require clarification to ensure accuracy of interpretation.*[1,6]

 - Determine availability and quality of family/SO(s) support. *Family is an important component of how an individual views self. The development of a positive sense of self depends on how the person relates to members of the family, as they are growing up and in the current situation.*[1,3]

- Identify family dynamics, present and past. *How family members interact affects an individual's development and sense of self-esteem. If family members are negative and nonsupportive, or positive and supportive, affects the needs of the client at this time.*[4,5]

- Be alert to client's concept of self in relation to cultural and religious ideal(s). *Composition and structure of nuclear family influences individual's sense of who they are in relation to others in the family and in society. For example, Mexican American culture dictates that family comes first, the father is the authority in the family, and the behavior of the individual reflects on the entire family.*[10]

- Determine degree of participation and cooperation with therapeutic regimen. *Maintaining scheduled medications (e.g., antidepressants, antipsychotics) and other aspects of the plan of care require ongoing evaluation and possible changes in regimen.*[1,2]

- Note willingness to seek assistance, motivation for change. *Determines client's degree of participation in adhering to therapeutic regimen.*[1,11]

NURSING PRIORITY NO. 2

To promote client's sense of self-esteem in dealing with situation:

- Develop therapeutic relationship. Be attentive, validate client's communication, provide encouragement for efforts, maintain open communication, use skills of Active-listening and I-messages. *Promotes trusting environment in which client is free to be open and honest with self and therapist so current situation can be dealt with most effectively.*[1,4,5]

- Collaborate in addressing/presenting medical issues and safety concerns. *Client's self-esteem may be affected by physical changes of current medical situation. Changes in body, such as weight loss or gain, chronic illness, amputation will affect how client sees self as a person. Attitude may contribute to feelings of depression and lack of attention to personal safety requiring evaluation and assistance.*[1,3,8]

- Accept client's perceptions or view of situation. Avoid threatening existing self-esteem. *Promotes trust and allows client to begin to look at options for improving self-esteem.*[2,9]

- Be aware that people are not programmed to be rational. *They must seek information—choosing to learn, to think, rather than merely accepting or reacting—in order to have respect for self, facts, honesty, and to develop positive self-esteem.*[1,3]

- Discuss client perceptions of self related to what is happening; confront misconceptions and negative self-talk. Address distortions in thinking, such as self-referencing (belief that others are focusing on individual's weaknesses or limitations), filtering (focusing on negative and ignoring positive), catastrophizing (expecting the worst outcomes). *Addressing these issues openly provides opportunity for change.*[1,3,11]

- Emphasize need to avoid comparing self with others. Encourage client to focus on aspects of self that can be valued. *Changing negative thinking can be effective in developing positive self-talk to enhance self-esteem.*[2,6]

- Have client list current and past successes and strengths. *Often in the depths of despair and sense of failure in current situation, individual forgets positive aspects of his or her life. Bringing them to mind can remind client of these successes, enhancing sense of self-esteem.*[3–5]

- Use positive I-messages rather than praise. *Praise may be heard as manipulative and insincere and be rejected. Use of positive I-messages communicates a feeling that is genuine and real and allows client to feel good about himself or herself, developing internal sense of self-esteem.*[4-6]

- Discuss what behavior does for client (positive intention) and what options are available to the client/SO(s). *Helping client begin to look at what rewards are gained from current actions and what actions might be taken to achieve the same rewards in a more positive way can provide a realistic and accurate self-appraisal, enhancing sense of competence and self-worth.*[1,3,11]
- Assist client to deal with sense of powerlessness. Refer to ND Powerlessness.
- Set limits on aggressive or problem behaviors such as acting out, suicide preoccupation, or rumination. Put self in client's place using empathy, not sympathy. *Preventing undesirable behavior prevents feelings of worthlessness. Suicidal thoughts need further evaluation and intervention. Use of empathy helps caregiver to understand client's feelings better.*[1,2]
- Give reinforcement for progress noted. *Positive words of encouragement promote continuation of efforts, supporting development of coping behaviors.*[2,4,5,12]
- Encourage client to progress at own rate. *Adaptation to a change in self-concept depends on its significance to individual, disruption to lifestyle, and length of crisis or condition.*[1,2,6]
- Assist client to recognize and cope with events, alterations, and sense of loss of control. *Incorporating changes accurately into self-concept enhances sense of self-worth.*[1,2,8]
- Involve in activities/exercise program, promote socialization. *Enhances sense of well-being and can help energize client*[1,6]

NURSING PRIORITY NO. 3

To promote wellness (Teaching/Discharge Considerations):

- Discuss inaccuracies in self-perception with client/SO(s). *Enables client and significant others to begin to look at misperceptions and accept reality and look at options for change to improve sense of self-worth.*[1,7,9]
- Model behaviors being taught, involving client in goal-setting and decision making. *Facilitates client's developing trust in their own unique strengths.*
- Prepare client for events or changes that are expected, when possible. *Providing time to adapt to changes allows client to prepare self and feel more confident in ability to manage the changes, enhancing sense of self-worth.*[1,2,8]
- Provide structure in daily routine and care activities. *Knowing what to expect promotes a sense of control and ability to deal with activities as they occur.*[1,2]
- Emphasize importance of grooming and personal hygiene. Assist in developing skills as indicated (e.g., makeup classes, dressing for success). *People feel better about themselves when they present a positive outer appearance.*[1,3,6]
- Assist client to identify goals that are personally achievable. Provide positive feedback for verbal and behavioral indications of improved self-view. *Increases likelihood of success and commitment to change.*[6,12]
- Refer to vocational or employment counselor, educational resources as appropriate. *Assists with development of social or vocational skills, promoting sense of competence and self-responsibility.*[1,2,4,6]
- Encourage participation in classes, activities, or hobbies that client enjoys or would like to experience. *Meaningful accomplishment, assuming self-responsibility, and participating in new activities engenders one's sense of competence and self-worth.*[9,13]
- Reinforce that this therapy is a brief encounter in overall life of the client/SO(s), with continued work and ongoing support being necessary to sustain behavior changes and personal growth. *Provides individual with information and encouragement to build on for the future.*[1,7,8]

● Refer to classes to assist with learning new skills (e.g., assertiveness training, positive self-image, communication skills). *These skills can help client develop a sense of competence through realistic and accurate self-appraisal promoting self-esteem.*[11]

 ● Refer to counseling or therapy, mental health or other special needs support groups as indicated. *May need additional intervention to develop needed changes.*[1,11,12]

DOCUMENTATION FOCUS

Assessment/Reassessment
• Individual findings, including early memories of negative evaluations (self and others), subsequent and precipitating failure events.
• Effects on interactions with others, family dynamics, lifestyle.
• Specific medical or safety issues.
• Cultural or religious factors.
• Motivation for and willingness to change.

Planning
• Plan of care and who is involved in planning.
• Teaching plan.

Implementation/Evaluation
• Responses to interventions, teaching, and actions performed.
• Attainment or progress toward desired outcome(s).
• Modifications to plan of care.

Discharge Planning
• Long-term needs and who is responsible for actions to be taken.
• Specific referrals made.

References

1. Townsend, M. C. (2006). *Psychiatric Mental Health Nursing Concepts of Care.* 5th ed. Philadelphia: F. A. Davis.
2. Doenges, M. E., Townsend, M. C., Moorhouse, M. F. (1998). *Psychiatric Care Plans: Guidelines for Individualizing Patient Care.* 3d ed. Philadelphia: F. A. Davis.
3. Doenges, M. E., Moorhouse, M. F., Geissler-Murr, A. C. (2004). *Nurse's Pocket Guide: Diagnoses, Interventions, and Rationales.* 9th ed. Philadelphia: F. A. Davis.
4. Gordon, T., Adams, L. *Family Effectiveness Training, Video Home Program.* Available at www.gordontraining.com.
5. Gordon, T. (2000). *Parent Effectiveness Training.* Updated ed. New York: Three River Press.
6. FAQs about self-esteem. National Association of Self-Esteem. Retrieved October 2009 from www.self-esteem-nase.org/faq.php.
7. Vasconcellos, J., et al. In defense of self-esteem. National Association for Self-Esteem. Retrieved January 2004 from www.self-esteem-nase.org.
8. Battle, J. (1990). *Self-Esteem: The New Revolution.* Edmonton, Alberta, Canada: James Battle & Associates.
9. Reasoner, R. (2000). *The True Meaning of Self-Esteem.* Palo Alto, CA: Consulting Psychologists Press.
10. Lipson, J. G., Dibble, S. L., Minarik, P. A. (1996). *Culture & Nursing Care: A Pocket Guide.* San Francisco: UCSF Nursing Press.
11. Peden, A. R., et al. (2000). Reducing negative thinking and depressive symptoms in college women. J Nurs Scholar, 32(2), 145–151.
12. Seligman, M., et al. (2005). *The Optimistic Child.* New York: Houghton Mifflin.
13. Branden, N. (1995). *The Six Pillars of Self-Esteem.* New York: Bantam Book.

situational low Self-Esteem

DEFINITION: Development of a negative perception of self-worth in response to a current situation (specify)

RELATED FACTORS

Developmental changes [e.g., maturational transitions, adolescence, aging]
Functional impairment; disturbed body image
Loss [e.g., loss of health status, body part, independent functioning; memory deficit or cognitive impairment]
Social role changes
Failures or rejections; lack of recognition [or rewards; feelings of abandonment by SO]
Behavior inconsistent with values

DEFINING CHARACTERISTICS

Subjective
Verbally reports current situational challenge to self-worth
Expressions of helplessness or uselessness
Evaluation of self as unable to deal with situations or events

Objective
Self-negating verbalizations
Indecisive or nonassertive behavior

Sample Clinical Applications: Traumatic injuries, surgery, pregnancy, newly diagnosed conditions (e.g., diabetes mellitus), adjustment disorders, substance use, stroke, dementia

DESIRED OUTCOMES/EVALUATION CRITERIA

Sample (NOC) linkages:
Self-Esteem: Personal judgment of self-worth
Psychosocial Adjustment: Life Change: Adaptive psychosocial response of an individual to a significant life change
Abuse Recovery: Emotional: Extent of healing of psychological injuries due to abuse

Client Will (Include Specific Time Frame)
• Verbalize understanding of individual factors that precipitated current situation.
• Identify feelings and underlying dynamics for negative perception of self.
• Express positive self-appraisal.
• Demonstrate behaviors to restore positive self-image.
• Participate in treatment regimen or activities to correct factors that precipitated crisis.

(continues on page 720)

situational low Self-Esteem (continued)
ACTIONS/INTERVENTIONS

Sample (NIC) linkages:
Self-Esteem Enhancement: Assisting a patient to increase his or her personal judgment of self-worth
Coping Enhancement: Assisting a patient to adapt to perceived stressors, changes, or threats that interfere with meeting life demands and roles
Support System Enhancement: Facilitation of support to patient by family, friends, and community

NURSING PRIORITY NO. 1

To assess causative/contributing factors:

- Determine individual situation (e.g., family crisis, termination of a relationship, loss of employment, physical disfigurement) related to low self-esteem in the present circumstances. *Many factors are involved in a person's self-esteem, and this information is essential for planning accurate care.*[1]
- Identify basic sense of self-esteem of client; image client has of self—existential, physical, and psychological. *The components of self-concept consist of the physical self or body image, the personal self or personal identity, and the self-esteem. Each aspect plays a role in the client's ability to deal with current situation/crisis.*[1]
- Assess degree of threat and perception of client concerning crisis. *How individuals perceive themselves is based on the self-judgments they make. How the client sees the current situation in relation to ability to cope will affect his or her sense of self-worth and needs to be acknowledged and planned for to help client deal with feelings of low self-esteem.*[1,2]
- Ascertain sense of control client has (or perceives to have) over self and situation. *Client's locus of control or degree of control client believes or perceives he or she has may be a critical factor in ability to deal with current situation or crisis. Individuals with internal locus of control tend to be more optimistic about their ability to deal with adversity even in the face of current difficulties. Individuals with external locus of control will look to others to solve problems and take care of them.*[1-3]
- Determine client's awareness of own responsibility for dealing with situation, personal growth, and so forth. *These factors enhance the ability of the client to effectively manage situation in a positive manner.*[4]
- Assess family/SO(s) dynamics and support of client. *How family members interact affects an individual's development and sense of self-esteem. Effective interactions among family members usually lead to positive support for the client in current situation. Dysfunctional interactions may be detrimental to client's ability to deal with what is happening.*[2,3]
- Verify client's concept of self in relation to cultural and religious ideals. *Self-esteem is developed by many factors, including genetics and environment. Cultural and religious influences during the individual's life affect beliefs about self, measure of worth, and ability to deal with current situation or crisis.*[1,5]
- Determine past coping skills in relation to current episode. *Trust is built over time, and past experiences with failure or success will affect client's expectations regarding the eventual outcome of dealing with current illness or crisis.*[8,9]
- Assess negative attitudes or self-talk. *An individual who is feeling unimportant, incompetent, and not in control often is unconsciously saying negative things to himself or herself that contribute to a loss of self-esteem and an attitude of despair, affecting current situation.*[1,7]

- Note nonverbal body language. *Incongruencies between verbal or nonverbal communication require clarification to assure accuracy of interpretation.*[1,2]
- Assess for self-destructive or suicidal thoughts or behavior. *Client who believes situation is hopeless often begins to consider suicide as an option.* Refer to ND risk for Suicide as appropriate.[1]
- Identify previous adaptations to illness or disruptive events in life. *May be predictive of current ability to deal with situation and suggest eventual outcome.*[1]
- Note availability and use of resources to address specific need (e.g., rehabilitation services, home-care support, job placement). *Individual may be unaware or have difficulty accessing community supports or assistance programs.*

NURSING PRIORITY NO. 2

To assist client to deal with loss/change and recapture sense of positive self-esteem:

- Assist with treatment of underlying condition when possible. *For example, cognitive restructuring and improved concentration in mild brain injury often result in restoration of positive self-esteem.*[1]
- Encourage expression of feelings, anxieties. Facilitate grieving the loss. *As client expresses feelings and anxieties, he or she begins to deal with the realities of the current situation and the loss that occurs with the changes of illness.*[1] (Refer to ND Grieving as appropriate.)
- Active-listen client's concerns or negative verbalizations without comment or judgment. *Conveys a message of acceptance and confidence in client's ability to deal with whatever occurs.*[6]
- Identify individual strengths, assets, and aspects of self that remain intact, can be valued. Reinforce positive traits, abilities, self-view. *Client may not see these in the anxiety and hopelessness of the immediate situation, and reminding client of own positive attributes can help him or her recover hope and develop a positive attitude about situation.*[1,7]
- Help client identify own responsibility and control or lack of control in situation. *Accepting responsibility enables client to look realistically at what is under own control and what is not. When client stops expending energy on issues that cannot be controlled, energy is freed up to concentrate on more productive avenues.*[1,8]
- Assist client to problem-solve situation, developing plan of action and setting goals to achieve desired outcome. *Personal involvement enhances commitment to plan, optimizing outcomes.*[6]
- Convey confidence in client's ability to cope with current situation. *Validation helps client accept own ability to deal with what is happening.*[1]
- Mobilize support systems; identify individuals in similar circumstances. *Feeling hopeless and alone lowers client's ability to manage care and concentrate on healing. Support systems can provide role modeling and the help needed to engender hope and enhance self-esteem.*[1,3]
- Provide opportunity for client to practice alternative coping strategies, including progressive socialization opportunities. *Involvement with others provides client with situation in which new actions can be tried out and validated or discarded to enhance feelings of self-worth.*[1,3]
- Encourage use of visualization, guided imagery, and relaxation. *These strategies promote a positive sense of self and general well-being, enhancing client's coping ability.*[1]
- Provide feedback about client's self-negating remarks or behavior, using I-messages. *Allows client to experience a different view. I-messages are a nonjudgmental way to let individual understand how behavior is perceived by or affecting others and self.*[6]
- Encourage involvement in decisions about care when possible. *Promotes sense of control over what is happening, enhancing feelings of self-worth.*[1,8]

- Give reinforcement for progress noted. *Positive words of encouragement promote continuation of efforts, supporting development of coping behaviors.*[6,10]

NURSING PRIORITY NO. 3

To promote wellness (Teaching/Discharge Considerations):

- Assist client to identify personally achievable goals. *Increases likelihood of client's success and commitment to change.*[2,10]
- Encourage client to look to the future and set long-range goals for achieving necessary lifestyle changes. *Supports view that this is an ongoing process, providing client with hope for the future.*[1,3]
- Support independence in activities of daily living (ADLs) and mastery of therapeutic regimen. *Individuals who are confident are more secure and positive in self-appraisal.*[1,2]
- Promote attendance in therapy or support group as indicated. *Provides opportunity to discuss own situation and hear how others are dealing with similar problems, promoting new ideas about own ability to deal with issues.*[1,9,10]
- Involve extended family/SO(s) in treatment plan as appropriate. *Enhances their understanding of what client wishes to accomplish, increasing likelihood they will provide appropriate support to client.*[1]
- Provide information and bibliotherapy, including reliable Web sites as appropriate. *Reinforces learning, allowing client to progress at own pace. Promotes opportunity for making informed decisions and improving ability to deal with situation.*[1,7]
- Refer to vocational or employment counselor, educational resources, as appropriate. *Assists with development of social or vocational skills, promoting sense of competence and self-responsibility.*[1,2]
- Suggest participation in group or community activities (e.g., assertiveness classes, volunteer work, support groups). *Provides opportunities for learning new information and being appreciated for contributions, enhancing sense of self-worth.*[1,2]
- Refer to counseling or therapy, mental health, or other special-needs support groups, as indicated. *May need additional support to deal with crisis.*[1,10]

DOCUMENTATION FOCUS

Assessment/Reassessment
- Individual findings, noting precipitating crisis, client's perceptions, effects on desired lifestyle/interaction with others.
- Cultural values or religious beliefs, locus of control.
- Family support, availability and use of resources.

Planning
- Plan of care and who is involved in planning.
- Teaching plan.

Implementation/Evaluation
- Responses to interventions, teaching, actions performed, and changes that may be indicated.
- Attainment or progress toward desired outcome(s).
- Modifications to plan of care.

Discharge Planning
- Long-term needs and goals and who is responsible for actions to be taken.
- Specific referrals made.

  Cultural   Collaborative   Community/Home Care   Diagnostic Studies   Pediatric/Geriatric/Lifespan   Medications

References

1. Townsend, M. C. (2003). *Psychiatric Mental Health Nursing Concepts of Care*. 4th ed. Philadelphia: F. A. Davis.
2. FAQs about self-esteem. National Association for Self-Esteem. Retrieved October 2009 from www.self-esteem-nase.org/faq.php.
3. Battle, J. (1990). *Self-Esteem: The New Revolution*. Edmonton, Alberta, Canada: James Battle & Associates.
4. Reasoner, R. (2000). *The True Meaning of Self-Esteem*. Palo Alto, CA: Consulting Psychologists Press.
5. Lipson, J. G., Dibble, S. L., Minarik, P. A. (1996). *Culture & Nursing Care: A Pocket Guide*. San Francisco: UCSF Nursing Press.
6. Gordon, T. (2000). *Parent Effectiveness Training*. Updated ed. New York: Three Rivers Press.
7. Peden, A., et al. (2000). Reducing negative thinking and depressive symptoms in college women. *J Nurs Scholarsh*, 32(2), 145–151.
8. Munson, P. J. (1991). Life's decisions—By chance or by choice? *Adapted from Winning Teachers, Teaching Winners*. Santa Cruz, CA: ETR Associates.
9. Vasconcellos, J., et al. In defense of self-esteem. National Association for Self-Esteem. Retrieved January 2004 from www.self-esteem-nase.org.
10. Seligman, M., et al. (1995). *The Optimistic Child*. New York: Houghton Mifflin.

risk for situational low Self-Esteem

DEFINITION: At risk for developing negative perception of self-worth in response to a current situation (specify)

RISK FACTORS

Developmental changes

Disturbed body image; functional impairment

Loss [e.g., loss of health status, body part, independent functioning; memory deficit/cognitive impairment]

Social role changes

Unrealistic self-expectations; history of learned helplessness

History of neglect, abuse, or abandonment

Behavior inconsistent with values

Lack of recognition; failures; rejections

Decreased control over environment

Physical illness

NOTE: A risk diagnosis is not evidenced by signs and symptoms, as the problem has not occurred; rather, nursing interventions are directed at prevention.

Sample Clinical Applications: Traumatic injuries, surgery, pregnancy, newly diagnosed conditions (e.g., diabetes mellitus, hypertension), adjustment disorders, substance use, stroke, dementia

(continues on page 724)

risk for situational low Self-Esteem (continued)
DESIRED OUTCOMES/EVALUATION CRITERIA

Sample NOC linkages:
Self-Esteem: Personal judgment of self-worth
Psychosocial Adjustment: Life Change: Adaptive psychosocial response of an individual to a significant life change
Abuse Recovery: Emotional: Extent of healing of psychological injuries due to abuse

Client Will (Include Specific Time Frame)
- Acknowledge factors that lead to possibility of feelings of low self-esteem.
- Verbalize view of self as a worthwhile, important person who functions well both interpersonally and occupationally.
- Demonstrate self-confidence by setting realistic goals and actively participating in life situation.

ACTIONS/INTERVENTIONS

Sample NIC linkages:
Self-Esteem Enhancement: Assisting a patient to increase his or her personal judgment of self-worth
Coping Enhancement: Assisting a patient to adapt to perceived stressors, changes, or threats that interfere with meeting life demands and roles
Support System Enhancement: Facilitation of support to patient by family, friends, and community

NURSING PRIORITY NO. 1

To assess causative/contributing factors:

- Determine individual factors that may contribute to diminished self-esteem. *Proactive information allows identification of appropriate interventions to deal with current situation.*[1,2]
- Identify basic sense of self-worth of client, image client has of self—existential, physical, psychological. *The components of self-concept consist of the physical self or body image, the personal self or personal identity, and the self-esteem, with each aspect playing a role in the client's ability to deal with anticipated changes.*[1]
- Note client's perception of threat to self in current situation. *Perception is more important than reality of what is happening. Some individuals view a potentially severe situation as something easily handled while another may view a minor problem with anxiety and catastrophizing.*[2,3]
- Ascertain sense of control client has (or perceives to have) over self and situation. *Individual with internal locus of control tends to perceive self in control of what is happening and will participate more actively in care and feel more sense of self-worth.*[7,8]
- Determine client awareness of own responsibility for dealing with situation, personal growth, and so forth. *Acceptance of responsibility for self enables client to feel more comfortable with treatment regime and participate more fully, promoting self-esteem.*[1,9]
- Assess family/SO(s) dynamics and support of client. *How family interacts with one another affects not only the development of self-esteem but also the maintenance of a sense of self-worth when client is facing an illness or crisis. Dysfunctional interactions may be detrimental to client's ability to deal with what is happening.*[1,5]

- Verify client's concept of self in relation to cultural or religious ideals. *Culture and religion play a major role in view individual has of self in relation to self-worth. Illness may interfere with this view; for instance, males in Mexican American culture are seen as the head of the household, and giving up this role because of illness can diminish self-esteem.*[4]
- Assess negative attitudes and/or self-talk. *Contributes to view of situation as hopeless, difficult.*[3,6]
- Listen for or note self-destructive or suicidal thoughts or behaviors. *Indicates high level of stress, need for further evaluation and referral for mental health services.*[1,6] Refer to ND risk for Suicide as appropriate.
- Note nonverbal body language. *Incongruencies between verbal and nonverbal communications require clarification to assure accuracy of interpretation.*[1]
- Identify previous adaptations to illness or disruptive events in life. *Provides information about how client handled those situations and may be predictive of current outcome.*[1]
- Determine availability and use of support systems. *Feeling hopeless and alone lowers client ability to manage care and concentrate on healing. Support systems can provide role modeling and the help needed to engender hope and enhance self-esteem.*[1]
- Note availability and use of resources to address specific need (e.g., rehabilitation services, home-care support, job placement). *Individual may be unaware or have difficulty accessing community supports or assistance programs.*
- Refer to NDs situational low Self-Esteem, and chronic low Self-Esteem as appropriate for additional nursing priorities and interventions.

DOCUMENTATION FOCUS

Assessment/Reassessment
- Individual findings, including individual expressions of lack of self-esteem, effects on interactions with others, lifestyle.
- Underlying dynamics and duration (situational or situational exacerbating chronic).
- Cultural values or religious beliefs, locus of control.
- Family support, availability and use of resources.

Planning
- Plan of care and who is involved in planning.
- Teaching plan.

Implementation/Evaluation
- Responses to interventions, teaching, actions performed, and changes that may be indicated.
- Attainment or progress toward desired outcome(s).
- Modifications to plan of care.

Discharge Planning
- Long-term needs and goals, and who is responsible for actions to be taken.
- Specific referrals made.

References

1. Townsend, M. C. (2003). *Psychiatric Mental Health Nursing Concepts of Care.* 4th ed. Philadelphia: F. A. Davis.
2. Battle, J. (1990). *Self-Esteem: The New Revolution.* Edmonton, Alberta, Canada: James Battle & Associates.
3. Reasoner, R. (2000). *The True Meaning of Self-Esteem.* Palo Alto, CA: Consulting Psychologists Press.

4. Lipson, J. G., Dibble, S. L., Minarik, P. A. (1996). *Culture & Nursing Care: A Pocket Guide*. San Francisco: UCSF Nursing Press.
5. Gordon, T. (2000). *Parent Effectiveness Training*. New York: Three Rivers Press.
6. Peden, A., et al. (2000). Reducing negative thinking and depressive symptoms in college women. *J Nurs Scholarsh*, 32(2), 145–151.
7. Munson, P. J. (1991). Life's decisions—By chance or by choice? *Adapted from Winning Teachers, Teaching Winners*. Santa Cruz, CA: ETR Associates.
8. Vasconcellos, J., et al. In defense of self-esteem. National Association for Self-Esteem. Retrieved January 2004 www.self-esteem-nase.org.
9. FAQs about self-esteem. *National Association for Self-Esteem*. Retrieved October 2009 from www.self-esteem-nase.org/faq.php.

Self-Mutilation

DEFINITION: Deliberate self-injurious behavior causing tissue damage with the intent of causing nonfatal injury to attain relief of tension

RELATED FACTORS

Adolescence; peers who self-mutilate; isolation from peers

Dissociation; depersonalization; psychotic state (e.g., command hallucinations); character disorder; borderline personality disorders; emotionally disturbed; developmentally delayed/autistic individual

History of self-injurious behavior, inability to plan solutions, inability to see long-term consequences

Childhood illness, surgery, or sexual abuse; battered child

Disturbed body image; eating disorders

Ineffective coping; perfectionism

Negative feelings (e.g., depression, rejection, self-hatred, separation anxiety, guilt, depersonalization); low self-esteem; unstable self-esteem or body image

Poor communication between parent and adolescent; lack of family confidant

Feels threatened with loss of significant relationship [loss of parent or parental relationship]

Disturbed interpersonal relationships; use of manipulation to obtain nurturing relationship with others

Family alcoholism or divorce; violence between parental figures; family history of self-destructive behaviors

Living in nontraditional settings (e.g., foster, group, or institutional care); incarceration

Inability to express tension verbally; mounting tension that is intolerable; needs quick reduction of stress

Irresistible urge to cut or damage self; impulsivity; labile behavior

Sexual identity crisis

Substance abuse

DEFINING CHARACTERISTICS

Subjective
Self-inflicted burns [e.g., eraser, cigarette]
Ingestion or inhalation of harmful substances or objects

Cultural   Collaborative   Community/Home Care   Diagnostic Studies   Pediatric/Geriatric/Lifespan   Medications

Objective
Cuts or scratches on body
Picking at wounds
Biting; abrading; severing
Insertion of object(s) into body orifice(s)
Hitting
Constricting a body part

Sample Clinical Applications: Borderline personality, dissociative disorders, bipolar disorder, developmental delay, autism, eating disorders, substance abuse, physical or psychological abuse, gender identity crisis

DESIRED OUTCOMES/EVALUATION CRITERIA

Sample NOC linkages:
Self-Mutilation Restraint: Personal actions to refrain from intentional self-inflicted injury (nonlethal)
Impulse Self-Control: Self-restraint of compulsive or impulsive behaviors
Distorted Thought Self-Control: Self-restraint of disruption in perception, thought processes, and thought content

Client Will (Include Specific Time Frame)
• Verbalize understanding of reasons for occurrence of behavior.
• Identify precipitating factors and awareness of arousal state that occurs prior to incident.
• Express increased self-concept or self-esteem.
• Seeks help when feeling anxious and having thoughts of harming self.

ACTIONS/INTERVENTIONS

Sample NIC linkages:
Behavior Management: Self-Harm: Assisting the patient to decrease or eliminate self-mutilating or self-abusive behavior
Environmental Management: Safety: Manipulation of the patient's surroundings for therapeutic benefit
Limit Setting: Establishing the parameters of desirable and acceptable patient behavior

NURSING PRIORITY NO. 1

To assess causative/contributing factors:

• Determine underlying dynamics of individual situation as listed in Related Factors. Note previous episodes of self-mutilation behavior. *Although some body piercing (e.g., ears) is generally accepted as decorative, piercing of multiple sites or industrial piercings are often an attempt to establish individuality, addressing issues of separation and belonging, but are not considered as self-injury or self-mutilating behaviors.*[1,7]
• Identify previous history of self-mutilative behavior and relationship to stressful events. *Self-injury is considered an attempt to alter a mood state, an outlet for negative emotions such as anger, shame. Information about previous behavior and precipitating factors is important to understanding and planning care in current situation.*[1,7,9]

- Determine presence of inflexible, maladaptive personality traits that reflect personality or character disorder. *Identification of impulsive, unpredictable, or inappropriate behaviors, intense anger, or lack of control of anger is important for planning appropriate interventions and plan of care. Clients who have been diagnosed as borderline personality disorder are often unstable and prone to self-injury and need a specific treatment plan to diminish these behaviors.*[1,9]

- Evaluate history of mental illness (e.g., borderline personality, identity disorder, bipolar disorder). *These illnesses may be the underlying cause of the self-injurious behavior.*[1,2]

- Note beliefs, cultural or religious practices that may be involved in choice of behavior. *Growing up in a family that did not allow feelings to be expressed, individual may believe that feelings are wrong or bad. Family dynamics may come out of religious or cultural expectations that support strict punishment for transgressions. Individuals may believe mental illness is the result of unacceptable actions, and feelings of guilt may lead to anxiety and subsequent self-injurious behaviors.*[4]

- Note use or abuse of addicting substances. *May be indicative of attempt to treat self and needs further evaluation and additional intervention.*[2,6]

- Review laboratory findings (e.g., blood alcohol, polydrug screen, glucose, and electrolyte levels). *Helpful for identifying drug use or medical problems that may be affecting behavior negatively.*[1]

NURSING PRIORITY NO. 2

To structure environment to maintain client safety:

- Assist client to identify feelings leading up to desire for self-mutilation. *Early recognition of recurring feelings provides opportunity to seek other ways of coping.*[5]

- Provide external controls or limit setting. *Decreasing the opportunity to self-mutilate helps the client learn to stop the behavior.*[4,8]

- Encourage appropriate expression of feelings. *Helps client to identify feelings and promote understanding of what leads to development of tension and subsequent injurious behavior.*[2]

- Keep client in continuous staff view and do special observation checks during inpatient stay. *Promotes safety by recognizing escalating behaviors and providing timely intervention.*[2,5]

- Structure inpatient milieu to maintain positive, clear, open communication among staff and clients, with an understanding that "secrets are not tolerated" and will be confronted. *Prevents manipulative behavior, so client does not pit one staff member against another to fulfill own desires.*[1,4,5]

- Note feelings of healthcare providers/family, such as frustration, anger, defensiveness, need to rescue. *Client may be manipulative, evoking defensiveness and conflict. These feelings need to be identified, recognized, and dealt with openly with staff/family and client.*[4]

- Provide care for client's wounds, when self-mutilation occurs, in a matter-of-fact manner. Refrain from offering sympathy or additional attention. *A matter-of-fact approach can convey empathy and concern but not undue concern that could provide reinforcement for maladaptive behavior and encourage its repetition.*[2]

- Discuss use of medication, such as clozapine. *This medication has been shown to reduce acts of self-injurious behavior and help client maintain a more stable mood.*[3]

- Develop schedule of or refer to alternative healthy, success-oriented activities. *Group or family therapy, or groups such as Eating Disorders or similar 12-step program based on individual needs, self-esteem activities, including positive affirmations, visiting with friends, and exercise helps client to practice new behaviors in a supportive environment.*[7]

NURSING PRIORITY NO. 3

To promote movement toward positive changes:

- Encourage client involvement in formulating plan of care and developing goals for preventing undesired behavior. *Being involved in own decisions can help to reestablish ego boundaries, enhances commitment to goals, optimizing outcomes and enhancing self-esteem.*[2,5]
- Develop a contract between client and counselor to enable the client to stay physically safe, such as "I will not cut or harm myself for the next 24 hours." Renew contract on a regular basis and have both parties sign and date each contract. *Making a commitment in writing helps client to think before acting and can prevent new incidents of self-injury.*[4]
- Provide avenues of communication for times when client needs to talk. *Having an opportunity to discuss anxieties helps client to avoid cutting or damaging self.*[4,6]
- Assist client to learn assertive behavior. Include the use of effective communication skills, focusing on developing self-esteem by replacing negative self-talk with positive comments. *Low self-esteem is a factor in this behavior, and by learning new ways of expressing self, client can begin to feel better and deal with anxieties in a more positive manner.*[2]
- Choose interventions that help the client to reclaim power in own life (e.g., experiential and cognitive). *Beginning to think in a positive manner and then translating that into action provides reinforcement for using power to stop injurious behaviors and develop a more productive lifestyle.*[2]

NURSING PRIORITY NO. 4

To promote wellness (Teaching/Discharge Considerations):

- Discuss commitment to safety and ways in which client will deal with precursors to undesired behavior. *Identifies specific precursors for individual and provides a plan for client to follow when anxiety becomes overwhelming.*[2,8]
- Promote the use of healthy behaviors, identifying the consequences and outcomes of current actions. *As client develops a more positive attitude and accepts the idea that current actions are being destructive to desired lifestyle, new behaviors can help make needed changes.*[2]
- Identify support systems. *Knowing who client can turn to when anxiety becomes a problem helps to avoid injurious behavior.*[1]
- Discuss living arrangements when client discharged from inpatient program. *May need assistance with transition to changes required to avoid recurrence of self-mutilating behaviors.*[2]
- Involve family/SO(s) in planning for discharge and involve in group therapies as appropriate. *Promotes coordination and continuation of plan, commitment to goals.*[2,6]
- Discuss the role neurotransmitters play in predisposing individual to beginning this behavior. *It is believed that problems in the serotonin system may make the person more aggressive and impulsive, combined with a home where they learned that feelings are bad or wrong leads to turning aggression on self.*[8]
- Provide information and discuss the use of medication as appropriate. *Antidepressant medications may be useful, but they need to be weighed against the potential for overdosing.*[1,3]
- Refer to NDs Anxiety; Self-Esteem (specify); impaired Social Interaction.

DOCUMENTATION FOCUS

Assessment/Reassessment
- Individual findings, including risk factors present, underlying dynamics, prior episodes.
- Cultural or religious practices.

- Laboratory test results.
- Substance use or abuse.

Planning
- Plan of care and who is involved in planning.
- Teaching plan.

Implementation/Evaluation
- Response to interventions, teaching, and actions performed.
- Attainment or progress toward desired outcome(s).
- Modifications to plan of care.

Discharge Planning
- Long-term needs and who is responsible for actions to be taken.
- Community resources, referrals made.

References

1. Townsend, M. C. (2006). *Psychiatric Mental Health Nursing Concepts of Care*. 5th ed. Philadelphia: F. A. Davis.
2. Doenges, M. E., Townsend, M. C., Moorhouse, M. F. (1998). *Psychiatric Care Plans: Guidelines for Individualizing Care*. 3d ed. Philadelphia: F. A. Davis.
3. Chengappa, K. N. (1999). Clozapine reduces severe self-mutilation and aggression in psychotic patients with borderline personality disorder. *J Clin Psychiatry*, 60(7), 477–484.
4. Clarke, L., Whittaker, M. (1998). Self-mutilation: Culture, contexts, and nursing responses. *J Clin Nurs*, 7(2), 129–137.
5. Dallam, S. J. (1997). The identification and management of self-mutilating patients in primary care. *Nurse Pract*, 22(5), 151–165.
6. Selekman, M. D. (2004). Adolescent self-harm: A growing epidemic. *Family Therapy Magazine*, 1(2), 34–40.
7. Cox, H. C., et. al (2002). *Clinical Applications of Nursing Diagnosis: Adult, Child, Women's, Psychiatric, Gerontic, and Home Health Considerations*. 4th ed. Philadelphia: F. A. Davis.
8. Focus Adolescent Services: Self-injury. (2001). Retrieved August 2007 from www.focusas.com/SelfInjury.html.
9. Frey, R. (2002, updated 2006). Self-mutilation. *Gale Encyclopedia of Medicine*. Retrieved October 2009 from www.encyclopedia.com/doc/1G2-3447200509.html.

risk for Self-Mutilation

DEFINITION: At risk for deliberate self-injurious behavior causing tissue damage with the intent of causing nonfatal injury to attain relief of tension

RISK FACTORS

Adolescence; peers who self-mutilate; isolation from peers
Dissociation; depersonalization; psychotic state (e.g., command hallucinations); character disorders; borderline personality disorders; emotionally disturbed child; developmentally delayed/autistic individuals
History of self-injurious behavior, inability to plan solutions, inability to see long-term consequences
Childhood illness, surgery, or sexual abuse; battered child

⊕ Cultural ⊛ Collaborative 🏠 Community/Home Care ✐ Diagnostic Studies ∞ Pediatric/Geriatric/Lifespan 💊 Medications

Disturbed body image; eating disorders

Ineffective coping; loss of control over problem-solving situations; perfectionism

Negative feelings (e.g., depression, rejection, self-hatred, separation anxiety, guilt); low or unstable self-esteem

Feels threatened with loss of significant relationship; loss of significant relationship; lack of family confidant

Disturbed interpersonal relationships; use of manipulation to obtain nurturing relationship with others

Family alcoholism or divorce; violence between parental figures; family history of self-destructive behaviors

Living in nontraditional settings (e.g., foster, group, or institutional care); incarceration

Inability to express tension verbally; mounting tension that is intolerable; needs quick reduction of stress; irresistible urge to damage self; impulsivity

Sexual identity crisis

Substance abuse

NOTE: A risk diagnosis is not evidenced by signs and symptoms, as the problem has not occurred; rather, nursing interventions are directed at prevention.

Sample Clinical Applications: Borderline personality, dissociative disorders, bipolar disorder, developmental delay, autism, eating disorders, substance abuse, physical/psychological abuse, gender identity crisis

DESIRED OUTCOMES/EVALUATION CRITERIA

Sample (NOC) linkages:

Self-Mutilation Restraint: Personal actions to refrain from intentional self-inflicted injury (nonlethal)

Impulse Self-Control: Self-restraint of compulsive or impulsive behaviors

Distorted Thought Self-Control: Self-restraint of disruption in perception, thought processes, and thought content

Client Will (Include Specific Time Frame)
- Verbalize understanding of reasons for occurrence of behavior.
- Identify precipitating factors and awareness of arousal state that occurs prior to incident.
- Express increased self-concept or self-esteem.
- Demonstrate self-control as evidenced by lessened (or absence of) episodes of self-mutilation.
- Engage in use of alternative methods for managing feelings and individuality.

ACTIONS/INTERVENTIONS

Sample (NIC) linkages:

Behavior Modification: Promotion of a behavior change

Calming Technique: Reducing anxiety in patient experiencing acute distress

Behavior Management: Self-Harm: Assisting the patient to decrease or eliminate self-mutilating or self-abusive behavior

NURSING PRIORITY NO. 1

To assess causative/contributing factors:

- Determine underlying dynamics of individual situation as listed in Risk Factors. Note the presence of conditions that may interfere with ability to control own behavior (e.g., psychotic state, mental retardation, autism) *that may lead to incidents of self-injury.*[1]
- Asses for inflexible, maladaptive personality traits. *May reflect personality or character disorder (e.g., impulsive, unpredictable, inappropriate behaviors, intense anger or lack of control of anger) that may lead to self-mutilative behaviors.*[1]
- Evaluate history of mental illness (e.g., borderline personality, identity disorder, bipolar disorder). *These illnesses may be the underlying cause of the self-injurious behavior.*[1,2]
- Identify previous episodes of self-mutilating behavior (e.g., cutting, scratching, bruising). *Self-injury is considered an attempt to alter a mood state, an outlet for negative emotions such as anger, shame. Information about previous behavior and precipitating factors is important to understanding and planning care in current situation.*[1,7,9] *Although some body piercing (e.g., ears) is generally accepted as decorative, piercing of multiple sites or industrial piercings are often an attempt to establish individuality, addressing issues of separation and belonging, but are not considered as self-injury or self-mutilating behaviors.*[2]
- Note beliefs, cultural or religious practices that may be involved in choice of behavior. *Growing up in a family that did not allow feelings to be expressed, individual may believe that feelings are wrong or bad. Family dynamics may come out of religious or cultural expectations that support strict punishment for transgressions. Individuals may believe mental illness is the result of unacceptable actions, and feelings of guilt may lead to anxiety and subsequent self-injurious behaviors.*[4]
- Determine use or abuse of addictive substances, including alcohol. *Individuals often use these substances to self-medicate feelings of anxiety and may increase the risk of suicide by sixfold.*[2,8]
- Note degree of impairment in social and occupational functioning. *May dictate treatment setting (e.g., specific outpatient program or short-stay inpatient when client is experiencing extreme anxiety).*[1,5]
- Review laboratory findings (e.g., blood alcohol, polydrug screen, glucose, and electrolyte levels). *Helpful for identifying drug use or medical problems that may be affecting behavior negatively.*[1]

NURSING PRIORITY NO. 2

To structure environment to maintain client safety:

- Assist client to identify feelings and behaviors that precede desire for self-mutilation. *Early recognition of recurring feelings provides client opportunity to seek other ways of coping, including asking for help.*[2,6]
- Provide external controls or limit-setting as indicated. *Decreases the opportunity to injure self and helps client think about reasons for actions and learn different ways to deal with them.*[1]
- Encourage client to recognize and appropriately express feelings verbally. *Learning to express feelings enables client not only to recognize them, but also to begin to find acceptable and appropriate ways to deal with them.*[6,7]
- Note feelings of healthcare providers/family, such as frustration, anger, defensiveness, distraction, despair and powerlessness, need to rescue. *Client may be manipulating or splitting providers/family members, which evokes defensiveness and resultant conflict. These feelings need to be identified, recognized, and dealt with openly with staff/family and client.*[1]

⊕ Cultural   Collaborative   Community/Home Care   Diagnostic Studies   ∞ Pediatric/Geriatric/Lifespan   Medications

- Refer to alternative healthy, success-oriented activities. *Groups such as Eating Disorders or similar 12-step program based on individual needs, self-esteem activities, including positive affirmations, visiting with friends, and exercise, help client to practice new behaviors in a supportive environment.*[6]

NURSING PRIORITY NO. 3

To promote movement toward positive actions:

- Encourage client involvement in formulating plan of care and developing goals for preventing undesired behavior. *Being involved in own decisions can help to reestablish ego boundaries, enhances commitment to goals, optimizing outcomes and enhancing self-esteem.*[2,5]
- Develop a contract between client and counselor to enable the client to stay physically safe, such as "I will not cut or harm myself for the next 24 hours." Renew contract on a regular basis, signed and dated by both parties. *Discussing the contract gets issues out in the open and conveys a sense of acceptance of the client, while placing some of the responsibility for safety on the client.*[1,2]
- Provide avenues of communication for times when client needs to talk. *Having an opportunity to discuss anxieties helps client to avoid cutting or damaging self.*[4,6]
- Choose interventions that help the client to reclaim power in own life (e.g., experiential and cognitive). *As client experiences new ways of interacting with others, he or she can begin to think more positively about self-worth and changing behaviors.*[2]
- Identify the consequences and outcomes of current actions: "Does this get you what you want?" "How does this behavior help you achieve your goals?" *Provides client with opportunity to look at own behaviors in a different way and begin to understand how they are harmful rather than helpful. Contrasting healthy behaviors versus current actions can help client decide to change them. Dialectic behavior therapy is effective in reducing injurious behavior along with the use of medication.*[1,3,6]
- Assist client to learn assertive behavior rather than nonassertive or aggressive behavior. Include use of effective communication skills, focusing on developing self-esteem by replacing negative self-talk with positive comments. *By learning these new skills, client interacts with others and gets needs met in positive, acceptable ways, promoting self-worth and lessening anxiety and risk of injurious actions.*[1,9]
- Discuss with client/family normalcy of adolescent task of separation and ways of achieving. *Helps individual members understand these actions and begin to recognize the normal from the ones that are of concern and need intervention.*[1,6]
- Involve client/family in group therapies as appropriate. *Group setting aids in promoting diffusion of anger; provides insight as to how negative, aggressive behavior affects others, making feedback easier to digest and understand.*[2]

NURSING PRIORITY NO. 4

To promote wellness (Teaching/Discharge Considerations):

- Discuss commitment to safety and ways in which client will deal with precursors to undesired behavior. *Helps client verbalize anger and anxiety and understand how these feelings lead to desire to injure self, and actions that can be taken to prevent this behavior.*[4,6]
- Mobilize support systems. *These individuals often come from abusive families, and unresolved feelings of abandonment remain into adulthood. Positive support by many people in their lives can help them begin to overcome these feelings.*[1,8]
- Arrange for continued involvement in group therapy after discharge from program. *Remaining in this supportive environment can help client maintain new behaviors as he or she begins to increase responsibility for self and own action.*[2]

- Discuss and provide information about the use of medication as appropriate. *Antidepressant medications may be useful, but use needs to be weighed against potential for overdosing. (Note: The antidepressant Effexor can cause hostility, suicidal ideas, and self-harm in adolescent or young adults.) Medications that stabilize moods, ease depression, and calm anxiety may be tried to reduce the urge to self-harm.*[1,3]
- Refer to NDs Anxiety; Self-Esteem (specify), impaired Social Interaction.

DOCUMENTATION FOCUS

Assessment/Reassessment
- Individual findings, including risk factors present, underlying dynamics, prior episodes.
- Cultural or religious practices.
- Laboratory test results.
- Substance use or abuse.

Planning
- Plan of care and who is involved in planning.
- Teaching plan.

Implementation/Evaluation
- Response to interventions, teaching, and actions performed.
- Attainment or progress toward desired outcome(s).
- Modifications to plan of care.

Discharge Planning
- Long-term needs and who is responsible for actions to be taken.
- Community resources, referrals made.

References

1. Townsend, M. C. (2006). *Psychiatric Mental Health Nursing Concepts of Care*. 4th ed. Philadelphia: F. A. Davis.
2. Doenges, M. E., Townsend, M. C., Moorhouse, M. F. (1998). *Psychiatric Care Plans: Guidelines for Individualizing Care*. 3d ed. Philadelphia: F. A. Davis.
3. Chengappa, K. N., (1999). Clozapine reduces severe self-mutilation and aggression in psychotic patients with borderline personality disorder. *J Clin Psychiatry*, 60(7), 477–484.
4. Clarke, L., Whittaker, M. (1998). Self-mutilation: Culture, contexts, and nursing responses. *J Clin Nurs*, 7(2), 129–137.
5. Dallam, S. J. (1997). The identification and management of self-mutilating patients in primary care. *Nurse Pract*, 22(5), 151–165.
6. Cox, H. C., et al. (2002). *Clinical Applications of Nursing Diagnosis: Adult, Child, Women's, Psychiatric, Gerontic, and Home Health Considerations*. 4th ed. Philadelphia: F. A. Davis.
7. Selekman, M. D. (2004). Adolescent self-harm: A growing epidemic. *Family Therapy Magazine*, 1(2), 34–40.
8. Focus Adolescent Services: Self-injury. (2001). Retrieved August 2007 from www.focusas.com/SelfInjury.html.
9. Frey, R. (2002, updated 2006). Self-mutilation. *Gale Encyclopedia of Medicine*. Retrieved October 2009 from www.encyclopedia.com/doc/1G2-3447200509.html.

disturbed Sensory Perception [specify: visual, auditory, kinesthetic, gustatory, tactile, olfactory]

DEFINITION: Change in the amount or patterning of incoming stimuli accompanied by a diminished, exaggerated, distorted, or impaired response to such stimuli

RELATED FACTORS

Insufficient environmental stimuli: [therapeutically restricted environments (e.g., isolation, intensive care, bedrest, traction, confining illnesses, incubator); socially restricted environment (e.g., institutionalization, homebound, aging, chronic/terminal illness, infant deprivation), stigmatized (e.g., mentally ill/developmentally delayed/handicapped)]

Excessive environmental stimuli: [excessive noise level, such as work environment, client's immediate environment (intensive care unit with support machinery)]

Altered sensory reception/transmission/integration: [neurological disease, trauma, or deficit; altered status of sense organs]

Biochemical imbalances [e.g., elevated blood urea nitrogen (BUN), elevated ammonia, hypoxia]; electrolyte imbalance; [drugs, e.g., stimulants or depressants, mind-altering drugs]

Psychological stress; [sleep deprivation]

DEFINING CHARACTERISTICS

Subjective

[Reported] change in sensory acuity [e.g., photosensitivity, hypoesthesias or hyperesthesias, diminished or altered sense of taste, inability to tell position of body parts (proprioception)]

Sensory distortions

Objective

[Measured] change in sensory acuity

Change in usual response to stimuli [e.g., rapid mood swings, exaggerated emotional responses, anxiety or panic state]

Change in behavior pattern; restlessness; irritability

Change in problem-solving abilities; poor concentration

Disorientation; hallucinations; [illusions]; [bizarre thinking]

Impaired communication

[Motor incoordination, altered sense of balance, falls (e.g., Ménière's syndrome)]

Sample Clinical Applications: Glaucoma, cataract, brain tumor, stroke, traumatic injury, amputation, surgery, immobility, peripheral neuropathy (e.g., diabetes), substance abuse, schizophrenia, developmental delay

DESIRED OUTCOMES/EVALUATION CRITERIA

Sample **NOC** linkages:

Sensory Function: Extent to which an individual correctly senses skin stimulation, sounds, proprioception, taste and smell, and visual images

Distorted Thought Self-Control: Self-restraint of disruptions in perception, thought processes, and thought content

Risk Control: Personal actions to prevent, eliminate, or reduce modifiable health threats

(continues on page 736)

disturbed Sensory Perception (continued)

Client Will (Include Specific Time Frame)
• Regain or maintain usual level of cognition.
• Recognize and correct or compensate for sensory impairments.
• Verbalize awareness of sensory needs and presence of overload and/or deprivation.
• Identify and modify external factors that contribute to alterations in sensory or perceptual abilities.
• Use resources effectively and appropriately.
• Be free of injury.

ACTIONS/INTERVENTIONS

Sample NIC linkages:
Communication Enhancement: Hearing [or] Vision Deficit: Assistance in accepting and learning alternative methods for living with diminished hearing [or] vision
Peripheral Sensation Management: Prevention or minimization of injury or discomfort in the patient with altered sensation
Hallucination [or] Delusion Management: Promoting the comfort, safety, and reality orientation of a patient experiencing hallucinations [or] false, fixed beliefs that have little or no basis in reality
Environmental Management: Manipulation of the patient's surroundings for therapeutic benefit, sensory appeal, and psychological well-being

NURSING PRIORITY NO. 1

To assess causative/contributing factors:

● Identify client with condition that can affect sensing, interpreting, and communicating stimuli, as noted in Related Factors. *Specific clinical concerns (e.g., neurological disease or trauma, intensive care unit confinement, surgery, pain, biochemical imbalances, psychosis, substance abuse, toxemia) have the potential for altering one or more of the senses, with resultant change in the reception, sensitivity, or interpretation of sensory input.*[1]
● Be aware of current diagnosis or treatments *(e.g., glaucoma, surgery, immobility, recent stroke, diabetes, mental illness; drug toxicity or side effects [e.g., halos around lights, ringing in ears]; middle-ear disturbances [altered sense of balance]) that can cause or exacerbate sensory problems.*
● Note age and developmental stage. *Problems with sensory perception may be known to client/caregiver (e.g., child wearing hearing aid, elderly adult with known macular degeneration), where compensatory interventions are in place. Screening or evaluation may be required if sensory impairments are suspected, but not obvious, as might occur when an infant is not progressing developmentally or an older individual has a gradual loss of sensory discrimination associated with aging; or sensory changes associated with a sudden neurological event.*[2,3,9]
● Evaluate medication regimen and determine possible use or misuse of drugs (prescription, over-the-counter [OTC], illicit) *to identify effects, side effects, adverse effects or drug interactions that may be causing or exacerbating sensory or perceptual problems.*
● Review results of sensory and motor neurological testing and laboratory studies (e.g., cognitive testing or laboratory values, such as electrolytes, chemical profile, arterial blood gases [ABGs], serum drug levels) *to note presence or possible cause of changes in response to sensory stimuli.*

🌐 Cultural   😊 Collaborative   🏠 Community/Home Care   ✏️ Diagnostic Studies   ∞ Pediatric/Geriatric/Lifespan   Medications

NURSING PRIORITY NO. 2

To determine degree of impairment:

- Assess ability to speak, hear, interpret, and respond to simple commands *to obtain an overview of client's mental and cognitive status and ability to interpret stimuli.*
- Evaluate sensory awareness (e.g., hot and cold, dull or sharp, smell, taste, visual acuity and hearing, gait, mobility, and location or function of body parts). *Screening can be done in clinic or facility may identify problems requiring more extensive evaluation.*
- Determine response to touch and painful stimuli *to note whether response is appropriate to stimulus and whether it is immediate or delayed. The sense of touch is usually maintained throughout life and may become more important if other senses are diminished. Different types of touch or contact are associated with different meanings (including communication of ideas, information, and emotion).*[3]
- Observe for behavioral responses (e.g., illusions, hallucinations, delusions; withdrawal, hostility, crying, inappropriate affect; confusion or disorientation) *that may indicate mental or emotional problems or chemical toxicity (as might occur with digoxin or other drug overdose or reaction) or be associated with brain or neurological trauma or infection.*
- Note inattention to body parts, segments of environment; lack of recognition of familiar objects or persons. *Loss of comprehension of auditory, visual, or other sensations may be indicative of unilateral neglect or inability to recognize and respond to environmental cues.*[10]
- Ascertain client's perception of problem or changes. Note SO's observations of changes that have occurred and client's responses to changes. *Client may or may not be aware of changes (e.g., diabetic with neuropathy may not realize he or she has lost discrimination for pain in feet; or parents may notice child's problem with coordination or difficulty with words).*
- Refer to additional NDs Anxiety; acute/chronic Confusion; disturbed Thought Processes; unilateral Neglect, as appropriate and based on findings.

NURSING PRIORITY NO. 3

To promote normalization of response to stimuli:

GENERAL INTERVENTIONS
- Note degree of alteration or involvement (single or multiple senses) *to determine scope and complexity of condition and needed interventions.*
- Ascertain and validate client's perceptions. Listen to and respect client's expressions of deprivation *to assist in planning of appropriate care, to identify inconsistencies in reception and integration of stimuli, and to provide compassionate regard for client's feelings.*[4]
- Provide means of communication as indicated by client's current situation.
- Document perceptual deficit in chart and code on wall in client's room, if needed, *so caregivers are aware of specific needs or limitations.*
- Avoid isolating client, physically or emotionally, *to prevent sensory deprivation and limit confusion.*
- Address client by name and have personnel wear name tags and reintroduce self, as needed, *to preserve client's sense of identity and orientation.*
- Reorient to time, place, and situation or events, as necessary, *to reduce confusion and provide sense of normalcy to client's daily life.*
- Explain procedures and activities, expected sensations, and outcomes. *Helpful in reducing anxiety associated with altered interpretation of environment.*

Nursing Diagnoses in Alphabetical Order

Sexual Dysfunction

DEFINITION: The state in which an individual experiences a change in sexual function during the sexual response phases of desire, excitation, and/or orgasm, which is viewed as unsatisfying, unrewarding, or inadequate

RELATED FACTORS

Ineffectual or absent role models; lack of SO
Lack of privacy
Misinformation or lack of knowledge
Vulnerability
Physical abuse; psychosocial abuse (e.g., harmful relationships)
Altered body function or structure (e.g., pregnancy, recent childbirth, drugs, surgery, anomalies, disease process, trauma, radiation, [effects of aging])
Biopsychosocial alteration of sexuality
Values conflict

DEFINING CHARACTERISTICS

Subjective
Verbalization of problem [e.g., loss of sexual desire, disruption of sexual response patterns such as premature ejaculation, dyspareunia, vaginismus]; alterations in achieving perceived sex role
Actual or perceived limitation imposed by disease or therapy
Alterations in achieving sexual satisfaction; inability to achieve desired satisfaction
Perceived deficiency of sexual desire or alteration in sexual excitation
Seeking confirmation of desirability [concern about body image]
Change of interest in self/others; [alteration in relationship with SO]

Sample Clinical Applications: Arthritis, cancer, major surgery, heart disease, hypertension, diabetes mellitus, spinal cord injury (SCI), multiple sclerosis (MS), traumatic injury, pregnancy, childbirth, abuse, depression

DESIRED OUTCOMES/EVALUATION CRITERIA

Sample NOC linkages:
Sexual Functioning: Integration of physical, socioemotional, and intellectual aspects of sexual expression and performance
Physical Aging: Normal physical changes that occur with the natural aging process
Abuse Recovery: Sexual: Extent of healing of physical and psychological injuries due to sexual abuse or exploitation

Client Will (Include Specific Time Frame)
• Verbalize understanding of sexual anatomy, function, and alterations that may affect function.
• Verbalize understanding of individual reasons for sexual problems.
• Identify stressors in lifestyle that may contribute to the dysfunction.
• Identify satisfying, acceptable sexual practices and alternative ways of dealing with sexual expression.
• Discuss concerns about body image, sex role, desirability as a sexual partner with partner/SO.

ACTIONS/INTERVENTIONS

Sample (NIC) linkages:

Sexual Counseling: Use of an interactive helping process focusing on the need to make adjustments to sexual practice or to coping with a sexual event/disorder

Teaching: Sexuality: Assisting individuals to understand physical and psychosocial dimensions of sexual growth and development

Values Clarification: Assisting another to clarify her/his own values in order to facilitate effective decision making

NURSING PRIORITY NO. 1

To assess causative/contributing factors:

- Perform a complete history and physical, including a sexual history, noting usual pattern of functioning and level of desire, issues of rape or abuse. *Establishes a database from which an individualized plan of care can be formulated.*[15]
- Note vocabulary and style of communication used by the individual/SO. *Maximizes communication and understanding of words and meaning in an area that individual may find difficult to discuss. Knowing that male and female brains are organized differently may help with recognizing different styles of communication.*[4]
- Have client describe problem in own words. *Sexual dysfunction is divided into four categories—sexual desire (decreased libido), arousal (erectile dysfunction [ED] or aversion or avoidance of sex), orgasm (delay, absence), or sexual pain disorders (dyspareunia, vaginismus).*[13,15] *Client's perception of the problem may differ from the care provider's, and plan of care needs to be based on client's perceptions for maximum effectiveness.*[1,9]
- Be alert to comments of client. *Sexual concerns are often disguised as humor, sarcasm, or offhand remarks. Many people are uncomfortable talking about sexual issues but want to discuss them with care provider, so they use this method to bring up the subject. It is important for the caregiver to recognize and acknowledge client's concern.*[2,5]
- Determine importance of sex to individual/partner and client's motivation for change. *Both individuals may have differing levels of desire and expectations that may create conflict in relationship.*[3,15]
- Assess client's/SO's knowledge of sexual anatomy, function, and effects of current situation or condition (e.g., client's concern about penis size, failure with performance). *Basic knowledge is essential for understanding the problem and how it is affecting the individual. Lack of knowledge may impact client's understanding of situation and expectation for return to previous norm or change for the future.*[3,7]
- Determine preexisting problems or conditions (e.g., illness, surgery, trauma) that may affect current situation and perception of individual/SO. *Physical conditions (e.g., arthritis, MS, hypertension, diabetes mellitus, fatigue, presence of a colostomy, urinary incontinence) can directly affect sexual functioning, or individual can believe that condition precludes sexual activity, such as recent myocardial infarction or heart surgery.*[3,6,7,13,16]
- Identify stress factors in individual situation (e.g., marital or job stress, role conflicts). *Interpersonal problems (marital and relationship), lack of trust and open communication between partners can contribute to difficulties. These factors may be producing enough anxiety to cause depression or other psychological reaction(s) that would cause physiological symptoms.*[6,11]
- Observe behavior and stage of grieving when related to body changes, loss of a body part, or change in function (e.g., pregnancy, obesity, amputation, mastectomy, hysterectomy,

menopause). *A change in body image can affect how individual views body in many aspects, but particularly in the sensitive area of sexual functioning and indicates need for information and additional support.*[7]

 • Discuss cultural values or religious beliefs and conflicts present. *Client may feel guilt or shame about sexual desires or difficulties because of family beliefs about sex and genital area of the body, and how sexuality was communicated to the client as he or she was growing up, or through religious teachings.*[1,2]

• Explore with client the meaning of client's behavior. *Masturbation, for instance, may have many meanings or purposes, such as for relief of anxiety, sexual deprivation, pleasure, a nonverbal expression of need to talk, a way of alienating.*[3] *Or, client's inhibitions may be diminished by changes in cognition.*[12]

• Review medication regimen and drug use (prescription, over-the-counter [OTC], illegal, alcohol) and cigarette use. *Antihypertensives may cause ED; monoamine oxidase inhibitors (MAOIs) and tricyclics can cause erection or ejaculation problems and anorgasmia in women; selective serotonin reuptake inhibtor (SSRI) antidepressants can cause decreased libido or orgasm disorders; antihistamines may cause temporary vaginal dryness (dyspareunia); narcotics and alcohol produce ED and inhibit orgasm; smoking creates vasoconstriction and may be a factor in ED. Evaluation of drug and individual response is important to determine accurate intervention.*[1,10,13,15]

• Review lab results (e.g., hormone levels, serum glucose, red blood cell [RBC] count, drug levels). *Testing may reveal undiagnosed conditions such as diabetes resulting in ED in men; anemia affecting arousal. Inappropriate drug levels or hormone deficiencies—decreased estrogen in women and decreased testosterone in men and women may result in decreased libido; hypothyroidism may impair sexual arousal.*[15]

• Assist with or review diagnostic studies to determine cause of erectile dysfunction. *More than half of the cases have a physical cause such as diabetes, vascular problems, and so on.* Monitor penile tumescence during rapid eye movement (REM) sleep *to determine physical ability. Men are embarrassed to bring up the subject with their healthcare provider even when they are seeing him or her for other conditions; unless the provider specifically asks, the subject is not addressed.*[6,8,9,13]

• Assist with or review diagnostic studies for female sexual disorders (e.g., vaginal photoplethysmography *to assess vaginal blood flow and engorgement*, vaginal pH *to identify infection or diminished secretions*, biothesiometer *to test sensitivity of clitoris and labia*).[16]

NURSING PRIORITY NO. 2

To assist client/SO(s) to deal with individual situation:

• Establish therapeutic nurse-client relationship. *Promotes treatment and facilitates sharing of sensitive information and feelings in a safe environment.*[1]

• Avoid making value judgments. *They do not help the client to cope with the situation. Nurse needs to be aware of and be in control of own feelings and response to client expressions and/or concerns. Client needs to be free to express concerns in whatever way is comfortable to individual.*[3] *And even clients with limited cognition have a right to engage in intimate behaviors.*[12]

• Assist with treatment of underlying medical conditions, including changes in medication regimen, weight management, cessation of smoking, and so forth. *Many conditions (e.g., cardiovascular, diabetes, arthritis) can affect sexual functioning, as well as medication side effects that may affect sexual ability.*[7,13-15]

• Collaborate with physical therapist to identify mechanical aides that may be useful for clients with physical conditions/disabilities.[15]

- Provide factual information about individual condition (e.g., premature ejaculation, female problems of dyspareunia; low sexual desire). *Accurate information helps client make informed decisions about own situation.*[2,8,10,15]
- Determine what client wants to know to tailor information to client needs. *Providing too much information may be overwhelming and result in client not remembering something that is essential. Information affecting client safety and consequences of actions may need to be reviewed or reinforced.*[1,7,9]
- Encourage and accept expressions of concern, anger, grief, fear. *Individuals need to be free to express these feelings and be accepted so they can begin to deal with situation and move on in a positive way.*[6,10,13]
- Assist client to be aware and deal with stages of grieving for loss or change. *Sexual dysfunction is often a result of losses such as breast cancer treatment, prostate surgery, and need to be addressed in the context of the whole. Healthcare providers need to be willing to help client understand grieving issues.*[2,7,11]
- Encourage client to share thoughts and concerns with partner and to clarify values or impact of condition on relationship. *Helps to identify issues in the relationship that may be related to the sexual dysfunction.*[3,11,15]
- Provide for or identify ways to obtain privacy to allow for sexual expression for individual or between partners without embarrassment or objections of others. *Often caregivers do not think about the importance of providing this basic need for couples, but in any setting, privacy may be difficult to provide unless it is thought about and planned for.*[6,12]
- Discuss client's rights regarding intimacy in residential or extended care settings with SO/family. Review appropriateness of home visits or provision for privacy for intimate contact. *Family members may not realize that the need for sexual expression is not limited by advancing age, declining cognition, or marital status. And they may be unaware that client has a right to engage in appropriate intimate behaviors.*[12]
- Assist client/SO(s) to problem-solve alternative ways of sexual expression. *When illness or condition, such as arthritis, paraplegia interfere with a couple's usual sexual activities, couple needs to learn new ways to achieve satisfaction.*[3]
- Discuss use of medications such as papaverine, sildenafil (Viagra), or vardenafil (Levitra) *for ED,* or lubricating gels, hormone creams, or possibly hormonal replacement therapy *for vaginal dryness and dyspareunia* as appropriate.[15,16]
- Provide information about availability of corrective measures such as reconstructive surgery (e.g., penile or breast implants), Eros Therapy (handheld device used to improve blood flow to clitoris and external labia to increase sensitivity of tissues), or behavioral therapies (e.g., self-stimulation, sensate focus exercises, Masters & Johnson treatment strategies), when indicated. *Sexual problems, such as ED, female orgasmic disorders, female sexual arousal disorders may respond to these interventions, providing more satisfactory sexual life.*[8,10,14–16]
- Refer to appropriate resources as need indicates (e.g., healthcare coworker with greater comfort level and/or knowledgeable clinical nurse specialist or professional sex therapist, family counseling). *Not all professionals are knowledgeable or comfortable dealing with sexual issues, and referrals to more appropriate resources can provide client/couple with accurate assistance.*[2,6,12]

NURSING PRIORITY NO. 3

To promote wellness (Teaching/Discharge Considerations):

- Provide sex education, explanation of normal sexual functioning when necessary. *Many individuals are not knowledgeable about these areas, and often providing accurate information can help assuage anxiety about unknowns, such as normal changes of aging, or provide an accurate basis for understanding problems being experienced.*[6,15,16]

🏠 ● Provide written material appropriate to individual needs. Include bibliotherapy and reliable Internet resources related to client's concerns. *Provides reinforcement for client to read and access at his or her leisure, when ready to deal with sensitive materials.*[3,6,7]

🏠 ● Encourage ongoing dialogue and take advantage of teachable moments that occur. *Within a therapeutic relationship, comfort is achieved and individual is encouraged to ask questions and be receptive to continuing conversation about sexual issues.*[1,2]

🏠 ● Demonstrate and assist client to learn relaxation or visualization techniques. *Stress is often a component of sexual dysfunction, and using these skills can help with resolution of problems.*[2,5]

🏠 ● Identify resources for assistive devices/sexual "aids." *These aids can enhance sex life of couple and prevent or help with problems of dysfunction.*[3,6]

🏠 ● Emphasize importance of engaging in regular self-examination as indicated (e.g., breast and testicular examinations). *Encourages client to participate in own health prevention activities, become more aware of potential problems, and become more comfortable with sexual self.*[3,5]

⊕ ● Identify community resources for further assistance, such as Reach for Recovery, Can-Surmount, Ostomy Association.[11]

⊕ ● Refer for further professional assistance concerning relationship difficulties, low sexual desire, other sexual concerns such as premature ejaculation, vaginismus, painful intercourse. *May need additional or continuing support to deal with individual situation or associated depression.*[3,15] *Note: Referral to counselor expert in trauma may be preferred to assist sexual abuse survivors overcome sexual difficulties.*[15]

DOCUMENTATION FOCUS

Assessment/Reassessment
- Individual findings, including nature of dysfunction, predisposing factors, perceived effect on sexuality and relationships.
- Cultural or religious factors, conflicts.
- Response of SO(s).
- Motivation for change.

Planning
- Plan of care and who is involved in planning.
- Teaching plan.

Implementation/Evaluation
- Response to interventions, teaching, and actions performed.
- Attainment or progress toward desired outcome(s).
- Modifications to plan of care.

Discharge Planning
- Long-term needs and who is responsible for actions to be taken.
- Community resources, specific referrals made.

References

1. Townsend, M. C. (2003). *Psychiatric Mental Health Nursing Concepts of Care.* 4th ed. Philadelphia: F. A. Davis.
2. Doenges, M. E., Townsend, M. C., Moorhouse, M. F. (1998). *Psychiatric Care Plans: Guidelines for Individualizing Care.* 3rd ed. Philadelphia: F. A. Davis.
3. Hyde, J., DeLamater, J. (2002). *Understanding Human Sexuality.* 7th ed. New York: McGraw-Hill.
4. Moir, A., Jessel, D. (1991). *Brain Sex: The Real Difference Between Men & Women.* New York: Dell.
5. Boston Women's Health Book Collective. (1998). *Our Bodies, Ourselves for the New Century.* 7th ed. Gloucester, MA: Peter Smith Publisher.
6. Harvard Medical School. (2003). *Sexuality in Midlife and Beyond: A Special Health Report from Harvard Medical School.* Cambridge, MA: Harvard Health Publications.
7. Stanley, M., Beare, P. G. (1999). *Gerontological Nursing.* 2d ed. Philadelphia: F. A. Davis.
8. Carver, C. (1998). Premature ejaculation: A common and treatable concern. *J Am Psy Nurs Assoc*, 4(6), 199–204.
9. McEnany, G. (1998). Sexual dysfunction in the pharmacologic treatment of depression: When "don't ask, don't tell" is an unsuitable approach to care. *J Am Psy Nurs Assoc*, 4(1), 24–29.
10. Phillips, N. A. (2000). Female sexual dysfunction: Evaluation and treatment. *Am Family Phys*, 62(1), 127–136, 141–142.
11. Cox, H. C., et al. (2002). *Clinical Applications of Nursing Diagnosis: Adult, Child, Women's, Psychiatric, Gerontic, and Home Health Considerations.* 4th ed. Philadelphia: F. A. Davis.
12. Sexuality in the Nursing Home. (1997): The Legal Center for People with Disabilities and Older People.
13. McDaniel, N. D. (2007). Beyond Viagra: The hidden roots and risks of erectile dysfunction. Retrieved August 2007 from www.lifescript.com/channels/healthy_living/Mens_Health/beyond_viagra_the_hidden_roots_and_risks_of_erectile_dysfunction.asp.
14. Male sexual health. (2005). Retrieved August 2007 from www.moderntherapy.com/male/sexual-health.html.
15. Ballas, P. (2006). Sexual problems overview. Retrieved August 2007 from www.nlm.nih.gov/medlineplus/ency/article/001951.htm.
16. Female sexual dysfunction. (2003). Retrieved August 2007 from www.womenshealthchannel.com/fsd/index.shtml.

(ineffective Sexuality Pattern)

DEFINITION: Expressions of concern regarding own sexuality

RELATED FACTORS

Knowledge or skill deficit about alternative responses to health-related transitions, altered body function or structure, illness or medical treatment

Lack of privacy

Impaired relationship with an SO; lack of SO

Ineffective or absent role models

Conflicts with sexual orientation or variant preferences

Fear of pregnancy or acquiring a sexually transmitted infection

(continues on page 748)

2. Workman, M. L. (2006). Interventions for clients with shock. In Inatavicius, D. D., Workman, M. L. (eds). *Medical-Surgical Nursing: Critical Thinking for Collaborative Care.* 5th ed. St. Louis, MO: Elsevier Saunders.

3. Spaniol, J. R., et al. (2007). Fluid resuscitation therapy for hemorrhagic shock. *J Trauma Nurs,* 14(13), 152–160.

4. Gorman, D., et al. (2008). Take a rapid treatment approach to cardiogenic shock. *Nurs Crit Care,* 3(4), 18–27.

5. Sharma, S. (2007). Septic shock. Retrieved March 2009 from http://emedicine.medscape.com/article/168402/.

6. Nelson, D. P., et al. (2009). Recognizing sepsis in the adult patient. *Am J Nurs,* 109(3), 40–50.

7. Sommers, M. S., Johnson, S. A., Beery, T. A. (2007). *Diseases and Disorders: A Nursing Therapeutics Manual.* 3d ed. Philadelphia: F. A. Davis.

8. Dellinger, R. P., et al. (2008). Surviving sepsis campaign: Guidelines for management for severe sepsis and septic shock. *Crit Care Med,* 32(3), 858–873.

9. Maier, R. V. (2005). Approach to the patient with shock. *Harrison's Principles of Internal Medicine.* Kasper, D. L., Harrison, T. R. 16th ed. New York: McGraw-Hill.

10. Adams, S. (2003). Shock, systemic inflammatory response and multiple organ dysfunction. In Brooker, C., Nicol, M. (eds). *Nursing Adults: The Practice of Caring.* Edinburgh: Mosby.

impaired Skin Integrity

DEFINITION: Altered epidermis and/or dermis

RELATED FACTORS

External
Hyperthermia; hypothermia
Chemical substance; radiation; medications
Physical immobilization
Humidity; moisture; [excretions, secretions]
Mechanical factors (e.g., shearing forces, pressure, restraint), [trauma: injury or surgery]
Extremes in age

Internal
Imbalanced nutritional state (e.g., obesity, emaciation); impaired metabolic state; changes in fluid status
Skeletal prominence; changes in turgor; [presence of edema]
Impaired circulation or sensation; changes in pigmentation
Developmental factors
Immunological deficit
[Psychogenic factors (e.g., obsessive compulsive behaviors)]

DEFINING CHARACTERISTICS

Subjective
[Reports of itching, pain, numbness of affected/surrounding area]

Objective
Disruption of skin surface [epidermis]
Destruction of skin layers [dermis]
Invasion of body structures

Sample Clinical Applications: Arteriosclerosis, venous insufficiency, hypertension, obesity, diabetes mellitus, malignant neoplasms, traumatic injury, surgery, chronic steroid use (e.g., chronic obstructive pulmonary disease [COPD], asthma), renal failure, burns, radiation therapy, malnutrition

DESIRED OUTCOMES/EVALUATION CRITERIA

Sample NOC linkages:
Tissue Integrity: Skin & Mucous Membranes: Structural intactness and normal physiological function of skin and mucous membranes
Wound Healing: Primary Intention: Extent of regeneration of cells and tissues following intentional closure
Wound Healing: Secondary Intention: Extent of regeneration of cells and tissues in an open wound

Client Will (Include Specific Time Frame)
• Display timely healing of skin lesions, wounds, or pressure sores without complication.
• Maintain optimal nutrition and physical well-being.
• Participate in prevention measures and treatment program.
• Verbalize feelings of increased self-esteem and ability to manage situation.

ACTIONS/INTERVENTIONS

Sample NIC linkages:
Wound Care: Prevention of wound complications and promotion of wound healing
Incision Site Care: Cleansing, monitoring, and promotion of healing in a wound that is closed with sutures, clips, or staples
Pressure Ulcer Care: Facilitation of healing in pressure ulcers

NURSING PRIORITY NO. 1

To assess causative/contributing factors:

• Identify underlying condition or pathology involved. *Skin integrity problems can be the result of (1) disease processes that affect circulation and perfusion of tissues (e.g., arteriosclerosis, venous insufficiency, hypertension, obesity, diabetes, malignant neoplasms); (2) medications (e.g., anticoagulants, corticosteroids, immunosuppressives, antineoplastics) that adversely affect or impair healing; (3) burns or radiation (can break down internal tissues as well as skin); and (4) nutrition and hydration (e.g., malnutrition deprives the body of protein and calories required for cell growth and repair, and dehydration impairs transport of oxygen and nutrients). Disruption in skin integrity can be intentional (e.g., surgical incision) or unintentional (e.g., accidental trauma, drug effect, allergic reaction), and closed (e.g., contusion, abrasion, rash) or open (e.g., laceration, penetrating wound, ulcerations).*[1,2,13]
• Note general health. *Many factors (e.g., debilitation; immobility; use of restraints; extremes of age; mental status; dehydration or malnutrition; presence of chronic disease;*

occupational, treatment, and environmental hazards) can all affect the ability of the skin to perform its functions (e.g., protection, sensation, movement and growth, chemical synthesis, immunity, thermoregulation and excretion).[3,4]

- Determine client's age and developmental factors or ability to care for self. *Newborn/ infant's skin is thin, provides ineffective thermal regulation and nails are thin.*[5] *Babies and children are prone to skin rashes associated with viral, bacterial, and fungal infections and allergic reactions. In adolescence, hormones stimulate hair growth and sebaceous gland activity. In adults, it takes longer to replenish epidermis cells, resulting in increased risk of skin cancers and infection. In older adults, there is decreased epidermal regeneration, fewer sweat glands, less subcutaneous fat, elastin, and collagen, causing skin to become thinner, drier, and less responsive to pain sensations.*[1,3,4,6,7]

- Evaluate client's skin care practices and hygiene issues. *Individual's skin may be oily, dry, or sensitive and is affected by bathing frequency (or lack of bathing), temperature of water, types of soap and other cleansing agents. Incontinence (urinary or bowel) and ineffective hygiene can result in serious skin impairment and discomfort.*

- Note presence of compromised vision, hearing, or speech *that may impact client's self-care as relates to skin care (e.g., diabetic with impaired vision probably cannot satisfactorily examine own feet).*[11]

- Ascertain allergy history. *Individual may be sensitive or allergic to substances (e.g., insects, grasses, medications, lotions, soaps, foods) that can adversely affect the skin.*

- Note distribution and scarcity of hair *(e.g., loss of hair on lower legs may indicate peripheral vascular disease).* Refer to ND risk for Peripheral Vascular Dysfunction for additional interventions.[5,14]

- Assess blood supply (e.g., capillary return time, color, and warmth) and sensation of skin surfaces and affected area on a regular basis *to provide comparative baseline and opportunity for timely intervention when problems are noted.*[3,9]

- Calculate ankle-brachial index (ABI) *to evaluate actual or potential for impairment of circulation to lower extremities. Result less than 0.9 indicates need for close monitoring or more aggressive intervention (e.g., tighter blood glucose and weight control in diabetic client).*[15]

- Determine treatment-related skin or tissue conditions (e.g., surgical incision, IV/invasive line insertion site, use of restraints). Assess surgical sites *for signs of infection (e.g., swelling, redness, pain)*; assess IV site *for infiltration (e.g., swelling, erythema, coolness, and pain, failure of infusion) or evidence of extravasation (e.g., blistering, blanching, skin sloughing).*[4] Evaluate skin surrounding restraints for abrasions, contusions, skin breaks, or skin color and temperature changes distal to restraints *suggesting impaired circulation.*

- Review laboratory results (e.g., hemoglobin/hematocrit [Hb/Hct], blood glucose, blood and/ or wound culture and sensitivities for infectious agents [viral, bacterial, fungal], albumin, protein) *to evaluate causative factors or ability to heal. Note: Albumin <3.5 correlates to decreased wound healing and increased incidence of pressure ulcers.*[1,15,16]

NURSING PRIORITY NO. 2

To assess extent of involvement/injury:

- Obtain a complete history of current skin condition(s) (especially in children where recurrent rash or lesions are common), including age at onset, date of first episode, duration, original site, characteristics of lesions, and any changes that have occurred. *Common skin manifestations of sensitivity or allergies are hives, eczema, and contact dermatitis. Contagious rashes include measles, rubella, roseola, chickenpox, and scarlet fever. Bacterial, viral, and fungal infections can also cause skin problems (e.g., impetigo, cellulitis, cold sores, shingles, athlete's foot, candidiasis diaper rashes).*[6]

- Perform routine skin inspections describing observed changes. Note color, temperature, surface changes, texture, and contours. Evaluate color changes in areas of least pigmentation (e.g., sclera, conjunctiva, nail beds, buccal mucosa, tongue, palms, and soles of feet). *Systematic inspection can identify improvement or changes for timely intervention.*[8]

GENERAL WOUNDS/LESIONS

- Describe rash or lesion, noting color, location, significant characteristics (e.g., flat or raised rash, weeping or painful blisters, itching wheal) and surrounding information (e.g., exposure to contagious disease, reaction to medication, recent insect bite, ingrown toenail, sexually transmitted disease) *to assist in diagnosing problem and needed interventions.*
- Determine anatomic location and depth of skin or tissue injury or damage (e.g., epidermis, dermis, and/or underlying issues) and describe (e.g., partial or full-thickness burn) *to provide baseline and document changes.*[3,10]
- Photograph lesion(s) as appropriate *to document status and provide visual baseline for future comparisons.*
- Note character and color of drainage, when present (e.g., blood, bile, pus, stoma effluent), *which can cause skin irritation or excoriation.*

PRESSURE ULCERS/DECUBITUS

- Determine and document (1) dimensions and depth in centimeters; (2) exudates—color, odor, and amount; (3) margins—fixed or unfixed; (4) tunneling or tracts; (5) evidence of necrosis (e.g., color gray to black) or healing (e.g., pink or red granulation tissue) *to establish comparative baseline and evaluate effectiveness of interventions.*[8,16,17]
- Classify pressure ulcer(s) using tool such as Waterlow, Braden, Norton (or similar) Ulcer Classification System. *Provides consistent terminology for assessment and documentation of pressure sores.*[8,16,17]
- Remeasure wound(s) regularly and periodically photograph, and observe incisions or wounds for complications *to monitor progress or failure of healing.*

NURSING PRIORITY NO. 3

To determine impact of condition:

- Determine if wound is acute (e.g., injury from surgery or trauma) or chronic (e.g., venous or arterial insufficiency), *which affects healing time and the client's emotional and physical responses. For example, an acute and noninfected wound can heal in about 4 weeks, while a chronic wound often does not progress through phases of healing in an orderly or timely fashion.*[10]
- Determine client's level of discomfort (e.g., can vary widely from minor itching or aching, to deep pain with burns, or excoriation associated with drainage) *to clarify intervention needs and priorities.*
- Ascertain attitudes of individual/SO(s) about condition (e.g., cultural values, stigma). Obtain or review psychological assessment of client's emotional status, noting potential or sexual problems arising from presence of condition. *The healthy wholeness and beauty of skin impacts the client's body image and self-esteem. Lesions or wounds that disfigure can be especially devastating.*

NURSING PRIORITY NO. 4

To assist client with correcting/minimizing condition and achieving optimal healing.

- Practice and instruct client/caregiver(s) in scrupulous hand hygiene and clean or sterile technique *to reduce incidence of contamination or infection.*

- Provide optimum nutrition (including adequate protein, lipids, calories, trace minerals and multivitamins [e.g., A, C, D, E]) *to promote skin health and healing, and to maintain general good health.*
- Provide adequate hydration (e.g., oral, tube feeding, IV, ambient room humidity) *to reduce and replenish transepidermal water loss.*
- Encourage client to verbalize feelings and discuss how or if condition affects self-concept. (Refer to NDs disturbed Body Image, situational low Self-Esteem.)
- Assist client to work through stages of grief and feelings associated with individual condition.
- Use touch, facial expressions, and tone of voice *to lend psychological support and acceptance of client.*

Promote wound healing:[1,5,9,12,14,17]

Keep surgical area(s) clean and dry; carefully dress wounds; support incision (e.g., use of Steri-Strips, splinting when coughing); and stimulate circulation to surrounding areas *to assist body's natural process of repair.*

Consult with physician or wound specialist as indicated *to assist with developing plan of care for problematic or potentially serious wounds.*

Assist with debridement or enzymatic therapy as indicated (e.g., burns, severe pressure sores) to remove nonviable, contaminated or infected tissue.[18]

Use body-temperature physiological solutions (e.g., isotonic saline) *to clean or irrigate wounds and prevent washout of electrolytes.*

Cleanse wound with irrigation syringe or gauze squares, avoiding cotton balls or other products *that shed fibers.*

Maintain appropriate moisture environment for particular wound (e.g., expose lesions or ulcer to air and light if excess moisture is impeding healing, or use occlusive dressings to maintain a moist environment for autolytic debridement of wound) as indicated.[18]

Use appropriate barrier dressings or wound coverings (e.g., semipermeable, occlusive, wet-to-damp, DuoDerm, Tegaderm, hydrocolloid, hydrofiber or gel, hydropolymers), drainage appliances, and skin-protective agents for open or draining wounds and stomas *to protect wound and surrounding tissues from excoriating secretions or drainage, and to promote wound healing.*[18]

Administer topical or systemic drugs as indicated *for individual situation.*

Prevent skin impairment:[3–5,7,9,12,14,17]

Maintain or instruct in overall skin hygiene (e.g., wash thoroughly, pat dry, gently massage with lotion or appropriate cream) *to provide barrier to infection, reduce risk of dermal trauma, improve circulation, and enhance comfort.*

Cleanse skin after incontinent or diaphoretic episodes *to restore normal skin pH and flora and limit potential for infection.*

Use proper turning and transfer techniques. Avoid movements *that cause friction or shearing (e.g., pulling client with parallel force, dragging movements).*

Encourage early ambulation or mobilization. *Reduces risks associated with immobility.*

Develop regularly timed repositioning schedule for client with mobility and sensation impairments, using turn sheet as needed; encourage or assist with periodic weight shifts for client in chair *to reduce stress on pressure points and encourage circulation to tissues.*

Use appropriate padding or pressure-reducing devices (e.g., heel rolls, foam boots, egg crate or gel pads), or pressure-relieving devices (e.g., air or water mattress) when indicated *to reduce pressure on and enhance circulation to compromised tissues.*

Avoid or limit use of plastic material (e.g., rubber sheet, plastic-backed linen savers), and remove wet or wrinkled linens promptly. *Moisture potentiates skin breakdown and increases risk for infection.*

Cultural   Collaborative   Community/Home Care   Diagnostic Studies   ∞ Pediatric/Geriatric/Lifespan   Medications

Remove adhesive products with care, removing on horizontal plane, and using mineral oil or Vaseline for softening, if needed, *to prevent abrasions or tearing of skin.*

Secure dressings with tape (e.g., elastic, paper tape, nonadherent dressings), or Montgomery straps when frequent dressing changes are required. Use stockinette, tubular or gauze wrap, or similar product instead of tape to secure dressings and drains *to limit dermal injury.*[13]

Apply hot and cold applications judiciously *to reduce risk of dermal injury in persons with circulatory and neurosensory impairments.*

Avoid use of latex products *when client has known or suspected sensitivity.* Refer to ND latex Allergy Response.

NURSING PRIORITY NO. 5

To promote wellness (Teaching/Discharge Considerations):

- Discuss importance of skin and measures to maintain proper skin functioning. *The integumentary system is the largest multifunctional organ of the body and thus merits special care.*
- Review benefits of following medical regimen. *Enhances commitment to plan, optimizing outcomes.*
- Encourage regular inspection and monitoring of skin for changes or failure to heal. *Early detection and reporting to healthcare providers promotes timely evaluation and intervention.*
- Identify safety measures for client with persistent sensation impairments. *Proper care of skin and extremities during cold or hot weather (e.g., wearing gloves, boots, clean, dry socks; properly fitting shoes or boots, face protection) reduces risk of injury.*[11,15]
- Encourage continued mobility, activity, and range of motion *to enhance circulation and promote health of skin and other organs.*
- Discuss avoidance of products containing perfumes, dyes, preservatives *(may cause dermatitis reactions)* or alcohol, povidone-iodine, hydrogen peroxide *(may hinder wound healing).*
- Encourage restriction or abstinence from tobacco, *which can cause vasoconstriction.*
- Review measures *to avoid spread or reinfection of communicable conditions.*
- Discuss proper and safe use of equipment or appliances (e.g., heating pad, ostomy appliances, padding straps of braces).
- Emphasize wisdom of limiting lengthy or unnecessary sun exposure, using high sun protection factor (SPF) sun block, and avoiding tanning beds.
- Assist client to learn stress reduction and alternate therapy techniques *to control feelings of helplessness and enhance coping ability.*
- Refer to dietitian or certified diabetes educator as appropriate *to manage general well-being, enhance healing, reduce risk of recurrence of diabetic ulcers.*

DOCUMENTATION FOCUS

Assessment/Reassessment
- Characteristics of lesion(s) or condition, ulcer classification.
- Causative or contributing factors.
- Impact of condition.

Planning
- Plan of care and who is involved in planning.
- Teaching plan.

Implementation/Evaluation
• Responses to interventions, teaching, and actions performed.
• Attainment or progress toward desired outcome(s).
• Modifications to plan of care.

Discharge Planning
• Long-term needs and who is responsible for actions to be taken.
• Specific referrals made.

References

1. Llewellyn, S. (2002). *Skin Integrity and Wound Care (lecture materials).* Chapel Hill, NC: Cape Fear Community College Nursing Program.
2. Colburn, L. (2001). Prevention for chronic wounds. In Krasner, D., Rodeheaver, G., Sibbald, R. G. (eds). *Chronic Wound Care: A Clinical Source Book for Healthcare Professionals.* 2d ed. Wayne, PA: HMP Communications.
3. Calianno, C. (2002). Patient hygiene, part 2—Skin care: Keeping the outside healthy. *Nursing,* 32(6).
4. Lund, C. H., Osborne, J. W., Culler, J. (2001). Neonatal skin care: Clinical outcomes of the AWHONN/NANN evidence-based clinical practice guideline. *J Neonatal Nurs,* 30(1), 30–40.
5. McGovern, C. (2003). Skin, hair and nail assessment. Unit 2 (lecture materials). Villanova University College of Nursing. Retrieved July 2007 from www.homepage.villanova.edu.
6. Engel, J. (2002). *Pocket Guide to Pediatric Assessment.* 4th ed. St. Louis, MO: Mosby, 99–112.
7. Wiersema, L. A., Stanley, M. (1999). The aging integumentary system. In Stanley, M., Beare, P. G. (eds). *Gerontological Nursing: A Health Promotion/Protection Approach.* 2d ed. Philadelphia: F. A. Davis, 102–111.
8. Krasner, D., Rodeheaver, G., Sibbald, R. G. (2001). Advanced wound caring for a new millennium. In Krasner, D., Rodeheaver, G., Sibbald, R. G. (eds). *Chronic Wound Care: A Clinical Source Book for Healthcare Professionals.* 2d ed. Wayne, PA: HMP Communications.
9. Doenges, M. E., Moorhouse, M. F., Geissler-Murr, A. C. (2002). ND: Skin Integrity, impaired. *Nursing Care Plans: Guidelines for Individualizing Patient Care.* 6th ed. Philadelphia: F. A. Davis.
10. Hahn, J. F., Wounds: Nursing care and product selection—Part 1 (CE offering). Nursing Spectrum. Retrieved September 2003 from http://nsweb.nursingspectrum.com/ce/ce80.htm.
11. Lawrance, D. P. *Diabetes FYI: Foot Care (Monograph 5 in series).* Champaign: University of Illinois, McKinley Diabetes Team.
12. Risk factors and prevention. Geriatric syndromes: Pressure ulcers. Novartis Foundation for Gerontology. Retrieved February 2004 from http://geriatricsyllabus.com.
13. Baranoski, S. (2003). Skin tears: Staying on guard against the enemy of frail skin. *Nursing,* 33(10), 14–20.
14. Hess, C. (2002). *Clinical Guide to Wound Care.* 4th ed. Philadelphia: Lippincott Williams & Wilkins.
15. Carrington, A. L., (2001). Peripheral vascular and nerve function associated with lower limb amputation in people with and without diabetes. *Clin Sci,* 101, 261–266.
16. Catania, K., et al. (2007). PUPPI: The pressure ulcer prevention protocol interventions. *Am J Nurs,* 107(4), 44–51.
17. Reddy, M., Gill, S. S., Rochon, P. A. (2006). Preventing pressure ulcers: A systematic review. *JAMA,* 296, 974–984.
18. Okan, K., Woo, K., Ayello, E. A. (2007). The role of moisture balance in wound healing. *Adv Skin Wound Care,* 20(1), 39–53.

risk for impaired Skin Integrity

DEFINITION: At risk for skin being adversely altered
Note: Risk should be determined by the use of a standardized risk assessment tool [e.g., Braden, Norton (or similar) Scale]

RISK FACTORS

External
Chemical substance; radiation
Hypothermia; hyperthermia
Physical immobilization
Excretions; secretions; humidity; moisture
Mechanical factors (e.g., shearing forces, pressure, restraint)
Extremes of age

Internal
Medications
Imbalanced nutritional state (e.g., obesity, emaciation), impaired metabolic state, [changes in fluid status]
Skeletal prominence; changes in skin turgor; [presence of edema]
Impaired circulation or sensation; change in pigmentation
Developmental factors
Psychogenic factors [e.g., obsessive compulsive behaviors]
Immunological factors

NOTE: A risk diagnosis is not evidenced by signs and symptoms, as the problem has not occurred; rather, nursing interventions are directed at prevention.
Sample Clinical Applications: Arteriosclerosis, venous insufficiency, hypertension, obesity, diabetes mellitus, systemic lupus, malignant neoplasms, chronic steroid use (e.g., chronic obstructive pulmonary disease [COPD], asthma), renal failure, malnutrition

DESIRED OUTCOMES/EVALUATION CRITERIA

Sample **NOC** linkages:
Risk Control: Personal actions to prevent, eliminate, or reduce modifiable health threats
Immobility Consequences: Physiological: Severity of compromise in physiological functioning due to impaired physical mobility
Tissue Integrity: Skin & Mucous Membranes: Structural intactness and normal physiological function of skin and mucous membranes

Client Will (Include Specific Time Frame)
• Identify individual risk factors.
• Verbalize understanding of treatment or therapy regimen.
• Demonstrate behaviors or techniques to prevent skin breakdown.

(continues on page 764)

risk for impaired Skin Integrity (continued)
ACTIONS/INTERVENTIONS

Sample **NIC** linkages:
Skin Surveillance: Collection and analysis of patient data to maintain skin and mucous membrane integrity
Pressure Management: Minimizing pressure to body parts
Pressure Ulcer Prevention: Prevention of pressure ulcers for a patient at high risk for developing them

NURSING PRIORITY NO. 1

To assess causative/contributing factors:

- Identify client with underlying conditions or problems that have potential for *skin integrity problems such as (1) disease processes that affect circulation and perfusion of tissues (e.g., arteriosclerosis, venous insufficiency, hypertension, obesity, diabetes, malignant neoplasms); (2) medications (e.g., anticoagulants, corticosteroids, immunosuppressives, antineoplastics) that adversely affect or impair healing; (3) radiation (can break down internal tissues as well as skin); and (4) nutrition and hydration (e.g., malnutrition deprives the body of protein and calories required for cell growth and repair, and dehydration impairs transport of oxygen and nutrients).*[1–5]
- Note general health. *Many factors (e.g., debilitation; immobility; use of restraints; extremes of age; mental status; dehydration or malnutrition; presence of chronic disease; occupational, treatment, and environmental hazards) can all affect the ability of the skin to perform its functions (e.g., protection, sensation, movement and growth, chemical synthesis, immunity, thermoregulation and excretion).*[1,6]
- Determine client's age and developmental factors or ability to care for self. *Newborn/infant's skin is thin. Babies and children are prone to skin rashes associated with viral, bacterial, and fungal infections and allergic reactions. In adolescence, hormones stimulate hair growth and sebaceous gland activity. In adults, it takes longer to replenish epidermis cells, resulting in increased risk of skin cancers and infection. In older adults there is decreased epidermal regeneration, fewer sweat glands, and less subcutaneous fat and elastin and collagen, causing skin to become thinner, drier, and less responsive to pain sensations.*[1,3,4,7–9]
- Perform risk assessment using a standardized tool (e.g., Braden Scale) *to determine pressure sore risk and appropriate interventions. Provides baseline for periodic comparison to note changes in risk status and need for alterations in the plan of care.*
- Evaluate client's skin care practices and hygiene issues. *Individual's skin may be oily, dry, or sensitive, and is affected by bathing frequency (or lack of bathing), temperature of water, and types of soap and other cleansing agents. Incontinence (urinary or bowel) and ineffective hygiene can result in serious skin impairment and discomfort.*
- Note presence of compromised vision, hearing, or speech *that may impact client's self-care as relates to skin care (e.g., diabetic with impaired vision probably cannot satisfactorily examine own feet).*[10]
- Ascertain allergy history. *Individual may be sensitive or allergic to substances (e.g., insects, grasses, medications, lotions, soaps, foods) that can adversely affect the skin.*
- Assess blood supply (e.g., capillary return time, color, warmth) and sensation of skin surfaces or affected area on a regular basis *to provide comparative baseline and opportunity for timely intervention when problems are noted.*[11]
- Calculate ankle-brachial index (ABI) *to evaluate actual or potential for impairment of circulation to lower extremities. Result less than 0.9 indicates need for close monitoring or*

more aggressive intervention (e.g., tighter blood glucose and weight control in diabetic client).[12,13]

- Review laboratory results (e.g., hemoglobin/hematocrit [Hb/Hct], blood glucose, albumin, protein) *to evaluate causative factors or ability to heal. Note: Albumin <3.5 correlates to decreased wound healing and increased incidence of pressure ulcers.*[14]

NURSING PRIORITY NO. 2

To maintain optimal skin integrity:[1,2,9,11]

- Perform routine skin inspections, assessing color, temperature, surface changes, texture, and contours. Evaluate color changes in areas of least pigmentation (e.g., sclera, conjunctiva, nailbeds, buccal mucosa, tongue, palms, soles of feet). Report potential problem areas (e.g., reddened/blanched areas or rashes) promptly. *Systematic inspection can identify developing problems; also promotes early intervention, thus reducing likelihood of progression to skin breakdown.*[15]
- Handle client gently (particularly infant, young child, elderly frail). *Epidermis of infants and very young children is thin and lacks subcutaneous depth that will develop with age. Skin of the older client is also thin, less elastic, and prone to injury, such as bruising and skin tears.*[5]
- Practice and instruct client/caregiver(s) in scrupulous hand hygiene and clean or sterile technique, as appropriate, *to reduce incidence of contamination or infection.*
- Maintain or instruct in good skin hygiene (e.g., wash thoroughly, pat dry, gently massage with lotion or appropriate cream) *to reduce risk of dermal trauma, improve circulation, and promote comfort.*
- Provide preventative skin care to incontinent client: change continence pads or diapers frequently; cleanse perineal skin daily and after each incontinence episode; apply skin protectant ointment *to minimize contact with irritants (urine, stool, excessive moisture).*[16]
- Cleanse skin after diaphoretic episodes *to maintain normal skin pH and flora and limit potential for infection.*
- Develop regularly timed repositioning schedule for client with mobility and sensation impairments, using turn sheet, as needed; encourage or assist with periodic weight shifts for client in chair *to reduce stress on pressure points and encourage circulation to tissues.*
- Use proper turning and transfer techniques. *Avoids movements that cause friction or shearing (e.g., pulling client with parallel force, dragging movements).*
- Pay special attention to bony prominences and other pressure points (e.g., heels, toes, elbows) when positioning client *to prevent pressure trauma and impaired circulation.*
- Provide foam, flotation, alternating pressure, or air mattress *to reduce or relieve pressure on skin, tissues, and lesions, decreasing tissue ischemia.*
- Use appropriate padding devices (e.g., egg crate, gel pads, heel rolls or foam boots) when indicated *to reduce pressure on and enhance circulation to compromised tissues.*
- Encourage early ambulation. *Promotes circulation and reduces risks associated with immobility.*
- Provide for safety measures during ambulation and other therapies *to reduce risk of dermal injury (e.g., assistive devices or sufficient personnel, grab bars, clear pathways, safe chairs, properly fitting hose and footwear, use of heating pads or lamps, restraints).*
- Avoid or limit use of plastic material (e.g., rubber sheet, plastic-backed linen savers), and remove wet or wrinkled linens promptly. *Moisture potentiates skin breakdown and increases risk for infection.*
- Use paper tape or a nonadherent dressing on frail skin and remove it gently, or use stockinette, tubular or gauze wrap, or other similar product instead of tape to secure dressings and drains *to limit dermal injury.*[5]

- Avoid use of latex products *when client has known or suspected sensitivity.* Refer to ND latex Allergy Response.
- Apply hot and cold applications judiciously *to reduce risk of dermal injury in persons with circulatory and neurosensory impairments.*
- Provide adequate clothing or covers; protect from drafts *to prevent vasoconstriction and reduction of circulation to skin.*
- Keep bedclothes dry, use nonirritating materials, and keep bed free of wrinkles, crumbs, and so forth *to prevent skin irritation.*
- Try colloidal bath, application of lotions, or careful use of ice pack *to decrease irritable itching.*
- Keep nails cut short, encouraging client *to refrain from scratching* or suggest use of/obtain order for mittens (considered a restraint), if necessary, *to prevent dermal injury from scratching.*
- Refer to ND impaired Skin Integrity for additional interventions, as indicated.

NURSING PRIORITY NO. 3

To promote wellness (Teaching/Discharge Considerations):

- Discuss importance of skin and measures to maintain proper skin functioning. *The integumentary system is the largest multifunctional organ of the body and thus merits special care.*
- Stress importance of regular inspection and monitoring of skin for changes and effective skin care in preventing skin problems. *Early detection and reporting to healthcare providers promotes timely evaluation and intervention.*
- Counsel diabetic and neurologically impaired client regarding the necessity of meticulous skin care, especially of lower extremities. *Healing of lower-extremity injuries tends to be more problematic in this population, resulting in increased incidence of amputation.*
- Avoid products containing perfumes, dyes, preservatives *(may cause dermatitis reactions)* or alcohol, povidone-iodine, hydrogen peroxide *(may hinder healing).*
- Instruct in care of skin and extremities during cold or hot weather (e.g., wearing gloves, boots, clean, dry socks; properly fitting shoes or boots, face protection) *to reduce risk of tissue damage, especially in clients with impaired sensation.*
- Recommend elevation of lower extremities when sitting *to enhance venous return and reduce edema formation.*
- Encourage continuation of regular exercise program (active or assistive) *to enhance circulation.*
- Discuss need for adequate nutritional intake (including adequate protein, lipids, calories, trace minerals, and multivitamins) *to promote skin health and healing and to maintain general good health.*
- Determine fluid needs and sources for hydration (e.g., oral, tube feeding, ambient room humidity) *to reduce and replenish transepidermal water loss.*
- Encourage restriction or abstinence from tobacco, *which can cause vasoconstriction.*
- Discuss importance of limiting lengthy or unnecessary sun exposure and avoiding use of tanning beds. Emphasize necessity of avoiding exposure to sunlight in specific conditions (e.g., systemic lupus, tetracycline or psychotropic drug use, radiation therapy) as well as potential for development of skin cancer.
- Advise use of high sun protection factor (SPF) sunblock or sunscreen, particularly on young child, client with fair skin (prone to burn), client using multiple medications, and so forth, *to limit skin damage (immediate and over time) associated with sun exposure.*

⊕ Cultural ⊛ Collaborative 🏠 Community/Home Care ⟋ Diagnostic Studies ∞ Pediatric/Geriatric/Lifespan Medications

DOCUMENTATION FOCUS

Assessment/Reassessment
- Individual findings, including individual risk factors.

Planning
- Plan of care and who is involved in planning.
- Teaching plan.

Implementation/Evaluation
- Responses to interventions, teaching, and actions performed.
- Attainment or progress toward desired outcome(s).
- Modifications to plan of care.

Discharge Planning
- Long-term needs and who is responsible for actions to be taken.

References

1. Calianno, C. (2002). Patient hygiene, part 2—Skin care: Keeping the outside healthy. *Nursing*, 32(6).
2. Neonatal skin care. Evidence-based clinical practice guideline. (2001). *Association of Women's Health, Obstetric and Neonatal Nurses (AWHONN)*. Retrieved September 2003 from www.guideline.gov.
3. Llewellyn, S. (2002). *Skin Integrity and Wound Care (lecture materials)*. Chapel Hill, NC: Cape Fear Community College Nursing Program.
4. Colburn, L. (2001). Prevention for chronic wounds. In Krasner, D., Rodeheaver, G., Sibbald, R. G. (eds). *Chronic Wound Care: A Clinical Source Book for Healthcare Professionals*. 2d ed. Wayne, PA: HMP Communications.
5. Baranoski, S. (2003). Skin tears: Staying on guard against the enemy of frail skin. *Nursing*, 33(10), 14–20.
6. Lund, C. H., Osborne, J. W., Culler, J. (2001). Neonatal skin care: Clinical outcomes of the AWHONN/NANN. Evidence-based clinical practice guideline. *J Neonatal Nurs*, 30(1), 30–40.
7. McGovern, C. (2003). Skin, hair and nail assessment, Unit 2 (lecture materials). Villanova University College of Nursing. Retrieved July 2007 from www.homepage.villanova.edu.
8. Engel, J. (2002). *Pocket Guide to Pediatric Assessment*. 4th ed. St. Louis, MO: Mosby, 99–112.
9. Wiersema, L. A., Stanley, M. (1999). The aging integumentary system. In Stanley, M., Beare, P. G. (eds). *Gerontological Nursing: A Health Promotion/Protection Approach*. 2d ed. Philadelphia: F. A. Davis, 102–111.
10. Lawrance, D. P. *Diabetes FYI-Foot Care (Monograph 5 in series)*. Champaign: University of Illinois, McKinley Diabetes Team.
11. Doenges, M. E., Moorhouse, M. F., Geissler-Murr, A. C. (2002). ND: Skin Integrity, impaired. *Nursing Care Plans: Guidelines for Individualizing Patient Care*. 6th ed. Philadelphia: F. A. Davis.
12. Murabito, J. M., et al. (2003). The ankle-brachial index in the elderly and risk of stroke, coronary disease and death. *Arch Intern Med*, 163, 1939–1942.
13. Carrington, A. L., et al. (2001). Peripheral vascular and nerve function associated with lower limb amputation in people with and without diabetes. *Clin Sci*, 101, 261–266.
14. Catania, K., et al. (2007). PUPPI. The pressure ulcer prevention protocol interventions. *Am J Nurs*, 107(4), 44–51.
15. Krasner, D., Rodeheaver, G., Sibbald, R. G. (2001). Advanced wound caring for a new millennium. *Chronic Wound Care: A Clinical Source Book for Healthcare Professionals*. 2d ed. Wayne, PA: HMP Communications.
16. Gray, M., Bliss, D. Z., Doughty, D. B., (2007). Incontinence-associated dermatitis: A consensus. *J Wound Ostomy Continence Nurs*, 34(1), 45–54.

Sleep Deprivation

DEFINITION: Prolonged periods of time without sleep (sustained natural, periodic suspension of relative consciousness)

RELATED FACTORS

Sustained environmental stimulation or uncomfortable sleep environment

Inadequate daytime activity; sustained circadian asynchrony; aging-related sleep stage shifts; non−sleep-inducing parenting practices

Sustained inadequate sleep hygiene; prolonged use of pharmacological or dietary anti-soporifics

Prolonged discomfort (e.g., physical, psychological); periodic limb movement (e.g., restless leg syndrome, nocturnal myoclonus); sleep-related enuresis or painful,erections

Nightmares; sleepwalking; sleep terror

Sleep apnea

Sundowner's syndrome; dementia

Idiopathic CNS hypersomnolence; narcolepsy; familial sleep paralysis

DEFINING CHARACTERISTICS

Subjective
Daytime drowsiness; decreased ability to function
Malaise; lethargy; fatigue
Anxiety
Perceptual disorders (e.g., disturbed body sensation, delusions, feeling afloat); heightened sensitivity to pain

Objective
Restlessness; irritability
Inability to concentrate; slowed reaction
Listlessness; apathy
Fleeting nystagmus; hand tremors
Acute confusion; transient paranoia; agitation; combativeness; hallucinations

Sample Clinical Applications: Chronic obstructive pulmonary disease (COPD), heart failure (nocturia), chronic pain, sleep apnea, pregnancy, postpartum, colic, dementia, Alzheimer's disease, anxiety disorders, posttraumatic stress disorder

DESIRED OUTCOMES/EVALUATION CRITERIA

Sample (NOC) linkages:
Sleep: Natural periodic suspension of consciousness during which the body is restored
Rest: Quantity and pattern of diminished activity for mental and physical rejuvenation
Pain Control: Personal actions to control pain

Client Will (Include Specific Time Frame)
• Identify individually appropriate interventions to promote sleep.
• Verbalize understanding of sleep disorder.
• Adjust lifestyle to accommodate chronobiological rhythms.
• Report improvement in sleep and rest pattern.

Sample (NOC) linkages:
• **Family Coping:** Family actions to manage stressors that tax an individual's resources

Family Will (Include Specific Time Frame)
• Deal appropriately with parasomnias.

ACTIONS/INTERVENTIONS

Sample (NIC) linkages:
Sleep Enhancement: Facilitation of regular sleep/wake cycles
Anxiety Reduction: Minimizing apprehension, dread, foreboding, or uneasiness related to an unidentified source or anticipated danger
Environmental Management: Comfort: Manipulation of the patient's surroundings for promotion of optimal comfort

NURSING PRIORITY NO. 1

To assess causative/contributing factors:

● Note client's age and developmental stage. *The average adult requires 7 to 8 hours sleep; pregnant women and new mothers, while needing more sleep, usually are sleep deprived; studies show that sleep disorders occur in 35% to 45% of children age 2 to 18 years;[16] adolescents and young adults don't get enough sleep, have irregular sleep patterns, and are at risk for problem sleepiness;[18] menopausal women often report interrupted sleep because of hot flashes or hormonal influences; elderly persons sleep fewer hours, report less restful sleep and need for more sleep.[1-5,15,16]*

● Determine presence of physical or psychological stressors: *These include multiple, varying factors, such as night-shift work hours or rotating shifts; pain (acute and chronic), current or recent illness, hospitalization, especially in intensive care unit; death of a spouse, loss of a job; new baby in the home, inadequate sleep-promoting behaviors, and so forth.*

● Note presence of diagnoses *that are known to affect sleep (e.g., mental confusion or dementias, certain brain infections [e.g., encephalitis], brain injury, narcolepsy, obsessive/compulsive disorder, anxiety, depression, and other major psychological disorders; drug or alcohol abuse; restless leg syndrome; sleep-induced respiratory disorders—obstructive sleep apnea, childhood snoring with sleep apnea).[6,7]*

● Evaluate medication regimen for products affecting sleep. *Diet pills or other stimulants, sedatives, antidepressants, antihypertensives, diuretics, narcotics, agents with anticholinergic effects, and need for medications requiring nighttime dosing can inhibit getting to sleep or remaining asleep.[8,9,20]*

● Note environmental factors affecting sleep *(e.g., unfamiliar or uncomfortable sleep environment, excessive noise and light, frequent checking of vital signs, uncomfortable temperature, roommate irritations or actions—snoring, watching television late at night). Note: Clients in critical care units are known to experience lack of sleep or frequent disruptions, often compounding their illness.[9]*

● Determine presence of parasomnias: nightmares or terrors, sleepwalking or talking, or other complex behaviors during sleep. *May occur at any age, with as many as 30% of children (peak age 4 to 8 years) having a sleep disorder at some time.[20] Note reports of terror, brief periods of paralysis, sense of body being disconnected from the brain. Occurrence of sleep paralysis, though not widely recognized in the United States, has been well documented elsewhere and may result in feelings of fear and reluctance to go to sleep. May require more extensive evaluation for serious sleep disorders.[10,17]*

NURSING PRIORITY NO. 2

To assess degree of impairment:

- Assess client's usual sleep patterns and current sleep disturbance, relying on client's/SO's report of problem. Incorporate screening information into in-depth sleep diary or testing if needed. *Usual sleep patterns are individual, but sleep loss has been shown to be the most common complaint reported in primary care settings;[4,11]therefore, screening for the problem should be routine. Data collected from a comprehensive assessment is needed to determine etiology of challenging sleep disturbances, including the stage of sleep that is impaired.[9,12]*
- Ascertain quality of sleep for bed partner/family members. *Loud irregular snoring (sleep apnea), periodic nightmares or sleep terrors, or sleep talking, sleepwalking, or involuntary muscle activity can interfere with sleep of bed partner/entire family.[20]*
- Determine client's sleep expectations. *Individual may have faulty beliefs or attitudes about sleep and unrealistic sleep expectations (e.g., "I must get 8 hours of sleep every night, or I can't accomplish anything").[11]*
- Ascertain duration of current problem and effect on life and functional ability. *Client may not get enough sleep and not realize that life functioning is being impaired (e.g., can't concentrate in school, falls asleep when stopped at a light while driving).[11]*
- Listen to subjective reports of sleep quality (e.g., "short, interrupted") and response from lack of good sleep (feeling foggy, sleepy, and woozy; fighting sleep; fatigue). *Helps clarify client's perception of sleep quantity and quality, and response to inadequate sleep.[11]*
- Observe for physical signs of fatigue. *Client may display restlessness, irritability, disorientation, frequent yawning, and/or other changes in mood, behavior or performance (e.g., inability to tolerate stress, problems with concentration or learning). Fatigue, daytime sleepiness, and functional impairment have been reported as significant problem in teens.[3,4,11,15,20]*
- Determine interventions client has tried to date. *Helps identify appropriate options and may reveal additional interventions that can be attempted.*
- Distinguish client's beneficial bedtime habits from detrimental ones *(e.g., drinking late-evening milk versus late-evening coffee).*
- Instruct client and/or bed partner to keep a sleep-wake log *to document symptoms and identify factors that are interfering with sleep.*
- Obtain a chronological chart *to determine client's peak performance rhythms.*
- Investigate anxious feelings *to help determine basis and appropriate anxiety-reduction techniques or behavioral therapy needs.[20]*

NURSING PRIORITY NO. 3

To assist client to establish optimal sleep pattern:[2,4,5,8,9,11,13,14]

- Review medications being taken and their effect on sleep, suggesting modifications in regimen, *if medications are found to be interfering.*
- Encourage client to restrict caffeine and other stimulating substances from late-afternoon and evening intake. Recommend avoidance of bedtime alcohol. *Both alcohol and some medications can produce immediate sleep followed by early awakening or difficulty remaining asleep.*
- Avoid eating large evening or late-night meals.
- Recommend light bedtime snack (protein, simple carbohydrate, and low fat) and/or glass of warm milk for individuals who feel hungry, ingested 15 to 30 minutes before retiring. *Sense of fullness and satiety can encourage sleep.*
- Limit evening fluid intake if nocturia is present *to reduce need for nighttime elimination.*

- Promote adequate physical exercise activity during day, finishing workout at least 3 hours before bedtime. *Enhances expenditure of energy and release of tension so that client feels ready for sleep or rest. Note: Rigorous exercise close to bedtime can delay onset of sleep.*
- Suggest abstaining from daytime naps, or napping in the morning *to improve ability to fall asleep at night.*
- Recommend quiet relaxing activities prior to bedtime such as reading, listening to soothing music, meditation *to reduce stimulation and promote relaxation.*
- Discuss or implement effective age-appropriate bedtime rituals (e.g., going to bed at same time each night, brushing teeth, reading, drinking warm milk, rocking, story reading, cuddling, favorite blanket or toy) *to enhance client's ability to fall asleep, reinforce that bed is a place to sleep, and promote sense of security for child.*
- Provide back massage or other therapeutic touching activities, as appropriate. *Touch can be relaxing and emotionally pleasing, given that the client has SO's undivided attention for a few moments.*
- Provide calm, quiet environment for hospitalized client, *to manage controllable sleep-disrupting factors (e.g., reduce noise and talking, dim lights, shut room door, adjust room temperature as needed, silence or reduce volume on phones, beepers, alarms, television, radios).*
- Administer pain medication first *to make sure client is pain-free,* and then sedatives or other sleep medications *(so that hypnotic will be more effective)* when indicated, noting client's response. Time pain medications for peak effect and duration *to reduce need for redosing during prime sleep hours.*
- Discuss appropriate use of benzodiazepines when indicated. *May be useful in some clients for reducing risk of injury associated with sleepwalking or for management of severe sleep terrors.*[20]
- Instruct client to get out of bed, leave bedroom, engage in relaxing activities *if unable to fall asleep,* and not return to bed until feeling sleepy.
- Recommend and instruct client in relaxation techniques (e.g., visualization, breathing, yoga).
- Refer for biofeedback, cognitive therapy, and so forth, *when measures that are more intensive are needed or desired to cope with stressors and promote relaxation.*
- Collaborate with healthcare team for evaluation and treatment of more serious sleep problems (e.g., obstructive sleep apnea, narcolepsy, sleep paralysis, bed-wetting, nocturnal leg cramps, restless leg syndrome).[16,17,19,20]
- Review with the client the physician's recommendations for managing obstructive sleep apnea such as medical or surgical treatment of obesity; medications, structural surgery (e.g., alteration of facial structures; removal of tonsils and adenoids in children),[19] or apnea/oxygenation therapy—continuous positive airway pressure (CPAP) such as Respironics—*when sleep apnea is severe as documented by sleep-disorder studies.*

NURSING PRIORITY NO. 4

To promote wellness (Teaching/Discharge Considerations):

- Review possibility of next-day drowsiness or "rebound" insomnia and temporary memory loss *that may be associated with sleep disorders and/or prescription sleep medications.*
- Discuss short-term use and appropriateness of over-the-counter (OTC) sleep medications or herbal supplements. Note possible side effects and drug interactions.
- Identify appropriate safety precautions (e.g., securing doors, windows and stairways, placing client bedroom on first floor), and attaching audible alarm to bedroom door *to alert parents when child is sleepwalking.*[19]

- Refer to support group or counselor *to help deal with psychological stressors (e.g., grief, sorrow).* (Refer to NDs Grieving, chronic Sorrow.)
- Encourage family counseling as indicated *to help deal with concerns arising from parasomnias (e.g., sleep talking, sleepwalking, night terrors).*
- Refer to sleep specialist for sleep studies *when problem is unresponsive to customary interventions.*

DOCUMENTATION FOCUS

Assessment/Reassessment
- Assessment findings, including specifics of sleep pattern (current and past) and effects on lifestyle/level of functioning.
- Medications used, interventions tried, previous therapies.
- Family history of similar problem.
- Effects of sleep disturbance on SO/family.

Planning
- Plan of care and who is involved in planning.
- Teaching plan.

Implementation/Evaluation
- Client's response to interventions, teaching, and actions performed.
- Attainment or progress toward desired outcome(s).
- Modifications to plan of care.

Discharge Planning
- Long-term needs and who is responsible for actions to be taken.
- Specific referrals made.

References

1. Cox, H. C., et al. (2002). ND: Sleep Deprivation (developmental considerations). *Clinical Applications of Nursing Diagnosis: Adult, Child, Women's, Psychiatric, Gerontic, and Home Health Considerations.* 4th ed. Philadelphia: F. A. Davis, 368–369.
2. Mindell, J. (1997). *Sleeping Through the Night: How Infants, Toddlers, and Their Parents Can Get a Good Night's Sleep.* New York: HarperCollins.
3. Adolescent sleep needs and patterns: Research report and resource guide. National Sleep Foundation. Retrieved July 2007 from www.sleepfoundation.org.
4. Women and sleep. National Sleep Foundation. Retrieved July 2007 from www.sleepfoundation.org.
5. Bahr, R. T., Sr. (1999). Sleep disturbances. In Stanley, M., Beare, P. G. (eds). *Gerontological Nursing: A Health Promotion/Protection Approach.* 2d ed. Philadelphia: F. A. Davis, 337–341.
6. Sateia, M. J., (2000). Evaluation of chronic insomnia: An American Academy of Sleep Medicine review. *Sleep*, 23(2), 243–308.
7. Subcommittee on Obstructive Sleep Apnea Syndrome, American Academy of Pediatrics Section on Pediatric Pulmonology. (2002). Clinical practice guideline: Diagnosis and management of childhood obstructive sleep apnea syndrome. *Pediatrics*, 109(4), 704–712.
8. Barroso, J. (2003). Living with illness: HIV-related fatigue. *Am J Nurs*, 102(5), 83.
9. Honkus, V. L. (2003). Sleep deprivation in critical care units. *Crit Care Nurs Quart*, 26(3), 179–191.
10. Cardinal, F. (2004). Sleep disorders—The basics. Retrieved July 2007 from http://sleepdisorders.about.com.

11. Cochran, H. (2003). Diagnose and treat primary insomnia *Nurse Pract*, 28(9), 13–27.
12. Spenceley, S. M. (1993). Sleep inquiry: A look with fresh eyes. *Image*, 25(3), 249–255.
13. Pronitis-Ruotolo, D. (2001). Surviving the night shift: Making Zeitgeber work for you. *Am J Nurs*, 101(7), 63.
14. Cmiel, C. A. (2004). Noise control: A nursing team's approach to sleep promotion. *Am J Nurs*, 104(2), 40–48.
15. National Agricultural Safety Database (NASD) (2002). Sleep deprivation: Cause and consequences. Fact sheet for Nebraska Rural Health and Safety Coalition. Retrieved August 2007 from www.cdc.gov/nasd/docs/d000701-d000800/d000705/d000705.html.
16. Connelly, K. P. (2006). Sleep disorders: Nightmares. Retrieved July 2007 from www.emedicine.com/ped/topic1609.htm.
17. Bruis, M. J. (2004, editorial review 2005). Sleep disorders: Parasomnias. Retrieved July 2007 from www.medicinenet.com/script/main/art.asp?articlekey=47489.
18. National Sleep Foundation Sleep and Teens Task Force. (2000). *Adolescent Sleep Needs and Patterns: Research Report and Resource Guide*. Washington, DC: National Sleep Foundation, 2–4.
19. Garcia, J., Wills, L. (2002). Sleep disorders in children and teens: Helping patients and their families get some sleep. *Postgrad Med*, 107(3), 161–188.
20. Schenck, C. H., Mahowald, M. W. (2002). Parasomnias: Managing bizarre sleep-related behavior disorders. *Postgrad Med*, 107(3), 145–160.

disturbed Sleep Pattern

DEFINITION: Time-limited interruptions of sleep amount and quality due to external factors

RELATED FACTORS

Ambient temperature, humidity; lighting; noise; noxious odors; physical restraint
Change in daylight-darkness exposure
Caregiving responsibilities
Lack of sleep privacy or control; sleep partner
Unfamiliar sleep surroundings
Interruptions (e.g., for therapeutics, monitoring, lab tests)

DEFINING CHARACTERISTICS

Subjective
Reports no difficulty falling asleep; reports being awakened
Verbal complaints of not feeling well rested; dissatisfaction with sleep

Objective
Change in normal sleep pattern
Decreased ability to function

Sample Clinical Applications: Hospitalized or long-term care client, ill family member

(continues on page 774)

disturbed Sleep Pattern (continued)
DESIRED OUTCOMES/EVALUATION CRITERIA

Sample (NOC) linkages:
Sleep: Natural periodic suspension of consciousness during which the body is restored
Comfort Status: Environment: Environmental ease, comfort, and safety of surroundings

Client Will (Include Specific Time Frame)
• Report improved sleep.
• Report increased sense of well-being and feeling rested.
• Identify individually appropriate interventions to promote sleep.

ACTIONS/INTERVENTIONS

Sample (NIC) linkages:
Sleep Enhancement: Facilitation of regular sleep-wake cycles
Environmental Management: Comfort: Manipulation of the patients surroundings for promotion of optimal comfort

NURSING PRIORITY NO. 1

To assess causative/contributing factors:

● Identify presence of factors known to interfere with sleep, including current illness, hospitalization; new baby or sick family member in home, and so forth. *Sleep problems can arise from internal and external factors and may require assessment over time to differentiate specific cause(s).*
  Note: *Unresolved long-term disturbances in sleep are thought to cause dysfunction of the immune system, interference with wound healing, neurological and behavioral changes, and significant impairment of quality of life.*[1] Refer to ND Sleep Deprivation.
● Ascertain presence of short-term alteration in sleep patterns, such as can occur with travel (jet-lag), sharing bed with new sleep partner, fighting with family member, crisis at work, loss of job, death in family. *Helps identify circumstances that are known to interrupt sleep acutely but do not necessarily represent long-term conditions. These situations may require short-term interventions but are often resolved over time.*[2]
● Note environmental factors, such as unfamiliar or uncomfortable room; excessive noise and light; uncomfortable temperature; frequent medical and monitoring interventions; and roommate actions (e.g., snoring, watching television late at night, wanting to talk). *These factors can reduce client's ability to rest and sleep at a time when more rest is needed.* Note: Clients in critical care units are known to experience lack of sleep or frequent disruptions, often compounding their illness.[3,4]

NURSING PRIORITY NO. 2

To evaluate sleep and degree of dysfunction:

● Assess client's usual sleep patterns and compare with current sleep disturbance, relying on client's/SO's report of problem *to ascertain intensity and duration of problems.*
● Listen to reports of sleep quality (e.g., "short, interrupted") and response from lack of good sleep (e.g., feeling foggy, sleepy, and woozy; fighting sleep; fatigue). *Helps clarify client's perception of sleep quantity and quality, and response to inadequate sleep.*[5]

- Determine client's sleep expectations. *Individual may have faulty beliefs or attitudes about sleep and/or unrealistic sleep expectations (e.g., "I must get 8 hours of sleep every night, or I can't accomplish anything").*[3,5]
- Observe for physical signs of fatigue (e.g., restlessness, hand tremors, thick speech, drooping eyes, inattention, lack of interest in activities).
- Incorporate screening information into in-depth sleep diary or testing if needed. *Information collected from a comprehensive assessment may be needed to evaluate the type and etiology of sleep disturbance and identify useful treatment options.*[5-7]

NURSING PRIORITY NO. 3

To assist client to establish optimal sleep/rest patterns:

- Manage environment for hospitalized client:[1,3,4,8-10]
  Adjust ambient lighting *to maintain daytime light and nighttime dark.*
  Provide privacy as indicated, such as requesting visitors to leave, closing room door, "quiet, patient sleeping" sign, etc.
  Encourage usual bedtime activities such as washing face and hands and brushing teeth.
  Provide HS care such as straightening bed sheets, changing damp linens or gown, back massage *to promote physical comfort.*
  Turn on soft music, calm TV program, or quiet environment, as client prefers, *to enhance relaxation.*
  Minimize sleep-disrupting factors (e.g., shut room door, adjust room temperature as needed, reduce talking and other disturbing noises such as phones, beepers, alarms). *Studies show that use of these interventions can promote readiness for sleep and improve sleep duration and quality.*[11]
  Perform monitoring and care activities without waking client whenever possible. *Allows for longer periods of uninterrupted sleep, especially during night.*
  Avoid or limit use of physical restraints in accordance with client's needs and facility policy.
- Refer to physician or sleep specialist as indicated *for specific interventions and/or therapies, including medications, biofeedback.*
- Refer to NDs Insomnia and Sleep Deprivation for related interventions and rationale.

NURSING PRIORITY NO. 4

To promote wellness (Teaching/Discharge Considerations):

- Assure client that occasional sleeplessness should not threaten health and that resolving time-limited situation can restore healthful sleep. *Knowledge that occasional insomnia is universal and usually not harmful may promote relaxation and relief from worry, which can perpetuate the problem.*[12]
- Problem-solve immediate needs. *Short-term solutions (e.g., sleeping in different rooms if partner's illness is keeping client awake, acquiring a fan if sleeping quarters are too warm, or getting a substitute to provide care to ill family member so client can get a good night's rest) may be needed until client adjusts to situation or crisis is resolved, with resulting return to more usual sleep pattern.*
- Encourage appropriate indoor light settings during day and night, avoidance of daytime napping as appropriate for age and situation, being active during day and more passive in evening. *Helps in promotion of normal sleep-wake patterns.*[8]
- Investigate use of aids to block out light and sound, such as sleep mask, room-darkening shades, earplugs, white noise.[3,10]

Nursing Diagnoses in Alphabetical Order

● Discuss use and appropriateness of over-the-counter (OTC) sleep medications or herbal supplements *to provide assistance in falling and staying asleep.*

DOCUMENTATION FOCUS

Assessment/Reassessment
- Assessment findings, including specifics of sleep pattern (current and past) and effects on lifestyle and level of functioning.
- Specific interventions, medications, or previously tried therapies.

Planning
- Plan of care and who is involved in planning.
- Teaching plan.

Implementation/Evaluation
- Response to interventions, teaching, and actions performed.
- Attainment or progress toward desired outcome(s).
- Modifications to plan of care.

Discharge Planning
- Long-term needs and who is responsible for actions to be taken.
- Available resources, specific referrals made.

References

1. Weinhouse, G. L., Schwab, R. J. (2006). Sleep in the critically ill patient. *Sleep*, 29(5), 707–716.
2. Sateia, M. J., et al. (2000). Evaluation of chronic insomnia: An American Academy of Sleep Medicine review. *Sleep*, 23(2), 243–308.
3. Doenges, M. E., Moorhouse, M. F., Murr, A. C. (2006). ND: disturbed Sleep Pattern. *Nurse's Pocket Guide: Diagnoses, Interventions and Rationales*. 10th ed. Philadelphia: F. A. Davis.
4. Patel, M., et al. (2008). Sleep in the intensive care setting. *Crit Care Nurs Q*, 31(4), 309–318.
5. Cochran, H. (2003). Diagnose and treat primary insomnia. *Nurse Pract*, 28(9), 13–27.
6. Honkus, V. L. (2003). Sleep deprivation in critical care units. *Crit Care Nurs Q*, 26(3), 179–191.
7. Spenceley, S. M. (1993). Sleep inquiry: A look with fresh eyes. *Image*, 25(3), 249–255.
8. Cole, C., Richards, K. (2007). Sleep disruption in older adults. *Am J Nurs*, 107(5), 40–49.
9. Richards, K. C. (1996). Sleep promotion. *Crit Care Clin North Am*, 8(1), 39–52.
10. Floyd, J. A. (2008). Sleep enhancement. In Ackley, B. J., Ladwig, G. B., Swan, B. A., Tucker, S. J. (eds). *Evidence-Based Nursing Care Guidelines: Medical-Surgical Interventions*. St. Louis, MO: Mosby Elsevier.
11. Olsen, D. M., et al. (2001). Quiet time: A nursing intervention to promote sleep in neurocritical care units. *Am J Crit Care*, 10(2), 74–78.
12. National Institute of Neurological Disorders and Stroke (NINDS). Brain basics. Understanding sleep. Retrieved March 2009 from www.ninds.nih.gov/disorders/brain_basics/understanding _sleep.htm.

 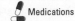

readiness for enhanced Sleep

DEFINITION: A pattern of natural, periodic suspension of consciousness that provides adequate rest, sustains a desired lifestyle, and can be strengthened

RELATED FACTORS

To be developed by nurse researchers and submitted to NANDA

DEFINING CHARACTERISTICS

Subjective
Expresses willingness to enhance sleep
Expresses a feeling of being rested after sleep
Follows sleep routines that promote sleep habits

Objective
Amount of sleep and rapid eye movement (REM) sleep is congruent with developmental needs
Occasional or infrequent use of medications to induce sleep

Sample Clinical Applications: Postoperative recovery, chronic pain, pregnancy—prenatal/postpartal period, sleep apnea

DESIRED OUTCOMES/EVALUATION CRITERIA

Sample NOC linkages:
Sleep: Natural periodic suspension of consciousness during which the body is restored
Rest: Quantity and pattern of diminished activity for mental and physical rejuvenation
Comfort Level: Extent of positive perception of physical and psychological ease

Client Will (Include Specific Time Frame)
• Identify individually appropriate interventions to promote sleep.
• Verbalize feeling rested after sleep.
• Adjust lifestyle to accommodate routines that promote sleep.

ACTIONS/INTERVENTIONS

Sample NIC linkages:
Sleep Enhancement: Facilitation of regular sleep-wake cycles
Relaxation Therapy: Use of techniques to encourage and elicit relaxation for the purpose of decreasing undesirable signs and symptoms such as pain, muscle tension, or anxiety
Environmental Management: Manipulation of the patient's surroundings for therapeutic benefit

NURSING PRIORITY NO. 1

To determine motivation for continued growth:

● Listen to client's reports of sleep quantity and quality. Determine client's perception of adequate sleep. *Reveals client's experience and expectations regarding sleep. Provides opportunity to address misconceptions or unrealistic expectations and plan for interventions.*

- Observe or obtain feedback from client/SO(s) regarding usual bedtime, number of hours of sleep, time of arising *to determine usual sleep pattern and provide comparative baseline for improvements.*
- Ascertain motivation and expectation for change. *Motivation to improve and high expectations can encourage client to make changes that will improve his or her life. However, unrealistic expectations may hamper efforts.*
- Note client report of potential for alteration of habitual sleep time (e.g., change of work pattern or rotating shifts) or change in normal bedtime (e.g., hospitalization). *Helps identify circumstances that are known to interrupt sleep patterns and that could disrupt the person's biological rhythms.*[1,2,8]

NURSING PRIORITY NO. 2

To assist client to enhance sleep/rest:

- Review client's usual bedtime rituals, routines, and environmental needs. *Provides information on client's management of the situation and identifies areas that might be modified when the need arises.*
- Discuss or implement effective age-appropriate bedtime rituals for infant/child (e.g., rocking, story reading, cuddling, favorite blanket or toy). *Rituals can enhance ability to fall asleep, reinforce that bed is a place to sleep, and promote sense of security for child.*[3]
- Provide quiet environment and comfort measures (e.g., back rub, washing hands and face, cleaning and straightening sheets) for client in facility. *Promotes relaxation and readiness for sleep.*
- Arrange care *to provide for uninterrupted periods for rest.* Explain necessity of disturbances for monitoring vital signs or other care when client is hospitalized. Do as much care as possible during night without waking client. *Allows for longer periods of uninterrupted sleep, especially during night.*
- Suggest limiting fluid intake in evening if nocturia or bed-wetting is a problem *to reduce need for nighttime elimination.*
- Provide instruction in use of necessary equipment. *Client may use oxygen or CPAP system to improve sleep/rest in presence of hypoxia or sleep apnea.*
- Discuss dietary matters, such as limiting chocolate, heavy meals, caffeine or alcoholic beverages prior to bedtime, *which are substances known to impair falling or staying asleep. Use of alcohol at bedtime may help individual fall asleep, but ensuing sleep is then fragmented.*[4]
- Explore or implement use of warm bath, intake of light protein snack before bedtime, comfortable room temperature, soothing music, favorite calming television show. *Nonpharmaceutical aids may enhance falling asleep without the undesired side effects associated with medications.*
- Investigate use of sleep mask, darkening shades or curtains, earplugs, low-level background (white) noise in situations *where sleep might not come easily or be disturbed by environmental factors.*
- Recommend continuing same schedule for sleep throughout week—including days off. *Maintaining sleep pattern helps sustain biological rhythms.*

NURSING PRIORITY NO. 3

To promote optimum wellness:

- Assure client that occasional sleeplessness should not threaten health. *Knowledge that occasional insomnia is universal and usually not harmful may promote relaxation and relief from worry.*[5]

- Encourage regular exercise during the day *to aid in stress control and release of energy. Note: Exercise at bedtime may stimulate rather than relax client and may actually interfere with sleep.*[7]
- Assist to develop individual program of relaxation (e.g., biofeedback, self-hypnosis, visualization, progressive muscle relaxation). *Reduces sympathetic response and stress to aid in inducing sleep.*[6]
- Address sleep management techniques that may be useful during stressful conditions or lifestyle changes (e.g., pregnancy, new baby, menopause, medical procedures, new job, moving, change in relationship, grief).
- Recommend periodic review of medications. *Many prescription and over-the-counter (OTC) drugs can disrupt sleep.*
- Advise using prescription or OTC sleep medications sparingly. These medications, while useful for promoting sleep in the short-term, can interfere with REM sleep.

DOCUMENTATION FOCUS

Assessment/Reassessment
- Assessment findings, including specifics of sleep pattern and effects on lifestyle/level of functioning.
- Any medications used, interventions tried, previous therapies.
- Motivation and expectations for change.

Planning
- Plan of care and who is involved in planning.
- Teaching plan.

Implementation/Evaluation
- Client's response to interventions, teaching, and actions performed.
- Attainment or progress toward desired outcome(s).
- Modifications to plan of care.

Discharge Planning
- Long-term needs and who is responsible for actions to be taken.
- Specific referrals made.

References

1. Cochran, H. (2003). Diagnose and treat primary insomnia. *Nurse Pract*, 28(9), 13–27.
2. Spenceley, S. M. (1993). Sleep inquiry: A look with fresh eyes. *Image*, 25(3), 249–255.
3. Mindell, J. (1997). *Sleeping Through the Night: How Infants, Toddlers, and Their Parents Can Get a Good Night's Sleep.* New York: HarperCollins.
4. Bahr, R. T., Sr. (1999). Sleep disturbances. In Stanley, M., Beare, P. G. (eds). *Gerontological Nursing: A Health Promotion/Protection Approach.* 2d ed. Philadelphia: F. A. Davis, 335–341.
5. National Institute of Neurological Disorders and Stroke (NINDS). Brain basics: Understanding sleep. Retrieved July 2007 from www.ninds.nih.gov.
6. Cox, H. C., et al. (2002). ND: Sleep Pattern, disturbed. *Clinical Applications of Nursing Diagnosis: Adult, Child, Women's, Psychiatric, Gerontic, and Home Health Considerations.* 4th ed. Philadelphia: F. A. Davis, 375–380.
7. Grandjean, C. K., Gibbons, S. W. (2000). Assessing ambulatory geriatric sleep complaints. *Nurse Pract: Am J Prim Health Care*, 25(9), 25.
8. Pronitis-Ruotolo, D. (2001). Surviving the night shift: Making Zeitgeber work for you. *Am J Nurs*, 101(7), 63.

impaired Social Interaction

DEFINITION: Insufficient or excessive quantity or ineffective quality of social exchange

RELATED FACTORS

Deficit about ways to enhance mutuality (e.g., knowledge, skills)
Communication barriers [including head injury, stroke, other neurological conditions affecting ability to communicate]
Self-concept disturbance
Absence of significant others
Limited physical mobility [e.g., neuromuscular disease]
Therapeutic isolation
Sociocultural dissonance
Environmental barriers
Disturbed thought processes

DEFINING CHARACTERISTICS

Subjective
Discomfort in social situations
Inability to communicate or receive a satisfying sense of social engagement (e.g., belonging, caring, interest, or shared history)
Family report of changes in interaction (e.g., style, pattern)

Objective
Use of unsuccessful social interaction behaviors
Dysfunctional interaction with others

Sample Clinical Applications: Brain injury, stroke, cancer, neuromuscular disease (e.g., multiple sclerosis [MS]), cerebral palsy, substance abuse, Alzheimer's disease, schizophrenia, autism

DESIRED OUTCOMES/EVALUATION CRITERIA

Sample NOC linkages:
Social Interaction Skills: Personal behaviors that promote effective relationships
Child Development: (specify age): Milestones of physical, cognitive, and psychosocial progression by [specify] months/years of age
Role Performance: Congruence of an individual's role behavior with role expectations

Client Will (Include Specific Time Frame)
• Verbalize awareness of factors causing or promoting impaired social interactions.
• Identify feelings that lead to poor social interactions.
• Express desire or be involved in achieving positive changes in social behaviors and interpersonal relationships.
• Give self positive reinforcement for changes that are achieved.
• Develop effective social support system; use available resources appropriately.

ACTIONS/INTERVENTIONS

Sample (NIC) linkages:
Socialization Enhancement: Facilitation of another person's ability to interact with others
Behavior Modification: Social Skills: Assisting the patient to develop or improve interpersonal social skills
Complex Relationship Building: Establishing a therapeutic relationship with a patient to promote insight and behavioral change

NURSING PRIORITY NO. 1

To assess causative/contributing factors:

- Review social history with client/SO(s) and go back far enough in time to note when changes in social behavior or patterns of relating occurred or began. *For example, loss or long-term illness of loved one; failed relationships; loss of occupation, financial, or political (power) position; change in status in family hierarchy (job loss, aging, illness); poor coping or adjustment to developmental stage of life, as with marriage, birth or adoption of child, or children leaving home are situations that may affect quality of social exchange.*[1]
- Ascertain ethnic, cultural, or religious implications for the client. *These factors can dictate choice of behaviors, may even script interactions with others. Client may perceive behaviors as normal because of belief system or may have conflict regarding behaviors that are not accepted by larger society, such as homosexuality or gender identity disorder.*[1,5,6]
- Review medical history, noting stressors of physical or long-term illness (e.g., stroke, cancer, MS, head injury, Alzheimer's disease), mental illness (e.g., schizophrenia), medications, substance use, debilitating accidents, learning disabilities (e.g., sensory integration difficulties, Asperger's disorder, autism spectrum disorder), and emotional disabilities. *Conditions such as these can isolate individual who feels disconnected from others, resulting in difficulty relating in social situations.*[3,4]
- Note presence of visual or hearing impairments. *Individuals with these conditions may find communication barriers are increased, social interaction is affected, and interventions need to be designed to promote involvement with others in positive ways.*[1,3]
- Determine family patterns of relating and social behaviors. Explore possible family scripting of behavioral expectations in the children and how the client was affected. *Parents are important in teaching their children social skills (e.g., sharing, taking turns, and allowing others to talk without interrupting). Family may not have effective patterns of relating to others, and the child learns these skills in this setting. Often child reflects family expectations rather than own desires, which may result in conforming or rebellious behaviors.*[2,6,9]
- Observe client while relating to family/SO(s) and note observations of prevalent patterns. *Identification of patterns will help with plan for change.*[2]
- Encourage client to verbalize feeling of discomfort about social situations. Note any causative factors, recurring precipitating patterns, and barriers to using support systems. *Identifies areas of concern and suggests possible ways to learn new skills.*[2]

NURSING PRIORITY NO. 2

To assess degree of impairment:

- Encourage client to verbalize perceptions of reasons for problems. Active-listen noting indications of hopelessness, powerlessness, fear, anxiety, grief, anger, feeling unloved or unlovable, problems with sexual identity, hate (directed or not). *These feelings arise from the anxiety that comes with the need to participate with others in social situations and begin to interfere with work, friendships, and life in general.*[5,7]

- Observe and describe social and interpersonal behaviors in objective terms, noting speech patterns, body language (1) in the therapeutic setting and (2) in normal areas of daily functioning (if possible): family, job, social or entertainment settings. *Provides information about extent of anxiety client experiences in different settings and suggests possible interventions.*[5,7]
- Determine client's use of coping skills and defense mechanisms. *Symptoms associated with social anxiety affect ability to be involved in social situations, making client's life miserable and seriously interfering with work, friendships, and family life.*[5,7]
- Evaluate possibility of client being the victim of or using destructive behaviors against self or others. (Refer to ND [actual/]risk for other-directed/self-directed Violence.) *Problems of poor communication lead to frustration and anger, leaving the individual with few coping skills and may result in destructive behaviors.*[1,2]
- Interview family, SO(s), friends, spiritual leaders, coworkers, as appropriate. *Obtaining observations of client's behavioral changes from others associated with the individual provides a broader view of actual problems and how behavior affects client's life/others.*[5]

NURSING PRIORITY NO. 3

To assist client/SO(s) to recognize/make positive changes in impaired social and interpersonal interactions:

- Establish therapeutic relationship using positive regard for the person, Active-listening, and providing safe environment for self-disclosure. *Client who is having difficulty interacting in social situations needs to feel comfortable and accepted before he or she is willing to talk about self and concerns.*[1,2]
- Have client list behaviors that cause discomfort. *Anxiety usually has physical symptoms (e.g., a racing heart, dry mouth, shaky voice, blushing, sweating, and nausea) and once recognized, client can choose to begin treatment to change.*[5,7]
- Have family/SO(s) list client's behaviors that are causing discomfort for them. *Anxiety is contagious, and by identifying specific behaviors, all members of the family can begin to deal appropriately with them so they are diminished.*[5,7]
- Review negative behaviors observed previously by caregivers, coworkers, and so forth. *Others may see behaviors and the problems associated with them, such as unwillingness to participate in necessary activities (eating in a public place, interviewing for a job) and may provide additional information needed to develop an appropriate plan of care.*[1]
- Compare lists and validate reality of perceptions. Help client prioritize those behaviors needing change. *Each individual may have a different view of what constitutes a problem, and by comparing lists, each person hears how others view the problems, enabling the client/family to identify behaviors or concerns to be dealt with.*[1,7]
- Explore with client and role-play means of making agreed upon changes in social interactions or behaviors (as determined earlier). *Client needs to learn social skills if he or she has never learned the elements of interacting with others in social settings. Role-playing one on one is less threatening and can help individual identify with another and practice new social skills.*[5]
- Role-play random social situations in therapeutically controlled environment with "safe" therapy group. Have group note behaviors, both positive and negative, and discuss these and any changes needed. *Having client participate in a controlled group environment provides opportunities to try out different behaviors in a built-in social setting where members can make friends and provide mutual advice and comfort.*[1,5]

Cultural   Collaborative   Community/Home Care   Diagnostic Studies   Pediatric/Geriatric/Lifespan   Medications

- Role-play changes and discuss impact. Include family/SO(s) as indicated. *Provides opportunity for person to recognize changes in feelings and behavior and enhances comfort with new behaviors.*[4]
- Provide positive reinforcement for improvement in social behaviors and interactions. *Encourages continuation of desired behaviors and efforts for change.*[5]
- Participate in multidisciplinary client-centered conferences *to evaluate progress.* Involve everyone associated with client's care, family members, SO(s), and therapy group. *These conferences have the advantage of providing information from and to each participant in an atmosphere of trust where questions can be asked, decisions can be made, and goals for the future can be agreed on.*[1]
- Work with the client to alleviate underlying negative self-concepts *because they often impede positive social interactions. By replacing negative thoughts with positive messages, client can reduce anxiety and develop a positive sense of self-esteem. While this is not an easy process, the rewards are great when client is willing to practice consistently.*[2]
- Involve neurologically impaired client in individual or group interactions as situation allows. *Individual may not be able to interact appropriately because of disabilities, but involvement in the group provides an opportunity to practice and relearn skills to enable reintegration into social situations.*[1,8]
- Refer for family therapy as indicated. *Social behaviors and interpersonal relationships involve more than the individual, and family may need additional help to resolve ongoing family problems.*[1,2]

NURSING PRIORITY NO. 4

To promote wellness (Teaching/Discharge Considerations):

- Encourage client to keep a daily journal in which social interactions of each day can be reviewed and the comfort or discomfort experienced noted with possible causes or precipitating factors. *Helps client to identify specific problem areas and begin to choose to take responsibility for own behavior(s).*[5,7]
- Assist the client to develop positive social skills through practice of skills in real social situations accompanied by a support person. Provide positive feedback with the use of I-messages during interactions with client. *Cognitive and behavioral methods can help individuals overcome fears with the help of a trusted person. I-messages convey a positive message, individual does not feel criticized, and is encouraged to continue new thinking and behaviors.*[1,5]
- Discuss the use of medications when indicated and monitor for effectiveness and side effects. *Several kinds of drugs have been found to be effective in the treatment of social anxiety problems, selective serotonin reuptake inhibitors (SSRIs), such as paroxetine (Paxil) and sertraline (Zoloft), are usually the first choice. Anti-anxiety drugs, such as clonazepam (Klonopin) and alprazolam (Xanax), can reduce anxiety and may be used alone or in conjunction with SSRIs. Propranolol (Inderal) has been found to be useful for performance anxiety, and when taken an hour before the scheduled event, may suppress the physical symptoms of anxiety.*[5,7]
- Seek community programs for client involvement that promote positive behaviors the client is striving to achieve. *Encouraging reading materials, attending classes, community support groups, and lectures for self-help can help to alleviate negative self-concepts that lead to impaired social interactions.*[2,5]
- Involvement in a music-based program, if available (e.g., the Listening Program). *There is a direct correlation between the musical portion of the brain and the language area, and the use of these programs may result in better communication skills.*[10]

- Encourage ongoing family or individual therapy as long as it is promoting growth and positive change. Be alert to possibility of therapy being used as a crutch. *While therapy groups can be useful, individuals can become dependent on the process and not move on to managing on their own.*[1]
- Provide for occasional follow-up for reinforcement of positive behaviors after professional relationship has ended. *Change is difficult and identifying problems that may arise during these contacts can enhance maintenance and enable client/family to continue to progress.*[2]
- Refer to psychiatric clinical nurse specialist when indicated. *May need additional assistance to promote long-term change.*[1]

DOCUMENTATION FOCUS

Assessment/Reassessment
- Individual findings, including factors affecting interactions, nature of social exchanges, specifics of individual behaviors, type of learning disability present.
- Cultural or religious beliefs and expectations.
- Perceptions and response of others.

Planning
- Plan of care and who is involved in the planning.
- Teaching plan.

Implementation/Evaluation
- Responses to interventions, teaching, and actions performed.
- Attainment or progress toward desired outcome(s).
- Modifications to plan of care.

Discharge Planning
- Long-term needs and who is responsible for actions to be taken.
- Community resources, specific referrals made.

References

1. Townsend, M. C. (2003). *Psychiatric Mental Health Nursing Concepts of Care.* 4th ed. Philadelphia: F. A. Davis.
2. Doenges, M. E., Townsend, M. C., Moorhouse, M. F. (1998). *Psychiatric Care Plans: Guidelines for Individualizing Care.* 3d ed. Philadelphia: F. A. Davis.
3. Cox, H. C., et al. (2002). *Clinical Applications of Nursing Diagnosis: Adult, Child, Women's, Psychiatric, Gerontic, and Home Health Considerations.* 4th ed. Philadelphia: F. A. Davis.
4. Drew, N. (1991). Combating the social isolation of chronic mental illness. *J Psychosoc Nurs,* 29(6), 14–17.
5. Beyond shyness and stage fright: Social anxiety disorder. (October 2003). *Harvard Mental Health Letter.*
6. Lipson, J. G., Dibble, S. L., Minarik, P. A. (1996). *Culture & Nursing Care: A Pocket Guide.* San Francisco: UCSF Nursing Press.
7. National Institute of Mental Health. (2000). Anxiety disorders. NIH Publication No. 00–3879. Retrieved August 2007 from www.medhelp.org/NIHlib/GF-222.html.
8. Bellis, T. J. (2002). *When the Brain Can't Hear: Unraveling the Mystery of Auditory Processing Disorder.* New York: Atria Books.
9. The development of social skills. Retrieved August 2007 from www.crediblehorizons.com/social-skills.htm.
10. The listening program. Retrieved August 2007 from www.thelisteningprogram.com/How_TLP_Works.asp.

Social Isolation

DEFINITION: Aloneness experienced by the individual and perceived as imposed by others and as a negative or threatened state

RELATED FACTORS

Factors contributing to the absence of satisfying personal relationships (e.g., delay in accomplishing developmental tasks); immature interests
Alterations in physical appearance or mental status
Altered state of wellness
Unaccepted social behavior or values
Inadequate personal resources
Inability to engage in satisfying personal relationships
[Traumatic incidents or events causing physical or emotional pain]

DEFINING CHARACTERISTICS

Subjective
Expresses feelings of rejection, or aloneness imposed by others
Insecurity in public
Inability to meet expectations of others; inadequate purpose in life
Developmentally inappropriate interests
Experiences feelings of differences from others; expresses values unacceptable to the dominant cultural group

Objective
Absence of supportive significant other(s)—[family, friends, group]
Sad or dull affect; uncommunicative; withdrawn; no eye contact
Evidence of handicap (e.g., physical/mental); illness
Developmentally inappropriate behaviors; repetitive or meaningless actions
Seeks to be alone; preoccupation with own thoughts
Shows behavior unaccepted by dominant cultural group; exists in a subculture; projects hostility

Sample Clinical Applications: Traumatic injuries, facial scarring/acne, chemotherapy, AIDS, dementia, major depression, conduct disorder, developmental delay, paranoid disorders, schizophrenia

DESIRED OUTCOMES/EVALUATION CRITERIA

Sample **NOC** linkages:
Social Involvement: Social interactions with persons, groups, or organizations
Loneliness Severity: Severity of emotional, social, or existential isolation response
Social Support: Reliable assistance from others

Client Will (Include Specific Time Frame)
• Identify causes and actions to correct isolation.
• Verbalize willingness to be involved with others.
• Participate in activities or programs at level of ability or desire.
• Express increased sense of self-worth.

(continues on page 786)

Social Isolation (continued)
ACTIONS/INTERVENTIONS

Sample (NIC) linkages:
Socialization Enhancement: Facilitation of another person's ability to interact with others
Visitation Facilitation: Promoting beneficial visits by family and friends
Normalization Promotion: Assisting parents and other family members of children with chronic diseases or disabilities in providing normal life experiences for their children and families

NURSING PRIORITY NO. 1

To assess causative/contributing factors:

- Determine presence of factors as listed in Related Factors and other concerns (e.g., elderly, female, adolescent, ethnic or racial minority, economically or educationally disadvantaged, hearing or visually impaired). *Identifying individual factors allows for developing an accurate plan of care for the client.*[5]
- Perform physical exam, paying particular attention to any illnesses identified. *Individuals who are isolated appear to be susceptible to health problems, especially coronary heart disease, although little is understood about why that is.*[10]
- Note onset of physical or mental illness and whether recovery is anticipated or condition is chronic or progressive. *Individual may withdraw from activities because of concern about how others view changes that occur due to illness, concern with own thoughts, alterations in physical appearance or mental status. Anticipated length of illness may dictate choice of interventions.*[1,4]
- Identify blocks to social contacts. *Reluctance to engage in social activities may be the result of problems such as physical immobility, sensory deficits, housebound for any reason, incontinence, financial constraints, transportation difficulties. Individual may be afraid of what others might think of her or him, be concerned with embarrassing self or with not having money or means of transportation for desired activities.*[1]
- Ascertain implications of cultural values or religious beliefs for the client *that may dictate choice of behaviors, may even script interactions with others. Client may perceive behaviors as normal because of belief system or may have conflict regarding behaviors that may be unacceptable to the larger society, such as homosexuality or gender identity disorder.*[1,5,6]
- Assess factors in client's life that may contribute to sense of helplessness. *Losses, such as a spouse, parent, or other, or presence of chronic pain or other disabling conditions may cause individual to withdraw, desire to be alone, and refuse to participate in therapeutic activities.*[1,3]
- Listen to comments of client regarding sense of isolation. Differentiate isolation from solitude and loneliness *that may be acceptable or by choice. Provides clues to what client is thinking and feeling about current situation. Client who chooses to be alone and is satisfied may not need further intervention.*[2,5]
- Assess client's feelings about self, sense of ability to control situation, sense of hope, and coping skills. *If client is isolating self because of negative feelings, lack of hope, and so forth, measures to promote self-esteem will need to be taken.*[5]
- Identify support systems available to the client, including presence of/relationship with extended family. *People with social anxiety often do not have support systems because of their withdrawal from contact with others. Often the family of origin may be anxious and does not provide the encouragement and support needed by a temperamentally inhibited*

child or may be too helpful, enabling client to withdraw further. It is difficult for these individuals to ask for help, because they are afraid to meet new people and often find support only when they seek help for other conditions, such as depression.[4,9]

- Identify behavior response of isolation. *Individual may display behaviors such as excessive sleeping or daydreaming, which also may potentiate isolation.*[7,10]
- Note drug use (prescription and illicit). *Individual may begin to use drugs such as alcohol or cocaine to control anxiety in social situations.*[7]
- Review history and elicit information about traumatic events that may have occurred. (Refer to ND Post-Trauma Syndrome.) *While little is known about the origins of social anxiety disorders, clients who have experienced a traumatic event may withdraw from contact and suffer from anxiety when faced with having to deal with social situations.*[1,5]

NURSING PRIORITY NO. 2

To alleviate conditions that contribute to client's sense of isolation:

- Establish therapeutic nurse-client relationship. *Promotes trust and acceptance, allowing client to feel safe and free to discuss sensitive matters without being judged.*[2]
- Spend time interacting with client and identify other resources available. *Getting to know client and identifying concerns about being involved in activities with others can lead to appropriate interventions. Other people such as a volunteer, social worker, chaplain may be able to spend time with client, enhancing circle of trusted people.*[4]
- Develop plan of action with client. Look at available resources; support risk-taking behaviors, financial planning, appropriate medical and self-care, and so forth. *Helping client to learn how to manage these issues of daily living can increase self-confidence and help individual to feel more comfortable in social settings.*[5]
- Introduce client to those with similar or shared interests and other supportive people. *Provides role models and encourages getting to know others who share feelings of anxiety, providing an opportunity to develop social skills and learn some ways of problem-solving to deal with anxiety.*[2,6]
- Promote participation in recreational or special-interest activities in setting that client views as safe. *These activities have the advantage of providing physical and mental stimulation for client who feels isolated and anxious in social settings.*[2,9]
- Provide positive reinforcement when client makes move(s) toward other(s). *Acknowledges and encourages continuation of efforts, helping client toward independence.*[1,7]
- Identify foreign language resources for client who speaks another language. *A professional interpreter is important to ensure accuracy of interpretation; newspaper, radio programming in appropriate foreign language helps client feel connected with own community.*[6,8]
- Assist client to problem solve solutions to short-term or imposed isolation. *Condition may require individual to be isolated from others for his or her protection as well as others', and working together to decide how to manage loneliness can promote successful outcome.*[1,3]
- Encourage open visitation when possible and/or telephone contacts. *Maintains involvement with others, promoting social involvement, especially when client is unable to go out to activities.*[3]
- Provide environmental stimuli when client is confined. *Open curtains in room, display pictures of family or views of nature, promote television and radio listening, Internet access to help client feel less isolated.*[3]
- Provide for placement in sheltered community when necessary. *The individual who is mentally impaired may be unable to learn to participate in society and display socially acceptable behaviors, and will benefit from an environment that offers structure and assistance.*[3]

Nursing Diagnoses in Alphabetical Order

NURSING PRIORITY NO. 3

To promote wellness (Teaching/Discharge Considerations):

- Assist client to learn social skills as needed. *Enhancing problem-solving, communication, social skills, and learning skills to manage ADLs will improve sense of self-esteem.*[4]

- Encourage and assist client to enroll in classes as appropriate. *Assertiveness, vocational, sex education classes may provide skills to improve ability to engage more effectively in social situations.*[5]

- Involve children and adolescents in age-appropriate programs or activities, as indicated. *Promotes socialization skills and peer contact to enable young person to learn by interacting with others.*[5]

- Help client differentiate between isolation and loneliness or aloneness and discuss how to avoid slipping into an undesired state. *Time for the individual to be alone is important to the maintenance of mental health, but the sadness created by isolation and loneliness needs different interventions.*[2]

- Involve client in programs directed to correction and prevention of identified causes of problem. *Activities such as senior citizen services, daily telephone contact, house sharing, pets, day-care centers, church resources can help individual move out of isolation and become involved in life.*[5,10]

- Discuss use of medications, as indicated. *Prescribed medications, such as selective serotonin reuptake inhibitors (SSRIs), can be very effective in treating social disorders.*[3,7]

- Refer to counselor or therapist, as appropriate. *Facilitates grief work, promotes relationship building, and provides opportunity to work toward improvement of individual issues affecting social interactions.*[1]

DOCUMENTATION FOCUS

Assessment/Reassessment
- Individual findings, including precipitating factors, effect on lifestyle, relationships, and functioning.
- Client's perception of situation.
- Cultural or religious factors.
- Availability and use of resources and support systems.

Planning
- Plan of care and who is involved in planning.
- Teaching plan.

Implementation/Evaluation
- Responses to intervention, teaching, and actions performed.
- Attainment or progress toward desired outcome(s).
- Modifications to plan of care.

Discharge Planning
- Long-term needs and who is responsible for actions to be taken.
- Available resources, specific referrals made.

References

1. Townsend, M. C. (2003). *Psychiatric Mental Health Nursing Concepts of Care.* 4th ed. Philadelphia: F. A. Davis.

2. Doenges, M. E., Townsend, M. C., Moorhouse, M. F. (1998). *Psychiatric Care Plans: Guidelines for Individualizing Care.* 3d ed. Philadelphia: F. A. Davis.
3. Cox, H. C., et al. (2002). *Clinical Applications of Nursing Diagnosis: Adult, Child, Women's, Psychiatric, Gerontic, and Home Health Considerations.* 4th ed. Philadelphia: F. A. Davis.
4. Drew, N. (1991). Combating the social isolation of chronic mental illness. *J Psychosoc Nurs*, 29(6), 14–17.
5. Beyond shyness and stage fright: Social anxiety disorder. (October 2003). *Harvard Mental Health Letter.*
6. Lipson, J. G., Dibble, S. L., Minarik, P. A. (1996). *Culture & Nursing Care: A Pocket Guide.* San Francisco: UCSF Nursing Press.
7. National Institute of Mental Health. (2000). Anxiety disorders. NIH Publication No. 00-3879. Retrieved August 2007 from www.medhelp.org/NIHlib/GF-222.html.
8. Andrulis, D. P. (2002). *What a Difference an Interpreter Can Make: Health Care Experiences of Uninsured with Limited English Proficiency. The Access Project.* Boston: Brandeis University.
9. McPherson, M., Smith-Lovin, L., Brashears, M. (June 2006). Social isolation in U.S.: Changes in core discussion networks over two decades. *Am Sociol Rev*, 71, 353–375.
10. House, J. (2001). Social isolation kills, but how and why? *Psychosom Med*, 63(2), 273–274.

chronic Sorrow

DEFINITION: Cyclical, recurring, and potentially progressive pattern of pervasive sadness experienced (by a parent or caregiver, individual with chronic illness or disability) in response to continual loss, throughout the trajectory of an illness or disability

RELATED FACTORS

Death of a loved one

Experiences chronic illness or disability (e.g., physical or mental); crises in management of the illness

Crises related to developmental stages; missed opportunities or milestones

Unending caregiving

DEFINING CHARACTERISTICS

Subjective

Expresses negative feelings (e.g., anger, being misunderstood, confusion, depression, disappointment, emptiness, fear, frustration, guilt, self-blame, helplessness, hopelessness, loneliness, low self-esteem, recurring loss, overwhelmed)

Expresses feelings of sadness (e.g., periodic, recurrent)

Objective

Expresses feelings that interfere with ability to reach highest level of personal or social well-being

Sample Clinical Applications: Cancer, multiple sclerosis (MS), Parkinson's disease, AIDS, amyotrophic lateral sclerosis (ALS), prematurity, genetic or congenital defects, infertility, dementia, Alzheimer's disease, bipolar disorder, schizophrenia, developmental delay

(continues on page 790)

chronic Sorrow (continued)
DESIRED OUTCOMES/EVALUATION CRITERIA

Sample (NOC) linkages:
Depression Level: Severity of level of melancholic mood and loss of interest in life events
Depression Self-Control: Personal actions to minimize melancholy and maintain interest in life events
Hope: Optimism that is personally satisfying and life-supporting

Client Will (Include Specific Time Frame)
• Acknowledge presence and impact of sorrow.
• Demonstrate progress in dealing with loss(es) as evidenced by recognizing positive aspects of situation.
• Participate in work and/or self-care activities of daily living (ADLs) as able.
• Verbalize a sense of progress toward resolution of sorrow and hope for the future.

ACTIONS/INTERVENTIONS

Sample (NIC) linkages:
Mood Management: Providing for safety, stabilization, recovery, and maintenance of a patient who is experiencing dysfunctionally depressed or elevated mood
Grief Work Facilitation: Assistance with the resolution of a significant loss
Hope Inspiration: Enhancing the belief in one's capacity to initiate and sustain actions

NURSING PRIORITY NO. 1

To assess causative/contributing factors and effect on life:

● Determine current or recent events or conditions contributing to client's state of mind, as listed in Related Factors (e.g., death of loved one, chronic physical or mental illness or disability). *Individual information is necessary when formulating a plan of care to address appropriate issues.*[1]

● Note cues of sadness. *Expressions of feelings of loss, such as sighing, faraway looks, unkempt appearance, inattention to conversation, and refusing food can be indicators of sorrow that is not being dealt with. Note: Chronic sorrow may be cyclical—at times deepening versus times of feeling somewhat better.*[4,5]

● Be aware of use of avoidance behaviors. *Anger, withdrawal, denial are part of the grieving process and may be used to avoid dealing with the reality of what has happened. However, in a situation that is unchangeable, such as developmentally disabled child or a child with diabetes, sorrow is seen as a normal response and will continue to be a factor even as the family copes with the condition.*[5,7]

● Identify cultural values or religious beliefs and possible conflicts. *Expressions of sorrow are influenced by these beliefs and may result in conflicts. For instance, the Mexican American culture believes genetic defects are the will of God, but individual may be angry at God because of occurrence. Or, individual/family may have difficulty living up to the expectations of others (e.g., "God does not give us more than we can handle").*[6]

● Ascertain response of family/SOs to client's situation and support provided. *Parents who have chronically ill children or premature babies, adults who have multiple sclerosis, elderly caregivers of spouses with dementia may continue to have feelings of sorrow even though they seem to be managing fairly well but due to cyclic nature of sorrow will require ongoing support/assistance from others to cope.*[4,7]

- Determine level of functioning, ability to care for self/others. Assess needs of family/SO. *Individual who is coping with chronic illness (e.g., Parkinson's disease, MS, HIV/AIDS) may exhibit chronic sorrow related to the illness, fear of death, poverty, and isolation associated with these conditions, which may lead to difficulty managing ADLs for self or meeting needs of family.*[2,3]
- Refer to NDs Caregiver Role Strain, ineffective Coping, complicated Grieving, as appropriate.

NURSING PRIORITY NO. 2

To assist client to move through sorrow:

- Encourage verbalization about situation. Active-listen feelings and be available for support and assistance. *Helpful in beginning resolution and acceptance. Individuals involved, client, and caregivers benefit from being able to talk freely about the situation. Active-listening conveys a message of acceptance and helps individual come to own resolution.*[1,5]
- Encourage expression of anger, fear, or anxiety. (Refer to appropriate NDs.) *Individual needs to deal with these feelings before she or he can move forward.*[1]
- Acknowledge reality of feelings of guilt or blame, including hostility toward spiritual power. (Refer to ND Spiritual Distress.) *It was believed that grief had an end stage, but research has shown that individuals in chronic conditions, such as diabetes mellitus, multiple sclerosis, disabling conditions, continue to experience chronic sorrow and lifelong recurring sadness. Understanding this can help individual accept that these feelings are real, and when they are validated, they can be dealt with.*[5,11,12]
- Provide comfort and availability as well as caring for physical needs. *The way healthcare professionals respond to families is important to helping them cope with the situation as physical care is given.*[5,9]
- Discuss ways individual has dealt with past losses and reinforce use of previously effective coping skills. *As client begins to look at how they have handled previous situations, effective coping skills can be recalled and applied to current situation.*[2,9,10]
- Instruct in and encourage use of visualization and relaxation skills. *Learning these stress-management skills can help the individual relax, enhancing ability to deal with feelings of sorrow regarding the long-term situation.*[5,8]
- Discuss use of medication when depression is interfering with ability to manage life. *Client may benefit from the short-term use of an antidepressant medication to help with dealing with situation.*[1]
- Assist SOs to cope with client response. *Family/SO may not be dysfunctional but may be intolerant and lack understanding of individual responses to long-term illness. Grief is unique to each individual and may not always follow a particular course to resolution that is understood by all.*[4,5,12]
- Include family/SO in setting realistic goals for meeting individual needs. *Inclusion of all family members ensures they all have the same information and are all working toward effective coping strategies.*[4,5]

NURSING PRIORITY NO. 3

To promote wellness (Teaching/Discharge Considerations):

- Discuss healthy ways of dealing with difficult situations. *Providing information about effective communication skills, understanding condition they are dealing with, and expectations of the course of the illness or condition can promote personal growth and lead to a positive outcome for the family.*[7,8]

⊕ ● Have client identify familial, religious, and cultural factors that have meaning for him or her. *May help bring loss or distressing situation into perspective and promote grief or sorrow understanding.*[6]

🏠 ● Encourage involvement in usual activities, exercise, and socialization within limits of physical and psychological state. *Energy is restored and individuals can go on with their lives when they are willing and able to continue activities.*[5,7]

🏠 ● Introduce concept of mindfulness (living in the moment), and encourage client to recognize and embrace moments of joy in own life. *Promotes feelings of capability and belief that this moment can be dealt with or enjoyed.*[8,12]

🔗 ● Refer to other resources (e.g., pastoral care, counseling, psychotherapy, respite care providers, support groups). *Provides additional help when needed to resolve situation, continue grief work, and move on with life.*[3]

DOCUMENTATION FOCUS

Assessment/Reassessment
• Individual findings, including nature of sorrow, effects on participation in treatment regimen.
• Physical and emotional response to conflict, expressions of sadness.
• Cultural or religious issues and conflicts.
• Reactions of family/SO.

Planning
• Plan of care and who is involved in planning.
• Teaching plan.

Implementation/Evaluation
• Response to interventions, teaching, and actions performed.
• Attainment or progress toward desired outcome(s).
• Modifications to plan of care.

Discharge Planning
• Long-term needs and who is responsible for actions to be taken.
• Available resources, specific referrals made.

References

1. Doenges, M. E., Moorhouse, M. F., Geissler-Murr, A. C. (2004). *Nurse's Pocket Guide Diagnoses: Interventions and Rationales.* 9th ed. Philadelphia: F. A. Davis.
2. Lindgren, C. L. (1996). Chronic sorrow in persons with Parkinson's and their spouse caregivers. *Sch Inq Nurs Pract,* 10(4), 351–366.
3. Lichtensten, B., Laska, M. K., Clair, J. M. (2002). Chronic sorrow in the HIV-positive patient: Issues of race, gender, and social support. *AIDS Patient Care STDs,* 16(1), 27–38.
4. Kearney, P. (2003). Chronic grief (or is it periodic grief?). Retrieved February 2004 from www.indiana.edu/~famlygrf/units/chronic.html.
5. Lowes, L., Lyne, P. (2000). Chronic sorrow in parents of children with newly diagnosed diabetes: A review of the literature and discussion of the implications for nursing practice. *J Adv Nurs,* 32(1), 41–48.
6. Lipson, J. G., Dibble, S. L., Minarik, P. A. (1996). *Culture & Nursing Care: A Pocket Guide.* San Francisco: UCSF Nursing Press.
7. Mallow, G. E., Bechtel, G. A. (1999). Chronic sorrow: The experience of parents with children who are developmentally disabled. *J Psychosoc Nurs,* 17(7), 31–43.
8. Kabat-Zinn, J. (1994). *Wherever You Go, There You Are.* New York: Hyperion.

9. Kearney, P. M., Griffin, T. (2001). Between joy and sorrow: Being a parent of a child with a developmental disability. *J Adv Nurs*, 34, 582–592.
10. Olansky, S. (1962). Chronic sorrow: A response to having a mentally defective child. *Soc Casework*, 43, 190–193.
11. Hobdell, E. (2004). Chronic sorrow and depression in parents of children with neural tube defects. *J Neurosci Nurs*, 36(2), 82, 94.
12. Kearney, P. (Updated 2006). Chronic grief (or is it periodic grief?). Grief in a Family Context. Retrieved May 2007 from www.indiana.edu/~famlygrf/units/chronic.html.

Spiritual Distress

DEFINITION: Impaired ability to experience and integrate meaning and purpose in life through a person's connectedness with self, others, art, music, literature, nature, and/or a power greater than oneself

RELATED FACTORS

Active dying
Loneliness; social alienation; self-alienation; sociocultural deprivation
Anxiety; pain
Life change
Chronic illness [of self or others]; death
[Challenged belief or value system (e.g., moral or ethical implications of therapy)]

DEFINING CHARACTERISTICS

Subjective
Connections to self:
Expresses lack of hope, meaning or purpose in life, serenity (e.g., peace), love, acceptance, forgiveness of self, courage
[Expresses] anger; guilt
Connections with others:
Refuses interactions with significant other(s) or spiritual leaders
Verbalizes being separated from support system
Expresses alienation
Connections with art, music, literature, nature:
Inability to express previous state of creativity (e.g., singing/listening to music/writing)
Disinterested in nature or reading spiritual literature
Connections with power greater than self:
Sudden changes in spiritual practices
Inability to pray or participate in religious activities, or to experience the transcendent
Expresses hopelessness, suffering, or having anger toward God
Expresses being abandoned
Request to see a religious leader

Objective
Connections to self: Poor coping
Connections with power greater than self: Inability to be introspective

(continues on page 794)

Spiritual Distress (continued)

Sample Clinical Applications: Chronic conditions (e.g., rheumatoid arthritis, multiple sclerosis [MS], systemic lupus erythematosus [SLE], amyotrophic lateral sclerosis [ALS]), cancer, traumatic brain injury vegetative state, fetal demise, infertility, sudden infant death syndrome (SIDS)

DESIRED OUTCOMES/EVALUATION CRITERIA

Sample NOC linkages:
Spiritual Health: Connectedness with self, others, higher power, all life, nature, and the universe that transcends and empowers the self
Hope: Optimism that is personally satisfying and life-supporting
Psychosocial Adjustment: Life Change: Adaptive psychosocial response of an individual to a significant life change

Client Will (Include Specific Time Frame)
• Verbalize increased sense of connectedness and hope for future.
• Demonstrate ability to help self and participate in care.
• Participate in activities with others, actively seek relationships.
• Discuss beliefs and values about spiritual issues.
• Verbalize acceptance of self as not deserving illness or situation: "No one is to blame."

ACTIONS/INTERVENTIONS

Sample NIC linkages:
Spiritual Support: Assisting the patient to feel balance and connection with a greater power
Hope Inspiration: Enhancing the belief in one's capacity to initiate and sustain actions
Grief Work Facilitation: Assistance with the resolution of a significant loss

NURSING PRIORITY NO. 1

To assess causative/contributing factors:

• Determine client's religious and spiritual orientation, current involvement, presence of conflicts. *Identification of individual spiritual practices and restrictions that may affect client care or create conflict between spiritual beliefs and treatment provides for more accurate interventions.*[1]
• Listen to client's/SO's reports or expressions of concern, anger, alienation from God, belief that illness or situation is a punishment for wrongdoing, and so forth. *Indicates depth of grieving process and possible need for spiritual advisor or other resource to address client's belief system if desired.*[2]
• Assess for influence of cultural beliefs and spiritual values that affect individual in this situation. *Circumstances of illness or situation may conflict with client's view of self, cultural background, and distress over values. For instance, many Mexican Americans are Catholic with strong beliefs in the relationship of illness and religious practices.*[5]
• Note recent changes in behavior (e.g., withdrawal from others and creative or religious activities, dependence on alcohol or medications). *Helpful in determining severity and duration of situation and possible need for additional referrals such as substance withdrawal.*[1,7]

- Assess sense of self-concept, worth, ability to enter into loving relationships. *Lack of connectedness with self or others impairs client's ability to trust others or feel worthy of trust from others, leading to difficulties in relationships with others.*[1,7]
- Observe behavior indicative of poor relationships with others (e.g., manipulative, nontrusting, demanding). *Manipulation is used for management of client's sense of powerlessness because of distrust of others, interfering with relationships with others.*[3,6]
- Determine support systems available to client/SO(s) and how they are used. *Provides insight to client's willingness to pursue outside resources.*[1,4]
- Determine sense of futility, feelings of hopelessness and helplessness, lack of motivation to help self. *Indicators that client may see no, or only limited, options, alternatives or personal choices available; that client lacks energy to deal with situation; and that further evaluation is needed.*[1]
- Note expressions of inability to find meaning in life, reason for living. Evaluate suicidal ideation *to refer for mental health evaluation and intervention as indicated. Crisis of the spirit or loss of will to live places client at increased risk for inattention to personal well-being and possible harm to self.*[1,7]

NURSING PRIORITY NO. 2

To assist client/SO(s) to deal with feelings/situation:

- Develop therapeutic nurse-client relationship. Ascertain client's views as to how care provider(s) can be most helpful. Convey acceptance of client's spiritual beliefs and concerns. *Promotes trust and comfort, encouraging client to be open about sensitive matters.*[6]
- Establish environment that promotes free expression of feelings and concerns. *Provides opportunity for client to explore own thoughts and make appropriate decisions regarding spiritual issues.*[4]
- Provide calm, peaceful setting when possible. *Promotes relaxation and enhances opportunity for reflection on situation/discussions with others, meditation.*[3]
- Encourage life-review by client. Support client in finding a reason for living. *Promotes sense of hope and willingness to continue efforts to improve situation.*[3]
- Be aware of influence of care provider's own belief system. *It is still possible to be helpful to client while remaining neutral and not espousing own beliefs, because client's beliefs and needs are what is important.*[6]
- Identify inappropriate coping behaviors currently being used and associated consequences and discuss with client. *Recognizing negative consequences of actions may enhance desire to change.*[2]
- Set limits on acting-out behavior that is inappropriate/destructive. *Promotes safety for client/others and helps prevent loss of self-esteem.*[2,7]
- Ascertain past successes and coping behaviors. *Helps to determine approaches used previously that may be effective in dealing with current situation, providing encouragement.*[6]
- Problem-solve solutions and identify areas for compromise. *May be useful in resolving conflicts that arise from feelings of anxiety regarding questioning of beliefs and current illness or situation.*[3]
- Assist in developing coping skills *to deal with stressors of illness and necessary changes in lifestyle.*[7,9]

NURSING PRIORITY NO. 3

To facilitate setting goals and moving forward:

- Use therapeutic communication skills of reflection and Active listening. *Conveys message of competence and helps client find own solutions to concerns.*[7]

- Involve client in refining healthcare goals and therapeutic regimen as appropriate. *Promotes feelings of control over what is happening, enhancing commitment to plan and optimizing outcomes.*[3]

 - Encourage client/family to ask questions. *Demonstrates support for individual's willingness to learn.*

- Discuss difference between grief and guilt and help client to identify and deal with each. Point out consequences of actions based on guilt. *Aids client in assuming responsibility for own actions and avoids acting out of false guilt.*[6]

- Identify role models (e.g., individual experiencing similar situation). *Provides opportunities for sharing of experiences and hope, and identifying new options to deal with situation.*[7]

- Assist client to learn use of meditation, mindfulness, and prayer, if desired. *Provides avenue for learning forgiveness to heal past hurts and developing a sense of peace.*[3,8]

- Provide information that anger with God is a normal part of the grieving process. *Realizing these feelings are not unusual can reduce sense of guilt, encourage open expression, and facilitate resolution of grief.*[3,7]

- Provide time and privacy to engage in spiritual growth or religious activities as desired (e.g., prayer, meditation, scripture reading, listening to music). *Allows client to focus on self and seek connectedness with spiritual beliefs and values.*[6]

- Encourage and facilitate outings to neighborhood park or nature walks. *Sunshine, fresh air, and activity can stimulate release of endorphins, promoting sense of well-being and encouraging connection with nature.*[6]

- Provide play therapy for child that encompasses spiritual data. *Interactive pleasurable activity promotes open discussion and enhances retention of information. Child will act out feelings in play therapy easier than talking. Provides opportunity for child to practice what has been learned and for therapist to evaluate child's progress.*[3]

- Abide by parents' wishes in discussing and implementing child's spiritual support. *Limits confusion for child and prevents conflict of values and beliefs.*[3]

- Refer to appropriate resources (e.g., pastoral or parish nurse or religious counselor, crisis counselor, hospice; psychotherapy; Alcoholics or Narcotics Anonymous). *Useful in dealing with immediate situation and identifying long-term resources for support to help foster sense of connectedness.*[7,8]

- Refer to NDs ineffective Coping, Powerlessness, Self-Esteem (specify), Social Isolation, risk for Suicide for additional interventions as indicated.

NURSING PRIORITY NO. 4

To promote wellness (Teaching/Discharge Considerations):

- Make time for nonjudgmental discussion of philosophical issues or questions about spiritual impact of illness or situation and/or treatment regimen. *Open communication can assist client in reality checks of perceptions and help to identify personal options.*[6]

- Assist client to develop long-term goals for dealing with future and illness situation. *Involvement in planning for desired outcomes enhances commitment to goal, optimizing outcomes.*[7]

- Suggest use of journaling. *Provides opportunity to write feelings and happenings; reviewing them over time can assist in clarifying values and ideas, recognizing and resolving feelings or situation.*[6,10]

- Assist client to identify SO(s)/others who could provide support as needed. *Ongoing support is important to enhance sense of connectedness and continue progress toward goals.*[6]

- Identify spiritual resources that could be helpful (e.g., contact spiritual advisor who has qualifications or experience in dealing with specific problems such as death/dying, relationship problems, substance abuse, suicide). *Provides answers to spiritual questions, assists in the journey of self-discovery, and can help client learn to accept and forgive self.*[6]

DOCUMENTATION FOCUS

Assessment/Reassessment
- Individual findings, including nature of spiritual conflict, effects of participation in treatment regimen.
- Physical and emotional responses to conflict.

Planning
- Plan of care and who is involved in planning.
- Teaching plan.

Implementation/Evaluation
- Responses to interventions, teaching, and actions performed.
- Attainment or progress toward desired outcome(s).
- Modifications to plan of care.

Discharge Planning
- Long-term needs and who is responsible for actions to be taken.
- Available resources, specific referrals made.

References

1. Fallot, R. D. (1998). Assessment of spirituality and implications for service planning. *New Dir Ment Health Serv*, 80, 13–23.
2. Moller, M. D. (1999). Meeting spiritual needs on an inpatient unit. *J Psychosoc Nurs*, 37(11), 5–10.
3. Baldacchino, D., Draper, P. (2001). Spiritual coping strategies: A review of the nursing research literature. *J Adv Nurs*, 34(6), 833–841.
4. Cox, H. C., et al. (2002). *Clinical Applications of Nursing Diagnosis*. 4th ed. Philadelphia: F. A. Davis.
5. Lipson, J. G., Dibble, S. L., Minarik, P. A. (1996). *Culture & Nursing Care: A Pocket Guide*. San Francisco: UCSF Nursing Press.
6. Ross, L. A. (1994). Spiritual aspects of nursing. *J Adv Nurs*, 19, 439–447.
7. Townsend, M. C. (2003). *Psychiatric Mental Health Nursing Concepts of Care*. 4th ed. Philadelphia: F. A. Davis.
8. Hospital and Palliative Nurses Association. (2005). Spiritual distress-patient/family teaching sheets. Retrieved May 2007 from www.hpna.org/pdf/PatientSheet_SpiritualDistress.pdf.
9. Savrock, J. (2006). Counseling distressed students may be improved by religious discussion. Retrieved May 2007 from www.ed.psu.edu/news/spiritual.asp.
10. Johnson, C. V., Hayes, J. A. (2003). Troubled spirits: Prevalence and predictors of religious and spiritual concerns among university students and counseling center clients. *J Couns Psychol*, 50, 409–419.

risk for Spiritual Distress

DEFINITION: At risk for an impaired ability to experience and integrate meaning and purpose in life through connectedness with self, others, art, music, literature, nature, and/or a power greater than oneself

RISK FACTORS

Physical
Physical or chronic illness, substance abuse

Psychosocial
Stress; anxiety; depression
Low self-esteem; poor relationships; blocks to experiencing love; inability to forgive; loss; separated support systems; racial or cultural conflict
Change in religious rituals or spiritual practices

Developmental
Life changes

Environmental
Environmental changes; natural disasters

NOTE: A risk diagnosis is not evidenced by signs and symptoms, as the problem has not occurred; rather, nursing interventions are directed at prevention.
Sample Clinical Applications: Chronic conditions (e.g., rheumatoid arthritis, multiple sclerosis [MS], systemic lupus erythematosus [SLE], amyotrophic lateral sclerosis [ALS]), cancer, traumatic brain injury, vegetative state, fetal demise, infertility, sudden infant death syndrome (SIDS)

DESIRED OUTCOMES/EVALUATION CRITERIA

Sample NOC linkages:
Spiritual Health: Connectedness with self, others, higher power, all life, nature, and the universe that transcends and empowers the self
Hope: Optimism that is personally satisfying and life-supporting
Psychosocial Adjustment: Life Change: Adaptive psychosocial response of an individual to a significant life change

Client Will (Include Specific Time Frame)
• Identify meaning and purpose in own life that reinforces hope, peace, and contentment.
• Verbalize acceptance of self as being worthy, not deserving of illness or situation, and so forth.
• Identify and use resources appropriately.

ACTIONS/INTERVENTIONS

Sample (NIC) linkages:
Spiritual Support: Assisting the patient to feel balance and connection with a greater power
Coping Enhancement: Assisting a patient to adapt to perceived stressors, changes, or threats which interfere with meeting life demands and roles
Forgiveness Facilitation: Assisting an individual to forgive and/or experience forgiveness in relationship with self, others, and higher power

NURSING PRIORITY NO. 1

To assess causative/contributing factors:

- Ascertain current situation (e.g., natural disaster, death of a spouse, personal injustice). *Identification of circumstances that put the individual at risk for loss of connectedness with spiritual beliefs is essential to plan for appropriate interventions.*[8]
- Listen to client's/SO's expressions of anger or concern, belief that illness or situation is a punishment for wrongdoing, and so forth. *Identifies need for client to talk about and be listened to in regard to concerns about potential loss of control over his or her life.*[3]
- Note reason for living and whether it is directly related to situation. *Tragic occurrences such as home and business washed away in a flood or lost in a fire, parent whose only child is terminally ill, loss of a spouse can cause individual to question previous beliefs, and how he or she has coped in the past and will cope in future.*[1,3]
- Determine client's religious or spiritual orientation, current involvement, presence of conflicts, especially in current circumstances. *Client may be a member of a religious organization, and whether he or she is active or whether conflicts have risen in relation to current illness or situation will indicate need for assistance from spiritual advisor, pastor, or other resource client would accept.*[1,9]
- Assess sense of self-concept, worth, ability to enter into loving relationships. *Lack of connectedness with self and others impairs client's ability to trust others or feel worthy of trust from others.*[1,7]
- Observe behavior indicative of poor relationships with others. *Client may be manipulative, nontrusting, and demanding because of distrust of self and others, interfering with relationships with others, indicating need for learning positive ways to interact with others.*[2,4]
- Determine support systems available to, and used by, client/SO(s). *Provides insight into individual's willingness to pursue outside resources.*[6,11]
- Ascertain substance use or abuse. *Complicates situation, affects ability to deal with problems in a positive manner, and identifies need for referral to appropriate treatment programs.*[4,10]
- Assess for influence of cultural beliefs and spiritual values that affect individual in this situation. *Circumstances of illness or situation may conflict with client's view of self, cultural background, and distress over values. For instance, many Mexican Americans are Catholic with strong beliefs in the relationship of illness and religious practices.*[5]

NURSING PRIORITY NO. 2

To assist client/SO(s) to deal with feelings/situation:

- Establish environment that promotes free expression of feelings and concerns. *Provides opportunity for client to explore own thoughts and make appropriate decisions regarding spiritual issues and conflicts.*[7,11]

- Use therapeutic communication skills of reflection and Active-listening. *Communicates confidence in client's ability to find own solutions to concerns.*[7]
- Have client identify and prioritize current or immediate needs. *Helps client focus on what needs to be done and identifies manageable steps to take to achieve goals.*[6]
- Discuss client's interest in the arts, music, and literature. *Provides insight into meaning of these issues and how they are integrated into individual's life.*
- Make time for nonjudgmental discussion of philosophical issues or questions about spiritual impact of illness or situation and/or treatment regimen. *Open communication can assist client to make reality checks of perceptions and begin to identify personal options.*[6]
- Discuss difference between grief and guilt and help client to identify and deal with each. *Helps client to assume responsibility for own actions, become aware of the consequences of acting out of false guilt.*[6]
- Review coping skills used and their effectiveness in current situation. *Identifies strengths to incorporate into plan and techniques needing revision.*[6]
- Identify role model (e.g., individual experiencing similar situation or disease). *Sharing of experiences and hope provides opportunity for client to look at options as modeled by others and to begin to deal with reality.*[7]
- ∞ Provide play therapy for child that encompasses spiritual data. *Interactive pleasurable activity promotes open discussion and enhances retention of information. Child will act out feelings in play therapy easier than talking. Provides opportunity for child to practice what has been learned and for therapist to evaluate child's progress.*[3]
- ∞ Abide by parents' wishes in discussing and implementing child's spiritual support. *Limits confusion for child and prevents conflict of values and beliefs.*[3]
- Refer to appropriate resources (e.g., crisis counselor, governmental agencies; pastoral or parish nurse or spiritual advisor who has qualifications or experience dealing with specific problems such as death/dying, relationship problems, substance abuse, suicide; hospice; psychotherapy; Alcoholics or Narcotics Anonymous). *Useful in dealing with immediate situation and identifying long-term resources for support to help foster sense of connectedness.*[7,9]

NURSING PRIORITY NO. 3

To promote wellness (Teaching/Discharge Considerations):

- Role-play new coping techniques. *Provides opportunity to practice and enhances integration of new skills or necessary lifestyle changes.*[4]
- Assist client to learn use of meditation, mindfulness, and prayer, if desired. *Provides avenue for learning forgiveness to heal past hurts and developing a sense of peace.*[3,9]
- Suggest use of journaling. *Provides opportunity to write feelings and happenings; reviewing them over time can assist in clarifying values and ideas, recognizing and resolving feelings or situation.*[6,10]
- Encourage individual to become involved in cultural activities of their choosing. *Art, music, plays, and other cultural activities provide a means of connecting with self and others.*
- Discuss possibilities of taking classes and becoming involved in discussion groups or community programs.
- Assist client to identify SO(s) and individuals/support groups who could provide ongoing support. *This is a daily need requiring lifelong commitment, and having sufficient support can help client maintain spiritual resolve.*[6]
- Discuss benefit of family counseling as appropriate. *Issues of this nature (e.g., situational losses, natural disasters, difficult relationships) affect family dynamics, and family may find it useful to discuss and resolve problems they are experiencing.*[7]

🌐 Cultural Ⓐ Collaborative 🏠 Community/Home Care ✏️ Diagnostic Studies ∞ Pediatric/Geriatric/Lifespan   Medications

DOCUMENTATION FOCUS

Assessment/Reassessment
- Individual findings, including risk factors, nature of current distress.
- Physical and emotional responses to distress.
- Access to and use of resources.

Planning
- Plan of care and who is involved in planning.
- Teaching plan.

Implementation/Evaluation
- Responses to interventions, teaching, and actions performed.
- Attainment or progress toward desired outcome(s).
- Modifications to plan of care.

Discharge Planning
- Long-term needs and who is responsible for actions to be taken.
- Available resources, specific referrals made.

References

1. Fallot, R. D. (1998). Assessment of spirituality and implications for service planning. *New Dir Ment Health Serv*, 80, 13–23.
2. Moller, M. D. (1999). J Psychosoc Nurs. *Meeting spiritual needs on an inpatient unit*, 37(11), 5–10.
3. Baldacchino, D., Draper, P. (2001). Spiritual coping strategies: A review of the nursing research literature. *J Adv Nurs*, 34(6), 833–841.
4. Cox, H. C., et al. (2002). *Clinical Applications of Nursing Diagnosis: Adult, Child, Women's, Psychiatric, Gerontic, and Home Health Considerations.* 4th ed. Philadelphia: F. A. Davis.
5. Lipson, J. G., Dibble, S. L., Minarik, P. A. (1999). *Culture & Nursing Care: A Pocket Guide.* San Francisco: UCSF Nursing Press.
6. Ross, L. A. (1994). Spiritual aspects of nursing. *J Adv Nurs*, 19, 439–447.
7. Townsend, M. C. (2003). *Psychiatric Mental Health Nursing Concepts of Care.* 4th ed. Philadelphia: F. A. Davis.
8. Doenges, M. E., Moorhouse, M. F., Murr, A. C. (2008). *Nurse's Pocket Guide: Diagnoses, Interventions, and Rationales.* 11th ed. Philadelphia: F. A. Davis.
9. Hospital and Palliative Nurses Association. (2005). Spiritual distress-patient/family teaching sheets. Retrieved May 2007 from www.hpna.org/pdf/PatientSheet_SpiritualDistress.pdf.
10. Savrock, J. (2006). Counseling distressed students may be improved by religious discussion. Retrieved May 2007 from www.ed.psu.edu/news/spiritual.asp.
11. Johnson, C. V., Hayes, J. A. (2003). Troubled spirits: Prevalence and predictors of religious and spiritual concerns among university students and counseling center clients. *J Couns Psychol*, 50, 409–419.

readiness for enhanced Spiritual Well-Being

DEFINITION: Ability to experience and integrate meaning and purpose in life through connectedness with self, others, art, music, literature, nature, and/or a power greater than oneself that can be strengthened

RELATED FACTORS

To be developed by nurse researchers and submitted to NANDA

DEFINING CHARACTERISTICS

Subjective
Connections to self:
Expresses desire for enhanced: acceptance, coping, courage, forgiveness of self, hope, joy, love, meaning or purpose in life, satisfying philosophy of life, surrender
Expresses lack of serenity (e.g., peace)
Meditation
Connections with others:
Requests interactions with significant others/spiritual leaders
Requests forgiveness of others
Connections with powers greater than self:
Participates in religious activities; prays
Expresses reverence or awe; reports mystical experiences

Objective
Connections with others: Provides service to others
Connections with art, music, literature, nature: Displays creative energy (e.g., writing, poetry, singing); listens to music; reads spiritual literature; spends time outdoors

Sample Clinical Applications: As a health-seeking behavior, the client may be healthy or this diagnosis can occur in any clinical condition

DESIRED OUTCOMES/EVALUATION CRITERIA

Sample NOC linkages:
Spiritual Health: Connectedness with self, others, higher power, all life, nature, and the universe that transcends and empowers the self
Hope: Optimism that is personally satisfying and life-supporting
Quality of Life: Extent of positive perception of current life circumstances

Client Will (Include Specific Time Frame)
• Acknowledge the stabilizing and strengthening forces in own life needed for balance and well-being of the whole person.
• Identify meaning and purpose in own life that reinforces hope, peace, and contentment.
• Verbalize a sense of peace or contentment and comfort of spirit.
• Demonstrate behavior congruent with verbalizations that lend support and strength for daily living.

ACTIONS/INTERVENTIONS

Sample **NIC** linkages:

Spiritual Growth Facilitation: Facilitation of growth in patient's capacity to identify, connect with, and call upon the source of meaning, purpose, comfort, strength, and hope in his or her life

Religious Ritual Enhancement: Facilitating participation in religious practices

Meditation Facilitation: Facilitating a person to alter his or her level of awareness by focusing specifically on an image or thought

NURSING PRIORITY NO. 1

To determine spiritual state/motivation for growth:

- Ascertain client's perception of current state or degree of connectedness and expectations. *Provides insight as to where client is currently and specific hopes for the future.*[1]
- Ascertain motivation and expectations for change. *Motivation to improve and high expectations can encourage client to make changes that will improve his or her life. However, unrealistic expectations may hamper efforts.*
- Review spiritual or religious history, activities, rituals, and frequency of participation. *Determines basis to build on for growth or change.*[1]
- Determine relational values of support systems to client's spiritual centeredness. *The client's family of origin may have differing beliefs from those espoused by the individual that may be a source of conflict for the client. Comfort can be gained when family and friends share client's beliefs and support the search for spiritual knowledge.*[2]
- Explore meaning or interpretation and relationship of spirituality, life and death, and illness to life's journey. *This information helps client strengthen personal belief system, enabling him or her to move forward and live life to the fullest.*[4]
- Clarify the meaning of client's spiritual beliefs or religious practice and rituals to daily living. *Discussing these issues allows client to explore spiritual needs and decide what fits own view of the world to enhance life.*[6]
- Explore ways that spirituality or religious practices have affected client's life and given meaning and value to daily living. Note consequences as well as benefits. *Promotes understanding and appreciation of the difference between spirituality and religion and how each can be used to enhance client's journey of self-discovery.*[3]
- Discuss life's or God's plan (when this is the person's belief) for the individual. *Helpful in determining individual goals and choosing specific options.*[2]

NURSING PRIORITY NO. 2

To assist client to integrate values and beliefs to achieve a sense of wholeness and optimum balance in daily living:

- Explore ways beliefs give meaning and value to daily living. *As client develops understanding of these issues, they will provide support for dealing with current and future concerns.*[1]
- Clarify reality and appropriateness of client's self-perceptions and expectations. *Necessary to provide firm foundation for growth. Unrealistic ideas can impede desired improvement.*[2]
- Determine influence of cultural beliefs or values. *Most individuals are strongly influenced by the spiritual or religious orientation of their family of origin, which can be a major determinate for client's choice of activities and receptiveness to various options.*[5]

- Discuss the importance and value of connections to client's daily life. *The contacts that one has with others sustains the feeling of belonging and connection, and promotes feelings of wholeness and well-being.*[4,6]
 - Identify ways to achieve connectedness or harmony with self, others, nature, higher power (e.g., meditation, prayer, talking or sharing self with others; being out in nature, gardening, or walking; attending religious activities). *This is a highly individual and personal decision, and no action is too trivial to be considered.*[4]

NURSING PRIORITY NO. 3

To enhance optimum spirituality:

- Encourage client to take time to be introspective in the search for peace and harmony. *Finding peace within oneself will carry over to relationships with others and own outlook on life.*[1]
- Discuss use of relaxation or meditative activities (e.g., yoga, tai chi, prayer). *Helpful in promoting general well-being and sense of connectedness with self, nature, and/or spiritual power.*[4,6]
- Suggest attendance or involvement in dream-sharing group *to develop and enhance learning of the characteristics of spiritual awareness and facilitate the individual's growth.*[1]
- Identify ways for spiritual or religious expression. *There are multiple options for enhancing spirituality through connectedness with self/others (e.g., volunteering time to community projects, mentoring, singing in the choir, painting, or spiritual writings).*[3,4]
- Encourage participation in desired religious activities, contact with minister or spiritual advisor. *Validating one's beliefs in an external way can provide support and strengthen the inner self.*[1,3]
- Discuss and role-play, as necessary, ways to deal with alternative view or conflict that may occur with family/SO(s)/society or cultural group. *Provides opportunity to try out different behaviors in a safe environment and be prepared for potentialities.*[3]
- Provide bibliotherapy, list of relevant resources (e.g., study groups, parish nurse, poetry society), and reliable Web sites *for later reference, self-paced learning, and ongoing support.*[3]

DOCUMENTATION FOCUS

Assessment/Reassessment
- Assessment findings, including client perception of needs and desire for growth.
- Cultural values or religious beliefs.
- Motivation and expectations for change.

Planning
- Plan for growth and who is involved in planning.

Implementation/Evaluation
- Response to activities, learning, and actions performed.
- Attainment or progress toward desired outcome(s).
- Modifications to plan.

Discharge Planning
- Long-term needs, expectations, and plan of action.
- Specific referrals made.

References

1. Fallot, R. D. (1998). Assessment of spirituality and implications for service planning. *New Dir Ment Health Serv*, 80, 13–23.

🌐 Cultural   Collaborative   🏠 Community/Home Care   Diagnostic Studies   ∞ Pediatric/Geriatric/Lifespan   Medications

2. Moller, M. D. (1999). Meeting spiritual needs on an inpatient unit. *J Psychosoc Nurs*, 37(11), 5–10.
3. Baldacchino, D., Draper, P. (2001). Spiritual coping strategies: A review of the nursing research literature. *J Adv Nurs*, 34(6), 833–841.
4. Cox, H. C., et al. (2002). *Clinical Applications of Nursing Diagnosis*. 4th ed. Philadelphia: F. A. Davis.
5. Lipson, J. G., Dibble, S. L., Minarik, P. A. (1996). *Culture & Nursing Care. A Pocket Guide*. San Francisco: UCSF Nursing Press.
6. Ross, L. A. (1994). Spiritual aspects of nursing. *J Adv Nurs*, 19, 439–447.

Stress Overload

DEFINITION: Excessive amounts and types of demands that require action

RELATED FACTORS

Inadequate resources (e.g., financial, social, education/knowledge level)
Intense, repeated stressors (e.g., family violence, chronic illness, terminal illness)
Multiple coexisting stressors (e.g., environmental threats/demands; physical threats/demands; social threats/demands)

DEFINING CHARACTERISTICS

Subjective
Expresses difficulty in functioning or problems with decision making
Expresses a feeling of pressure or tension
Expresses increased feelings of impatience or anger
Reports negative impact from stress (e.g., physical symptoms, psychological distress, feeling of "being sick" or of "going to get sick")
Reports situational stress as excessive (e.g., rates stress level as a 7 or above on a 10-point scale)

Objective
Demonstrates increased feelings of impatience or anger

Sample Clinical Applications: Chronic illness (e.g., multiple sclerosis [MS], diabetes, Parkinson's disease), terminal illness (e.g., ovarian cancer, amyotrophic lateral sclerosis [ALS]), abusive situations, bipolar disorder, depression, social phobia

DESIRED OUTCOMES/EVALUATION CRITERIA

Sample (NOC) linkages:
Stress Level: Severity of manifested physical or mental tension resulting from factors that alter an existing equilibrium
Anxiety Self-Control: Personal actions to eliminate or reduce feelings of apprehension, tension, or uneasiness from an unidentifiable source
Leisure Participation: Use of relaxing, interesting, and enjoyable activities to promote well being

(continues on page 806)

Stress Overload (continued)

Client Will (Include Specific Time Frame)
- Assess current situation accurately.
- Identify ineffective stress-management behaviors and consequences.
- Meet psychological needs as evidenced by appropriate expression of feelings, identification of options, and use of resources.
- Verbalize or demonstrate reduced stress reaction.

ACTIONS/INTERVENTIONS

Sample (NIC) linkages:
Emotional Support: Provision of reassurance, acceptance, and encouragement during times of stress
Coping Enhancement: Assisting a patient to adapt to perceived stressors, changes, or threats that interfere with meeting life demands and roles
Resiliency Promotion: Assisting individuals, families, and communities in development, use, and strengthening of protective factors to be used in coping with environmental and societal stressors

NURSING PRIORITY NO. 1

To identify causative/precipitating factors and degree of impairment:

- Ascertain what events have occurred (e.g., family violence, death of loved one; separation from living partner/parent; change in financial status or living conditions; chronic or terminal illness, workplace stress, loss of job or retirement; major trauma; catastrophic natural or man-made event) over remote and recent past *to assist in determining number, duration, and intensity of events causing perception of overwhelming stress.*
- Evaluate client's report of physical or emotional problems (e.g., fatigue, aches and pains, irritable bowel, skin rashes, frequent colds, sleeplessness, crying spells, anger, feeling overwhelmed or numb, compulsive behaviors) *that can be representing body's response to stress.*[1]
- Determine client's/SO's understanding of events, noting differences in viewpoints.
- Note client's gender, age, and developmental level of functioning. *Women, children, young adults, divorced and separated persons tend to have higher stress levels. Multiple stressors can weaken immune system and tax physical and emotional coping mechanisms of persons of any age, but particularly the elderly.*[1–3]
- Note cultural values or religious beliefs *that may affect client's expectation for self in dealing with situation, ability to ask for help from others, and expectations placed on client by SO/family.*[7]
- Identify client locus of control: internal (expressions of responsibility for self and ability to control outcomes—"I didn't quit smoking") or external (expressions of lack of control over self and environment—"Nothing ever works out"). *Knowing client's locus of control will help in developing a plan of care reflecting client's ability to realistically make changes that will help to manage stress better.*[7]
- Assess emotional responses and coping mechanisms being used.
- Determine stress feelings and self-talk client is engaging in. *Negative self-talk, all or nothing or pessimistic thinking, exaggeration, unrealistic expectations will contribute to stress overload.*[2]

- Assess degree of mastery client has exhibited in life. *Passive individual may have more difficulty being assertive and standing up for rights.*
- Determine presence or absence and nature of resources (e.g., whether family/SO are supportive, lack money, problems with relationship or social functioning).
- Note change in relationships with SO(s). *Conflict in the family, loss of a family member, divorce can result in a change in support client is accustomed to and impair ability to manage situation.*
- Evaluate stress level using appropriate tool (e.g., Stress & Depression, Self-Assessment Tool) to help identify areas of most distress. *While most stress seems to come from disastrous events in individual's life, positive events can also be stressful.*
- Review lab results to identify physiological conditions (e.g., thyroid or other hormone imbalance, anemia, unstable glucose levels, kidney or liver disease) *that may be causing or exacerbating stress.*[1]

NURSING PRIORITY NO. 2

To assist client to deal with current situation:

- Discuss situation or condition in simple, concise manner. *May help client to express emotions, grasp situation, and feel more in control.*
- Active-listen concerns and provide empathetic presence, using talk and silence as needed.
- Deal with the immediate issues first (e.g., treatment of physical injury, meet safety needs, removal from traumatic or violent environment).
- Collaborate in treatment of underlying conditions (e.g., diabetes, hormone imbalance, depression).[1]
- Provide or encourage restful environment where possible.
- Assist client in determining whether or not he or she can change stressor or response. *May help client to sort out things over which he or she has control and determine responses that can be modified.*
- Allow client to react in own way without judgment. Provide support and diversion as indicated.
- Help client to set limits on acting-out behaviors and learn ways to express emotions in an acceptable manner. *Promotes internal locus of control, enabling client to maintain self-concept and feel more positive about self.*
- Address use of ineffective or dangerous coping mechanisms (e.g., substance use or abuse, self-/other-directed violence) and refer for counseling as indicated.

NURSING PRIORITY NO. 3

To promote wellness (Teaching/Discharge Considerations):

- Use client's locus of control to develop individual plan of care *(e.g., for client with internal control, encourage client to take control of own care; for those with external control, begin with small tasks and add as tolerated).*[4]
- Incorporate strengths, assets, and past coping strategies that were successful for client. *Reinforces that client is able to deal with difficult situations.*
- Encourage strengthening of positive SO/family routines and interactions *that support and provide assistance in managing stress.*[5]
- Provide information about stress and exhaustion phase, which occurs when person is experiencing chronic or unresolved stress. *Release of cortisol can contribute to reduction in immune function, resulting in physical illness, mental disability, and life dysfunction.*

🏠 ● Review stress management and coping skills that client can use:[1,2,4-6]

Practice behaviors that may help *reduce negative consequences*—change thinking by focusing on positives, reframing thoughts, changing lifestyle.

Learn to read own body signs (e.g., shakiness, irritability, sleep disturbances, fatigue).

Take a step back, reduce obligations; simplify life; learn to say no *to reduce sense of being overwhelmed*.

Practice exchanging stresses (i.e., when a new stress comes into play, eliminate or postpone another stress) *to keep total stress level below overstress level*.

Seek help or assistance in meeting obligations, delegate tasks as appropriate.

Learn to control and redirect anger.

Develop and practice positive self-esteem skills.

Rest, sleep, and exercise on regular schedule or set times *to recuperate and rejuvenate self*.

Postpone changes in living situation (e.g., moving, remodeling) if possible.

Participate in self-help actions (e.g., deep breathing, find time to be alone, get involved in recreation or desired activity, plan something fun, develop humor) *to actively relax*.

Eliminate possible food or environmental allergens and toxins.

Eat nutritious meals; avoid junk food and excessive sugars.

Avoid excessive caffeine, alcohol or other drugs, and nicotine *to balance body chemicals and support general health*.

Take a multivitamin, mineral, trace element preparation.

Develop spiritual self (e.g., meditate or pray; block negative thoughts; learn to give and take, speak and listen, forgive and move on).

Interact socially, reach out, nurture self and others *to reduce loneliness or sense of isolation*.

💊 ● Review proper medication use *to manage exacerbating conditions (e.g., depression, mood disorders)*.

🄰 ● Identify community resources (e.g., vocational counseling, educational programs, child or elder care, Women, Infants, and Children [WIC] program or food stamps, home or respite care) *that can help client manage lifestyle and environmental stress*.

🄰 ● Refer for therapy, as indicated (e.g., medical treatment, psychological counseling; hypnosis, massage, biofeedback).

DOCUMENTATION FOCUS

Assessment/Reassessment
• Individual findings, noting specific stressors, individual's perception of the situation, locus of control.
• Specific cultural or religious factors.
• Availability and use of support systems and resources.

Planning
• Plan of care and who is involved in planning.
• Teaching plan.

Implementation/Evaluation
• Responses to interventions, teaching, and actions performed.
• Attainment or progress toward desired outcome(s).
• Modifications to plan of care.

Discharge Planning
• Long-term needs and who is responsible for actions to be taken.
• Specific referrals made.

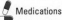

References

1. Burns, S. L. (1997). The medical basis of stress, depression, anxiety, sleep problems and drug use. Retrieved August 2007 from www.teahhealth.com.
2. Klimes, R. (2007). Managing stress: Living without stress overload. Retrieved April 2007 from www.learnwell.org/stress.htm.
3. Woolston, C. (2006). Stress and aging. Retrieved July 2007 from www.yourhealthconnection.com/topic/stressaging.
4. Donatelle, R. (2003). Managing stress: Coping with life's challenges. *Health: The Basics*. 5th ed. San Francisco: Benjamin Cummings.
5. Beckett, C. (2000). Family theory as a framework for assessment. Retrieved August 2007 from http://jan.ucc.nau.edu/~nur350-c/class/2_family/theory/lesson2-1-3.html.
6. Harvard Medical School. (2007). *Stress Control: Techniques for Preventing and Easing Stress*. Boston: Harvard Health Publications.
7. Lipson, J. G., Dibble, S. L., Minarik, P. A. (1996). *Culture & Nursing Care: A Pocket Guide*. San Francisco: UCSF Nursing Press.

risk for Suffocation

DEFINITION: Accentuated risk of accidental suffocation (inadequate air available for inhalation)

RISK FACTORS

Internal
Reduced olfactory sensation
Reduced motor abilities
Lack of safety education or precautions
Cognitive or emotional difficulties [e.g., altered consciousness/mentation]
Disease or injury process

External
Pillow or propped bottle placed in an infant's crib
Hanging a pacifier around infant's neck
Playing with plastic bags; inserting small objects into airway
Leaving children unattended in water
Discarded refrigerators without removed doors
Vehicle warming in closed garage [faulty exhaust system]; use of fuel-burning heaters not vented to outside
Household gas leaks; smoking in bed
Low-strung clothesline
Eating large mouthfuls [or pieces] of food

NOTE: A risk diagnosis is not evidenced by signs and symptoms, as the problem has not occurred; rather, nursing interventions are directed at prevention.
Sample Clinical Applications: Substance use or abuse, spinal cord injury, crushing chest injury, obesity, near-drowning, burn or inhalation injury, sleep apnea, seizure disorder

(continues on page 810)

risk for Suffocation (continued)
DESIRED OUTCOMES/EVALUATION CRITERIA

Sample (NOC) linkages:
Risk Control: Personal actions to prevent, eliminate, or reduce modifiable health threats
Aspiration Prevention: Personal actions to prevent the passage of fluid and solid particles into the lung
Personal Safety Behavior: Personal actions that prevent physical injury to self

Client/Caregiver Will (Include Specific Time Frame)
• Verbalize knowledge of hazards in the environment.
• Identify interventions appropriate to situation.
• Correct hazardous situations to prevent or reduce risk of suffocation.
• Demonstrate CPR skills and how to access emergency assistance.

ACTIONS/INTERVENTIONS

Sample (NIC) linkages:
Airway Management: Facilitation of patency of air passages
Aspiration Precautions: Prevention or minimization of risk factors in the patient at risk for aspiration
Teaching Infant Safety: Instruction on safety during first year of life

NURSING PRIORITY NO. 1

To assess causative/contributing factors:

● Determine client's/SO's knowledge of individual safety concerns and environmental hazards present *to identify misconceptions and educational needs. Suffocation can be caused by (1) spasm of airway (e.g., food or water going down wrong way, irritant gases, asthma); (2) airway obstruction (e.g., foreign body, tongue falling back in unconscious person, swelling of tissues from burn injury or allergic reaction); (3) airway compression (e.g., tying rope or band tightly around neck, hanging, throttling, smothering); (4) conditions affecting the respiratory mechanism (e.g., epilepsy, tetanus, rabies, nerve diseases causing paralysis of chest wall or diaphragm); (5) conditions affecting respiratory center in brain (e.g., electric shock; stroke or other brain trauma; medications such as morphine, barbiturates); and (6) compression of the chest (e.g., crushing as might occur with cave-in, motor vehicle crash, pressure in a massive crowd).*[1,7,8]

● Identify level of concern or awareness and motivation of client/SO(s) to correct safety hazards and improve individual situation. *Lack of commitment may limit growth or willingness to make changes, placing dependent individuals at risk.*

∞ ● Determine age, developmental level, and mentation (e.g., infant/young child, frail elder, person with developmental delay, altered level of consciousness, or cognitive impairments or dementia) *to identify individuals unable to be responsible for or protect self.*

● Assess neurological status and note history of conditions such as stroke, cerebral palsy, multiple sclerosis (MS), amyotrophic lateral sclerosis (ALS), *that have potential to compromise airway or affect ability to swallow.*[4]

● Determine presence of seizure disorder, noting use of antiepileptics and how well condition is controlled. *Seizure activity (and especially status epileptics) is a major risk factor for respiratory inhibition or arrest.*[4]

⊕ Cultural 🅐 Collaborative 🏠 Community/Home Care ⬛ Diagnostic Studies ∞ Pediatric/Geriatric/Lifespan   Medications

- Note reports of sleep disturbance and daytime fatigue. *May be indicative of sleep apnea (airway obstruction) requiring referral for evaluation.* Refer to NDs Insomnia, Sleep Deprivation.
- Review medication regimen *to note potential for oversedation and respiratory failure (e.g., central nervous system [CNS] depressants, analgesics, sedatives, antidepressants).*[10]
- Assess for allergies to medications, foods, environmental factors *that could result in severe reaction or anaphylaxsis resulting in respiratory arrest.*
- Be alert to and carefully monitor those individuals who are severely depressed, mentally ill, or aggressive and in restraints. *These individuals could be at risk for suicide by suffocation (e.g., inhaled carbon monoxide or death by strangling or hanging).*[2] Refer to ND risk for Suicide.
- Note signs of respiratory distress (e.g., cough, stridor, wheezing, increased work of breathing) *that could indicate swelling or obstruction of airways.*[3] Refer to NDs ineffective Airway Clearance, risk for Aspiration, ineffective Breathing Pattern, impaired spontaneous Ventilation, as appropriate, for additional interventions.

NURSING PRIORITY NO. 2

To reverse/correct contributing factors:

- Discuss with client/SO(s) identified environmental or work-related safety hazards and problem-solve methods for resolution (e.g., need for smoke and carbon monoxide alarms, vents for household heater, clean chimney, properly strung clothesline, proper venting of machinery exhaust, monitoring of stored chemicals, bracing trench walls when digging).
- Protect airway at all times, especially if client unable to protect self:[2,4,7,11]
  Use proper positioning, suctioning, use of airway adjuncts, as indicated, *for comatose or cognitively impaired individual or client with swallowing impairment or obstructive sleep apnea.*
  Provide seizure precautions and antiseizure medication, as indicated.
- Administer medications when client is sitting or standing upright and can swallow without difficulty.
  Emphasize importance of chewing carefully, taking small amounts of food, and using caution *to prevent aspiration when talking or drinking while eating.*
  Provide diet modifications as indicated by specific needs (e.g., developmental level; presence/degree of swallowing disability, impaired cognition) *to reduce risk of aspiration.*
  Avoid physical and mechanical restraints, including vest or waist restraint, side rails, choke hold. *Increases agitation and risk of partial escape, resulting in entrapment of head and hanging.*
- Emphasize with client/SO the importance of getting help when beginning to choke or feel respiratory distress (e.g., staying with people instead of leaving table, make gestures across throat; making sure someone recognizes the emergency) *in order to provide timely intervention such as abdominal thrusts and calling 911.*
- Refrain from smoking in bed; supervise smoking materials (use, disposal, and storage) for impaired individuals. Keep smoking materials out of reach of children.
- Avoid idling automobile (or using fuel-burning heaters) in closed or unvented spaces.
- Emphasize importance of periodic evaluation and repair of gas appliances and furnace, automobile exhaust system *to prevent exposure to carbon monoxide.*
- Review child protective measures:[2,5,6,9,11]
  Place infant in supine position for sleep. Refer to ND sudden infant Death Syndrome.
  Do not prop baby bottles in infant crib.
  Attach pacifier to clothing—not around neck; remove bib before putting baby in bed.

Store or dispose of plastic bags (e.g., shopping, garbage, dry cleaning, and shipping) out of reach of infants/young children.

Avoid use of plastic mattress or crib covers.

Avoid placing infant to sleep on soft surfaces (e.g., beanbag chair, basket with soft sides, soft pillow or comforter, water bed) *that baby can sink into or be unable to free face.*

Use a crib with slats that are no more than 2 3/8 inches apart *so that baby cannot get head trapped or slip body through slats.*

Refrain from bedsharing with infant/young child *to prevent accidental smothering.*

Provide constant supervision of young children in bathtub or swimming pool.

Make certain that blind and curtain cords, drawstrings on clothing, and so forth, are out of reach of small children *to prevent accidental hanging.*

Observe young child/impaired individual for objects put in mouth (e.g., food such as raw carrots, nuts, seeds, popcorn, hot dogs; toy parts; buttons; balloons; batteries; coins) *that can get lodged in airway and cause choking.*

Lock or remove lid or door of chests, trunks, old refrigerators or freezers *to prevent child from being trapped in airless environment.*

NURSING PRIORITY NO. 3

To promote wellness (Teaching/Discharge Considerations):

🏠 ● Review safety factors identified in individual situation and methods for remediation.

🏠 ● Develop plan with client/caregiver for long-range management of situation to avoid risks. *Enhances commitment to plan, optimizing outcomes.*

🏠 ● Discuss possibility of choking resulting from relaxation of throat muscle and impaired judgment *when combining drinking alcohol with eating.*

🏠 ● Involve family members in learning and practicing rescue techniques (e.g., treating of choking or breathing problems, cardiopulmonary resuscitation [CPR]) *to deal with emergency situations (especially when at-home client is at risk on a regular basis).*

🏠 ● Encourage individuals to read package labels and identify and remove safety hazards such as toys with small parts, and monitor Web sites for product recalls.

🏠 ● Promote water and swimming pool safety, vigilance, and use of approved flotation equipment, fencing and locked gates, alarm system, and so forth.

🏠 ● Discuss fire safety and concerns regarding use of heaters, household gas appliances, and old, discarded appliances. Encourage home fire safety drills yearly.

🏠 ● Promote public education in techniques for clearing blocked airways (e.g., Heimlich maneuver, CPR).

🔵∞ ● Collaborate in community public health education regarding hazards for children (e.g., appropriate toy size for young child; discussing dangers of "huffing" [inhalants] and playing choking or hanging games with preteens; how to spot potential for depression and risk of suicidal gestures in adolescent) *to reduce potential for accidental or intentional suffocation.*[12]

DOCUMENTATION FOCUS

Assessment/Reassessment
• Individual risk factors, including individual's cognitive status and level of knowledge.
• Level of concern and motivation for change.
• Equipment or airway adjunct needs.

Planning
- Plan of care and who is involved in planning.
- Teaching plan.

Implementation/Evaluation
- Responses to interventions, teaching, and actions performed.
- Attainment or progress toward desired outcome(s).
- Modifications to plan of care.

Discharge Planning
- Long-term needs, appropriate preventive measures, and who is responsible for actions to be taken.
- Specific referrals made.

References

1. Suffocation and artificial respiration. (2000). Fact sheet for WebHealthCentre. Retrieved July 2007 from http://webhealthcentre.com.
2. Masters, K. J., et al. (2001). Summary of the practice parameter for the prevention and management of aggressive behavior in child and adolescent psychiatric institutions with special reference to seclusion and restraint. *J Am Acad Child Adoles Psychiatry*, 40(11), 1356–1358.
3. Kline, A. (2003). Pinpointing the cause of pediatric respiratory distress. *Nursing*, 33(9), 58–63.
4. Doenges, M. E., Moorhouse, M. F., Geissler-Murr, A. C. (2002). ND: Suffocation, risk for in Seizure Disorders. *Nursing Care Plans: Guidelines for Individualizing Patient Care*. 6th ed. Philadelphia: F. A. Davis, 201–203.
5. Task Force on Infant Sleep Position and Sudden Infant Death Syndrome. (2000). Changing concepts of sudden infant death syndrome: Implications for infant sleeping environment and sleep position. *Pediatrics*, 105(3), 650–656.
6. Suffocation. *Doctors Book of Home Remedies for Children*. Retrieved July 2007 from www.mothernature.com.
7. Green, P. M. (1993). High risk for suffocation. In McFarland, G. K., McFarlane, E. A. (eds). *Nursing Diagnosis and Interventions*. St. Louis, MO: Mosby.
8. Suffocation. Health Sciences Centre. Retrieved July 2007 from www.hsc.mb.ca/impact/suffocation.htm.
9. Preventing strangulation and suffocation among infants and children. SAFEUSA. Retrieved July 2007 from http://safeusa.org.
10. Apnea: Handbook of signs and symptoms. 3d ed. Retrieved July 2007 from www.wrongdiagnosis.com/s/suffocation/book-diseases-5a.htm.
11. Homeir, B. P. (2004). Household safety: Preventing suffocation. Retrieved April 2007 from www.kidshealth.org/parent/positive/family/safety_suffocation.html.
12. Dowshen, S. (2005). Kids and dangerous "suffocation games." Retrieved April 2007 from www.kidshealth.org/research/suffocation.html.

risk for Suicide

DEFINITION: At risk for self-inflicted, life-threatening injury

RISK FACTORS

Behavioral
History of prior suicide attempt
Buying a gun; stockpiling medicines
Making or changing a will; giving away possessions
Sudden euphoric recovery from major depression
Impulsiveness; marked changes in behavior, attitude, or school performance

Demographic
Age (e.g., elderly, young adult males, adolescents)
Race (e.g., Caucasian, Native American)
Male gender
Divorced; widowed

Physical
Physical or terminal illness; chronic pain

Psychological
Family history of suicide; abuse in childhood
Substance use or abuse
Psychiatric illness or disorder (e.g., depression, schizophrenia, bipolar disorder)
Guilt
Gay or lesbian youth

Situational
Living alone; retired; economic instability; relocation; institutionalization
Loss of autonomy or independence
Presence of gun in home
Adolescents living in nontraditional settings (e.g., juvenile detention center, prison, halfway house, group home)

Social
Loss of important relationship; disrupted family life; poor support systems; social isolation
Grief, loneliness
Hopelessness; helplessness
Legal or disciplinary problems
Cluster suicides

Verbal
Threats of killing oneself; states desire to die [or end it all]

NOTE: A risk diagnosis is not evidenced by signs and symptoms, as the problem has not occurred; rather, nursing interventions are directed at prevention.

Sample Clinical Applications: Acute or chronic brain syndrome, hormonal imbalances (e.g., premenstrual syndrome [PMS], postpartum psychosis), substance use or abuse, chronic or terminal illness (e.g., amyotrophic lateral sclerosis [ALS], cancer), major depression, schizophrenia, bipolar disorder, panic state

DESIRED OUTCOMES/EVALUATION CRITERIA

Sample NOC linkages:
Suicide Self-Restraint: Personal actions to refrain from gestures and attempts at killing self
Coping: Personal actions to manage stressors that tax an individual's resources
Hope: Optimism that is personally satisfying and life-supporting

Client Will (Include Specific Time Frame)
• Acknowledge difficulties perceived in current situation.
• Identify current factors that can be dealt with.
• Be involved in planning course of action to correct existing problems.
• Make decision that suicide is not the answer to perceived or real problems.

ACTIONS/INTERVENTIONS

Sample NIC linkages:
Suicide Prevention: Reducing the risk for self-inflicted harm with intent to end life
Behavior Management: Self-Harm: Assisting the patient to decrease or eliminate self-mutilating or self-abusive behavior
Patient Contracting: Negotiating an agreement with an individual that reinforces a specific behavior change

NURSING PRIORITY NO. 1

To assess causative/contributing factors and degree of risk:

● Identify degree of risk or potential for suicide and seriousness of threat. Use a scale of 1 to 10 and prioritize according to severity of threat, availability of means. *Most people who are contemplating suicide send a variety of signals indicating their intent, and recognizing these warning signs allows for immediate intervention.*[4]
● Note behaviors indicative of intent. *Individual may not make statements of intent, but gestures (e.g., threats, giving away possessions), presence of means (e.g., guns), previous attempts, and presence of hallucinations or delusions may provide clues to intent.*[3,6]
● Ask directly if person is thinking of acting on thoughts or feelings to determine intent. *Most individuals want someone to see what desperate straits they are in, and by bringing the issue into the open, discussion can begin and plans made to keep the person safe.*[3,7]
● Note withdrawal from usual activities, lack of social interactions. *These are classic behaviors of the individual who is feeling depressed and sad and may be having negative thoughts of worthlessness.*[6]
● Identify losses client has experienced and meaning of those losses. *Unresolved issues may be contributing to thoughts of hopelessness, feelings of despair, and suicidal ideation.*[3,6]
∞ ● Note age and gender. *While women talk about suicide more frequently, men usually succeed more often. Risk of suicide is greater in teens and the elderly, but there is a rising awareness of risk in early childhood.*[4,8,10]

- Determine cultural or religious beliefs that may be affecting client's thinking about life and death. *Family of origin and culture in which individual grew up influence attitudes toward taking one's own life; for instance, Protestants commit suicide more frequently than Catholics or Jews, and whites are at highest risk, followed by Native Americans, African Americans, Hispanic Americans, and Asian Americans.*[2,3,10]
- Identify conditions such as acute or chronic brain syndrome, panic state, hormonal imbalance (e.g., PMS, postpartum psychosis, drug-induced). *These conditions may interfere with ability to control own behavior leading to impulsive actions that may put client at risk.*[1,10]
- Review laboratory results (e.g., blood alcohol, serum glucose, arterial blood gases [ABGs], electrolytes, renal function tests). *Identifies factors that may affect reasoning ability, interfering with ability to think clearly about issues that are leading to thoughts of suicide.*[1,3,5]
- Assess physical complaints. *Sleeping difficulties, lack of appetite can be indicators of depression and suicidal ideation requiring further evaluation.*[3,4]
- Review family history for suicidal behavior. *Individual risk is increased when other family members have committed suicide or exhibited symptoms of depression. Studies have shown a possible genetic link toward suicidal behavior.*[3]
- Assess coping behaviors presently used. *Client's current negative thinking may preclude looking at positive behaviors that have been used in the past that would help in the current situation. Client may believe there is no alternative except suicide.*[6,7]
- Ascertain presence of SO(s)/friends available for support. *Individuals who have positive support systems whom they can rely on during a crisis situation are less likely to commit suicide and are more apt to return to a successful life.*[3]
- Determine drug use or "self"-medication. *The use of alcohol, especially the combination of alcohol and barbiturates, increases the risk of suicide.*
- Note history of disciplinary problems or involvement with judicial system. *Feelings of despair over problems with the legal system and lack of hope about outcome can lead to belief that the only solution is suicide.*[3,10]

NURSING PRIORITY NO. 2

To assist clients to accept responsibility for own behavior and prevent suicide:

- Develop therapeutic nurse-client relationship, providing consistent care provider. *Promotes sense of trust, allowing individual to discuss feelings openly. Collaborating with the client to better understand the problem affirms the client's ability to solve the current situation.*[3,6]
- Maintain straightforward communication. *By being direct and honest and acknowledging need for attention, care provider can avoid reinforcing manipulative behavior.*[6]
- Explain concern for safety and willingness to help client stay safe. *Clients often believe their concerns will not be taken seriously, and stating clearly that they will be listened to sends a clear message of support and caring.*[6]
- Encourage expression of feelings and make time to listen to concerns. *Acknowledges reality of feelings and that they are okay. Helps individual sort out thinking and begin to develop understanding of situation.*[3,6]
- Give permission to express angry feelings in acceptable ways and let client know someone will be available to assist in maintaining control. *Promotes acceptance and sense of safety while client is regaining own control.*[3,4]
- Acknowledge reality of suicide as an option. Discuss consequences of actions if they follow through on intent. Ask how it will help individual to resolve problems. *Can help client to focus on consequences of actions and begin to discuss the possibility of other options.*[5,7]
- Help client identify more appropriate solutions/behaviors. *Alternative activities, such as exercise, can lessen sense of anxiety and associated physical manifestations.*[3]

- Maintain observation of client and check environment for hazards that could be used to commit suicide. *Increases client safety and reduces risk of impulsive behavior when client is hospitalized.*[3]
- Discuss use of antidepressant medications, especially when there may be a significant organic component to the suicidal ideation. *While the use of medications may be helpful in the short term, there are some drawbacks, namely, the length of time it takes for most medications to take effect, and the potential for giving a client a means of suicide because of the possibility of a lethal overdose.*[6,9,10]
- Reevaluate potential for suicide periodically at key times (e.g., mood changes, increasing withdrawal), as well as when client is feeling better and planning for discharge becomes active. *The highest risk is when the client has both suicidal ideation and sufficient energy with which to act.*[5,6]

NURSING PRIORITY NO. 3

To assist client to plan course of action to correct/deal with existing situation:

- Gear interventions to individual involved. *Age, relationships, and current situation determine what is needed to help client deal with feelings of despair and hopelessness.*[6,10]
- Negotiate contract with client regarding willingness not to do anything lethal for a stated period of time. Specify what care provider will be responsible for and what client responsibilities are. *Making a contract in which the individual agrees to stay alive for a specified period of time, from day one through the entire course of treatment and written and signed by each party, may help the client to follow through with therapy to find reason for living. Although there is little research on the effectiveness of these contracts, they are frequently used.*[6]
- Specify alternative actions necessary if client is unwilling to negotiate contract. *Client may be willing to agree to other actions (i.e., calling therapist if feelings are overwhelming), even though he or she is not willing to commit to a contract.*[6]
- Provide directions for actions client can take, avoiding negative statements such as "do nots." *Providing opportunity for client to have control over circumstances can promote a positive attitude and give client some hope for the future.*[3,5]

NURSING PRIORITY NO. 4

To promote wellness (Teaching/Discharge Considerations):

- Promote development of internal control. *Helping the client look at new ways to deal with problems can provide a sense of own ability to solve problems, improve situation, and hope for the future.*[3]
- Assist with learning problem-solving, assertiveness training, and social skills. *By learning these new skills, client can begin to feel more confidence in own ability to handle problems that arise and deal with the current situation.*[3,5]
- Engage in physical activity programs. *Promotes release of endorphins and feelings of self-worth, improving sense of well-being and giving client hope.*[3]
- Determine nutritional needs and help client to plan for meeting them. *Enhances general well-being and energy level.*[1,10]
- Review use of antidepressants noting that it takes 4 to 8 weeks for effects of medication to be observed, and different medications may need to be tried to obtain maximum benefit. Stress importance of continuing medication after symptoms of depression resolve. *Studies of older adults age 70 and over reveal significant decrease in relapse when antidepressant continued for 2 years beyond becoming symptom-free.*[10]

🏠 • Involve family/SO in planning. *Improves understanding and support when family knows the facts and has a part in planning for rehabilitation efforts for the client.*[1,5]

 • Refer to formal resources as indicated. *May need assistance with referrals to individual, group, or marital psychotherapy; substance abuse treatment program, or social services when situation involves mental illness, family disorganization.*[3,5,10]

DOCUMENTATION FOCUS

Assessment/Reassessment
• Individual findings, including nature of concern (e.g., suicidal or behavioral risk factors and level of impulse control, plan of action and means to carry out plan).
• Client's perception of situation, motivation for change.
• Cultural or religious beliefs influencing attitudes about life and suicide.
• Availability of family and other support systems.

Planning
• Plan of care and who is involved in the planning.
• Details of contract regarding suicidal ideation or plans.
• Teaching plan.

Implementation/Evaluation
• Actions taken to promote safety.
• Response to interventions, teaching, and actions performed.
• Attainment or progress toward desired outcome(s).
• Modifications to plan of care.

Discharge Planning
• Long-term needs and who is responsible for actions to be taken.
• Available resources, specific referrals made.

References

1. Cox, H. C., et al. (2002). *Clinical Applications of Nursing Diagnosis: Adult, Child, Women's, Psychiatric, Gerontic, and Home Health Considerations.* 4th ed. Philadelphia: F. A. Davis.
2. Lipson, J. G., Dibble, S. L., Minarik, P. A. (1996). *Culture & Nursing Care: A Pocket Guide.* San Francisco: UCSF Nursing Press.
3. Townsend, M. C. (2003). *Psychiatric Mental Health Nursing Concepts of Care.* 4th ed. Philadelphia: F. A. Davis.
4. Doenges, M. E., Moorhouse, M. F., Murr, A. G. (2004). *Nurse's Pocket Guide: Diagnoses, Interventions, and Rationales.* 9th ed. Philadelphia: F. A. Davis.
5. Doenges, M., Townsend, M., Moorhouse, M. (1998). *Psychiatric Care Plans: Guidelines for Individualizing Care.* 3d ed. Philadelphia: F. A. Davis.
6. Jurich, A. P. (2003). The nature of suicide. *Clinical Update (insert in Family Therapy Magazine),* 3(6), 1–8.
7. Gettinger-Dinner, L. (2007). Suicide risk assessment: What providers need to know. Retrieved May 2007 from http://news.nurse.com/apps/pbcs.dll/article?AID=/20070430/CA09/304300012&SearchID=73281745058190.
8. Whetstone, L., Morrissey, S. (2007). Children at risk: The association between perceived weight status and suicidal thoughts and attempts in middle school youth. *J School Health,* 77(2), 59–66.
9. Sherman, C. (2002). Antisuicidal effect of psychotropics remains uncertain. *Clin Psychiatry News,* 30(8). Retrieved October 2009 from http://findarticles.com/p/articles/mi_hb4345/is_8_30/ai_n28939004/.

10. National Institute of Mental Health. (April 2007). Older adults. Depression & suicide facts. NIH Publication no. 4593. Retrieved May 2007 from www.nimh.nih.gov/publicat/elderlydepsuicide.cfm.

delayed Surgical Recovery

DEFINITION: Extension of the number of postoperative days required to initiate and perform activities that maintain life, health, and well-being

RELATED FACTORS

Extensive or prolonged surgical procedure
Pain
Obesity
Preoperative expectations
Postoperative surgical site infection

DEFINING CHARACTERISTICS

Subjective
Perception that more time is needed to recover
Report of pain or discomfort; fatigue
Loss of appetite with or without nausea
Postpones resumption of work or employment activities

Objective
Evidence of interrupted healing of surgical area (e.g., red, indurated, draining, immobilized)
Difficulty in moving about; requires help to complete self-care

Sample Clinical Applications: Major surgical procedures, traumatic injuries with surgical intervention, chronic conditions (e.g., diabetes mellitus, cancer, HIV/AIDS, chronic obstructive pulmonary disease [COPD])

DESIRED OUTCOMES/EVALUATION CRITERIA

Sample NOC linkages:
Wound Healing: Primary Intention: Extent of regeneration of cells and tissues following intentional closure
Self-Care: Activities of Daily Living (ADL): Ability to perform the most basic physical tasks and personal care activities independently with or without assistive device
Endurance: Capacity to sustain activity

Client Will (Include Specific Time Frame)
• Display complete healing of surgical area.
• Perform desired self-care activities.
• Report increased energy, able to participate in usual (work or employment) activities.

(continues on page 820)

delayed Surgical Recovery (continued)
ACTIONS/INTERVENTIONS

Sample NIC linkages:
Self-Care Assistance: Assisting another to perform ADLs
Energy Management: Regulating energy use to treat or prevent fatigue and optimize function
Wound Care: Prevention of wound complications and promotion of wound healing

NURSING PRIORITY NO. 1

To assess causative/contributing factors:

- Identify factors affecting ability to care for self and meet own needs (e.g., low socioeconomic status or poverty; lack of insurance; inadequate transportation; lack of family or support system; severe trauma or prolonged hospitalization with multiple complicating factors; client with severe anxiety about diagnosis or outcome) *that increase risk for adverse outcomes.*[7]
- Determine age, developmental level, and general state of health *to help determine time that may be required for client to resume ADLs and other activities, or expectation of time needed for healing. Note: The older adult undergoing surgical treatment is at greater risk for delayed recovery because of age-related changes in numerous systems and protective mechanisms that increase the potential for complications.*[1,8]
- Note underlying condition or pathology (e.g., cancer, burns, diabetes, hypothyroidism, obesity, steroid therapy, major trauma, infections, radiation therapy, cardiopulmonary disorders, debilitating illness) *that can adversely affect healing and prolong recuperation time.*[4,9]
- Determine the length of operative procedure or time under anesthesia (e.g., typical or lengthy); type and severity of perioperative complications (e.g., trauma or other conditions requiring multiple surgeries; heavy bleeding during procedure); type of surgical wound (e.g., clean, clean-contaminated, or grossly contaminated, acutely infected); and development of postoperative complications (e.g., surgical site infection, suture reactions, dehiscence, ventilator-associated pneumonia, deep vein thrombosis [DVT]) *that can affect the pace of healing or prolong recovery.*[3,4]
- Assess circulation and sensation in surgical area *to evaluate for (1) internal bleeding that compromises wound integrity; or (2) loss of blood flow to area, resulting in decreased oxygen supply to tissues, or nerve damage delaying healing.*[2,3]
- Note use of plastics (e.g., incontinence pads or moisture barriers) or latex materials. *Plastics retain heat and enhance growth of pathogens in wound. Client sensitivity to latex can cause skin or tissue reactions that delay healing.* Refer to ND latex Allergy Response.
- Review client's preoperative medication regimen *to ascertain that none could impede healing processes (e.g., aspirin and NSAIDs increase bleeding time, alcohol—a potent vasodilator—and some herbals such as garlic and ginkgo biloba can also be associated with bleeding complications)*[3]
- Determine nutritional status and current intake *to ascertain if nutrition is adequate to support healing. Client may have preexisting nutritional concerns (e.g., elderly person with anorexia, person with morbid obesity) or may have been fasting for several days perioperatively or experienced nausea, vomiting, and loss of appetite postoperatively, depending on the surgical procedure performed and client's reactions to medications (e.g., pain medications, antibiotics).*[2,3,8]
- Note lifestyle factors (e.g., obesity, cigarette smoking, sedentary lifestyle) *that may impede recovery.*

- Perform pain assessment *to ascertain whether pain management is adequate to meet client's needs during recovery.*
- Review results of laboratory tests (e.g., complete blood count [CBC], blood/wound cultures, serum glucose) *to assess for presence and type of infections, metabolic or endocrine dysfunction, or other conditions affecting body's ability to heal.*
- Evaluate client's cognitive and emotional state, noting presence of postoperative changes, including confusion, depression, apathy, expressions of helplessness *to determine need for further assessment of possible physical or psychological interferences.*
- Ascertain attitudes and cultural values of individual about condition. *Family beliefs and cultural values, stress and fear related to surgery (and the reason for it), possible stigma about relative condition or disease, or change in body image; or motivation to return to usual role and activities all impact rate and expectations for sick role and recovery.*[6]

NURSING PRIORITY NO. 2

To determine impact of delayed recovery:

- Note length of illness or hospitalization, time of discharge, and progress to date *to compare with general expectations for procedure and situation.*
- Determine client's/SO's expectations for recovery and specific stressors related to delay (e.g., return to work or school, home responsibilities, child care, financial difficulties, limited support system).
- Determine energy level and current participation in ADLs *to compare with usual level of function.*
- Ascertain whether client usually requires assistance in home setting and who provides it, and individual's current availability and capability.
- Note client/SO reports of helplessness or inability to cope with situation.
- Obtain psychological assessment of client's emotional status, noting potential problems arising from current situation.

NURSING PRIORITY NO. 3

To promote optimal recovery:

- Practice and instruct client/caregiver(s) in proper hand hygiene and aseptic technique for incisional care *to reduce incidence of contamination and infection.*[5]
- Administer or discuss use of medications to manage postoperative discomforts (e.g., pain, nausea, vomiting) and other concurrent or underlying conditions, such as diabetes, osteoporosis, heart failure, COPD. *Client may require antibiotics, insulin to support tissue repair, or management of chronic pain to improve mobility and tissue recovery.*[2]
- Instruct client/SO in necessary self-care of incisions and specific symptom management. *With short hospital stays, client/SO are usually expected to provide a great deal of postoperative care and monitoring at home.*[7]
- Provide wound care expectations and instructions in verbal and written forms *to facilitate self-care and reduce likelihood of misinterpretation of information when client/SO is providing care at home.*[3]
- Instruct client/SO in routine inspection of incision or wound and to report changes in wound indicative of failure to heal (e.g., deepening wound, local or systemic fever, exudates [noting color, amount, and odor], loss of approximation of wound edges) *to establish comparative baseline and allow for early intervention (e.g., antimicrobial therapy, wound irrigation or packing).*
- Avoid or limit use of plastics or latex materials in wound care, as appropriate. *Can delay healing and cause skin breakdown.*

Nursing Diagnoses in Alphabetical Order

- Collaborate in treatment and assist with wound care, as indicated. *May require surgical debridement, barrier dressings, skin-protective agents, wound vac for open or draining wounds.* Include wound care specialist or stomal therapist, as appropriate, *to troubleshoot healing difficulties.*
- Provide optimal nutrition with adequate protein *to provide a positive nitrogen balance, which aids in healing and contributes to general good health.*
- Encourage adequate fluid and electrolyte intake *to avoid dehydration of tissues and to promote optimal cellular and organ function.*[2]
- Encourage early ambulation and regular exercise *to promote circulation, improve muscle strength and overall endurance, and reduce risks associated with immobility.*[2]
- Recommend pacing (alternating activity with adequate rest periods) *to reduce fatigue and allow weakened muscles and tissues to recuperate.*[2]
- Employ nonpharmacological healing measures, as indicated (e.g., breathing exercises, listening to music, relaxation tapes, biofeedback, hot or cold applications) *to promote relaxation of muscles and tissue healing as well as improve coping and outlook for positive healing experience.*[2]
- Refer for outpatient or follow-up care, as indicated (e.g., telephone monitoring, home visit, wound care clinic, pain management program).

NURSING PRIORITY NO. 4

To promote wellness (Teaching/Discharge Considerations):

- Discuss reality of recovery process and client's/SO's expectations. *Individuals are often unrealistic regarding energy and time required for healing and own abilities and responsibilities to facilitate process.*
- Involve client/SO(s) in setting incremental goals. *Enhances commitment to plan and reduces likelihood of frustration, thus blocking progress.*
- Demonstrate self-care skills, provide client/SO with health-related information and psychosocial support *to manage symptoms and pain, thus enhancing well-being.*
- Refer to physical or occupational therapist, as indicated *to address exercise program and home-care needs and identify assistive devices to facilitate independence in ADLs.*
- Identify suppliers for dressings and wound care items, and assistive devices, as needed.
- Consult nutritionist for individual dietary plan *to meet increased nutritional needs that reflect personal situation and resources.*
- Evaluate home situation (e.g., lives alone, bedroom or bathroom on second floor, availability of assistance). *Identifies necessary adjustments, such as moving bedroom to first floor, arranging for commode during recovery, and obtaining an in-home emergency call system.*
- Discuss alternative placement (e.g., convalescent or rehabilitation center, as appropriate). *Brief stay with concentrated support and therapy may speed recovery and return to home.*
- Identify community resources (e.g., visiting nurse, home healthcare agency, Meals on Wheels, respite care). *Facilitates adjustment to home setting.*
- Refer for counseling or support. *May need additional help to overcome feelings of discouragement, deal with changes in life.*

DOCUMENTATION FOCUS

Assessment/Reassessment
- Assessment findings, including individual concerns, family involvement and support factors, availability of resources.

- Cultural expectations.
- Assistive device use or need.

Planning
- Plan of care and who is involved in planning.
- Teaching plan.

Implementation/Evaluation
- Responses of client/SO(s) to plan, interventions, teaching, and actions performed.
- Attainment or progress toward desired outcome(s).
- Modifications to plan of care.

Discharge Planning
- Long-term needs and who is responsible for actions to be taken.
- Specific referrals made.

References

1. Cox, H. C., et al. (2002). ND: Surgical Recovery, delayed. *Clinical Applications of Nursing Diagnosis: Adult, Child, Women's, Psychiatric, Gerontic, and Home Health Considerations.* 4th ed. Philadelphia: F. A. Davis.
2. Post-surgical rehabilitation and healing: Benefits of RECOVERY. Surgery, Treatments and Wound Healing with Biostructural Medicine. Retrieved July 2007 from www.recoverymedicine.com/post_surgical_healing.htm.
3. Semchyshyn, N., Sengelmann, R. D. (2002, update 2006). Surgical complications. Retrieved July 2007 from www.emedicine.com/derm/topic829.htm.
4. Odom-Forren, J. (2006). Preventing surgical site infections. *Nursing*, 36(6), 59–63.
5. Stadelmann, W. K., Degenis, A. G., Tobin, G. R. (1998). Impediments to wound healing. *Am J Surg*, 176(2A suppl), 39S.
6. Purnell, L., Paulanka, B. (1998). *Transcultural Health Care: A Culturally Diverse Approach.* 2d ed. Philadelphia: F. A. Davis.
7. Pieper, B., et al. (2006). Discharge information needs of patients after surgery. *J Wound Ostomy Continence Nurs*, 33(3), 281–290.
8. Dunn, D. (2006). Age-smart care: Preventing perioperative complications in older adults. *Nursing Made Incredibly Easy!*, 4(3), 30–39.
9. Dunn, D. (2005). Preventing perioperative complications in special populations. *Nursing*, 35(1), 36–43.

(impaired Swallowing)

DEFINITION: Abnormal functioning of the swallowing mechanism associated with deficits in oral, pharyngeal, or esophageal structure or function

RELATED FACTORS

Congenital Deficits
Upper airway anomalies; mechanical obstruction (e.g., edema, tracheostomy tube, tumor); history of tube feeding
Neuromuscular impairment (e.g., decreased or absent gag reflex, decreased strength or excursion of muscles involved in mastication, perceptual impairment, facial paralysis); conditions with significant hypotonia

(continues on page 824)

impaired Swallowing (continued)

Respiratory disorders; congenital heart disease

Behavioral feeding problems; self-injurious behavior

Failure to thrive; protein energy malnutrition

Neurological Problems

Nasal or nasopharyngeal cavity defects; oropharynx or laryngeal anomalies; tracheal, laryngeal, or esophageal defects

Gastroesophageal reflux disease; achalasia

Traumas; acquired anatomic defects; cranial nerve involvement; traumatic head injury

Prematurity; developmental delay; cerebral palsy

DEFINING CHARACTERISTICS

Subjective

Esophageal phase impairment:

Complaints [reports] of "something stuck"; odynophagia

Food refusal; volume limiting

Heartburn; epigastric pain

Nighttime coughing or awakening

Objective

Oral phase impairment:

Weak suck resulting in inefficient nippling

Slow bolus formation; lack of tongue action to form bolus; premature entry of bolus

Incomplete lip closure; food pushed out of or falls from mouth

Lack of chewing

Coughing, choking, or gagging before a swallow

Piecemeal deglutition; abnormality in oral phase of swallow study

Inability to clear oral cavity; pooling in lateral sulci; nasal reflux; sialorrhea or drooling

Long meals with little consumption

Pharyngeal phase impairment:

Food refusal

Altered head positions; delayed or multiple swallows

Inadequate laryngeal elevation; abnormality in pharyngeal phase by swallow study

Choking; coughing; gagging; nasal reflux; gurgly voice quality

Unexplained fevers; recurrent pulmonary infections

Esophageal phase impairment:

Observed evidence of difficulty in swallowing (e.g., stasis of food in oral cavity, coughing/choking); abnormality in esophageal phase by swallow study

Hyperextension of head (e.g., arching during or after meals)

Repetitive swallowing; bruxism

Unexplained irritability surrounding mealtime

Acidic-smelling breath; regurgitation of gastric contents (wet burps); vomitus on pillow; vomiting; hematemesis

Sample Clinical Applications: Brain injury/stroke, neuromuscular conditions (e.g., muscular dystrophy, cerebral palsy, Parkinson's disease, amyotrophic lateral sclerosis [ALS], Guillain-Barré syndrome), facial trauma, head/neck cancer, radical neck surgery/laryngectomy, cleft lip/palate, tracheoesophageal fistula, gastroesophageal reflux disease (GERD), dementia

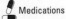

DESIRED OUTCOMES/EVALUATION CRITERIA

Sample (NOC) linkages:
Swallowing Status: Safe passage of fluids and solids from the mouth to the stomach
Self-Care: Eating: Ability to prepare and ingest food and fluid independently with or without assistive device

Client Will (Include Specific Time Frame)
- Pass food and fluid from mouth to stomach safely.
- Maintain adequate hydration as evidenced by good skin turgor, moist mucous membranes, and individually appropriate urine output.
- Achieve or maintain desired body weight.

Sample (NOC) linkage:
Risk Control: Personal actions to prevent, eliminate, or reduce modifiable health threats

Client/Caregiver Will (Include Specific Time Frame)
- Verbalize understanding of causative/contributing factors.
- Identify individually appropriate interventions/actions to promote intake and prevent aspiration.
- Demonstrate feeding methods appropriate to the individual situation.
- Demonstrate emergency measures in the event of choking.

ACTIONS/INTERVENTIONS

Sample (NIC) linkages:
Swallowing Therapy: Facilitating swallowing and preventing complications of impaired swallowing
Aspiration Precautions: Prevention or minimization of risk factors in the patient at risk for aspiration
Airway Suctioning: Removal of airway secretions by inserting a suction catheter into the patient's oral airway or trachea

NURSING PRIORITY NO. 1

To assess causative/contributing factors and degree of impairment:

- Evaluate client's potential for swallowing problems, noting age and medical conditions (e.g., Parkinson's disease, multiple sclerosis [MS], myasthenia gravis, or other neuromuscular conditions). *Swallowing disorders are especially common in the elderly, possibly due to coexistence of variety of neurological, neuromuscular, or other conditions. Infants at risk include those born prematurely, or with tracheoesophageal fistula, or lip and palate malformation. Persons with traumatic brain injuries often exhibit swallowing impairments, regardless of gender or age.*[1-4]
- Determine current situation (e.g., intubation, surgery of head, neck, or jaw; cervical spine injury, vocal cord paralysis, problems with saliva production or management; pain with swallowing; mental or anxiety disorder).[12]
- Assess client's cognitive and sensory-motor functional status. *Sensory awareness, orientation, concentration, and motor coordination affect desire and ability to swallow safely and effectively.*[7]
- Note voice quality and speech. *Abnormal voice (dysphonia) and abnormal speech patterns (dysarthria) are signs of motor dysfunction of structures involved in oral and pharyngeal swallowing.*[1]

- Note symmetry of facial structures and muscle tone. Assess strength and excursion of muscles involved in chewing and swallowing. Evaluate ability to swallow using small sips of water.
- Note hyperextension of head or arching of neck during or after meals, or repetitive swallowing, *which suggests inability to complete swallowing process.*
- Determine infant's ability to initiate and sustain effective suck. *Weak suck results in inefficient nippling, suggesting ineffective movement of tongue and mouth muscles, impairing ability to swallow.*
- Ascertain presence and strength of cough and gag reflex. *Although absence of gag reflex is not necessarily predictive of client's eventual ability to swallow safely, it does increase client's potential for aspiration (overt or silent).*[1,4] *Coughing, drooling, double swallowing, decreased ability to move food in mouth, and throat clearing with or after swallowing is indicative of swallowing dysfunction and increases risk for aspiration.*[1,8,9]
- Auscultate breath sounds *to evaluate the presence of aspiration, especially if client is coughing with intake or has a "gurgly" or "gargly" voice.*[8]
- Inspect oropharyngeal cavity for edema, inflammation, altered integrity of oral mucosa or structures (e.g., lesions or tumors of the mouth or oral cavity and throat).[1,6]
- Evaluate state of dentition (e.g., poor or missing teeth, ill-fitting dentures) and adequacy of oral hygiene.
- Review medications *that may affect oropharyngeal function (e.g., benzodiazapines, neuroleptics, anticonvulsants, anticholinergics, opioids, antidepressants, antineoplastics, diuretics), thus impairing swallowing by means of sedation, pharyngeal weakness, dry mouth, and so forth.*[1,5]
- Review laboratory test results for underlying problems (e.g., *Candida* or other infections; Cushing's disease or other metabolic conditions) *that can affect swallowing.*[5]
- Prepare for or assist with diagnostic testing of swallowing activity (e.g., transnasal or esophageal endoscopy, videofluorographic swallow studies [VFSS]; fiber-optic endoscopic examination of swallowing techniques [FEEST]) *to identify the pathophysiology of swallowing disorder.*[1,6,13]

NURSING PRIORITY NO. 2

To prevent aspiration and maintain airway patency:

- Withhold oral feedings until appropriate diagnostic workup is completed *to determine client's individual factors causing impaired swallowing and identify specific needs.*
- Consult with physician or dietitian regarding meeting current nutritional needs. *May need enteral (preferably by gastrostomy [PEG] tube) or parenteral feedings in order to obtain nutrition, while reducing risk of aspiration that could accompany nasogastric feedings.*[10]
- Move client to chair for meals, snacks, and drinks when possible; if client must be in bed, raise head of bed as upright as possible with head in anatomic alignment and slightly flexed forward during feeding. Keep head of bed elevated for 30 to 45 minutes after feeding, if possible, *to reduce risk of regurgitation and aspiration.*[12,14]
- Instruct client to cough and expectorate *when secretion management is of concern.*
- Have suction equipment available during initial feeding attempts and as indicated. Suction oral cavity if client cannot clear secretions *to prevent aspiration.*
- Instruct client in self-suctioning techniques, when appropriate (e.g., for drooling, frequent choking, structural changes in mouth or throat). *Promotes independence and sense of control.*

NURSING PRIORITY NO. 3

To enhance swallowing ability to meet fluid and caloric body requirements:

- Consult with physician, speech pathologist, dysphagia specialist, gastroenterologist, or rehabilitation team, as indicated. *Therapies may consist of dietary modification, compensatory movements, medical or surgical procedures, and so forth. For example, medications may help with underlying condition (e.g., swallowing problem associated with Parkinson's disease), surgery (e.g., reconstructive facial surgery following trauma or to correct structural defect in infant), or esophageal dilatation when impaired sphincter function or esophageal strictures impede swallowing. Client/SO may learn specific retraining or compensatory techniques (e.g., modifying head and neck posture, strengthening of swallowing muscles, or techniques of food placement in mouth).*[1,6,13-15]
- Encourage a rest period before meals *if fatigue is interfering with efforts.*
- Provide analgesics (with caution) before feeding, as indicated, *to enhance comfort, but avoiding decreasing awareness or sensory perception.*
- Implement dietary modifications as indicated:[1,6,13-15]
  - Provide proper consistency of food and fluids. *Foods that can be formed into a bolus before swallowing such as gelatin desserts prepared with less water than usual, pudding, and custard; thickened liquids (addition of thickening agent, or yogurt, cream soups prepared with less water), thinned purees (hot cereal with water added) or thick drinks such as nectars or fruit juices that have been frozen into "slush" consistency, medium-soft boiled or scrambled eggs, canned fruit, soft-cooked vegetables are most easily swallowed.*
  - Feed one consistency or texture of food at a time. *Single textured foods (e.g., pudding, hot cereal, pureed food) should be tolerated well before advancing to soft table foods.*[10]
  - Avoid milk products and chocolate, *which may thicken oral secretions and impair swallowing,* and sticky foods (e.g., peanut butter, white bread) *that are difficult to swallow or need fluids to completely swallow.*[10]
  - Ensure temperature (hot or cold versus tepid) of foods and fluids, *which will stimulate sensory receptors.*
  - Avoid pouring liquid into the mouth or "washing food down" with liquid. *May cause client to lose control of food bolus, increasing risk of aspiration. Note: To avoid posterior head tilting while drinking, some people find drinking from a straw easier than sipping from a cup (if a straw is easier, consider using a flexible one-way straw); if a cup is easier, consider using a "nosey" cup that is double handled and made of durable plastic.*
  - Feed smaller, more frequent meals *to limit fatigue associated with eating efforts and to promote adequate nutritional intake.*
  - Determine food preferences of client and present foods in an appealing, attractive manner. *Client may make effort to overcome swallowing problems when food is appealing and desired.*
- Provide or encourage use of proper food placement, chewing, and swallowing techniques:[1,6,13-15]
  - Provide cognitive cues and specific directions (e.g., remind client to "open mouth, chew, or swallow now"), as indicated, *to enhance concentration and performance of swallowing sequence.*
  - Focus attention on feeding and swallowing activity by decreasing environmental stimuli, *which may be distracting during feeding. Also, if client is talking or laughing while eating, risk of aspiration is increased.*[11]

Position client on the unaffected side when appropriate, placing food in this side of mouth and having client use the tongue *to assist with managing the food when one side of the mouth is affected (e.g., hemiplegia).*

Manage size of bites—use a small spoon or cut all solid foods into small pieces (e.g., *small bites 1/2 tsp or less are usually easier to swallow).*

Place food midway in oral cavity *to adequately trigger the swallowing reflex.*

Massage the laryngopharyngeal musculature (sides of trachea and neck) gently *to stimulate swallowing.*

Observe oral cavity after each bite and have client check around cheeks with tongue for remaining or unswallowed food *to prevent overloading mouth with food and reduce risk of aspiration.*

Allow ample time for eating (feeding). Incorporate client's eating style and pace when feeding *to avoid fatigue and frustration with process.*

Remain with client during meal *to reduce anxiety and provide assistance if needed.*

Provide positive feedback for client's efforts. *Encourages continuation of efforts and attainment of goals.*

Discontinue feeding and remove any food from mouth if client choking or unable to swallow *to reduce potential for aspiration.*

- Provide oral hygiene following each feeding. *To clear mouth of retained food particles, reduce risk of infection and dental carries.*
- Monitor intake, output, and body weight *to evaluate adequacy of fluid and caloric intake and need for changes to therapeutic regimen.*
- Discuss use of tube feedings or parenteral solutions as indicated *for the client unable to achieve adequate nutritional intake.*
- Refer to lactation counselor or support group (e.g., La Leche League) *for breastfeeding guidance and problem-solving.* Refer to NDs ineffective Breastfeeding; ineffective Infant Feeding Pattern for additional interventions for infants.

NURSING PRIORITY NO. 4

To promote wellness (Teaching/Discharge Considerations):

- Consult with nutritionist *to establish optimum dietary plan considering specific pathology, nutritional needs, available resources.* (Refer to ND risk for imbalanced Nutrition: less than body requirements.)
- Establish routine schedule for obtaining weight (same time of day and same clothes) and specific weight loss or gain to be reported to primary care provider. *Facilitates timely intervention to change regimen as needed.*
- Consult with pharmacist *to determine if pills may be crushed or if liquids or capsules are available.* Administer medication in gelatin, jelly, or puddings as appropriate.
- Instruct client and/or SO in specific feeding and swallowing techniques. *Enhances client safety and independence.*
- Instruct client/SO in emergency measures in event of choking *to prevent aspiration or more serious complications.*
- Encourage continuation of facial exercise program *to maintain or improve muscle strength.*
- Recommend avoiding food intake within 3 hours of bedtime, eliminating alcohol and caffeine intake, reducing weight if needed, using stress-reduction techniques, and elevating head of bed during sleep *to limit potential for gastric reflux and aspiration.*

DOCUMENTATION FOCUS

Assessment/Reassessment
• Individual findings, including degree and characteristics of impairment, current weight and recent changes, and nutritional status.
• Effects on lifestyle and socialization.

Planning
• Plan of care and who is involved in planning.
• Teaching plan.

Implementation/Evaluation
• Response to interventions, teaching, and actions performed.
• Attainment or progress toward desired outcome(s).
• Modifications to plan of care.

Discharge Planning
• Long-term needs and who is responsible for actions to be taken.
• Available resources and specific referrals made.

References

1. Palmer, J. B., Drennan, J. C., Baba, M. (2000). Evaluation and treatment of swallowing impairments. Retrieved July 2007 from www.aafp.org/afp/20000415/2453.html.
2. Engel, J. (2002). *Pocket Guide to Pediatric Assessment*. 4th ed. St. Louis, MO: Mosby, 158.
3. Kosta, J. C., Mitchell, C. A. (1998). Current procedures for diagnosing dysphagia in elderly clients. *Geriatr Nurs*, 19(4), 195.
4. Leder, S. B. (1999). Fiberoptic endoscopic evaluation of swallowing in patients with acute traumatic brain injury. *J Head Trauma Rehabil*, 14(5), 448–453.
5. American Gastroenterological Association. (1999). Medical position statement on management of oropharyngeal dysphagia. *Gastroenterology*, 116(2), 452–454.
6. Swallowing problems (dysphagia). College of Physicians and Surgeons, Department of Otolaryngology/Head and Neck Surgery. Retrieved July 2007 from www.entcolumbia.org/dysphag.htm.
7. Poertner, L. C., Coleman, R. F. (1998). Swallowing therapy in adults. *Otolaryngol Clin North Am*, 31(3), 56.
8. Lugger, K. F. (1994). Dysphagia in the elderly stroke patient. *J Neurosci Nurs*, 26, 78.
9. Baker, D. M. (1993). Assessment and management of impairments in swallowing. *Nurs Clin North Am*, 28, 793.
10. Fine, R., Ackley, B. J. (2002). ND: Impaired Swallowing. In Ackley, B. J., Ladwig, G. B. (eds). *Nursing Diagnosis Handbook: A Guide to Planning Care*. 5th ed. St. Louis, MO: Mosby, 735, 736.
11. Galvan, T. J. (2001). Dysphagia: Going down and staying down. *Am J Nurs*, 101(1), 37–42.
12. Haines, C. (2006). Digestive diseases: Swallowing problems. Retrieved April 2007 from www.medicinctnet.com/swallowing/.
13. National Institute for Neurological Disorders and Stroke (NINDS). (2007). Swallowing disorders information page. Retrieved April 2007 from www.ninds.nih.gov.
14. Searle, J. Eating and swallowing: Fact sheet regarding Huntington's disease. Retrieved April 2007 from http://huntingtondisease.tripod.com/swallowing/id22.html.
15. McCarron, K. (2006). The shakedown on Parkinson's disease. *Nursing Made Incredibly Easy!*, 4(6), 40–49.

effective Therapeutic Regimen Management [retired from Taxonomy 2009]

DEFINITION: Pattern of regulating and integrating into daily living a program for treatment of illness and its sequelae that is satisfactory for meeting specific health goals

RELATED FACTORS

To be developed by nurse researchers and submitted to NANDA
[Complexity of healthcare management; therapeutic regimen]
[Added demands made on individual or family]
[Adequate social supports]

DEFINING CHARACTERISTICS

Subjective
Verbalizes desire to manage the treatment of illness or prevention of sequelae
Verbalizes intent to reduce risk factors for progression of illness and sequelae

Objective
Appropriate choices of daily activities for meeting the goals of a treatment or prevention program
Illness symptoms that are within a normal range of expectation

Sample Clinical Applications: Chronic conditions (e.g., asthma, arthritis, systemic lupus), genetic/congenital conditions (e.g., sickle cell anemia, spina bifida)

DESIRED OUTCOMES/EVALUATION CRITERIA

Sample NOC linkages:
Symptom Control: Personal actions to minimize perceived adverse changes in physical and emotional functioning
Knowledge: Treatment Regimen: Extent of understanding conveyed about a specific treatment regimen
Participation in Health Care Decisions: Personal involvement in selecting and evaluating healthcare options to achieve desired outcome

Client Will (Include Specific Time Frame)
• Develop plan to address individual risk factors for progression of illness or sequelae.
• Demonstrate effective problem-solving in integrating changes of therapeutic regimen into lifestyle.
• Identify and use available resources.
• Remain free of preventable complications or progression of illness and sequelae.

ACTIONS/INTERVENTIONS

Sample (NIC) linkages:

Health System Guidance: Facilitating a patient's location and use of appropriate health services

Health Education: Developing and providing instruction and learning experiences to facilitate voluntary adaptation of behavior conducive to health in individuals, families, groups, or communities

Anticipatory Guidance: Preparation of patient for an anticipated developmental or situational crisis

NURSING PRIORITY NO. 1

To assess situation and individual needs:

- Ascertain client's knowledge and understanding of condition and treatment needs. Note specific health goals. *Provides a basis for determining direction client wants to go and planning individualized care.*[1]
- Identify individual's perceptions of adaptation to treatment and anticipated changes. *How client sees the situation is important to discussing what is happening in regard to the treatment regimen and planning for the future.*[1]
- Note treatments added to present regimen and client's/SO's associated learning needs. *As changes are made, client needs to understand what the new medication or treatment is for and what to expect, as well as how it fits into the current regimen. Understanding these issues helps client feel confident in incorporating new treatments.*[3]
- Determine client's/family's health goals, patterns of healthcare, and associated cultural or religious beliefs. *Provides information about current behaviors, possible misperceptions, and areas of potential conflict such as values, cultural mores, religious beliefs, or financial concerns.*[1]
- Discuss present resources used by client, and possible need for change. *Continuing to monitor needs, such as hours of home-care assistance, access to case manager, and making changes as indicated, supports complex or long-term program.*[3]

NURSING PRIORITY NO. 2

To assist client/SO(s) in developing strategies to meet increased demands of therapeutic regimen:

- Identify steps necessary to reach desired health goal(s). *Promotes understanding that goal(s) can only be reached by knowing what needs to be done as treatment regimen progresses.*[5]
- Accept client's evaluation of own strengths/limitations while working together to improve abilities. *Promotes sense of self-esteem and confidence to continue efforts.*[3]
- Provide information about individual healthcare needs, using client's/SO's preferred learning style and tools (e.g., books, articles, television reports, pictures, audiovideo, computer databases). *Promotes sense of control and confidence in own ability to be able to learn about illness or condition and to be in charge of own treatment regimen.*[5]
- Encourage client/SO to ask questions, check information with their own healthcare provider, *who can recommend articles, books, or reliable Web sites. Remind client that not all information is written by qualified medical experts.*[6]

● Acknowledge individual's efforts, capabilities, and skills to acquire/maintain interpersonal, self-care, and coping skills. *Reinforces client's movement toward attainment of desired outcomes.*[5,7]

NURSING PRIORITY NO. 3

To promote optimum wellness (Teaching/Discharge Considerations):

● Promote client/caregiver choices and involvement in planning and implementing added tasks or responsibilities. *Individuals gain self-esteem by being involved in the daily planning of care when they have sufficient support and are given options about what they can do.*[3]

● Provide for follow-up contact (e.g., clinic or home visit, telephone or e-mail) as appropriate. *Encourages continuation of therapeutic regimen and opportunity to help client/family identify needs and solutions as they arise, preventing untoward complications.*[3,7]

● Assist in implementing strategies for monitoring progress or responses to therapeutic regimen. *Promotes proactive problem-solving to maintain effectiveness of regimen.*[5]

● Mobilize support systems, including peers, family/SO(s), social, financial, and so forth. *When client gets the support needed to master and sustain self-management, there are potential benefits for individual health and the overall healthcare system. When these issues are managed well, client/family can attend to the process of recovery or (in the case of chronic illness) learn to live well with situation.*[1,4,8]

● Refer to community support systems, as indicated, *for assistance with lifestyle or relationship issues, finances, housing, or legal concerns (e.g., advance directives, healthcare choices).*[2]

DOCUMENTATION FOCUS

Assessment/Reassessment
• Findings, including dynamics of individual situation.
• Individual strengths and additional needs.
• Cultural or religious beliefs and expectations.

Planning
• Plan of care and who is involved in planning.
• Teaching plan.

Implementation/Evaluation
• Response to interventions, teaching, and actions performed.
• Attainment or progress toward desired outcome(s).
• Modifications to plan of care.

Discharge Planning
• Short- and long-term needs and who is responsible for actions.
• Available resources, specific referrals made.

References

1. Cox, H. C., et al. (2002). *Clinical Applications of Nursing Diagnosis: Adult, Child, Women's, Psychiatric, Gerontic, and Home Health Considerations.* 4th ed. Philadelphia: F. A. Davis.
2. *Healthy People 2010 Toolkit: A Field Guide to Health Planning.* (2002). Washington, DC: Public Health Foundation.
3. Stuifbergen, A. (1997). Health promotion: An essential component of rehabilitation for persons with chronic disabling conditions. *Adv Nurs Sci*, 19(4), 147–148.

⊕ Cultural   Collaborative   🏠 Community/Home Care   ✎ Diagnostic Studies   ∞ Pediatric/Geriatric/Lifespan    Medications

4. Larsen, L. S. (1998). Effectiveness of counseling intervention to assist family caregivers of chronically ill relatives. *J Psychosoc Nurs*, 36(8), 26–32.
5. Lai, S. C., Cohen, M. N. (1999). Promoting lifestyle changes. *Am J Nurs*, 99(4), 63–67,
6. National Institute of Arthritis and Musculoskeletal and Skin Diseases (NIAMS). How to find medical information. Retrieved July 2007 from www.niams.nih.gov/hi/topics/howto/howto.htm.
7. New York State Office of Mental Health Wellness. Self-management: Evidenced based practices. Retrieved July 2007 from www.omh.state.ny.us/omhweb/ebp/adult_wellness.htm.
8. Heisler, M. (2006). Building peer support programs to manage chronic disease: Seven models for success. Retrieved July 2007 from www.chcf.org/topics/chronicdisease/index.cfm?itemID =127997.

ineffective community Therapeutic Regimen Management [retired from Taxonomy 2009]

DEFINITION: Pattern of regulating and integrating into community processes programs for treatment of illness and the sequelae of illness that are unsatisfactory for meeting health-related goals

RELATED FACTORS

To be developed by nurse researchers and submitted to NANDA
[Lack of safety for community members]
[Economic insecurity]
[Healthcare not available]
[Unhealthy environment]
[Education not available for all community members]
[Lack of means to meet human needs for recognition, fellowship, security, and membership]

DEFINING CHARACTERISTICS

Subjective
[Community members or agencies verbalize overburdening of resources or inability to meet therapeutic needs of all members]

Objective
Deficits in advocates for aggregates
Deficit in community activities for prevention
Illness symptoms above the norm expected for the population; unexpected acceleration of illness
Insufficient healthcare resources (e.g., people, programs); unavailable healthcare resources for illness care
[Deficits in community for collaboration and development of coalitions to address needs]

Sample Clinical Applications: HIV/AIDS, substance abuse, sexually transmitted diseases, teen pregnancy, prematurity, acute lead poisoning, influenza, severe acute respiratory syndrome (SARS)

(continues on page 834)

ineffective community Therapeutic Regimen Management [retired from Taxonomy 2009] (continued)
DESIRED OUTCOMES/EVALUATION CRITERIA

Sample (NOC) linkages:
Community Competence: Capacity of a community to collectively problem-solve to achieve community goals
Community Health Status: General state of well-being of a community or population
Community Risk Control: Communicable Disease: Community actions to eliminate or reduce the spread of infectious agents that threaten public health

Community Will (Include Specific Time Frame)
• Identify both strengths and limitations affecting community treatment programs for meeting health-related goals.
• Participate in problem-solving of factors interfering with regulating and integrating community programs.
• Report unexpected acceleration or illness symptoms near norm expected for the incidence or prevalence of disease(s).

ACTIONS/INTERVENTIONS

Sample (NIC) linkages:
Community Health Development: Facilitating members of a community to identify a community's health concerns, mobilize resources, and implement solutions
Program Development: Planning, implementing, and evaluating a coordinated set of activities designed to enhance wellness, or to prevent, reduce, or eliminate one or more health problems of a group or community
Health Policy Monitoring: Surveillance and influence of government and organization regulations, rules, and standards that affect nursing systems and practices to ensure quality care of patients

NURSING PRIORITY NO. 1

To identify causative/precipitating factors:

• Evaluate community healthcare resources for illness or sequelae of illness. *Identifying current available resources provides a starting point to determine needs of the community and plan for future needs.*[1]
• Note reports from members of the community regarding ineffective or inadequate community functioning. *Provides feedback from people who live in the community and avail themselves of resources, thus presenting a realistic picture of problem areas.*[2]
• Determine areas of conflict among members of community. *Cultural or religious beliefs, values, social mores, and lack of a shared vision may limit dialogue or creative problem-solving if not addressed.*[4]
• Investigate unexpected acceleration of illness in the community. *Prompt identification of illness, such as West Nile virus, H1N1, or tuberculosis allows community to develop plan of care and intervene to prevent further spread with possibility of becoming epidemic.*[2]
• Identify strengths and limitations of community resources and community commitment to change. *Knowledge of these factors is important for developing a plan for community improvement. Without this information, any plan will have difficulty succeeding.*[2]

Cultural   Collaborative   Community/Home Care   Diagnostic Studies   Pediatric/Geriatric/Lifespan   Medications

- Ascertain effect of related factors on community activities. *Issues of safety, poor air quality, lack of education or information, lack of sufficient healthcare facilities affect citizens and how they view their community—whether it is a healthy, positive environment in which to live or lacks adequate healthcare or safety resources.*[1]
- Determine knowledge and understanding of treatment regimen. *Citizens need to know and understand what is being proposed to correct the identified deficiencies, before they are willing to be involved and actively support goals of the treatment regimen.*[1]
- Note use of resources available to community for developing and funding programs. *May require creative program planning to utilize resources to meet multiple needs.*

NURSING PRIORITY NO. 2

To assist community to develop strategies to improve community functioning and management:

- Foster cooperative spirit of community without negating individuality of members/groups. *As individuals feel valued and respected, they are more willing to work together with others to develop plan for identifying and improving healthcare for the community.*[2]
- Involve community in determining healthcare goals and prioritizing them to facilitate planning process. *The goal is healthy people in a healthy community, and as community members become involved and see that by prioritizing the identified goals, progress can be seen as individuals become healthier and needed services become readily available.*[2]
- Plan together with community health and social agencies to problem-solve solutions identified and anticipated problems and needs. *Working together promotes a sense of involvement and control, helping people implement more effective problem-solving.*[3]
- Identify specific populations at risk or underserved to actively involve them in process. *Populations, such as low-income and poverty level families; migrant, immigrant, and homeless; and racial and ethnic minorities, need to be involved in problem identification and solutions, because they are closely involved in the issues they face on a daily basis and can provide important facts to be considered. Being part of the solution empowers these groups and promotes continued participation in the process.*[3,5]
- Create teaching plan, form speakers' bureau. *Disseminating information to community members regarding value of treatment or preventive programs helps people know and understand the importance of these actions and be willing to support the programs.*[3]

NURSING PRIORITY NO. 3

To promote wellness (Teaching/Discharge Considerations):

- Assist community to develop a plan for continued assessment of community needs and functioning (e.g., access to adequate healthcare; education regarding disease prevention, public health threats, and immunization; local warning system and evacuation plan in event of disaster; emergency contact numbers; planning for community members with special needs [including elderly, handicapped, low-income]; violence prevention, personal or property protection; water, sanitation, and toxic substance management, mobilization of local, state, and national resources). *Promotes proactive approach in planning for the future and continuation of efforts to improve healthy behaviors and necessary services.*[1,5]
- Encourage community to form partnerships within the community and between the community and the larger society. *Aids in long-term planning for anticipated and projected needs and concerns to assure the quality and accessibility of health services.*[1]

DOCUMENTATION FOCUS

Assessment/Reassessment
• Assessment findings, including members' perceptions of community problems, healthcare resources.
• Community use of available resources.

Planning
• Plan and who is involved in planning process.
• Teaching plan.

Implementation/Evaluation
• Community's response to plan, interventions, and actions performed.
• Attainment or progress toward desired outcome(s).
• Modifications to plan.

Discharge Planning
• Long-term goals and who is responsible for actions to be taken.
• Specific referrals made.

References

1. American Public Health Association. Environmental Health Competency Project: Draft recommendations for non-technical competencies at the local level. Retrieved July 2007 from www.apha.org/programs/standards/healthcompproject/.
2. American Public Health Association. (1994). Public health in America. Retrieved July 2007 from www.health.gov/phfunctions/public.
3. *Healthy People 2010 Toolkit: A Field Guide to Health Planning.* (2002). Washington, DC: Public Health Foundation.
4. Cox, H. C., et al. (2002). *Clinical Applications of Nursing Diagnosis: Adult, Child, Women's, Psychiatric, Geronic, and Home Health Considerations.* 4th ed. Philadelphia: F. A. Davis.
5. U.S. Department of Human Services, Centers for Disease Control and Prevention. CDC health protection goals. Retrieved July 2007 from www.cdc.gov/index.htm.

(ineffective family Therapeutic Regimen Management)

DEFINITION: Pattern of regulating and integrating into family processes a program for treatment of illness and the sequelae of illness that is unsatisfactory for meeting specific health goals

RELATED FACTORS

Complexity of therapeutic or healthcare system
Decisional conflicts
Economic difficulties
Excessive demands; family conflicts

DEFINING CHARACTERISTICS

Subjective
Verbalizes difficulty with therapeutic regimen
Verbalizes desire to manage the illness

⊕ Cultural Collaborative 🏠 Community/Home Care Diagnostic Studies ∞ Pediatric/Geriatric/Lifespan 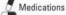 Medications

Objective
Inappropriate family activities for meeting health goals
Acceleration of illness symptoms of a family member
Failure to take action to reduce risk factors; lack of attention to illness

Sample Clinical Applications: Chronic conditions (e.g., chronic obstructive pulmonary disease [COPD], multiple sclerosis [MS], arthritis, chronic pain, substance abuse, end-stage liver or renal failure) or new diagnoses necessitating lifestyle changes

DESIRED OUTCOMES/EVALUATION CRITERIA

Sample (NOC) linkages:
Family Health Status: Overall health and social competence of family unit
Family Participation in Professional Care: Family involvement in decision making, delivery, and evaluation of care provided by healthcare personnel
Family Functioning: Capacity of the family to meet the needs of its members during developmental transitions

Family Will (Include Specific Time Frame)
• Identify individual factors affecting regulation/integration of treatment program.
• Participate in problem-solving of identified factors.
• Verbalize acceptance of need or desire to change actions to achieve agreed-on outcomes or health goals.
• Demonstrate behaviors/changes in lifestyle necessary to maintain therapeutic regimen.

ACTIONS/INTERVENTIONS

Sample (NIC) linkages:
Family Involvement Promotion: Facilitating family participation in the emotional and physical care of the patient
Family Mobilization: Utilizing family strengths to influence patient's health in a positive direction
Health System Guidance: Facilitating a patient's location and use of appropriate health services

NURSING PRIORITY NO. 1

To identify causative/precipitating factors:

• Ascertain family's perception of efforts to date. *Perceptions are more important than facts, and by getting family's point of view, realistic goals can be set and family can look to the future.*[2]
• Evaluate family functioning and activities as related to appropriateness. *Looking at frequency and effectiveness of family communication, promotion of autonomy, adaptation to meet changing needs, health of home environment and lifestyle, problem-solving abilities, ties to community provides information about current problem areas and need for specific interventions.*[1]
• Note family health goals and agreement of individual members. *Presence of conflict interferes with problem-solving and needs to be addressed before family can move forward to meet goals.*[2]

- Determine understanding and value of the treatment regimen to the family. *Individual members may misunderstand either the cause of the illness or the prescribed regimen and may disagree with what is happening, thereby promoting dissension within the family group and causing distress for the identified client.*[1]
- Identify cultural values and religious beliefs affecting view of situation and willingness to make necessary changes. *May influence choice of interventions.*
- Identify availability and use of resources. *Knowing who is available to help and support the family will help in planning care to maximize positive outcomes.*[2]

NURSING PRIORITY NO. 2

To assist family to develop strategies to improve management of therapeutic regimen:

- Provide information to aid family in understanding the value of the treatment program. *Accurate information helps individuals make decisions based on that knowledge, see the connection between illness and treatment, and may improve adherence to therapeutic regimen.*[3]
- Assist family members to recognize inappropriate family activities. Help the members identify both togetherness and individual needs and behavior. *Effective interactions can be enhanced and perpetuated when these factors are identified and used to improve family behaviors.*[2]
- Make a plan jointly with family members to deal with complexity of healthcare regimen or system and other related factors. *Enhances commitment to plan, optimizing outcomes when family and caregivers work together to plan therapeutic regimen.*[2,5]
- Identify community resources as needed using the three strategies of education, problem-solving, and resource-linking to address specific deficits. *Providing information, helping family members learn effective problem-solving techniques, and how to access needed resources can help them deal successfully with the chronically ill family member.*[4]

NURSING PRIORITY NO. 3

To promote wellness as related to future health and well-being of family members:

- Help family identify criteria to promote ongoing self-evaluation of situation and effectiveness, and family progress. *Involvement promotes sense of control and provides the opportunity to be proactive in meeting needs.*[2]
- Make referrals to and/or jointly plan with other health, social, and community resources. *Problems often are multifaceted, requiring involvement of numerous providers or agencies to plan appropriate regimen to meet family/individual needs.*[3]
- Provide contact person or case manager for one-on-one assistance as needed. *Having a single contact to coordinate care, provide support, and assist with problem-solving maintains continuity and prevents misunderstandings and errors in managing the family's regimen.*[1]
- Refer to NDs Caregiver Role Strain, ineffective self Health Management, as indicated.

DOCUMENTATION FOCUS

Assessment/Reassessment
- Individual findings, including nature of problem and degree of impairment, family values, health goals, and level of participation and commitment of family members.
- Cultural values, religious beliefs.
- Availability and use of resources.

🌐 Cultural ⊕ Collaborative 🏠 Community/Home Care ⟋ Diagnostic Studies ∞ Pediatric/Geriatric/Lifespan 💊 Medications

Planning
- Plan of care and who is involved in planning.
- Teaching plan.

Implementation/Evaluation
- Response to interventions, teaching, and actions performed.
- Attainment or progress toward desired outcome(s).
- Modifications of plan of care.

Discharge Planning
- Long-term needs, plan for meeting and who is responsible for actions.
- Specific referrals made.

References

1. Cox, H. C., et al. (2002). *Clinical Applications of Nursing Diagnosis: Adult, Child, Women's, Psychiatric, Gerontic, and Home Health Considerations.* 4th ed. Philadelphia: F. A. Davis.
2. *Healthy People 2010 Toolkit: A Field Guide to Health Planning.* (2002). Washington, DC: Public Health Foundation.
3. Stuifbergen, A. (1997). Health promotion: An essential component of rehabilitation for persons with chronic disabling conditions. *Adv Nurs Sci*, 19(4), 147–148.
4. Larsen, L. S. (1998). Effectiveness of counseling intervention to assist family caregivers of chronically ill relatives. *J Psychosoc Nurs*, 36(8), 26–32.
5. Gance-Cleveland, B. (2005). Motivational interviewing as a strategy to increase families' adherence to treatment regimens. *J Spec Pediatr Nurs*, 10(3), 151–155.

(ineffective Thermoregulation)

DEFINITION: Temperature fluctuation between hypothermia and hyperthermia

RELATED FACTORS

Trauma; illness [e.g., cerebral edema, cerebrovascular accident (CVA), intracranial surgery, or head injury]
Immaturity; aging [e.g., loss or absence of brown adipose tissue]
Fluctuating environmental temperature
[Changes in hypothalamic tissue causing alterations in emission of thermosensitive cells and regulation of heat loss and production]
[Changes in metabolic rate or activity; changes in level or action of thyroxine and catecholamines]
[Chemical reactions in contracting muscles]

DEFINING CHARACTERISTICS

Objective
Fluctuations in body temperature above and below the normal range
Tachycardia
Reduction in body temperature below normal range; cool skin; moderate pallor; mild shivering; piloerection; cyanotic nail beds; slow capillary refill; hypertension

(continues on page 840)

ineffective Thermoregulation (continued)

Warm to touch; flushed skin; increased respiratory rate; seizures

Sample Clinical Applications: Prematurity, brain injury, CVA, intracranial surgery (cerebral edema), infection or sepsis, major surgical procedures

DESIRED OUTCOMES/EVALUATION CRITERIA

Sample **NOC** linkages:
Thermoregulation: Balance among heat production, heat gain, and heat loss
Thermoregulation: Newborn: Balance among heat production, heat gain, and heat loss during the first 28 days of life

Client/Caregiver Will (Include Specific Time Frame)
• Verbalize understanding of individual factors and appropriate interventions.
• Demonstrate techniques or behaviors to correct underlying condition or situation.
• Maintain body temperature within normal limits.

ACTIONS/INTERVENTIONS

Sample **NIC** linkages:
Temperature Regulation: Attaining or maintaining body temperature within a normal range
Temperature Regulation: Intraoperative: Attaining or maintaining body temperature within a normal range
Fever Treatment: Management of a patient with hyperpyrexia caused by nonenvironmental factors

NURSING PRIORITY NO. 1

To identify causative/contributing factors:

● Obtain history concerning present symptoms, correlate with previous episodes or family history, and diagnostic studies. *Thermoregulation is a controlled process that maintains the body's core temperature in the range at which most biochemical processes work best (99°F–99.6°F [37.2°C–37.6°C]).*[1,2] *Exercise, behavioral impulses, metabolic and hormonal changes influence changes in body temperature, leading to loss or gain of heat.*

● Determine specific factors involved in current temperature fluctuation (e.g., environmental factors, surgery, infectious process, effects of drugs or toxins, brain or spinal cord injury). *Thermoregulation is affected in two ways: (1) endogenous factors (via diseases or conditions of body/organ systems) and (2) exogenous factors (via environmental exposures, medications, and nutrition).*[2] *Helps to determine the scope of interventions that may be needed (e.g., simple addition of warm blankets after surgery, or hypothermia therapy following brain trauma).*[4,6]

∞ ● Note client's age (e.g., premature neonate, young child, or aging individual), *as it can directly impact ability to maintain or regulate body temperature and respond to changes in environment.*[3,5]

● Review laboratory results (e.g., tests indicative of infection, thyroid or other endocrine tests, drug screens) *to identify potential internal causes of temperature imbalances.*

NURSING PRIORITY NO. 2

To assist with measures to correct/treat underlying cause:

- Monitor temperature by appropriate route (e.g., tympanic, rectal, oral), noting variation from client's usual or normal temperature. *Rectal and tympanic temperatures most closely approximate core temperature; however, shell temperatures (oral, axillary, touch) are often measured at home and are predictive of fever or subnormal temperatures. Rectal temperature measurement may be the most accurate but is not always expedient (e.g., client declines, is agitated, has rectal lesions or surgery). Abdominal temperature monitoring may be done in the premature neonate.*
- Have cooling and warming equipment and supplies readily available during and following procedures or surgery.
- Initiate emergent or immediate interventions, such as cooling or warming measures, fluids, electrolytes, nutrients, and medications (e.g., antipyretics, antibiotics, neoplastics), as indicated, *to restore or maintain body temperature within normal range and optimize organ function.*[1-8]
- Maintain ambient temperature in comfortable range *to prevent or compensate for client's heat production or heat loss (e.g., may need to add or remove clothing or blankets, avoid drafts, reduce or increase room temperature and humidity).*
- Place newborn infant under radiant warmer, cover infant's head with cap, use layers of lightweight blankets. *Newborns/infants can have temperature instability. Heat loss is greatest through the head and by evaporation and convection.*[5]
- Refer to NDs risk for imbalanced Body Temperature, Hypothermia, or Hyperthermia for additional interventions.

NURSING PRIORITY NO. 3

To promote wellness (Teaching/Discharge Considerations):

- Review causative or related factors with client/SO(s). *Provides information about what, if any, measures can be implemented to protect client from harm or limit potential for problems associated with ineffective thermoregulation.*
- Discuss appropriate dressing with client/caregivers, such as:[1]
  Wearing layers of clothing that can be removed or added as needed
  Donning hat and gloves in cold weather
  Using water-resistant outer gear to protect from wet weather chill
  Dressing in light, loose protective clothing in hot weather
- Review home management of temperature fluctuations in special population (e.g., newborn infant, person with spinal cord injury (SCI), frail elder). *Measures could include use of heating pads, ice bag; heaters or fans; adding or removing clothing or blankets, cool or warm liquids and bathwater; skin-to-skin contact in newborn, and so forth.*[5-8]
- Provide oral and written information concerning client's disease processes, current therapies, and postdischarge precautions, as appropriate to situation. *Allows for review of instructions for early intervention and implementation of preventive or corrective measures*
- Refer to teaching section in NDs risk for imbalanced Body Temperature, Hypothermia, or Hyperthermia, as appropriate.

DOCUMENTATION FOCUS

Assessment/Reassessment
• Individual findings, including nature of problem, degree of impairment or fluctuations in temperature.

Planning
• Plan of care and who is involved in planning.
• Teaching plan.

Implementation/Evaluation
• Responses to interventions, teaching, and actions performed.
• Attainment or progress toward desired outcome(s).
• Modifications to plan of care.

Discharge Planning
• Long-term needs and who is responsible for actions to be taken.
• Specific referrals made.

References

1. Worfolk, J. (1997). Keep frail elders warm! *Geriatr Nurs*, 18(1), 7–11.
2. Kneis, R. C. (1996). Geriatric trauma: What you need to know. *Int J Traum Nurs*, 2(3), 85–91.
3. Cox, H. C., et al. (2002). *Clinical Applications of Nursing Diagnosis: Adult, Child, Women's, Psychiatric, Gerontic, and Home Health Considerations.* 4th ed. Philadelphia: F. A. Davis.
4. Doenges, M. E., Moorhouse, M. F., Geissler-Murr, A. C. (2002). ND: Surgical Intervention. *Nursing Care Plans: Guidelines for Individualizing Patient Care.* 6th ed. Philadelphia: F. A. Davis.
5. Suggested guidelines for early discharge of term, healthy newborns. (Revised 1998). Retrieved July 2007 from http://depts.washington.edu/nicuweb/NICU-WEB/earlydis.stm.
6. Hoppe, J., Sinert, R. (2006). Heat exhaustion and heatstroke. Retrieved March 2007 from www.emedicine.com/emerg/topic236.htm.
7. Galligan, M. (2006). Proposed guidelines for skin-to-skin treatment of neonatal hypothermia. *Amer J Matern Child Nurs*, 31(5), 298–304.
8. Jones, T. S. (2005). A bolt out of the blue: Dealing with the aftermath of spinal cord injury. *Nursing Made Incredibly Easy!*, 3(6), 14–28.

disturbed Thought Processes [retired from Taxonomy 2009]

DEFINITION: Disruption in cognitive operations and activities

RELATED FACTORS

To be developed by nurse researchers and submitted to NANDA
[Physiological changes, aging, hypoxia, head injury, malnutrition, infections]
[Biochemical changes, medications, substance abuse]
[Sleep deprivation]
[Psychological conflicts, emotional changes, mental disorders]

DEFINING CHARACTERISTICS

Subjective
[Ideas of reference, hallucinations, delusions]

Objective
Inaccurate interpretation of environment
Inappropriate thinking; egocentricity
Memory deficit; [confabulation]
Hypervigilance; hypovigilance
Cognitive dissonance [decreased ability to grasp ideas, make decisions, problem-solve, use abstract reasoning or conceptualize, calculate; disordered thought sequencing]
Distractibility; [altered attention span]
[Inappropriate social behavior]

Sample Clinical Applications: Brain injury, cerebrovascular accident (CVA), central nervous system (CNS) infections, anorexia nervosa, substance abuse, septicemia, cirrhosis of liver, delirium, dementia, schizophrenia, dissociative disorders, paranoid disorder, obsessive-compulsive disorder

DESIRED OUTCOMES/EVALUATION CRITERIA

Sample (NOC) linkages:
Distorted Thought Self-Control: Self-restraint of disruptions in perception, thought processes, and thought content
Cognition: Ability to execute complex mental processes
Memory: Ability to cognitively retrieve and report previously stored information

Client Will (Include Specific Time Frame)
• Recognize changes in thinking and behavior.
• Verbalize understanding of causative factors when known and as able.
• Identify interventions to deal effectively with situation.
• Demonstrate behaviors or lifestyle changes to prevent or minimize changes in mentation.
• Maintain usual reality orientation.

ACTIONS/INTERVENTIONS

Sample (NIC) linkages:
Dementia Management: Provision of a modified environment for the patient who is experiencing a chronic confusional state
Delusion Management: Promoting the comfort, safety, and reality orientation of a patient experiencing false, fixed beliefs that have little or no basis in reality
Environmental Management: Safety: Manipulation of the patient's surroundings for therapeutic benefit

NURSING PRIORITY NO. 1

To assess causative/contributing factors:

● Identify underlying condition. *Disturbances in thinking can be the result of a wide variety of conditions (e.g., recent stroke, CNS infections; dementias, retardation; traumatic brain*

---

injury with increased intracranial pressure, anoxic event; acute urinary infections [especially in elderly]; malnutrition, metabolic problems [e.g., acid-base imbalances, diabetes, renal or hepatic failure]; sensory deprivation or overstimulation; toxins, including drug interactions/reactions, drug overdose, accidental exposures; emotional or psychiatric illness [e.g., schizophrenia]).[2,8–10]

- Interview SO(s)/caregiver(s) to determine client's usual cognitive ability, changes in behavior, length of time problem has existed, and other pertinent information *to provide baseline for comparison.*[6,10]

- Determine alcohol or other drug use (prescription, over-the-counter [OTC], illicit, and herbal). *Drugs can have direct effects on the brain or have dose-related effects that alter thought processes and sensory perception.*[2,8,9]

- Note schedule of medication administration. *May be significant when evaluating cumulative effects and interactions.*

- Assess for presence and severity of pain, as well as use of or need for analgesics. *Both pain and the treatments for pain can diminish the acuity of client's thinking processes. Untreated pain can increase confusion and agitation.*[1,7]

- Assess dietary intake and nutritional status. *Good nutrition is essential for optimal brain functioning. Persons with anorexia, major depression, substance use, and chronic debilitating conditions may have problems with thinking related to deficits in nutrients, vitamins, electrolytes, and minerals.*[2,8–10]

- Evaluate impact of environment. *Excessive noise, multiple people in client's surroundings, chaotic lifestyle, rapid changes in routines, and so forth, can result in overstimulation/confusion, clouding client's thinking and impairing coping abilities.*

- Monitor laboratory results. *Abnormalities such as metabolic alkalosis, hypokalemia, anemia, elevated ammonia levels, infections, drug toxicity, and so forth, may be affecting thought processes.*

- Assist with and review results of diagnostic testing (e.g., magnetic resonance imaging [MRI], computed tomography [CT] scan, spinal tap) *to help identify etiology of thinking impairment.*

NURSING PRIORITY NO. 2

To assess degree of impairment:

- Evaluate mental status using appropriate tools *(establishes baseline and comparative functional level according to age, developmental stage, and neurological status)*, noting:[5,11]
  Extent of impairment in thinking ability. *Varies widely, with impairments being overt or difficult to identify. Long time periods and sophisticated neuropsychiatric testing may be required to more fully identify nature of this impairment.*
  Remote and recent memory. *Remote memory is often intact, while recent or short-term memory may be lost or impaired.*
  Orientation to person, place, and time. *Confusion may be short term, long term, or permanent and can be stable or progressive.* (Refer to NDs acute/chronic Confusion.)
  Insight and judgment. *Client may/may not be aware of changes in these areas, but family, friends or colleagues may report concerns.*[8,11]
  Changes in personality or response to stimuli. *Can range from lethargy and withdrawal to anger, agitation, and violent responses.*[9,10]
  Attention span, distractibility, and ability to make decisions or problem-solve. *Determines ability to participate in planning and executing care.*
  Ability to receive, send, and appropriately interpret communications. Note absence of speech or changes in speech patterns (e.g., slowing and/or slurring of speech, problems

with word finding, presence of aphasia). *Speech and communication difficulties are both indicators and consequences of impaired thought processes.*[9]

Client's anxiety level (from mild to panic level) *that both causes and potentiates alterations in thought processes.*[2,9,10] Refer to ND Anxiety.

Occurrence of paranoia and delusions, hallucinations. *Can occur with brain injury, mental illness, metabolic and electrolyte disturbances, alcohol or other drug use or overdose, dementias, and so forth, reflecting escalation of thought disturbances.*[2]

- Assist with in-depth testing of specific cognitive abilities and executive brain functions, as appropriate.

NURSING PRIORITY NO. 3

To prevent further deterioration, maximize level of function:

- Perform periodic neurological and behavioral assessments as indicated and compare with baseline. Note changes in level of consciousness and cognition (e.g., increased lethargy, confusion, drowsiness, irritability; changes in ability to communicate or appropriateness of thinking and behavior). Have client write name periodically; keep this record for comparison and report differences. *Early recognition of changes promotes proactive modifications to plan of care.*[2]

- Assist with treatment for underlying problems such as anorexia, brain injury—increased intracranial pressure, sleep disorders, biochemical imbalances. *Cognition and thinking often improves with treatment or correction of medical or psychiatric problems.*[6]

- Establish alternate means for self-expression if unable to communicate verbally. *Provides way of determining thinking ability.* Refer to ND impaired verbal Communication.

- Reorient to person, place, and time as needed *to reinforce or maintain reality of the moment. Note: Inability to maintain orientation is a sign of deterioration.*

- Encourage family/SO(s) to participate in reorientation and provide ongoing input (e.g., current news and family happenings). *Promotes sense of normalcy, maintains contact with family.*

- Stay with client when agitated, frightened. *Support may provide calming effect, reducing anxiety and risk of injury.*[2]

- Note behavior indicative of potential for violence and take appropriate actions to prevent harm to client/others. *Clients with brain injuries often have lowered impulse control, problems with anger management, and the potential for violent outbursts, requiring specific interventions designed to help the client learn to control these behaviors.*[7] Refer to ND risk for other-directed Violence.

- Provide safety measures (e.g., side rails, padding as necessary; bed in low position or on floor, close supervision, seizure precautions) as indicated. *May help to prevent accidents and injury to client.*[2]

- Schedule structured activity and rest periods. *Provides stimulation without undue fatigue, helping to maintain orientation and sense of reality.*[3]

- Encourage or provide opportunities for adequate sleep. *Sleep deprivation can increase confusion. Regular sleep routine reinforces the idea of bedtime, and adequate rest can enhance clarity of thinking.*[6] Refer to ND Sleep Deprivation.

- Monitor medication regimen, limit use of sedatives and drugs affecting the nervous system *that have shown correlation with episodes of confusion.*[1–3,8]

- Refer to appropriate rehabilitation providers. *Cognitive retraining program, speech therapist, psychosocial resources, biofeedback, counselor may help client to enhance degree of functioning.*[6]

NURSING PRIORITY NO. 4

To create therapeutic milieu and assist client/SO(s) to develop coping strategies (especially when condition is irreversible):

- Provide opportunities for SO(s)/caregiver(s) to ask questions and obtain information. *SOs frequently have difficulty accepting and dealing with client's aberrant behavior and may require assistance in understanding and coping with the situation.*[2]
- Listen with regard to client's verbalizations in spite of speech pattern and content *to convey interest and worth to individual, enhancing self-esteem and encouraging continued efforts.*[3]
- Maintain a pleasant, quiet environment and approach client in a slow, calm manner. *Client may respond with anxious or aggressive behaviors if startled or overstimulated.*
- Maintain reality-oriented relationship and environment. *Using aids such as clocks, calendars, personal items, and seasonal decorations helps individual maintain current reality.*[6]
- Present reality concisely and briefly and do not challenge illogical thinking. *Helps client stay focused on the present. Client may react defensively if thinking is challenged.*[6]
- Give simple directions, using short words and simple sentences. *Provides for processing of basic communication when thinking is impaired.*[3]
- Reduce provocative stimuli, negative criticism, arguments, and confrontations *to avoid triggering fight-or-flight responses.*
- Refrain from forcing activities and communications. *Client may feel threatened and may withdraw or rebel.*
- Respect individuality and personal space. *Conveys concern for the person regardless of the circumstances.*[3]
- Use touch judiciously, respecting personal needs and cultural beliefs, but keeping in mind physical and psychological importance of touch. *Touch is a powerful communication tool that can elicit positive or negative reactions. Appropriate touch is defined by family practices, societal expectations, and cultural environment.*[5]
- Provide nutritionally well-balanced diet incorporating client's preferences as able. Encourage client to eat, provide pleasant environment, and allow sufficient time to eat. *Enhances intake, improving nutritional status and general well-being.*[6]
- Provide ample time for client to respond to questions or comments and make simple decisions. *Processing information takes more time when thinking is impaired, and allowing more time promotes communication and client's sense of self-esteem.*[6]
- Inform family/caregiver of the meaning of and reasons for common behaviors observed in client with disturbed thought processes, as well as the probable course of disease process and plan of care. *Helps them to understand and cope with situation and assists them in providing a safe environment for the client.*[4]
- Support client/SO(s) with grieving for loss of self and abilities, as in Alzheimer's disease. *Progressive loss of mental abilities is difficult for family members to deal with as they grieve the loss of the person they knew. Providing opportunity for individuals to talk about feelings of grief will promote coping abilities.*[4] Refer to ND Grieving.
- Encourage participation in resocialization activities or groups as appropriate. *Can help the individual maintain or regain some degree of social skills. Even in conditions of dementia, client can benefit from these activities.*[6]

NURSING PRIORITY NO. 5

To promote wellness (Teaching/Discharge Considerations):

- Assist in identifying ongoing treatment needs or rehabilitation program for the individual *to maintain gains and continue progress if able.*[6]

⊕ Cultural ⊛ Collaborative 🏠 Community/Home Care ✎ Diagnostic Studies ∞ Pediatric/Geriatric/Lifespan 💊 Medications

- Emphasize importance of cooperation with therapeutic regimen. *Client and SOs benefit from maintaining regimen as agreed on, and working together benefits everyone.*[6]
- Promote socialization within individual limitations. *Client may have difficulty tolerating large (or even small) groups of people, and unfamiliar or noisy surroundings.* Refer to ND disturbed Sensory Perception.
- Identify problems related to aging that are remediable and assist client/SO(s) to seek appropriate assistance and access resources. *Encourages problem solving to improve condition when possible rather than accept the status quo.*
- Help client/SO(s) develop plan of care when problem is progressive or long term. *Advance planning addressing home care, transportation, assistance with care activities, support and respite for caregivers enhances management of client in home setting.* Refer to NDs risk for Caregiver Role Strain; Self-Care Deficit (specify) for related interventions.
- Refer to community resources (e.g., social services, day-care programs, support groups, drug or alcohol rehabilitation; mental health treatment program) *to provide assistance and support for client/caregivers.*
- Refer to NDs acute/chronic Confusion; impaired Environmental Interpretation Syndrome; Grieving; impaired Memory; Self-Care Deficit; disturbed Sensory Perception as appropriate for additional interventions.

DOCUMENTATION FOCUS

Assessment/Reassessment
- Individual findings, including nature of problem, current and previous level of function, effect on independence and lifestyle.
- Results of laboratory tests, diagnostic studies, and mental status or cognitive evaluations.
- SO/family support and participation.
- Availability and use of resources.

Planning
- Plan of care and who is involved in planning.
- Teaching plan.

Implementation/Evaluation
- Response to interventions, teaching, and actions performed.
- Attainment or progress toward desired outcome(s).
- Modifications to plan of care.

Discharge Planning
- Long-term needs and who is responsible for actions to be taken.
- Available resources, specific referrals made.

References

1. Foreman, M. (1989). Complexities of acute confusion. *Geriatr Nurs*, 3, 136–139.
2. Doenges, M. E., Moorhouse, M. F., Geissler-Murr, A. C. (2002). ND: Thought Processes, disturbed. *Nursing Care Plans: Guidelines for Individualizing Patient Care*. 6th ed. Philadelphia: F. A. Davis, 217, 369, 410, 535, 715, 773.
3. Dellasaga, C., Stricklin, M. L. (1993). Cognitive impairment in the elderly home health clients. *Home Health Care Serv Q*, 14, 81–92.
4. Smart, G., Sundeen, S. (1991). *Pocket Guide to Psychiatric Assessment*. St. Louis, MO. Mosby.

5. Doenges, M. E., Townsend, M. C., Moorhouse, M. F. (1998). *Psychiatric Care Plans: Guidelines for Individualizing Care*. 3d ed. Philadelphia: F. A. Davis.

6. Cox, H. C., et al. (2002). *Clinical Applications of Nursing Diagnosis: Adult, Child, Women's, Psychiatric, Gerontic, and Home Health Considerations*. 4th ed. Philadelphia: F. A. Davis.

7. Johnson, G. (1998). Traumatic brain injury survival guide. Retrieved July 2007 from www.tbiguide.com.

8. Naylor, M. D., et al. (2005). Cognitively impaired older adults. *Am J Nurs*, 105(2), 52–61.

9. Palmer, R. M. (2006). Management of common clinical disorders in geriatric patients: Delerium. Retrieved May 2007 from www.medscape.com/viewarticle/53466.

10. Simon, J. H. (2004). Schizophrenia. Hardin Memorial Hospital. Retrieved May 2007 from www.hmh.net/adam/patientreports/000047.htm.

11. Holm, K., Foreman, M. (2006). Analysis of measures of functional and cognitive ability for aging adults with cardiac and vascular disease. *J Cardiovasc Nurs*, 21(5 suppl), 40–45.

impaired Tissue Integrity

DEFINITION: Damage to mucous membrane, corneal, integumentary, or subcutaneous tissues

RELATED FACTORS

Altered circulation
Nutritional factors (e.g., deficit or excess); [metabolic/endocrine dysfunction]
Fluid deficit or excess
Knowledge deficit
Impaired physical mobility
Chemical irritants (including body excretions, secretions, medications); radiation (including therapeutic radiation)
Temperature extremes
Mechanical (e.g., pressure, shear, friction), [surgery]
Knowledge deficit
[Infection]

DEFINING CHARACTERISTICS

Objective
Damaged tissue (e.g., cornea, mucous membrane, integumentary, subcutaneous)
Destroyed tissue

Sample Clinical Applications: Trauma, burns, diabetes mellitus, peripheral vascular disease, venous insufficiency, AIDS, cancer, radiation therapy, sickle cell crisis, cocaine use, scleroderma, infections, borderline personality or obsessive-compulsive disorder

DESIRED OUTCOMES/EVALUATION CRITERIA

Sample NOC linkages:
Tissue Integrity: Skin & Mucous Membranes: Structural intactness and normal physiological function of skin and mucous membranes
Tissue Perfusion: Peripheral: Adequacy of blood flow through the small vessels of the extremities to maintain tissue function

Client/Caregiver Will (Include Specific Time Frame)
- Verbalize understanding of condition and causative factors.
- Identify interventions appropriate for specific condition.
- Demonstrate behaviors or lifestyle changes to promote healing and prevent complications or recurrence.

Sample (NOC) linkage:
Wound Healing: Secondary Intention: Extent of regeneration of cells and tissues in an open wound

Client Will (Include Specific Time Frame)
- Display progressive improvement in wound or lesion healing.

ACTIONS/INTERVENTIONS

Sample (NIC) linkages:
Wound Care: Prevention of wound complications and promotion of wound healing
Incision Site Care: Cleansing, monitoring, and promotion of healing in a wound that is closed with sutures, clips, or staples
Pressure Ulcer Care: Facilitation of healing in pressure ulcers

NURSING PRIORITY NO. 1

To identify causative/contributing factors:

- Identify underlying condition or pathology involved in tissue injury (e.g., diabetic neuropathies, peripheral arterial disorders; sensory or perceptual deficits; cognitive impairments, developmental delay; frail elder; emotional or psychological problems; surgery, traumatic injuries; debilitating illness, long-term immobility). *Suggests treatment options, desire and ability to protect self, and potential for recurrence of tissue damage.*
- Assess skin and tissue color, temperature, and sensation *for adequacy of blood supply and nerve innervation.*
- Observe trauma or surgical client for tissue bleeding or spread of hematoma formation in injured areas, *which can result in compressed blood vessels and impaired circulation, aggravating injury to tissues.*[1,2]
- Assess for individual factors *that increase risk of circulatory insufficiency or occlusion and can impede healing; for example: (1) trauma to extremity that causes internal tissue damage (e.g., burns, high-velocity and penetrating trauma); fractures (especially long-bone fractures) with hemorrhage; (2) external pressures (e.g., from tight dressings, splints or casting, burn eschar); (3) immobility (e.g., long-term bedrest, traction/cast); (4) presence of conditions affecting peripheral circulation and sensation (e.g., atherosclerosis, diabetes, venous insufficiency); (5) lifestyle factors (e.g., smoking, obesity, and sedentary lifestyle); (6) use of medications (e.g., anticoagulants, corticosteroids, immunosuppressives, antineoplastics) that adversely affect healing; (7) vigorous sports or exercise; (8) malnutrition (deprives the body of protein and calories required for cell growth and repair); and (9) dehydration (impairs transport of oxygen and nutrients).*[1-5,11,14,17]
- Evaluate skin and mucous membranes for hydration status; note presence and degree of edema (1+ to 4+), urine characteristics and output. *Determines presence of fluid deficit or overload that can adversely affect cell or tissue strength and organ function. Note: Edematous tissues are prone to breakdown.* Refer to ND risk for imbalanced Fluid Volume.

- Evaluate pulses, calculate ankle-brachial index *to evaluate actual or potential for impairment of circulation to lower extremities. Result less than 0.9 indicates need for close monitoring or more aggressive intervention (e.g., tighter blood glucose and weight control in diabetic client).*[7]

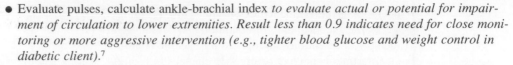

- Determine race and ethnic background, family history for genetic factors *that may make individual vulnerable to particular conditions (e.g., sickle cell disease impairs circulation),* and cultural or religious beliefs and practices regarding use of folk remedies or customs *that may damage tissues or impact choice of treatment options.*
- Determine nutritional status and impact of malnutrition on situation (e.g., pressure points on emaciated or elderly client, obesity, lack of activity, slow healing or failure to heal).
- Evaluate client's health and safety practices noting lack of cleanliness, poor oral care, lack of foot and toenail care, unsafe sexual practices, failure to use safety equipment for occupational or sports-related activities, and unprotected exposure to sun or toxic substances *that can place client at risk for injury to tissues or impaired function.*
- Note use of prosthetic, diagnostic, or external devices (e.g., artificial limbs, contacts, dentures, endotracheal airways, indwelling catheters, esophageal dilators), *which can cause pressure on/injure delicate tissues or provide entry point for infectious agents.*

NURSING PRIORITY NO. 2

To assess degree of impairment:

- Obtain history of condition (e.g., pressure, venous, or diabetic wound; eye or oral lesions), including whether condition is acute or recurrent, original site and characteristics of wound, and duration of problem and changes that have occurred over time.
- Assess skin and tissues, bony prominences, and pressure areas, noting color, texture, and turgor. Assess areas of least pigmentation for color changes (e.g., sclera, conjunctiva, nailbeds, buccal mucosa, tongue, palms, and soles of feet).
- Assess wound/lesion, documenting (1) location; (2) dimensions and depth in cm; (3) exudates—color, odor, and amount; (4) margins-fixed or unfixed; (5) tunneling/tracts—*(full extent of lesions of mucous membranes or subcutaneous tissue may not be visually discernible);* (6) evidence of necrosis (e.g., color gray to black) or healing (e.g., pink or red granulation tissue) *in order to clarify treatment needs and establish a comparative baseline.*[4,5]
- Classify pressure ulcer(s) using such tools as Waterlow, Braden, Norton (or similar) Ulcer Classification System. *Provides consistent terminology for assessment and documentation of pressure ulcers.*[6]
- Remeasure and photograph wound(s) periodically *to evaluate progress, development of complications or delayed healing.*
- Review diagnostic studies (e.g., x-rays, imaging scans, biopsies). *May be necessary to determine cause for and extent of impairment.*
- Obtain specimens of wound exudate or lesions for culture and sensitivity, when appropriate, *to identify effective antimicrobial therapies.*
- Monitor laboratory studies (e.g., complete blood count [CBC], electrolytes, glucose, cultures) *for systemic changes indicative of infection or other systemic complications.*
- Determine psychological effects of condition on the client and family. *Can be devastating for client's body or self-image and esteem—especially if condition is severe, disfiguring, or chronic—as well as costly and burdensome for SO/caregiver.*

NURSING PRIORITY NO. 3

To facilitate healing:

GENERAL[10,11,13,14]

- Modify or eliminate factors contributing to condition, if possible. Assist with treatment of underlying condition(s), as appropriate.
- Provide or encourage optimum nutrition (including adequate protein, lipids, calories, trace minerals, and multivitamins) *to promote tissue health/healing* and adequate hydration *to reduce and replenish cellular water loss and enhance circulation.*
- Encourage adequate periods of rest and sleep *to promote healing and meet comfort needs.*
- Promote early mobility. Assist with or encourage position changes, active or passive and assistive exercises *to promote circulation and prevent excessive tissue pressure.*

INCISIONS/WOUNDS[10,11,13–15]

- Inspect lesions or wounds daily for changes (e.g., signs of infection, complications, or healing). *Promotes timely intervention and revision of plan of care.*
- Keep surgical area(s) clean and dry, change dressings or drainage appliances frequently, as indicated, *to prevent accumulation of secretions or excretions that can cause skin and tissue excoriation.*
- Practice aseptic technique for cleansing, dressing, and medicating wounds or lesions. *Reduces risk of cross-contamination.*
- Protect incision or wound approximation (e.g., use of Steri-Strips, splinting when coughing) and stimulate circulation to surrounding areas *to assist body's natural process of repair.*
- Collaborate with other healthcare providers (e.g., physician, wound specialist, or ostomy nurse), as indicated, *to assist with developing plan of care for problematic or potentially serious wounds.*
- Apply appropriate barrier dressings or wound coverings (e.g., semipermeable, occlusive, wet-to-damp, hydrocolloid, hydrogel), drainage appliances, and skin-protective agents for open or draining wounds and stomas *to protect the wound and surrounding tissues from excoriating secretions or drainage and to enhance healing.*[14,16]
- Assist with débridement or enzymatic therapy, as indicated (e.g., burns, severe pressure ulcer).
- Provide appropriate protective and healing devices (e.g., eye pads or goggles; heel protectors, padding, cushions, gel pads; therapeutic beds and mattresses; splints, chronic ulcer dressings, compression wrap).
- Refer to NDs dependent on individual situation (e.g., risk for perioperative positioning Injury, impaired physical/bed Mobility, impaired Skin Integrity, disturbed visual Sensory Perception, ineffective peripheral tissue Perfusion, risk for Trauma, risk for Infection) *for related interventions.*

NURSING PRIORITY NO. 4

To correct hazards/minimize impairment:[4–6,8–12]

- Assess IV sites on regular basis for erythema, edema, tenderness, burning, and so forth, *which indicate infiltration or phlebitis, requiring immediate discontinuation of site use or interventions to heal the area.*
- Use appropriate catheter (e.g., peripheral or central venous) when infusing anticancer or other toxic drugs, and ascertain that IV is patent and infusing well *to prevent infiltration and extravasation with resulting tissue damage.*
- Inspect skin and tissues routinely around incisions and cast edges and traction devices *to ensure proper application and function; note possible development of pressure points.*

- Remove adhesive products with care, removing on horizontal plane and using mineral oil or Vaseline for softening, if needed, *to prevent abrasions or tearing of skin and damage to underlying tissues.*
- Monitor for correct placement of tubes, catheters, and other devices, and assess skin tissues around these devices for effects of tape or fasteners, or pressure from the devices *to prevent damage to skin and tissues as a result of pressure, friction, or shear forces.*
- Develop regularly timed repositioning schedule for client with mobility and sensation impairments, using turn sheet as needed; encourage and assist with periodic weight shifts for client in chair *to reduce stress on pressure points and encourage circulation to tissues.*
- Use or demonstrate proper turning and transfer techniques *to avoid movements that cause friction or shearing (e.g., pulling client with parallel force, dragging movements).*
- Provide appropriate mattress (e.g., foam, flotation, alternating pressure, or air mattress) and appropriate padding devices (e.g., foam boots, heel protectors, ankle rolls), when indicated, *to reduce tissue pressure and enhance circulation to compromised tissues.*[16]
- Limit use of plastic material (e.g., rubber sheet, plastic-backed linen savers), and remove wet or wrinkled linens promptly. *Moisture potentiates skin and underlying tissues, increasing risk of breakdown and infection.*
- Avoid or restrict use of restraints; use adequate padding and evaluate circulation, movement, and sensation of extremity frequently, when restraints are required. *Reduces risk of impaired circulation and tissue ischemia.*
- Elevate linens over affected extremity with bed cradle *to reduce pressure on and irritation of compromised tissues.*
- Encourage physical activity and exercise *to stimulate circulation, enhance organ function, and prevent/limit potential complications of immobility.*
- Provide or assist with oral care (e.g., oral and dental hygiene, avoiding extremes of hot or cold, change position of endotracheal/nasogastric tubes, lubricate lips) *to prevent damage to oral mucous membranes.* Refer to ND impaired Oral Mucous Membrane for additional interventions.
- Encourage use of adequate clothing or covers; protect from drafts *to prevent vasoconstriction that can compromise circulation.*
- Provide or instruct in proper care of extremities during cold or hot weather. *Individuals with impaired sensation or young children/individuals unable to verbalize discomfort require special attention to deal with extremes in weather (e.g., dressing in layers, wearing gloves, boots, clean, dry socks; properly fitting shoes or boots, face mask in winter; or use of sunscreen and light clothing to protect from dermal injury in summer).*
- Advise smoking cessation and refer for resources, if indicated. *Smoking causes vasoconstriction/interferes with healing.*

NURSING PRIORITY NO. 5

To promote wellness (Teaching/Discharge Considerations):

- Encourage verbalizations of feelings and expectations regarding condition and potential for recovery of structure and function.
- Help client and family to identify and implement successful coping skills *to reduce pain or discomforts and to improve quality of life.*
- Discuss importance of follow-up care (e.g., diabetic foot care clinic, wound care specialist, enterostomal therapist) as appropriate, self-monitoring and reporting of changes in condition or pain characteristics. *Promotes early intervention and reduces potential for complications.*
- Review medical regimen (e.g., proper use of topical sprays, creams, ointments, soaks, or irrigations).

- 🏠 ● Instruct in dressing changes (technique and frequency) and proper disposal of soiled dressings *to prevent spread of infectious agent.*
- 🏠 ● Identify required changes in lifestyle, occupation, or environment *necessitated by limitations imposed by condition or to avoid causative factors.*
- Ⓐ ● Refer to community or governmental resources as indicated (e.g., Public Health Department, Occupational Safety and Health Administration [OSHA], National Association for the Prevention of Blindness) *for information regarding specific conditions and to report hazards.*

DOCUMENTATION FOCUS

Assessment/Reassessment
- Individual findings, including history of condition, characteristics of wound or lesion, evidence of other organ or tissue involvement.
- Impact on functioning and lifestyle.
- Availability and use of resources.

Planning
- Plan of care and who is involved in planning.
- Teaching plan.

Implementation/Evaluation
- Responses to interventions, teaching, and actions performed.
- Attainment or progress toward desired outcome(s).
- Modifications to plan of care.

Discharge Planning
- Long-term needs and who is responsible for actions to be taken.
- Specific referrals made.

References

1. Fort, C. W. (2003). How to combat 3 deadly trauma complications. *Nursing*, 33(5), 58–63.
2. Paula, R. (2002, update 2006). Compartment syndrome, extremity. Retrieved July 2007 from www.emedicine.com/emerg/topic739.htm.
3. Peripheral vascular disease. (Public information sheet). Retrieved January 2004 from http://ivillagehealth.com.
4. Llewellyn, S. (2002). *Skin integrity and wound care. (Lecture materials).* Chapel Hill, NC: Cape Fear Community College Nursing Program.
5. Colburn, L., et al. (2001). Prevention for chronic wounds. *Chronic Wound Care: A Clinical Source Book for Healthcare Professionals.* 2d ed. Wayne, PA: Health Management Publications.
6. Risk factors and prevention. Geriatric syndromes: Pressure ulcers. Retrieved February 2004 from http://geriatricsyllabus.com.
7. Murabito, J. M., et al. (2003). The ankle-brachial index in the elderly and risk of stroke, coronary disease and death. *Arch Intern Med*, 163, 1939–1942.
8. Calianno, C. (2002). Patient hygiene, part 2—Skin care: Keeping the outside healthy. *Nursing*, 32(6). June Clinical suppl.
9. Wiersema, L. A., Stanley, M. (1999). The aging integumentary system. In Stanley, M., Beare, P. G. (eds). *Gerontological Nursing: A Health Promotion/Protection Approach.* 2d ed. Philadelphia: F. A. Davis, 102–111.
10. Doenges, M. E., Moorhouse, M. F., Geissler-Murr, A. C. (2002). NDs: Skin Integrity, impaired and Tissue Integrity, impaired. *Nursing Care Plans: Guidelines for Individualizing Patient Care.* 6th ed. Philadelphia: F. A. Davis.

11. McGovern, C. (2003). Skin, hair and nail assessment. Unit 2. (Lecture materials). Retrieved July 2007 from www.homepage.villanova.edu/.

12. Faller, N., Beitz, J. (2001). When a wound isn't a wound: Tubes, drains, fistulas and draining wounds. In Krasner, D., Rodeheaver, G., Sibbald, R. G. (eds). *Chronic Wound Care: A Clinical Source Book for Healthcare Professionals*. 2d ed. Wayne, PA: Health Management Publications.

13. Peripheral arterial occlusive disease. (Fact sheet). Retrieved January 2004 from www.fpnotebook.com.

14. Wound Ostomy and Continence Nurses Society (WOCN). (2002). Guideline for management of wounds in patients with lower-extremity arterial disease. Clinical practice guideline series, no. 1. Retrieved July 2007 from www.guideline.gov/summary/summary.aspx?doc_id=3290.

15. Okan, K., Woo, K., Ayello, E. A., (2007). The role of moisture balance in wound healing. *Adv Wound Care*, 20(1), 39–53.

16. Sieggreen, N. Y. (2006). Getting a leg up on managing venous ulcers. *Nursing Made Incredibly Easy!*, 4(6), 52–60.

17. Stotts, N. A., Wipke-Tevis, D. D., Hopf, H. W. (2007). Cofactors in impaired wound healing [excerpts]. Chronic Wound Care. 4th ed. Retrieved August 2007 from www.chronicwoundcarebook.com/.

impaired Transfer Ability

DEFINITION: Limitation of independent movement between two nearby surfaces

RELATED FACTORS

Insufficient muscle strength; deconditioning; neuromuscular impairment; musculoskeletal impairment (e.g., contractures)
Impaired balance
Pain
Obesity
Impaired vision
Lack of knowledge; cognitive impairment
Environment constraints (e.g., bed height, inadequate space, wheelchair type, treatment equipment, restraints)

DEFINING CHARACTERISTICS

Subjective or Objective
Inability to transfer from bed to chair or chair to bed; from chair to car or car to chair; from chair to floor or floor to chair; on or off a toilet or commode; in or out of tub or shower; from bed to standing or standing to bed; from chair to standing or standing to chair; from standing to floor or floor to standing; between uneven levels
Note: Specify level of independence using a standardized functional scale—[refer to ND impaired physical Mobility for suggested functional level classification]

Sample Clinical Applications: Arthritis, fractures, amputation, neuromuscular diseases (e.g., multiple sclerosis [MS], amyotrophic lateral sclerosis [ALS], Guillain-Barré syndrome), paralysis, glaucoma, macular degeneration, dementias

Cultural Collaborative Community/Home Care Diagnostic Studies Pediatric/Geriatric/Lifespan Medications

DESIRED OUTCOMES/EVALUATION CRITERIA

Sample (NOC) linkages:
Transfer Performance: Ability to change body location independently with or without assistive device
Balance: Ability to maintain body equilibrium
Body Positioning: Self-Initiated: Ability to change own body position independently with or without assistive device

Client/Caregiver Will (Include Specific Time Frame)
• Verbalize understanding of situation and appropriate safety measures.
• Master techniques of transfer successfully.
• Make desired transfer safely.

ACTIONS/INTERVENTIONS

Sample (NIC) linkages:
Transfer: Moving a patient with limitation of independent movement
Body Mechanics Promotion: Facilitating the use of posture and movement in daily activities to prevent fatigue and musculoskeletal strain or injury
Exercise Promotion: Strength Training: Facilitating regular physical exercise to maintain or advance to a higher level of fitness and health

NURSING PRIORITY NO. 1

To assess causative/contributing factors:

• Determine presence of conditions that contribute to transfer problems. *Neuromuscular and musculoskeletal problems, such as MS, fractures, back injuries, knee/hip replacement surgery, amputation, quadriplegia or paraplegia, contractures or spastic muscles, agedness (arthritis, decreased muscle mass, tone, or strength), and effects of dementias, brain injury, and so forth, can seriously impact balance and physical and psychological well-being.*[1,5]
• Evaluate perceptual and cognitive impairments and ability to follow directions. *Plan of care and choice of interventions is dependent upon nature of condition—acute, chronic, progressive; for example, client with severe brain injury may have permanent limitations because of impaired cognition affecting memory, judgment, problem-solving, and motor coordination, requiring more intensive inpatient and long-term care.*
• Note factors complicating current situation. *Recent surgery, traction apparatus; debilitating illness, weakness; mechanical ventilation, multiple IV/indwelling tubings can restrict movement.*
• Review medication regimen and schedule *to determine possible side effects or drug interactions impairing balance and/or muscle tone.*

NURSING PRIORITY NO. 2

To assess functional ability:

• Perform "Get-up and Go" test, as indicated, *to assess client's basic ability to transfer and ambulate safely. In this test, the client is asked to get up from a seated position in a chair, stand still momentarily, walk forward 10 feet, turn around, walk back to the chair, turn, and sit down. Factors assessed include sitting balance, ability to transfer from sitting to*

---

standing and back to sitting, the pace and stability of ambulation, and the ability to turn without staggering. If the client is not safe with ambulation, assistance may also be required with transfers.[2] *Note: Client may perform this test adequately and still have difficulty with some transfers, such as in or out of a car or bathtub or from floor to chair.*

- Determine degree of impairment in relation to 0 to 4 scale, noting muscle strength and tone, joint mobility, cardiovascular status, balance, and endurance. *Identifies strengths and deficits (e.g., ability to ambulate with assistive devices or problems with balance, failure to attend to one side, inability to bear weight [client is nonweight-bearing or partial weight-bearing]) and may provide information regarding potential for recovery.*[5]
- Observe movement when client is unaware of observations *to note any incongruence with reported abilities.*
- Note emotional and behavioral responses of client/SO to problems of immobility. *Restrictions or limitations imposed by immobility can cause physical, social, emotional, and financial difficulties for everyone.*

NURSING PRIORITY NO. 3

To promote optimal level of movement:

- Assist with treatment of underlying condition causing dysfunction. *Treatment of condition (e.g., surgery for hip replacement, therapy for unilateral neglect following stroke) can alleviate or improve difficulties with transfer activity.*
- Consult with physical and occupational therapists, or rehabilitation team *to develop general and specific muscle strengthening and range-of-motion exercises, transfer training and techniques, as well as recommendations and provision of balance, gait, and mobility aids or adjunctive devices.*[2]
- Position devices (e.g., call light, bed-positioning switch) in easy reach on the bed or chair. *Facilitates transfer and allows client to obtain assistance for transfer as needed.*
- Use appropriate number of people to assist with transfers and correct equipment *to safely transfer the client in a particular situation (e.g., chair to bed, chair to car, in or out of shower or tub).*[6,7]
- Demonstrate and assist with use of side rails or stand pole, overhead trapeze, transfer or sit-to-stand hoist; specialty slings; cane, walker, wheelchair, crutches, as necessary, *to protect client or care providers from injury during transfers and movements.*[6,7]
- Provide instruction and reinforce information for client and caregivers regarding body and equipment positioning *to improve or maintain balance during transfers.*
- Monitor body alignment, posture, and balance and encourage wide base of support *when standing to transfer.*
- Use full-length mirror, as needed, *to facilitate client's view of own postural alignment.*

NURSING PRIORITY NO. 4

To promote wellness (Teaching/Discharge Considerations):

- Instruct client/caregiver in appropriate safety measures. *Actions (e.g., proper use of transfer board; locking wheels on bed or chair; correct placement of equipment for optimal body mechanics of client and caregivers(s); use of gait belt, supportive nonslip footwear; good lighting; clearing floor of clutter), are important to facilitating transfers and reducing the possibility of fall and subsequent injury to client and caregiver.*[3]
- Discuss need for and sources of care or supervision. *Home-care agency, before- and after-school programs, elderly day care, personal companions, and so forth, may be required to assist with or monitor activity.*[4]

- Refer to appropriate community resources *for evaluation and modification of environment (e.g., roll-in-shower or tub, correction of uneven floor surfaces and steps, installation of ramps, use of standing tables or lifts).*
- Refer also to NDs impaired bed/physical/wheelchair Mobility, unilateral Neglect, or impaired Walking for additional interventions.

DOCUMENTATION FOCUS

Assessment/Reassessment
- Individual findings, including level of function and ability to participate in desired transfers.
- Mobility aides and transfer devices used.

Planning
- Plan of care and who is involved in the planning.
- Teaching plan.

Implementation/Evaluation
- Responses to interventions, teaching, and actions performed.
- Attainment or progress toward desired outcome(s).
- Modifications to plan of care.

Discharge Planning
- Discharge and long-term needs, noting who is responsible for each action to be taken.
- Specific referrals made.
- Sources of and maintenance for assistive devices.

References

1. Mass, M. L. (1989) *Impaired physical mobility*. (Unpublished manuscript). Cited in research article for National Institutes for Health.
2. Cruise, C. M., Koval, K. J. (1998). Rehabilitation of the elderly. *Arch Am Acad Orthop Surg*, 2(1), 103–107.
3. Patient safety during transfers. (2000). *Policy/Operations Manual*. Galveston, TX: UTMB Department of Rehabilitation Services.
4. Hogue, C. C. (1984). Falls and mobility late in life. An ecological model. *J Am Geriatr Soc*, 32, 858–861.
5. Tinetti, M. E., Williams, T. F., Mayewski, R. (1986). Fall risk index for elderly patients based on number of chronic disabilities. *Am J Med*, 80, 429–434.
6. Parsons, K. S., Galinsky, T. L., Waters, T. (2006). Suggestions for preventing musculoskeletal disorders in home healthcare workers, Part 1: Lift and transfer assistance for partially weight-bearing home care patients. *Home Healthc Nurs*, 24(3), 158–164.
7. Parsons, K. S., Galinsky, T. L., Waters, T. (2006). Suggestions for preventing musculoskeletal disorders in home healthcare workers, Part 2: Lift and transfer assistance for non-weight-bearing home care patients. *Home Healthcare Nurse*, 24(4), 227–233.

risk for Trauma

DEFINITION: Accentuated risk of accidental tissue injury (e.g., wound, burn, fracture)

RISK FACTORS

Internal
Weakness; balancing difficulties; reduced muscle or hand-eye coordination
Poor vision
Reduced sensation
Lack of safety education or precautions
Insufficient finances
Cognitive or emotional difficulties
History of previous trauma

External [Includes But Is Not Limited To]:
Slippery floors (e.g., wet or highly waxed); unanchored rugs or electric wires
Bathtub without antislip equipment
Use of unsteady ladder or chairs
Obstructed passageways; entering unlighted rooms
Inadequate stair rails; children playing without gates at top of stairs
High beds; inappropriate call-for-aid mechanisms for bedresting client
Unsafe window protection in homes with young children
Pot handles facing toward front of stove; bathing in very hot water (e.g., unsupervised bathing of young children)
Potential igniting gas leaks; delayed lighting of gas appliances
Wearing flowing clothes around open flames; flammable children's clothing or toys
Smoking in bed or near oxygen; grease waste collected on stoves
Children playing with dangerous objects; accessibility of guns
Playing with explosives; experimenting with chemicals; inadequately stored combustibles (e.g., matches, oily rags) or corrosives (e.g., lye); contact with corrosives
Overloaded fuse boxes; faulty electrical plugs; frayed wires; defective appliances; overloaded electrical outlets
Exposure to dangerous machinery; contact with rapidly moving machinery
Struggling with restraints
Contact with intense cold; lack of protection from heat source; overexposure to radiation
Large icicles hanging from the roof
Use of cracked dishware; knives stored uncovered
High-crime neighborhood
Driving a mechanically unsafe vehicle; driving at excessive speeds; driving without necessary visual aids; driving while intoxicated
Children riding in the front seat of car; nonuse or misuse of seat restraints
Unsafe road or walkways; physical proximity to vehicle pathways (e.g., driveways, lanes, railroad tracks)
Misuse[or nonuse] of necessary headgear [e.g., for bicycles, motorcycles, skateboarding, skiing]

NOTE: A risk diagnosis is not evidenced by signs and symptoms, as the problem has not occurred; rather, nursing interventions are directed at prevention.

Sample Clinical Applications: Substance intoxication or abuse, peripheral neuropathy, cataracts, glaucoma, macular degeneration, Parkinson's disease, seizure disorder, dementia, major depression, developmental delay

DESIRED OUTCOMES/EVALUATION CRITERIA

Sample **NOC** linkages:
Physical Injury Severity: Severity of injuries from accidents and trauma
Abuse Protection: Protection of self or dependent others from abuse
Knowledge: Personal Safety: Extent of understanding conveyed about prevention of unintentional injuries

Client/Caregiver Will (Include Specific Time Frame)
• Identify and correct potential risk factors in the environment.
• Demonstrate appropriate lifestyle changes to reduce risk of injury.
• Identify resources to assist in promoting a safe environment.
• Recognize need for and seek assistance to prevent accidents/injuries.

ACTIONS/INTERVENTIONS

This ND is a compilation of a number of situations that can result in injury. Refer to specific NDs, such as risk for imbalanced Body Temperature; risk for Contamination; impaired Environmental Interpretation Syndrome; risk for Falls; impaired Home Maintenance; Hyperthermia; Hypothermia; risk for Injury; impaired physical Mobility; risk for impaired Parenting; risk for Poisoning; disturbed Sensory Perception; impaired Skin Integrity; risk for Suffocation; disturbed Thought Processes; impaired Tissue Integrity; risk for self-/other-directed Violence; impaired Walking, as appropriate, for more specific interventions.

Sample **NIC** linkages:
Environmental Management: Safety: Manipulation of the patient's surroundings for therapeutic benefit
Environmental Management: Worker Safety: Monitoring and manipulation of the worksite environment to promote safety and health of workers
Teaching: Infant [or] Toddler Safety [specify age]: Instruction on safety during first/second and third years of life
Surveillance: Safety: Purposeful and ongoing collection and analysis of information about the patient and the environment for use in promoting and maintaining patient safety

NURSING PRIORITY NO. 1

To assess causative/contributing factors:

● Determine factors related to individual situation and extent of risk for trauma. *Influences scope and intensity of interventions to manage threats to safety, which are dynamic and constants in every life and situation. Clients interfacing with the healthcare system are at higher risk for trauma for any number of reasons (e.g., illness state, cognitive function, family structure, information and training) and require protection in numerous ways.*[1]

∞ ● Note client's age, gender, developmental stage, decision-making ability, level of cognition and competence *to determine client's ability to recognize danger and to protect self.*

● Ascertain client's/SO's knowledge of safety needs, injury prevention, and ways of looking at and improving own environment. *Lack of appreciation of significance of individual hazards increases risk of traumatic injury.*[1]

● Assess influence of stressors (e.g., physical, mental, work-related, financial) *that can impair judgment and greatly increase client's potential for injury.*

● Assess mood, coping abilities, personality styles (i.e., temperament, aggression, impulsive behavior, level of self-esteem). *May result in careless or increased risk-taking without consideration of consequences.*[13,14]

● Evaluate individual's emotional and behavioral response to violence in surroundings (e.g., neighborhood, television, peer group). *May affect client's view of and regard for own/others' safety.*[13–15]

🏠 ● Evaluate environment (home, work, transportation) *for obvious safety hazards, as well as situations that can exacerbate injury or adversely affect client's well-being. Unsafe factors include a vast array of possibilities (e.g., unsafe heating appliances, smoking materials, toxic substances and chemicals, open flames, knives, improperly stored guns, overloaded electrical outlets, dangerous neighborhoods, unsupervised children).*[1]

🏠 ● Review potential occupational risk factors (e.g., works with dangerous tools and machinery, electricity, explosives; police, fire, emergency medical service [EMS] officers; working with hazardous chemicals, various inhalants, or radiation).

● Note history of accidents during specific period of time, noting circumstances of the accident (e.g., time of day that falls occur, activities going on, who was present). *Investigation of such events can provide clues for client's risk for subsequent events and potential for enhanced safety by a change in the people or environment involved (e.g., client may need assistance when getting up at night, or increased playground supervision may be required).*

🏠 ● Determine potential for abusive behavior by family members/SO(s)/peers. *Anyone, but especially child/frail elder, may require placement if incurring repeated injuries in family/community setting.*

🏠 ● Note socioeconomic status, availability and use of resources. *Lack of resources, including financial, may limit ability to meet safety needs (e.g., proper child safety seat, appliance repairs, window grates).*

🔬 ● Review diagnostic studies and laboratory results, noting impairments or imbalances *that may result in or exacerbate conditions, such as confusion, tetany, pathological fractures, and so forth.*

NURSING PRIORITY NO. 2

To enhance safety in healthcare environment:

● Perform thorough assessments regarding safety issues when planning for client care and discharge. *Failure to accurately assess and intervene or refer regarding these issues can place the client at needless risk and creates negligence issues for the healthcare practitioner.*[12]

● Monitor client's therapeutic regimen on a continual basis (e.g., client's vital signs, medications, treatment modalities, infusions, nutrition, physical environment) *to prevent healthcare-related injuries.*[12]

🤝 ● Collaborate in treatment of underlying medical, surgical, or psychiatric conditions *to improve cognition and thinking processes, musculoskeletal function, awareness of own safety needs, and general well-being.*

🤝 ● Refer to physical or occupational therapist as appropriate *to identify high-risk tasks, conduct site visits, select, create, or modify equipment; and provide education about body mechanics and musculoskeletal injuries, as well as provide needed therapies.*[3]

- Emphasize with client importance of obtaining assistance when weak or sedated and when problems of balance, coordination, or postural hypotension are present *to reduce risk of syncope and falls.*
- Provide quiet environment and reduced stimulation as indicated. *Helps limit confusion or overstimulation for clients at risk for such conditions as seizures, tetany, autonomic hyperreflexia.*
- Demonstrate and encourage use of techniques to reduce or manage stress and vent emotions such as anger, hostility *to reduce risk of violence to self/others.*
- Provide for routine safety needs:[2–11]

  Provide adequate supervision and frequent observation.

  Place young children, confused client/person with dementia near nurses' station.

  Provide for appropriate communication tools (e.g., call light, writing implements and paper; alphabet picture board).

  Demonstrate use and place call bell/light or phone within client's reach.

  Orient or reorient client to environment as needed.

  Encourage client's use of corrective vision and hearing aids.

  Keep bed in low position or place mattress on floor as appropriate.

  Maintain correct body alignment and mechanics.

  Provide positioning as required by situation (e.g., immobilization of fractures).

  Implement appropriate measures to maintain skin and tissue health.

  Protect client (with sensory impairments) from injury due to heat and cold.

  Provide seizure precautions when indicated.

  Lock wheels on bed, wheelchair, and movable furniture.

  Assist with activities and transfers as needed.

  Provide well-fitting, nonskid footwear.

  Demonstrate and monitor use of assistive devices, such as cane, walker, crutches, wheelchair, safety bars.

  Clear travel paths, pick up small items from floor; keep furniture in one place and door in one position (completely open or closed).

  Provide adequate area lighting.

  Follow facility protocol and closely monitor use of restraints when required (e.g., vest, limb, belt, mitten).
- Administer treatments, medications and therapies in a therapeutic manner.

  Dispose of sharp implements in appropriate container.

NURSING PRIORITY NO. 3

To enhance safety for client in community care setting:

- Provide information to caregivers regarding client's specific disease or condition(s) and associated risks. *For example, postural hypotension, muscle weakness (e.g., multiple sclerosis [MS]), dementia, osteoporosis, head injury can impair function or cognition, impacting client's ability to protect self.*
- Identify interventions and safety devices to promote safe physical environment and individual safety:[7,8,11–14]

  Recommend wearing visual or hearing aids *to maximize sensory input.*

  Ensure availability of communication devices (e.g., telephone, computer, alarm system or medical emergency alert device).

  Install and maintain electrical and fire safety devices, extinguishers, and alarms.

  Review oxygen safety rules.

Identify environmental needs (e.g., decals on glass doors; *to show when they are closed*, adequate lighting of stairways, handrails, ramps, bathtub safety tapes *to reduce risk of falls*; lowering temperature on hot water heater *to prevent accidental burns*; creation of ergonomic workstation).

Obtain seat raisers for chairs; ergonomic beds or chairs.

Encourage participation in back-safety classes; injury-prevention exercises, mobility or transfer device training.

Install childproof cabinets for medications and toxic household substances, use tamper-proof medication containers.

Review proper storage and disposal of volatile liquids; installation of proper ventilation for use when mixing or using toxic substances; use of safety glasses or goggles.

Stress importance of appropriate use of car restraints, bicycle, skating, or skiing helmets.

Discuss swimming pool fencing and supervision; attending first-aid and cardiopulmonary resuscitation (CPR) classes.

Obtain trigger locks or gun safes for firearms.

- Initiate appropriate teaching *if reckless behavior is occurring or likely to occur (e.g., smoking in bed, driving without safety belts, working with chemicals without safety goggles)*.
- Encourage participation in self-help programs *to address individual risks (e.g., assertiveness training, positive self-image to enhance self-esteem, smoking cessation, weight management)*.
- Refer to counseling or psychotherapy, as needed, *especially when individual is "accident-prone" or self-destructive behavior is noted*. Refer to NDs [actual/]risk for self-directed Violence.

NURSING PRIORITY NO. 4

To promote wellness (Teaching/Discharge Considerations):

- Discuss importance of self-monitoring of conditions or emotions that can contribute to occurrence of injury to self/others (e.g., fatigue, anger, irritability). *Client/SO may be able to modify risk through monitoring of actions, or postponement of certain actions, especially during times when client is likely to be highly stressed.*
- Review expectations caregivers have of children, cognitively impaired, or elderly family members *to identify needed information, required assistance with care, follow-up that may be needed to provide safe environment for client.*
- Problem-solve with client/parent *to provide adequate child supervision after school, during working hours, and on school holidays.*
- Discuss need for and sources of adult supervision (e.g., elderly day care, home health aide or companion).
- Encourage client's family to identify neighbors or friends willing *to assist elderly/individuals with disabilities in providing such things as checking on client who lives alone, removing snow and ice from walks and steps, assisting with structural maintenance, and so forth.*
- Explore behaviors related to use of alcohol, tobacco, and recreational drugs and other substances. *Provides opportunity to review consequences of previously determined risk factors (e.g., increase in oral cancer among teenagers using smokeless tobacco, potential consequences of illegal activities, effects of smoking on health of family members as well as fire danger; occurrence of spontaneous abortion, fetal alcohol syndrome or neonatal addiction in prenatal women using tobacco, alcohol, and other drugs).*[13-15]
- Encourage development of fire safety program. *Participation in family fire drills, use of smoke detectors, yearly chimney cleaning, purchase of fire-retardant clothing (especially*

children's nightwear), fireworks safety, safe use of in-home oxygen or propane sources, and so forth, enhances home safety.

- Recommend use of seat belts, approved infant seat, fitted helmets for cyclists, wearing necessary visual aids; driver training course for new and mature drivers; avoidance of hitchhiking; substance abuse program as indicated *to promote transportation safety.*
- Identify community resources (e.g., financial, volunteer) *to assist with necessary home improvements or equipment purchases.*
- Refer to other resources as indicated (e.g., counseling/psychotherapy, parenting classes, budget counseling).
- Provide client/caregiver with emergency contact numbers as individually indicated (e.g., doctor, 911, poison control, police).
- Provide client/caregiver with bibliotherapy and written resources *for later review and self-paced learning.*
- Encourage involvement in community awareness programs and problem-solving of identified community needs:

  Participate in self-help programs (e.g., Neighborhood Watch, Helping Hand, after-school activities). *Programs based on identified needs enhances support of community members and potential funding sources.*

  Promote educational opportunities *geared toward increasing awareness of safety measures (e.g., firearms safety) and resources available to the individual.*

  Seek out and involve businesses in volunteer outreach activities such as building safe playgrounds, community or street cleanup, home repair or improvement for frail elders, and so forth.

  Advocate for and promote solutions for problems of design of buildings, equipment, transportation, and workplace practices *that contribute to accidents.*

DOCUMENTATION FOCUS

Assessment/Reassessment
- Individual risk factors, past and recent history of injuries, awareness of safety needs.

Planning
- Plan of care and who is involved in the planning.
- Teaching plan.

Implementation/Evaluation
- Responses to interventions, teaching, and actions performed.
- Attainment or progress toward desired outcome(s).
- Modifications to plan of care.

Discharge Planning
- Long-term needs and who is responsible for actions to be taken.
- Available resources, specific referrals made.

References

1. Ebright, P. R., Patterson, E. S., Render, M. L. (2002). The "New Look" approach to patient safety: A guide for clinical specialist leadership. *Clin Nurs Spec*, 16(5), 247–253.
2. Doenges, M. E., Moorhouse, M. F., Geissler-Murr, A. C. (2002). ND: Trauma, risk for. *Nurse's Pocket Guide: Diagnoses, Interventions, and Rationales.* 8th ed. Philadelphia: F. A. Davis.

3. Nelson, A., (2003). Safe patient handling & movement. *Am J Nurs*, 103(3), 32–43.
4. Walton, J. (2001). Helping high-risk surgical patients beat the odds. *Nursing*, 31(3), 54.
5. Mion, L. C., Mercurio, A. T. (1992). Methods to reduce restraints: Process, outcomes and future directions. *J Gerontol Nurs*, 20(10), 5.
6. Wright, A. (1998). Nursing interventions with advanced osteoporosis. *Home Healthcare Nurse*, 16(3), 145.
7. Kedlaya, D., Kuang, T. (2002, update 2007). Assistive devices to improve independence. Retrieved July 2007 from www.emedicine.com/pmr/topic210.htm.
8. Safety for older consumers' home safety checklist. Consumer Product Safety Commission (CPSC). Retrieved July 2007 from www.cpsc.gov.
9. Doenges, M. E., Moorhouse, M. F., Geissler-Murr, A. C. (2002). Nursing care plan: Extended care, falls, risk for. *Nursing Care Plans: Guidelines for Individualizing Patient Care* (CD-ROM). 6th ed. Philadelphia: F. A. Davis.
10. Daus, C. (1999). Maintaining mobility: Assistive equipment helps the geriatric population stay active and independent. *Rehabil Manage*, 12(5), 58–61.
11. Horn, L. B. (2000). Reducing the risk of falls in the elderly. *Rehabil Manage*, 13(3), 36–38.
12. Keepnews, D., Mitchell, P. H. (2003). Health systems' accountability for patient safety. *Online J Issues Nurs*, 8(3), 2.
13. Gorman-Smith, D., Tolan, P. (1998). The role of exposure to community violence and developmental problems among inner city youth. *Dev Psychopathol*, 10(1), 101.
14. Youth violence in the United States. National Center for Injury Prevention and Control. Retrieved July 2007 from www.cdc.gov/ncipc/factsheets/yvfacts.htm.
15. Schwebel, D. C., Barton, B. K. (2005). Contributions of multiple risk factors to child injury. *J of Pediatr Psychol*, 30(7), 553–561.

risk for vascular Trauma

DEFINITION: At risk for damage to a vein and its surrounding tissues related to the presence of a catheter and/or infused solutions

RISK FACTORS

Insertion site; impaired ability to visualize the insertion site
Catheter type; catheter width
Nature of solution (e.g., concentration, chemical irritant, temperature, pH); infusion rate; length of insertion time

NOTE: A risk diagnosis is not evidenced by signs and symptoms, as the problem has not occurred; rather, nursing interventions are directed at prevention.
Sample Clinical Applications: Surgery, trauma, cancer/chemotherapy, pneumonia, sepsis, dehydration, heat stroke

DESIRED OUTCOMES/EVALUATION CRITERIA

Sample NOC linkages:
Symptom Control: Personal actions to minimize perceived adverse changes in physical and emotional functioning
Knowledge: Treatment Procedure: Extent of understanding conveyed about a procedure required as part of a treatment regimen

⊕ Cultural   ⊛ Collaborative   🏠 Community/Home Care   ▱ Diagnostic Studies   ∞ Pediatric/Geriatric/Lifespan   ⚗ Medications

Client Will (Include Specific Time Frame)
• Identify sign/symptoms to report to healthcare provider.
• Be free of signs/symptoms associated with infusion phlebitis or local infection.
• Develop plan for home therapy and demonstrate appropriate procedures as indicated.

ACTIONS/INTERVENTIONS

Sample **NIC** linkages:
Intravenous (IV) Insertion: Insertion of a needle into a peripheral vein for the purpose of administering fluids, blood, or medications
Intravenous (IV) Therapy: Administration and monitoring of intravenous fluids and medications

NURSING PRIORITY NO. 1

To assess risk factors:

• Determine presence of medical condition(s) requiring IV therapy, such as dehydration, trauma, surgery; long-term antibiotic treatment of severe infections; cancer therapies; pain management when oral drugs not effective or practical.

∞ • Note client's age, body size, and weight. *Very young and elderly clients are at risk because of lack of subcutaneous tissue surrounding veins, and veins may be fragile or ropy, causing difficulties with insertion. Forearm veins may be difficult to see in obese, edematous, or dark-skinned individual.*[3,4]

• Identify particular issues such as client's emotional state including fear of needles, mental or developmental status that might interfere with client's ability to cooperate with procedures, IV site choices that interfere with client's mobility *to prevent or limit potential for vascular damage.*[3]

• Determine type(s) of solutions being used or planned. *Certain infusates are associated with greater risk of vein irritation and pain (e.g., potassium); others are associated with of tissue injury, especially upon infiltration into surrounding tissues, including certain antibiotics (e.g., nafcillin, vancomycin). Hyperosmolar solutions such as total parenteral nutrition (TPN) can cause tissue damage by altering osmotic pressure. Most cancer chemotherapeutic agents cause direct cellular toxicity after extravasation, and some have potential for causing substantial tissue necrosis (e.g., doxorubicin, vincristine).*[5] *Note: Therapies not appropriate for peripheral short catheters include continuous vesicant therapy, parenteral nutrition, infusates with a pH less than 5 or greater than 9, and solutions with an osmolarity greater than 600 mOsm/L.*[6,7]

• Assess peripheral IV site, when one is already in place, to determine potential for complications. *Reddened, blanched, tight, translucent, or cool skin; swelling; pain; numbness; streak formation; a palpable venous cord or purulent drainage are indicative of problem with IV requiring immediate intervention.*[1]

• Assess central venous access device (CVAD), if present, to determine potential for complications. *Inability to aspirate, slowed or absent solution flow, site pain; engorged veins or swelling in upper arm, chest wall, neck, or jaw on side of catheter insertion may indicate vein or catheter-related thrombus, requiring immediate intervention.*[1,2]

NURSING PRIORITY NO. 2

To reduce potential complications:

- Determine appropriate site choice:

  Identify extremities and sites that have impaired circulation or injury, such as lymphedema, postoperative swelling, recent trauma, hematoma, axillary lymph node dissection, open wounds, and so forth.[4] *Note: Leg veins should be avoided in adults due to potential for thrombophlebitis. Anticubital veins should be avoided for peripheral catheters where possible because they limit client's movement and are easily dislodged.*[6]

  Inspect and palpate chosen veins to determine size and condition. *Vein that is scarred, lumpy, or small and fragile not only can cause problems upon cannulation but also can impede effectiveness of infusion.*[1,6]

  Avoid inserting needle in vein valve site. *Damage to this area can cause blood pooling and increase risk of thrombosis.*[3]

- Use best-practice approach to IV insertion and therapies:

  Determine best type of access when IV therapy is to be initiated. *Peripheral catheter in forearm is recommended for short-duration, nonirritating solutions of less than 7 days' duration. CVAD placed so that tip is in or near the superior vena cava, is appropriate for infusing many kinds of solutions over long periods of time.*[4,8,9]

  Choose appropriate needle or catheter for situation considering planned length and type of therapy, avoiding steel butterfly needles when possible *to reduce risk of vein injury and infiltration.*[1,2,4] *Over-the-needle catheter for hand or forearm may be ideal for most solutions over a short length of time, while midline catheter may be chosen for chemotherapy or when antibiotic therapy is planned for 1 to 4 weeks; central venous catheter (CVC) is used for infusates and other substances that are too irritating to peripheral veins, when client has suffered multiple peripheral sticks, or when one extremity is not available (e.g., amputation, dialysis shunt in one arm).*[4,8]

  Use appropriate needle gauge. *Size should be smallest diameter possible for chosen vein and solution to be infused to deliver solution at appropriate rate, to promote hemodilution of fluid(s) at the catheter tip, and to reduce mechanical and chemical irritation to vein wall.*[1,3,4]

  Clean site and inject 1% lidocaine per agency protocol *to reduce risk of infection and pain with needle or cannula insertion.*

  Stretch and immobilize skin and tissues *to stabilize vein and prevent rolling, requiring multiple sticks.*

  Insert needle bevel up, during insertion and hold at 3- to 10-degree angle *to prevent "blowing" the vein by piercing the back wall.*[2]

  Release tourniquet immediately when insertion is complete *to prevent intravascular pressure from causing bleeding into surrounding tissues.*[1]

  Observe for hematoma development and/or reports of pain and discomfort during insertion, *indicating vein damage with bleeding into tissues.*[4]

  Secure needle or cannula with tape or other securement device *to prevent dislodging and extend catheter dwell time.*[6]

  Avoid placing tape entirely around arm to anchor catheter. *This may impede venous return and cause venous stasis, pooling of fluid, infiltration or extravasation into surrounding tissues.*[4]

  Utilize transparent dressing over insertion site *to protect from external contaminants, and to easily observe for potential complications.*

  Adhere to recommended infusions, dilutions, and administration rates for medications or irritating substances such as potassium, *to reduce incidence of tissue irritation and sloughing.*[2,4,6]

 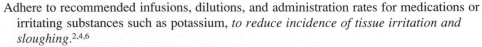

- Consult with IV nurse or other medical provider *to problem-solve issues that arise with IVs and/or when different access should be considered (e.g., midline catheter for continuous infusion of irritating solutions, peripheral intravenous central catheter [PICC] for parenteral nutrition), or for evaluation and interventions for complications such as thrombus development in central catheter tip or in the vein around the catheter.*[4,9]

NURSING PRIORITY NO. 3

To promote optimum therapeutic effect:

- Observe IV site on a regular basis and instruct client/caregiver to report any discomfort, bruising, redness, swelling, bleeding or other fluid leaking from site *to allow for prompt intervention and limit serious complications.*
- Replace peripheral catheters every 72 to 96 hours (or per agency policy) *to prevent thrombophlebitis and catheter-related infections.*[4]
- Apply pressure to site when IV is discontinued for sufficient time *to prevent bleeding, especially in client with coagulopathies or on anticoagulants.*[4]
- Adhere to specific protocols related to infection control *to promote safe infusion of solutions or medications and prevent complications.* Refer to ND risk for Infection.
- Identify community resources and suppliers *to support home therapy regimen.*

DOCUMENTATION FOCUS

Assessment/Reassessment
- Assessment findings pre- and postinsertion, site choice, use of local anesthetic, type and gauge of needle or cannula inserted, number of sticks required, dressing applied.
- Type, amount, and rate of solution administered, presence of additives.
- Client's response to procedure.

Planning
- Plan of care, specific interventions, and who is involved in the planning.
- Teaching plan as appropriate.

Implementation/Evaluation
- Attainment or progress toward desired outcome(s).
- Modifications to plan of care.

Discharge Planning
- Long-range needs, identifying who is responsible for actions to be taken.
- Community resources for equipment and supplies for home therapy.
- Specific referrals made.

References

1. Hadaway, L. C. (2005). Reopen the pipeline for I.V. therapy. *Nursing,* 35(8), 54–61.
2. Hadaway, L. C., Millam, D. A. (2007). On the road to successful I.V. starts. *Nursing,* 37(8 suppl), 1–14.
3. Rosenthal, K. (2005). Tailor your I.V. insertion techniques for special populations. *Nursing,* 35(5), 36–41.
4. Camp-Sorrell, D., Cope, D. G. (2004). *Access Device Guidelines: Recommendations for Nursing Practice and Education.* 2d ed. Pittsburgh, PA: Oncology Nursing Society.
5. Buck, M. L. (1998). Treatment of intravenous extravasations. Adapted from *Pediatric Pharm* 4(1). Retrieved March 2009 from www.medscape.com/viewarticle/416651/.

6. Infusion Nurses Society. (2006). Infusion nursing standards of practice. *J Infus Nurs*, 29(1 suppl), S1–S92.
7. Gorski, L. A. (2008). Intravenous therapy. In Ackley, B. J., et al. (eds). *Evidence-Based Nursing Care Guidelines: Medical-Surgical Interventions*. St. Louis, MO: Mosby Elsevier.
8. Cook, L. S. (2007). Choosing the right intravenous catheter. *Home Healthcare Nurse*, 25(8), 523–531.
9. Hadaway, L. C. (2008). Targeting therapy with central venous access devices. *Nursing*, 38(6), 34–40.

impaired Urinary Elimination

DEFINITION: Dysfunction in urine elimination

RELATED FACTORS

Multiple causality; sensory motor impairment; anatomical obstruction; urinary tract infection (UTI); [mechanical trauma; fluid/volume states; psychogenic factors; surgical diversion]

DEFINING CHARACTERISTICS

Subjective
Frequency; urgency
Hesitancy
Dysuria
Nocturia, [enuresis]

Objective
Incontinence
Retention

Sample Clinical Applications: UTI, prostate disease (BPH), bladder cancer, interstitial cystitis, spinal cord injury (SCI), multiple sclerosis (MS), pregnancy, childbirth, pelvic trauma, abdominal surgery, dementia, Alzheimer's disease

DESIRED OUTCOMES/EVALUATION CRITERIA

Sample NOC linkages:
Urinary Elimination: Collection and drainage of urine
Urinary Continence: Control of the elimination of urine from the bladder
Self-Care: Toileting: Ability to toilet self independently with or without assistive device

Client Will (Include Specific Time Frame)
• Verbalize understanding of condition.
• Identify specific causative factors.
• Achieve normal elimination pattern or participate in measures to correct or compensate for defects.
• Demonstrate behaviors or techniques to prevent urinary infection.
• Manage care of urinary catheter or stoma and appliance following urinary diversion.

ACTIONS/INTERVENTIONS

Sample (NIC) linkages:

Urinary Elimination Management: Maintenance of an optimum urinary elimination pattern

Urinary Catheterization: Insertion of a catheter into the bladder for temporary or permanent drainage of urine

Perineal Care: Maintenance of perineal skin integrity and relief of perineal discomfort

NURSING PRIORITY NO. 1

To assess causative/contributing factors:

- Note presence of physical diagnoses that may be involved, such as UTI, dehydration; surgery (including urinary diversion); neurological conditions (e.g., MS, stroke, Parkinson's disease; paraplegia, tetraplegia); mental or emotional dysfunction (e.g., impaired cognition, delirium, confusion, depression, Alzheimer's disease); prostate disorders; recent or multiple pregnancies; pelvic trauma.[1]
- Determine pathology of bladder dysfunction relative to identified medical diagnosis (e.g., in neurological or demyelinating diseases, such as MS, problem may be failure to store urine, empty bladder, or both). *Identifies direction for further evaluation and treatment options to discover specifics of individual situation.*[2,3,9]
- Note client's age and gender. Incontinence and UTIs are more prevalent in women and older adults; painful bladder syndrome or interstitial cystitis (PBS/IC) is more common in women.[5,10]
- Perform physical examination (e.g., cough test *for incontinence*, palpation *for bladder retention and masses*, prostate size, observation for urethral stricture).[11]
- Investigate pain, noting location, duration, intensity; presence of bladder spasms; back or flank pain *to assist in differentiating between bladder and kidney cause of dysfunction. Note: Bladder pain located suprapubically, vaginally, in the perineum, low back, or medial aspects of the thighs that is relieved by voiding and often recurs with bladder filling suggests presence of PBS/IC.*[10]
- Have client complete standardized self-report tool, such as Pelvic Pain and Urgency/Frequency (PUF) client symptom survey, as indicated. *Helpful in evaluating the presence and severity of PBS/IC symptoms.*[10]
- Note reports of exacerbations (flare-ups) and spontaneous remissions of symptoms of urgency and frequency, which may/may not be accompanied by pain, pressure, or spasm. *Clients with PBS/IC void approximately 16 times per day with voided volumes usually less than normal.*[10]
- Determine client's usual daily fluid intake (both amount and beverage choices and use of caffeine). Note condition of skin and mucous membranes, color of urine *to determine level of hydration.*[5]
- Review medication regimen to identify drugs that can alter bladder or kidney function (e.g., some antihypertensive agents [e.g. angiotensin-converting enzyme—ACE inhibitors, beta-blockers]; anticholinergics [e.g. antihistamines, antiparkinsonian drugs]; antidepressants, antipsychotics; sedatives, hypnotics, opioids; caffeine; and alcohol).[12]
- Send urine specimen (midstream clean-voided or catheterized) for culture and sensitivities in presence of signs of UTI—cloudy, foul odor; bloody urine.
- Obtain specimen for antibody-coated bacteria assay. *Diagnosis of bacterial infection of the kidney or prostate is important for immediate treatment to prevent damage to these organs.*[3]

- Strain all urine for calculi and describe stones expelled or send to laboratory for analysis. *Retrieval of calculi allows identification of type of stone and influences choice of therapy.*[3]
- Review laboratory tests *for hyperglycemia, hyperparathyroidism, or other metabolic conditions; changes in renal function, presence of infection/sexually transmitted disease (STD), cytology revealing cancer.*
- Rule out gonorrhea in men. *This infection needs to be considered when urethritis with a penile discharge is present and there are no bacteria in the urine.*[3]
- Assist with or perform potassium sensitivity test (instillation of potassium solution into bladder). *Eighty percent of clients with PBS/IC will react positively.*[10]
- Review results of other diagnostic studies (e.g., uroflowmetry; cystometogram; postvoid residual, pressure flow, and leak point pressure measurement; videourodynamics; electromyography; kidneys, ureters, and bladder [KUB] imaging) *to identify presence and type of elimination problem.*[13]

NURSING PRIORITY NO. 2

To assess degree of interference/disability:

- Ascertain client's previous pattern of elimination and compare with current situation. Note reports of problems (e.g., frequency, urgency, painful urination; leaking or incontinence; changes in size or force of urinary stream; problems emptying bladder completely; nocturia, enuresis) *to assist in identification and treatment of particular dysfunction.*
- Ascertain client's/SO's perception of problem, degree of disability, and impact on self-image (e.g., client may be restricting social, employment, or travel activities; having sexual or relationship difficulties; experiencing depression).
- Note influence of culture or ethnicity, or gender on client's view of problems of incontinence. *Limited evidence exists to understand and help people cope with the physical and psychosocial consequences of this chronic, socially isolating, and potentially devastating disorder.*[6]
- Have client keep a voiding diary for 3 days to record fluid intake, voiding times, precise urine output, and dietary intake. *Helps determine baseline symptoms, the severity of frequency/urgency; and whether diet is a factor if symptoms worsen.*

NURSING PRIORITY NO. 3

To assist in treating/preventing urinary alteration:

- Encourage fluid intake up to 2000 to 3000 mL/day (within cardiac tolerance), including cranberry juice. *Maintains renal function, prevents infection and formation of urinary stones, avoids encrustation around indwelling catheter, or may be used to flush urinary diversion appliance.*[5]
- Discuss possible dietary restrictions (e.g., especially coffee, alcohol, carbonated drinks, citrus, tomatoes, and chocolate) based on individual symptoms.[10]
- Assist with developing toileting routines (e.g., timed voiding, bladder training, prompted voiding, habit retraining) as appropriate. *For adults who are cognitively intact and physically capable of self-toileting, bladder training, timed voiding, and habit retraining may be beneficial.*[5,14] *However, bladder retraining is not recommended for clients with PBS.*[10]
- Encourage client to verbalize fear or concerns (e.g., disruption in sexual activity, inability to work, concern about involvement in social activities). *Open expression allows client to talk about, deal with feelings, and begin to solve the identified problems.*[6]
- Implement and monitor interventions for specific elimination problem (e.g., pelvic floor exercises or other bladder retraining modalities; medication regimen, antimicrobials [single

dose is frequently being used for UTI], sulfonamides, antispasmodics). Evaluate client's response *to modify treatment as needed.*[3]

- Discuss possible surgical procedures and medical regimen as indicated (e.g., client with benign prostatic hypertrophy, bladder or prostatic cancer, PBS/IC). *For example, cystoscopy with bladder hydrodistention for PBS/IC, or an electrical stimulator may be implanted to treat chronic urinary urge incontinence, nonobstructive urinary retention, and symptoms of urgency and frequency.*[6,10]
- Refer to specific NDs Urinary Incontinence (specify); [acute/chronic] Urinary Retention for additional interventions/treatment regimens.

NURSING PRIORITY NO. 4

To assist in management of long-term urinary alterations:

- Keep bladder deflated by use of an indwelling catheter connected to closed drainage. Investigate alternatives when possible. *Measures such as intermittent catheterization, surgical interventions, urinary drugs, voiding maneuvers, condom catheter may be preferable to the indwelling catheter to provide more effective control and prevent possibility of recurrent infections.*[3,7]
- Provide latex-free catheter and care supplies. *Reduces risk of developing sensitivity to latex, which can develop in individuals requiring frequent catheterization or who have long-term indwelling catheters.*[8]
- Check frequently for bladder distention and observe for overflow. *Requires immediate intervention to reduce risk of infection or autonomic hyperreflexia.*[3]
- Maintain acidic environment of the bladder by the use of agents such as vitamin C, Mandelamine when appropriate. *There is some evidence that the acidic environment discourages bacterial growth by preventing bacteria from adhering to the bladder wall.*[3]
- Adhere to a regular bladder or diversion appliance emptying schedule. *Avoids accidents and prevents embarrassment to the individual.*[4]
- Provide for routine diversion appliance care, and assist client to recognize and deal with problems such as alkaline salt encrustation, ill-fitting appliance, malodorous urine, infection, and so forth. *Provides information and promotes competence in care, increasing self-confidence in dealing with appliance on a regular basis.*[4]

NURSING PRIORITY NO. 5

To promote wellness (Teaching/Discharge Considerations):

- Emphasize importance of keeping perineal area clean and dry. *Reduces risk of infection or skin breakdown.*[3]
- Instruct female clients with urinary tract infection to drink large amounts of fluid, void immediately after intercourse, wipe from front to back, promptly treat vaginal infections, and take showers rather than tub baths as appropriate. *These measures can limit risk of or avoid reinfection.*[5]
- Recommend smoking cessation program as appropriate. *Cigarette smoking can be a source of bladder irritation.*
- Encourage SO(s) who participate in routine care to recognize complications (including latex allergy) necessitating medical follow-up. *Client may be embarrassed to discuss symptoms, and caregivers need to be alert to changes that necessitate evaluation and treatment.*[6]
- Instruct in proper application and care of appliance for urinary diversion. Encourage liberal fluid intake, avoidance of foods and medications that produce strong odor, use of white

vinegar or deodorizer in pouch to promote odor control. *These measures help to ensure patency of device and prevent embarrassing situations for client.*[4]

- Identify sources for supplies, programs or agencies providing financial assistance. *Lack of access to necessities can be a barrier to management of incontinence and having help to obtain needed equipment can assist with daily care.*[6]
- Recommend avoidance of gas-forming foods in presence of ureterosigmoidostomy. *Flatus can cause urinary incontinence.*[2]
- Recommend use of silicone catheter. *These catheters are more comfortable and have fewer problems with infection when permanent or long-term catheterization is required.*[3]
- Demonstrate proper positioning of catheter drainage tubing and bag. *Facilitates drainage and prevents reflux and complications of infection.*[2]
- Refer client/SO(s) to appropriate community resources such as ostomy specialist, support group, sex therapist, psychiatric clinical nurse specialist, and so on. *May be necessary to deal with changes in body image and function.*[6]

DOCUMENTATION FOCUS

Assessment/Reassessment
- Individual findings, including previous and current pattern of voiding, nature of problem, effect on desired lifestyle.
- Cultural factors or concerns.

Planning
- Plan of care and who is involved in planning.
- Teaching plan.

Implementation/Evaluation
- Response to interventions, teaching, and actions performed.
- Attainment or progress toward desired outcome(s).
- Modifications to plan of care.

Discharge Planning
- Long-term needs and who is responsible for actions to be taken.
- Available resources and specific referrals made.
- Individual equipment needs and sources.

References

1. Doenges, M. E., Moorhouse, M. F., Murr, A. C. (2004). ND: Urinary Elimination, impaired. *Nurse's Pocket Guide: Diagnoses, Interventions, and Rationales.* 9th ed. Philadelphia: F. A. Davis.
2. Cox, H. C., et al. (2002). *Clinical Applications of Nursing Diagnosis: Adult, Child, Women's, Psychiatric, Gerontic, and Home Health Considerations.* 4th ed. Philadelphia: F. A. Davis.
3. Doenges, M. E., Moorhouse, M. F., Geissler-Murr, A. C. (2002). ND: Urinary Elimination, impaired. *Nursing Care Plans: Guidelines for Individualizing Patient Care.* 6th ed. Philadelphia: F. A. Davis.
4. Colwell, J. C. (2001). The state of the standard diversion. *J Wound Ostomy Continence Nurs,* 28(1), 6–17.
5. Wyman, J. F. (2003). Treatment of urinary incontinence in men and older women: The evidence shows the efficacy of a variety of techniques. *Am J Nurs,* 103(suppl), 26–35.
6. Newman, D. K., Palmer, M. H. (eds). (2003). The state of the science on urinary incontinence. *Am J Nurs,* 103(suppl), 20.

Cultural Collaborative Community/Home Care Diagnostic Studies Pediatric/Geriatric/Lifespan Medications
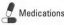

7. Beers, M. H., Berkow, R. (eds). (1999). *The Merck Manual of Diagnosis and Therapy*. 17th ed. Whitehouse Station, NJ: Merck Research Laboratories.

8. Statement on natural latex allergies and SB latex. Retrieved July 2007 from www.regnet.com/sblc/html/body_sbvsnat.html.

9. Gray, M. (2005). Overactive bladder: An overview. *J Wound Ostomy Continence Nurs*, 32(3 suppl), 1–5.

10. Panzera, A. K. (2007). Interstitial cystitis/painful bladder syndrome. *Urol Nurs*, 27(1), 13–19.

11. Bates, B. (2007). Simple questions can help uncover urinary incontinence. (Women's health). *Family Practice News*. Retrieved May 2007 from www.highbeam.com/doc/1G1-160480576 .html.

12. Newman, D. K. (2005). Assessment of the patient with an overactive bladder. *J Wound Ostomy Continence Nurs*, 32(3 suppl), 5–10.

13. Albo, M., Richter, H. E. (2006). Urodynamic testing. Fact sheet for National Kidney and Urologic Diseases Information Clearinghouse. Retrieved August 2007 from http://kidney.niddk .nih.gov/kudiseases/pubs/urodynamic/index.htm.

14. Milne, J. L., Krissovich, M. (2004). Behavioral therapies at the primary care level: The current state of knowledge. *J Wound Ostomy Continence Nurs*, 31(6), 367–376.

readiness for enhanced Urinary Elimination

DEFINITION: A pattern of urinary functions that is sufficient for meeting eliminatory needs and can be strengthened

RELATED FACTORS

To be developed by nurse researchers and submitted to NANDA

DEFINING CHARACTERISTICS

Subjective
Expresses willingness to enhance urinary elimination
Positions self for emptying of bladder

Objective
Urine is straw-colored, odorless
Amount of output or specific gravity is within normal limits
Fluid intake is adequate for daily needs

Sample Clinical Applications: Spinal cord injury (SCI), multple sclerosis (MS), pregnancy, childbirth, pelvic trauma, abdominal surgery, prostate disease

DESIRED OUTCOMES/EVALUATION CRITERIA

Sample **NOC** linkages:
Urinary Continence: Control of the elimination of urine from the bladder
Knowledge: Disease Process: Extent of understanding conveyed about a specific disease process
Urinary Elimination: Collection and drainage of urine

(continues on page 874)

readiness for enhanced Urinary Elimination (continued)

Client Will (Include Specific Time Frame)
• Verbalize understanding of condition that has potential for altering elimination.
• Achieve normal or acceptable elimination pattern, emptying bladder and voiding in appropriate amounts.
• Alter lifestyle or environment to accommodate individual needs.

ACTIONS/INTERVENTIONS

Sample (NIC) linkages:
Urinary Elimination Management: Maintenance of an optimum urinary elimination pattern
Prompted Voiding: Promotion of urinary continence through the use of timed verbal toileting reminders and positive social feedback for successful toileting
Urinary Habit Training: Establishing a predictable pattern of bladder emptying to prevent incontinence for persons with limited cognitive ability who have urge, stress, or functional incontinence

NURSING PRIORITY NO. 1

To assess situation and adaptive skills being used by client:

● Note presence of physical diagnoses (e.g., surgery, childbirth, recent or multiple pregnancies, pelvic trauma, neurogenic bladder from central nervous disorders or neuropathies [stroke, SCI, diabetes], mental or emotional dysfunction, prostate disease or surgery) *that can impact client's elimination patterns.*[1]
● Determine client's usual or previous pattern of elimination and compare with current situation *to determine how pattern can be improved.*[1]
● Observe current voiding pattern and time, color and amount voided, as indicated (e.g., postsurgical client), *to document normalization of elimination.*[1]
● Ascertain methods of self-management (e.g., limiting or increasing liquid intake, acting on urge in timely manner, establishing voiding schedule, regularly spaced catheterization) *to identify strengths and areas of concern in elimination management.*[2]
● Determine client's usual daily fluid intake. *Both amount and beverage choices are important in managing elimination.*[2–4]
● Ascertain motivation and expectations for change. *Motivation to improve and high expectations can encourage client to make changes that will improve his or her life. However, unrealistic expectations may hamper efforts.*

NURSING PRIORITY NO. 2

To assist client to strengthen management of urinary elimination:

● Encourage fluid intake, including water and cranberry juice, *to help maintain renal function, prevent infection.*[1]
● Regulate liquid intake at prescheduled times *to promote predictable voiding pattern.*[2,3]
● Suggest restricting fluid intake 2 to 3 hours before bedtime *to reduce voiding during the night.*[2,4,5]
● Assist with modifying current routines, as appropriate. *Client may benefit from additional information, such as regarding cues and urge to void, adjusting schedule of voiding or*

catheterization (shorter or longer), relaxation or distraction techniques, standing or sitting upright during voiding, to ensure that bladder is completely empty, or practicing pelvic muscle strengthening exercises.[2,4–6]

- Provide assistance or devices as indicated. *Having means of summoning assistance; placement of bedside commode, urinal, or bedpan within client's reach; use of elevated toilet seats or mobility devices enhance client's ability to maintain urinary function.*[5]
- Modify or recommend dietary changes if indicated. *Client may benefit from reduction of caffeine because of its bladder-irritant effect, or weight loss may help reduce overactive bladder symptoms and incontinence by decreasing pressure on the bladder.*[2,4–6]
- Modify medication regimens as appropriate. For example, administer prescribed diuretics in the morning *to lessen nighttime voiding*; reduce or eliminate use of hypnotics, if possible, *as client may be too sedated to recognize or respond to urge to void.*[5]
- Refer to appropriate resources (e.g., medical supply company, ostomy nurse, rehabilitation team) *for assistance, as desired or needed, to promote self-care.*

NURSING PRIORITY NO. 3

To promote optimum wellness:

- Encourage continuation of successful toileting program and identify possible alterations to meet individual needs (e.g., use of adult briefs for extended outing or travel with limited access to toilet). *Promotes proactive problem-solving and supports self-esteem and normalization of social interactions and desired lifestyle activities.*[1]
- Instruct client/SO/caregivers in cues that client needs (e.g., voiding on routine schedule; showing client location of the bathroom; providing adequate room lighting, signs, color coding of door) *to assist client in continued continence, especially when in unfamiliar surroundings.*[3–5]
- Review expectations and prognosis of underlying condition (e.g., MS, prostate disease). *Provides information to assist client/SO to make informed decisions and plan for possible changes.*
- Review with client/SO the signs and symptoms of urinary complications and need for medical follow-up. *Promotes timely intervention to limit or prevent adverse events.*

DOCUMENTATION FOCUS

Assessment/Reassessment
- Findings including previous and current voiding pattern, impact on lifestyle, and adaptive skills being used.
- Motivation and expectation for change.

Planning
- Plan of care and who is involved in planning.
- Teaching plan.

Implementation/Evaluation
- Responses to treatment plan, interventions, and actions performed.
- Attainment or progress toward desired outcome(s).
- Modifications to plan of care.

Discharge Planning
- Available resources, equipment needs and sources.

References

1. Doenges, M. E., Moorhouse, M. F., Murr, A. C. (2004). ND: Urinary Elimination, readiness for enhanced. *Nurse's Pocket Guide: Diagnoses, Interventions and Rationales.* 9th ed. Philadelphia: F. A. Davis.
2. Sampselle, C. M. (2003). Behavioral interventions in young and middle-age women: Simple interventions to combat a complex problem. *Am J Nurs*, 103(suppl), 9–19.
3. Lyons, S. S., Specht, J. K. P. (1999). Prompted voiding for persons with urinary incontinence. University of Iowa Gerontological Nursing Interventions Research Center. Retrieved June 2003 from www.guideline.gov.
4. Wyman, J. F. (1998). Comparative efficacy of behavioral interventions in the management of female urinary incontinence. *Am J Obstet Gynecol*, 179(4), 999–1007.
5. Wyman, J. F. (2003). Treatment of urinary incontinence in men and older women: The evidence shows the efficacy of a variety of techniques. *Am J Nurs*, 103(suppl), 26–35.
6. Burgio, K. L., Stutzman, R. E., Engel, B. T. (1989). Behavioral training for post-prostatectomy urinary incontinence. *J Urol*, 141(2), 303–306.
7. Pringle-Specht, J. K. (2005). Nine myths of incontinence in older adults. *Am J Nurs*, 105(6), 58–68.

functional Urinary Incontinence

DEFINITION: Inability of usually continent person to reach toilet in time to avoid unintentional loss of urine

RELATED FACTORS

Altered environmental factors [e.g., poor lighting or inability to locate bathroom]
Neuromuscular limitations
Weakened supporting pelvic structures
Impaired vision
Psychological factors; impaired cognition; [dementia; reluctance to request assistance or use bedpan]
[Increased urine production]

DEFINING CHARACTERISTICS

Subjective
Senses need to void
[Voiding in large amounts]

Objective
Loss of urine before reaching toilet; amount of time required to reach toilet exceeds length of time between sensing urge and uncontrolled voiding
Able to completely empty bladder
May only be incontinent in early morning

Sample Clinical Applications: Diabetes mellitus, congestive heart failure (CHF) (diuretic use), arthritis, bladder prolapse or cystocele, stroke

functional Urinary Incontinence (continued)
DESIRED OUTCOMES/EVALUATION CRITERIA

Sample **NOC** linkages:
Urinary Elimination: Collection and drainage of urine
Urinary Continence: Control of the elimination of urine from the bladder
Self-Care: Toileting: Ability to toilet self independently with or without assistive device

Client/Caregiver Will (Include Specific Time Frame)
• Verbalize understanding of condition and identify interventions to prevent incontinence.
• Alter environment to accommodate individual needs.
• Report voiding in individually appropriate amounts.
• Void at acceptable times and places.

ACTIONS/INTERVENTIONS

Sample **NIC** linkages:
Prompted Voiding: Promotion of urinary continence through the use of timed verbal toileting reminders and positive social feedback for successful toileting
Urinary Habit Training: Establishing a predictable pattern of bladder emptying to prevent incontinence for persons with limited cognitive ability who have urge, stress, or functional incontinence
Self-Care Assistance: Toileting: Assisting another with elimination

NURSING PRIORITY NO. 1

To assess causative/contributing factors:

● Identify or differentiate client with functional incontinence (e.g., bladder and urethra are functioning normally, but client either cannot get to toilet or has impaired mental function that interferes with recognizing need to urinate and getting to toilet on time) from other types of incontinence.[5]
● Determine if client is voluntarily postponing urination. *Often the demands of the work setting (because of restrictions on bathroom breaks, working alone [e.g., pharmacist, nurse, teacher], demands of the job [heavy workload and unable to find time for a bathroom break]) make it difficult for individuals to go to the bathroom when the need arises, resulting in frequent urinary tract infections and incontinence.*[1]
● Evaluate cognition. *Disease process or medications can affect mental status—orientation to place, recognition of urge to void, or its significance.*[1]
● Note presence and type of functional impairments (e.g., poor eyesight, mobility difficulties, dexterity problems, self-care deficits) *that can hinder ability to get to bathroom.*[6]
● Identify environmental conditions that interfere with timely access to bathroom or successful toileting process. *Unfamiliar surroundings, poor lighting, improperly fitted chair walker, low toilet seat, absence of safety bars, and travel distance to toilet may affect self-care ability.*
● Review medical history for conditions known to increase urine output or alter bladder tone. *For example, diabetes mellitus, prolapsed bladder, MS can affect frequency of urination and ability to hold urine until individual can reach the bathroom.*[1]
● Note use of medications or agents that can increase urine formation. *Diuretics, alcohol, caffeine are several factors that can increase amount and frequency of voiding.*

Nursing Diagnoses in Alphabetical Order

- Test urine for presence of glucose. *Hyperglycemia can cause polyuria and overdistention of the bladder, resulting in problem with continence.*

NURSING PRIORITY NO. 2

To assess degree of interference/disability:

- Determine the frequency and timing of continent and incontinent voids. *Information will be used to plan program to manage incontinence.*[3]
- Initiate voiding diary. Note time of day or night when incontinence occurs as well as timing issues (e.g., difference between the time it takes to get to bathroom, remove clothing, and involuntary loss of urine).
- Measure or estimate amount of urine voided or lost with incontinent episodes *to help determine options for managing problem.*
- Ascertain effect on lifestyle (including socialization and sexuality) and self-esteem. *There is a general belief that incontinence is an inevitable result of aging and that nothing can be done about it. However, those with incontinence problems are often embarrassed, withdraw from social activities and relationships, and hesitate to discuss the problem—even with their healthcare provider.*[1]

NURSING PRIORITY NO. 3

To assist in treating/preventing incontinence:

- Remind client to void when needed and schedule voiding times (e.g., cognitive decline, client who ambulates slowly because of physical limitations) *to reduce incontinence episodes and promote comfort.*[6]
- Administer prescribed diuretics in the morning. *The effect of these medications diminishes by bedtime, thus resulting in less nighttime voidings.*[2]
- Reduce or eliminate use of hypnotics, if possible. *Client may be too sedated to recognize or respond to urge to void.*[4]
- Provide means of summoning assistance. *Ready placement of a call light when hospitalized or a bell in the home setting enables client to obtain toileting help, as needed.*[4]
- Use night-lights to mark bathroom location. *Elderly person may become confused upon arising and be unable to locate bathroom in the dark, and lighting will facilitate access, reducing the possibility of accidents.*[4]
- Provide cues such as adequate room lighting, signs, and color coding of door. *Assists disoriented client to find the bathroom.*[4]
- Remove throw rugs, excess furniture in travel path to bathroom. *Reduces risk of falls, facilitates access to bathroom, and avoids loss of urine.*[4]
- Adapt clothes for quick removal. *Velcro fasteners, full skirts, crotchless panties or no panties, suspenders or elastic waists instead of belts on pants facilitate toileting once urge to void is noted.*[4]
- Raise chair or toilet seat or provide bedside commode, urinal, or bedpan as indicated. *Facilitates toileting when individual has difficulty with movement.*[1]
- Schedule voiding on regular time schedule (e.g., every 3 hours). *Emptying bladder on a regular schedule minimizes pressure, reducing overflow voiding.*[1]
- Restrict fluid intake 2 to 3 hours before bedtime. *Reduces need to waken to void during the night.*[1]
- Include physical or occupational therapist in determining ways to alter environment, appropriate assistive devices. *Useful in meeting individual needs of client.*[1]

NURSING PRIORITY NO. 4

To promote wellness (Teaching/Discharge Considerations):

- Discuss with client/SO need for prompted and scheduled voidings *to manage continence when client is unable to respond immediately to urge to void.*[1]
- Suggest limiting intake of coffee, tea, and alcohol. *Diuretic effect of these substances impacts voiding pattern and can contribute to incontinence.*[1]
- Maintain positive regard when incontinence occurs. *Reduces embarrassment associated with incontinence, need for assistance, use of bedpan.*[1]
- Promote participation in developing long-term plan of care. *Encourages involvement in follow-through of plan, thus increasing possibility of success and confidence in own ability to manage program.*[1]
- Refer to NDs reflex/stress/total/or urge Urinary Incontinence for additional interventions, as appropriate.

DOCUMENTATION FOCUS

Assessment/Reassessment
- Current elimination pattern, assessment findings, and effect on lifestyle and self-esteem.

Planning
- Plan of care and who is involved in planning.
- Teaching plan.

Implementation/Evaluation
- Response to interventions, teaching, and actions performed.
- Attainment or progress toward desired outcome(s).
- Modifications to plan of care.

Discharge Planning
- Long-term needs and who is responsible for actions to be taken.
- Specific referrals made.

References

1. Newman, D. K., Palmer, M. H. (eds). (2003). The state of the science on urinary incontinence. *Am J Nurs*, 103(suppl), 20.
2. Doenges, M. E., Moorhouse, M. F., Geissler-Murr, A. C. (2002). *Nursing Care Plans: Guidelines for Individualizing Patient Care.* 6th ed. Philadelphia: F. A. Davis.
3. Wyman, J. F. (2003). Treatment of urinary incontinence in men and older women: The evidence shows the efficacy of a variety of techniques. *Am J Nurs*, 103(suppl), 26–35.
4. Cox, H. C., et. al. (2002). *Clinical Applications of Nursing Diagnosis: Adult, Child, Women's, Psychiatric, Gerontic, and Home Health Considerations.* 4th ed. Philadelphia: F. A. Davis.
5. American Geriatrics Society Foundation for Health in Aging. (2004). Incontinence. Eldercare at Home, Chapter 10. Retrieved August 2007 from http://healthinaging.org/public_education/eldercare/10.xml.
6. Pringle-Specht, J. K. (2005). Nine myths of incontinence in older adults. *Am J Nurs*, 105(6), 58–68.

overflow Urinary Incontinence

DEFINITION: Involuntary loss of urine associated with overdistention of the bladder

RELATED FACTORS

Bladder outlet obstruction; fecal impaction
Urethral obstruction; severe pelvic prolapse
Detrusor external sphincter dyssynergia; detrusor hypocontractility
Side effects of anticholinergic or decongestant medications; calcium channel blockers

DEFINING CHARACTERISTICS

Subjective
Reports involuntary leakage of small volumes of urine
Nocturia

Objective
Bladder distention
High postvoid residual volume
Observed involuntary leakage of small volumes of urine

Sample Clinical Applications: Uterine prolapse, benign prostatic hypertrophy, diabetes mellitus, multiple sclerosis (MS), spinal cord injury (SCI), pelvic fractures, urinary stones

DESIRED OUTCOMES/EVALUATION CRITERIA

Sample NOC linkages:
Urinary Continence: Control of elimination of urine from the bladder
Urinary Elimination: Collection and drainage of urine
Knowledge: Disease Process: Extent of understanding conveyed about a specific disease process

Client Will (Include Specific Time Frame)
• Verbalize understanding of causative factors and appropriate interventions for individual situation.
• Demonstrate techniques or behaviors to alleviate or prevent overflow incontinence.
• Void in sufficient amounts with no palpable bladder distention; experience no postvoid residuals greater than 50 mL; have no dribbling or overflow.

ACTIONS/INTERVENTIONS

Sample NIC linkages:
Urinary Incontinence Care: Assistance in promoting continence and maintaining perineal skin integrity
Urinary Catheterization: Intermittent: Regular periodic use of a catheter to empty the bladder

NURSING PRIORITY NO. 1

To assess causative/contributing factors:

- Review client's history for (1) bladder outlet obstruction (e.g., prostatic hypertrophy, urethral stricture, urinary stones or tumors); (2) nonfunctioning detrusor muscle (i.e., sensory or motor paralytic bladder due to underlying neurological disease); or (3) atonic bladder that has lost its muscular tone (i.e., chronic overdistention) *to identify potential for or presence of conditions associated with overflow incontinence.*[5]
- Note client's age and gender. *Urinary incontinence due to overflow bladder is more common in older men because of the prevalence of obstructive prostate gland enlargement.*[1,4,5]
- Review medication regimen *for drugs that can cause or exacerbate retention and overflow incontinence (e.g., anticholinergics, calcium channel blockers, psychotropics, anesthesia, opiates, sedatives, alpha- and beta-blockers, antihistamines, neuroleptics).*[2–4,6]

NURSING PRIORITY NO. 2

To determine degree of interference/disability:

- Note client reports of symptoms common to overflow incontinence:[3,4]
  Feeling no need to urinate, while simultaneously losing urine
  Feeling the urge to urinate but not being able to
  Feeling as though the bladder is never completely empty
  Passing a dribbling stream of urine, even after spending a long time at the toilet
  Frequently getting up at night to urinate
- Prepare for or assist with urodynamic testing (e.g., uroflowmetry *to assess urine speed and volume;* cystometrogram *to measure bladder pressure and volume;* bladder scan *to measure retention or postvoid residual, leak point pressure).*[1]

NURSING PRIORITY NO. 3

To assist in treating/preventing overflow incontinence:

- Collaborate in treatment of underlying conditions (e.g., medications or surgery for prostatic hypertrophy; use of medication, such as terazosin, to relax urinary sphincter; altering dose or discontinuing medications contributing to retention). *If the underlying cause of the overflow problem can be treated or eliminated, client may be able to return to normal voiding pattern.*
- Demonstrate and encourage use of gentle massage over bladder (Credé's maneuver). *May facilitate bladder emptying when cause is detrusor weakness.*
- Implement intermittent or continuous catheterization. *Short-term use may be required while acute conditions are treated (e.g., infection, surgery for enlarged prostate); long-term use is required for permanent conditions (e.g., SCI or other neuromuscular conditions resulting in permanent bladder dysfunction).*
- Refer to NDs urge Urinary Incontinence, stress Urinary Incontinence, [acute/chronic] Urinary Retention for additional interventions.

NURSING PRIORITY NO. 4

To promote wellness (Teaching/Discharge Considerations):

- Establish regular schedule for bladder emptying whether voiding or using catheter.
- Stress need for adequate fluid intake, including use of acidifying fruit juices or ingestion of vitamin C *to discourage bacterial growth and stone formation.*

Nursing Diagnoses in Alphabetical Order

• Instruct client/SO(s) in clean intermittent self-catheterization (CISC) techniques *to prevent reflux or increased renal pressures, and to enhance independence.*

 • Review signs/symptoms of complications requiring prompt medical evaluation *to promote timely intervention and prevent complications.*

DOCUMENTATION FOCUS

Assessment/Reassessment
• Current elimination pattern, assessment findings, and effect on lifestyle and sleep.

Planning
• Plan of care and who is involved in planning.
• Teaching plan.

Implementation/Evaluation
• Response to interventions, teaching, and actions performed.
• Attainment or progress toward desired outcome(s).
• Modifications to plan of care.

Discharge Planning
• Long-term needs and who is responsible for actions to be taken.
• Specific referrals made.

References

1. Weiss, B. D. (1998). Diagnostic evaluation of urinary incontinence in geriatric patients. *Am Fam Physician*, 57(11), 2688–2690.
2. National Association for Continence (NAFC). (2005). The four basic types of urinary incontinence. Fact sheet. Retrieved August 2007 from www.nafc.org/about_incontinence/types/htm.
3. Gray, M. (2005). Overactive bladder: An overview. *J Wound Ostomy Continence Nurs*, 32(3 suppl), 1–5.
4. American Geriatrics Society Foundation for Health in Aging. (2004). Incontinence. Eldercare at Home, Chapter 10. Retrieved August 2007 from http://healthinaging.org/public_education/eldercare/10.xml.
5. Urinary incontinence [section 3, chapter 57]. (1995–2007). The Merck Manual of Health & Aging (online). Retrieved August 2007 from www.merck.com/pubs/mmanual_ha/sec3/ch57/ch57a.html.
6. Goode, P. S., Burgio, K. L. (2001). Managing incontinence in the geriatric patient. In Kursh, E. D., Ulchaker, J. C. (eds). *Office Urology: The Clinician's Guide*. Totawa, NJ: Humana Press.

(reflex Urinary Incontinence)

DEFINITION: Involuntary loss of urine at somewhat predictable intervals when a specific bladder volume is reached

RELATED FACTORS

Tissue damage (e.g., due to radiation cystitis, inflammatory bladder conditions, radical pelvic surgery)
Neurological impairment above level of sacral or pontine micturition center

Cultural   Collaborative   Community/Home Care   Diagnostic Studies   Pediatric/Geriatric/Lifespan   Medications

DEFINING CHARACTERISTICS

Subjective

No sensation of bladder fullness, urge to void, or voiding

Sensation of urgency without voluntary inhibition of bladder contraction

Sensations associated with full bladder (e.g., sweating, restlessness, abdominal discomfort)

Objective

Predictable pattern of voiding

Inability to voluntarily inhibit or initiate voiding

Complete emptying with [brain] lesion above pontine micturition center

Incomplete emptying with [spinal cord] lesion above sacral micturition center

Sample Clinical Applications: Spinal cord injury (SCI), multiple sclerosis (MS), bladder or pelvic cancer, Parkinson's disease, dementia

DESIRED OUTCOMES/EVALUATION CRITERIA

Sample (NOC) linkages:

Urinary Continence: Control of the elimination of urine from the bladder

Neurological Status: Autonomic: Ability of the autonomic nervous system to coordinate visceral and hemostatic function

Urinary Elimination: Collection and discharge of urine

Client Will (Include Specific Time Frame)

- Verbalize understanding of condition or contributing factors.
- Establish bladder regimen appropriate for individual situation.
- Demonstrate behaviors or techniques to control condition and prevent complications.
- Void at acceptable times and places.

ACTIONS/INTERVENTIONS

Sample (NIC) linkages:

Urinary Bladder Training: Improving bladder function for those with urge incontinence by increasing the bladder's ability to hold urine and the patient's ability to suppress urination

Urinary Catheterization: Intermittent: Regular periodic use of a catheter to empty the bladder

Urinary Incontinence Care: Assistance in promoting continence and maintaining perineal skin integrity

NURSING PRIORITY NO. 1

To assess degree of interference/disability:

- Identify pathology of problem (e.g., pelvic cancer, central nervous system [CNS] disorder, SCI, stroke, Parkinson's disease, brain tumor) *that results in either hypotonic or spastic neurogenic bladder, thereby affecting bladder storage, emptying, and control.*[1,1-9]

- Note whether client experiences any sense of bladder fullness or awareness of incontinence. *Individuals with reflex incontinence have little to no awareness of need to void. Loss of sensation of bladder filling can result in overfilling, inadequate emptying (retention), and/or constant dribbling.*[2,3,6,9] (Refer to NDs [acute/chronic] Urinary Retention and overflow Urinary Incontinence for additional interventions.)
- Review voiding diary, if available, or record frequency and time of urination. Compare timing of voidings, particularly in relation to liquid intake and medications. *Aids in targeting interventions to meet individual situation.*[4]
- Measure amount of each voiding. *Incontinence often occurs once a specific bladder volume is reached and may indicate need for insertion of a permanent or intermittent catheter.*[5]
- Evaluate for concomitant urinary retention; determine actual bladder volume (via bladder scan) in client with incomplete emptying or on scheduled catheterization *when attempting toilet training and to avoid unnecessary catheterizations.*[10] *Note: Often the bladder is not completely emptied, because there is no voluntary control of the bladder.*[2]
- Measure or scan postvoid residuals, catheterization volumes. *Determines frequency for emptying bladder and reduces incontinence episodes.*[10]
- Evaluate client's ability to manipulate or use urinary collection device or catheter. *Type and degree of neurological impairment (i.e., SCI, MS, dementia) may interfere with client's ability to be self-sufficient.*[3]
- Determine availability and use of resources or assistance.
- Refer to urologist or appropriate specialist for testing. *Urinalysis, ultrasound, radiographs, and urine flowmetry are standard to measure urine flow. A urodynamic evaluation measuring bladder capacity, pressure, and rate of urinary flow may also be indicated.*[6]

NURSING PRIORITY NO. 2

To assist in managing incontinence:

- Collaborate in treatment of underlying cause or management of incontinence. *Degree of impairment, potential for improvement, client's capabilities and availability of assistance, if needed, must be considered in order to develop a comprehensive plan.*
- Involve client/SO/caregiver in creating plan of care *to develop mutually agreed upon goals and ensure individual needs are met, enhancing commitment to plan.*
- Encourage minimum of 1500 to 2000 mL of fluid intake daily. Regulate liquid intake at prescheduled times (with and between meals). *Promotes a predictable voiding pattern to help with treatment regimen.*[6]
- Restrict fluids 2 to 3 hours before bedtime. *Can reduce need to void during the night, preventing incontinence and interruption of sleep.*[6]
- Instruct client to void or take to toilet before the expected time of incontinence *in an attempt to stimulate the reflex for voiding.*[4]
- Instruct in measures such as pouring warm water over perineum, running water in sink, stimulating or massaging tissues over bladder, lower abdomen, thighs. *May stimulate voiding reflexes and voiding, preventing loss of urine at unpredictable times.*[7]
- Set alarm to awaken during night to maintain schedule, or use external catheter or collection device, as appropriate. *Developing a regular time for voiding will empty the bladder, preventing incontinence during the night.*[3,6]
- Implement continuous or intermittent catheterization schedule, if condition indicates, *to prevent bladder overdistention and detrusor muscle damage.*[4,8]

NURSING PRIORITY NO. 3

To promote wellness (Teaching/Discharge Considerations):

● Encourage continuation of regular toileting or bladder program. *May be able to establish a schedule that takes advantage of whatever ability remains, even though the neurological impairment is affecting bladder sensation.*[6]

● Suggest use of incontinence pads/pants during day and with social contact, if appropriate. *Depending on client's activity level, amount of urine loss, manual dexterity, and cognitive ability, these devices provide security and comfort and protect the skin and clothing from urine leakage, reduce odor, and are generally unnoticeable under clothing.*[6]

● Stress importance of perineal care following voiding and frequent changing of incontinence pads, if used. *Maintains cleanliness and prevents skin irritation or breakdown and odor.*[6]

● Encourage limited intake of coffee, tea, and alcohol. *Diuretic effect of these substances may affect predictability of voiding pattern.*[2]

● Instruct in proper care of catheter and cleaning techniques. *Reduces risk of infection.*[3]

● Review signs/symptoms of urinary complications and need for medical follow-up. *Provides immediate attention preventing exacerbation of problem or extension of infection into kidneys.*

DOCUMENTATION FOCUS

Assessment/Reassessment
• Findings including degree of disability and effect on lifestyle.
• Availability of resources or support person.

Planning
• Plan of care and who is involved in planning.
• Teaching plan.

Implementation/Evaluation
• Responses to treatment plan, interventions, and actions performed.
• Attainment or progress toward desired outcome(s).
• Modifications to plan of care.

Discharge Planning
• Long-term needs and who is responsible for actions to be taken.
• Available resources, equipment needs and sources.

References

1. Doenges, M. E., Moorhouse, M. F., Murr, A. C. (2004). ND: Urinary Incontinence, reflex. *Nurse's Pocket Guide: Diagnoses, Interventions, and Rationales.* 9th ed. Philadelphia: F. A. Davis.
2. Incontinence/overactive bladder. (Updated 2006). Retrieved August 2007 from www.webmd.com/urinary-incontinence-oab/womens-guide/Urinary-Incontinence-in-Women-Topic-Overview.
3. Doenges, M. E., Moorhouse, M. F., Geissler-Murr, A. C. (2002). *Nursing Care Plans: Guidelines for Individualizing Patient Care.* 6th ed. Philadelphia: F. A. Davis.
4. Newman, D. K., Palmer, M. H. (eds). (2003). The state of the science on urinary incontinence. *Am J Nurs,* 103(suppl), 20.
5. Cox, H. C., et al. (2002). *Clinical Applications of Nursing Diagnosis: Adult, Child, Women's, Psychiatric, Gerontic, and Home Health Considerations.* 4th ed. Philadelphia: F. A. Davis.

6. Urinary incontinence. Penn State Health and Disease Information: A–Z Topics. Retrieved August 2007 from www.hmc.psu.edu/healthinfo/uz/urinaryincontinence.htm.
7. Beers, M. H., Berkow, R. (eds). (1999). *The Merck Manual of Diagnosis and Therapy*. 17th ed. Whitehouse Station, NJ: Merck Research Laboratories.
8. Gray, M. (2005). Assessment and management of urinary incontinence. *Nurse Pract*, 30(7), 32–43.
9. Rackley, R., Vasavada, S. P. (2006). Incontinence, urinary: Nonsurgical therapies. Retrieved April 2007 from www.emedicine.com/med/topic3085.htm.
10. Newman, D. K. (2006). Using the BladderScan™ for bladder volume assessment. Retrieved May 2007 from www.seekwellness.com/incontinence/using_the_bladderscan.htm.

risk for urge Urinary Incontinence

DEFINITION: At risk for an involuntary loss of urine associated with a sudden, strong sensation or urinary urgency

RISK FACTORS

Effects of medications, caffeine, or alcohol
Detrusor hyperreflexia (e.g., from cystitis, urethritis, tumors, renal calculi, central nervous system [CNS] disorders above pontine micturition center)
Impaired bladder contractility; involuntary sphincter relaxation
Ineffective toileting habits
Small bladder capacity

NOTE: A risk diagnosis is not evidenced by signs and symptoms, as the problem has not occurred; rather, nursing interventions are directed at prevention.
Sample Clinical Applications: Multiple sclerosis (MS), benign prostatic hypertrophy (BPH), recurrent urinary tract infections (UTIs), renal calculi, pelvic surgery or radiation, Guillain-Barré syndrome, dementia, major depression

DESIRED OUTCOMES/EVALUATION CRITERIA

Sample **NOC** linkages:
Urinary Continence: Control of elimination of urine from the bladder
Risk Control: Personal actions to prevent, eliminate, or reduce modifiable health threats
Neurological Status: Autonomic: Ability of the autonomic nervous system to coordinate visceral and hemostatic function

Client Will (Include Specific Time Frame)
• Identify individual risk factors and appropriate interventions.
• Demonstrate behaviors or lifestyle changes to prevent development of problem.

ACTIONS/INTERVENTIONS

Sample **NIC** linkages:
Urinary Habit Training: Establishing a predictable pattern of bladder emptying to prevent incontinence for persons with limited cognitive ability who have urge, stress, or functional incontinence

Self-Care Assistance: Toileting: Assisting another with elimination
Prompted Voiding: Promotion of urinary continence through the use of timed verbal toileting reminders and positive social feedback for successful toileting

NURSING PRIORITY NO. 1

To assess potential for developing incontinence:

- Note presence of diagnoses often associated with urgent voiding. *Such conditions as stroke, brain injury, MS, Parkinson's disease, spinal cord injury (SCI); delirium or dementias; pelvic inflammatory disease, abdominal or pelvic surgery; obesity, abdominal distention; acute bladder infection, kidney stones can affect bladder capacity, pelvic, bladder, or urethral musculature tone, and/or innervation.*[1-3,10]
- Note factors that may affect ability to respond to urge to void. *Impaired mobility due to aging, chronic conditions, sedation, acute injuries, lack of access to toilet, impaired awareness (either cognition or sensation), or use of restraints can all affect client's ability to respond in a timely manner.*[2,4,10]
- Determine use or presence of bladder irritants. *A significant intake of alcohol or caffeine can result in increased output or concentrated urine and contribute to the possibility of incontinence.*[5]
- Review client's medications and other drugs for affect bladder function, such as beta-blockers and cholinergic drugs *(can increase detrusor tone)*; neuroleptics, antidepressants, sedatives, opiates *(can cause detrusor relaxation)*; muscle relaxants and psychoactive drugs *(can cause sphincter relaxation)*; diuretics *(can increase urine production)*.[12]
- Measure amount of urine voided, especially noting amounts less than 100 mL or greater than 550 mL. *Provides information about amount of urine required to initiate desire to void, as well as potential for dehydration or excessive fluid loss if large voidings are frequent.*[6]
- Prepare for and assist with appropriate testing (e.g., urinalysis, noninvasive bladder scanning, urine culture, urine and serum glucose, voiding cystometrogram). *Accurate assessment and diagnosis can determine voiding pattern and identify pathology that may lead to the development of incontinence.*[2,4,13]

NURSING PRIORITY NO. 2

To prevent occurrence of problem:

- Assist in treatment of underlying conditions that may contribute to urge incontinence.
- Record intake and frequency and degree of urgency of voiding. *May reveal developing incontinence problem when need to void is more frequent and urgent in relation to normal fluid intake.*[7]
- Ascertain client's awareness and concerns about developing problem and whether lifestyle is affected (e.g., daily activities, socialization, sexual patterns). *Provides information regarding the degree of concern client is experiencing and need for preventive measures to be instituted.*[8]
- Regulate liquid intake at prescheduled times (with and between meals). *Promotes a predictable voiding pattern to establish a bladder-training program to prevent incontinence.*[5]
- Establish schedule for voiding (habit training) based on client's usual voiding pattern. *Can successfully reduce risk for incontinence.*[8]
- Provide assistance or devices, as indicated, for clients who are mobility impaired. *Providing means of summoning assistance and placing bedside commode, urinal, or bedpan within client's reach can promote sense of control in self-managing voiding.*[9]

Nursing Diagnoses in Alphabetical Order

🏠 • Encourage regular pelvic floor strengthening exercises (Kegel exercises or use of vaginal cones). *Can improve pelvic musculature tone and strength, preventing progression of incontinence problem.*[5]

NURSING PRIORITY NO. 3

❋ To promote wellness (Teaching/Discharge Considerations):

🏠 • Provide information to client/SO about potential for urge incontinence and lifestyle measures to prevent development of incontinence, as individually indicated.

🏠 • Recommend limiting intake of coffee, tea and alcohol. *These substances have an irritating effect on the bladder and may contribute to incontinence.*[7]

🏠 • Suggest wearing loose-fitting or especially adapted clothing. *Facilitates response to voiding urge, especially in elderly or infirm individuals, enabling them to reach the toilet without loss of urine.*[10]

🏠 • Emphasize importance of perineal care after each voiding. *Reduces risk of ascending infection.*[11]

DOCUMENTATION FOCUS

Assessment/Reassessment
• Individual findings, including specific risk factors and pattern of voiding.

Planning
• Plan of care, specific interventions, and who is involved in planning.
• Teaching plan.

Implementation/Evaluation
• Response to interventions, teaching, and actions performed.
• Attainment or progress toward desired outcome(s).
• Modifications to plan of care.

Discharge Planning
• Discharge needs and who is responsible for actions to be taken.
• Specific referrals made.

References

1. Guerrero, P., Sinert, R. (2002). Urinary incontinence. Retrieved August 2007 from www.emedicine.com/emerg/topic791.htm.
2. Booth, C. (2002). Introduction to urinary incontinence. *Hosp Pharmacist*, 9(3), 65–68.
3. Association of Women's Health, Obstetric and Neonatal Nurses (AWHONN). (2000). Evidence-based clinical practice guideline—Continence for women. Retrieved January 2004 from www.guideline.gov.
4. American Medical Directors Association (AMDA). (1996). Urinary incontinence. Retrieved September 2003 from www.guideline.gov.
5. Newman, D. K., Palmer, M. H. (eds). (2003). The state of the science on urinary incontinence. *Am J Nurs*, 103(Suppl), 20.
6. Doenges, M. E., Moorhouse, M. F., Geissler-Murr, A. C. (2004). *Nurse's Pocket Guide: Diagnoses, Interventions, and Rationales*. 9th ed. Philadelphia: F. A. Davis.
7. What is urinary incontinence? Retrieved September 2003 from http://ourworld.compuserve.com/homepages/nacs/INCONT.HTM.
8. Ford-Martin, P. A. (1999). Urinary incontinence. *Gale Encyclopedia of Medicine*. Retrieved August 2007 from http://findarticles.com/p/articles/mi_g2601/is_0014/ai_2601001430/pg_3.

9. Cox, H. C., et al. (2002). ND: Urinary Incontinence. *Clinical Applications of Nursing Diagnosis: Adult, Child, Women's, Psychiatric, Gerontic, and Home Health Considerations.* 4th ed. Philadelphia: F. A. Davis.
10. Wyman, J. F. (2003). Treatment of urinary incontinence in men and older women: The evidence shows the efficacy of a variety of techniques. *Am J Nurs*, 103(suppl), 26–35.
11. Doenges, M. E., Moorhouse, M. F., Geissler-Murr, A. C. (2002). *Nursing Care Plans: Guidelines for Individualizing Patient Care.* 6th ed. Philadelphia: F. A. Davis.
12. Kidney and urinary tract disorders: Urinary incontinence. (2003). The Merck Manuals Online Medical Library. Retrieved August 2007 from www.merck.com/mmhe/sec11/ch147/ch147a.html.
13. Newman, D. K. (2006). Using the BladderScan™ for bladder volume assessment. Retrieved May 2007 from www.seekwellness.com/incontinence/using_the_bladderscan.htm.

stress Urinary Incontinence

DEFINITION: Sudden leakage of urine with activities that increase intra-abdominal pressure

RELATED FACTORS

Degenerative changes in pelvic muscles; weak pelvic muscles
High intra-abdominal pressure [e.g., obesity, gravid uterus]
Intrinsic urethral sphincter deficiency

DEFINING CHARACTERISTICS

Subjective
Reported involuntary leakage of small amounts of urine on exertion [e.g., lifting, impact aerobics]; with sneezing, laughing, or coughing; in the absence of detrusor contraction or an overdistended bladder

Objective
Observed involuntary leakage of small amounts of urine on exertion [e.g., lifting, impact aerobics]; with sneezing, laughing, or coughing; in the absence of detrusor contraction or an overdistended bladder

DESIRED OUTCOMES/EVALUATION CRITERIA

Sample NOC linkages:
Urinary Continence: Control of elimination of urine from the bladder
Symptom Control: Personal actions to minimize perceived adverse changes in physical and emotional functioning

Client Will (Include Specific Time Frame)
- Verbalize understanding of condition and interventions for bladder conditioning.
- Demonstrate behaviors or techniques to strengthen pelvic floor musculature.
- Remain continent even with increased intra-abdominal pressure.

(continues on page 890)

stress Urinary Incontinence (continued)
ACTIONS/INTERVENTIONS

Sample (NIC) linkages:
Pelvic Muscle Exercise: Strengthening and training the levator ani and urogenital muscles through voluntary repetitive contraction to decrease stress, urge, or mixed types of urinary incontinence
Urinary Incontinence Care: Assistance in promoting continence and maintaining perineal skin integrity
Urinary Habit Training: Establishing a predictable pattern of bladder emptying to prevent incontinence for persons with limited cognitive ability who have urge, stress, or functional incontinence

NURSING PRIORITY NO. 1

To assess causative/contributing factors:

- Identify physiological causes of increased intra-abdominal pressure (e.g., obesity, gravid uterus; repeated heavy lifting [occupational risk]); contributing history, such as multiple births, bladder or pelvic trauma/fractures; surgery (e.g., radical prostatectomy, bladder or other pelvic surgeries that may damage sphincter muscles); and participation in high-impact athletic or military field activities (particularly women). *Identification of specifics of individual situation provides for developing an accurate plan of care.*[1,4,10,15]

- Assess for urine loss (usually in small amounts) with coughing, sneezing, or sports activities; relaxed pelvic musculature and support, noting inability to start and stop stream while voiding, bulging of perineum when bearing down. *Severity of symptoms may indicate need for more specialized evaluation.*

- Review client's medications for those that may cause or exacerbate stress incontinence (e.g., alpha-blockers, angiotensin-converting enzyme [ACE] inhibitors, loop diuretics).[16]

- Assess for mixed incontinence (consisting of two or more kinds of incontinence), noting whether bladder irritability, reduced bladder capacity, or voluntary overdistention is present. *Concomitant urge or reflex incontinence often occurs with stress incontinence and impacts treatment choices.*[6] (Refer to NDs Urinary Incontinence [specify urge, reflex], [acute/chronic], Urinary Retention.)

NURSING PRIORITY NO. 2

To assess degree of interference/disability:

- Observe voiding patterns, time and amount voided, and note the stimulus provoking incontinence. Review voiding diary if available. *Provides information that can help determine type of incontinence and type of treatment indicated.*[6]

- Prepare for and assist with testing or refer to urology specialist as indicated. *Diagnosing urinary incontinence often requires comprehensive evaluation (e.g., measuring bladder filling and capacity, leak-point pressure, rate of urinary flow, pelvic ultrasound, cystogram/other scans) to differentiate stress incontinence from other types.*[2–4,7,17]

- Determine effect on lifestyle (including daily activities, participation in sports or exercise and recreation, socialization, sexuality) and self-esteem. *Untreated incontinence can have emotional and physical consequences. Client may limit or abstain from sports or recreational activities. Urinary tract infections, skin rashes, and sores can occur. Self-esteem is affected and the client may suffer from depression and withdraw from social functions.*[6,15]

Cultural   Collaborative   Community/Home Care   Diagnostic Studies   Pediatric/Geriatric/Lifespan   Medications

- Ascertain methods of self-management. *Client may already be limiting liquid intake, voiding before any activity, or using undergarment protection.*[6]
- Perform bladder scan to determine postvoid residuals as indicated. *Presence of volumes greater than 100 mL (or 150 mL in elder clients) suggests incomplete emptying of bladder, requiring further evaluation.*[17]

NURSING PRIORITY NO. 3

To assist in treating/preventing incontinence:

- Suggest/implement self-help techniques:
  Practice timed voidings (e.g., every 3 hours during the day) *to keep bladder relatively empty.*
  Delay voiding to 3- to 4-hour intervals between voids. *May improve bladder capacity and retention time, and acceptable time between bathroom breaks.*[6]
  Restrict fluid intake 2 to 3 hours before bedtime. *Decreasing the amount of evening fluid intake reduces the need for awakening to void, resulting in more restful sleep.*[5]
  Limit use of coffee, tea and alcohol. *Diuretic effect of these substances may lead to bladder distention, increasing likelihood of incontinence.*[12]
  Encourage weight loss as indicated *to reduce pressure on intra-abdominal and pelvic organs.*[7]
  Void before physical exertion such as exercise or sports activities *to reduce potential for incontinence.*[18]
  Encourage regular pelvic floor strengthening exercises (Kegel exercises). *These exercises involve tightening the muscles of the pelvic floor and need to be done numerous times throughout the day.*[6,10]
  Avoid or limit heavy lifting and high-impact aerobics or sports *to decrease incontinence associated with elevated intra-abdominal pressures.*[12]
  Incorporate "bent-knee sit-ups" into exercise program. *Increasing abdominal muscle tone can help relieve stress incontinence.*[11]
- Assist with medical treatment of underlying urological condition, as indicated. *Stress incontinence may be treated with surgical intervention (e.g., bladder neck suspension, pubovaginal sling to reposition bladder and strengthen pelvic musculature; or prostate surgery) and nonsurgical therapies (e.g., use of pessary, vaginal cones; electrical stimulation; biofeedback).*[8,9,18–20]
- Administer medications, as indicated, such as sympathomimetics (propantheline or Pro-Banthine); antispasmodics (oxybutynin or Ditropan). *May improve bladder tone and increase effectiveness of bladder sphincter and proximal urethra contractions.*[6,9,14]

NURSING PRIORITY NO. 4

To promote wellness (Teaching/Discharge Considerations):

- Suggest use of incontinence pads or pants as needed. *Considering client's activity level, amount of urine loss, physical size, manual dexterity, and cognitive ability to determine specific product choices best suited to individual situation and needs may be necessary when leakage continues to occur in spite of other measures.*[9,13]
- Emphasize importance of perineal care following voiding and frequent changing of incontinence pads. Recommend application of oil-based emollient. *Prevents infection and protects skin from irritation.*[13]
- Discuss participation in incontinence management for activities such as heavy lifting, strenuous sports activities that increase intra-abdominal pressure. *Substituting swimming,*

Nursing Diagnoses in Alphabetical Order

bicycling, or low-impact exercise if possible may help reduce frequency of incontinence and maintain active life.

 • Recommend or refer for behavioral training, as indicated. *Research indicates that combining pelvic floor muscle exercises with biofeedback is more effective than simple verbal or written instructions.*[21]

DOCUMENTATION FOCUS

Assessment/Reassessment
- Findings including pattern of incontinence and physical factors present.
- Effect on lifestyle and self-esteem.
- Client understanding of condition.

Planning
- Plan of care and who is involved in the planning.
- Teaching plan.

Implementation/Evaluation
- Responses to interventions, teaching, actions performed, and changes that are identified.
- Attainment or progress toward desired outcome(s).
- Modifications to plan of care.

Discharge Planning
- Long-term needs, referrals, and who is responsible for specific actions.
- Specific referrals made.

References

1. Doenges, M. E., Moorhouse, M. F., Geissler-Murr, A. C. (2004). *Nurse's Pocket Guide: Diagnoses, Interventions, and Rationales.* 9th ed. Philadelphia: F. A. Davis.
2. Urinary incontinence. Penn State Health & Disease Information. Retrieved July 2007 from www.hmc.psu.edu/healthinfo/uz/urinaryincontinence.htm.
3. Urinary incontinence. (1996). *American Medical Directors Association (AMDA).* Retrieved September 2003 from www.guideline.gov.
4. Guerrero, P., Sinert, R. (2002, update 2006). Urinary incontinence. Retrieved August 2007 from www.emedicine.com/emerg/topic791.htm.
5. Doenges, M. E., Moorhouse, M. F., Geissler-Murr, A. C. (2002). *Nursing Care Plans: Guidelines for Individualizing Patient Care.* 6th ed. Philadelphia: F. A. Davis.
6. Ford-Martin, P. A. (1999, update 2002). Urinary catheterization. *Gale Encyclopedia of Medicine.* Gale Research. Retrieved August 2007 from www.lifesteps.com/gm/Atoz/ency/urinary_catheterization.jsp.
7. Beers, M. H., Berkow, R. (eds). (1999). *The Merck Manual of Diagnosis and Therapy.* 17th ed. Whitehouse Station, NJ: Merck Research Laboratories.
8. Choe, J. M. (2003). Incontinence, urinary: Surgical therapies. Retrieved July 2007 from www.emedicine.com/emerg/topic3084.htm.
9. Choe, J. M. (2002). Incontinence, urinary: Nonsurgical therapies. Retrieved July 2007 from www.emedicine.com/emerg/topic3085.htm.
10. Wyman, J. F. (2003). Treatment of urinary incontinence in men and older women: The evidence shows the efficacy of a variety of techniques. *Am J Nurs*, 103(suppl), 26–35.
11. Cox, H. C., et al. (2002). ND: Urinary Incontinence, stress. *Clinical Applications of Nursing Diagnosis: Adult, Child, Women's, Psychiatric, Gerontic, and Home Health Considerations.* 4th ed. Philadelphia: F. A. Davis.

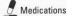

12. Newman, D. K., Palmer, M. H. (eds). (2003). The state of the science on urinary incontinence. *Am J Nurs*, 103(suppl), 20.
13. What is urinary incontinence? Retrieved September 2003 from http://ourworld.compuserve.com/homepages/nacs/INCONT.HTM.
14. Booth, C. (2002). Introduction to urinary incontinence. *Hosp Pharmacist*, 9(3), 65–68.
15. Carls, C. (2007). The prevalence of stress urinary incontinence in high school and college-age female athletes in the Midwest: Implications for education and prevention. *Urol Nurs*, 27(1), 21–24, 39.
16. Resnick, N. M. (2003). Urinary incontinence. In Cassel, C. K., et al. (eds). *Geriatric Medicine: An Evidence-Based Approach*. New York: Springer.
17. Newman, D. K. (2006). Using the BladderScan™ for bladder volume assessment. Retrieved May 2007 from www.seekwellness.com/incontinence/using_the_bladderscan.htm.
18. Bray, B., Van Sell, S. L., Miller-Anderson, M. (2007). Stress incontinence: It's no laughing matter. *RN*, 70(4), 25–29.
19. Rackley, R., Vasavada, S. P. (2006). Incontinence, urinary: Nonsurgical therapies. Retrieved May 2007 from www.emedicine.com/med/topic3085.htm.
20. National Kidney and Urologic Diseases Information Clearing House (NKUDIC). (2003). Treatments for urinary incontinence in women. Retrieved August 2007 from http://kidney.niddk.nih.gov/kudiseases/pubs/treatmentsuiwomen/index.htm.
21. Bump, R. C., Hurt, W. G., Fantl, J. A. (1991). Assessment of Kegel pelvic muscle exercise performance after brief verbal instruction. *Am J Obstet Gynecol*, 165, 322–327.

total Urinary Incontinence [retired from Taxonomy 2009]

DEFINITION: Continuous and unpredictable loss of urine

RELATED FACTORS

Neuropathy preventing transmission of reflex [signals to the reflex arc] indicating bladder fullness
Neurological dysfunction [e.g., cerebral lesions]
Independent contraction of detrusor reflex
Trauma or disease affecting spinal cord nerves [destruction of sensory or motor neurons below the injury level]
Anatomic (fistula)

DEFINING CHARACTERISTICS

Subjective
Constant flow of urine at unpredictable times without uninhibited bladder contractions/spasm or distention
Nocturia
Lack of bladder or perineal filling [awareness]
Unawareness of incontinence

(continues on page 894)

total Urinary Incontinence [retired from Taxonomy 2009] (continued)

Objective
Unsuccessful incontinence refractory treatments

Sample Clinical Applications: Spinal cord injury (SCI) or nerve compression, spina bifida, myelomeningocele, Guillain-Barré syndrome, brain injury, stroke, hydrocephalus, multiple sclerosis (MS), cerebral palsy, Parkinson's disease, diabetes mellitus, abdominal trauma, dementia

DESIRED OUTCOMES/EVALUATION CRITERIA

Sample NOC linkages:
Urinary Continence: Control of elimination of urine from the bladder
Self-Care: Toileting: Ability to toilet self independently with or without assistive device
Tissue Integrity: Skin & Mucous Membranes: Structural intactness and normal physiological function of skin and mucous membranes

Client/Caregiver Will (Include Specific Time Frame)
• Verbalize awareness of causative or contributing factors.
• Establish bladder regimen for individual situation.
• Demonstrate behaviors, techniques to manage condition and to prevent complications.
• Manage incontinence so that social functioning is regained or maintained.

ACTIONS/INTERVENTIONS

Sample NIC linkages:
Urinary Incontinence Care: Assistance in promoting continence and maintaining perineal skin integrity
Urinary Catheterization: Insertion of a catheter into the bladder for temporary or permanent drainage of urine
Perineal Care: Maintenance of perineal skin integrity and relief of perineal discomfort

NURSING PRIORITY NO. 1

To assess causative/contributing factors:

• Identify client with condition(s) causing actual/potential for total incontinence as listed in Related Factors. *High-risk persons include frail elderly, women, presence of brain lesions or disease (e.g., stroke, cancer, Parkinson's disease, cerebral palsy, hydrocephalus, dementia); SCI (e.g., quadriplegia, paraplegia, herniated disk, pelvic crush injury); chronic neurological diseases (e.g., MS, child with myelomeningocele); pregnancy, prolonged labor, early postpartum period; genitourinary surgery or trauma (e.g., radical hysterectomy, abdominoperineal resection); peripheral neuropathy (e.g., diabetes mellitus, AIDS, poliomyelitis, Guillain-Barré syndrome); and lifestyle issues (e.g., certain medications, irritating foods, fluid intake, mobility limitations).*[1,2]
• Note effect of global neurological impairment, neuromuscular trauma after surgery, radiation therapy, or childbirth; or presence of fistula. *Injury to the nerves supplying the bladder can result in constant loss of urine because of loss of integrity of lower urinary tract function. Presence of vesicovaginal fistula may also cause incontinence.*[3]
• Determine if client is aware of incontinence. *Cognitive, developmental issues, or medical conditions can impair client's awareness and sensory perception of voiding need, process, and incontinence.*[3]

- Check for perineal sensation and fecal impaction *to determine whether sensation and reflexes are impaired when neurological condition is present.*[1,4]
- Determine concomitant chronic retention (e.g., palpate bladder, scan or catheterize for urine volume and residual). *Rather than relaxing when the bladder contracts, the outlet contracts, leading to severe outlet obstruction and urine retention.*[3]
- Observe for overflow incontinence *due to chronic urinary retention or secondary to flaccid bladder associated with obstructive or neuropathic lesion.*[1,2] Refer to ND overflow Incontinence for related interventions.
- Assist with diagnostic procedures and tests (e.g., postvoid residual, urine flowmetry, pressure studies, cystoscopy, filling and voiding cystogram) *to establish diagnosis and identify needed interventions.*[1,5]

NURSING PRIORITY NO. 2

To assess degree of interference/disability:

- Have client/caregivers keep an incontinence chart. Note times of voiding and incontinence. *Determines pattern of urination and whether there is any control.*[1,4]
- Determine client's particular symptoms (e.g., continuous dribbling superimposed upon an otherwise normal voiding pattern, or high-volume urine loss that replaces any detectable pattern of bladder filling, storage, and voiding). *Influences choice of interventions.*[11]
- Review past interventions *to ascertain cause for continence failure (e.g., client unable to sustain behavioral management of bladder training program, medical conditions do not allow for success in voiding efforts).*
- Ascertain effect of condition on lifestyle and self-esteem. *Incontinence is embarrassing and distressing and may severely affect the quality of life for the individual and even the family members.*[6]
- Inspect skin for areas of erythema or excoriation. *Constant loss of urine can abrade the skin, causing breakdown if not cared for frequently.*[5]

NURSING PRIORITY NO. 3

To assist in preventing/managing incontinence:

- Collaborate in treatment of underlying conditions (e.g., neurological disorders, prostate problems, chronic urinary tract infections [UTIs], psychiatric disorders) *that contribute to incontinence.*
- Implement bladder training and/or incontinence management, as indicated:
  Provide ready access to bathroom, commode, bedpan, or urinal.
  Encourage adequate fluid and regulate time of intake *to ensure sufficient fluid intake and to prevent dehydration and promote a predictable voiding pattern where possible.*[4]
  Establish voiding or bladder emptying schedule by toileting at same time as recorded voidings and 30 minutes earlier than recorded time of incontinence. *Bladder training may be an effective strategy when neurological impairment is not extensive.*[6]
  Use condom catheter or other external collecting device during daytime and absorptive pads during the night if external device is not tolerated. *Maintains dry clothing and bedding, preventing skin irritation, odor with resultant embarrassment.*[4]
- Implement and instruct client/SO in techniques of clean intermittent self-catheterization (CISC) using small-lumen straight catheter (or Mitrofanoff continent urinary channel *for clients not able to catheterize themselves*) as indicated. *In the presence of neurological damage and when client is cognitively competent, these measures can assure a successful management program.*[8,9]

- Implement continuous urine collection (e.g., indwelling urethral or suprapubic catheter) when dictated by client's conditions (*e.g., severely impaired individual in whom other interventions [e.g., bladder training, self-catheterization] are not an option; or person lives alone and cannot provide own supportive care*).[2]
- Prepare for surgical intervention, when indicated. *Many forms of surgical repair have been developed, depending on underlying cause (e.g., to treat urethral hypermobility, to suspend the bladder, to repair vaginal walls, remove obstructions; provide artificial sphincter or bladder reservoir*).[7,10]
- Refer to ND functional/stress/reflex Urinary Incontinence for additional interventions specific to diagnosis.

NURSING PRIORITY NO. 4

To promote wellness (Teaching/Discharge Considerations):

- Assist client to identify regular period of time for bladder program *that meets individual physical and psychosocial needs*.[6,12]
- Suggest use of incontinence pads or adult briefs, as indicated (e.g., during social contacts and work hours). *Provides protection and enhances confidence when other measures have not been successful*.[7,12]
- Emphasize importance of pericare after voiding (using alcohol-free products) and application of oil-based emollient. *Protects the skin from irritation from the constant flow of urine*.[5]
- Instruct in proper care of catheter and clean technique. *Reduces risk of infection when client is using catheterization on a regular basis*.[6]
- Recommend use of silicone catheter. *When long-term or continuous placement is indicated after other measures and bladder training have failed, use of a silicone catheter has fewer problems with deterioration and infection than latex products*.[5]
- Encourage self-monitoring of catheter patency and avoidance of reflux of urine. *Reduces risk of infection*.[5]
- Suggest intake of acidifying juices, such as cranberry. *Discourages bacterial growth and adherence to bladder wall, preventing recurrent infections*.[5]

DOCUMENTATION FOCUS

Assessment/Reassessment
- Current elimination pattern.
- Assessment findings, including effect on lifestyle and self-esteem.

Planning
- Plan of care, specific interventions, and who is involved in planning.
- Teaching plan.

Implementation/Evaluation
- Response to interventions, teaching, and actions performed.
- Attainment or progress toward desired outcome(s).
- Modifications to plan of care.

Discharge Planning
- Discharge plan, long-term needs, and who is responsible for actions to be taken.
- Specific referrals made.

References

1. Guerrero, P., Sinert, R. (2002). Urinary incontinence. Retrieved August 2007 from www.emedicine.com/emerg/topic791.htm.
2. Choe, J. M., Mardovin, W. Neurogenic bladder. Retrieved September 2003 from www.emedicine.com.
3. Beers, M. H., Berkow, R. (eds). (1999). *The Merck Manual of Diagnosis and Therapy.* 17th ed. Whitehouse Station, NJ: Merck Research Laboratories.
4. Cox, H. C., et al. (2002). ND: Urinary incontinence. *Clinical Applications of Nursing Diagnosis: Adult, Child, Women's, Psychiatric, Gerontic, and Home Health Considerations.* 4th ed. Philadelphia: F. A. Davis.
5. Doenges, M. E., Moorhouse, M. F., Geissler-Murr, A. C. (2002). *Nursing Care Plans: Guidelines for Individualizing Patient Care.* 6th ed. Philadelphia: F. A. Davis.
6. Newman, D. K., Palmer, M. H. (eds). (2003). The state of the science on urinary incontinence. *Am J Nurs,* 103(suppl), 20.
7. Booth, C. (2002). Introduction to urinary incontinence. *Hosp Pharmacist,* 9(3), 65–68.
8. Understanding female urinary incontinence. (Update 2005). Family Doctor Series, pamphlet. Retrieved July 2007 from www.patient.co.uk/showdoc/23068768/.
9. Choe, J. M. (2003). Incontinence, urinary: Surgical therapies. Retrieved July 2007 from www.emedicine.com/emerg/topic3084.htm.
10. Choe, J. M. (2002). Incontinence, urinary: Nonsurgical therapies. Retrieved July 2007 from www.emedicine.com/emerg/topic3085.htm.
11. Gray, M. (2004). Stress urinary incontinence in women. *J Am Acad Nurse Pract,* 16(5), 188–190, 192–199.
12. Santos, A., Hunt, M. (2005). Managing incontinence: Once a cause of isolation and embarrassment, incontinence does not have to limit quality of life. *Paraplegia News,* 59(11).

urge Urinary Incontinence

DEFINITION: Involuntary passage of urine occurring soon after a strong sense of urgency to void

RELATED FACTORS

Decreased bladder capacity
Bladder infection; atrophic urethritis or vaginitis
Alcohol or caffeine intake; [increased fluids]
Use of diuretics
Fecal impaction
Detrusor hyperactivity with impaired bladder contractility

DEFINING CHARACTERISTICS

Subjective
Reports urinary urgency; involuntary loss of urine with bladder contractions or spasms; inability to reach toilet in time to avoid urine loss

Objective
Observed inability to reach toilet in time to avoid urine loss

(continues on page 898)

urge Urinary Incontinence (continued)
Sample Clinical Applications: Abdominal trauma/surgery, pelvic inflammatory disease (PID), recurrent urinary tract infections (UTIs), brain injury, stroke, multiple sclerosis (MS), Parkinson's disease, diabetes mellitus, dementia

DESIRED OUTCOMES/EVALUATION CRITERIA

Sample NOC linkages:
Urinary Continence: Control of elimination of urine from the bladder
Cognition: Ability to execute complex mental processes
Self-Care: Toileting: Ability to toilet self independently with or without assistive device

Client Will (Include Specific Time Frame)
• Verbalize understanding of condition.
• Demonstrate behaviors or techniques to control or correct situation.
• Report increase in interval between urge and involuntary loss of urine.
• Void every 3 to 4 hours in individually appropriate amounts.

ACTIONS/INTERVENTIONS

Sample NIC linkages:
Urinary Habit Training: Establishing a predictable pattern of bladder emptying to prevent incontinence for persons with limited cognitive ability who have urge, stress, or functional incontinence
Urinary Incontinence Care: Assistance in promoting continence and maintaining perineal skin integrity
Perineal Care: Maintenance of perineal skin integrity and relief of perineal discomfort

NURSING PRIORITY NO. 1

To assess causative/contributing factors:

● Note presence of conditions often associated with urgent voiding (e.g., stroke, MS, Parkinson's disease, spinal cord injury [SCI], Alzheimer's disease, obesity; pelvic inflammatory disease; abdominal or pelvic surgeries, recent or lengthy use of indwelling urinary catheter) *affecting bladder capacity, pelvic musculature tone, or innervation.*
● Ask client about urgency (more than just normal desire to void). *Urgency (also sometimes called overactive bladder syndrome) is a sudden, compelling need to void that is difficult to defer and may be accompanied by leaking or incontinence.*[10,11]
● Note factors that may affect ability to respond to urge to void in timely manner. *Impaired mobility, use of sedation, or cognitive impairments may result in client not recognizing need to void, or moving too slowly to make it to the bathroom, with subsequent loss of urine.*[3]
● Review client's medications and substance use (e.g., diuretics, antipsychotics, sedatives; caffeine, alcohol) *for agents that increase urine production or exert a bladder irritant effect.*[2]
● Assess for cloudy, odorous urine associated with acute, painful urgency symptoms. *Incontinence often leads to or reflects UTIs.*[1]
● Test urine for glucose. *Presence of glucose in urine causes polyuria, resulting in overdistention of the bladder and inability to hold urine until reaching the bathroom.*[4]

- Assist with appropriate diagnostic testing (e.g., pre- and postvoid bladder scanning; pelvic examination *for strictures, impaired perineal sensation or musculature*; urinalysis, uroflowmetry voiding pressures; cystoscopy, cystometrogram) *to determine anatomic and functional status of bladder and urethra.*[5–5,12]
- Assess for concomitant stress or functional incontinence. *Older women often have a mix of stress and urge incontinence, whereas individuals with dementia or disabling neurological disorders tend to have urge and functional incontinence.* (Refer to NDs stress/functional Urinary Incontinence for additional interventions.)

NURSING PRIORITY NO. 2

To assess degree of interference/disability:

- Measure amount of urine voided, especially noting amounts less than 100 mL or greater than 550 mL. *Bladder capacity may be impaired, or bladder contractions facilitating emptying may be ineffective.*[6] (Refer to ND [acute/chronic] Urinary Retention.)
- Record frequency of voiding during a typical day and typical night. *Maintaining a voiding diary identifies degree of difficulty being experienced by client.*[7]
- Note length of warning time between initial urge and loss of urine. *Overactivity or irritability decreases the length of time between urge and loss and helps clarify the type of incontinence.*[2]
- Ascertain if client experiences triggers (e.g., sound of running water, putting hands in water, seeing a restroom sign, "key-in-the lock" syndrome).[12]
- Ascertain effect on lifestyle (including daily activities, socialization, sexuality) and self-esteem. *There is a considerable reduction in the quality of life of individuals with an incontinence problem, affecting socialization and view of themselves as sexual beings and sense of self-esteem.*[4]

NURSING PRIORITY NO. 3

To assist in treating/preventing incontinence:

- Implement continence management interventions:
  Establish voiding schedule (habit and bladder training) based on client's usual voiding pattern. *Bladder retraining program is often successful in the control of urge incontinence.*[7,13]
  Recommend consciously delaying voiding by using distraction (e.g., slow, deep breathing); self-statements (e.g., "I can wait"); and contracting pelvic muscles when exposed to triggers. *Behavioral techniques for urge suppression.*[4,13,14]
- Encourage regular pelvic floor strengthening exercise (Kegel exercises) or use of vaginal cones. Combine activity with biofeedback, as appropriate. *Enhances effectiveness of training and success at controlling incontinence.*[7,13,15]
  Instruct client to tighten pelvic floor muscles before arising from bed. *Helps prevent loss of urine as abdominal pressure changes.*[7]
  Set alarm to awaken during night, if indicated. *May be necessary to continue voiding schedule.*[7]
  Increase fluid intake to 1500 to 2000 mL/day (or as indicated) *to prevent dehydration and promote good urine flow.*[7] *Note: Too much fluid can also increase bladder irritation, so amount of intake needs to be determined by individual response.*[19]
  Regulate liquid intake at prescheduled times, and limit fluids 2 to 3 hours prior to bedtime. *Promotes a predictable voiding pattern and can help limit nocturia.*[8]

Modify diet, as indicated (e.g., reduce acidic/citrus juices, carbonated beverages, spicy foods, artificial sweeteners), *to reduce bladder irritants.*[19]

Suggest limiting intake of coffee, tea and alcohol *to reduce urge symptoms and nighttime incontinence.*[2,19]

Manage bowel elimination *to prevent urinary problems associated with constipation or fecal impaction.*

- Offer assistance to cognitively impaired client (e.g., prompt client or take to bathroom on regularly timed schedule) *to reduce frequency of incontinence episodes and promote comfort.*

- Provide assistance or devices, as indicated, for clients who are mobility impaired. *Providing means of summoning assistance, placing bedside commode, urinal, or bedpan within reach helps to avoid unintended loss of urine and promotes sense of control over situation.*[7]

- Collaborate in treating underlying cause. *Urgency symptoms may resolve with treatment of medical problem (e.g., infection, recovery from surgery, childbirth, or pelvic trauma) or may be resistant to resolution (e.g., incontinence associated with neurogenic bladder).*

- Refer to specialist or treatment program, as indicated, for additional or specialized interventions (e.g., biofeedback, use of vaginal cones, electronic stimulation therapy). *Significant reduction in incontinence episodes is reported with use of combined therapies (e.g., electronic stimulation therapy plus pelvic muscle exercises).*[18]

- Administer medications (e.g., antibiotics, antimuscarinics [oxybutynin, tolterodine]) *to reduce incidence of UTIs and reduce voiding frequency and urgency by blocking overactive detrusor contractions.*[10,16]

- Discuss possible surgical interventions to change position of or enlarge the bladder, add support to weakened pelvic muscles, replace the urinary sphincter, or implantation of a sacral nerve stimulator that acts as a bladder pacemaker. *When other options have failed, different surgical interventions have been developed to cure various forms of incontinence and minimize surgical trauma, thus decreasing the length of hospitalization.*[4,17]

NURSING PRIORITY NO. 4

To promote wellness (Teaching/Discharge Considerations):

- Encourage comfort measures (e.g., use of incontinence pads or adult briefs, wearing loose-fitting or especially adapted clothing) *to prepare for or manage urge incontinence symptoms over the long-term as well as to enhance sense of security and confidence in abilities to be socially active.*[8]

- Emphasize importance of perineal care after each voiding. *Prevents skin irritation and reduces potential for bladder infection.*[9]

- Identify signs/symptoms indicating urinary complications and need for medical follow-up care. *Helps client be aware and seek intervention in a timely manner to prevent more serious problems from developing.*[7]

DOCUMENTATION FOCUS

Assessment/Reassessment
- Individual findings, including pattern of incontinence, effect on lifestyle and self-esteem.

Planning
- Plan of care, specific interventions, and who is involved in planning.
- Teaching plan.

Implementation/Evaluation
- Response to interventions, teaching, and actions performed.
- Attainment or progress toward desired outcome(s).
- Modifications to plan of care.

Discharge Planning
- Discharge needs and who is responsible for actions to be taken.
- Specific referrals made.

References

1. Wyman, J. F. (2003). Treatment of urinary incontinence in men and older women: The evidence shows the efficacy of a variety of techniques. *Am J Nurs*, 103(suppl), 26–35.
2. What is urinary incontinence? Retrieved September 2003 from http://ourworld.compuserve.com/homepages/nacs/INCONT.HTM.
3. Urinary incontinence. Penn State Health & Disease Information. Retrieved August 2007 from www.hmc.psu.edu/healthinfo/uz/urinaryincontinence.htm.
4. Booth, C. (2002). Introduction to urinary incontinence. *Hosp Pharmacist*, 9(3), 65–68.
5. Beers, M. H., Berkow, R. (eds). (1999). *The Merck Manual of Diagnosis and Therapy*. 17th ed. Whitehouse Station, NJ: Merck Research Laboratories.
6. Doenges, M. E., Moorhouse, M. F., Geissler-Murr, A. C. (2004). *Nurse's Pocket Guide: Diagnoses, Interventions, and Rationales*. 9th ed. Philadelphia: F. A. Davis.
7. Newman, D. K., Palmer, M. H. (eds). (2003). The state of the science on urinary incontinence. *Am J Nurs*, 103(suppl), 20.
8. Ford-Martin, P. A. (1999). Urinary incontinence. *Gale Encyclopedia of Medicine*. Retrieved August 2007 from http://findarticles.com/p/articles/mi_g2601/is_0014/ai_2601001430/pg_3.
9. Cox, H. C., et al. (2002). ND: Urinary incontinence. *Clinical Applications of Nursing Diagnosis: Adult, Child, Women's, Psychiatric, Gerontic, and Home Health Considerations*. 4th ed. Philadelphia: F. A. Davis.
10. Gray, M. (2005). Assessment and management of urinary incontinence. *Nurse Pract*, 30(7), 32–43.
11. Gray, M. (2005). Overactive bladder: An overview. *J Wound Ostomy Continence Nurs*, 32(3 suppl), 1–5.
12. Newman, D. K. (2005). Assessment of the patient with an overactive bladder. *J Wound Ostomy Continence Nurs*, 32(3 suppl), 5–10.
13. Wyman, J. F. (2005). Behavioral interventions for the patient with overactive bladder. *J Wound Ostomy Continence Nurs*, 32(3 suppl), 11–15.
14. Urinary incontinence [section 3, chapter 57]. (1995–2007). The Merck Manual of Health & Aging (online). Retrieved August 2007 from www.merck.com/pubs/mmanual_ha/sec3/ch57/ch57a.html.
15. Bump, R. C., Hurt, W. G., Fantl, J. A., (1999). Assessment of Kegel pelvic muscle exercise performance after brief verbal instruction. *Am J Obstet Gynecol*, 165, 322–327.
16. Mauk, K. L. (2005). Medications for management of overactive bladder. *ARN*, (June/July). 3–7.
17. Mayo Clinic. Surgical treatments for urinary incontinence. Retrieved August 2007 from www.mayoclinic.org/urinary-incontinence/surgery.html.
18. Incontinence—Biofeedback and electrical stimulation. (February 2007). Retrieved August 2007 from www.emedicinehealth.com/incontinence/page8_em.htm.
19. Incontinence—Nonsurgical treatment: Dietary measures. (February 2007). Retrieved August 2007 from www.emedicinehealth.com/incontinence/page6_em.htm.

[acute/chronic] Urinary Retention

DEFINITION: Incomplete emptying of the bladder

RELATED FACTORS

High urethral pressure
Inhibition of reflex arc
Strong sphincter; blockage [e.g., benign prostatic hypertrophy (BPH), perineal swelling]
[Habituation of reflex arc]
[Infections; neurological diseases or trauma]
[Use of medications with side effect of retention (e.g., atropine, belladonna, psychotropics, antihistamines, opiates)]

DEFINING CHARACTERISTICS

Subjective
Sensation of bladder fullness
Dribbling
Dysuria

Objective
Bladder distention
Small or frequent voiding; absence of urine output
Residual urine [150 mL or more]
Overflow incontinence
[Reduced stream]

Sample Clinical Applications: BPH, prostatitis, cancer, perineal surgery, birth trauma, urethral calculi, multiple sclerosis (MS), spinal cord compression, urinary tract infection (UTI), genital herpes

DESIRED OUTCOMES/EVALUATION CRITERIA

Sample NOC linkages:
Urinary Elimination: Collection and discharge of urine
Symptom Control: Personal actions to minimize perceived adverse changes in physical and emotional functioning
Knowledge: Disease Process: Extent of understanding conveyed about a specific disease process

Client Will (Include Specific Time Frame)
• Verbalize understanding of causative factors and appropriate interventions for individual situation.
• Demonstrate techniques or behaviors to alleviate or prevent retention.
• Void in sufficient amounts with no palpable bladder distention; experience no postvoid residuals greater than 50 mL; have no dribbling or overflow.

ACTIONS/INTERVENTIONS

Acute Retention
Sample (NIC) linkages:
Urinary Catheterization: Insertion of a catheter into the bladder for temporary or permanent drainage of urine
Fluid Monitoring: Collection and analysis of patient data to regulate fluid balance

NURSING PRIORITY NO. 1

To assess causative/contributing factors:

- Note presence of pathological conditions such as neurological injury or disease, kidney or bladder infection or stone formation, and reaction to medications, diagnostic dye, or anesthesia *that can cause mechanical obstruction, nerve dysfunction, ineffective contraction, or decompensation of detrusor musculature, resulting in ineffective emptying of the bladder and urine retention.*[1,7]
- Investigate reports of sudden loss of ability to pass urine, great difficulty passing urine, pain with urination, blood in urine. *May indicate UTI or obstruction.*[7]
- Review results of laboratory tests, such as urinalysis for presence of red and white blood cells, nitrates, glucose, bacteria, and cultures, as indicated; blood may be tested for infection, electrolyte imbalance, and (in men) prostate-specific antigen (PSA) *to determine presence of treatable conditions.*[3,4]
- Review medication regimen *for drugs that can cause or exacerbate retention (e.g., psychotropics, opiates, sedatives, alpha- and beta-blockers, anticholinergics, antihistamines, neuroleptics, anesthesia).*[2,7]
- Determine anxiety level. *Client may be too embarrassed to void in presence of others or talk about problem with care providers.*[2]
- Examine for fecal impaction, pelvic or perineal surgical site swelling, postpartal edema, vaginal or rectal packing, enlarged prostate, or other "mechanical" factors *that may produce a blockage of the urethra.*[2]
- Strain urine for presence of stones or calculi *that may be causing outlet obstruction, or to note when treatments are being effective in stone breakup and removal.*[1,7]

NURSING PRIORITY NO. 2

To determine degree of interference/disability:

- Ascertain if client can empty bladder completely, partially, or not at all, in spite of urge to urinate. *Signs of urinary retention caused by (1) blockage of the urethra or (2) disruption of complex system of nerves that connects the urinary tract with the brain. In men, blockage is most commonly caused by enlargement of the prostate, cancer, stones, and urethral stricture. Causes that can occur in both genders include scar tissue, injury (as in car crash or fall), blood clots, infection, tumors, and stones (rare). Disruption of nerves, or nerve transmission, or interpretation of signals can be caused by injury (e.g., spinal cord injury [SCI] or tumor, herniated disk, stroke), pelvic infections, surgery, and certain medications.*[3,5,7]
- Determine if there has been any significant urine output in the previous 6 to 8 hours. *Small amount of urine may leak out of bladder but generally not enough to relieve symptoms.*[3]
- Note recent amount and type of fluid intake. *Fluids may initially need to be restricted to prevent bladder distention until adequate urine flow is established.*[1]
- Palpate height of the bladder. Ascertain whether client has sensation of bladder fullness, level of discomfort. *Sensation and discomfort can vary, depending on underlying cause of*

retention. Most people with acute retention also feel pain in lower abdomen (pelvis). Back pain, fever, and painful urination may be present with retention if the cause is urinary tract infection.[3]

- Catheterize, or perform bladder scan or ultrasound, for bladder residual after voiding *to determine presence and degree of urine retention.*[1]

- Review results of diagnostic tests. *Urine flow rate, bladder capacity, and postvoid residual scanning may be done. Ultrasound, computed tomography (CT) scan, intravenous pyelogram (IVP) and cystoscopy can help locate the source of obstruction (e.g., lower or upper tract). Lumbar spine radiographs, CT scan, or magnetic resonance imaging (MRI) may be done when retention is thought to be due to an acute spinal problem (e.g., herniated disk, spinal cord disruption, infection).*[3,4,7,8]

NURSING PRIORITY NO. 3

To assist in treating/preventing retention:

- Assist in treatment to relieve mechanical obstruction (e.g., removal of blockage—vaginal packing, bowel impaction; application of ice *to reduce perineal swelling) that is restricting urinary flow.*[2]

- Administer medications as indicated (e.g., antibiotics, stool softeners, pain relievers) *to treat underlying cause, promote muscle relaxation.*[2]

- Provide privacy *to reduce retention caused by embarrassment or anxiety.*

- Assist client to sit upright on bedpan or commode, or stand *to provide functional position of voiding.*[2]

- Encourage warm sitz bath or shower, voiding in tub or shower if need be. *Warm water stimulates bladder to relax and may facilitate voiding.*[2]

- Use ice techniques, spirits of wintergreen, stroking inner thigh, running water in sink, or warm water over perineum *to stimulate reflex arc.*[2]

- Instruct client with mild or moderate obstructive symptoms to "double void" by urinating, resting on toilet for 3 to 5 minutes, and then making a second attempt to urinate. *Promotes more efficient bladder evacuation by allowing the detrusor to contract initially, then rest and contract again.*[5]

- Drain bladder with straight catheter per agency protocol or catheterize with intermittent or indwelling catheter *to resolve acute retention.*[2] *Note: References are mixed as to need for fractional drainage in increments of 200 mL at a time to prevent possibility of bladder spasm, syncope or hypotension.*[6]

- Encourage adequate fluid intake, including use of acidifying fruit juices or ingestion of vitamin C or Mandelamine *to discourage bacterial growth and stone formation.*[2]

- Adjust fluid intake and timing if indicated, *to prevent bladder distention.*

- Prepare for more aggressive intervention (e.g., reconstructive surgery, lithotripsy, prostatectomy) as indicated *to remove source of obstruction, reconstruct sphincter, or provide for urinary diversion.*[2]

NURSING PRIORITY NO. 4

To promote wellness (Teaching/Discharge Considerations):

- Stress good voiding habits (e.g., four to six times/day). *Repeated holding of urination for prolonged periods can, over time, overstretch and weaken bladder muscles.*

- Encourage client to report problems immediately *so treatment can be instituted promptly.*[2]

- Emphasize need for adequate fluid intake.

Chronic Retention
Sample (NIC) linkages:
Urinary Retention Care: Assistance in relieving bladder distention
Exercise Therapy: Muscle Control: Use of specific activity or exercise protocols to enhance or restore controlled body movement

NURSING PRIORITY NO. 1

To assess causative/contributing factors:

- Review medical history for diagnoses, such as congenital defects, neurological disorders (e.g., MS, polio); prostatic hypertrophy or surgery; birth canal injury or scarring; spinal cord injury with lower motor neuron injury *that may cause detrusor muscle atrophy or chronic overdistention because of outlet obstruction.*[2,6]
- Determine presence of weak or absent sensory or motor impulses (as with CVAs, spinal injury, or diabetes) *that predispose client to compromised enervation or interpretation of sensory signals resulting in impaired urination.*[2]
- Evaluate customary fluid intake.
- Assess client's medication regimen (e.g., psychotropic, antihistamines, atropine, belladonna) *to consult with primary care provider regarding client's continued use of drugs that are known to potentiate urinary retention.*[2]

NURSING PRIORITY NO. 2

To determine degree of interference/disability:

- Ascertain effect of condition on functioning and lifestyle. *Chronic urinary retention can limit client's desired lifestyle (e.g., daily activities, social functioning), and can lead to chronic incontinence and life-threatening complications (e.g., intractable UTIs, kidney failure).*[3,9]
- Instruct client/SO to maintain voiding log noting frequency and timing of voiding, or dribbling *to determine severity of condition.*[5]
- Determine presence and severity (0 to 10 scale) of bladder spasms, pelvic pain, and other discomforts.
- Assist with urodynamic testing (e.g., uroflowmetry to assess urine speed and volume, cystometrogram to measure bladder pressure and volume, bladder scan to measure retention or postvoid residual, leak point pressure).[7]

NURSING PRIORITY NO. 3

To assist in treating/preventing retention:

- Collaborate in treatment of underlying conditions (e.g., BPH, reducing or eliminating medications responsible for retention, repairing perineal scarring or outlet obstruction), *which may correct or reduce severity of retention and associated overflow or total incontinence.*
- Instruct client/SO in management of voiding problems as indicated:
  Attempt voiding in complete privacy *to reduce embarrassment and distractions.*[2]
  Void on frequent, timed schedule *to maintain low bladder pressure and prevent overdistention of bladder.*[2]
  Maintain consistent fluid intake *to wash out bacteria, avoid infections, and limit bladder stone formation.*[9]
  Adjust fluid amount and timing if indicated *to prevent bladder distention.*

Perform Credé's or Valsalva's maneuver if appropriate *to facilitate emptying of the bladder.*[2]

 • Establish regular self-catheterization program, as indicated, *to prevent reflux and increased renal pressures and to improve client's quality of life (e.g., ability to participate in desired or needed activities and social interactions). Note: Clean intermittent catheterization (CIC) is a treatment option for individuals who can urinate but cannot completely empty their bladder.*[3,9]

 • Consult with urologist and prepare for more aggressive intervention (e.g., reconstructive surgery, lithotripsy, prostatectomy) as indicated *to remove source of obstruction, reconstruct sphincter, or provide for urinary diversion.*[2]

• Refer for consideration of advanced or research-based therapies (e.g., implanted sacra, tibial, or pelvic electrical stimulating device) for long-term management of retention.[9]

NURSING PRIORITY NO. 4

To promote wellness (Teaching/Discharge Considerations):

• Establish regular schedule for bladder emptying whether voiding or using catheter.

• Instruct SO/caregiver(s) in clean intermittent catheterization techniques *so that more than one individual is able to assist the client in care of elimination needs.*[2]

• Instruct client/SO in care when client has indwelling (urethral or suprapubic catheter) or urinary diversion device (e.g., clean technique, emptying and cleaning of leg bag or drainage bag; irrigation and replacement) *to promote self-care, enhance independence, and prevent complications.*[2]

• Stress need for adequate fluid intake, including use of acidifying fruit juices or ingestion of vitamin C or Mandelamine *to discourage bacterial growth and bladder stone formation.*[2]

• Discuss appropriate use of herbal products *such as saw palmetto to improve symptoms of BPH.*

• Review signs/symptoms of complications *to promote timely contact with healthcare provider for evaluation and intervention.*

DOCUMENTATION FOCUS

Assessment/Reassessment
• Individual findings, including nature of problem, degree of impairment, and whether client is incontinent.

Planning
• Plan of care and who is involved in planning.
• Teaching plan.

Implementation/Evaluation
• Response to interventions.
• Attainment or progress toward desired outcome(s).
• Modifications to plan of care.

Discharge Planning
• Long-term needs and who is responsible for actions to be taken.
• Specific referrals made.

References

1. Doenges, M. E., Moorhouse, M. F., Geissler-Murr, A. C. (2002). ND: Urinary retention. *Nursing Care Plans: Guidelines for Individualizing Patient Care.* 6th ed. Philadelphia: F. A. Davis.

2. Doenges, M. E., Moorhouse, M. F., Murr, A. C. (2004). ND: Urinary retention. *Nurse's Pocket Guide: Diagnoses, Interventions, and Rationales.* 9th ed. Philadelphia: F. A. Davis.

3. Gaynes, S. M. (2001). Urinary retention: Inability to urinate. Retrieved August 2007 from www.emedicine.com/aaem/topic466.htm.

4. American Urological Association. (2003). The management of benign prostatic hyperplasia. Retrieved August 2007 from www.guideline.gov.

5. Gray, M. (2000). Urinary retention: Management in the acute care setting (part 2). *Am J Nurs,* 100(8), 36–44.

6. Policastro, M. A., Sinert, R., Guerrero, P. (2007). Urinary obstruction. Retrieved May 2007 from www.emedicine.com/emerg/topic624.htm.

7. Newman, D. K. (2005). Assessment of the patient with an overactive bladder. *Journal Wound Ostomy Continence Nurs,* 32(3 suppl), 5–10.

8. Albo, M., Richter, H. E. (2006). Urodynamic testing. Fact sheet for National Kidney and Urologic Diseases Information Clearinghouse. Retrieved August 2007 from http://kidney.niddk.nih.gov/kudiseases/pubs/urodynamic/index.htm.

9. Santos, A., Hunt, M. (2005). Managing incontinence: Once a cause of isolation and embarrassment, incontinence does not have to limit quality of life. *Paraplegia News,* 59(11).

impaired spontaneous Ventilation

DEFINITION: Decreased energy reserves that results in an individual's inability to maintain breathing adequate to support life

RELATED FACTORS

Metabolic factors; [hypermetabolic state (e.g., infection), nutritional deficits or depletion of energy stores]
Respiratory muscle fatigue
[Airway size or resistance; inadequate secretion management]

DEFINING CHARACTERISTICS

Subjective
Dyspnea
Apprehension

Objective
Increased metabolic rate
Increased heart rate
Increased restlessness; decreased cooperation
Increased use of accessory muscles
Decreased tidal volume
Decreased PO_2/SaO_2; increased PCO_2

Sample Clinical Applications: Chronic obstructive pulmonary disease (COPD), asthma, pulmonary embolus, acute respiratory distress syndrome, brain injury, chest trauma or surgery, Guillain-Barré syndrome, amyotrophic lateral sclerosis (ALS)

(continues on page 908)

impaired spontaneous Ventilation (continued)
DESIRED OUTCOMES/EVALUATION CRITERIA

Sample (NOC) linkages:
Mechanical Ventilation Response: Adult: Alveolar exchange and tissue perfusion supported by mechanical ventilation
Respiratory Status: Ventilation: Movement of air in and out of the lungs
Endurance: Capacity to sustain activity

Client Will (Include Specific Time Frame)
• Reestablish and maintain effective respiratory pattern via ventilator, with absence of retractions or use of accessory muscles, cyanosis, or other signs of hypoxia; and with arterial blood gases (ABGs)/SaO$_2$ within acceptable range.
• Participate in efforts to wean (as appropriate) within individual ability.

Sample (NOC) linkage:
Energy Conservation: Personal actions to manage energy for initiating and sustaining activity

Caregiver Will (Include Specific Time Frame)
• Demonstrate behaviors necessary to maintain client's respiratory function.

ACTIONS/INTERVENTIONS

Sample (NIC) linkages:
Ventilation Assistance: Promotion of an optimal spontaneous breathing pattern that maximizes oxygen and carbon dioxide exchange in the lungs
Mechanical Ventilation Management: Invasive: Use of an artificial device to help patient breathe
Respiratory Monitoring: Collection and analysis of patient data to ensure airway patency and adequate gas exchange

NURSING PRIORITY NO. 1

To determine degree of impairment:

• Identify client with impending respiratory failure (e.g., developing apnea or slow, shallow breathing; declining mentation or obtunded with need for airway protection).[10]
• Assess spontaneous respiratory pattern, noting rate, depth, rhythm, symmetry of chest movement, and use of accessory muscles. *Tachypnea, shallow breathing, demonstrated or reports of dyspnea (using 0 to 10 scale); increased heart rate, dysrhythmias; pallor or cyanosis; and intercostal retractions and use of accessory muscles indicate increased work of breathing or gas exchange impairment.*[3,10]
• Auscultate breath sounds, noting presence or absence and equality of breath sounds, adventitious breath sounds (e.g., wheezing) *to evaluate presence and degree of ventilatory impairment.*
• Evaluate ABGs or pulse oximetry and capnography *to determine presence and degree of arterial hypoxemia (<55%) and hypercapnia (CO$_2$ > 45%) resulting in impaired ventilation requiring support.*[11,12]
• Obtain or review results of pulmonary function studies (e.g., lung volumes, inspiratory and expiratory pressures, and forced vital capacity), as appropriate, *to assess presence and degree of respiratory insufficiency.*

- Investigate etiology of respiratory failure (e.g., exacerbation of COPD, pneumonia, pulmonary embolus, heart failure, trauma) *to determine client's ventilation needs and most appropriate type of ventilatory support.*[1]
- Review serial chest x-rays and imaging scans (e.g., magnetic resonance imaging [MRI], computed tomography [CT]) that may be performed *to diagnose disorder and monitor response to treatment.*
- Note response to current measures and respiratory therapy (e.g., bronchodilators, supplemental oxygen, intermittent positive pressure breathing [IPPB] treatments). *Client may already be receiving treatments to maintain airway patency and enhance gas exchange or may have respiratory failure associated with sudden event (e.g., severe trauma, sudden onset respiratory illness, surgery with complications).*[1]
- Ascertain desires of client/SO(s) regarding plan for treatment of respiratory failure, as indicated. *Client may have advance directives, prior stated decisions about the level of therapy aggressiveness that he or she desires if situation is chronic or long term. Family members may help in decision-making processes if client is a minor or is incapacitated.*[2]

NURSING PRIORITY NO. 2

To provide/maintain ventilatory support:

- Collaborate with physician, respiratory care practitioners regarding effective mode of ventilation (e.g., noninvasive oxygenation) or intubation and mechanical ventilation (e.g., continuous mandatory [CMV], assist control [ACV], intermittent mandatory [IMV], pressure support [PSV]). *Specific mode is determined by client's respiratory requirements, presence of underlying disease process, and the extent to which client can participate in ventilatory efforts.*
- Ensure effective ventilation:[1,4,8,12]
  Observe overall breathing pattern, distinguishing between spontaneous respirations and ventilator breaths. *Client may be completely dependent on the ventilator or able to take breaths but have poor oxygen saturation without the ventilator. The client on noncontrolled ventilation mode can still experience hyper or hypoventilation or "air hunger" and attempt to correct deficiency by overbreathing.*[1,12]
  Verify that client's respirations are in phase with the ventilator. *Decreases work of breathing, maximizes O_2 delivery when client is not fighting the ventilator.*
  Inflate tracheal or endotracheal tube cuff properly using minimal leak or occlusive technique *to ensure adequate ventilation and delivery of desired tidal volume.*
  Check cuff inflation periodically per facility protocol and whenever cuff is deflated then reinflated *to prevent risks associated with under or overinflation.*
  Check tubings for obstruction (e.g., kinking or accumulation of water) *that can impede flow of oxygen.* Drain tubing, as indicated; refrain from draining toward the client or back into the reservoir, *which can result in contamination and provide medium for growth of bacteria.*
  Check ventilator alarms for proper functioning. Do not turn off alarms, even for suctioning. Verify that alarms can be heard in the nurses' station by care providers *to ensure care provider is alerted to emergent situation, ventilator disconnect.*
  Suction, as needed, *to clear secretions if client is coughing excessively, has visible secretions, or is tripping high-pressure alarm on ventilator.*
  Remove from ventilator and ventilate manually *if source of ventilator alarm cannot be quickly identified and rectified.*
  Verify that oxygen line is in proper outlet or tank; monitor inline oxygen analyzer or perform periodic oxygen analysis *to deliver an acceptable oxygen percentage and saturation for client's specific needs.*

Assess ventilator settings routinely and readjust, as indicated, *according to client's primary disease and results of diagnostic testing.*

Verify tidal volume set to volume needed for individual situation and proper functioning of spirometer, bellows, or computer readout of delivered volume *to reduce risk of complications associated with alteration in lung compliance or leakage through machine or around tube cuff.*

Monitor airway pressure for developing complications or equipment problems (e.g., increased airway resistance, retained secretions, decreased lung compliance, client out of phase or off ventilator).

Promote periodic maximal ventilation of alveoli; check sigh rate intervals (usually 1 1/2 to 2 times tidal volume). *Reduces risk of atelectasis, helps mobilize secretions.*

Note inspired humidity and temperature; maintain hydration *to prevent excessive drying of mucosa and secretions.*

- Auscultate breath sounds periodically. Note frequent crackles or rhonchi that do not clear with coughing or suctioning. *May indicate developing complications (e.g., atelectasis, pneumonia, acute bronchospasm, pulmonary edema).*
- Note changes in chest symmetry. *May indicate improper placement of ET tube, development of barotrauma.*
- Keep resuscitation bag at bedside *to allow for manual ventilation whenever indicated (e.g., if client is removed from ventilator or troubleshooting equipment problems).*
- Administer and monitor response to medications that promote airway patency and gas exchange *to determine efficacy and need for change.*
- Administer sedation, as required, *to synchronize respirations and reduce work of breathing and energy expenditure.*
- Refer to NDs ineffective Airway Clearance, ineffective Breathing Pattern, and impaired Gas Exchange for related interventions.

NURSING PRIORITY NO. 3

To prepare for/assist with weaning process if appropriate:

- Determine client's physical and psychological readiness to wean. Weaning readiness testing should begin soon after intubation, whenever possible, *to limit complications associated with long-term mechanical ventilation.* Weaning parameters include (1) evidence for some reversal of the underlying cause of respiratory failure; (2) adequate oxygenation and normal pH; (3) hemodynamic stability; (4) capability and willingness to initiate inspiratory effort; (5) absence of excessive secretions; and (6) nutritional status sufficient *to maintain work of breathing.*[1,4–7,10]
- Determine mode for weaning. *Recent studies indicate that pressure support mode or multiple daily T-piece trials may be superior to IMV; low-level pressure support may be beneficial for unassisted breathing trials; and early extubation and institution of noninvasive positive pressure ventilation may have substantial benefits in alert, cooperative client.*[5,7,10]
- Explain to client/SO weaning activities and techniques, individual plan, and expectations. *Reduces fear of unknown, provides opportunities to deal with concerns, clarifies reality of fears, and helps reduce anxiety to a more manageable level.*[1,6,8,12]
- Engage client in specialized exercise program *to enhance respiratory muscle strength and general endurance.*
- Maximize weaning effort:
  Elevate head of bed/place in orthopedic chair, if possible, or position *to alleviate dyspnea and to facilitate oxygenation.*

Coach client in "taking control" of breathing during weaning periods (e.g., to take slower, deeper breaths, practice abdominal or pursed-lip breathing, assume position of comfort) *to maximize respiratory function and reduce anxiety.*

Instruct in or assist client to perform effective coughing techniques. *Necessary for secretion management after extubation.*

Provide quiet environment, calm approach, and undivided attention of nurse. *Promotes relaxation, decreasing energy and oxygen requirements.*

Involve family/SO(s) as appropriate. Provide diversionary activity. *Helps client focus on something other than breathing.*

Instruct client in use of energy-saving techniques during care activities *to limit oxygen consumption and fatigue associated with work of breathing.*

- Acknowledge and provide ongoing encouragement for client's efforts. Communicate hope for successful weaning response (even partial). *Emotional support can enhance client's commitment to continue weaning activity, maximizing outcomes.*[1]

NURSING PRIORITY NO. 4

To prepare for discharge on ventilator when indicated:

- Ascertain plan for discharge placement (e.g., return home, short-term admission to subacute or rehabilitation center, or permanent placement in extended-care facility). *Helps to determine care needs and fiscal impact of home care versus extended-care facility.*[8]
- Review layout of home, noting size of rooms, doorways, placement of furniture, number and type of electrical outlets *to identify necessary modifications and safety needs.*
- Determine specific equipment needs and resources for equipment and maintenance. Arrange for delivery before client discharge *to allow SO/caregivers to prepare for transfer.*
- Allow sufficient opportunity for SO(s)/family to practice new skills. Role-play potential crisis situations *to enhance confidence in ability to handle client's needs.*
- Demonstrate airway management techniques and proper equipment cleaning practices *to reduce risk of infection.*
- Instruct SO(s)/caregivers in other pulmonary physiotherapy measures (e.g., chest physiotherapy), as indicated. Refer for home respiratory therapy support, as needed.
- Provide positive feedback and encouragement for efforts of SO(s)/caregivers. *Promotes continuation of desired behaviors.*
- List names and phone numbers for identified contact persons and resources. *Can reduce sense of isolation and enhance likelihood of obtaining assistance and support when needed.*
- Review and provide written or audiovisual materials regarding proper ventilator management, maintenance, and safety for reference in home setting. *Provides information to enhance client's/SO's level of comfort with challenging tasks.*
- Identify signs/symptoms requiring prompt medical evaluation or intervention. *Timely treatment may prevent progression of problem or untoward complications.*
- Obtain no-smoking signs to be posted in home, and remind family members to refrain from smoking *to reduce risk of fire.*
- Have family/SO(s) notify utility company and fire department of presence of ventilator in home. *Client will be placed in high-risk list for follow-up in case of power outage or fire.*[9]

NURSING PRIORITY NO. 5

To promote wellness (Teaching/Discharge Considerations):

- Discuss impact of specific activities on respiratory status and problem-solve solutions *to maximize weaning effort or to reduce incidence of respiratory distress or failure.*

- ● Monitor health of visitors, persons involved in care *to protect client from sources of infection.*
- ● Encourage time-out or respite for caregivers *so they may attend to personal needs, wellness, and growth.* Refer to ND risk for Caregiver Role Strain.
- ● Provide opportunities for client/SO(s) to discuss advance directives. *Clarifies parameters for termination of therapy or other end-of-life decisions, as desired.*
- ● Recommend involvement in support group; introduce to other ventilator-dependent individuals who are successfully managing home ventilation, if desired, *to answer questions, provide role model, assist with problem-solving, and offer encouragement and hope for the future.*

DOCUMENTATION FOCUS

Assessment/Reassessment
- Baseline findings, subsequent alterations in respiratory function.
- Results of diagnostic testing.
- Individual risk factors and concerns.

Planning
- Plan of care and who is involved in planning.
- Teaching plan.

Implementation/Evaluation
- Client's/other's responses to interventions, teaching, and actions performed.
- Skill level and assistance needs of SO(s)/family.
- Attainment or progress toward desired outcome(s).
- Modifications to plan of care.

Discharge Planning
- Discharge plan, including appropriate referrals, action taken, and who is responsible for each action.
- Equipment needs and source.
- Resources for support persons or home-care providers.

References

1. Doenges, M. E., Moorhouse, M. F., Geissler-Murr, A. C. (2002). CP: Ventilatory assistance (mechanical). *Nursing Care Plans: Guidelines for Individualizing Patient Care.* 6th ed. Philadelphia: F. A. Davis, 167–179.
2. Campbell, M., Thill-Baharozian, M. (1994). Impact of the DNR therapeutic plan on patient care requirements. *Am J Crit Care*, 3, 202–207.
3. Gift, A., Narsavage, G. (1998). Validity of the numeric rating scale as a measure of dyspnea. *Am J Crit Care*, 7(3), 200–204.
4. Epstein, S. K. (2002). Weaning from mechanical ventilation. *Respir Care*, 47(4), 454–466.
5. MacIntyre, N. R. (2001). Evidence-based guidelines for weaning and discontinuation of ventilatory support. (Collective task force facilitated by the American College of Chest Physicians; the American Association for Respiratory Care; and the American College of Critical Care Medicine). *Chest*, 120(6 suppl), 385S–484S.
6. Tasota, F. J., Dobbin, D. (2000). Weaning your patient from mechanical ventilation. *Nursing*, 30(10), 41–46.
7. Cook, D. J., Meade, M., Guyatt, G., et al. (2000). *Criteria for Weaning from Mechanical Ventilation.* Rockville, MD: Agency for Healthcare Research and Quality.

8 Lysaght, L. (2002). Ventilation, impaired spontaneous. In Ackley, B. J., Ladwig, G. B. (eds). *Nursing Diagnosis Handbook: A Guide to Planning Care*. 5th ed. St. Louis, MO: Mosby.

9. Humphrey, C. (1994). *Home Care Nursing Handbook*. 2d ed. Gaithersburg, MD: Aspen.

10. Sharma, S., Hayes, J. A. (2006). Hypoventilation syndromes. Retrieved May 2007 from www.emedicine.com/emerg/topic3470.htm.

11. D'Arcy, Y. (2007). Eye on capnography. *Men Nurs*, 2(2), 25–29.

12. Amitai, A., Sinert, D. (2006). Ventilator management. Retrieved May 2007 from www.emedicine.com/emerg/topic788.htm.

dysfunctional Ventilatory Weaning Response

DEFINITION: Inability to adjust to lowered levels of mechanical ventilator support that interrupts and prolongs the weaning process

RELATED FACTORS

Physiological
Ineffective airway clearance
Sleep pattern disturbance
Inadequate nutrition
Uncontrolled pain or discomfort
[Muscle weakness or fatigue, inability to control respiratory muscles; immobility]

Psychological
Knowledge deficit of the weaning process
Client's perceived inefficacy about the ability to wean
Decreased motivation or self-esteem
Anxiety; fear; insufficient trust in the nurse [or care provider]
Hopelessness; powerlessness
[Unprepared for weaning attempt]

Situational
Uncontrolled episodic energy demands
Inappropriate pacing of diminished ventilator support
Inadequate social support
Adverse environment (e.g., noisy, active environment; negative events in the room, low nurse-client ratio; unfamiliar nursing staff)
History of ventilator dependence >4 days
History of multiple unsuccessful weaning attempts

DEFINING CHARACTERISTICS

Mild DVWR
Subjective
Expressed feelings of increased need for O_2; breathing discomfort; fatigue, warmth
Queries about possible machine malfunction

(continues on page 914)

dysfunctional Ventilatory Weaning Response (continued)

Objective
Restlessness
Slight increase of respiratory rate from baseline
Increased concentration on breathing

Moderate DVWR
Subjective
Apprehension
Objective
Slight increase from baseline blood pressure (<20 mm Hg)/heart rate (<20 beats/min)
Baseline increase in respiratory rate (<5 breaths/min); slight respiratory accessory muscle use; decreased air entry on auscultation
Hypervigilance to activities; wide-eyed look
Inability to cooperate or respond to coaching
Diaphoresis
Color changes; pale, slight cyanosis

Severe DVWR
Objective
Agitation; decreased level of consciousness
Deterioration in arterial blood gases from current baseline
Increase from baseline blood pressure (>20 mm Hg)/heart rate (>20 beats/min)
Respiratory rate that increases significantly from baseline; full respiratory accessory muscle use; shallow or gasping breaths; paradoxical abdominal breathing
Adventitious breath sounds, audible airway secretions
Asynchronized breathing with the ventilator
Profuse diaphoresis
Cyanosis

Sample Clinical Applications: Traumatic brain injury, stroke, substance overdose, chronic obstructive pulmonary disease (COPD), crushing chest trauma, respiratory or cardiac arrest

DESIRED OUTCOMES/EVALUATION CRITERIA

Sample NOC linkages:
Mechanical Ventilation Weaning Response: Adult: Respiratory and psychological adjustment to progressive removal of mechanical ventilation
Respiratory Status: Ventilation: Movement of air in and out of the lungs
Respiratory Status: Gas Exchange: Alveolar exchange of carbon dioxide and oxygen to maintain arterial blood gas (ABG)concentrations

Client Will (Include Specific Time Frame)
• Actively participate in the weaning process.
• Reestablish independent respiration with ABGs within client's normal range and be free of signs of respiratory failure.
• Demonstrate increased tolerance for activity and participate in self-care within level of ability.

ACTIONS/INTERVENTIONS

Sample **NIC** linkages:
Mechanical Ventilation Management: Invasive: Use of an artificial device to assist a patient to breathe
Mechanical Ventilatory Weaning: Assisting the patient to breathe without the aid of a mechanical ventilator
Energy Management: Regulating energy use to treat or prevent fatigue and optimize function

NURSING PRIORITY NO. 1

To identify contributing factors/degree of dysfunction:

- Determine extent and nature of underlying disorders or factors (e.g., preexisting cardiopulmonary diseases, significant trauma, neuromuscular disorders; complications from surgical procedures) *that contribute to client's reliance on mechanical support, thus affecting weaning efforts.*[9]
- Note length of time client has been on ventilator. Review previous episodes of extubation and reintubation. *Previous unsuccessful weaning attempts (e.g., due to inability to protect airway or clear secretions; oxygen saturation <50% on room air) can influence weaning interventions. Although most individuals remain on the ventilator for 7 days or less, some require support for several weeks or more. Weaning is more difficult in those clients and may require multiple attempts.*[1,10]
- Complete Burns Weaning Assessment Program (BWAP) or similar checklist (e.g., stability of vital signs, factors that increase metabolic rate [e.g., sepsis, fever]; hydration status; need for or recent use of analgesia or sedation; nutritional state, muscle strength, and activity level) *to assess systemic parameters that may affect readiness for weaning.*[1–3,11,12]
- Ascertain client's alertness and understanding of weaning process, expectations, and concerns. *Client/SO may need specific and repeated instructions during process to allay fears and enhance cooperation. Unrealistic expectations or unvoiced concerns can impair weaning process or willingness to participate.*
- Determine psychological readiness, presence/degree of anxiety. *Weaning provokes anxiety regarding ability to breathe on own and likelihood of ventilator dependence. The client must be highly motivated, be able to actively participate in the weaning process, and be physically comfortable enough to work at weaning.*[4]
- Review laboratory studies, such as CBC, *to determine number and integrity of red blood cells for O_2 transport*; electrolytes; and nutritional markers, such as serum protein and albumin, *to determine if client has sufficient nutritional stores to meet demands of weaning.*[1,12]
- Review chest radiograph, pulse oximetry or ABGs, and/or capnometry. *Before weaning attempts, chest radiograph should show clear lungs or marked improvement in pulmonary congestion. ABGs should document satisfactory oxygenation on an FIO_2 of 40% or less.*[4] *Capnometry measures end-tidal carbon dioxide values and can be used to confirm correct placement of endotracheal (ET) tube and monitor integrity of ventilation equipment.*[5,10]

NURSING PRIORITY NO. 2

To support weaning process:

- Discuss with client/SO individual plan and expectations. *May reduce client's anxiety about process and ultimate outcome and support willingness to work at spontaneous breathing.*[1,2]

- Consult with dietitian, nutritional support team for adjustments in composition of diet prior to weaning *to prevent excessive production of CO_2, which could alter respiratory drive. Individuals on long-term ventilation may require tube-feeding through enteral feedings with high intake of carbohydrates, protein, and calories to improve respiratory muscle function.*[4,10]
- Collaborate in implementing weaning protocols and mode (e.g., spontaneous breathing trials with T-piece, partial client support by means of synchronized intermittent mandatory ventilation [SIMV], or pressure support ventilation [PSV] during client's spontaneous breathing) *to determine if client can assume the full work of breathing and to provide support for spontaneous ventilation. Indeed, an increasing body of research suggests that the key to successful weaning lies not in the use of a particular method but, rather, through a coordinated approach by a skilled multidisciplinary team.*[6,9,12]
- Note response to activity or client care during weaning and limit, as indicated. Provide undisturbed rest or sleep periods. Avoid stressful procedures or situations and nonessential activities *to prevent excessive O_2 consumption or demand with increased possibility of weaning failure.*[4]
- Discuss impact of specific activities on respiratory status, and problem-solve solutions to maximize weaning effort.
- Time medications during weaning efforts *to minimize sedative effects.*
- Provide quiet room, calm approach, and undivided attention. *Enhances relaxation, thereby conserving energy.*
- Involve SO(s)/family, as appropriate (e.g., sit at bedside, provide encouragement, and help monitor client status).
- Provide diversionary activity (e.g., watching TV, reading aloud) *to focus attention away from breathing when not actively working at breathing exercises.*
- Acknowledge and provide ongoing encouragement for client's efforts.
- Minimize setbacks, focus client attention on gains and progress to date *to reduce frustration that may further impair progress.*
- Suspend weaning (take a "holiday") periodically as individually appropriate (e.g., initially may rest 45 or 50 minutes each hour, progressing to a 20-minute rest period every 4 hours, then weaning during daytime and resting during night).[9]

NURSING PRIORITY NO. 3

To prepare for discharge on ventilator when indicated:

- Prepare client/SO for alternative actions when client is unable to resume spontaneous ventilation (e.g., tracheostomy with long-term ventilation support in alternate care setting or home, palliative care or end-of-life procedures).[7]
- Ascertain that all needed equipment is in place, caregivers are trained, and safety concerns have been addressed (e.g., alternative power source, backup equipment, client call or alarm system) *to ease the transfer when client is going home on ventilator.*[4]
- Evaluate caregiver capabilities and burden when client requires long-term ventilator in the home *to determine potential or presence of skill-related problems or emotional issues (e.g., caregiver overload, burnout, or depression).*[8]
- Refer to ND impaired spontaneous Ventilation for additional interventions.

NURSING PRIORITY NO. 4

To promote wellness (Teaching/Discharge Considerations):

- Encourage client/SO(s) to evaluate impact of ventilatory dependence on their lifestyle and what changes they are willing or unwilling to make, when client is discharged on ventilator.

Quality-of-life issues must be examined and resolved by the ventilator dependent client and SO(s); all parties need to understand that ventilatory support is a 24-hour job that ultimately affects everyone.[1] Findings may dictate alternative placement such as foster care or extended-care facility.

🏠 • Discuss importance of time for self and identify appropriate sources for respite care. *Initially, caregivers have limited understanding of the magnitude of the demands on their time and energy. Knowing support is available enhances coping abilities.* Refer to ND risk for Caregiver Role Strain.

🏠 • Emphasize to client/SO(s) importance of monitoring health of visitors and persons involved in care, avoiding crowds during flu season, obtaining immunizations, and so forth, *to protect client from sources of infection.*

⚕ • Engage in rehabilitation program *to enhance respiratory muscle strength and general endurance.*

🏠 • Encourage client/SO(s) to discuss advance directives. *Clarifies parameters for termination of therapy or other end-of-life decisions, as desired.*

🏠 • Recommend involvement in support group; introduce to other ventilator-dependent individuals who are successfully managing home ventilation, if desired, *to answer questions, provide role model, assist with problem-solving, and offer encouragement and hope for the future.*

⚕ • Identify conditions requiring immediate medical intervention *to treat developing complications and prevent respiratory failure.*

DOCUMENTATION FOCUS

Assessment/Reassessment
• Baseline findings and subsequent alterations.
• Results of diagnostic testing and procedures.
• Individual risk factors.

Planning
• Plan of care, specific interventions, and who is involved in the planning.
• Teaching plan.

Implementation/Evaluation
• Client response to interventions.
• Attainment or progress toward desired outcome(s).
• Modifications to plan of care.

Discharge Planning
• Status at discharge, long-term needs and referrals, indicating who is to be responsible for each action.
• Equipment needs and supplier.

References

1. Tasota, F. J., Dobbin, K. (2000). Weaning your patient from mechanical ventilation. *Nursing*, 30(10), 41.
2. Weaning from mechanical ventilation: Protocols and beyond. Retrieved August 2007 from www.ed4nurse.com/weaning.htm.
3. MacIntyre, N. R., et al. (2001). Evidence-based guidelines for weaning and discontinuation of ventilatory support. A collective task force facilitated by the American College of Chest Physicians; the American Association for Respiratory Care; and the American College of Critical Care Medicine. *Chest*, 120(6 suppl), 385S–484S.

4. Doenges, M. E., Moorhouse, M. F., Geissler-Murr, A. C. (2002). CP: Ventilatory assistance (mechanical). *Nursing Care Plans: Guidelines for Individualizing Patient Care.* 6th ed. Philadelphia: F. A. Davis, 167–179.
5. Frakes, M. A. (2001). Measuring end-tidal carbon dioxide: Clinical applications and usefulness. *Crit Care Nurse*, 21(5), 23–35.
6. Henneman, E. A. (2001). Liberating patients from mechanical ventilation: A team approach. *Crit Care Nurse*, 21(3), 25–33.
7. Iregui, M., et al. (2002). Determinants of outcome for patients admitted to a long-term ventilator unit. *South Med J*, 95(3), 310–317.
8. Douglas, S. L., Daly, B. J. (2003). Caregivers of long-term ventilator patients: Physical and psychological outcomes. *Chest*, 123, 1073–1081.
9. Forrette, T. L. (2006). Transitioning from mechanical ventilation. Retrieved May 2007 from www.medscape.com/viewprogram/5230_pnt.
10. McLean, S. E., et al. (2006). Improving adherence to a mechanical ventilation weaning protocol for critically ill adults: Outcomes after an implementation program. *Am J Crit Care*, 15(3), 299–309.
11. Burns, S. M. (2005). Mechanical ventilation of clients with acute respiratory distress syndrome and patents requiring weaning: The evidence guiding practice. *Crit Care Nurse*, 25(4), 14–24.
12. Epstein, C. D., Peerless, J. R. (2006). Weaning readiness and fluid balance in older critically ill surgical clients. *Am J of Crit Care*, 15(1), 54–64.

risk for[/actual] other-directed Violence

DEFINITION: At risk for behaviors in which an individual demonstrates that he or she can be physically, emotionally, or sexually harmful to others

RISK FACTORS[/INDICATORS] FOR OTHER-DIRECTED VIOLENCE*

History of:

Violence against others (e.g., hitting, kicking, scratching, biting, or spitting; throwing objects at someone; attempted rape, rape, sexual molestation; urinating/defecating on a person)

Threats (e.g., verbal threats against property/person, social threats, cursing, threatening notes/letters, threatening gestures, sexual threats)

Violent antisocial behavior (e.g., stealing, insistent borrowing, insistent demands for privileges, insistent interruption of meetings; refusal to eat/take medication, ignoring instructions)

Indirect violence (e.g., tearing off clothes, urinating/defecating on floor, stamping feet, temper tantrum, running in corridors, yelling, writing on walls, ripping objects off walls, throwing objects, breaking a window, slamming doors, sexual advances)

History of childhood abuse or witnessing family violence

[Although a risk diagnosis does not have defining characteristics (signs and symptoms), the factors identified here can be used to denote an actual diagnosis or as indicators of risk for/escalation of violence.]

🌐 Cultural 👥 Collaborative 🏠 Community/Home Care ✎ Diagnostic Studies ∞ Pediatric/Geriatric/Lifespan 💊 Medications

Neurological impairment (e.g., positive electroencephalogram [EEG], computed tomography [CT], or magnetic resonance imaging [MRI]; neurological findings; head trauma; seizure disorders)

Cognitive impairment (e.g., learning disabilities, attention deficit disorder, decreased intellectual functioning); [organic brain syndrome]

Cruelty to animals; fire-setting

Prenatal or perinatal complications

History of substance abuse; pathological intoxication; [toxic reaction to medication]

Psychotic symptomatology (e.g., auditory, visual, command hallucinations; paranoid delusions; loose, rambling, or illogical thought processes); [panic states; rage reactions; catatonic or manic excitement]

Motor vehicle offenses (e.g., frequent traffic violations, use of a motor vehicle to release anger)

Suicidal behavior; impulsivity; availability of weapon(s)

Body language (e.g., rigid posture, clenching of fists and jaw, hyperactivity, pacing, breathlessness, threatening stances)

[Hormonal imbalance (e.g., premenstrual syndrome—PMS, postpartal depression or psychosis)]

[Expressed intent or desire to harm others directly or indirectly]

[Almost continuous thoughts of violence]

Sample Clinical Applications: Psychotic conditions (e.g., schizophrenia, paranoia), antisocial personality disorder, dementia, substance abuse (e.g., phencyclidine [PCP], delirium tremens), postpartum psychosis, premenstrual syndrome [PMS], brain injured

NANDA has separated the diagnosis of Violence into its two elements: "directed at others" and "self-directed." However, the interventions in general address both situations and have been left in one block following the definition and supporting data of the two diagnoses.

risk for[/actual] self-directed Violence

DEFINITION: At risk for behaviors in which an individual demonstrates that he or she can be physically, emotionally, or sexually harmful to self

RISK FACTORS[/INDICATORS] FOR SELF-DIRECTED VIOLENCE

Age 15 to 19; over 45

Marital status (single, widowed, divorced)

Employment problems (e.g., unemployed, recent job loss/failure); occupation (executive, administrator/owner of business, professional, semiskilled worker)

Conflictual interpersonal relationships

Family background (e.g., chaotic or conflictual, history of suicide)

Sexual orientation (bisexual [active], homosexual [inactive])

Physical health problems (e.g., hypochondriac, chronic or terminal illness)

Mental health problems (e.g., severe depression, [bipolar disorder] psychosis, severe personality disorder, alcoholism or drug abuse)

(continues on page 920)

risk for[/actual] self-directed Violence (continued)

Emotional problems (e.g., hopelessness, [lifting of depressed mood], despair, increased anxiety, panic, anger, hostility); history of multiple suicide attempts; suicidal ideation; suicidal plan

Lack of personal resources (e.g., poor achievement, poor insight, affect unavailable and poorly controlled)

Lack of social resources (e.g., poor rapport, socially isolated, unresponsive family)

Verbal clues (e.g., talking about death, "better off without me," asking questions about lethal dosages of drugs)

Behavioral clues (e.g., writing forlorn love notes, directing angry messages at a significant other who has rejected the person, giving away personal items, taking out a large life insurance policy)

NOTE: A risk diagnosis is not evidenced by signs and symptoms, as the problem has not occurred; rather, nursing interventions are directed at prevention.

Sample Clinical Applications: Major depression, postpartum depression/psychosis, Munchausen syndrome, psychosis, substance abuse (e.g., phencyclidine [PCP]), abuse or neglect

DESIRED OUTCOMES/EVALUATION CRITERIA (FOR OTHER-/SELF-DIRECTED VIOLENCE)

Sample **NOC** linkages:

Aggression Self-Control: Self-restraint of assaultive, combative, or destructive behaviors toward others

Abusive Behavior Self-Restraint: Self-restraint of abusive and neglectful behaviors toward others

Impulse Self-Control: Self-restraint of compulsive or impulsive behaviors

Depression Self-Control: Personal actions to minimize melancholy and maintain interest in life events

Client Will (Include Specific Time Frame)
• Acknowledge realities of the situation.
• Verbalize understanding of why behavior occurs.
• Identify precipitating factors in individual situation.
• Express realistic self-evaluation and increased sense of self-esteem.
• Participate in care and meet own needs in an assertive manner.
• Demonstrate self-control as evidenced by relaxed posture, nonviolent behavior or verbalizations.
• Use resources and support systems in an effective manner.

ACTIONS/INTERVENTIONS (ADDRESSES BOTH OTHER- AND SELF-DIRECTED)

Sample **NIC** linkages:

Anger Control Assistance: Facilitation of the expression of anger in an adaptive, nonviolent manner

Environmental Management: Violence Prevention: Monitoring and manipulation of the physical environment to decrease the potential for violent behavior directed toward self, others, or environment

Behavior Modification: Self-Harm: Assisting the patient to decrease or eliminate self-mutilating or self-abusive behavior

NURSING PRIORITY NO. 1

To assess causative/contributing factors:

- Determine underlying dynamics as listed in Risk Factors.
- Identify conditions, such as acute or chronic brain syndrome, panic state, hormonal imbalance, premenstrual syndrome (PMS), postpartum psychosis, drug-induced psychotic states, postanesthesial or postseizure confusion *that may interfere with ability to control own behavior and lead to violent episodes.*[1,13]
- Review laboratory findings (e.g., blood alcohol, blood glucose, arterial blood gases [ABGs], electrolytes, renal function tests). *Provides information about possible treatable sources of behavior.*[2,6]
- Ascertain client's perception of self and situation. Note use of defense mechanisms. *Individuals who are prone to violent behavior may see themselves as victims (denial), blaming others (projection), not following social norms, and impulsive.*[1]
- Observe and listen for early cues of distress or increasing anxiety. *Behaviors, such as irritability, lack of cooperation, demanding behavior, body posture or expression may signal escalating potential for violent behavior and need for immediate intervention.*[16]
- Observe for signs of suicidal or homicidal intent. *Perceived morbid or anxious feelings while with the client; warning from the client, "It doesn't matter," "I'd/They'd be better off dead"; mood swings; "accident-prone" or self-destructive behavior; possession of alcohol or other drug(s) in known substance abuser needs to be noted, taken seriously, and treated appropriately.*[1,6,9] Refer to ND risk for Suicide.
- Note family history of suicidal or homicidal behavior. *Dynamics in family of origin and current family, parental deprivation or abuse in the early years of an individual's life may contribute to violent behavior in current situation as individual uses violence as a means of solving problems.*[1,9,10]
- Ask directly if the person is thinking of acting on thoughts or feelings. *Can determine reality and urgency of violent intent and importance of immediate intervention.*[6,11]
- Determine availability of suicidal or homicidal means. *Identifies urgency of situation and need to intervene by removing lethal means, possibly hospitalizing client, or instituting other measures to ensure safety of client and others.*[1,6,8]
- Assess client coping behaviors. *Client believes there are no alternatives other than violence and has been dealing with frustration and anger in unacceptable ways (yelling, hitting, other violent behaviors) and needs to learn alternative coping skills.*[1,9]
- Identify risk factors and assess for indicators of child abuse or neglect (e.g., unexplained or frequent injuries, failure to thrive). *Visible evidence of physical abuse or neglect makes it more easily recognized; however, behaviors of withdrawal, acting out may also signal the presence of abuse.*[6,9,12]
- Determine presence, extent, and acceptance of violence in the client's culture. *Youth violence has become a national concern with widely publicized school shootings and an increase in arrests of both boys and girls for violent crimes and weapons violations. Young people who are at risk for violence need to be identified, and positive programs aimed at promoting emotional wellness need to be instituted in schools, parent education meetings, churches, and community centers.*[3,7,12]

NURSING PRIORITY NO. 2

To assist client to accept responsibility for impulsive behavior and potential for violence:

- Develop therapeutic nurse-client relationship. Provide consistent caregiver when possible. *Promotes sense of trust, allowing client to discuss feelings openly and to begin to identify sources of anger and more acceptable ways of dealing with it.*[1,6]

- Maintain straightforward communication. *Avoids reinforcing manipulative behavior. Manipulation is used for management of powerlessness because of distrust of others, fear of loss of power or control, fear of intimacy, and search for approval.*[4,6]
- Discuss motivation for change (e.g., failing relationships, job loss, involvement with judicial system). *Crisis situation can provide impetus for change but requires timely therapeutic intervention to sustain efforts.*[7,8]
- Make time to listen to expressions of feelings. Acknowledge reality of client's feelings and that feelings are okay. (Refer to ND Self-Esteem, specify.) *Promotes understanding of how feelings lead to actions and that individual is responsible for controlling behavior in acceptable ways.*[5,6]
- Help client recognize that own actions may be in response to own fear (may be afraid of own behavior, loss of control), dependency, and feeling of powerlessness. *Promotes understanding of self and ability to deal with feelings in acceptable ways.*[6,14]
- Confront client's tendency to minimize situation or behavior. *Individuals often want to say that things "are not as bad" as portrayed or "It was just a small argument" and "I didn't think I hit her (or him) that hard." By confronting this minimalization, the reality of the situation can be brought out and discussed, leading to better understanding of the situation and changes in behavior.*[1,6,11]
- Identify feelings or events (e.g., individual's view of self, hallucinations, individual/family or peer conflict, aggressive behavior) involved in precipitating violent behavior. *By identifying the factors involved in current situation, an appropriate plan can be made to change actions to prevent future violent behavior.*[1,7,11]
- Discuss impact of behavior on others and consequences of actions. *Discussing these issues openly can help client to develop empathy and understand other person's reactions and begin to change behaviors that can lead to violence.*[5,8]
- Acknowledge reality of suicide or homicide as an option. Discuss consequences of actions if they were to follow through on intent. Ask how it will help client to resolve problems. *Acknowledging the reality of individual's thoughts provides opportunity to look at how actions would affect others, ability to control own behavior, and make choices to live and make a better life for self.*[6,12]
- Accept client's anger without reacting on emotional basis. Give permission to express angry feelings in acceptable ways and let client know that staff will be available to assist in maintaining control. *Promotes acceptance and sense of safety. Client's anger is usually directed at the situation and not at the caregiver, and by remaining separate, the therapist can be more helpful for resolution of the anger.*[6,9]
- Help client identify more appropriate solutions/behaviors. *Motor activities or exercise can lessen sense of anxiety and associated physical manifestations, thus diminishing feelings of anger.*[8]
- Provide directions for actions client can take, avoiding negatives, such as "do nots." *Discussing positive ideas to help client begin to look toward a better future can provide hope that violent behaviors can be changed, promoting feelings of self-worth and belief in control of own self.*[5,14]

NURSING PRIORITY NO. 3

To assist client in controlling behavior:

- Contract with client regarding safety of self/others. *Making a contract in which the individual agrees to refrain from any violent behavior for a specified period of time, from day one through the entire course of treatment, and written and signed by each party may help the client to follow through with therapy to find more effective ways of resolving conflict.*

Cultural   Collaborative   Community/Home Care   Diagnostic Studies   Pediatric/Geriatric/Lifespan   Medications

Although there is little research on the effectiveness of these contracts, they are frequently used.[6,7]

- Give client as much control as possible within constraints of individual situation. *Because control issues are a factor in violent behavior, giving client control in appropriate ways can enhance self-esteem, promote confidence in ability to change behavior.*[7]
- Be truthful when giving information and dealing with individual. *Builds trust, enhancing therapeutic relationship, and prevents manipulative behavior.*[5]
- Identify current and past successes and strengths. Discuss effectiveness of coping techniques used and possible changes. Refer to ND ineffective Coping. *Client is often not aware of positive aspects of life, and once recognized, they can be used as a basis for change.*[8]
- Give positive reinforcement for client's efforts. *Encourages continuation of desired behaviors.*[1]
- Assist client to distinguish between reality and hallucinations or delusions. *Violent behavior in clients with major mental disorders (schizophrenia, mania) may be in response to command hallucinations and may require more aggressive treatment or hospitalization until behavior is under control.*[1,6]
- Approach in positive manner, acting as if the client has control and is responsible for own behavior. Be aware, though, that the client may not have control, especially if under the influence of drugs (including alcohol). *Individuals will often respond to a positive expectation, reducing threatening actions. Staff needs to be trained in management of this behavior and be prepared to take control of the situation if client is out of control.*[1,6]
- Maintain distance and do not touch client when situation indicates client does not tolerate such closeness. *Individuals who have experienced traumatic events, such as rape, or suffer from posttrauma response may fear close contact even with trusted persons.*[1,6]
- Remain calm and state limits on inappropriate behavior (including consequences) in a firm manner. *Calm manner enables client to de-escalate anger, and knowing what the consequences will be gives an opportunity to choose to change behavior and deal appropriately with situation. Consequences need to be decided beforehand and agreed to by client, or they may sound like punishment and be counterproductive.*[1,6,13]
- Direct client to stay in view of staff. *Intervention may be needed to maintain safety of client and others.*[1,6] Refer to ND risk for Suicide.
- Administer prescribed medications (e.g., anti-anxiety or antipsychotic), taking care not to oversedate client. *May be least restrictive way to help client control violent behaviors while learning new coping skills to handle anger and impulsive behavior. The chemistry of the brain is changed by early violence and has been shown to respond to serotonin as well as related neurotransmitter systems, which play a role in restraining aggressive impulses.*[1,6,9]
- Monitor for possible drug interactions, cumulative effects of drug regimen (e.g., anticonvulsants, antidepressants). *May be contributing factor in violent behavior.*[1,6]

NURSING PRIORITY NO. 4

To assist client/SO(s) to correct/deal with existing situation:

- Gear interventions to individual(s) involved, based on age, relationship, and so forth. *Conflict resolution skills can be learned by all age groups when age-appropriate materials are used.*[5,8]
- Maintain calm, matter-of-fact, nonjudgmental attitude. *Decreases defensive response, allowing individual to think about own responsibility in the conflict and choose positive behaviors instead of usual angry reaction.*[4,5,8]
- Notify potential victims in the presence of serious homicidal threat in accordance with legal and ethical guidelines. *Various Tarasoff statutes exist in many states requiring therapists/ healthcare providers to report specific threats to both the individual named and law*

enforcement when client expresses homicidal intent overtly or covertly in addition to helping the client realize that the proposed action is not wise or in his or her own best interest.[1]

- Discuss situation with abused or battered person, providing accurate information about choices and effective actions that can be taken. *Promotes understanding of options, giving hope and support for planning for a violence-free future.*[2]
- Assist individual to understand that angry, vengeful feelings are appropriate in the situation and need to be expressed but not acted on. (Refer to ND Post-Trauma Syndrome, as psychological responses may be very similar.) *Helps client accept feelings as natural and begin to learn effective coping skills, and promotes sense of control over situation.*[2,11]
- Identify resources available for assistance (e.g., battered women's shelter, social services, financial). *Helps client to manage immediate needs such as food, shelter, and safety with a long-range goal of attaining or maintaining independence and violence-free life.*[2]

NURSING PRIORITY NO. 5

To promote safety in event of violent behavior:

- Provide a safe, quiet environment and remove items from the client's environment that could be used to inflict harm to self/others. *Reducing stimuli can help client to calm down, and removing articles provides for safety of client and staff.*[1,6]
- Maintain distance from client who is striking out or hitting and take evasive or controlling actions, as indicated. *Staff safety is of prime importance, and avoiding physical confrontation until client regains control or takedown team is assembled can prevent injury.*[6]
- Call for additional staff/security personnel. *Having sufficient people available to handle the situation may defuse client's anger, allowing situation to calm down without further action. All personnel need to be trained in takedown techniques.*[6]
- Approach aggressive or attacking client from the front, just out of reach, in a commanding posture with palms down. *Safety is a prime concern, and these actions may defuse the situation.*[6]
- Tell client *"Stop"* in a firm voice. *This may be sufficient to help client control own actions.*[6]
- Maintain direct and constant eye contact when appropriate. *Assists in identifying client's intentions and conveys sense of caring. Eye contact may be perceived as threatening, so it needs to be used cautiously.*[2,6]
- Speak in a low, commanding voice. *Tone of voice conveys message of control and concern and can help to calm the client's anger.*[6]
- Provide client with a sense that caregiver is in control of the situation. *Client is feeling out of control, and seeing that staff are in control provides a feeling of safety.*[6]
- Maintain clear route for staff and client and be prepared to move quickly. *Safety for all is of prime importance, and staff may need to leave the room to regroup while continuing to protect the client. Takedown needs to be done quickly to gain control of the individual.*[6]
- Hold client, using restraints or seclusion when necessary until client regains self-control. *Brief period of physical restraint may be required until client regains control or other therapeutic interventions take effect.*[6]
- Administer medication, as indicated. *Client may require chemical restraint until control is regained.*[1,6]
- Discuss event with client after situation is calmed down and control is regained. *Helping client to understand how feelings of anger had gotten out of control and what can be done to prevent a recurrence can provide a learning opportunity for the individual.*[2,6]

NURSING PRIORITY NO. 6

To promote wellness (Teaching/Discharge Considerations):

- Promote client involvement in planning care within limits of situation, allowing for meeting own needs for enjoyment. *Individuals often believe they are not entitled to pleasure and good things in their lives and need to learn how to meet these needs in acceptable ways.*[6,14]
- Assist client to learn assertive behaviors. *Manipulative, nonassertive, or aggressive behaviors lead to anger, which can result in violence. Learning assertiveness skills can facilitate change, increase self-esteem, and promote interpersonal relationships.*[1,14]
- Provide information about conflict-resolution skills and help client learn how to use them effectively. *Conflict is always present in human relationships, and learning how to manage conflict is one of the most important tools we can use to solve disagreements and improve relationships.*[4,5,8]
- Discuss reasons for client's behavior with SO(s). Determine desire and commitment of involved parties to sustain current relationships. *Family members may believe individual is purposefully behaving in angry ways, and understanding underlying reasons for behavior can defuse feelings of anger on their part, leading to willingness to resolve problems.*[1,4]
- Develop strategies to help parents learn more effective parenting skills. *Participating in parenting classes and learning appropriate ways of dealing with frustrations can improve family relationships and prevent angry interactions and the possibility of violent behavior.*[4,5]
- Identify support systems. *Presence of family/friends, clergy who can serve as mentors, listen to individual nonjudgmentally, can help client defuse angry feelings and learn appropriate ways of dealing with them.*[1] *Note: Not just the client needs help, but those around them need to learn how to provide positive role models and display a broader array of skills for resolving problems.*
- Refer to formal resources, as indicated. *May need individual or group psychotherapy, substance abuse treatment program, anger management class, social services, safe house to facilitate change.*[1]
- Promote violence prevention and emotional literacy programs in the schools and community. *These programs are based on the premise that intelligent management of emotions is critical to successful living. Aggressive youth lack skills in arousal management and nonviolent problem-solving, which can be learned in programs and reinforced by the adults in their lives.*[7,12,14]
- Refer to NDs impaired Parenting, family Coping, [specify]; Post-Trauma Syndrome.

DOCUMENTATION FOCUS

Assessment/Reassessment
- Individual findings, including nature of concern (e.g., suicidal, homicidal), behavioral risk factors, and level of impulse control, plan of action and means to carry out plan.
- Client's perception of situation, motivation for change.
- Family history of violence.
- Availability and use of resources.

Planning
- Plan of care and who is involved in the planning.
- Details of contract regarding violence to self/others.
- Teaching plan.

Implementation/Evaluation
- Actions taken to promote safety, including notification of parties at risk.
- Response to interventions, teaching, and actions performed.

• Attainment or progress toward desired outcome(s).
• Modifications to plan of care.

Discharge Planning
• Long-term needs and who is responsible for actions to be taken.
• Available resources, specific referrals made.

References

1. Townsend, M. C. (2003). *Psychiatric Mental Health Nursing Concepts of Care*. 4th ed. Philadelphia: F. A. Davis.
2. Cox, H. C., et al. (2002). *Clinical Applications of Nursing Diagnosis: Adult, Child, Women's, Psychiatric, Gerontic, and Home Health Considerations*. 4th ed. Philadelphia: F. A. Davis.
3. Lipson, J. G., Dibble, S. L., Minarik, P. A. (1996). *Culture & Nursing Care: A Pocket Guide*. San Francisco: UCSF Nursing Press.
4. Gordon, T. (1989). *Teaching Children Self-Discipline: At Home and At School*. New York: Random House.
5. Gordon, T. (2000). *Family Effectiveness Training Video*. Solana Beach, CA: Gordon Training International.
6. Doenges, M. E., Townsend, M. C., Moorhouse, M. F. (1998). *Psychiatric Care Plans: Guidelines for Individualizing Care*. 3d ed. Philadelphia: F. A. Davis.
7. Thomas, S. P. (2003). Identifying and intervening with girls at risk for violence. *J School Nurs*, 19(3), 130–139.
8. Porter-O'Grady, T. (2003). Managing conflict in the workplace. *NSNA/Imprint*, 48(4), 66–68.
9. Goleman, D. (October 3, 1995). Early violence leaves its mark on the brain. *New York Times*. Retrieved August 2007 from www.cirp.org/library/psych/goleman/.
10. What is neuroscience? (2007). Society for Neuroscience. Retrieved August 2007 from www.sfn.org/index.cfm?pagename=whatIsNeuroscience.
11. Cooper, S. Sylvia's inquiry into violence and the brain. Retrieved August 2007 from http://serendip.brynmawr.edu/local/suminst/bbi01/projects/cooper/.
12. Hyman, S. E. (August 3, 1998; updated 1999). Thinking about violence in our schools, discussion at the White House. National Institute of Mental Health. Retrieved August 2007 from www.medhelp.org/NIHlib/GF-376.html.
13. Eby, N., Car, M. (2004). Violence and brain injuries. Quality Matters. Brain Injury Association of Montana. Retrieved August 2007 from www.biamt.org/publications/violence.htm.
14. Goleman, D. (2006). *Emotional Intelligence Why It Matters More Than IQ*. 10th Anniversary ed. New York: Bantam.

impaired Walking

DEFINITION: Limitation of independent movement within the environment on foot (Note: Specify level of independence using a standardized functional scale.)

RELATED FACTORS

Insufficient muscle strength; neuromuscular impairment; musculoskeletal impairment (e.g., contractures)
Limited endurance; deconditioning
Fear of falling; impaired balance
Impaired vision
Pain

Obesity
Depressed mood; cognitive impairment
Lack of knowledge
Environmental constraints (e.g., stairs, inclines, uneven surfaces, unsafe obstacles, distances, lack of assistive devices or persons, restraints)

DEFINING CHARACTERISTICS

Subjective or Objective
Impaired ability to walk required distances, walk on an incline or decline, walk on uneven surfaces, navigate curbs, climb stairs

Sample Clinical Applications: Arthritis, obesity, amputation, brain injury, stroke, traumatic injury, fractures, chronic pain, peripheral vascular disease (PVD), spinal nerve compression, multiple sclerosis (MS), cerebral palsy, Parkinson's disease, macular degeneration, dementia

DESIRED OUTCOMES/EVALUATION CRITERIA

Sample NOC linkages:
Ambulation: Ability to walk from place to place independently with or without assistive device
Mobility: Ability to move purposefully in own environment independently with or without assistive device
Balance: Ability to maintain body equilibrium

Client Will (Include Specific Time Frame)
• Be able to move about within environment as needed or desired within limits of ability or with appropriate adjuncts.
• Verbalize understanding of situation, risk factors, and safety measures.

ACTIONS/INTERVENTIONS

Sample NIC linkages:
Exercise Therapy: Ambulation: Promotion and assistance with walking to maintain or restore autonomic and voluntary body functions during treatment and recovery from illness or injury
Body Mechanics Promotion: Facilitating the use of posture and movement in daily activities to prevent fatigue and musculoskeletal strain or injury
Exercise Therapy: Balance: Use of specific activities, postures, and movements to maintain, enhance, or restore balance
Refer also to NDs impaired Mobility [specify] for additional assessments and interventions.

NURSING PRIORITY NO. 1

To assess causative/contributing factors:

● Identify conditions or diagnoses (e.g., advanced age, vision impairments, pain, chronic fatigue, cognitive dysfunction, acute illness with weakness, *chronic illness* [e.g., cardiopulmonary disorders, cancer], musculoskeletal injuries [e.g., fractures, tendon or ligament injury, amputation], *balance problems* [e.g., inner ear infection, brain injury, stroke], *nerve disorders* [e.g., MS, Parkinson's disease, cerebral palsy], *spinal abnormalities* [disease, trauma, degeneration], *neuropathies* [e.g., peripheral, diabetic, alcoholic], *degenerative muscle disorders* [e.g., muscular dystrophy, myositis], *foot conditions* [e.g., plantar warts, bunions, ingrown toenails, pressure ulcers]) *that contribute to walking impairment and identify specific needs and appropriate interventions.*[1-10]

- Determine ability to follow directions and presence of emotional or behavioral responses *that may be affecting client's ability or desire to engage in activity.*
- Note client's particular symptoms (e.g., unable to bear weight, can't walk usual distance, limping, staggering, stiff leg, leg pain, shuffling, asymmetric or unsteady gait). *Influences choice of interventions.*[7,10,11]

NURSING PRIORITY NO. 2

To assess functional ability:

- Perform "Get Up and Go" test, as indicated, to assess client's basic ability to ambulate safely. Factors assessed include sitting balance, ability to transfer from sitting to standing and back to sitting, the pace and stability of ambulation, and the ability to turn without staggering. Additional testing is indicated for individuals requiring more than 20 seconds to complete the test.[12]
- Determine muscle strength and tone, joint mobility, cardiovascular status, balance, endurance, and use of assistive device. *Identifies strengths and deficits (e.g., ability to ambulate with/without assistive devices) and may provide information regarding potential for recovery (e.g., client with severe brain injury may have permanent limitations because of impaired cognition affecting memory, judgment, problem-solving and motor planning, requiring more intensive inpatient and long-term care).*
- Note whether impairment is temporary or permanent. *Condition may be caused by reversible condition (e.g., weakness associated with acute illness or fractures/surgery with weight-bearing restrictions); or walking impairment can be permanent (e.g., congenital anomalies, amputation, severe rheumatoid arthritis).*[1,8]
- Assist with or review results of mobility testing (e.g., timing of walking over fixed distance, distance walked over set period of time [endurance], limb movement analysis, leg strength and speed of walking, ambulatory activity monitoring) *for differential diagnosis and to guide treatment interventions.*[11,12]
- Note emotional or behavioral responses of client/SO to problems of mobility. *Can negatively affect self-concept and self-esteem, autonomy, and independence. Social, occupational, and relationship roles can change, leading to isolation, depression, and economic consequences.*[8,9]

NURSING PRIORITY NO. 3

To promote safe, optimal level of independence in walking:

- Assist with treatment of underlying condition as needed or indicated by individual situation. *Treatment can often reverse or limit dysfunction.*
- Consult with physical therapist, occupational therapist, or rehabilitation team *to develop individual program (e.g., to improve general conditioning, coordination and balance, range-of-motion exercises, specific muscle strengthening), to instruct in specific tasks (e.g., stair-climbing or gait-training), and to identify and develop appropriate adjunctive devices (e.g., shoe insert, leg brace for proper foot alignment; customized cane, crutches, or walker).*[2]

- Monitor client's cardiopulmonary tolerance for walking. *Increased pulse rate, chest pain, breathlessness, irregular heartbeat is indicative of need to reduce level of activity.* Refer to ND Activity Intolerance; decreased Cardiac Output for related interventions.
- Encourage adequate rest and gradual increase in walking *to reduce fatigue or leg pain associated with walking and improve stamina.*[6,7] Refer to NDs Fatigue; risk for Peripheral Neurovascular Dysfunction.
- Administer medication, as indicated, *to manage pain and maximize level of functioning.* Refer to NDs acute/chronic Pain.
- Implement fall precautions for high-risk clients (e.g., frail or ill elderly, visually or cognitively impaired, person on multiple medications, presence of balance disorders) *to reduce risk of accidental injury.*[1,6] Refer to NDs risk for Falls; risk for Disuse Syndrome for related interventions.
- Instruct in proper application of prostheses, immobilizers (e.g., walking cast or boot), and braces before walking *to maintain joint stability or immobilization or to maintain alignment during movement.*[3,4]
- Demonstrate and remind client to properly use assistive devices (e.g., cane, crutches, walker) *prescribed to improve balance, reduce limb pain and dysfunction, and provide support during ambulation.*[2]
- Use adequate personnel and safety devices (e.g., gait belt, nonslip shoes, handrail) when ambulating *to prevent injury to client or caregivers.*[2,6]
- Limit distractions, provide safe environment. *Allows client to concentrate on walking activities or learning use of assistive devices.*[2]
- Provide cueing as indicated. *Client may need reminders (e.g., lift foot higher, look where going, walk tall) to concentrate on/perform tasks of walking, especially when balance or cognition is impaired.*[5]
- Provide ample time to perform mobility-related tasks *to reduce risk of falling and manage fatigue or pain.*
- Provide positive, constructive feedback *to encourage continuation of efforts and enhance client's self-sufficiency.*[6]
- Assist client to obtain needed information, such as handicapped sticker for close-in parking, sources for mobility scooter, or special public transportation options, when indicated, *to deal with temporary or permanent disability access.*

NURSING PRIORITY NO. 4

To promote wellness (Teaching/Discharge Considerations):

- Evaluate client's home (or work) environment for barriers to walking (e.g., uneven surfaces, many steps, no ramps, long distances between places client needs to walk) *to determine needed changes, make recommendations for client safety.*
- Involve client/SO in problem-solving, assisting them to learn ways of managing deficits, *to enhance safety for client with long-term or permanent impairments.*
- Encourage participation in regular active and passive exercise program. Advance levels of exercise, as able, *to improve muscle tone and strength, and increase stamina and endurance.*
- Discuss appropriate use of electric scooter, if indicated. *Enhances mobility, especially over distances to maintain independence and socialization.*
- Identify appropriate resources for obtaining and maintaining appliances, equipment, and environmental modifications *to promote safe mobility.*
- Instruct client/SO in safety measures in home, as individually indicated (e.g., maintaining safe travel pathway, proper lighting, wearing glasses, handrails on stairs, grab bars in

bathroom, using walker instead of cane when sleepy or walking on uneven surface) *to reduce risk of falls.*

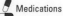 • Discuss need for emergency call/support system (e.g., Lifeline, HealthWatch) *to provide immediate assistance for falls, other home emergencies when client lives alone.*

DOCUMENTATION FOCUS

Assessment/Reassessment
• Individual findings, including level of function and ability to participate in specific or desired activities.
• Equipment and assistive device needs.

Planning
• Plan of care and who is involved in the planning.
• Teaching plan.

Implementation/Evaluation
• Responses to interventions, teaching, and actions performed.
• Attainment or progress toward desired outcome(s).
• Modifications to plan of care.

Discharge Planning
• Discharge and long-term needs, noting who is responsible for each action to be taken.
• Specific referrals made.
• Sources of and maintenance for assistive devices.

References

1. Doenges, M. E., Moorhouse, M. F., Geissler-Murr, A. C. (2002). ND: Walking impaired. *Nursing Care Plans: Guidelines for Individualizing Patient Care.* 6th ed. Philadelphia: F. A. Davis.
2. Kuang, T., Kedlaya, D. (2002, update 2007). Assistive devices to improve independence. Retrieved August 2007 from www.emedicine.com/pmr/topic210.htm.
3. Teplicky, R., Law, M., Russell, D. (2002). The effectiveness of casts, orthotics, and splints for children with neurological disorders. *Infants Young Child,* 15(1), 42–50.
4. Wilson, G. B. (1988). Progressive mobilization. In Sine, R. D., et al. (eds). *Basic Rehabilitation Techniques: A Self-Instructional Guide.* 3d ed. Gaithersburg, MD: Aspen.
5. Gee, Z. I., Passarella, P. M. (1985). *Nursing Care of the Stroke Patient: A Therapeutic Approach.* Pittsburgh, PA: AREN.
6. Jitramontree, N. (2001). *Evidence-Based Protocol. Exercise Promotion: Walking in Elders [Research Dissemination Core, 53].* Iowa City: University of Iowa Gerontological Nursing Interventions Research Center.
7. Eberhardt, R. T. (2002). Exercise for intermittent claudication: Walking for life? [Editorial]. *J Cardiopulm Rehabil,* 22(3), 199–200.
8. Mass, M. L. (1989). Impaired physical mobility. Unpublished manuscript. Cited in research article for National Institutes for Health.
9. Hogue, C. C. (1984). Falls and mobility late in life: An ecological model. *J Am Geriatr Soc,* 32, 858–861.
10. Symptom: Walking symptoms. Retrieved April 2007 from http://wrongdiagnosis.com/sym/walking_symptoms.htm.
11. Pearsen, O. R., Busse, M. E., van Deuresn, R. W. M. (2004). Quantification of walking mobility in neurological disorders. *Q J Med,* 97, 463–475.
12. Baer, H. R., Wolf, S. L. (2001). Modified Emory Functional Ambulation Profile: An outcome measure for the rehabilitation of poststroke gait dysfunction. *Stroke,* 32, 973–979.

Wandering [specify: sporadic or continual]

DEFINITION: Meandering, aimless, or repetitive locomotion that exposes the individual to harm; frequently incongruent with boundaries, limits, or obstacles

RELATED FACTORS

Cognitive impairment (e.g., memory and recall deficits, disorientation, poor visuoconstructive or visuospatial ability, language defects); sedation
Cortical atrophy
Premorbid behavior (e.g., outgoing, sociable personality; premorbid dementia)
Separation from familiar environment; overstimulating environment
Emotional state (e.g., frustration, anxiety, boredom, depression, agitation)
Physiological state or need (e.g., hunger, thirst, pain, urination, constipation)
Time of day

DEFINING CHARACTERISTICS

Objective
Frequent or continuous movement from place to place, often revisiting the same destinations
Persistent locomotion in search of something; scanning or searching behaviors
Haphazard locomotion; fretful locomotion or pacing; long periods of locomotion without an apparent destination
Locomotion into unauthorized or private spaces; trespassing
Locomotion resulting in unintended leaving of a premise
Inability to locate significant landmarks in a familiar setting; getting lost
Locomotion that cannot be easily dissuaded; shadowing a caregiver's locomotion
Hyperactivity
Periods of locomotion interspersed with periods of nonlocomotion (e.g., sitting, standing, sleeping)

Sample Clinical Applications: Brain injury, dementias, developmental delays, major depression, substance abuse, amnesia, fugue

DESIRED OUTCOMES/EVALUATION CRITERIA

Sample NOC linkage:
Physical Injury Severity: Severity of injuries from accidents and trauma

Client Will (Include Specific Time Frame)
• Be free of injury, or unplanned exits.

Sample NOC linkages:
Safe Home Environment: Physical arrangements to minimize environmental factors that might cause physical harm or injury in the home
Safe Wandering: Safe, socially acceptable moving about without apparent purpose in an individual with cognitive impairment

(continues on page 932)

Wandering (continued)

Caregiver(s) Will (Include Specific Time Frame)
• Modify environment, as indicated, to enhance safety.
• Provide for maximal independence of client.

ACTIONS/INTERVENTIONS

Sample (NIC) linkages:
Elopement Precautions: Minimizing the risk of a patient leaving a treatment setting without authorization when departure presents a threat to the safety of patient or others
Area Restriction: Limitation of patient mobility to a specified area for purposes of safety or behavior management
Environmental Management: Safety: Manipulation of the patient's surroundings for therapeutic benefit

NURSING PRIORITY NO. 1

To assess degree of impairment/stage of disease process:

• Ascertain history of client's memory loss and cognitive changes.
• Review responses of collaborative diagnostic examinations (e.g., cognition, functional capacity, behavior, memory impairments, reality orientation, general physical health and quality of life). *A combination of tests is often needed to complete an evaluation of client's overall condition relating to chronic or irreversible condition. These tests include (but are not limited to) Mini-Mental State Examination (MMSE), Alzheimer's Disease Assessment Scale cognitive subsection (ADAS-cog), Functional Assessment Questionnaire (FAQ), Clinical Global Impression of Change (CGIC), Neuropsychiatric Inventory (NPI).*[1]
• Evaluate client's past history (e.g., individual was very active physically and socially or reacted to stress with physical activity rather than emotional reactions) *to help identify likelihood of wandering.*[2]
• Determine presence of depression. *Research supports the idea that wandering develops more often in depressed client with Alzheimer's disease.*[2]
• Evaluate client's mental status during both daytime and nighttime, noting when client's confusion is most pronounced and when and how long client sleeps. *Information about cognition and behavioral habits can reveal circumstances under which client is likely to wander.*[3]
• Identify client's reason for wandering, if possible. Client may demonstrate searching behavior (e.g., looking for lost item, pursuing certain unattainable activity), inexhaustible drive to do things and remain busy, or be experiencing sensations (e.g., hunger, thirst, or discomfort) without ability to express the actual need.[2]
• Determine bowel and bladder elimination pattern, timing of incontinence, presence of constipation *for possible correlation to wandering behavior.*
• Note timing and pattern of wandering behavior. *Client attempting to leave at 5:00 p.m. every day may believe he is going home from work; client may be goal directed (e.g., searching for person or object) or nongoal directed (wandering aimlessly). Knowledge of patterns can prompt caregivers to anticipate need for personal attention.*[3,6,8]
• Ascertain if client has delusions due to shadows, lights, and noises *to determine necessary changes to environment.*

🌐 Cultural 👥 Collaborative 🏠 Community/Home Care ⚗ Diagnostic Studies ∞ Pediatric/Geriatric/Lifespan 💊 Medications

- Evaluate usual travel patterns. *Activity may be (1) direct (from one location to another without diversion), (2) random (random direction with no obvious stopping point), (3) pacing (back and forth within limited area), or (4) lapping (circling large areas).*[2,6,7]
- Assist with or review results of specific testing (e.g., Algase Wandering Scale [AWS], Need-Driven Dementia-Compromised Behavior [NDB] or similar tool), as indicated. *Researchers are using adjunct tools for clinical assessment, which quantify wandering in several domains (as reported by caregivers) to determine individual risks and safety needs.*[2,7]
- Monitor client's need for and use of assistive devices, such as glasses, hearing aids, cane, safe walking shoes, comfortable clothing, and so forth. *Wandering client is at high risk for falls due to cognitive impairments and the fatigue related to functional decline or forgetting necessary assistive devices or how to properly use them.*[4]

NURSING PRIORITY NO. 2

To assist client/caregiver to deal with situations:

- Provide a structured daily routine:
  Encourage participation in family activities and familiar routines, such as folding laundry, listening to music, or shared-walking time outdoors. *Activities and exercises may reduce anxiety, depression, and restlessness. Note: Repetitive activity (e.g., rocking, folding laundry, or paperwork) may help client with "lapping," wandering to reduce energy expenditure and fatigue.*[3]
  Offer food, fluids, toileting on a regular schedule when client is unable to verbalize, *as agitation, pacing, or wandering may be associated with these basic needs.*[3]
  Sit with client and talk *when client is socially gregarious, enjoys conversation, or reminiscence is calming.*
  Provide television, radio or music, *which may be more effective than talking or reading to decrease wandering.*[1]
  Monitor activities, loud conversations, number of visitors at one time *to prevent overstimulation or increased agitation.*
  Remove items from immediate environment (e.g., coat, hat, keys) *to reduce stimulus for leaving the site.*[3]
- Provide safe place for client to wander:
  Remove environmental safety hazards such as hot water faucets, knobs on kitchen stove; gate or block open stairways, and so forth.[1-3]
  Keep area free of clutter, place comfortable furniture and other items against the wall or out of travel path *to accommodate safe walking and promote rest periods during times of continual lapping.*[1]
  Install safety locks or latches on doors and windows; *door latches are complex and less accessible;* equip exits with alarms (that are always turned on).[1-3]
  Provide for 24-hour supervision, as indicated. *Client can be awake at any time and fail to recognize day or night routines.*
- Register client with community and national resources such as SafeReturn Program administered by the Alzheimer's Association. *Program registers persons with dementia and operates a 24-hour help line to facilitate the return of lost persons (800-272-3900).*[5,6]
- Monitor activity when hospitalized or admitted to facility:
  Place in room near monitoring station; check client location on frequent basis.
  Assign consistent staff as much as possible.
  Create "Wanderer's lounge," or large safe walking area with inaccessible exits or outside gated area.[1-3]

Avoid overstimulation from activities or new partner/roommate during rest periods.

🏠 ● Use technology to promote safety:

Provide pressure-sensitive bed or chair alarms *to alert caregivers of movement, especially when client frequently gets up at night or when no one is present.*

Provide client ID bracelet or necklace with updated photograph, client name, and emergency contact *to assist with identification efforts, particularly when progressive dementia produces marked changes in client's appearance.*[3,5]

Obtain electronic locator devices *to find client when there is the potential for client to get lost or go missing.*[4,5]

Install verbal door alarm system. *Voice command is more effective at redirecting client and less likely to increase agitation than loud sound.*[1]

🏠 ● Use universal symbols, large-print signs, portrait-like photographs, pictures, and signs *to assist client in finding way, especially when client has diminished ability or has lost ability to read.*[3]

🏠 ● Avoid using physical or chemical restraints (sedatives) to control wandering behavior. *May increase agitation, sensory deprivation, and falls, and can aggravate wandering behavior.*

NURSING PRIORITY NO. 3

To promote wellness (Teaching/Discharge Considerations):

🏠 ● Identify problems that are remediable and assist client/SO to seek appropriate assistance and access resources. *Encourages problem-solving to improve condition rather than accept the status quo.*

🏠 ● Notify neighbors about client's condition and request that they contact client's family or local police if they see client outside alone. *Community awareness can prevent or reduce risk of client being lost or hurt.*

🏠 ● Help client/SO and family members develop plan of care when problem is progressive. *Client may initially need part-time assistance at home, progressing to enrollment in day-care program, then full-time home care or placement in care facility.*

🏠 ● Refer to community resources, such as day-care programs, support groups, respite care, and so forth. *Caregiver(s) will require access to multiple kinds of assistance and opportunities to promote problem-solving, enhance coping, and obtain necessary respite.*

● Refer to NDs acute/chronic Confusion; impaired Environmental Interpretation Syndrome; risk for Falls; risk for Injury; disturbed Sensory Perception (specify); impaired Thought Processes.

DOCUMENTATION FOCUS

Assessment/Reassessment
• Assessment findings, including individual concerns, family involvement, and support factors.
• Availability and use of resources.

Planning
• Plan of care and who is involved in planning.
• Teaching plan.

Implementation/Evaluation
• Responses of client/SO(s) to plan interventions and actions performed.
• Attainment or progress toward desired outcome(s).
• Modifications to plan of care.

Discharge Planning

• Long-term needs and who is responsible for actions to be taken.

• Specific referrals made.

References

1. About Alzheimer's (various educational materials). (2003). Physicians and Care Professionals. Retrieved August 2007 from www.alz.org.
2. Futrell, M., Melillo, K. D. (2002). Wandering: Evidence-based protocol. University of Iowa Gerontological Nursing Interventions Research Center, Research Dissemination Core. Retrieved August 2007 from www.guideline.gov/summary/summary.aspx?doc_id=3250.
3. Cox, H. C., et al. (2002). ND: Wandering. *Clinical Applications of Nursing Diagnosis: Adult, Child, Women's, Psychiatric, Gerontic, and Home Health Considerations*. 4th ed. Philadelphia: F. A. Davis.
4. Brody, E., et al. (1984). Predictors of falls among institutionalized females with Alzheimer's disease. *J Am Geriatr*, 32, 877–882.
5. Rowe, M. A. (2003). People with dementia who become lost. *Am J Nurs*, 103(7), 32–39.
6. Alzheimer's disease and related disorders SAR research: Wandering overview. Retrieved August 2007 from www.dbs-sar.com/SAR_Research/wandering.htm.
7. Algase, D. L., Beel-Bates, C., Beattie, E. (2003). Wandering in long term care. *Ann Long Term Care*, 11(1), 33–39.
8. Mayo Clinic Staff. (2005). Alzheimer's: Understand and control wandering. Retrieved May 2007 from www.mayoclinic.com/health/alzheimers/HQ00218.

CHAPTER 6

Health Conditions and Client Concerns With Associated Nursing Diagnoses

This chapter presents 850 disorders/health conditions and life situations reflecting all specialty areas, with associated nursing diagnoses written as client problem/need statements that include the "related to" and "evidenced by" components.

This section facilitates and helps validate the assessment and diagnosis steps of the nursing process. Because the nursing process is perpetual and ongoing, other nursing diagnoses may be appropriate based on changing individual situations. Therefore, the nurse must continually assess, identify, and validate new client needs and evaluate subsequent care.

To facilitate access to the health conditions/concerns and nursing diagnoses, the client needs are listed alphabetically and coded to identify nursing specialty areas.

MS: Medical-Surgical
PED: Pediatric
OB/GYN: Obstetric/Gynecological
CH: Community/Home
PSY: Psychiatric/Behavioral

There is no separate category for geriatrics because concerns and conditions in this population are subsumed under the other specialty areas and because elderly persons are susceptible to the majority of these problems.

Abdominal hysterectomy	MS

Refer to Hysterectomy

Abdominal perineal resection	MS

Also refer to Surgery, general

disturbed Body Image may be related to presence of surgical wounds, possibly evidenced by verbalizations of feelings or perceptions, fear of reaction by others, preoccupation with change.

risk for Constipation: risk factors may include decreased physical activity and gastric motility, abdominal muscle weakness, insufficient fluid intake, change in usual foods or eating pattern.

risk for Sexual Dysfunction: risk factors may include altered body structure or function, radical resection or treatment procedures, vulnerability, psychological concern about response of significant other(s) [SO(s)], and disruption of sexual response pattern (e.g., erection difficulty).

Abortion, elective termination   OB

risk for decisional Conflict: risk factors may include unclear personal values or beliefs, lack of experience or interference with decision making, information from divergent sources, deficient support system.

deficient Knowledge [Learning Need] regarding reproduction, contraception, self-care, and Rh factor may be related to lack of exposure or recall or misinterpretation of information, possibly evidenced by request for information, statement of misconception, inaccurate follow-through of instructions, development of preventable events or complications.

risk for Spiritual Distress/moral Distress: risk factors may include perception of moral or ethical implications of therapeutic procedure, time constraints for decision making.

Anxiety [specify level] may be related to situational or maturational crises, unmet needs, unconscious conflict about essential values or beliefs possibly evidenced by increased tension, apprehension, fear of unspecific consequences, sympathetic stimulation, focus on self.

acute Pain/impaired Comfort may be related to after-effects of procedure, drug effect, possibly evidenced by verbal report, distraction behaviors, changes in muscle tone, changes in vital signs.

risk for maternal Injury: risk factors may include surgical procedure, effects of anesthesia or medications.

Abortion, spontaneous termination   OB

risk for Bleeding: risk factors may include abnormal blood profile—decreased hemoglobin, altered clotting factors.

risk for Spiritual Distress: risk factors may include need to adhere to personal religious beliefs and practices, blame for loss directed at self or God.

deficient Knowledge [Learning Need] regarding cause of abortion, self-care, contraception, and future pregnancy may be related to lack of familiarity with new self healthcare needs, sources for support, possibly evidenced by requests for information and statement of concern or misconceptions, development of preventable complications.

Grieving related to perinatal loss, possibly evidenced by crying, expressions of sorrow, or changes in eating habits or sleep patterns.

risk for Sexual Dysfunction: risk factors may include increasing fear of pregnancy or repeat loss, impaired relationship with SO(s), self-doubt regarding own femininity.

Abruptio placentae   OB

Also refer to Hemorrhage, prenatal

risk for Bleeding: risk factors may include pregnancy-related complication—abruptio placentae.

Fear related to threat of death (perceived or actual) to fetus/self, possibly evidenced by verbalization of specific concerns, increased tension, sympathetic stimulation.

acute Pain may be related to collection of blood between uterine wall and placenta, possibly evidenced by verbal reports, abdominal guarding, muscle tension, or alterations in vital signs.

impaired fetal Gas Exchange may be related to altered uteroplacental oxygen transfer, possibly evidenced by alterations in fetal heart rate and movement.

Abscess, brain (acute)   MS

acute Pain may be related to inflammation, edema of tissues, possibly evidenced by reports of headache, restlessness, irritability, and moaning.

risk for Hyperthermia: risk factors may include inflammatory process, hypermetabolic state, and dehydration.

acute Confusion may be related to physiological changes (e.g., cerebral edema, altered perfusion, fever), possibly evidenced by fluctuation in cognition or level of consciousness, increased agitation, restlessness, hallucinations.

risk for Suffocation/Trauma: risk factors may include development of clonic/tonic muscle activity and changes in consciousness (seizure activity).

Abscess, gingival   CH

impaired Dentition may be related to ineffective oral hygiene, access/economic barriers to professional care possibly evidenced by toothache, root caries, purulent drainage.

risk for imbalanced Nutrition: less than body requirements: risk factors may include decreased intake.

Abscess, skin/tissue   CH/MS

impaired Skin/Tissue Integrity may be related to immunological deficit/infection, possibly evidenced by disruption of skin, destruction of skin layers or tissues, invasion of body structures.

risk for Infection [spread]: risk factors may include broken skin, traumatized tissues, chronic disease, malnutrition, insufficient knowledge.

Abuse, physical   CH/PSY

Also refer to Battered child syndrome

risk for Trauma: risk factors may include vulnerable client, recipient of verbal threats, history of physical abuse.

Powerlessness may be related to abusive relationship, lifestyle of helplessness as evidenced by verbal expressions of having no control, reluctance to express true feelings, apathy, passivity.

chronic low Self-Esteem may be related to continual negative evaluation of self or capabilities, personal vulnerability, willingness to tolerate possible life-threatening domestic violence as evidenced by self-negative verbalization, evaluation of self as unable to deal with events, rejects positive feedback about self.

ineffective Coping may be related to situational or maturational crisis, overwhelming threat to self, personal vulnerability, inadequate support systems, possibly evidenced by verbalized concern about ability to deal with current situation, chronic worry, anxiety, depression, poor self-esteem, inability to problem-solve, high illness rate, destructive behavior toward self/others.

Sexual Dysfunction may be related to ineffectual or absent role model, vulnerability, physical abuse possibly evidenced by verbalizations, change in sexual behaviors or activities, inability to achieve desired satisfaction.

Abuse, psychological   CH/PSY

ineffective Coping may be related to situational or maturational crisis, overwhelming threat to self, personal vulnerability, inadequate support systems, possibly evidenced by verbalized concern about ability to deal with current situation, chronic worry, anxiety, depression, poor self-esteem, inability to problem-solve, high illness rate, destructive behavior toward self/others.

Powerlessness may be related to abusive relationship, lifestyle of helplessness as evidenced by verbal expressions of having no control, reluctance to express true feelings, apathy, passivity.

Sexual Dysfunction may be related to ineffectual or absent role model, vulnerability, psychological abuse (harmful relationship), possibly evidenced by reported difficulties, inability to achieve desired satisfaction, conflicts involving values, seeking confirmation of desirability.

Achalasia (cardiospasm)   MS

impaired Swallowing may be related to neuromuscular impairment, possibly evidenced by observed difficulty in swallowing or regurgitation.

imbalanced Nutrition: less than body requirements may be related to inability or reluctance to ingest adequate nutrients to meet metabolic demands or nutritional needs, possibly evidenced by reported or observed inadequate intake, weight loss, and pale conjunctiva and mucous membranes.

acute Pain may be related to spasm of the lower esophageal sphincter, possibly evidenced by reports of substernal pressure, recurrent heartburn, or gastric fullness (gas pains).

Anxiety [specify level]/Fear may be related to recurrent pain, choking sensation, altered health status, possibly evidenced by verbalizations of distress, apprehension, restlessness, or insomnia.

risk for Aspiration: risk factors may include regurgitation or spillover of esophageal contents.

deficient Knowledge [Learning Need] regarding condition, prognosis, self-care, and treatment needs may be related to lack of familiarity with pathology and treatment of condition, possibly evidenced by requests for information, statement of concern, or development of preventable complications.

Acidosis, metabolic   MS
Refer to underlying cause/condition, e.g., Diabetic ketoacidosis; Renal dialysis

Acidosis, respiratory   MS
(Also refer to underlying cause/condition)

impaired Gas Exchange may be related to ventilation perfusion imbalance (decreased oxygen-carrying capacity of blood, altered oxygen supply, alveolar-capillary membrane changes), possibly evidenced by dyspnea with exertion, tachypnea, changes in mentation, irritability, tachycardia, hypoxia, hypercapnia.

Acne   CH/PED
impaired Skin Integrity may be related to secretion, infectious process as evidenced by disruptions of skin surface.

disturbed Body Image may be related to change in visual appearance as evidenced by fear of rejection of others, focus on past appearance, negative feelings about body, change in social involvement.

situational low Self-Esteem may be related to adolescence, negative perception of appearance as evidenced by self-negating verbalizations, expressions of helplessness.

Acoustic neuroma   MS
Also refer to Surgery, general

disturbed auditory Sensory Perception may be related to altered sensory reception (compression of eighth cranial nerve), possibly evidenced by unilateral sensorineural hearing loss, tinnitus.

risk for Falls: risk factors may include hearing difficulties, dizziness, sense of unsteadiness.

Acquired immune deficiency syndrome   CH
Refer to AIDS

Acromegaly   CH
chronic Pain may be related to soft tissue swelling, joint degeneration, peripheral nerve compression, possibly evidenced by verbal reports, altered ability to continue previous activities, changes in sleep pattern, fatigue.

disturbed Body Image may be related to biophysical illness and changes, possibly evidenced by verbalization of feelings or concerns, fear of rejection or of reaction of others, negative comments about body, actual change in structure and appearance, change in social involvement.

risk for Sexual Dysfunction: risk factors may include altered body structure, changes in libido.

Acute respiratory distress syndrome   MS
Refer to Respiratory distress syndrome, acute

Adams-Stokes syndrome   CH
Refer to Dysrhythmia

ADD   PED
Refer to Attention deficit disorder

Addiction   CH/PSY
Refer to specific substance used; Substance dependence/abuse rehabilitation

Addison's disease   MS
deficient Fluid Volume [hypotonic] may be related to vomiting, diarrhea, increased renal losses, possibly evidenced by delayed capillary refill, poor skin turgor, dry mucous membranes, report of thirst.

risk for Electrolyte Imbalance: risk factors may include vomiting, diarrhea, endocrine dysfunction.

decreased Cardiac Output may be related to hypovolemia and altered electrical conduction (dysrhythmias) or diminished cardiac muscle mass, possibly evidenced by alterations in vital signs, changes in mentation, and irregular pulse or pulse deficit.

CH

Fatigue may be related to decreased metabolic energy production, altered body chemistry (fluid, electrolyte, and glucose imbalance), possibly evidenced by unremitting overwhelming lack of energy, inability to maintain usual routines, decreased performance, impaired ability to concentrate, lethargy, and disinterest in surroundings.

disturbed Body Image may be related to changes in skin pigmentation, mucous membranes, loss of axillary and pubic hair, possibly evidenced by verbalization of negative feelings about body and decreased social involvement.

risk for impaired physical Mobility: risk factors may include neuromuscular impairment (muscle wasting, weakness) and dizziness, syncope.

imbalanced Nutrition: less than body requirements may be related to glucocorticoid deficiency; abnormal fat, protein, and carbohydrate metabolism; nausea, vomiting, anorexia, possibly evidenced by weight loss, muscle wasting, abdominal cramps, diarrhea, and severe hypoglycemia.

risk for impaired Home Maintenance: risk factors may include effects of disease process, impaired cognitive functioning, and inadequate support systems.

Adenoidectomy   PED/MS
Anxiety [specify level]/Fear may be related to separation from supportive others, unfamiliar surroundings, and perceived threat of injury or abandonment, possibly evidenced by crying, apprehension, trembling, and sympathetic stimulation (pupil dilation, increased heart rate).

risk for ineffective Airway Clearance: risk factors may include sedation, collection of secretions and blood in oropharynx, and vomiting.

risk for deficient Fluid Volume: risk factors may include operative trauma to highly vascular site, hemorrhage.

acute Pain may be related to physical trauma to oronasopharynx, presence of packing, possibly evidenced by restlessness, crying, and facial mask of pain.

Adjustment disorder   PED/PSY

Refer to Anxiety disorders—PED

Adoption/loss of child custody   PSY

risk for complicated Grieving: risk factors may include actual loss of child, expectations for future of child/self, thwarted grieving response to loss.

    risk for Powerlessness: risk factors may include perceived lack of options, no input into decision process, no control over outcome.

Adrenal crisis, acute   MS

Also refer to Addison's disease; Shock

    deficient Fluid Volume [hypotonic] may be related to failure of regulatory mechanism (damage to or suppression of adrenal gland), inability to concentrate urine, possibly evidenced by decreased venous filling, pulse volume and pressure; hypotension, dry mucous membranes, changes in mentation, decreased serum sodium.

    acute Pain may be related to effects of disease process and metabolic imbalances, decreased tissue perfusion, possibly evidenced by reports of severe pain in abdomen, lower back, or legs.

    impaired physical Mobility may be related to neuromuscular impairment, decreased muscle strength and control, possibly evidenced by generalized weakness, inability to perform desired activities or movements.

    risk for Hyperthermia: risk factors may include presence of illness or infectious process, dehydration.

    risk for ineffective Protection: risk factors may include hormone deficiency, drug therapy, nutritional or metabolic deficiencies.

Adrenalectomy   MS

ineffective tissue Perfusion (specify) may be related to hypovolemia and vascular pooling of blood (vasodilation), possibly evidenced by diminished pulse, pallor or cyanosis, hypotension, and changes in mentation.

    risk for Infection: risk factors may include inadequate primary defenses (incision, traumatized tissues), suppressed inflammatory response, invasive procedures.

    deficient Knowledge [Learning Need] regarding condition, prognosis, self-care, and treatment needs may be related to unfamiliarity with long-term therapy requirements, possibly evidenced by request for information and statement of concern or misconceptions.

Adrenal insufficiency   CH

Refer to Addison's disease

Affective disorder   PSY

Refer to Bipolar disorder; Depressive disorders, major

Affective disorder, seasonal   PSY

Also refer to Depressive disorders, major

    intermittent ineffective Coping may be related to situational crisis (fall-winter season), disturbance in pattern of tension release, and inadequate resources available, possibly evidenced by verbalizations of inability to cope, changes in sleep pattern (too little or too much), reports of lack of energy or fatigue, lack of resolution of problem, behavioral changes (irritability, discouragement).

    risk for imbalanced Nutrition: more/less than body requirements: risk factors may include eating in response to internal cues other than hunger, alteration in usual coping patterns, change in usual activity level, decreased appetite, lack of energy or interest to prepare food.

Agoraphobia   PSY
Also refer to Phobia

Anxiety [panic] may be related to contact with feared situation (public place, crowds), possibly evidenced by tachycardia, chest pain, dyspnea, gastrointestinal distress, faintness, sense of impending doom.

Agranulocytosis   MS
risk for Infection: risk factors may include suppressed inflammatory response.

risk for impaired Oral Mucous Membrane: risk factors may include infection.

risk for imbalanced Nutrition: less than body requirements: risk factors may include inability to ingest food or fluids (lesions of oral cavity).

AIDS (acquired immunodeficiency syndrome)   MS
Also refer to HIV infection

risk for Infection, [progression to sepsis/onset of new opportunistic infection]: risk factors may include depressed immune system, use of antimicrobial agents, inadequate primary defenses, broken skin, traumatized tissue, malnutrition, environmental exposure, invasive procedures, and chronic disease processes.

risk for deficient Fluid Volume: risk factors may include excessive losses—copious diarrhea, profuse sweating, vomiting, hypermetabolic state or fever; and restricted intake—nausea, anorexia, lethargy.

acute/chronic Pain may be related to tissue inflammation or destruction: infections, internal or external cutaneous lesions, rectal excoriation, malignancies, necrosis, peripheral neuropathies, myalgias and arthralgias, possibly evidenced by verbal reports, narrowed focus, alteration in muscle tone, paresthesias, paralysis, guarding behaviors, changes in vital signs (acute), autonomic responses, and restlessness.

risk for ineffective Breathing Pattern/impaired Gas Exchange: risk factors may include muscular impairment—wasting of respiratory musculature, decreased energy, fatigue, decreased lung expansion; retained secretions (tracheobronchial obstruction), infectious or inflammatory process, pain, ventilation perfusion imbalance—*Pneumocystis carinii* pneumonia, other pneumonias, anemia.

CH

imbalanced Nutrition: less than body requirements may be related to altered ability to ingest, digest, or absorb nutrients (nausea, vomiting, hyperactive gag reflex, gastrointestinal disturbances, fatigue); increased metabolic rate and nutritional needs (fever, infection), possibly evidenced by weight loss, decreased subcutaneous fat or muscle mass; lack of interest in food, aversion to eating, altered taste sensation; abdominal cramping, hyperactive bowel sounds, diarrhea, sore and inflamed buccal cavity, abnormal laboratory results—vitamin, mineral, and protein deficiencies; electrolyte imbalances.

Fatigue may be related to decreased metabolic energy production, increased energy requirements (hypermetabolic state), overwhelming psychological or emotional demands, altered body chemistry (side effects of medication, chemotherapy), sleep deprivation, possibly evidenced by unremitting or overwhelming lack of energy, inability to maintain usual routines, decreased performance, impaired ability to concentrate, lethargy, listlessness, and disinterest in surroundings.

ineffective Protection may be related to chronic disease affecting immune and neurological systems, inadequate nutrition, drug therapies, possibly evidenced by deficient immunity, impaired healing, neurosensory alterations, maladaptive stress response, fatigue, anorexia, disorientation.

Social Isolation may be related to changes in physical appearance, mental status, state of wellness; perceptions of unacceptable social or sexual behavior or values, physical isolation, phobic fear of others (transmission of disease), possibly evidenced by expressed feelings of aloneness or rejection, absence of supportive SO(s), and withdrawal from usual activities.

disturbed Thought Processes/chronic Confusion may be related to physiological changes (hypoxemia, central nervous system infection by HIV, brain malignancies, or disseminated systemic opportunistic infection); altered drug metabolism and excretion, accumulation of toxic elements (renal failure, severe electrolyte imbalance, hepatic insufficiency), possibly evidenced by clinical evidence of organic impairment, altered attention span, distractibility, memory deficit, disorientation, cognitive dissonance, delusional thinking, impaired ability to make decisions or problem-solve, inability to follow complex commands/mental tasks, loss of impulse control and altered personality.

AIDS dementia   CH
Also refer to Dementia, HIV

impaired Environmental Interpretation Syndrome may be related to dementia, depression, possibly evidenced by consistent disorientation, inability to follow simple directions or instructions, loss of social functioning from memory decline.

ineffective Protection may be related to chronic disease affecting immune and neurological systems, inadequate nutrition, drug therapies, possibly evidenced by deficient immunity, impaired healing, neurosensory alterations, maladaptive stress response, fatigue, anorexia, disorientation.

Alcohol abuse/withdrawal   CH/MS/PSY
Refer to Alcohol intoxication, acute; Delirium tremens; Substance dependency/abuse rehabilitation

Alcohol intoxication, acute   MS
Also refer to Delirium tremens

acute Confusion may be related to substance abuse, hypoxemia, possibly evidenced by hallucinations, exaggerated emotional response, fluctuation in cognition or level of consciousness, increased agitation.

risk for ineffective Breathing Pattern: risk factors may include direct effect of alcohol toxicity on respiratory center and/or sedative drugs given to decrease alcohol withdrawal symptoms, tracheobronchial obstruction, presence of chronic respiratory problems, inflammatory process, decreased energy, fatigue.

risk for Aspiration: risk factors may include reduced level of consciousness, depressed cough or gag reflexes, delayed gastric emptying.

Alcoholism   CH
Refer to Substance dependency/abuse rehabilitation

Aldosteronism, primary   MS
deficient Fluid Volume [isotonic] may be related to increased urinary losses, possibly evidenced by dry mucous membranes, poor skin turgor, dilute urine, excessive thirst, weight loss.

impaired physical Mobility may be related to neuromuscular impairment, weakness, and pain, possibly evidenced by impaired coordination, decreased muscle strength, paralysis, and positive Chvostek's and Trousseau's signs.

---

risk for decreased Cardiac Output: risk factors may include hypovolemia and altered electrical conduction—dysrhythmias.

Alkalosis, metabolic   MS
Refer to underlying cause/condition, e.g., Renal dialysis

Alkalosis, respiratory   MS
(Also refer to underlying cause/condition.)

impaired Gas Exchange may be related to ventilation perfusion imbalance (decreased oxygen-carrying capacity of blood, altered oxygen supply, alveolar-capillary membrane changes), possibly evidenced by dyspnea, tachypnea, changes in mentation, tachycardia, hypoxia, hypocapnia.

Allergies, seasonal   CH
Refer to Hay fever

Alopecia   CH
disturbed Body Image may be related to effects of illness, therapy or aging process, change in appearance, possibly evidenced by verbalization of feelings or concerns, fear of rejection or reaction of others, focus on past appearance, preoccupation with change, feelings of helplessness.

ALS   CH
Refer to Amyotrophic lateral sclerosis

Alzheimer's disease   CH
Also refer to Dementia, presenile/senile

risk for Injury/Trauma: risk factors may include inability to recognize or identify danger in environment, disorientation, confusion, impaired judgment, weakness, muscular incoordination, balancing difficulties, altered perception, and seizure activity.

chronic Confusion, related to physiological changes (neuronal degeneration), possibly evidenced by inaccurate interpretation of or response to stimuli, progressive or long-standing cognitive impairment, short-term memory deficit, impaired socialization, altered personality, and clinical evidence of organic impairment.

disturbed Sensory Perception (specify) may be related to altered sensory reception, transmission, or integration (neurological disease, deficit), socially restricted environment (homebound or institutionalized), sleep deprivation, possibly evidenced by changes in usual response to stimuli, change in problem-solving abilities, exaggerated emotional responses (anxiety, paranoia, hallucinations), inability to tell position of body parts, diminished or altered sense of taste.

Sleep Deprivation may be related to sensory impairment, changes in activity patterns, psychological stress (neurological impairment), possibly evidenced by wakefulness, disorientation (day/night reversal), increased aimless wandering, inability to identify need or time for sleeping, changes in behavior, lethargy, dark circles under eyes, and frequent yawning.

ineffective Health Maintenance may be related to deterioration affecting ability in all areas, including coordination, communication, and cognition; ineffective individual or family coping, possibly evidenced by reported or observed inability to take responsibility for meeting basic health practices, lack of equipment/financial or other resources, and impairment of personal support system.

PSY
risk for Stress Overload: risk factors may include inadequate resources, chronic illness, physical demands, threats of violence.

compromised family Coping/Caregiver Role Strain may be related to disruptive behavior of client, family grief about their helplessness watching loved one deteriorate, prolonged disease or disability progression that exhausts the supportive capacity of SO or family, highly ambivalent family relationships, possibly evidenced by verbalizations of frustrations in dealing with day-to-day care, reports of conflict, feelings of depression, expressed anger/guilt directed toward client, and withdrawal from interaction with client or social contacts.

risk for Relocation Stress Syndrome: Risk factors may include little or no preparation for transfer to a new setting, changes in daily routine, sensory impairment, physical deterioration, separation from support systems.

Amenorrhea (secondary or pathological)   GYN
Also refer to Anorexia nervosa

imbalanced Nutrition: less than body requirements may be related to inability to ingest or digest food or absorb nutrients, possibly evidenced by verbal reports, aversion to eating, lack of interest in food, weight loss, excessive hair growth or lanugo, pale conjunctiva and mucous membranes, abnormal lab studies.

risk for Sexual Dysfunction: risk factors may include altered body function.

Amphetamine abuse   PSY
Refer to Stimulant abuse

Amputation   MS
risk for ineffective peripheral tissue Perfusion: risk factors may include reduced arterial or venous blood flow, tissue edema, hematoma formation, hypovolemia.

acute Pain may be related to tissue and nerve trauma, psychological impact of loss of body part, possibly evidenced by reports of incisional or phantom pain, guarding or protective behavior, narrowed or self-focus, and autonomic responses.

impaired physical Mobility may be related to loss of limb (primarily lower extremity), altered sense of balance, pain or discomfort, possibly evidenced by reluctance to attempt movement, impaired coordination; decreased muscle strength, control, and mass.

situational low Self-Esteem may be related to loss of a body part, change in functional abilities, possibly evidenced by verbalization of feelings of powerlessness; grief; preoccupation with loss; negative feelings about body; focus on past strength, function, or appearance; change in usual patterns of responsibility or physical capacity to resume role; fear of rejection or reaction by others; and unwillingness to look at or touch residual limb.

Amyotrophic lateral sclerosis (ALS)   MS
impaired physical Mobility may be related to muscle wasting, weakness, possibly evidenced by impaired coordination, limited range of motion, and impaired purposeful movement.

ineffective Breathing Pattern/impaired spontaneous Ventilation may be related to neuromuscular impairment, decreased energy, fatigue, tracheobronchial obstruction, possibly evidenced by shortness of breath, fremitus, respiratory depth changes, and reduced vital capacity.

impaired Swallowing may be related to muscle wasting and fatigue, possibly evidenced by recurrent coughing, choking, and signs of aspiration.

PSY

Powerlessness may be related to chronic and debilitating nature of illness, lack of control over outcome, possibly evidenced by expressions of frustration about inability to care for self and depression over physical deterioration.

Grieving may be related to perceived potential loss of self and physiopsychosocial well-being, possibly evidenced by sorrow, choked feelings, expression of distress, changes in eating habits/sleeping patterns, altered communication patterns, and changes in libido.

---

impaired verbal Communication may be related to physical barrier (neuromuscular impairment), possibly evidenced by impaired articulation, inability to speak in sentences, and use of nonverbal cues (changes in facial expression).

risk for Caregiver Role Strain: risk factors may include illness severity of care receiver, complexity and amount of home-care needs, duration of caregiving required, caregiver is spouse, family/caregiver isolation, lack of respite or recreation for caregiver.

Anaphylaxis   CH
Also refer to Shock

ineffective Airway Clearance may be related to airway spasm (bronchial), laryngeal edema, possibly evidenced by diminished or adventitious breath sounds, cough ineffective or absent, difficulty vocalizing, wide-eyed.

decreased Cardiac Output may be related to decreased preload—increased capillary permeability (third spacing) and vasodilation, possibly evidenced by tachycardia/palpitations, changes in blood pressure, anxiety, restlessness.

Anemia   CH
Activity Intolerance may be related to imbalance between oxygen supply and demand, possibly evidenced by reports of fatigue and weakness, abnormal heart rate or blood pressure response, decreased exercise or activity level, and exertional discomfort or dyspnea.

imbalanced Nutrition: less than body requirements may be related to failure to ingest or inability to digest food or absorb nutrients necessary for formation of normal red blood cells, possibly evidenced by weight loss or weight below normal for age, height, body build; decreased triceps skinfold measurement, changes in gums and oral mucous membranes; decreased tolerance for activity, weakness, and loss of muscle tone.

deficient Knowledge [Learning Need] regarding condition, prognosis, self-care, and treatment needs may be related to inadequate understanding or misinterpretation of dietary or physiological needs, possibly evidenced by inadequate dietary intake, request for information, and development of preventable complications.

Anemia, iron-deficiency   CH
Also refer to Anemia

Fatigue may be related to anemia, malnutrition, possibly evidenced by feeling tired, inability to maintain usual routines or level of physical activity.

risk for deficient Fluid Volume: risk factors may include active or chronic blood loss.

risk for impaired Oral Mucous Membrane: risk factors may include dehydration, malnutrition, vitamin deficiency.

Anemia, pernicious   CH
Also refer to Anemia

disturbed kinesthetic/visual Sensory Perception may be related to changes in reception or perception, possibly evidenced by paresthesia, inability to tell position of extremities (proprioception), loss of vibratory sensation, changes in sensory acuity (yellow-blue color blindness).

risk for Constipation/Diarrhea: risk factors may include muscular weakness, changes in gastrointestinal motility, neurological impairment.

risk for Injury/Falls: risk factors may include generalized weakness, paresthesia of extremities, loss of proprioception, ataxia.

Anemia, sickle cell   MS

impaired Gas Exchange may be related to decreased oxygen-carrying capacity of blood, reduced red blood cell life span or premature destruction, abnormal red blood cell structure, increased blood viscosity, pulmonary congestion—impairment of surface phagocytosis, predisposition to bacterial pneumonia and pulmonary infarcts, possibly evidenced by dyspnea, use of accessory muscles, signs of hypoxia—cyanosis, tachycardia, changes in mentation, and restlessness.

ineffective tissue Perfusion (specify) may be related to stasis, vaso-occlusive nature of sickling, inflammatory response, atrioventricular shunts in pulmonary and peripheral circulation, myocardial damage (small infarcts, iron deposits, fibrosis), possibly evidenced by signs and symptoms dependent on system involved; for example, renal—decreased specific gravity and pale urine in face of dehydration; cerebral—paralysis and visual disturbances; peripheral—distal ischemia, tissue infarctions, ulcerations, bone pain; cardiac—angina, palpitations.

CH

acute/chronic Pain may be related to intravascular sickling with localized vascular stasis, occlusion, infarction or necrosis and deprivation of oxygen and nutrients, accumulation of noxious metabolites, possibly evidenced by reports of localized, generalized, or migratory joint or abdominal/back pain; guarding and distraction behaviors (moaning, crying, restlessness); facial grimacing; narrowed focus; and autonomic responses.

deficient Knowledge [Learning Need] regarding disease process, genetic factors, prognosis, self-care, and treatment needs may be related to lack of exposure or recall, misinterpretation of information, unfamiliarity with resources, possibly evidenced by questions, statement of concern or misconceptions, exacerbation of condition, inadequate follow-through of therapy instructions, and development of preventable complications.

risk for sedentary Lifestyle: risk factors may include lack of interest or motivation, resources; lack of training or knowledge of specific exercise needs, safety concerns, fear of injury.

PED

delayed Growth and Development may be related to effects of physical condition, possibly evidenced by altered physical growth and delay or difficulty performing skills typical of age group.

compromised family Coping may be related to chronic nature of disease and disability, family disorganization, presence of other crises or situations impacting significant person or parent, lifestyle restrictions, possibly evidenced by SO expressing preoccupation with own reaction and displaying protective behavior disproportionate to client's ability or need for autonomy.

Anencephaly   OB
Also refer to Fetal demise

Anxiety [specify level] may be related to situational crisis, threat of fetal death, interpersonal transmission or contagion, possibly evidenced by increased tension, apprehension, feelings of inadequacy, somatic complaints, difficulty sleeping.

risk for decisional Conflict [specify]: risk factors may include threat to value/belief system, multiple or divergent sources of information, support system deficit, feelings of guilt (particularly regarding ethical issues such as termination of pregnancy, organ donation).

Aneurysm, abdominal aortic   MS
Refer to Aortic aneurysm, abdominal

Health Conditions and Client Concerns With Associated Nursing Diagnoses

Aneurysm, cerebral   MS
Refer to Cerebrovascular accident

Aneurysm, ventricular   MS
decreased Cardiac Output may be related to altered stroke volume (decreased contractility, increased systemic vascular resistance), changes in heart rate or rhythm, possibly evidenced by dyspnea, adventitious breath sounds, S_3/S_4 heart sounds, changes in hemodynamic measurements, dysrhythmias.

ineffective tissue Perfusion (specify) may be related to decreased arterial blood flow, possibly evidenced by blood pressure changes, diminished pulses, edema, dyspnea, dysrhythmias, altered mental status, decreased renal function.

Activity Intolerance may be related to imbalance between oxygen supply and demand, possibly evidenced by weakness, fatigue, abnormal heart rate/blood pressure response to activity, electrocardiogram changes (dysrhythmias, ischemia).

Angina pectoris   MS
acute Pain may be related to decreased myocardial blood flow, increased cardiac workload and oxygen consumption, possibly evidenced by verbal reports, narrowed focus, distraction behaviors (restlessness, moaning), and autonomic responses (diaphoresis, changes in vital signs).

risk for decreased Cardiac Output: risk factors may include inotropic changes such as transient or prolonged myocardial ischemia and effects of medications, alterations in rate, rhythm and electrical conduction.

Anxiety [specify level] may be related to situational crises, change in health status or threat of death, negative self-talk, possibly evidenced by verbalized apprehension, expressed concerns, association of condition with loss of abilities, facial tension, extraneous movements, and focus on self.

                                                                           CH
Activity Intolerance may be related to imbalance between oxygen supply and demand, possibly evidenced by exertional dyspnea, abnormal pulse/blood pressure response to activity, and electrocardiogram changes.

deficient Knowledge [Learning Need] regarding condition, prognosis, self-care, and treatment needs may be related to lack of exposure, inaccurate/misinterpretation of information, possibly evidenced by questions, request for information, statement of concern, and inaccurate follow-through of instructions.

risk for sedentary Lifestyle: risk factors may include lack of training or knowledge of specific exercise needs, safety concerns, fear of myocardial injury.

risk for risk-prone health Behavior: risk factors may include condition requiring long-term therapy/change in lifestyle, multiple stressors, assault to self-concept, and altered locus of control.

Anorexia nervosa   MS
imbalanced Nutrition: less than body requirements may be related to psychological restrictions of food intake or excessive activity, laxative abuse, possibly evidenced by weight loss, poor skin turgor and muscle tone, denial of hunger, unusual hoarding or handling of food, amenorrhea, electrolyte imbalance, cardiac irregularities, hypotension.

risk for deficient Fluid Volume: risk factors may include inadequate intake of food and liquids, chronic laxative or diuretic use.

                                                                          PSY
disturbed Thought Processes may be related to severe malnutrition or electrolyte imbalance, psychological conflicts, possibly evidenced by impaired ability to make decisions,

problem-solve, nonreality-based verbalizations, ideas of reference, altered sleep patterns, altered attention span, distractibility; perceptual disturbances with failure to recognize hunger, fatigue, anxiety, and depression.

disturbed Body Image/chronic low Self-Esteem may be related to morbid fear of obesity, negative perception of body or self, perceived loss of control in some aspect of life, unmet dependency needs, personal vulnerability, dysfunctional family system, possibly evidenced by distorted view of body as fat even in presence of severe emaciation, use of denial, feeling powerless to prevent or make changes, expressions of shame or guilt, overly conforming, dependent on others' opinions.

impaired Parenting may be related to issues of control in family, situational or maturational crises, history of inadequate coping methods, possibly evidenced by enmeshed family; dissonance among family members; focus on "identified patient"; family developmental tasks not being met; family members acting as enablers; ill-defined family rules, functions, and roles.

Anthrax, cutaneous   MS/CH

impaired Skin/Tissue Integrity may be related to infectious agent, possibly evidenced by disruption of skin surface, damage to tissues.

impaired Comfort may be related to local edema, effects of circulating toxins, possibly evidenced by reports of headache, muscle aches, nausea, malaise.

risk for Infection [spread/sepsis]: risk factors may include broken skin, tissue destruction, lack of immunity, presence of infective agent.

Anthrax, gastrointestinal   MS

Anxiety [moderate to severe]/Fear may be related to situational crisis, change in health status, threat of death, interpersonal transmission or contagion, possibly evidenced by expressed concerns, apprehension, uncertainty, fearful, increased tension, restlessness, blocking of thought.

risk for deficient Fluid Volume: risk factors may include decreased intake (nausea), excessive loss—bloody vomit or diarrhea, hypermetabolic state.

imbalanced Nutrition: less than body requirements may be related to inability to ingest food or absorb nutrients, increased metabolic demands, possibly evidenced by reports of loss of appetite, nausea, abdominal pain, vomiting, diarrhea.

impaired Oral Mucous Membranes may be related to effects of infection, dehydration, possibly evidenced by oropharyngeal ulcerations, oral pain, difficulty swallowing.

Anthrax, inhalation (pulmonary)   MS

Also refer to Ventilator assist/dependence

impaired Comfort may be related to effects of inflammatory response, possibly evidenced by fever, malaise, weakness, fatigue, mild chest pain.

Anxiety [moderate to severe]/Fear may be related to situational crisis, change in health status/threat of death, interpersonal transmission or contagion, possibly evidenced by expressed concerns, apprehension, uncertainty, fearfulness, increased tension, restlessness, blocking of thought.

impaired Gas Exchange may be related to alveolar-capillary membrane changes (fluid collection or shifts into interstitial space or alveoli), possibly evidenced by dyspnea, restlessness, irritability, abnormal rate or depth of respirations, cyanosis, hypoxia, lethargy, confusion.

risk for impaired spontaneous Ventilation: risk factors may include problems with secretion management, mechanical compression of lungs (widening of mediastinum), depletion of energy stores.

Antisocial personality disorder   PSY

risk for other directed Violence: risk factors may include contempt for authority or rights of others, inability to tolerate frustration, need for immediate gratification, easy agitation, vulnerable

---

self-concept, inability to verbalize feelings, use of maladjusted coping mechanisms, including substance use.

ineffective Coping may be related to very low tolerance for external stress, lack of experience of internal anxiety (e.g., guilt, shame), personal vulnerability, unmet expectations, multiple life changes, possibly evidenced by choice of aggression and manipulation to handle problems or conflicts, inappropriate use of defense mechanisms (e.g., denial, projection), chronic worry, anxiety, destructive behaviors, high rate of accidents.

chronic low Self-Esteem may be related to lack of positive or repeated negative feedback, unmet dependency needs, retarded ego development, dysfunctional family system, possibly evidenced by acting-out behaviors (e.g., substance abuse, sexual promiscuity, feelings of inadequacy, nonparticipation in therapy).

compromised/disabled family Coping may be related to family disorganization or role changes, highly ambivalent family relationships, client providing little support in turn for the primary person(s), history of abuse or neglect in the home, possibly evidenced by expressions of concern or complaints, preoccupation of primary person with own reactions to situation, display of protective behaviors disproportionate to client's abilities or need for autonomy.

impaired Social Interaction may be related to inadequate personal resources (shallow feelings), immature interests, underdeveloped conscience, unaccepted social values, possibly evidenced by difficulty meeting expectations of others, lack of belief that rules pertain to self, sense of emptiness or inadequacy covered by expressions of self-conceit, arrogance, contempt; behavior unaccepted by dominant cultural group.

Anxiety disorder, generalized   PSY

Anxiety [specify level]/Powerlessness may be related to real or perceived threat to physical integrity or self-concept (may or may not be able to identify the threat), unconscious conflict about essential values or beliefs and goals of life, unmet needs, negative self-talk, possibly evidenced by sympathetic stimulation, extraneous movements (foot shuffling, hand or arm fidgeting, rocking movements, restlessness), persistent feelings of apprehension and uneasiness, a general anxious feeling that client has difficulty alleviating, poor eye contact, focus on self, impaired functioning, free-floating anxiety, impaired functioning, and nonparticipation in decision making.

ineffective Coping may be related to level of anxiety being experienced by the client, personal vulnerability; unmet expectations, unrealistic perceptions, inadequate coping methods or support systems, possibly evidenced by verbalization of inability to cope or problem-solve, excessive compulsive behaviors (e.g., smoking, drinking), and emotional tension, alteration in societal participation, high rate of accidents.

Insomnia may be related to psychological stress, repetitive thoughts, possibly evidenced by reports of difficulty in falling asleep, awakening earlier or later than desired, reports of not feeling rested, dark circles under eyes, and frequent yawning.

risk for compromised family Coping: risk factors may include inadequate or incorrect information or understanding by a primary person, temporary family disorganization and role changes, prolonged disability that exhausts the supportive capacity of SO(s).

impaired Social Interaction/Social Isolation may be related to low self-concept, inadequate personal resources, misinterpretation of internal or external stimuli, hypervigilance, possibly evidenced by discomfort in social situations, withdrawal from or reported change in pattern of interactions, dysfunctional interactions; expressed feelings of difference from others; sad, dull affect.

Anxiety disorders   PED/PSY

Anxiety [severe/panic] may be related to situational or maturational crisis, internal transmission or contagion, threat to physical integrity or self-concept, unmet needs, dysfunctional family system, independence conflicts, possibly evidenced by somatic complaints, nightmares, excessive psychomotor activity, refusal to attend school, persistent worry, fear of catastrophic doom to family/self.

ineffective Coping may be related to maturational crisis, multiple life changes or losses, personal vulnerability, lack of self-confidence, possibly evidenced by inability to problem-solve, persistent or overwhelming fears, inability to meet role expectations, social inhibition, panic attacks.

Impaired Social Interaction may be related to excessive self-consciousness, inability to interact with unfamiliar people, altered thought processes possibly evidenced by verbalized or observed discomfort in social situations, inability to receive or communicate a satisfying sense of social engagement—belonging, caring, interest; use of unsuccessful social interaction behaviors.

risk for Self-Mutilation/self-directed Violence: risk factors may include panic states, dysfunctional family, history of self-destructive behaviors, emotional disturbance, increasing motor activity.

compromised/disabled family Coping may be related to situational or developmental crisis (e.g., divorce, addition to family, midlife crisis), unrealistic parental expectations, frequent disruptions in living arrangements, high-risk family situations (neglect or abuse, substance abuse), possibly evidenced by SO reports of frustration with clinging behaviors, emotional lability, harsh or punitive response to tyrannical behaviors, disproportionate protective behaviors.

Anxiolytic abuse   PSY
Refer to Depressant abuse

Aortic aneurysm, abdominal (AAA)   MS
risk for ineffective peripheral tissue Perfusion: risk factors may include interruption of arterial blood flow [embolus formation, spontaneous blockage of aorta].

risk for Infection: risk factors may include turbulent blood flow through arteriosclerotic lesion.

acute Pain may be related to vascular enlargement-dissection or rupture, possibly evidenced by verbal coded reports, guarding behavior, facial mask, change in abdominal muscle tone.

Aortic aneurysm repair, abdominal   MS
Also refer to Surgery, general
Fear related to threat of injury or death, surgical intervention, possibly evidenced by verbal reports, apprehension, decreased self-assurance, increased tension, changes in vital signs.

risk for Bleeding: risk factors may include weakening of vascular wall, failure of vascular repair.

risk for ineffective renal/peripheral tissue Perfusion: risk factors may include interruption of arterial blood flow, hypovolemia.

Aortic insufficiency   MS/CH
Refer to Valvular heart disease

Aortic stenosis   MS
Also refer to Valvular heart disease
decreased Cardiac Output may be related to structural changes of heart valve, left ventricular outflow obstruction, alteration of afterload (increased left ventricular end-diastolic pressure and systemic vascular resistance), alteration in preload—increased atrial pressure and

venous congestion, alteration in electrical conduction, possibly evidenced by fatigue, dyspnea, changes in vital signs and hemodynamic parameters, and syncope.

risk for impaired Gas Exchange: risk factors may include alveolar-capillary membrane changes, congestion.

CH

risk for acute Pain: risk factors may include episodic ischemia of myocardial tissues and stretching of left atrium.

Activity Intolerance may be related to imbalance between oxygen supply and demand (decreased or fixed cardiac output), possibly evidenced by exertional dyspnea, reported fatigue, weakness, and abnormal blood pressure or electrocardiogram changes, dysrhythmias in response to activity.

Aplastic anemia   **CH**
Also refer to Anemia

risk for ineffective Protection: risk factors may include abnormal blood profile (leukopenia, thrombocytopenia), drug therapies (antineoplastics, antibiotics, NSAIDs, anticonvulsants).

Fatigue may be related to anemia, disease states, malnutrition, possibly evidenced by verbalization of overwhelming lack of energy, inability to maintain usual routines or level of physical activity, tired, decreased libido, lethargy, increase in physical complaints.

Appendectomy   **MS**
Also refer to Surgery, general

risk for Infection: risk factors may include release of pathogenic organisms into peritoneal cavity (prior to or at time of surgery).

Appendicitis   **MS**
acute Pain may be related to distention of intestinal tissues by inflammation, possibly evidenced by verbal reports, guarding behavior, narrowed focus, and autonomic responses (diaphoresis, changes in vital signs).

risk for deficient Fluid Volume: risk factors may include nausea, vomiting, anorexia, and hypermetabolic state.

risk for Infection: risk factors may include release of pathogenic organisms into peritoneal cavity.

ARDS   **MS**
Refer to Respiratory distress syndrome, acute

Arrhythmia, cardiac   **MS/CH**
Refer to Dysrhythmia, cardiac

Arterial occlusive disease, peripheral   **CH**
ineffective peripheral tissue Perfusion may be related to decreased arterial blood flow, possibly evidenced by skin discolorations, temperature changes, altered sensation, claudication, delayed healing.

risk for impaired Walking: risk factors may include presence of circulatory problems, pain with activity.

risk for impaired Skin/Tissue Integrity: risk factors may include altered circulation and sensation.

Arthritis, gouty   **CH**
Refer to Gout

Arthritis, juvenile rheumatoid   PED/CH

Also refer to Arthritis, rheumatoid

risk for delayed Development: risk factors may include effects of physical disability and required therapy.

risk for Social Isolation: risk factors may include delay in accomplishing developmental task, altered state of wellness, and changes in physical appearance.

Arthritis, rheumatoid   CH

acute/chronic Pain may be related to accumulation of fluid, inflammatory process, degeneration of joint, and deformity, possibly evidenced by verbal reports, narrowed focus, guarding or protective behaviors, and physical and social withdrawal.

impaired physical Mobility may be related to musculoskeletal deformity, pain or discomfort, decreased muscle strength, possibly evidenced by limited range of motion, impaired coordination, reluctance to attempt movement, and decreased muscle strength, control, and mass.

Self-Care Deficit [specify] may be related to musculoskeletal impairment, decreased strength and endurance, limited range of motion, pain on movement, possibly evidenced by inability to manage activities of daily living.

disturbed Body Image/Role Performance, ineffective may be related to change in body structure and function, impaired mobility or ability to perform usual tasks, focus on past strength, function, or appearance, possibly evidenced by negative self-talk, feelings of helplessness, change in lifestyle and physical abilities, dependence on others for assistance, decreased social involvement.

Arthritis, septic   CH

acute Pain may be related to joint inflammation, possibly evidenced by verbal or coded reports, guarding behaviors, restlessness, narrowed focus.

impaired physical Mobility may be related to joint stiffness, pain or discomfort, reluctance to initiate movement, possibly evidenced by limited range of motion, slowed movement.

Self-Care Deficit [specify] may be related to musculoskeletal impairment, pain or discomfort, decreased strength, impaired coordination, possibly evidenced by inability to perform desired activities of daily living.

risk for Infection, spread: risk factors may include presence of infectious process, chronic disease states, invasive procedures.

Arthroplasty   MS

risk for Infection: risk factors may include breach of primary defenses (surgical incision), stasis of body fluids at operative site, and altered inflammatory response.

risk for Bleeding: risk factors may include surgical procedure, trauma to vascular area.

impaired physical Mobility may be related to decreased strength, pain, musculoskeletal changes, possibly evidenced by impaired coordination and reluctance to attempt movement.

acute Pain may be related to tissue trauma, local edema, possibly evidenced by verbal reports, narrowed focus, guarded movement, and autonomic responses (diaphoresis, changes in vital signs).

Arthroscopy, knee   MS

deficient Knowledge [Learning Need] regarding procedure, outcomes, and self-care needs may be related to unfamiliarity with information or resources, misinterpretations, possibly evidenced by questions and requests for information, misconceptions.

risk for impaired Walking: risk factors may include joint stiffness, discomfort, prescribed movement restrictions, use of assistive device for ambulation.

Health Conditions and Client Concerns With Associated Nursing Diagnoses

Asbestosis   CH

impaired Gas Exchange may be related to alveolar-capillary membrane changes, ventilation perfusion imbalance, possibly evidenced by dyspnea, tachypnea, restlessness, clubbing of fingers, abnormal arterial blood gases.

Activity Intolerance may be related to imbalance between oxygen supply and demand, possibly evidenced by exertional dyspnea, decreased exercise tolerance, abnormal cardiopulmonary response to activity.

ineffective Airway Clearance may be related to inflammatory response to inhaled foreign body (asbestos fibers), smoking or secondhand smoke, infection, possibly evidenced by dyspnea, adventitious breath sounds, increased sputum.

risk for Infection: risk factors may include decrease in ciliary action, stasis of body fluids, chronic disease, malnutrition, insufficient knowledge to avoid exposure.

acute Pain may be related to inflammation or irritation of the parietal pleura, possibly evidenced by verbal reports, guarding or distraction behaviors, self-focus, and autonomic responses (changes in vital signs).

Asperger's disorder   PED/PSY

impaired Social Interaction may be related to skill deficit about ways to enhance mutuality, communication barriers (poor pragmatic language skills), preoccupations, compulsions, repetitive motor mannerisms, possibly evidenced by observed discomfort in social situations, dysfunctional interactions with others, inability to receive or communicate satisfying sense of belonging.

risk for Injury: risk factors may include rituals, repetitive motor mannerisms, clumsiness, poor coordination, vulnerability to manipulation or peer pressure.

Aspiration, foreign body   CH

ineffective Airway Clearance may be related to presence of foreign body, possibly evidenced by dyspnea, ineffective cough, diminished or adventitious breath sounds.

Anxiety [specify] may be related to situational crisis, perceived threat of death, possibly evidenced by apprehension, fearfulness, pupil dilation, increased tension.

risk for Suffocation: risk factors may include lack of safety education or precautions, eating large mouthfuls or pieces of food.

Asthma   MS

Also refer to Emphysema

ineffective Airway Clearance may be related to increased production and retained pulmonary secretions, bronchospasm, decreased energy, fatigue, possibly evidenced by wheezing, difficulty breathing, changes in depth and rate of respirations, use of accessory muscles, and persistent ineffective cough with or without sputum production.

impaired Gas Exchange may be related to altered delivery of inspired oxygen, air trapping, possibly evidenced by dyspnea, restlessness, reduced tolerance for activity, cyanosis, and changes in arterial blood gases and vital signs.

Anxiety [specify level] may be related to perceived threat of death, possibly evidenced by apprehension, fearful expression, and extraneous movements.

                                                          CH

Activity Intolerance may be related to imbalance between oxygen supply and demand, possibly evidenced by fatigue and exertional dyspnea.

risk for Contamination: risk factors may include presence of atmospheric pollutants, environmental contaminants in the home (e.g., smoking or secondhand tobacco smoke).

Atelectasis   MS

impaired Gas Exchange may be related to inflammatory process, stasis of secretions affecting oxygen exchange across alveolar membrane, and hypoventilation, possibly evidenced by restlessness, changes in mentation, dyspnea, tachycardia, pallor, cyanosis, and arterial blood gases/oximetry evidence of hypoxia.

Atherosclerosis   CH/MS

Refer to Coronary artery disease, Peripheral vascular disease

Athlete's foot   CH

impaired Skin Integrity may be related to fungal invasion, humidity, secretions, possibly evidenced by disruption of skin surface, reports of painful itching.

risk for Infection [spread]: risk factors may include multiple breaks in skin, exposure to moist, warm environment.

Atrial fibrillation   CH

Also refer to Dysrhythmias

Activity Intolerance may be related to imbalance between oxygen supply and demand, possibly evidenced by dyspnea, dizziness, presyncope or syncopal episodes.

risk for ineffective cerebral tissue Perfusion: risk factors may include interruption of arterial flow (microemboli).

Atrial flutter   CH

Also refer to Dysrhythmias

Anxiety [specify] may be related to threat to or change in health status, possibly evidenced by expressed concerns, apprehension, awareness of physiological symptoms (palpitations, dizziness, presyncope or syncopal episodes), focus on self.

Atrial tachycardia   CH

Refer to Dysrhythmias

Attention deficit disorder   PED/PSY

ineffective Coping may be related to situational or maturational crisis, retarded ego development, low self-concept, possibly evidenced by easy distraction by extraneous stimuli, shifting between uncompleted activities.

chronic low Self-Esteem may be related to retarded ego development, lack of positive or repeated negative feedback, negative role models, possibly evidenced by lack of eye contact, derogatory self-comments, hesitance to try new tasks, inadequate level of confidence.

deficient Knowledge [Learning Need] regarding condition, prognosis, and therapy may be related to misinformation or misinterpretations, unfamiliarity with resources, possibly evidenced by verbalization of problems or misconceptions, poor school performance, unrealistic expectations of medication regimen.

Autistic disorder   PED/PSY

impaired Social Interaction may be related to abnormal response to sensory input, inadequate sensory stimulation, organic brain dysfunction; delayed development of secure attachment or trust, lack of intuitive skills to comprehend and accurately respond to social cues, disturbance in self-concept, possibly evidenced by lack of responsiveness to others, lack of eye contact or facial responsiveness, treating persons as objects, lack of awareness of feelings in others, indifference or aversion to comfort, affection, or physical contact; failure to develop cooperative social play and peer friendships in childhood.

impaired verbal Communication may be related to inability to trust others, withdrawal into self, organic brain dysfunction, abnormal interpretation or response to or inadequate sensory stimulation, possibly evidenced by lack of interactive communication mode, no use of gestures or spoken language, absent or abnormal nonverbal communication; lack of eye contact or facial expression; peculiar patterns of speech (form, content, or speech production), and impaired ability to initiate or sustain conversation despite adequate speech.

risk for Self-Mutilation: risk factors may include organic brain dysfunction, inability to trust others, disturbance in self-concept, inadequate sensory stimulation, or abnormal response to sensory input (sensory overload); history of physical, emotional, or sexual abuse; and response to demands of therapy, realization of severity of condition.

disturbed personal Identity may be related to organic brain dysfunction, lack of development of trust, fixation at presymbiotic phase of development, possibly evidenced by lack of awareness of the feelings or existence of others, increased anxiety resulting from physical contact with others, absent or impaired imitation of others, repeating what others say, persistent preoccupation with parts of objects, obsessive attachment to objects, marked distress over changes in environment; autoerotic or ritualistic behaviors, self-touching, rocking, swaying.

compromised/disabled family Coping may be related to family members unable to express feelings; excessive guilt, anger, or blaming among family members regarding child's condition; ambivalent or dissonant family relationships, prolonged coping with problem exhausting supportive ability of family members, possibly evidenced by denial of existence or severity of disturbed behaviors, preoccupation with personal emotional reaction to situation, rationalization that problem will be outgrown, attempts to intervene with child are achieving increasingly ineffective results, family withdraws from or becomes overly protective of child.

Bacteremia   MS
Refer to Sepsis

Barbiturate abuse   CH/PSY
Refer to Depressant abuse

Battered child syndrome   PED/CH
Also refer to Abuse

risk for Trauma: risk factors may include dependent position in relationship(s), vulnerability (e.g., congenital problems/chronic illness), history of previous abuse or neglect, lack or nonuse of support systems by caregiver(s).

delayed Growth and Development may be related to inadequate caretaking or neglect, indifference, inconsistent responsiveness, environmental or stimulation deficiencies, possibly evidenced by delay or difficulty in performing age-appropriate skills, altered physical growth, loss of previously acquired skills, precocious or accelerated sexual awareness, flat affect, decreased responses.

interrupted Family Processes/impaired Parenting may be related to poor role model, unrealistic expectations, presence of stressors, and lack of support, possibly evidenced by verbalization of negative feelings, inappropriate caretaking behaviors, and evidence of physical or psychological trauma to child.

PSY

chronic low Self-Esteem may be related to deprivation and negative feedback of family members, personal vulnerability, feelings of abandonment, possibly evidenced by lack of eye contact, withdrawal from social contacts, discounting own needs, nonassertive or passive, indecisive, or overly conforming behaviors.

Post-Trauma Syndrome may be related to sustained or recurrent physical or emotional abuse, possibly evidenced by acting-out behavior, development of phobias, poor impulse control, and emotional numbness.

Bedsores   CH/MS
Refer to Ulcer, pressure

Bed-wetting   PED
Refer to Enuresis

Benign prostatic hyperplasia   CH/MS
[acute/chronic] Urinary Retention/overflow Urinary Incontinence may be related to mechanical obstruction (enlarged prostate), decompensation of detrusor musculature, inability of bladder to contract adequately, possibly evidenced by frequency, hesitancy, inability to empty bladder completely, incontinence or dribbling, nocturia, bladder distention, residual urine.

acute Pain may be related to mucosal irritation, bladder distention, colic, urinary infection, and radiation therapy, possibly evidenced by verbal reports of bladder or rectal spasm, narrowed focus, altered muscle tone, grimacing, distraction behaviors, restlessness, and autonomic responses.

risk for deficient Fluid Volume/Electrolyte Imbalance: risk factors may include active fluid volume loss—postobstructive diuresis, endocrine or renal dysfunction.

Fear/Anxiety [specify level] may be related to change in health status (possibility of surgical procedure, malignancy); embarrassment, loss of dignity associated with genital exposure before, during, and after treatment, and concern about sexual ability, possibly evidenced by increased tension, apprehension, worry, expressed concerns regarding perceived changes, and fear of unspecific consequences.

Besnier-Boeck disease   CH
Refer to Sarcoidosis

Biliary calculus   CH/MS
Refer to Cholelithiasis

Biliary cancer   MS
Also refer to Cancer

imbalanced Nutrition: less than body requirements may be related to inability to ingest or absorb nutrients (anorexia, nausea, indigestion), abdominal discomfort, possibly evidenced by aversion to eating, observed lack of intake, muscle wasting, weight loss, and imbalances in nutritional studies.

risk for impaired Skin Integrity: risk factors may include accumulation of bile salts in skin, poor skin turgor, skeletal prominence.

death Anxiety may be related to lack of successful treatment options, poor prognosis, possibly evidenced by fear of the process of dying, leaving SO/family alone after death, negative death images, concern of overworking caregiver, deep sadness.

Binge-eating disorder   PSY
Refer to Bulimia nervosa

Bipolar disorder   PSY
risk for other-directed Violence: risk factors may include irritability, impulsive behavior; delusional thinking; angry response when ideas are refuted or wishes denied; manic excitement, with possible indicators of threatening body language or verbalizations, increased motor activity, overt and aggressive acts, hostility.

imbalanced Nutrition: less than body requirements may be related to inadequate intake in relation to metabolic expenditures, possibly evidenced by body weight 20% or more below ideal weight, observed inadequate intake, inattention to mealtimes, and distraction from task of eating; laboratory evidence of nutritional deficits or imbalances.

risk for Poisoning [lithium toxicity]: risk factors may include narrow therapeutic range of drug, client's ability (or lack of) to follow through with medication regimen and monitoring, and denial of need for information or therapy.

Insomnia may be related to psychological stress, lack of recognition of fatigue/need to sleep, hyperactivity, possibly evidenced by denial of need to sleep, interrupted nighttime sleep, one or more nights without sleep, changes in behavior and performance, increasing irritability, restlessness, and dark circles under eyes.

disturbed Sensory Perception (specify)/Stress Overload may be related to decrease in sensory threshold, endogenous chemical alteration, psychological stress, sleep deprivation, possibly evidenced by increased distractibility and agitation, anxiety, disorientation, poor concentration, auditory or visual hallucination, bizarre thinking, and motor incoordination.

interrupted Family Processes may be related to situational crises (illness, economics, change in roles); euphoric mood and grandiose ideas or actions of client, manipulative behavior and limit-testing, client's refusal to accept responsibility for own actions, possibly evidenced by statements of difficulty coping with situation, lack of adaptation to change, or not dealing constructively with illness; ineffective family decision-making process, failure to send and receive clear messages, and inappropriate boundary maintenance.

Bladder cancer   MS
Also refer to Cancer; Urinary diversion

impaired Urinary Elimination may be related to presence of tumor, possibly evidenced by frequency, burning, dysuria.

acute/chronic Urinary Retention may be related to blockage of urethra, possibly evidenced by sensation of fullness, bladder distention, residual urine, dysuria.

Body dysmorphic disorder   PSY
Refer to Hypochondriasis

Bone cancer   MS/CH
Also refer to Myeloma, multiple; Amputation

acute Pain may be related to bone destruction, pressure on nerves, possibly evidenced by verbal or coded report, protective behavior, autonomic responses.

risk for Trauma: risk factors may include increased bone fragility, general weakness, balancing difficulties.

Bone marrow transplantation   MS/CH
Also refer to Transplantation, recipient

risk for Injury: risk factors may include immune dysfunction or suppression, abnormal blood profile, action of donor T cells.

deficient Diversional Activity may be related to hospitalization or length of treatment, restriction of visitors, limitation of activities, possibly evidenced by expressions of boredom, restlessness, withdrawal, and requests for something to do.

risk for imbalanced Nutrition: less than body requirements: risk factors may include increased metabolic needs for healing, altered ability to ingest nutrients—nausea, vomiting, loss of appetite, taste changes, oral lesions.

Borderline personality disorder   PSY

risk for self/other-directed Violence/Self-Mutilation: risk factors may include use of projection as a major defense mechanism, pervasive problems with negative transference, feelings of guilt or need to "punish" self, distorted sense of self, inability to cope with increased psychological or physiological tension in a healthy manner.

Anxiety [severe to panic] may be related to unconscious conflicts (experience of extreme stress), perceived threat to self-concept, unmet needs, possibly evidenced by easy frustration and feelings of hurt, abuse of alcohol or other drugs, transient psychotic symptoms, and performance of self-mutilating acts.

chronic low Self-Esteem/disturbed Personal Identity may be related to lack of positive feedback, unmet dependency needs, retarded ego development—fixation at an earlier level of development, possibly evidenced by difficulty identifying self or defining self-boundaries, feelings of depersonalization, extreme mood changes, lack of tolerance of rejection or of being alone, unhappiness with self, striking out at others, performance of ritualistic self-damaging acts, and belief that punishing self is necessary.

Social Isolation may be related to immature interests, unaccepted social behavior, inadequate personal resources, and inability to engage in satisfying personal relationships, possibly evidenced by alternating clinging and distancing behaviors, difficulty meeting expectations of others, experiencing feelings of difference from others, expressing interests inappropriate to developmental age, and exhibiting behavior unaccepted by dominant cultural group.

Botulism (food-borne)   MS

deficient Fluid Volume [isotonic] may be related to active losses (vomiting, diarrhea, decreased intake), nausea, dysphagia, possibly evidenced by reports of thirst; dry skin or mucous membranes, decreased blood pressure and urine output, change in mental state, increased hematocrit.

impaired physical Mobility may be related to neuromuscular impairment, possibly evidenced by limited ability to perform gross or fine motor skills.

Anxiety [specify level]/Fear may be related to threat of death, interpersonal transmission, possibly evidenced by expressed concerns, apprehension, awareness of physiological symptoms, focus on self.

risk for impaired spontaneous Ventilation: risk factors may include neuromuscular impairment, presence of infectious process.

            CH

Contamination may be related to lack of proper precautions in food storage or preparation as evidenced by gastrointestinal and neurological effects of exposure to biological agent.

Bowel obstruction   MS
Refer to Ileus

Bowel resection   CH
Refer to Intestinal surgery [without diversion]

BPH   CH/MS
Refer to Benign prostatic hyperplasia

Brachytherapy (radioactive implants)   MS
risk for Injury: risk factors may include radiation emitted by client (depending on type of procedure), accidental dislodgement or removal of radiation source.

---

risk for impaired physical Mobility: risk factors may include prescribed restrictions (48 hours for low-dose implants), reluctance to move (fear of dislodging implants), decreased strength or endurance, depressed mood.

Bradycardia   CH
Refer to Dysrhythmia, cardiac

Brain tumor   MS
Also refer to Cancer

acute Pain may be related to pressure on brain tissues, possibly evidenced by reports of headache, facial mask of pain, narrowed focus, and autonomic responses (changes in vital signs).

disturbed Thought Processes may be related to altered circulation to or destruction of brain tissue, possibly evidenced by memory loss, personality changes, impaired ability to make decisions or conceptualize, and inaccurate interpretation of environment.

disturbed Sensory Perception (specify) may be related to compression or displacement of brain tissue, disruption of neuronal conduction, possibly evidenced by changes in visual acuity, alterations in sense of balance, gait disturbance, and paresthesia.

risk for deficient Fluid Volume: risk factors may include recurrent vomiting from irritation of vagal center in medulla and decreased intake.

Self-Care Deficit [specify] may be related to sensory or neuromuscular impairment interfering with ability to perform tasks, possibly evidenced by unkempt or disheveled appearance, body odor, and verbalization or observation of inability to perform activities of daily living.

Breast cancer   MS/CH
Also refer to Cancer

Anxiety [specify level] may be related to change in health status, threat of death, stress, interpersonal transmission, possibly evidenced by expressed concerns, apprehension, uncertainty, focus on self, diminished productivity.

deficient Knowledge [Learning Need] regarding diagnosis, prognosis, and treatment options may be related to lack of exposure or unfamiliarity with information resources, information misinterpretation, cognitive limitation, anxiety, possibly evidenced by verbalizations, statements of misconceptions, inappropriate behaviors.

risk for disturbed Body Image: risk factors may include significance of body part with regard to sexual perceptions.

risk for Sexual Dysfunction: risk factors may include health-related changes, medical treatments, concern about relationship with SO.

Bronchitis   CH
ineffective Airway Clearance may be related to excessive, thickened mucous secretions, possibly evidenced by presence of rhonchi, tachypnea, and ineffective cough.

Activity Intolerance [specify level] may be related to imbalance between oxygen supply and demand, general weakness, exhaustion—interruption in usual sleep pattern due to cough, discomfort, dyspnea, possibly evidenced by reports of fatigue, dyspnea, and abnormal vital sign response to activity.

acute Pain may be related to inflammation of lung parenchyma, persistent cough, cellular reactions to circulating toxins, possibly evidenced by reports of pleuritic chest pain, guarding affected area, distraction behaviors, and restlessness.

Bronchogenic carcinoma   MS/CH
Also refer to Cancer

impaired Gas Exchange may be related to ventilation perfusion imbalance (bronchial narrowing with air trapping, atelectasis), presence of inflammatory exudate possibly evidenced by dyspnea, diminished or adventitious breath sounds, decreased chest expansion (depth of breathing), abnormal arterial blood gases.

risk for ineffective Airway Clearance: risk factors may include retained secretions, inflammatory exudate, bronchial narrowing, pain, smoking or secondhand smoke, infection.

risk for Infection: risk factors may include stasis of body fluids, tissue destruction, chronic disease, malnutrition.

Bronchopneumonia   MS/CH
Also refer to Bronchitis

ineffective Airway Clearance may be related to tracheal bronchial inflammation, edema formation, increased sputum production, pleuritic pain, decreased energy, fatigue, possibly evidenced by changes in rate and depth of respirations, abnormal breath sounds, use of accessory muscles, dyspnea, cyanosis, cough with or without sputum production.

impaired Gas Exchange may be related to inflammatory alveolar-capillary membrane changes, ventilation-perfusion mismatch—collection of secretions affecting oxygen exchange across alveolar membrane, hypoventilation, altered release of oxygen at cellular level—fever, shifting oxyhemoglobin curve, possibly evidenced by restlessness, changes in mentation, dyspnea, tachycardia, pallor, cyanosis, and arterial blood gas or oximetry evidence of hypoxia.

risk for Infection [spread]: risk factors may include decreased ciliary action, stasis of secretions, presence of existing infection, immunosuppression, chronic disease, malnutrition.

Brown-Sequard syndrome   MS/CH
Also refer to Paraplegia; Quadriplegia

impaired physical Mobility may be related to neuromuscular and sensoriperceptual impairment, possibly evidenced by limited motion, weakness, or paralysis (hemiparaplegia).

disturbed kinesthetic/tactile Sensory Perception may be related to altered sensory transmission (e.g., neurological trauma, ischemia, inflammation, infection), possibly evidenced by reported change in sensory acuity—loss of touch, vibration, and position on one side of the body, loss of pain and temperature sensation on opposite side of body (hemianesthesia).

Buck's traction   MS
Refer to Traction

Buerger's disease   CH
Refer to Peripheral vascular disease

Bulimia nervosa   PSY/MS
Also refer to Anorexia nervosa

impaired Dentition may be related to dietary habits, poor oral hygiene, chronic vomiting, possibly evidenced by erosion of tooth enamel, multiple caries, abraded teeth.

impaired Oral Mucous Membrane may be related to malnutrition or vitamin deficiency, poor oral hygiene, chronic vomiting, possibly evidenced by sore, inflamed buccal mucosa; swollen salivary glands; ulcerations of mucosa; reports of constant sore mouth or throat.

risk for deficient Fluid Volume: risk factors may include consistent self-induced vomiting, excessive laxative or diuretic use, esophageal erosion or tear (Mallory-Weiss syndrome).

deficient Knowledge [Learning Need] regarding condition, prognosis, complications, and treatment may be related to lack of exposure or recall, unfamiliarity with information about condition, learned maladaptive coping skills, possibly evidenced by verbalization of misconception of relationship of current situation and bingeing and purging behaviors, distortion of body image, verbalization of the problem.

Bunion CH

impaired Walking may be related to inflammation and degeneration of joint, inappropriate footwear, possibly evidenced by inability to walk required distances.

Bunionectomy MS

Also refer to Surgery, general; Postoperative recovery period

impaired Walking may be related to surgical intervention, restrictive therapy, possibly evidenced by inability to walk required distances, navigate curbs, climb stairs.

Burns (dependent on type, degree, and severity of the injury) MS/CH

risk for deficient Fluid Volume/Bleeding: risk factors may include loss of fluids through wounds, capillary damage and evaporation, hypermetabolic state, insufficient intake, hemorrhagic losses.

risk for ineffective Airway Clearance: risk factors may include tracheobronchial obstruction—mucosal edema and loss of ciliary action with smoke inhalation; circumferential fullthickness burns of the neck, thorax, and chest, with compression of the airway or limited chest excursion, trauma—direct upper airway injury by flame, steam, chemicals or gases; fluid shifts, pulmonary edema, decreased lung compliance.

risk for Infection: risk factors may include loss of protective dermal barrier, traumatized tissue, necrosis, decreased hemoglobin, suppressed inflammatory response, environmental exposure/invasive procedures.

acute/chronic Pain may be related to destruction of skin, tissue, and nerves; edema formation; and manipulation of injured tissues, possibly evidenced by verbal reports, narrowed focus, distraction and guarding behaviors, facial mask of pain, and changes in vital signs.

risk for imbalanced Nutrition: less than body requirements: risk factors may include hypermetabolic state as much as 50%–60% higher than normal proportional to the severity of injury, protein catabolism, anorexia, restricted oral intake.

Post-Trauma Syndrome may be related to life-threatening event, possibly evidenced by reexperiencing the event, repetitive dreams or nightmares, psychic or emotional numbness, and sleep disturbance.

ineffective Protection may be related to extremes of age, inadequate nutrition, anemia, impaired immune system, possibly evidenced by impaired healing, deficient immunity, fatigue, anorexia.

PED

deficient Diversional Activity may be related to long-term hospitalization, frequent lengthy treatments, and physical limitations, possibly evidenced by expressions of boredom, restlessness, withdrawal, and requests for something to do.

risk for delayed Development: risk factors may include effects of physical disability, separation from SO(s), and environmental deficiencies.

Bursitis CH

acute/chronic Pain may be related to inflammation of affected joint, possibly evidenced by verbal reports, guarding behavior, and narrowed focus.

impaired physical Mobility may be related to inflammation and swelling of joint and pain, possibly evidenced by diminished range of motion, reluctance to attempt movement, and imposed restriction of movement by medical treatment.

CABG MS

Refer to Coronary artery bypass surgery

CAD CH/MS

Refer to Coronary artery disease

Calculi, urinary CH/MS

acute Pain may be related to increased frequency or force of ureteral contractions, tissue trauma, edema formation, cellular ischemia, possibly evidenced by reports of sudden, severe, colicky pains; guarding and distraction behaviors; self-focus; and autonomic responses.

impaired Urinary Elimination may be related to stimulation of the bladder by calculi, renal or ureteral irritation, mechanical obstruction of urinary flow, inflammation, possibly evidenced by urgency and frequency, oliguria, hematuria.

risk for deficient Fluid Volume: risk factors may include stimulation of renal intestinal reflexes causing nausea, vomiting, and diarrhea; changes in urinary output, postobstructive diuresis.

risk for Infection: risk factors may include stasis of urine.

deficient Knowledge [Learning Need] regarding condition, prognosis, self-care, and treatment needs may be related to lack of exposure or recall and information misinterpretation, possibly evidenced by requests for information, statements of concern, and recurrence or development of preventable complications.

Cancer MS

Also refer to Chemotherapy; Radiation therapy

Fear/death Anxiety may be related to situational crises, threat to or change in health, socioeconomic status, role functioning, or interaction patterns; threat of death, separation from family, interpersonal transmission of feelings, possibly evidenced by expressed concerns, feelings of inadequacy/helplessness, insomnia; increased tension, restlessness, focus on self, sympathetic stimulation.

Grieving may be related to potential loss of physiological well-being (body part or function), change in lifestyle, perceived potential death, possibly evidenced by anger, sadness, withdrawal, choked feelings, changes in eating or sleep patterns, activity level, libido, and communication patterns.

acute/chronic Pain may be related to the disease process (compression of nerve tissue, infiltration of nerves or their vascular supply, obstruction of a nerve pathway, inflammation), or side effects of therapeutic agents, possibly evidenced by verbal reports, self-focusing or narrowed focus, alteration in muscle tone, facial mask of pain, distraction or guarding behaviors, autonomic responses, and restlessness.

Fatigue may be related to decreased metabolic energy production, increased energy requirements—hypermetabolic state; overwhelming psychological or emotional demands, and altered body chemistry—side effects of medications, chemotherapy, radiation therapy, biotherapy, possibly evidenced by unremitting or overwhelming lack of energy, inability to maintain usual routines, decreased performance, impaired ability to concentrate, lethargy, listlessness, and disinterest in surroundings.

impaired Home Maintenance may be related to debilitation, lack of resources, or inadequate support systems, possibly evidenced by verbalization of problem, request for assistance, and lack of necessary equipment or aids.

PED

risk for interrupted Family Processes: risk factors may include situational or transitional crises long-term illness, change in roles or economic status; developmental—anticipated loss of a family member.

readiness for enhanced family Coping may be related to individual's needs being sufficiently gratified and adaptive tasks effectively addressed enabling goals of self-actualization to surface, possibly evidenced by verbalizations of impact of crisis on own values, priorities, goals, or relationships.

Candidiasis CH
Also refer to Thrush

impaired Skin/Tissue Integrity may be related to infectious lesions, possibly evidenced by disruption of skin surfaces and mucous membranes.

acute Pain/impaired Comfort may be related to exposure of irritated skin and mucous membranes to excretions (urine, feces), possibly evidenced by verbal or coded reports, restlessness, guarding behaviors.

risk for Sexual Dysfunction: risk factors include presence of infectious process, vaginal discomfort.

Cannabis abuse CH
Refer to Depressant abuse

Carbon monoxide poisoning MS
impaired Gas Exchange may be related to altered oxygen-carrying capacity of blood, possibly evidenced by headache, confusion, somnolence, elevated carbon monoxide levels.

Activity Intolerance may be related to imbalance between oxygen supply and demand, possibly evidenced by fatigue, exertional dyspnea.

risk for Injury: risk factors may include therapeutic intervention (hyperbaric oxygen therapy).

risk for Trauma/Suffocation: risk factors may include cognitive limitations, altered consciousness, loss of large- or small-muscle coordination (seizure).

CH
disturbed Thought Processes may be related to period of hypoxia—altered affinity of hemoglobin for oxygen, possibly evidenced by memory disturbances, difficulty concentrating.

Cardiac catheterization MS
Anxiety [specify] may be related to threat to or change in health status, stress, family heredity, possibly evidenced by expressed concerns, apprehension, uncertainty, focus on self.

risk for decreased Cardiac Output: risk factors may include altered heart rate or rhythm (vasovagal response, ventricular dysrhythmias), decreased myocardial contractility (ischemia).

risk for ineffective tissue Perfusion (specify): risk factors may include mechanical reduction of arterial blood flow, local hematoma formation, thrombosis, emboli, allergic dye response.

Cardiac conditions, prenatal OB
Also refer to Pregnancy, high-risk

risk for Cardiac Output [decompensation]: risk factors may include increased circulating volume, dysrhythmias, altered myocardial contractility, inotropic changes in the heart.

risk for excess Fluid Volume: risk factors may include increasing circulating volume, changes in renal function, dietary indiscretion.

risk for ineffective uteroplacental tissue Perfusion: risk factors may include changes in circulating volume, right-to-left shunt.

risk for Activity Intolerance: risk factors may include presence of circulatory problems, previous episodes of intolerance, deconditioned status.

Cardiac inflammatory disease MS
Refer to Endocarditis; Myocarditis; Pericarditis

Cardiac surgery MS/PED
risk for decreased Cardiac Output: risk factors may include altered myocardial contractility secondary to temporary factors—ventricular wall surgery, recent myocardial infarction, response

to certain medications or drug interactions; altered preload—hypovolemia, and afterload—systemic vascular resistance; altered heart rate or rhythm—dysrhythmias

risk for Bleeding/deficient Fluid Volume: risk factors may include intraoperative bleeding with inadequate blood replacement; bleeding related to insufficient heparin reversal, fibrinolysis, or platelet destruction; or volume depletion effects of intraoperative or postoperative diuretic therapy.

risk for impaired Gas Exchange: risk factors may include alveolar-capillary membrane changes (atelectasis), intestinal edema, inadequate function or premature discontinuation of chest tubes, and diminished oxygen-carrying capacity of the blood.

acute Pain/impaired Comfort may be related to tissue inflammation or trauma, edema formation, intraoperative nerve trauma, and myocardial ischemia, possibly evidenced by reports of incisional discomfort or pain in chest and donor site; paresthesia or pain in hand, arm, shoulder, anxiety, restlessness, irritability; distraction behaviors, and changes in heart rate and blood pressure.

impaired Skin/Tissue Integrity related to mechanical trauma (surgical incisions, puncture wounds) and edema evidenced by disruption of skin surface and tissues.

Cardiogenic shock   MS
Refer to Shock, cardiogenic

Cardiomyopathy   CH/MS
decreased Cardiac Output may be related to altered contractility, possibly evidenced by dyspnea, fatigue, chest pain, dizziness, syncope.

Activity Intolerance may be related to imbalance between oxygen supply and demand, possibly evidenced by weakness, fatigue, dyspnea, abnormal heart rate or blood pressure response to activity, electrocardiogram changes.

ineffective Role Performance may be related to changes in physical health, stress, demands of job and life, possibly evidenced by change in usual patterns of responsibility, role strain, change in capacity to resume role.

Carotid endarterectomy   MS
Also refer to Surgery, general
risk for ineffective cerebral tissue Perfusion: risk factors may include interruption of arterial flow (wound hematoma, emboli), pressure changes with edema formation (hyperperfusion syndrome).

Carpal tunnel syndrome   CH/MS
acute/chronic Pain may be related to pressure on median nerve, possibly evidenced by verbal reports, reluctance to use affected extremity, guarding behaviors, expressed fear of reinjury, altered ability to continue previous activities.

impaired physical Mobility may be related to neuromuscular impairment and pain, possibly evidenced by decreased hand strength, weakness, limited range of motion, and reluctance to attempt movement.

risk for Peripheral Neurovascular Dysfunction: risk factors may include mechanical compression (e.g., brace, repetitive tasks or motions), immobilization.

deficient Knowledge [Learning Need] regarding condition, prognosis, and treatment and safety needs may be related to lack of exposure or recall, information misinterpretation, possibly evidenced by questions, statements of concern, request for information, inaccurate follow-through of instructions, development of preventable complications.

Casts   CH/MS
Also refer to Fractures
risk for Peripheral Neurovascular Dysfunction: risk factors may include presence of fracture(s), mechanical compression (cast), tissue trauma, immobilization, vascular obstruction.

risk for impaired Skin Integrity: risk factors may include pressure of cast, moisture or debris under cast, objects inserted under cast to relieve itching, or altered sensation or circulation.

Self-Care Deficit [specify] may be related to impaired ability to perform self-care tasks, possibly evidenced by statements of need for assistance and observed difficulty in performing activities of daily living.

Cataract   CH

disturbed visual Sensory Perception may be related to altered sensory reception or status of sense organs, possibly evidenced by diminished acuity, visual distortions, and change in usual response to stimuli.

risk for Trauma: risk factors may include poor vision, reduced hand-eye coordination.

Anxiety [specify level]/Fear may be related to alteration in visual acuity, threat of permanent loss of vision and independence, possibly evidenced by expressed concerns, apprehension, and feelings of uncertainty.

deficient Knowledge [Learning Need] regarding ways of coping with altered abilities, therapy choices, and lifestyle changes may be related to lack of exposure or recall, misinterpretation, or cognitive limitations, possibly evidenced by requests for information, statement of concern, inaccurate follow-through of instructions, development of preventable complications.

Cataract extraction (postoperative care)   MS

risk for Injury: risk factors may include increased intraocular pressure, intraocular hemorrhage, vitreous loss.

risk for Infection: risk factors may include invasive procedure, surgical manipulation, presence of chronic disease.

disturbed visual Sensory Perception may be related to altered sensory reception (use of eyedrops, cataract glasses), therapeutically restricted environment (surgical procedure, patching), possibly evidenced by visual distortions or blurring, visual confusion, change in depth perception.

Cat scratch disease   CH

acute Pain may be related to effects of circulating toxins (fever, headache, and lymphadenitis), possibly evidenced by verbal reports, guarding behavior, and autonomic response (changes in vital signs).

Hyperthermia may be related to inflammatory process, possibly evidenced by increased body temperature, flushed warm skin, tachypnea, and tachycardia.

Celiac disease   CH

imbalanced Nutrition: less than body requirements may be related to inability to absorb nutrients (mucosal damage, loss of villi, proliferation of crypt cells, shortened transit time through gastrointestinal tract), possibly evidenced by weight loss, abdominal distention, steatorrhea, evidence of anemia, vitamin deficiencies.

Diarrhea may be related to irritation, malabsorption, possibly evidenced by abdominal pain, hyperactive bowel sounds, at least three loose stools per day.

risk for deficient Fluid Volume: risk factors may include mild to massive steatorrhea, diarrhea.

Cellulitis   CH/MS

risk for Infection [abscess, bacteremia]: risk factors may include broken skin, chronic disease, presence of pathogens, insufficient knowledge to avoid exposure to pathogens.

acute Pain/impaired Comfort may be related to inflammatory process, circulating toxins, possibly evidenced by reports of localized pain, headache, guarding behaviors, restlessness, autonomic responses.

impaired Tissue Integrity may be related to trauma, inflammation, or invasion of tissues by infectious bacterial agent, or altered circulation, possibly evidenced by redness, warmth, edema, tenderness or pain under the surface of skin or deep in tissues.

Cerebral embolism MS/CH
Refer to Cerebrovascular accident

Cerebral palsy PED/CH
Refer to Palsy, cerebral

Cerebrovascular accident MS
ineffective cerebral tissue Perfusion may be related to interruption of blood flow (occlusive disorder, hemorrhage, cerebral vasospasm or edema), possibly evidenced by altered level of consciousness, changes in vital signs, changes in motor or sensory responses, restlessness, memory loss; sensory, language, intellectual, and emotional deficits.

impaired physical Mobility may be related to neuromuscular involvement (weakness, paresthesia, flaccid or hypotonic paralysis, spastic paralysis), perceptual or cognitive impairment, possibly evidenced by inability to purposefully move involved body parts, limited range of motion; impaired coordination or decreased muscle strength or control.

impaired verbal [or written] Communication may be related to impaired cerebral circulation, neuromuscular impairment, loss of facial or oral muscle tone and control; generalized weakness, fatigue, possibly evidenced by impaired articulation, does not or cannot speak (dysarthria); inability to modulate speech, find or name words, identify objects, or inability to comprehend written/spoken language; inability to produce written communication.

Self-Care Deficit [specify] may be related to neuromuscular impairment, decreased strength or endurance, loss of muscle control or coordination, perceptual or cognitive impairment, pain, discomfort, and depression, possibly evidenced by stated or observed inability to perform activities of daily living, requests for assistance, disheveled appearance, and incontinence.

risk for impaired Swallowing: risk factors may include muscle paralysis and perceptual impairment.

risk for unilateral Neglect: risk factors may include sensory loss of part of visual field with perceptual loss of corresponding body segment.

CH
impaired Home Maintenance may be related to condition of individual family member, insufficient finances/family organization or planning, unfamiliarity with resources, and inadequate support systems, possibly evidenced by members expressing difficulty in managing home in a comfortable manner, requesting assistance with home maintenance, disorderly surroundings, and overtaxed family members.

situational low Self-Esteem/disturbed Body Image/ineffective Role Performance may be related to biophysical, psychosocial, and cognitive or perceptual changes, possibly evidenced by actual change in structure or function, change in usual patterns of responsibility or physical capacity to resume role, and verbal or nonverbal response to actual or perceived change.

Cervix, dysfunctional OB
Refer to Dilation of Cervix, premature

Cesarean birth OB
Also refer to Cesarean birth, unplanned/postpartal

deficient Knowledge [Learning Need] regarding surgical procedure, expectation, postoperative routines and therapy, and self-care needs may be related to lack of information or misinterpretation, possibly evidenced by statements of concern, questions, and misconceptions.

risk for deficient Fluid Volume/Bleeding: risk factors may include restrictions of oral intake, blood loss.

risk for impaired Attachment: risk factors may include separation, existing health conditions maternal/infant, lack of privacy.

Cesarean birth, postpartal   OB
Also refer to Postpartal period

risk for impaired Attachment: risk factors may include developmental transition—gain of a family member, situational crisis (e.g., surgical intervention, physical complications interfering with initial acquaintance or interaction, negative self-appraisal).

acute Pain/impaired Comfort may be related to surgical trauma, effects of anesthesia, hormonal effects, bladder or abdominal distention, possibly evidenced by verbal reports (e.g., incisional pain, cramping, afterpains, spinal headache), guarding or distraction behaviors, irritability, facial mask of pain.

risk for situational low Self-Esteem: risk factors may include perceived "failure" at life event, maturational transition, perceived loss of control in unplanned delivery.

risk for Injury: risk factors may include biochemical or regulatory functions (e.g., orthostatic hypotension, development of pregnancy-induced hypertension or eclampsia), effects of anesthesia, thromboembolism, abnormal blood profile (anemia, excessive blood loss, rubella sensitivity, Rh incompatibility), tissue trauma.

risk for Infection: risk factors may include tissue trauma, broken skin, decreased hemoglobin, invasive procedures or increased environmental exposure, prolongs rupture of amniotic membranes, malnutrition.

Self-Care Deficit (specify) may be related to effects of anesthesia, decreased strength and endurance, physical discomfort, possibly evidenced by verbalization of inability to perform desired activities of daily living.

Cesarean birth, unplanned   OB
Also refer to Cesarean birth, postpartal

deficient Knowledge [Learning Need] regarding underlying procedure, pathophysiology, and self-care needs may be related to incomplete or inadequate information, possibly evidenced by request for information, verbalization of concerns or misconceptions, and inappropriate or exaggerated behavior.

Anxiety [specify level] may be related to actual or perceived threat to mother/fetus, emotional threat to self-esteem, unmet needs, expectations, interpersonal transmission, possibly evidenced by increased tension, apprehension, feelings of inadequacy, sympathetic stimulation, and narrowed focus, restlessness.

Powerlessness may be related to interpersonal interaction, perception of illness-related regimen, lifestyle of helplessness, possibly evidenced by verbalization of lack of control, lack of participation in care or decision making, passivity.

risk for impaired fetal Gas Exchange: risk factors may include altered blood flow to placenta or through umbilical cord.

risk for acute Pain: risk factors may include increased or prolonged contractions, psychological reaction.

risk for Infection: risk factors may include invasive procedures, rupture of amniotic membranes, break in skin, decreased hemoglobin, exposure to pathogens.

Chemical dependence   PSY/CH
Refer to specific agents; Substance dependency/abuse rehabilitation

Chemotherapy   MS/CH
Also refer to Cancer

risk for deficient Fluid Volume: risk factors may include gastrointestinal losses (vomiting), interference with adequate intake (stomatitis, anorexia), losses through abnormal routes (indwelling tubes, wounds, fistulas), hypermetabolic state.

imbalanced Nutrition: less than body requirements may be related to inability to ingest adequate nutrients (nausea, stomatitis, gastric irritation, taste distortions, and fatigue), hypermetabolic state, poorly controlled pain, possibly evidenced by weight loss (wasting), aversion to eating, reported altered taste sensation, sore, inflamed buccal cavity; diarrhea or constipation.

impaired Oral Mucous Membrane may be related to side effects of therapeutic agents or radiation, dehydration, and malnutrition, possibly evidenced by ulcerations, leukoplakia, decreased salivation, and reports of pain.

disturbed Body Image may be related to anatomical or structural changes; loss of hair and weight, possibly evidenced by negative feelings about body, preoccupation with change, feelings of helplessness, hopelessness, and change in social environment.

ineffective Protection may be related to inadequate nutrition, drug therapy, radiation, abnormal blood profile, disease state (cancer), possibly evidenced by impaired healing, deficient immunity, anorexia, fatigue.

readiness for enhanced Hope may be related to expectations of therapeutic interventions, results of diagnostic procedures as evidenced by expressed desire to enhance belief in possibilities or sense of meaning to life.

Chickenpox   CH/PED
Refer to Measles

Chlamydia trachomatis infection   CH
Refer to Sexually transmitted disease

Cholecystectomy   MS
acute Pain may be related to interruption in skin and tissue layers with mechanical closure (sutures, staples) and invasive procedures including T-tube/nasogastric tube, possibly evidenced by verbal reports, guarding or distraction behaviors, and autonomic responses—changes in vital signs.

ineffective Breathing Pattern may be related to pain, muscular impairment, decreased energy, fatigue, ineffective cough, possibly evidenced by fremitus, tachypnea, decreased respiratory depth and vital capacity, holding breath, reluctance to cough.

risk for deficient Fluid Volume/Bleeding: risk factors may include losses from vomiting or nasogastric aspiration, medically restricted intake, altered coagulation.

Cholelithiasis   CH
acute Pain may be related to obstruction or ductal spasm, inflammatory process, tissue ischemia, necrosis, possibly evidenced by verbal reports, guarding or distraction behaviors, self or narrowed focus, and changes in vital signs.

risk for imbalanced Nutrition: less than body requirements: risk factors may include self-imposed or prescribed dietary restrictions, nausea and vomiting, dyspepsia, pain; loss of nutrients; impaired fat digestion—obstruction of bile flow

deficient Knowledge [Learning Need] regarding pathophysiology, therapy choices, and self-care needs may be related to lack of information or recall, misinterpretation, possibly evidenced by verbalization of concerns, questions, and recurrence of condition.

Cholera   CH/MS

deficient Fluid Volume [isotonic] may be related to active volume loss—profuse watery diarrhea, vomiting, possibly evidenced by intense thirst, marked loss of tissue turgor, decreased urine output (oliguria, anuria), change in mental state, hemoconcentration.

    risk for Shock: risk factors may include hypotension, hypovolemia, sepsis.

Christmas disease   CH
Refer to Hemophilia

Chronic obstructive lung disease   CH/MS

ineffective Airway Clearance may be related to bronchospasm, increased production of tenacious secretions, retained secretions, and decreased energy, fatigue, possibly evidenced by presence of wheezes, crackles, tachypnea, dyspnea, changes in depth of respirations, use of accessory muscles, persistent cough, and chest radiograph findings.

    impaired Gas Exchange may be related to altered oxygen delivery (obstruction of airways by secretions/bronchospasm, air trapping) and alveoli destruction, possibly evidenced by dyspnea, restlessness, confusion, abnormal arterial blood gas values—hypoxia, hypercapnia, changes in vital signs, and reduced tolerance for activity.

    Activity Intolerance may be related to imbalance between oxygen supply and demand, and generalized weakness, possibly evidenced by verbal reports of fatigue, exertional dyspnea, and abnormal vital sign response.

    imbalanced Nutrition: less than body requirements may be related to inability to ingest adequate nutrients (dyspnea, fatigue, medication side effects, sputum production, anorexia), possibly evidenced by weight loss, reported altered taste sensation, decreased muscle mass and subcutaneous fat, poor muscle tone, and aversion to eating or lack of interest in food.

    risk for Infection: risk factors may include decreased ciliary action, stasis of secretions, and debilitated state, malnutrition.

Circumcision   PED

deficient Knowledge [Learning Need] regarding surgical procedure, prognosis, and treatment may be related to lack of exposure, misinterpretation, unfamiliarity with information resources, possibly evidenced by request for information, verbalization of concern or misconceptions, inaccurate follow-through of instructions.

    acute Pain may be related to trauma to and edema of tender tissues, possibly evidenced by crying, changes in sleep pattern, refusal to eat.

    impaired urinary Elimination may be related to tissue injury, inflammation, development of urethral fistula, possibly evidenced by edema, difficulty voiding.

    risk for Bleeding: risk factors may include circumcision, decreased clotting factors immediately after birth, previously undiagnosed problems with bleeding or clotting.

    risk for Infection: risk factors may include immature immune system, invasive procedure/tissue trauma, environmental exposure.

Cirrhosis   MS
Also refer to Substance dependence/abuse rehabilitation; Hepatitis, acute viral

    risk for impaired Liver Function: risk factors may include viral infection, alcohol abuse.

CH

imbalanced Nutrition: less than body requirements may be related to inability to ingest or absorb nutrients (anorexia, nausea, indigestion, early satiety), abnormal bowel function, impaired storage of vitamins, possibly evidenced by aversion to eating, observed lack of intake, muscle wasting, weight loss, and imbalances in nutritional studies.

excess Fluid Volume may be related to compromised regulatory mechanism (syndrome of inappropriate antidiuretic hormone, decreased plasma proteins, malnutrition) and excess sodium or fluid intake, possibly evidenced by generalized or abdominal edema, weight gain, dyspnea, blood pressure changes, positive hepatojugular reflex, change in mentation, altered electrolytes, changes in urine specific gravity, and pleural effusion.

risk for impaired Skin Integrity: risk factors may include altered circulation or metabolic state, poor skin turgor, skeletal prominence, and presence of edema, ascites, accumulation of bile salts in skin.

risk for Bleeding: risk factors may include abnormal blood profile, altered clotting factors—decreased production of prothrombin, fibrinogen, and factors VIII, IX, and X; impaired vitamin K absorption; release of thromboplastin, portal hypertension, development of esophageal varices.

risk for acute Confusion: risk factors may include alcohol abuse, increased serum ammonia level, and inability of liver to detoxify certain enzymes and drugs.

Self-Esteem (specify)/disturbed Body Image may be related to biophysical changes, altered physical appearance, uncertainty of prognosis, changes in role function, personal vulnerability, self-destructive behavior (alcohol-induced disease), possibly evidenced by verbalization of changes in lifestyle, fear of rejection or reaction of others, negative feelings about body or abilities, and feelings of helplessness, hopelessness, powerlessness.

Cleft lip/palate   PED/MS
Also refer to Newborn, special needs

ineffective Infant Feeding Pattern may be related to anatomical abnormality, possibly evidenced by inability to sustain an effective suck, inability to coordinate sucking, swallowing, and breathing.

risk for Aspiration: risk factors may include impaired swallowing, regurgitation.

risk for impaired verbal Communication: risk factors may include anatomic defect, developmental delay.

risk for disturbed Body Image/Social Isolation: risk factors may include altered appearance, anatomic deficit, significance of body part (face).

Cocaine hydrochloride poisoning, acute   MS
Also refer to Stimulant abuse; Substance dependence/abuse rehabilitation

ineffective Breathing Pattern may be related to pharmacological effects on respiratory center of the brain, possibly evidenced by tachypnea, altered depth of respiration, shortness of breath, and abnormal arterial blood gases.

risk for decreased Cardiac Output: risk factors may include drug effect on myocardium (degree dependent on drug purity/quality used); alterations in electrical rate, rhythm, or conduction; preexisting myocardiopathy.

                                                            CH

risk for impaired Liver Function: risk factors may include cocaine abuse.

Coccidioidomycosis (San Joaquin Valley/Valley Fever)   CH
acute Pain may be related to inflammation, possibly evidenced by verbal reports, distraction behaviors, and narrowed focus.

Fatigue may be related to decreased energy production, states of discomfort, possibly evidenced by reports of overwhelming lack of energy, inability to maintain usual routine, emotional lability, irritability, impaired ability to concentrate, and decreased endurance, decreased libido.

deficient Knowledge [Learning Need] regarding nature and course of disease, therapy, and self-care needs may be related to lack of information, possibly evidenced by statements of concern and questions.

Colectomy   MS
Refer to Intestinal surgery [without diversion]

Colitis, ulcerative   MS
Diarrhea may be related to inflammation or malabsorption of the bowel, presence of toxins or segmental narrowing of the lumen, possibly evidenced by increased bowel sounds and peristalsis; urgency; frequent, watery stools (acute phase); abdominal pain; urgency; cramping.

acute/chronic Pain may be related to inflammation of the intestines, hyperperistalsis, prolonged diarrhea, and anal or rectal irritation, fissures, fistulas, possibly evidenced by verbal reports, guarding or distraction behaviors—restlessness, self-focusing.

risk for deficient Fluid Volume: risk factors may include continued gastrointestinal losses—severe diarrhea, vomiting; capillary plasma loss, restricted intake—nausea, anorexia, hypermetabolic state (inflammation, fever).

CH
imbalanced Nutrition: less than body requirements may be related to altered intake or absorption of nutrients (medically restricted intake, fear that eating may cause diarrhea) and hypermetabolic state, possibly evidenced by weight loss, decreased subcutaneous fat or muscle mass, poor muscle tone, hyperactive bowel sounds, steatorrhea, pale conjunctiva and mucous membranes, and aversion to eating.

ineffective Coping may be related to chronic nature and indefinite outcome of disease, multiple stressors (repeated over time), personal vulnerability, severe pain, inadequate sleep, lack of or ineffective support systems, possibly evidenced by verbalization of inability to cope, discouragement, anxiety; preoccupation with physical self, chronic worry, emotional tension; depression and recurrent exacerbation of symptoms.

risk for Powerlessness: risk factors may include unresolved dependency conflicts, feelings of insecurity, resentment, repression of anger and aggressive feelings; lacking a sense of control in stressful situations, sacrificing own wishes for others, and retreating from aggression or frustration.

Collagen disorders   CH
Refer to Arthritis, rheumatoid/juvenile rheumatoid; Lupus erythematosus, systemic; Polyarteritis nodosa; Temporal arteritis

Colorectal cancer   MS
Refer to Cancer; Colostomy

Colostomy   MS
risk for impaired Skin Integrity: risk factors may include absence of sphincter at stoma, character and flow of effluent and flatus from stoma, reaction to product or removal of adhesive, and improperly fitting appliance.

risk for Diarrhea/Constipation: risk factors may include interruption or alteration of normal bowel function (placement of ostomy), changes in dietary or fluid intake, and effects of medication.

deficient Knowledge [Learning Need] regarding changes in physiological function and self-care/treatment needs may be related to lack of exposure or recall, information misinterpretation, possibly evidenced by questions, statement of concern, inaccurate follow-through of instruction or performance of ostomy care, development of preventable complications.

disturbed Body Image may be related to biophysical changes (presence of stoma, loss of control of bowel elimination) and psychosocial factors (altered body structure, disease process/associated treatment regimen), possibly evidenced by verbalization of change in perception of self, negative feelings about body, fear of rejection or reaction of others, not touching or looking at stoma, and refusal to participate in care.

impaired Social Interaction may be related to fear of embarrassing situation secondary to altered bowel control with loss of contents, odor, possibly evidenced by reduced participation and verbalized or observed discomfort in social situations.

risk for Sexual Dysfunction: risk factors may include altered body structure and function, radical resection and treatment procedures, vulnerability, psychological concern about response of SO(s), and disruption of sexual response pattern (e.g., erection difficulty).

Coma   MS

risk for Suffocation: risk factors may include cognitive impairment, loss of protective reflexes and purposeful movement.

risk for deficient Fluid Volume/imbalanced Nutrition: less than body requirements: risk factors may include inability to ingest food or fluids, increased needs—hypermetabolic state.

total Self-Care Deficit may be related to cognitive impairment and absence of purposeful activity, evidenced by inability to perform activities of daily living.

risk for ineffective cerebral tissue Perfusion: risk factors may include reduced or interrupted arterial or venous blood flow (direct injury, edema formation, space-occupying lesions), metabolic alterations, effects of drug or alcohol overdose, hypoxia or anoxia.

risk for Infection: risk factors may include stasis of body fluids (oral, pulmonary, urinary), invasive procedures, and nutritional deficits.

Coma, diabetic   MS
Refer to Diabetic ketoacidosis

Compartment syndrome, abdominal   MS
acute Pain may be related to increasing abdominal distention and edema formation, inflammation, possibly evidenced by reports of pain, guarding behaviors, restlessness, narrowed focus.

risk for ineffective gastrointestinal Perfusion: risk factors may include trauma, abdominal aortic aneurysm, liver dysfunction, sepsis, increasing abdominal pressure.

ineffective Breathing Pattern may be related to abdominal distention, pain possibly evidenced by dyspnea, tachypnea, altered chest excursion.

risk for Shock: risk factors may include hypotension, hypovolemia.

Compartment syndrome, extremity   MS
acute Pain may be related to increasing pressure within muscle, possibly evidenced by reports of progressing pain distal to injury unrelieved by routine analgesics.

ineffective peripheral tissue Perfusion may be related to interruption of arterial blood flow, elevated tissue pressures, possibly evidenced by absent or diminished distal pulses, erythema, pain.

risk for Peripheral Neurovascular Dysfunction: risk factors may include reduction or interruption of blood flow (direct vascular injury, tissue trauma, excessive edema, elevated tissue pressures, hypovolemia).

Complex regional pain syndrome   CH

acute/chronic Pain may be related to continued nerve stimulation, possibly evidenced by verbal reports, distraction or guarding behaviors, narrowed focus, changes in sleep pattern, and altered ability to continue previous activities.

ineffective peripheral tissue Perfusion may be related to reduction of arterial blood flow (arteriole vasoconstriction), possibly evidenced by reports of pain, decreased skin temperature and pallor, diminished arterial pulsations, and tissue swelling.

disturbed tactile Sensory Perception may be related to altered sensory reception (neurological deficit, pain), possibly evidenced by change in usual response to stimuli—abnormal sensitivity of touch, physiological anxiety, and irritability.

risk for ineffective Role Performance: risk factors may include situational crisis, chronic disability, debilitating pain.

risk for compromised family Coping: risk factors may include temporary family disorganization or role changes, and prolonged disability that exhausts the supportive capacity of SO(s).

Concussion, brain   CH
Also refer to Postconcussion syndrome

acute Pain may be related to trauma to/edema of cerebral tissue, possibly evidenced by reports of headache, guarding or distraction behaviors, and narrowed focus.

risk for deficient Fluid Volume: risk factors may include vomiting, decreased intake, and hypermetabolic state (fever).

risk for disturbed Thought Processes: risk factors may include trauma to and edema of cerebral tissue.

deficient Knowledge [Learning Need] regarding condition, treatment, safety needs, and potential complications may be related to lack of recall, misinterpretation, cognitive limitation, possibly evidenced by questions, statement of concerns, development of preventable complications.

Conduct disorder (childhood, adolescence)   PSY/PED

risk for self-/other-directed Violence: risk factors may include retarded ego development, antisocial character, poor impulse control, dysfunctional family system, loss of significant relationships, history of suicidal or acting-out behaviors.

defensive Coping may be related to inadequate coping strategies, maturational crisis, multiple life changes/losses, lack of control of impulsive actions, and personal vulnerability, possibly evidenced by inappropriate use of defense mechanisms; inability to meet role expectations; poor self-esteem; failure to assume responsibility for own actions; hypersensitivity to slight or criticism; and excessive smoking, drinking, or drug use.

disturbed Thought Processes may be related to physiological changes, lack of appropriate psychological conflict, biochemical changes, as evidenced by tendency to interpret the intentions or actions of others as blaming and hostile; deficits in problem-solving skills, with physical aggression the solution most often chosen.

chronic low Self-Esteem may be related to life choices perpetuating failure, personal vulnerability, possibly evidenced by self-negating verbalizations, anger, rejection of positive feedback, frequent lack of success in life events.

compromised/disabled family Coping may be related to excessive guilt, anger, or blaming among family members regarding child's behavior; parental inconsistencies; disagreements regarding discipline, limit setting, and approaches; and exhaustion of parental resources (prolonged coping with disruptive child), possibly evidenced by unrealistic parental expectations; rejection or overprotection of child; and exaggerated expressions of anger, disappointment, or despair regarding child's behavior or ability to improve or change.

impaired Social Interaction may be related to retarded ego development, developmental state (adolescence), lack of social skills, low self-concept, dysfunctional family system, and neurological impairment, possibly evidenced by dysfunctional interaction with others (difficulty waiting turn in games or group situations, not seeming to listen to what is being said), difficulty playing quietly and maintaining attention to task or play activity, often shifting from one activity to another and interrupting or intruding on others.

Congestive heart failure　　　　　　　　　　MS
Refer to Heart failure, chronic

Conjunctivitis, bacterial　　　　　　　　　　CH
acute Pain/impaired Comfort may be related to inflammation, ocular irritation, edema, possibly evidenced by verbal reports, irritability, guarding behavior.

risk for Infection [spread]: risk factors may include purulent discharge, insufficient knowledge to avoid spread.

risk for ineffective self Health Management: risk factors may include length of therapy, perceived benefit.

Connective tissue disease　　　　　　　　　　CH
Refer to Arthritis, rheumatoid/juvenile rheumatoid; Lupus erythematosus, systemic; Polyarteritis nodosa; Temporal arteritis

Conn's syndrome　　　　　　　　　　MS/CH
Refer to Aldosteronism, primary

Constipation　　　　　　　　　　CH
Constipation may be related to weak abdominal musculature, gastrointestinal obstructive lesions, pain on defecation, medications, diagnostic procedures, pregnancy, possibly evidenced by change in character and frequency of stools, feeling of abdominal or rectal fullness or pressure, changes in bowel sounds, abdominal distention.

acute Pain may be related to abdominal fullness or pressure, straining to defecate, and trauma to delicate tissues, possibly evidenced by verbal reports, reluctance to defecate, and distraction behaviors.

deficient Knowledge [Learning Need] regarding dietary needs, bowel function, and medication effect may be related to lack of information, misconceptions, possibly evidenced by development of problem and verbalization of concerns, questions.

Conversion disorder　　　　　　　　　　PSY
Refer to Somatoform disorders

Convulsions　　　　　　　　　　CH
Refer to Seizure disorder

COPD　　　　　　　　　　　　　　　　　　　　　　**CH**
Refer to Chronic obstructive lung disease

Corneal transplantation　　　　　　　　　　　　　**MS**
risk for Injury: risk factors may include intraocular hemorrhage, edema/swelling, changes in visual acuity, increased intraocular pressure, glaucoma.

risk for Infection: risk factors may include surgical manipulation, use of corticosteroids, presence of chronic disease.

disturbed visual Sensory Perception may be related to altered sensory reception (use of eyedrops, edema, swelling), therapeutically restricted environment (patching), possibly evidenced by visual distortions, blurring, change in acuity.

Coronary artery bypass surgery　　　　　　　　　**MS**
risk for decreased Cardiac Output: risk factors may include decreased myocardial contractility, diminished circulating volume (preload), alterations in electrical conduction, and increased systemic vascular resistance (afterload).

acute Pain may be related to direct chest tissue and bone trauma, invasive tubes and lines, donor site incision, tissue inflammation, edema formation, intraoperative nerve trauma, possibly evidenced by verbal reports, changes in vital signs, distraction behaviors, restlessness, irritability.

disturbed Sensory Perception (specify) may be related to restricted environment (postoperative), sleep deprivation, effects of medications, continuous environmental sounds and activities, and psychological stress of procedure, possibly evidenced by disorientation, alterations in behavior, exaggerated emotional responses, and visual or auditory distortions.

　　　　　　　　　　　　　　　　　　　　　　　　CH
ineffective Role Performance may be related to situational crises (dependent role), recuperative process, uncertainty about future, possibly evidenced by delay or alteration in physical capacity to resume role, change in usual role or responsibility, change in self-/others' perception of role.

Coronary artery disease　　　　　　　　　　　　　**CH**
Activity Intolerance may be related to imbalance between oxygen supply and demand, sedentary lifestyle, possibly evidenced by exertional discomfort, pain, fatigue, abnormal heart rate response, electrocardiogram changes—dysrhythmias, ischemia.

risk for decreased Cardiac Output: risk factors may include altered heart rate or rhythm, altered contractility, increased peripheral vascular resistance.

Cor pulmonale　　　　　　　　　　　　　　　　　**CH/MS**
Also refer to Heart failure, chronic; Chronic obstructive lung disease

Activity Intolerance may be related to imbalance between oxygen supply and demand, generalized weakness, chest pain, possibly evidenced by exertional dyspnea, fatigue, cyanosis.

excess Fluid Volume may be related to compromised regulatory mechanism, possibly evidenced by shortness of breath, dependent edema, jugular vein distention, positive hepatojugular reflux, abnormal breath sounds, change in mental status.

impaired Gas Exchange may be related to ventilation perfusion imbalance (heart failure), possibly evidenced by dyspnea, restlessness, lethargy, cyanosis, abnormal arterial blood gas values (hypoxemia, hypercapnia, acidosis), polycythemia.

Cradle cap　　　　　　　　　　　　　　　　　　　**CH**
Refer to Dermatitis, seborrheic

Craniotomy　　　　　　　　　　　　　　　　　　　**MS**
Also refer to Surgery, general

risk for decreased Intracranial Adaptive Capacity: risk factors may include brain injuries, surgical procedure, systemic hypotension with intracranial hypertension.

disturbed Sensory Perception (specify) may be related to altered sensory reception, transmission or integration (neurological deficit), possibly evidenced by disorientation to time, place, person; motor incoordination, altered communication patterns, restlessness, irritability, change in behavior pattern.

risk for disturbed Thought Processes: risk factors may include trauma to or manipulation of brain tissue, changes in circulation or perfusion, increased intracranial pressure.

risk for Infection: risk factors may include traumatized tissues, broken skin, invasive procedures, nutritional deficits, altered integrity of closed system (cerebrospinal fluid leak).

Creutzfeldt-Jakob disease   CH

impaired Memory may be related to neurological deficits, possibly evidenced by observed experiences of forgetting, inability to perform previously learned skills, inability to recall factual information or recent or past events.

Fear may be related to decreases in functional abilities, progressive deterioration, lack of treatment options, possibly evidenced by apprehension, irritability, defensiveness, suspiciousness, aggressive behavior, social isolation.

impaired Walking may be related to changes in muscle coordination and balance, visual changes, impaired judgment, myoclonic seizures, possibly evidenced by inability to walk desired distances, climb stairs, navigate uneven surfaces.

disturbed visual Sensory Perception may be related to altered sensory reception or integration (neurological disease), possibly evidenced by change in sensory acuity (visual field defects, diplopia, dimness, blurring, visual agnosia), change in usual response to stimuli.

total Self-Care Deficit may be related to cognitive decline, physical limitations, frustration over loss of independence, depression, possibly evidenced by impaired ability to perform activities of daily living, unkempt appearance, poor hygiene, apathy.

risk for Caregiver Role Strain: risk factors may include illness severity of care receiver, duration of caregiving required, care receiver exhibiting deviant or bizarre behavior; family/caregiver isolation, lack of respite or recreation, spouse is caregiver.

Crohn's disease   MS/CH
Also refer to Colitis, ulcerative

imbalanced Nutrition: less than body requirements may be related to intestinal pain after eating, decreased transit time through bowel, fear that eating may cause diarrhea, possibly evidenced by weight loss, decreased subcutaneous fat and muscle mass, poor muscle tone, aversion to eating, and observed lack of intake.

Diarrhea may be related to inflammation of small intestines, presence of toxins, irritation—particular dietary intake, malabsorption of the bowel, segmental narrowing of the lumen, possibly evidenced by hyperactive bowel sounds, increased peristalsis, cramping, and frequent loose liquid stools.

deficient Knowledge [Learning Need] regarding condition, nutritional needs, and prevention of recurrence may be related to misinterpretation of information, lack of recall, unfamiliarity with resources, possibly evidenced by statements of concern, questions, inaccurate follow-through of instructions, and development of preventable complications or exacerbation of condition.

Croup   PED/CH

ineffective Airway Clearance may be related to presence of thick, tenacious mucus and swelling or spasms of the epiglottis, possibly evidenced by harsh, brassy cough; tachypnea; use of accessory breathing muscles; and presence of wheezes.

deficient Fluid Volume [isotonic] may be related to decreased ability or aversion to swallowing, presence of fever, and increased respiratory losses, possibly evidenced by dry mucous membranes; poor skin turgor; and scanty, concentrated urine.

Croup membranous   PED/CH
Also refer to Croup

risk for Suffocation: risk factors may include inflammation of larynx with formation of false membrane.

Anxiety [specify level]/Fear may be related to change in environment, perceived threat to self (difficulty breathing), and transmission of anxiety of adults, possibly evidenced by restlessness, facial tension, glancing about, and sympathetic stimulation.

C-section   OB
Refer to Cesarean birth, unplanned

Cubital tunnel syndrome   CH
acute/chronic Pain may be related to pressure on ulnar nerve at elbow, possibly evidenced by verbal reports, reluctance to use affected extremity, guarding behaviors, expressed fear of reinjury, altered ability to continue previous activities.

impaired physical Mobility may be related to neuromuscular impairment and pain, possibly evidenced by decreased pinch or grasp strength, hand fatigue, and reluctance to attempt movement.

risk for Peripheral Neurovascular Dysfunction: risk factors may include mechanical compression (e.g., brace, repetitive tasks or motions), immobilization.

Cushing's syndrome   CH/MS
risk for excess Fluid Volume: risk factors may include compromised regulatory mechanism (fluid and sodium retention).

risk for Infection: risk factors may include immunosuppressed inflammatory response, skin and capillary fragility, and negative nitrogen balance.

imbalanced Nutrition: less than body requirements may be related to inability to utilize nutrients (disturbance of carbohydrate metabolism), possibly evidenced by decreased muscle mass and increased resistance to insulin.

Self-Care Deficit [specify] may be related to muscle wasting, generalized weakness, fatigue, and demineralization of bones, possibly evidenced by statements of or observed inability to complete or perform activities of daily living.

disturbed Body Image may be related to change in structure or appearance (effects of disease process, drug therapy), possibly evidenced by negative feelings about body, feelings of helplessness, and changes in social involvement.

Sexual Dysfunction may be related to loss of libido, impotence, and cessation of menses, possibly evidenced by verbalization of concerns or dissatisfaction with and alteration in relationship with SO.

risk for Trauma [fractures]: risk factors may include increased protein breakdown, negative protein balance, demineralization of bones.

CVA   MS/CH
Refer to Cerebrovascular accident

Cyclothymic disorder   PSY
Refer to Bipolar disorder

Cystic fibrosis   CH/PED

ineffective Airway Clearance may be related to excessive production of thick mucus and decreased ciliary action, possibly evidenced by abnormal breath sounds, ineffective cough, cyanosis, and altered respiratory rate and depth.

risk for Infection: risk factors may include stasis of respiratory secretions and development of atelectasis.

imbalanced Nutrition: less than body requirements may be related to impaired digestive process and absorption of nutrients, possibly evidenced by failure to gain weight, muscle wasting, and retarded physical growth.

deficient Knowledge [Learning Need] regarding pathophysiology of condition, medical management, and available community resources may be related to insufficient information, misconceptions, possibly evidenced by statements of concern, questions; inaccurate follow-through of instructions, development of preventable complications.

compromised family Coping may be related to chronic nature of disease and disability, inadequate or incorrect information or understanding by a primary person, and possibly evidenced by SO attempting assistive or supportive behaviors with less than satisfactory results, protective behavior disproportionate to client's abilities or need for autonomy.

Cystitis   CH

acute Pain may be related to inflammation and bladder spasms, possibly evidenced by verbal reports, distraction behaviors, and narrowed focus.

impaired Urinary Elimination may be related to inflammation or irritation of bladder, possibly evidenced by frequency, nocturia, and dysuria.

deficient Knowledge [Learning Need] regarding condition, treatment, and prevention of recurrence may be related to inadequate information, misconceptions, possibly evidenced by statements of concern and questions; recurrent infections.

Cytomegalic inclusion disease   CH

Refer to Cytomegalovirus infection

Cytomegalovirus (CMV) infection   CH

risk for disturbed visual Sensory Perception: risk factors may include inflammation of the retina.

risk for fetal Infection: risk factors may include transplacental exposure, contact with blood or body fluids.

D&C   OB/GYN

Refer to Dilation and curettage

Deep vein thrombosis   CH/MS

Refer to Thrombophlebitis

Degenerative disc disease   CH/MS

Refer to Herniated nucleus pulposus

Degenerative joint disease   CH

Refer to Arthritis, rheumatoid

(Although this is a degenerative process versus the inflammatory process of rheumatoid arthritis, nursing concerns are the same.)

Dehiscence, abdominal wound   MS

impaired Skin Integrity may be related to altered circulation, altered nutritional state (obesity, malnutrition), and physical stress on incision, possibly evidenced by poor or delayed wound healing and disruption of skin surface or wound closure.

risk for Infection: risk factors may include inadequate primary defenses (separation of incision, traumatized intestines, environmental exposure).

risk for impaired Tissue Integrity: risk factors may include exposure of abdominal contents to external environment.

Fear/Anxiety [severe] may be related to crises, perceived threat of death, possibly evidenced by fearfulness, restless behaviors, and sympathetic stimulation.

deficient Knowledge [Learning Need] regarding condition, prognosis and treatment needs may be related to lack of information or recall and misinterpretation of information, possibly evidenced by development of preventable complications, requests for information, and statement of concern.

Dehydration   PED/CH

deficient Fluid Volume [specify] may be related to etiology as defined by specific situation, possibly evidenced by dry mucous membranes, poor skin turgor, decreased pulse volume and pressure, and thirst.

risk for impaired Oral Mucous Membrane: risk factors may include dehydration and decreased salivation.

deficient Knowledge [Learning Need] regarding fluid needs may be related to lack of information/misinterpretation, possibly evidenced by questions, statement of concern, and inadequate follow-through of instructions, development of preventable complications.

Delirium tremens   MS/PSY

Also refer to Alcohol intoxication, acute

Anxiety [severe/panic]/Fear may be related to cessation of alcohol intake, physiological withdrawal, threat to self-concept, perceived threat of death, possibly evidenced by increased tension; apprehension; feelings of inadequacy, shame, self-disgust, or remorse; fear of unspecified consequences; identifies object of fear.

disturbed Sensory Perception (specify) may be related to exogenous (alcohol consumption and sudden cessation) or endogenous factors (electrolyte imbalance, elevated ammonia and blood urea nitrogen) chemical alterations, sleep deprivation, and psychological stress, possibly evidenced by disorientation, restlessness, irritability, exaggerated emotional responses, bizarre thinking, and visual and auditory distortions or hallucinations.

risk for decreased Cardiac Output: risk factors may include direct effect of alcohol on heart muscle, altered systemic vascular resistance, presence of dysrhythmias.

risk for Trauma: risk factors may include alterations in balance, reduced muscle coordination, cognitive impairment, and involuntary clonic/tonic muscle activity.

imbalanced Nutrition: less than body requirements may be related to poor dietary intake, effects of alcohol on organs involved in digestion, interference with absorption or metabolism of nutrients and amino acids, possibly evidenced by reports of inadequate food intake, altered taste sensation, lack of interest in food, debilitated state, decreased subcutaneous fat or muscle mass, signs of mineral or electrolyte deficiency, including abnormal laboratory findings.

Delivery, precipitous/out of hospital   OB

Also refer to Labor, precipitous; Labor stages I–IV

risk for deficient Fluid Volume: risk factors may include presence of nausea/vomiting, lack of intake, excessive vascular loss.

risk for Infection: risk factors may include broken or traumatized tissue, increased environmental exposure, rupture of amniotic membranes.

risk for fetal Injury: risk factors may include rapid descent, pressure changes, compromised circulation, environmental exposure.

Delusional disorder   PSY

risk for self-/other-directed Violence: risk factors may include perceived threats of danger, increased feelings of anxiety, acting out in an irrational manner.

[severe] Anxiety may be related to inability to trust, possibly evidenced by rigid delusional system, frightened of other people and own hostility.

Powerlessness may be related to lifestyle of helplessness, feelings of inadequacy, interpersonal interaction, possibly evidenced by verbal expressions of no control or influence over situation(s), use of paranoid delusions, aggressive behavior to compensate for lack of control.

disturbed Thought Processes may be related to psychological conflicts, increasing anxiety or fear, possibly evidenced by interference with ability to think clearly and logically, fragmentation and autistic thinking, delusions, beliefs and behaviors of suspicion/violence.

impaired Social Interaction may be related to mistrust of others, delusional thinking, lack of knowledge or skills to enhance mutuality, possibly evidenced by discomfort in social situations, difficulty in establishing relationships with others, expression of feelings of rejection, no sense of belonging.

Dementia, HIV   CH/PSY

Also refer to Dementia, presenile/senile

acute/chronic Confusion may be related to direct central nervous system infection with HIV, disseminated systemic opportunistic infection, hypoxemia, brain malignancies, cerebrovascular accident, vasculitis, altered drug metabolism and excretion, electrolyte imbalance, sleep deprivation, possibly evidenced by fluctuation of cognition, progressive cognitive impairment, increased agitation, restlessness, altered interpretation or response to stimuli, clinical evidence of organic impairment.

[mild to severe] Anxiety may be related to threat to self-concept, unmet needs, perceived threat to or change in health status, interpersonal transmission or contagion, possibly evidenced by reports of feeling scared, shaky, increased tension, loss of control—"going crazy," apprehension, increased wariness, extraneous movements, tremors, increased somatic complaints.

compromised family Coping (specify) may be related to prolonged disease progression that exhausts the supportive capacity of SOs, highly ambivalent family relationship, sense of shame or guilt related to diagnosis, other crises SOs may be facing, possibly evidenced by intolerance, rejection, abandonment, neglectful relationships with other family members, SO preoccupied with personal reaction, distortion of reality of health problem.

Dementia, presenile/senile   CH/PSY

Also refer to Alzheimer's disease

impaired Memory may be related to neurological disturbances, possibly evidenced by observed experiences of forgetting, inability to determine if a behavior was performed, inability to perform previously learned skills, inability to recall factual information or recent or past events.

Fear may be related to decreases in functional abilities, public disclosure of disabilities, further mental or physical deterioration, possibly evidenced by social isolation, apprehension, irritability, defensiveness, suspiciousness, aggressive behavior.

Self-Care Deficit [specify] may be related to cognitive decline, physical limitations, frustration over loss of independence, depression, possibly evidenced by impaired ability to perform activities of daily living.

risk for Trauma: risk factors may include changes in muscle coordination/balance, impaired judgment, seizure activity.

risk for Caregiver Role Strain: risk factors may include illness severity of care receiver, duration of caregiving required, complexity or amount of caregiving tasks, care receiver exhibiting deviant or bizarre behavior; family/caregiver isolation, lack of respite or recreation, spouse is caregiver.

Grieving may be related to awareness of something "being wrong," predisposition for anxiety and feelings of inadequacy, family perception of potential loss of loved one, possibly evidenced by expressions of distress, anger at potential loss, choked feelings, crying, alteration in activity level, communication patterns, eating habits, and sleep patterns.

Dementia, vascular   CH/PSY
Refer to Alzheimer's disease

Depersonalization disorder   PSY
Refer to Dissociative disorders

Depressant abuse   CH/PSY
Also refer to Drug overdose, acute [depressants]

ineffective Denial may be related to weak underdeveloped ego, unmet self-needs, possibly evidenced by inability to admit impact of condition on life, minimizes symptoms or problem, refuses healthcare attention.

ineffective Coping may be related to weak ego, possibly evidenced by abuse of chemical agents, lack of goal-directed behavior, inadequate problem-solving, destructive behavior toward self.

imbalanced Nutrition: less than body requirements may be related to use of substance in place of nutritional food, possibly evidenced by loss of weight, pale conjunctiva and mucous membranes, electrolyte imbalances, anemias.

risk for Injury: risk factors may include changes in sleep, decreased concentration, loss of inhibitions.

Depression, major   PSY
risk for self-directed Violence: risk factors may include depressed mood and feelings of worthlessness and hopelessness.

[moderate to severe] Anxiety/disturbed Thought Processes may be related to psychological conflicts, unconscious conflict about essential values or goals of life, unmet needs, threat to self-concept, sleep deprivation, interpersonal transmission or contagion, possibly evidenced by reports of nervousness or fearfulness, feelings of inadequacy; agitation, angry or tearful outbursts, rambling, discoordinated speech; restlessness, hand rubbing or wringing, tremulousness; poor memory or concentration, decreased ability to grasp ideas, impaired ability to make decisions, numerous or repetitious physical complaints without organic cause, ideas of reference, hallucinations, delusions.

Insomnia may be related to biochemical alterations (decreased serotonin), unresolved fears and anxieties, and inactivity, possibly evidenced by difficulty in falling or remaining asleep, early morning awakening or awakening later than desired, reports of not feeling rested, physical signs (e.g., dark circles under eyes, excessive yawning); hypersomnia (using sleep as an escape).

Social Isolation/impaired Social Interaction may be related to alterations in mental status or thought processes (depressed mood), inadequate personal resources, decreased energy, inertia, difficulty engaging in satisfying personal relationships, feelings of worthlessness or low self-concept, inadequacy in or absence of significant purpose in life, and knowledge or skill deficit about social interactions, possibly evidenced by decreased involvement with others, expressed feelings of difference from others, remaining in home or bed, refusing invitations of social involvement, and dysfunctional interaction with peers, family, or others.

interrupted Family Processes may be related to situational crises of illness of family member with change in roles or responsibilities, developmental crises (e.g., loss of family member or relationship), possibly evidenced by statements of difficulty coping with situation, family system not meeting needs of its members, difficulty accepting or receiving help appropriately, ineffective family decision-making process, and failure to send and to receive clear messages.

risk for Injury [effects of electroconvulsive therapy]: risk factors may include effects of therapy on the cardiovascular, respiratory, musculoskeletal, and nervous systems; and pharmacological effects of anesthesia.

Depression, postpartum   OB/PSY
Also refer to Depressive disorders

risk for impaired Attachment: risk factors may include anxiety associated with the parent role, inability to meet personal needs, perceived guilt regarding relationship with infant.

risk for other-directed Violence: risk factors may include hopelessness, increased anxiety, mood swings, despondency, severe depression, psychosis.

Depressive disorders   PSY
Refer to Depression, major, Bipolar disorder, Premenstrual Dysphoric disorder

de Quervain's syndrome   CH
acute/chronic Pain may be related to inflammation of tendon sheath at base of thumb, swelling, possibly evidenced by verbal reports, reluctance to use affected hand, guarding behaviors, expressed fear of reinjury, altered ability to continue previous activities.

impaired physical Mobility may be related to musculoskeletal impairment, swelling, pain, numbness of thumb and index finger, possibly evidenced by decreased grasp or pinch strength, weakness, limited range of motion of thumb, and reluctance to attempt movement.

Dermatitis, contact   CH
acute Pain/impaired Comfort may be related to cutaneous inflammation and irritation, possibly evidenced by verbal reports, irritability, and scratching.

impaired Skin Integrity may be related to exposure to chemicals or environmental allergens, pruritus, possibly evidenced by inflammation, epidermal edema, development of vesicles or bullae.

risk for Infection: risk factors may include broken skin and tissue trauma.

Social Isolation may be related to alterations in physical appearance, possibly evidenced by expressed feelings of rejection and decreased interaction with peers.

Dermatitis, seborrheic   CH
impaired Skin Integrity may be related to chronic inflammatory condition of the skin, possibly evidenced by disruption of skin surface with dry or moist scales, yellowish crusts, erythema, and fissures.

Developmental disorders, pervasive   PED/PSY
Refer to Autistic disorder; Rett's syndrome; Asperger's disorder

Diabetes, gestational   OB
Also refer to Diabetes mellitus

risk for unstable blood Glucose Level: risk factors may include pregnancy, dietary intake, lack of diabetes management, inadequate blood glucose monitoring.

risk for disturbed Maternal/Fetal Dyad: risk factors may include impaired glucose metabolism, compromised oxygen transport—changes in circulation; treatment related side effects.

deficient Knowledge [Learning Need] regarding diabetic condition, prognosis, and self-care treatment needs may be related to lack of resources or exposure to information, misinformation, lack of recall, possibly evidenced by questions, statements of misconception, inaccurate follow-through of instructions, development of preventable complications.

Diabetes insipidus   MS/CH

deficient Fluid Volume [hypertonic] may be related to failure of regulatory mechanisms and hormone imbalance (e.g., brain injury, medication, sickle cell anemia, hypothyroidism), possibly evidenced by urinary frequency, thirst, polydipsia, dilute urine, dry skin and mucous membranes, decreased skin turgor, nocturia, increased serum sodium.

  risk for ineffective self Health Management: risk factors may include complexity of medication regimen, presence of side effects, economic difficulties, inadequate knowledge, perceived seriousness and benefits.

Diabetes, juvenile   PED

Also refer to Diabetes mellitus

  risk-prone health Behavior may be related to inadequate comprehension, negative attitude toward healthcare, multiple stressors and life changes, possibly evidenced by failure to take action that prevents health problems, minimizes health status change, failure to achieve optimal sense of control.

  risk for Injury: risk factors may include ineffective control or swings in serum glucose level, changes in mentation, developmental age, risk-taking behaviors.

  ineffective Coping may be related to maturational crisis (desire to be like peers), inadequate level of perception of control, gender differences in coping strategies, possibly evidenced by use of forms of coping that impede adaptive behavior, inadequate problem-solving, risk-taking, destructive behavior toward self (loss of or inadequate diabetic control).

  compromised family Coping may be related to inadequate or incorrect information or understanding by primary person(s), other situational or developmental crises or situations the SO(s) may be facing, lifelong condition requiring behavioral changes impacting family, possibly evidenced by family expressions of confusion about what to do, verbalizations that they are having difficulty coping with situation; family does not meet physical or emotional needs of its members; SO(s) preoccupied with personal reaction (e.g., guilt, fear), display protective behavior disproportionate (too little or too much) to client's abilities or need for autonomy.

Diabetes mellitus   CH/PED

deficient Knowledge [Learning Need] regarding disease process/treatment and individual care needs may be related to unfamiliarity with information, lack of recall, misinterpretation, possibly evidenced by requests for information, statements of concern, misconceptions, inadequate follow-through of instructions, and development of preventable complications.

  risk for unstable blood Glucose Level: risk factors may include lack of adherence to diabetes management, medication management, inadequate blood glucose monitoring, physical activity level, health status, stress, rapid growth periods.

  risk for ineffective self Health Management: risk factors may include complexity and duration of treatment, perceived excessive demands made on individual, powerlessness, perceived susceptibility to complications.

  risk for Infection: risk factors may include decreased leukocyte function, circulatory changes, and delayed healing.

  risk for disturbed Sensory Perception (specify): risk factors may include endogenous chemical alteration (glucose, insulin or electrolyte imbalance).

Diabetes mellitus, intrapartum   OB

Also refer to Diabetes mellitus

  risk for Trauma/impaired fetal Gas Exchange: risk factors may include inadequate maternal diabetic control, presence of macrosomia or intrauterine growth retardation.

risk for maternal Injury: risk factors may include inadequate diabetic control (hypertension, severe edema, ketoacidosis, uterine atony or overdistention, dystocia).

[mild to moderate] Anxiety may be related to situational "crisis," threat to health status (maternal/fetus), possibly evidenced by increased tension, apprehension, fear of unspecific consequences, sympathetic stimulation.

Diabetes mellitus, postpartum   OB

risk for unstable blood Glucose Level: risk factors may include deficient knowledge of diabetes, medication management, dietary intake, increased metabolic demands (recuperation, lactation).

risk for Injury: risk factors may include biochemical or regulatory complications—uterine atony/hemorrhage, pregnancy-induced hypertension, hyperglycemia).

risk for impaired Attachment: risk factors may include interruption in bonding process, physical illness, changes in physical abilities.

Diabetic ketoacidosis   CH/MS

deficient Fluid Volume [specify] may be related to hyperosmolar urinary losses, gastric losses, and inadequate intake, possibly evidenced by increased urinary output, dilute urine; reports of weakness, thirst; sudden weight loss; hypotension; tachycardia; delayed capillary refill; dry mucous membranes; poor skin turgor.

unstable blood Glucose Level may be related to medication management, lack of diabetes management, inadequate blood glucose monitoring, presence of infection, possibly evidenced by elevated serum glucose level, presence of ketones in urine, nausea, weight loss, blurred vision, irritability.

Fatigue may be related to decreased metabolic energy production, altered body chemistry (insufficient insulin), increased energy demands (hypermetabolic state, infection), possibly evidenced by overwhelming lack of energy, inability to maintain usual routines, decreased performance, impaired ability to concentrate, listlessness.

risk for Infection: risk factors may include high glucose levels, decreased leukocyte function, stasis of body fluids, invasive procedures, alteration in circulation and perfusion.

Dialysis, general   CH

Also refer to Dialysis, peritoneal; hemodialysis

imbalanced Nutrition: less than body requirements may be related to inadequate ingestion of nutrients—dietary restrictions, anorexia, nausea, vomiting, stomatitis, sensation of feeling full with continuous ambulatory peritoneal dialysis; loss of peptides and amino acids (building blocks for proteins) during dialysis, possibly evidenced by reported inadequate intake, aversion to eating, altered taste sensation, poor muscle tone, weakness, sore and inflamed buccal cavity, pale conjunctiva and mucous membranes.

Grieving may be related to actual or perceived loss, chronic or fatal illness, and thwarted grieving response to a loss, possibly evidenced by verbal expression of distress or unresolved issues, denial of loss; altered eating habits, sleep and dream patterns, activity levels, libido; crying, labile affect; feelings of sorrow, guilt, and anger.

disturbed Body Image/situational low Self-Esteem may be related to situational crisis and chronic illness with changes in usual roles and body image, possibly evidenced by verbalization of changes in lifestyle, focus on past function, negative feelings about body, feelings of helplessness, powerlessness, extension of body boundary to incorporate environmental objects (e.g., dialysis setup), change in social involvement, overdependence on others for care, not taking responsibility for self-care, lack of follow-through, and self-destructive behavior.

Self-Care Deficit [specify] may be related to perceptual or cognitive impairment (accumulated toxins); intolerance to activity, decreased strength and endurance; pain, discomfort, possibly evidenced by reported inability to perform activities of daily living, disheveled, unkempt appearance, strong body odor.

Powerlessness may be related to illness-related regimen and healthcare environment, possibly evidenced by verbal expression of having no control, depression over physical deterioration, nonparticipation in care, anger, and passivity.

compromised/disabled family Coping may be related to inadequate or incorrect information or understanding by a primary person, temporary family disorganization and role changes, client providing little support in turn for the primary person, and prolonged disease or disability progression that exhausts the supportive capacity of significant persons, possibly evidenced by expressions of concern or reports about response of SO(s)/family to client's health problem, preoccupation of SO(s) with own personal reactions, display of intolerance or rejection, and protective behavior disproportionate (too little or too much) to client's abilities or need for autonomy.

Dialysis, peritoneal   MS/CH

Also refer to Dialysis, general

risk for excess Fluid Volume: risk factors may include inadequate osmotic gradient of dialysate, fluid retention—malpositioned, kinked, or clotted catheter; bowel distention, peritonitis, scarring of peritoneum; excessive PO/IV intake.

risk for Trauma: risk factors may include improper placement during insertion or manipulation of catheter.

acute Pain/impaired Comfort may be related to catheter irritation, improper catheter placement, presence of edema, abdominal distention, inflammation, or infection; rapid infusion or infusion of cold or acidic dialysate, possibly evidenced by verbal reports, guarding or distraction behaviors, and self-focus.

risk for Infection [peritonitis]: risk factors may include contamination of catheter or infusion system, skin contaminants, sterile peritonitis—response to composition of dialysate.

risk for ineffective Breathing Pattern: risk factors may include increased abdominal pressure restricting diaphragmatic excursion, rapid infusion of dialysate, pain or discomfort, inflammatory process (e.g., atelectasis/pneumonia).

Diaper rash   PED

Refer to Candidiasis

Diaphragmatic hernia   CH/MS

Refer to Hernia, hiatal

Diarrhea   PED/CH

deficient Knowledge [Learning Need] regarding causative or contributing factors and therapeutic needs may be related to lack of information, misconceptions, possibly evidenced by statements of concern, questions, and development of preventable complications.

risk for deficient Fluid Volume: Risk factors may include excessive losses through gastrointestinal tract, altered intake.

acute Pain may be related to abdominal cramping and irritation or excoriation of skin, possibly evidenced by verbal reports, facial grimacing, and autonomic responses.

impaired Skin Integrity may be related to effects of excretions on delicate tissues, possibly evidenced by reports of discomfort and disruption of skin surface, destruction of skin layers.

DIC   MS

Refer to Disseminated intravascular coagulation

Diffuse axonal (brain) injury   **MS**

Refer to Traumatic brain injury; Cerebrovascular accident

Digitalis toxicity   **MS/CH**

decreased Cardiac Output may be related to altered myocardial contractility and electrical conduction, properties of digitalis (long half-life and narrow therapeutic range), concurrent medications, age and general health status, and electrolyte/acid-base balance, possibly evidenced by changes in rate, rhythm, and conduction (development or worsening of dysrhythmias), changes in mentation, worsening of heart failure, elevated serum drug levels.

    risk for imbalanced Fluid Volume: risk factors may include excessive losses from vomiting or diarrhea, decreased intake, nausea, decreased plasma proteins, malnutrition, continued use of diuretics; excess sodium and fluid retention.

    deficient Knowledge [Learning Need] regarding condition, therapy and self-care needs may be related to information misinterpretation and lack of recall, possibly evidenced by inaccurate follow-through of instructions and development of preventable complications.

    risk for disturbed Thought Processes: risk factors may include physiological effects of toxicity, reduced cerebral perfusion.

Dilation and curettage   **OB/GYN**

Also refer to Abortion, elective or spontaneous termination

    deficient Knowledge [Learning Need] regarding surgical procedure, possible postprocedural complications, and therapeutic needs may be related to lack of exposure or unfamiliarity with information, possibly evidenced by requests for information and statements of concern, misconceptions.

Dilation of cervix, premature   **OB**

Also refer to Preterm labor

    Anxiety [specify level] may be related to situational crisis, threat of death or fetal loss, possibly evidenced by increased tension, apprehension, feelings of inadequacy, sympathetic stimulation, and repetitive questioning.

    risk for disturbed Maternal/Fetal Dyad: risk factors may include surgical intervention, use of tocolytic drugs.

    Grieving may be related to perceived potential fetal loss, possibly evidenced by expression of distress, guilt, anger, choked feelings.

Dislocation/subluxation of joint   **CH**

acute Pain may be related to lack of continuity of bone/joint, muscle spasms, edema, possibly evidenced by verbal or coded reports, guarded or protective behaviors, narrowed focus, autonomic responses.

    risk for Injury: risk factors may include nerve impingement, improper fitting of splint device.

    impaired physical Mobility may be related to immobilization device, activity restrictions, pain, edema, decreased muscle strength, possibly evidenced by limited range of motion, limited ability to perform motor skills, gait changes.

Disruptive behavior disorder   **PED/PSY**

Refer to Oppositional defiant disorder

Disseminated intravascular coagulation   **MS**

risk for Shock: risk factors may include failure of regulatory mechanism (coagulation process) and active loss, hemorrhage.

---

ineffective tissue Perfusion (specify) may be related to alteration of arterial or venous flow (microemboli throughout circulatory system, and hypovolemia), possibly evidenced by changes in respiratory rate and depth, changes in mentation, decreased urinary output, and development of acral cyanosis and focal gangrene.

Anxiety [specify level]/Fear may be related to sudden change in health status/threat of death, interpersonal transmission/contagion, possibly evidenced by sympathetic stimulation, restlessness, focus on self, and apprehension.

risk for impaired Gas Exchange: risk factors may include reduced oxygen-carrying capacity, development of acidosis, fibrin deposition in microcirculation, and ischemic damage of lung parenchyma.

acute Pain may be related to bleeding into joints/muscles, with hematoma formation, and ischemic tissues with areas of acral cyanosis and focal gangrene, possibly evidenced by verbal reports, narrowed focus, alteration in muscle tone, guarding or distraction behaviors, restlessness, autonomic responses.

Dissociative disorders   PSY

[severe/panic] Anxiety/Fear may be related to a maladaptation or ineffective coping continuing from early life, unconscious conflict(s), threat to self-concept, unmet needs, or phobic stimulus, possibly evidenced by maladaptive response to stress (e.g., dissociating self, fragmentation of the personality), increased tension, feelings of inadequacy, and focus on self, projection of personal perceptions onto the environment.

risk for self-/other-directed Violence: risk factors may include dissociative state, conflicting personalities, depressed mood, panic states, and suicidal or homicidal behaviors.

disturbed Personal Identity may be related to psychological conflicts (dissociative state), childhood trauma or abuse, threat to physical integrity and self-concept, and underdeveloped ego, possibly evidenced by alteration in perception or experience of the self, loss of one's own sense of reality and the external world, poorly differentiated ego boundaries, confusion about sense of self, purpose or direction in life; memory loss, presence of more than one personality within the individual.

compromised family Coping may be related to multiple stressors repeated over time, prolonged progression of disorder that exhausts the supportive capacity of significant person(s), family disorganization and role changes, high-risk family situation, possibly evidenced by family/SO(s) describing inadequate understanding or knowledge that interferes with assistive or supportive behaviors; relationship and marital conflict.

Diverticulitis   CH

acute Pain may be related to inflammation of intestinal mucosa, abdominal cramping, and presence of fever and chills, possibly evidenced by verbal reports, guarding or distraction behaviors, autonomic responses, and narrowed focus.

Diarrhea/Constipation may be related to altered structure and function, and presence of inflammation, possibly evidenced by signs and symptoms dependent on specific problem (e.g., increase or decrease in frequency of stools and change in consistency).

deficient Knowledge [Learning Need] regarding disease process, potential complications, therapy, and self-care needs may be related to lack of information, misconceptions, possibly evidenced by statements of concern, request for information, and development of preventable complications.

risk for Powerlessness: risk factors may include chronic nature of disease process and recurrent episodes despite cooperation with medical regimen.

Down syndrome   PED/CH
Also refer to Mental delay (formerly retardation)

delayed Growth and Development may be related to effects of physical and mental disability, possibly evidenced by altered physical growth; delay or inability in performing skills and self-care or self-control activities appropriate for age.

    risk for Trauma: risk factors may include cognitive difficulties and poor muscle tone or coordination, weakness.

    imbalanced Nutrition: less than body requirements may be related to poor muscle tone and protruding tongue, possibly evidenced by weak and ineffective sucking or swallowing and observed lack of adequate intake with weight loss or failure to gain.

    interrupted Family Processes may be related to situational or maturational crises requiring incorporation of new skills into family dynamics, possibly evidenced by confusion about what to do, verbalized difficulty coping with situation, unexamined family myths.

    risk for complicated Grieving: risk factors may include loss of "the perfect child," chronic condition requiring long-term care, and unresolved feelings.

    risk for impaired Attachment: risk factors may include ill infant/child who is unable to effectively initiate parental contact due to altered behavioral organization, inability of parents to meet the personal needs.

    risk for Social Isolation: risk factors may include withdrawal from usual social interactions and activities, assumption of total child care, and becoming overindulgent or overprotective.

Dressler's syndrome   CH

acute Pain may be related to tissue inflammation and presence of effusion, possibly evidenced by verbal reports of chest pain affected by movement or position and deep breathing, guarding or distraction behaviors, self-focus, and changes in vital signs.

    Anxiety [specify level] may be related to threat to or change in health status, possibly evidenced by increased tension, apprehension, restlessness, and expressed concerns.

    risk for ineffective Breathing Pattern: risk factors may include pain on inspiration.

    risk for impaired Gas Exchange: risk factors may include ventilation perfusion imbalance—pleural effusion, pulmonary infiltrates.

Drug overdose, acute (depressants)   MS/PSY

Also refer to Substance dependence/abuse rehabilitation

    ineffective Breathing Pattern/impaired Gas Exchange may be related to neuromuscular impairment, central nervous system depression, decreased lung expansion, possibly evidenced by changes in respirations, cyanosis, and abnormal arterial blood gases.

    risk for Trauma/Suffocation/Poisoning: risk factors may include central nervous system depression, agitation, hypersensitivity to the drug(s), psychological stress.

    risk for self-/other-directed Violence: risk factors may include suicidal behaviors, toxic reactions to drug(s).

    risk for Infection: risk factors may include drug injection techniques, impurities in injected drugs, localized trauma; malnutrition, altered immune state.

Drug withdrawal   CH/MS

disturbed Thought Processes may be related to substance abuse and cessation, sleep deprivation, malnutrition, possibly evidenced by inaccurate interpretation of environment, inappropriate or nonreality-based thinking, paranoia.

    risk for Injury: risk factors may include central nervous system agitation (depressants).

    risk for Suicide: risk factors may include alcohol or substance abuse, legal or disciplinary problems, depressed mood (stimulants).

    acute Pain/impaired Comfort may be related to biochemical changes associated with cessation of drug use, possibly evidenced by reports of muscle aches, fever, diaphoresis, rhinorrhea, lacrimation, malaise.

Self-Care Deficit (specify) may be related to perceptual or cognitive impairment, therapeutic management (restraints), possibly evidenced by inability to meet own physical needs.

Insomnia may be related to cessation of substance use, fatigue, possibly evidenced by reports of insomnia or hypersomnia, decreased ability to function, increased irritability.

Fatigue may be related to altered body chemistry (drug withdrawal), sleep deprivation, malnutrition, poor physical condition, possibly evidenced by verbal reports of overwhelming lack of energy, inability to maintain usual level of physical activity, inability to restore energy after sleep, compromised concentration.

DTs   **MS/PSY**
Refer to Delirium tremens

Duchenne's muscular dystrophy   **PED/CH**
Refer to Muscular dystrophy [Duchenne's]

Duodenal ulcer   **MS/CH**
Refer to Ulcer, peptic

DVT   **CH/MS**
Refer to Thrombophlebitis

Dysmenorrhea   **GYN**
acute Pain may be related to exaggerated uterine contractibility, possibly evidenced by verbal reports, guarding or distraction behaviors, narrowed focus, and changes in vital signs.

risk for Activity Intolerance: risk factors may include severity of pain and presence of secondary symptoms (nausea, vomiting, syncope, chills), depression.

ineffective Coping may be related to chronic, recurrent nature of problem; anticipatory anxiety, and inadequate coping methods, possibly evidenced by muscular tension, headaches, general irritability, chronic depression, and verbalization of inability to cope, report of poor self-concept.

Dyspareunia   **GYN/PSY**
Sexual Dysfunction may be related to physical or psychological alteration in function (menopausal involution, allergy to contraceptive, abnormalities of genital tract, guilt, control issues), possibly evidenced by verbalization of problem, inability to achieve desired satisfaction, sexual aversion, alteration in relationship with SO.

Anxiety [specify] may be related to situational crisis, stress, unconscious conflict about essential values, unmet needs, possibly evidenced by expressed concerns, distressed, feelings of inadequacy.

Dysrhythmia, cardiac   **CH/MS**
risk for decreased Cardiac Output: risk factors may include altered electrical conduction and reduced myocardial contractility.

deficient Knowledge [Learning Need] regarding medical condition and therapy needs may be related to lack of information, misinterpretation and unfamiliarity with information resources, possibly evidenced by questions, statement of misconception, failure to improve on previous regimen, and development of preventable complications.

risk for Activity Intolerance: risk factors may include imbalance between myocardial oxygen supply and demand, and cardiac depressant effects of certain drugs (beta-blockers, antidysrhythmics).

risk for Poisoning [digitalis toxicity]: risk factors may include limited range of therapeutic effectiveness, lack of education or proper precautions, reduced vision, cognitive limitations.

Dysthymic disorder   PSY/CH
Refer to Depression, major

Dystocia   OB
Also refer to Labor, stage I [latent/active phases]

risk for maternal Injury: risk factors may include alteration of muscle tone/contractile pattern, mechanical obstruction to fetal descent, maternal fatigue.

risk for fetal Injury: risk factors may include prolonged labor, fetal malpresentations, tissue hypoxia and acidosis, abnormalities of the maternal pelvis, cephalopelvic disproportion.

risk for deficient Fluid Volume: risk factors may include hypermetabolic state, vomiting, profuse diaphoresis, restricted oral intake, mild diuresis associated with oxytocin administration.

ineffective Coping may be related to situational crisis, personal vulnerability, unrealistic expectations or perceptions, inadequate or exhausted support systems, possibly evidenced by verbalizations and behavior indicative of inability to cope (loss of control, inability to problem-solve, or meet role expectations), irritability, reports of fatigue, increased tension.

Eating disorders   CH/PSY
Refer to Anorexia nervosa; Bulimia nervosa

Ebola   MS
Also refer to Disseminated intravascular coagulation; Multiple organ dysfunction syndrome

acute Pain/impaired Comfort may be related to infectious process, possibly evidenced by reports of headache, myalgia, abdominal or chest pain, sore throat, fever.

Hyperthermia may be related to inflammatory process, possibly evidenced by increased body temperature, warm skin, headache.

risk for deficient Fluid Volume: risk factors may include inadequate intake (nausea, painful swallowing, abdominal pain), increased losses (vomiting, diarrhea, hemorrhage/disseminated intravascular coagulation), hypermetabolic state (fever).

risk for [spread of or secondary] Infection: risk factors may include mode of transmission, invasive monitoring and procedures, debilitated state, malnutrition, insufficient knowledge or resources to avoid exposure to pathogens.

acute Confusion may be related to infectious process, hypoxemia, possibly evidenced by fluctuations in cognition, agitation, change in level of consciousness (stupor, coma).

Eclampsia   OB
Also refer to Pregnancy-induced hypertension

Anxiety [specify]/Fear may be related to situational crisis, threat of change in health status or death (self/fetus), separation from support system, interpersonal contagion, possibly evidenced by expressed concerns, apprehension, increased tension, decreased self-assurance, difficulty concentrating.

risk for maternal Injury: risk factors may include tissue edema, hypoxia, tonic clonic convulsions, abnormal blood profile or clotting factors.

impaired physical Mobility may be related to prescribed bedrest, discomfort, anxiety, possibly evidenced by difficulty turning, postural instability.

risk for Self-Care Deficit (specify): risk factors may include weakness, discomfort, physical restrictions.

ECT   **PSY**
Refer to Electroconvulsive therapy

Ectopic pregnancy (tubal)   **OB**
Also refer to Abortion, spontaneous termination

acute Pain may be related to distention/rupture of fallopian tube, possibly evidenced by verbal reports, guarding or distraction behaviors, facial mask of pain, diaphoresis, and changes in vital signs.

risk for Bleeding/deficient Fluid Volume [isotonic]: risk factors may include pregnancy-related complication, hemorrhagic losses, and decreased or restricted intake.

Anxiety [specify level]/Fear may be related to threat of death and possible loss of ability to conceive, possibly evidenced by increased tension, apprehension, sympathetic stimulation, restlessness, and focus on self.

Eczema   **CH**
Refer to Dermatitis, contact/seborrheic

acute Pain/impaired Comfort may be related to cutaneous inflammation and irritation, possibly evidenced by verbal reports, irritability, and scratching.

risk for Infection: risk factors may include broken skin and tissue trauma.

Social Isolation may be related to alterations in physical appearance, possibly evidenced by expressed feelings of rejection and decreased interaction with peers.

Edema, pulmonary   **MS**
excess Fluid Volume may be related to decreased cardiac functioning, excessive fluid and sodium intake, possibly evidenced by dyspnea, presence of crackles (rales), pulmonary congestion on radiograph, restlessness, anxiety, and increased central venous pressure and pulmonary pressures.

impaired Gas Exchange may be related to altered blood flow and decreased alveolar-capillary exchange (fluid collection or shifts into interstitial space and alveoli), possibly evidenced by hypoxia, restlessness, and confusion.

Anxiety [specify level]/Fear may be related to perceived threat of death (inability to breathe), possibly evidenced by responses ranging from apprehension to panic state, restlessness, and focus on self.

Elder abuse   **CH/PSY**
Refer to Abuse, physical/psychological

Electrical injury   **MS**
Also refer to Burns

risk for decreased Cardiac Output: risk factors may include altered heart rate and rhythm (ventricular fibrillation, asystole).

impaired [internal] Tissue Integrity may be related to thermal injury (along path of current), altered circulation (massive edema), possibly evidenced by damaged or destroyed tissue, necrosis.

risk for impaired peripheral tissue Perfusion: risk factors may include reduction of venous or arterial blood flow (vein coagulation, muscle edema), increased tissue pressure (compartment syndrome).

risk for Trauma/Suffocation: risk factors may include muscle paralysis (central nervous system damage), loss of large- or small-muscle coordination (seizures).

Electroconvulsive therapy   **PSY**
decisional Conflict may be related to lack of relevant or multiple and divergent sources of information, mistrust of regimen or healthcare personnel, sense of powerlessness, support system deficit.

risk for Injury [effects of electroconvulsive therapy]: risk factors may include effects of therapy on the cardiovascular, respiratory, musculoskeletal, and nervous systems, and pharmacological effects of anesthesia.

acute Confusion may be related to central nervous system effects of electric shock, medications, and anesthesia, possibly evidenced by fluctuation in cognition, agitation.

impaired Memory may be related to neurological disturbance (electrical shock), possibly evidenced by reported or observed experiences of forgetting, difficulty recalling recent events or factual information.

Emphysema   CH/MS

impaired Gas Exchange may be related to alveolar capillary membrane changes or destruction, possibly evidenced by dyspnea, restlessness, changes in mentation, abnormal arterial blood gas values.

ineffective Airway Clearance may be related to increased production and retained tenacious secretions, decreased energy level, and muscle wasting, possibly evidenced by abnormal breath sounds (rhonchi), ineffective cough, changes in rate and depth of respirations, and dyspnea.

Activity Intolerance may be related to imbalance between oxygen supply and demand, possibly evidenced by reports of fatigue or weakness, exertional dyspnea, and abnormal vital sign response to activity.

imbalanced Nutrition: less than body requirements may be related to inability to ingest food (shortness of breath, anorexia, generalized weakness, medication side effects), possibly evidenced by lack of interest in food, reported altered taste, loss of muscle mass and tone, fatigue, and weight loss.

risk for Infection: risk factors may include inadequate primary defenses (stasis of body fluids, decreased ciliary action), chronic disease process, and malnutrition.

Powerlessness may be related to illness-related regimen and healthcare environment, possibly evidenced by verbal expression of having no control, depression over physical deterioration, nonparticipation in therapeutic regimen, anger, and passivity.

Encephalitis   MS

risk for ineffective cerebral tissue Perfusion: risk factors may include cerebral edema altering or interrupting cerebral arterial or venous blood flow, hypovolemia, exchange problems at cellular level (acidosis).

Hyperthermia may be related to increased metabolic rate, illness, and dehydration, possibly evidenced by increased body temperature; flushed, warm skin; and increased pulse and respiratory rates.

acute Pain may be related to inflammation or irritation of the brain and cerebral edema, possibly evidenced by verbal reports of headache, photophobia, distraction behaviors, restlessness, and changes in vital signs.

risk for Trauma/Suffocation: risk factors may include restlessness, clonic-tonic activity, altered sensorium, cognitive impairment, generalized weakness, ataxia, vertigo.

Encopresis   PSY/PED

Bowel Incontinence may be related to situational or maturational crisis, psychogenic factors (predisposing vulnerability, threat to physical integrity—child/sexual abuse), possibly evidenced by involuntary passage of stool at least once monthly, strong odor of feces on client, hiding soiled clothing in inappropriate places.

disturbed Body Image/chronic low Self-Esteem may be related to negative view of self, maturational expectations, social factors, stigma attached to loss of body function in public, family's belief condition is volitional, shame related to body odor, possibly evidenced by angry outbursts or oppositional behavior, verbalization of powerlessness, reluctance to engage in social activities.

compromised family Coping may be related to inadequate or incorrect information or understanding of condition, belief that behavior is volitional, disagreement regarding treatment or coping strategies, possibly evidenced by attempts to intervene with child are increasingly ineffective, significant person describes preoccupation with personal reaction (excessive guilt, anger, blame regarding child's condition or behavior), overprotective behavior.

Endocarditis   MS

risk for decreased Cardiac Output: risk factors may include inflammation of lining of heart and structural change in valve leaflets.

Anxiety [specify level] may be related to change in health status and threat of death, possibly evidenced by apprehension, expressed concerns, and focus on self.

acute Pain may be related to generalized inflammatory process and effects of embolic phenomena, possibly evidenced by verbal reports, narrowed focus, distraction behaviors, and autonomic responses (changes in vital signs).

risk for Activity Intolerance: risk factors may include imbalance between oxygen supply and demand, debilitating condition.

risk for ineffective tissue Perfusion (specify): risk factors may include embolic interruption of arterial flow (embolization of thrombi or valvular vegetations).

End-of-life care   CH
Refer to Hospice care

Endometriosis   GYN

acute/chronic Pain may be related to pressure of concealed bleeding, formation of adhesions, possibly evidenced by verbal reports (pain between and with menstruation), guarding or distraction behaviors, and narrowed focus.

Sexual Dysfunction may be related to pain secondary to presence of adhesions, possibly evidenced by verbalization of problem and altered relationship with partner.

deficient Knowledge [Learning Need] regarding pathophysiology of condition and therapy needs may be related to lack of information, misinterpretations, possibly evidenced by statements of concern and misconceptions.

Enteral feeding   MS/CH

imbalanced Nutrition: less than body requirements may be related to conditions that interfere with nutrient intake or increase nutrient need or metabolic demand—cancer and associated treatments, anorexia, surgical procedures, dysphagia, or decreased level of consciousness, possibly evidenced by body weight 10% or more under ideal, decreased subcutaneous fat or muscle mass, poor muscle tone, changes in gastric motility and stool characteristics.

risk for Infection: risk factors may include invasive procedure, surgical placement of feeding tube, malnutrition, chronic disease.

risk for Aspiration: risk factors may include presence of feeding tube, bolus tube feedings, increased intragastric pressure, delayed gastric emptying, medication administration.

risk for imbalanced Fluid Volume: risk factors may include active loss or failure of regulatory mechanisms (specific to underlying disease process or trauma), inability to obtain or ingest fluids.

Fatigue may be related to decreased metabolic energy production, increased energy requirements (hypermetabolic state, healing process), altered body chemistry (medications, chemotherapy), possibly evidenced by overwhelming lack of energy, inability to maintain usual routines or accomplish routine tasks, lethargy, impaired ability to concentrate.

Enteritis   MS/CH
Refer to Colitis, ulcerative; Crohn's disease

Enuresis   PSY/PED
impaired Urinary Elimination may be related to situational or maturational crisis, psychogenic factors (predisposing vulnerability, threat to physical integrity—abuse), possibly evidenced by nocturnal or diurnal enuresis, strong odor of urine on client, hiding soiled clothing in inappropriate places

    disturbed Body Image/chronic low Self-Esteem may be related to negative view of self, maturational expectations, social factors, stigma attached to loss of body function in public, family's belief condition is volitional, shame related to body odor, possibly evidenced by angry outbursts or oppositional behavior, verbalization of powerlessness, reluctance to engage in social activities.

    compromised family Coping may be related to inadequate or incorrect information or understanding of condition, belief that behavior is volitional, disagreement regarding treatment or coping strategies, possibly evidenced by attempts to intervene with child are increasingly ineffective, SO describes preoccupation with personal reaction (excessive guilt, anger, blame regarding child's condition or behavior), overprotective behavior.

Epididymitis   MS
acute Pain may be related to inflammation, edema formation, and tension on the spermatic cord, possibly evidenced by verbal reports, guarding or distraction behaviors (restlessness), and changes in vital signs.

    risk for Infection [spread]: risk factors may include presence of inflammation and infectious process, insufficient knowledge to avoid spread of infection.

    deficient Knowledge [Learning Need] regarding pathophysiology, outcome, and self-care needs may be related to lack of information, misinterpretations, possibly evidenced by statements of concern, misconceptions, and questions.

Epilepsy   CH
Refer to Seizure disorder

Episiotomy   OB
acute Pain may be related to tissue trauma, edema, surgical incision, possibly evidenced by verbalizations, guarding behavior, self-focusing.

    risk for Infection: risk factors may include broken skin, traumatized tissue, body excretions, inadequate hygiene.

    risk for Sexual Dysfunction: risk factors may include recent childbirth, presence of incision.

Epistaxis   CH
[mild to moderate] Anxiety may be related to situational crisis, threat to health status, interpersonal transmission, possibly evidenced by expressed concerns, apprehension, anxiety.

    risk for Aspiration: risk factors may include uncontrolled nasal bleeding.

Epstein-Barr virus   CH
Refer to Mononucleosis, infectious

Erectile dysfunction   CH/PSY
Sexual Dysfunction may be related to altered body function, side effects of medication, possibly evidenced by reports of disruption of sexual response pattern, inability to achieve desired satisfaction.

---

situational low Self-Esteem may be related to functional impairment, perceived failure to perform satisfactorily, rejection of other(s), possibly evidenced by self-negating verbalizations, expressions of helplessness, powerlessness.

Esophageal reflux disease   CH
Refer to Gastroesophageal reflux disease

Esophageal varices   CH/MS
Refer to Varices, esophageal

Esophagitis   CH
Refer to Gastroesophageal reflux disease; Achalasia

ETOH withdrawal   MS/CH
Refer to Alcohol intoxication, acute; Substance dependence/abuse rehabilitation

Evisceration   MS
Refer to Dehiscence, abdominal

Facial reconstructive surgery   MS/CH
Also refer to Surgery, general; Intermaxillary fixation
   risk for ineffective Airway Clearance: risk factors may include soft tissue edema, airway trauma, retained secretions.
   impaired Skin Integrity may be related to traumatic injury, surgical procedure (incisions/grafts), edema, altered circulation, possibly evidenced by disruption or destruction of skin layers.
   Fear/Anxiety may be related to situational crisis, memory of traumatic event, threat to self-concept (disfigurement), possibly evidenced by expressed concerns, apprehension, uncertainty, decreased self-assurance, restlessness.
   disturbed Body Image may be related to traumatic event, disfigurement, possibly evidenced by negative feelings about self, fear of rejection reaction by others, preoccupation with change, change in social involvement.
   risk for Social Isolation: risk factors may include change in physical appearance.

Failure to thrive, adult   CH/MS
adult Failure to Thrive may be related to depression, apathy, aging process, fatigue, degenerative condition, possibly evidenced by expressed lack of appetite, difficulty performing self-care tasks, altered mood state, inadequate intake, weight loss, physical decline.
   ineffective Protection may be related to inadequate nutrition, anemia, extremes of age, possibly evidenced by fatigue, weakness, deficient immunity, impaired healing, pressure sores.

Failure to thrive, infant/child   PED
imbalanced Nutrition: less than body requirements may be related to inability to ingest, digest, or absorb nutrients (defects in organ function or metabolism, genetic factors); physical deprivation; psychosocial factors, possibly evidenced by lack of appropriate weight gain or weight loss, poor muscle tone, pale conjunctiva, and laboratory tests reflecting nutritional deficiency.
   delayed Growth and Development may be related to inadequate caretaking (physical or emotional neglect or abuse), indifference, inconsistent responsiveness, multiple caretakers, environmental and stimulation deficiencies, possibly evidenced by altered physical growth, flat affect, listlessness, decreased response; delay or difficulty in performing skills or self-control activities appropriate for age group.

risk for impaired Parenting: risk factors may include lack of knowledge, inadequate bonding, unrealistic expectations for self/infant, and lack of appropriate response of child to relationship.

deficient Knowledge [Learning Need] regarding pathophysiology of condition, nutritional needs, growth/development expectations, and parenting skills may be related to lack of information, misinformation or misinterpretation, possibly evidenced by verbalization of concerns, questions, misconceptions; or development of preventable complications.

Fat embolism syndrome   MS
Refer to Pulmonary embolism; Respiratory distress syndrome, acute

Fatigue syndrome, chronic   CH
Fatigue may be related to disease state, inadequate sleep, possibly evidenced by verbalization of unremitting or overwhelming lack of energy, inability to maintain usual routines, listlessness, compromised concentration.

chronic Pain may be related to chronic physical disability, possibly evidenced by verbal reports of headache, sore throat, arthralgias, abdominal pain, muscle aches, altered ability to continue previous activities, changes in sleep pattern.

Self-Care Deficit [specify] may be related to tiredness, pain, discomfort, possibly evidenced by reports of inability to perform desired activities of daily living.

risk for ineffective Role Performance: risk factors may include health alterations, stress.

Febrile seizure   PED
Hyperthermia may be related to illness, dehydration, decreased ability to perspire, possibly evidenced by increase in body temperature; flushed, warm skin; seizures.

Fecal diversion   MS/CH
Refer to Colostomy

Fecal impaction   CH
Constipation may be related to irregular defecation habits, decreased activity, dehydration, abdominal muscle weakness, neurological impairment, possibly evidenced by inability to pass stool, abdominal distention, tenderness or pain, nausea, vomiting, anorexia.

Femoral popliteal bypass   MS
Also refer to Surgery, general

risk for ineffective peripheral tissue Perfusion: risk factors may include interruption of arterial blood flow, hypovolemia.

risk for Peripheral Neurovascular Dysfunction: risk factors may include vascular obstruction, immobilization, mechanical compression, dressings.

impaired Walking may be related to surgical incisions, dressings, possibly evidenced by inability to walk desired distance, climb stairs, negotiate inclines.

Fetal alcohol syndrome   PED
risk for Injury [central nervous system damage]: risk factors may include external chemical factors (alcohol intake by mother), placental insufficiency, fetal drug withdrawal in utero or postpartum, and prematurity.

disorganized Infant Behavior may be related to prematurity, environmental overstimulation, lack of containment or boundaries, possibly evidenced by change from baseline physiological measures, tremors, startles, twitches, hyperextension of arms and legs, deficient self regulatory behaviors, deficient response to visual or auditory stimuli.

risk for impaired Parenting: risk factors may include mental or physical illness, inability of mother to assume the overwhelming task of unselfish giving and nurturing, presence of stressors (financial or legal problems), lack of available or ineffective role model, interruption of bonding process, lack of appropriate response of child to relationship.

PSY

ineffective [maternal] Coping may be related to personal vulnerability, low self-esteem, inadequate coping skills, and multiple stressors (repeated over period of time), possibly evidenced by inability to meet basic needs, fulfill role expectations, or problem-solve; and excessive use of drug(s).

dysfunctional Family Processes may be related to lack of or insufficient support from others, mother's drug problem and treatment status, together with poor coping skills, lack of family stability, overinvolvement of parents with children and multigenerational addictive behaviors, possibly evidenced by abandonment, rejection, neglectful relationships with family members, and decisions and actions by family that are detrimental.

Fetal demise OB
Refer to Perinatal loss/death of child

Fetal transfusion syndrome OB
Refer to Twin-twin transfusion syndrome

Fibrocystic breast disease CH
[mild to moderate] Anxiety may be related to situational crisis, threat to health status, family heredity, interpersonal transmission, possibly evidenced by expressed concerns, apprehension, uncertainty, fearfulness, focus on self, increased tension.

acute/chronic Pain may be related to physical agents (edema formation, nerve irritation), possibly evidenced by verbal reports, guarded or protective behavior, expressive behavior, self-focusing.

risk for ineffective Coping: risk factors may include situational crisis, perceived high degree of threat, inadequate resources or social supports.

Fibroids, uterine GYN
Refer to Uterine myomas

Fibromyalgia syndrome, primary CH
acute/chronic Pain may be related to idiopathic diffuse condition, possibly evidenced by reports of achy pain in fibrous tissues (muscles, tendons, ligaments), muscle stiffness or spasm, disturbed sleep, guarding behaviors, fear of reinjury or exacerbation, restlessness, irritability, self-focusing, reduced interaction with others.

Fatigue may be related to disease state, stress, anxiety, depression, sleep deprivation, possibly evidenced by verbalization of overwhelming lack of energy, inability to maintain usual routines or level of physical activity, tired, feelings of guilt for not keeping up with responsibilities, increase in physical complaints, listlessness.

risk for Hopelessness: risk factors may include chronic debilitating physical condition, prolonged activity restriction (possibly self-induced), creating isolation, lack of specific therapeutic cure, prolonged stress.

Flail chest MS
Refer to Hemothorax; Pneumothorax

Food poisoning   CH/MS
Refer to Gastroenteritis

Fractures   MS/CH
Also refer to Casts; Traction
  risk for Trauma [additional injury]: risk factors may include loss of skeletal integrity, movement of skeletal fragments, use of traction apparatus.
  acute Pain may be related to muscle spasms, movement of bone fragments, tissue trauma, edema, traction or immobility device, stress, and anxiety, possibly evidenced by verbal reports, distraction behaviors, self-focusing or narrowed focus, facial mask of pain, guarding or protective behavior, alteration in muscle tone, and changes in vital signs.
  risk for Peripheral Neurovascular Dysfunction: risk factors may include reduction or interruption of blood flow (direct vascular injury, tissue trauma, excessive edema, thrombus formation, hypovolemia).
  impaired physical Mobility may be related to neuromuscular or skeletal impairment, pain, discomfort, restrictive therapies (bedrest, extremity immobilization), and psychological immobility, possibly evidenced by inability to purposefully move within the physical environment, imposed restrictions, reluctance to attempt movement, limited range of motion, and decreased muscle strength or control.
  risk for impaired Gas Exchange: risk factors may include altered blood flow, blood or fat emboli, alveolar-capillary membrane changes (interstitial or pulmonary edema, congestion).
  deficient Knowledge [Learning Need] regarding healing process, therapy requirements, potential complications, and self-care needs may be related to lack of exposure or recall, misinterpretation of information, possibly evidenced by statements of concern, questions, and misconceptions.

Frostbite   MS/CH
impaired Tissue Integrity may be related to altered circulation and thermal injury, possibly evidenced by damaged or destroyed tissue.
  acute Pain may be related to diminished circulation with tissue ischemia or necrosis and edema formation, possibly evidenced by verbal reports, guarding or distraction behaviors, narrowed focus, and changes in vital signs.
  risk for Infection: risk factors may include traumatized tissue, tissue destruction, altered circulation, and compromised immune response in affected area.

Fusion, cervical   MS
Refer to Laminectomy, cervical

Fusion, lumbar   MS
Refer to Laminectomy, lumbar

Gallstones   CH
Refer to Cholelithiasis

Gangrene, dry   MS
ineffective peripheral tissue Perfusion may be related to interruption in arterial flow, possibly evidenced by cool skin temperature, change in color (black), atrophy of affected part, and presence of pain.
  acute Pain may be related to tissue hypoxia and necrotic process, possibly evidenced by verbal reports, guarding or distraction behaviors, narrowed focus, and changes in vital signs.

Gangrene, gas   MS

impaired Tissue Integrity may be related to trauma, surgery, infection, altered circulation, possibly evidenced by edema, brown or serous exudate, bronze or blackish green skin color, gas bubbles or crepitation, pain.

[severe] Anxiety/Fear may be related to situational crisis, interpersonal transmission, threat of death, possibly evidenced by expressed concerns, distress, apprehension, fearfulness, restlessness, irritability, focus on self.

risk for impaired renal Perfusion: risk factors may include effects of circulating toxins, altered circulation, shock.

risk for Injury: risk factors may include therapeutic intervention (hyperbaric oxygen therapy).

Gas, lung irritant   MS/CH

ineffective Airway Clearance may be related to irritation or inflammation of airway, possibly evidenced by marked cough, abnormal breath sounds (wheezes), dyspnea, and tachypnea.

risk for impaired Gas Exchange: risk factors may include irritation or inflammation of alveolar membrane (dependent on type of agent and length of exposure).

Anxiety [specify level] may be related to change in health status and threat of death, possibly evidenced by verbalizations, increased tension, apprehension, and sympathetic stimulation.

Gastrectomy, subtotal   MS

Also refer to Surgery, general

risk for imbalanced Nutrition: less than body requirements: risk factors may include restricted oral intake, early satiety, change in digestive process, malabsorption of nutrients, fear of complications (e.g., dumping syndrome, reactive hypoglycemia).

risk for Fatigue: risk factors may include malnutrition, anemia.

risk for Diarrhea: risk factors may include malabsorption.

Gastric partitioning   MS

Refer to Gastroplasty

Gastric resection   MS

Refer to Gastrectomy, subtotal

Gastric ulcer   MS/CH

Refer to Ulcer, peptic

Gastrinoma   MS/CH

Refer to Zollinger-Ellison syndrome

Gastritis, acute   MS

acute Pain may be related to irritation or inflammation of gastric mucosa, possibly evidenced by verbal reports, guarding or distraction behaviors, and changes in vital signs.

risk for deficient Fluid Volume [isotonic]/Bleeding: risk factors may include excessive losses through vomiting and diarrhea, continued bleeding, reluctance to ingest or restrictions of oral intake.

Gastritis, chronic   CH

risk for imbalanced Nutrition: less than body requirements: risk factors may include inability to ingest adequate nutrients (prolonged nausea, vomiting, anorexia, epigastric pain).

deficient Knowledge [Learning Need] regarding pathophysiology, psychological factors, therapy needs, and potential complications may be related to lack of information or recall, unfamiliarity with information resources, information misinterpretation, possibly evidenced by verbalization of concerns, questions, and continuation of problem or development of preventable complications.

Gastroenteritis   CH/MS

Diarrhea may be related to toxins, contaminants, travel, infectious process, parasites, possibly evidenced by at least three loose liquid stools per day, hyperactive bowel sounds, abdominal pain.

risk for deficient Fluid Volume: risk factors may include excessive losses (diarrhea, vomiting), hypermetabolic state (infection), decreased intake (nausea, anorexia), extremes of age or weight.

risk for Infection [transmission]: risk factors may include insufficient knowledge to prevent contamination (inappropriate hand hygiene and food handling).

Gastroesophageal reflux disease (GERD)   CH

acute/chronic Pain may be related to acidic irritation of mucosa, muscle spasm, recurrent vomiting, possibly evidenced by reports of heartburn, distraction behaviors.

impaired Swallowing may be related to GERD, esophageal defects, achalasia, possibly evidenced by reports of heartburn or epigastric pain, "something stuck" when swallowing, food refusal or volume limiting, nighttime coughing or awakening.

risk for imbalanced Nutrition: less than body requirements: risk factors may include limited intake, recurrent vomiting.

risk for Insomnia: risk factors may include nighttime heartburn, regurgitation of stomach contents.

risk for Aspiration: risk factors may include incompetent lower esophageal sphincter, regurgitation of gastric acid.

Gastrointestinal hemorrhage   MS

Refer to Gastritis, acute or chronic; Ulcer, peptic; Colitis, ulcerative; Crohn's disease; Varices, esophageal

Gastroplasty   MS

Also refer to Surgery, general

ineffective Breathing Pattern may be related to decreased lung expansion, pain, anxiety, decreased energy, fatigue, tracheobronchial obstruction, possibly evidenced by dyspnea, tachypnea, changes in respiratory depth, reduced vital capacity, wheezes, rhonchi, abnormal arterial blood gases.

risk for ineffective peripheral tissue Perfusion: risk factors may include diminished blood flow, hypovolemia, immobility or bedrest, interruption of venous blood flow (thrombus).

risk for deficient Fluid Volume: risk factors may include excessive gastric losses, nasogastric suction, diarrhea, reduced intake.

risk for imbalanced Nutrition: less than body requirements: risk factors may include decreased intake, dietary restrictions, early satiety, increased metabolic rate (healing), malabsorption of nutrients, impaired absorption of vitamins.

Diarrhea may be related to changes in dietary fiber and bulk, inflammation, irritation, malabsorption of bowel, possibly evidenced by loose or liquid stools, increased frequency, hyperactive bowel sounds.

Gender identity disorder PSY

(For individuals experiencing persistent and marked distress regarding uncertainty about issues relating to personal identity, e.g., sexual orientation and behavior.)

Anxiety [specify level] may be related to unconscious or conscious conflicts about essential values or beliefs (ego-dystonic gender identification), threat to self-concept, unmet needs, possibly evidenced by increased tension, helplessness, hopelessness, feelings of inadequacy, uncertainty, insomnia and focus on self, and impaired daily functioning.

ineffective Role Performance/disturbed Personal Identity may be related to crisis in development in which person has difficulty knowing or accepting to which sex he or she belongs or is attracted, sense of discomfort and inappropriateness about anatomic sex characteristics, possibly evidenced by confusion about sense of self, purpose, or direction in life, sexual identification or preference, verbalization of desire to be or insistence that person is the opposite sex, change in self-perception of role, and conflict in roles.

ineffective Sexuality Pattern may be related to ineffective or absent role models and conflict with sexual orientation or preferences, lack of or impaired relationship with an SO, possibly evidenced by verbalizations of discomfort with sexual orientation or role, and lack of information about human sexuality.

risk for compromised/disabled family Coping: risk factors may include inadequate or incorrect information or understanding, SO unable to perceive or to act effectively in regard to client's needs, temporary family disorganization and role changes, and client providing little support in turn for primary person.

readiness for enhanced family Coping may be related to individual's basic needs being sufficiently gratified and adaptive tasks effectively addressed to enable goals of self-actualization to surface, possibly evidenced by family member(s) attempts to describe growth or impact of crisis on own values, priorities, goals, or relationships; family member(s) moving in direction of health-promoting and enriching lifestyle that supports client's search for self; and choosing experiences that optimize wellness.

Genetic disorder CH/OB

Anxiety may be related to presence of specific risk factors (e.g., exposure to teratogens), situational crisis, threat to self-concept, conscious or unconscious conflict about essential values and life goals, possibly evidenced by increased tension, apprehension, uncertainty, feelings of inadequacy, expressed concerns.

deficient Knowledge [Learning Need] regarding purpose and process of genetic counseling may be related to lack of awareness of ramifications of diagnosis, process necessary for analyzing available options, and information misinterpretation, possibly evidenced by verbalization of concerns, statement of misconceptions, request for information.

risk for interrupted Family Processes: risk factors may include situational crisis, individual/family vulnerability, difficulty reaching agreement regarding options.

Grieving may be related to anticipatory or actual loss (e.g., childbearing or reproductive issues), possibly evidenced by suffering, blame, despair, change in usual routines and activities of daily living.

Spiritual Distress may be related to intense inner conflict about the outcome, normal grieving for the loss of the perfect child, anger that is often directed at God/greater power, religious beliefs or moral convictions, possibly evidenced by verbalization of inner conflict about beliefs, questioning of the moral and ethical implications of therapeutic choices, viewing situation as punishment, anger, hostility, and crying.

Genital herpes CH

Refer to Herpes simplex; Sexually transmitted disease

Genital warts (human papillomavirus)　　　　　CH
Refer to Sexually transmitted disease

GERD　　　　　CH
Refer to Gastroesophageal reflux disease

GI bleeding　　　　　MS
Refer to Gastritis, acute or chronic; Ulcer, peptic

Gigantism　　　　　CH
Refer to Acromegaly

Gingivitis　　　　　CH
impaired Oral Mucous Membrane may be related to ineffective oral hygiene, ill-fitting dentures, decreased salivation, hormonal changes, possibly evidenced by edema, gingival bleeding, hyperplasia, oral pain.

Glaucoma　　　　　CH
disturbed visual Sensory Perception may be related to altered sensory reception and altered status of sense organ (increased intraocular pressure, atrophy of optic nerve head), possibly evidenced by progressive loss of visual field.

Anxiety [specify level] may be related to change in health status, presence of pain, possibility or reality of loss of vision, unmet needs, and negative self-talk, possibly evidenced by apprehension, uncertainty, and expressed concern regarding changes in life event.

Glomerulonephritis　　　　　PED
excess Fluid Volume may be related to failure of regulatory mechanism (inflammation of glomerular membrane inhibiting filtration), possibly evidenced by weight gain, edema, anasarca, intake greater than output, and blood pressure changes.

acute Pain may be related to effects of circulating toxins and edema or distention of renal capsule, possibly evidenced by verbal reports, guarding or distraction behaviors, and changes in vital signs.

imbalanced Nutrition: less than body requirements may be related to anorexia and dietary restrictions, possibly evidenced by aversion to eating, reported altered taste, weight loss, and decreased intake.

deficient Diversional Activity may be related to treatment modality and restrictions, fatigue, and malaise, possibly evidenced by statements of boredom, restlessness, and irritability.

risk for disproportionate Growth: risk factors may include infection, malnutrition, chronic illness.

Gluten sensitive enteropathy　　　　　CH
Refer to Celiac disease

Goiter　　　　　CH
disturbed Body Image may be related to visible swelling in neck, possibly evidenced by verbalization of feelings, fear of reaction of others, actual change in structure, change in social involvement.

Anxiety may be related to change in health status, progressive growth of mass, perceived threat of death.

risk for imbalanced Nutrition: less than body requirements: risk factors may include decreased ability to ingest or difficulty swallowing.

risk for ineffective Airway Clearance: risk factors may include tracheal compression or obstruction.

Gonorrhea   CH

Also refer to Sexually transmitted disease

risk for Infection [dissemination/bacteremia]: risk factors may include presence of infectious process in highly vascular area and lack of recognition of disease process.

acute Pain may be related to irritation or inflammation of mucosa and effects of circulating toxins, possibly evidenced by verbal reports of genital or pharyngeal irritation, perineal or pelvic pain, guarding or distraction behaviors.

deficient Knowledge [Learning Need] regarding disease cause, transmission, therapy, and self-care needs may be related to lack of information, misinterpretation, denial of exposure, possibly evidenced by statements of concern, questions, misconceptions, and inaccurate follow-through of instructions, development of preventable complications.

Gout   CH

acute Pain may be related to inflammation of joint(s), possibly evidenced by verbal reports, guarding or distraction behaviors, and changes in vital signs.

impaired physical Mobility may be related to joint pain, edema, possibly evidenced by reluctance to attempt movement, limited range of motion, and therapeutic restriction of movement.

deficient Knowledge [Learning Need] regarding cause, treatment, and prevention of condition may be related to lack of information, misinterpretation, possibly evidenced by statements of concern, questions, misconceptions, and inaccurate follow-through of instructions.

Grand mal seizures   CH/PED

Refer to Seizure disorder

Grave's disease   CH

Refer to Hyperthyroidism

Guillain-Barré syndrome (acute polyneuritis)   MS

risk for ineffective Breathing Pattern/Airway Clearance: risk factors may include weakness or paralysis of respiratory muscles, impaired gag or swallow reflexes, decreased energy, fatigue.

disturbed Sensory Perceptual (specify) may be related to altered sensory reception, transmission, or integration (altered status of sense organs, sleep deprivation); therapeutically restricted environment; endogenous chemical alterations (electrolyte imbalance, hypoxia); and psychological stress, possibly evidenced by reported or observed change in usual response to stimuli, altered communication patterns, and measured change in sensory acuity and motor coordination.

impaired physical Mobility may be related to neuromuscular impairment, pain, discomfort, possibly evidenced by impaired coordination, partial or complete paralysis, decreased muscle strength or control.

Anxiety [specify level]/Fear may be related to situational crisis, change in health status, threat of death, possibly evidenced by increased tension, restlessness, helplessness, apprehension, uncertainty, fearfulness, focus on self, and sympathetic stimulation.

risk for Disuse Syndrome: risk factors may include paralysis and pain.

Gulf War syndrome   CH/MS

[chronic] Fatigue may be related to unknown environmental exposure, stress, anxiety, disease state, possibly evidenced by overwhelming lack of energy, inability to maintain usual routines or level of physical activity, lethargic, compromised concentration.

Anxiety [specify] may be related to exposure to toxins, change in health status, threat of death, change in role function or economic status, unmet needs, possibly evidenced by expressed concerns, apprehension, uncertainty, fear of unspecific consequences, sleep disturbance, irritability, preoccupation.

impaired Memory may be related to neurological disturbances, possibly evidenced by reported or observed experiences of forgetting, inability to recall recent events.

chronic Pain may be related to chronic physical condition, possibly evidenced by verbal reports of muscle or joint pain, headaches, altered ability to continue previous activities, fatigue, reduced interaction with others.

Diarrhea may be related to environmental exposure to toxins, high stress levels/anxiety, possibly evidenced by liquid stools, abdominal pain.

disturbed visual Sensory Perception may be related to altered sensory reception, possibly evidenced by blurred vision, photosensitivity.

Hallucinogen abuse   CH/PSY
Also refer to Substance dependence/abuse rehabilitation

disturbed Thought Processes may be related to physiological changes associated with drug use, impaired judgment, memory loss, possibly evidenced by inaccurate interpretation of environment, bizarre thinking, disorientation, inability to make decisions, unpredictable behavior, distractibility, nonreality-based thinking.

Anxiety/Fear may be related to situational crisis, threat to or change in health status, perceived threat of death, inexperience or unfamiliarity with effects of drug, possibly evidenced by assumptions of "losing my mind/control," apprehension, preoccupation with feelings of impending doom, sympathetic stimulation.

Self-Care Deficit (specify) may be related to perceptual or cognitive impairment, therapeutic management (restraints), possibly evidenced by inability to meet own physical needs.

Hand-foot-mouth disease   PED/CH
Also refer to Meningitis

impaired Oral Mucous Membrane may be related to infection, dehydration, possibly evidenced by oral lesions, ulcers, pain, difficulty eating.

risk for Infection [transmission]: risk factors may include insufficient knowledge to avoid exposure to pathogens, inadequate acquired immunity.

risk for deficient Fluid Volume: risk factors may include deviations affecting intake (oral ulcers and pain), increased fluid needs (hypermetabolic state, fever).

Hansen's disease   CH
impaired Skin/Tissue integrity may be related to altered circulation, sensation, pigmentation and [invasion of tissues by bacterial infection], possibly evidenced by symmetric skin lesions lighter than normal color, nodules, plaques, thickened dermis with loss of sensation, and frequent involvement of the nasal mucosa resulting in nasal congestion and epistaxis.

risk for Infection [spread/transmission]: risk factors may include inadequate primary or secondary defenses, insufficient knowledge to avoid exposure to/early treatment of infectious bacterial [*Mycobacterium leprae*] agent.

impaired physical Mobility may be related to neuromuscular and sensoriperceptual impairments, possibly evidenced by muscular weakness, or numbness or absence of sensation in hands, arms, legs, feet.

disturbed Body Image may be related to biophysical illness, trauma, possibly evidenced by permanent nerve damage, [cosmetic damage], actual change in structure, missing body part, fear of reaction or rejection by others.

Hantavirus   **MS**

Refer to Hantavirus pulmonary syndrome

Hantavirus pulmonary syndrome   **MS**

Also refer to Disseminated intravascular coagulation

 acute Pain/impaired Comfort may be related to inflammatory process, circulating toxins, possibly evidenced by reports of headache, myalgia, gastrointestinal distress, fever.

 impaired Gas Exchange may be related to alveolar-capillary membrane changes (fluid collection or shifts into interstitial space or alveoli), possibly evidenced by dyspnea, restlessness, irritability, abnormal rate or depth of respirations, lethargy, confusion.

 [moderate to severe] Anxiety may be related to change in health status, threat of death, interpersonal transmission, possibly evidenced by expressed concerns, distressed, apprehension, extraneous movement.

 risk for impaired spontaneous Ventilation: risk factors may include respiratory muscle fatigue, problems with secretion management.

Hashimoto's thyroiditis   **CH**

Refer to Hypothyroidism; Goiter

Hay fever   **CH**

impaired Comfort/acute Pain may be related to irritation or inflammation of upper airway mucous membranes and conjunctiva, possibly evidenced by verbal reports, irritability, and restlessness.

 deficient Knowledge [Learning Need] regarding underlying cause, appropriate therapy, and required lifestyle changes may be related to lack of information, possibly evidenced by statements of concern, questions, and misconceptions.

Headache   **CH/MS**

Also refer to Temporal arteritis

 acute/chronic Pain may be related to stress, tension, nerve irritation or pressure, vasospasm, increased intracranial pressure, possibly evidenced by verbal or coded reports, pallor, facial mask of pain, guarding or distraction behaviors, restlessness, self-focusing, changes in sleep pattern or appetite, preoccupation with pain.

 risk for ineffective Coping: risk factors may include situational crisis, personal vulnerability, inadequate support systems, work overload, no vacations, inadequate relaxation, severe pain, overwhelming threat to self.

 deficient Knowledge [Learning Need] regarding condition, prognosis, and treatment needs may be related to lack of exposure or recall, unfamiliarity with information or resources, cognitive limitations, possibly evidenced by request for information, statement of misconceptions, inaccurate follow-through of instructions, development of preventable complications.

Head injury   **MS/CH**

Refer to Traumatic brain injury

Heart attack   **MS**

Refer to Myocardial infarction

Heart failure, chronic   **MS**

decreased Cardiac Output may be related to altered myocardial contractility, inotropic changes; alterations in rate, rhythm, and electrical conduction; and structural changes (valvular defects, ventricular aneurysm), possibly evidenced by tachycardia, dysrhythmias, changes in blood pressure, extra heart sounds, decreased urine output, diminished peripheral pulses, cool and ashen skin, orthopnea, crackles; dependent or generalized edema and chest pain.

excess Fluid Volume may be related to reduced glomerular filtration rate, increased antidiuretic hormone production, and sodium/water retention, possibly evidenced by orthopnea and abnormal breath sounds, S_3 heart sound, jugular vein distention, positive hepatojugular reflex, weight gain, hypertension, oliguria, generalized edema.

risk for impaired Gas Exchange: risk factors may include alveolar-capillary membrane changes—fluid collection or shifts into interstitial space and alveoli.

CH

Activity Intolerance may be related to imbalance between oxygen supply and demand, generalized weakness, and prolonged bedrest or sedentary lifestyle, possibly evidenced by reported or observed weakness, fatigue; changes in vital signs, presence of dysrhythmias; dyspnea, pallor, and diaphoresis.

risk for impaired Skin Integrity: risk factors may include prolonged chair or bedrest, edema, vascular pooling, decreased tissue perfusion.

deficient Knowledge [Learning Need] regarding cardiac function, disease process, therapy, and self-care needs may be related to lack of information, misinterpretation, possibly evidenced by questions, statements of concern or misconceptions; development of preventable complications or exacerbations of condition.

Heart transplantation   MS/CH
Refer to Cardiac surgery; Transplantation, recipient

Heat exhaustion   CH/MS
deficient Fluid Volume may be related to excessive losses (profuse sweating), hypermetabolic state (core temperature 101°F–105°F [38.3°C–40.6°C]), lack of intake, extremes of age, possibly evidenced by weakness, fatigue, slow pulse, decreased blood pressure, changes in mentation.

Heatstroke   MS
Hyperthermia may be related to prolonged exposure to hot environment, vigorous activity with failure of regulating mechanism of the body, possibly evidenced by high body temperature (>105°F [40.6°C]), flushed/hot skin, tachycardia, and seizure activity.

decreased Cardiac Output may be related to functional stress of hypermetabolic state, altered circulating volume and venous return, and direct myocardial damage secondary to hyperthermia, possibly evidenced by decreased peripheral pulses, dysrhythmias, tachycardia, and changes in mentation.

Hematoma, epidural   MS
acute Confusion may be related to head injury, possibly evidenced by fluctuation in cognition or level of consciousness.

risk for decreased Intracranial Adaptive Capacity: risk factors may include brain injuries, decreased cerebral perfusion pressure, systemic hypotension with intracranial hypertension.

risk for ineffective Breathing Pattern: risk factors may include neuromuscular dysfunction (injury to respiratory center of brain), perception or cognitive impairment.

risk for deficient Fluid Volume: risk factors may include restricted oral intake, hypermetabolic state, loss of fluid through normal or abnormal routes.

Hematoma, subdural-acute   MS
Refer to Traumatic brain injury

Hematoma, subdural-chronic CH

acute/chronic Pain may be related to physical agent (space-occupying clot), possibly evidenced by reports of increasing daily headache.

acute/chronic Confusion may be related to head injury, alcohol abuse, possibly evidenced by fluctuations in cognition, increased agitation, restlessness, misperceptions, inappropriate responses.

impaired physical Mobility may be related to neuromuscular impairment (hemiparesis), decreased muscle strength, cognitive impairment, possibly evidenced by limited ability to perform gross or fine motor skills, gait changes, postural instability.

Hemiplegia, spastic PED/CH

Refer to Palsy, cerebral

Hemodialysis MS/CH

Also refer to Dialysis, general

risk for Injury [loss of vascular access]: risk factors may include clotting or thrombosis, infection, disconnection, hemorrhage.

risk for deficient Fluid Volume: risk factors may include excessive fluid losses or shifts via ultrafiltration, fluid restrictions, altered coagulation, disconnection of shunt.

risk for excess Fluid Volume: risk factors may include rapid or excessive fluid intake—IV, blood, plasma expanders, or saline given to support blood pressure during procedure.

ineffective Protection may be related to chronic disease state, drug therapy, abnormal blood profile, inadequate nutrition, possibly evidenced by altered clotting, impaired healing, deficient immunity, fatigue, anorexia.

Hemophilia PED

risk for Bleeding/deficient Fluid Volume [isotonic]: risk factors may include impaired coagulation, inherent coagulopathies, trauma, hemorrhagic losses.

risk for acute/chronic Pain: risk factors may include nerve compression from hematomas, nerve damage or hemorrhage into joint space.

risk for impaired physical Mobility: risk factors may include joint hemorrhage, swelling, degenerative changes, and muscle atrophy.

ineffective Protection may be related to abnormal blood profile, possibly evidenced by altered clotting.

compromised family Coping may be related to prolonged nature of condition that exhausts the supportive capacity of significant person(s), possibly evidenced by protective behaviors disproportionate to client's abilities or need for autonomy.

Hemorrhage, postpartum OB

risk for Shock: risk factors may include hypovolemia—postpartum complications, disseminated intravascular coagulation.

risk for Injury: risk factors may include decreased hemoglobin, tissue hypoxia.

[moderate] Anxiety may be related to situational crisis, threat of change in health status or death, interpersonal transmission or contagion, physiological response (catecholamine release), possibly evidenced by increased tension, apprehension, feelings of inadequacy or helplessness, sympathetic stimulation, self-focus.

risk for Infection: risk factors may include traumatized tissue, stasis of body fluids (lochia), decreased hemoglobin, invasive procedures.

risk for impaired Attachment: risk factors may include interruption in bonding process, physical condition, perceived threat to own survival.

Hemorrhage, prenatal   OB

risk for Shock: risk factors may include hypovolemia—ectopic or molar pregnancy, abruptio placentae.

risk for disturbed Maternal/Fetal Dyad: risk factors may include compromised oxygen transport—hypovolemia.

Fear may be related to threat of death [perceived or actual] to self/fetus, possibly evidenced by verbalizations of specific concerns, increased tension, sympathetic stimulation.

acute Pain may be related to muscle contractions, cervical dilation, tissue trauma (fallopian tube rupture), possibly evidenced by reports, distraction behaviors, and change in blood pressure/pulse.

risk for imbalanced Fluid Volume: risk factors may include excessive or rapid replacement of fluid losses.

Hemorrhagic fever, viral   MS

Refer to Ebola; Hantavirus pulmonary syndrome

Hemorrhoidectomy   MS/CH

acute Pain may be related to edema or swelling and tissue trauma, possibly evidenced by verbal reports, guarding or distraction behaviors, focus on self, and changes in vital signs.

risk for Urinary Retention: risk factors may include perineal trauma, edema or swelling, and pain.

deficient Knowledge [Learning Need] regarding therapeutic treatment and potential complications may be related to lack of information, misconceptions, possibly evidenced by statements of concern and questions.

Hemorrhoids   CH/OB

acute Pain may be related to inflammation and edema of prolapsed varices, possibly evidenced by verbal reports and guarding or distraction behaviors.

Constipation may be related to pain on defecation and reluctance to defecate, possibly evidenced by frequency, less than usual pattern, and hard, formed stools.

Hemothorax   MS

Also refer to Pneumothorax

risk for Trauma/Suffocation: risk factors may include concurrent disease or injury process, dependence on external device (chest drainage system), and lack of safety education or precautions.

Anxiety [specify level] may be related to change in health status and threat of death, possibly evidenced by increased tension, restlessness, expressed concern, sympathetic stimulation, and focus on self.

Hepatitis, acute viral   MS/CH

impaired Liver Function related to viral infection as evidenced by jaundice, hepatic enlargement, abdominal pain, marked elevations in serum liver function tests.

Fatigue may be related to decreased metabolic energy production, discomfort, altered body chemistry—changes in liver function, effect on target organs, possibly evidenced by reports of lack of energy, inability to maintain usual routines, decreased performance, and increased physical complaints.

imbalanced Nutrition: less than body requirements may be related to inability to ingest adequate nutrients (nausea, vomiting, anorexia); hypermetabolic state, altered absorption and metabolism—reduced peristalsis, bile stasis, possibly evidenced by aversion to eating or lack of interest in food, altered taste sensation, observed lack of intake, and weight loss.

---

acute Pain/impaired Comfort may be related to inflammation and swelling of the liver, arthralgias, urticarial eruptions, and pruritus, possibly evidenced by verbal reports, guarding or distraction behaviors, focus on self, and changes in vital signs.

risk for Infection: risk factors may include inadequate secondary defenses and immunosuppression, malnutrition, insufficient knowledge to avoid exposure to pathogens or spread to others.

risk for impaired Tissue Integrity: risk factors may include bile salt accumulation in the tissues.

risk for impaired Home Management: risk factors may include debilitating effects of disease process and inadequate support systems—family, financial, role model.

deficient Knowledge [Learning Need] regarding disease process and transmission, treatment needs, and future expectations may be related to lack of information or recall, misinterpretation, unfamiliarity with resources, possibly evidenced by questions, statement of concerns, misconceptions, inaccurate follow-through of instructions, and development of preventable complications.

Hepatorenal syndrome   MS
Refer to Cirrhosis; Renal failure, acute

Hernia, hiatal   CH
chronic Pain may be related to regurgitation of acidic gastric contents, possibly evidenced by verbal reports, facial grimacing, and focus on self.

deficient Knowledge [Learning Need] regarding pathophysiology, prevention of complications, and self-care needs may be related to lack of information, misconceptions, possibly evidenced by statements of concern, questions, and recurrence of condition.

Hernia, inguinal   MS
Refer to Herniorrhaphy

Herniated nucleus pulposus   CH/MS
acute/chronic Pain may be related to nerve compression or irritation and muscle spasms, possibly evidenced by verbal reports, guarding or distraction behaviors, preoccupation with pain, self-focus, narrowed focus, changes in vital signs when pain is acute, altered muscle tone or function, changes in eating or sleeping patterns and libido, and physical or social withdrawal.

impaired physical Mobility may be related to pain (muscle spasms), therapeutic restrictions (e.g., rest, braces or traction), muscular impairment, and depressive mood state, possibly evidenced by reports of pain on movement, reluctance to attempt or difficulty with purposeful movement, decreased muscle strength, impaired coordination, and limited range of motion.

deficient Diversional Activity may be related to length of recuperation period and therapy restrictions, physical limitations, pain and depression, possibly evidenced by statements of boredom, disinterest, "nothing to do," and restlessness, irritability, withdrawal.

Herniorrhaphy   MS/PED
acute Pain may be related to disruption of skin, tissue, and muscle integrity, possibly evidenced by verbal or coded reports, alteration in muscle tone, distraction or guarding behaviors, narrowed focus, and autonomic responses.

risk for Injury: risk factors may include surgical repair, insertion of graft, increased intra-abdominal pressure (straining at stool, heavy lifting, strenuous activity).

Heroin abuse   CH
risk for Infection: risk factors may include injection, reuse or sharing of needles, malnutrition, environmental exposure, insufficient knowledge or motivation to avoid pathogens.

imbalanced Nutrition: less than body requirements may be related to inadequate intake, possibly evidenced by anorexia, lack of food or methods to prepare food, economic difficulties, weight loss, poor muscle tone, decreased muscle mass.

risk for Trauma: risk factors may include personal vulnerability, cigarette smoking, lack of safety precautions, driving impaired or under the influence, high-crime neighborhood.

risk for ineffective Protection: risk factors may include effects of substance use, malnutrition, chronic disease, lifestyle choices, unhealthy environment.

Heroin withdrawal   CH/MS

acute Pain/impaired Comfort may be related to cessation of drug, muscle tremors or twitching, possibly evidenced by reports of muscle aches, hot and cold flashes, diaphoresis, lacrimation, rhinorrhea, drug cravings.

[severe] Anxiety may be related to central nervous system hyperactivity, possibly evidenced by apprehension, pervasive anxious feelings, jittery, restlessness, weakness, insomnia, anorexia.

risk for ineffective self Health Management: risk factors may include protracted withdrawal, economic difficulties, family or social support deficits, perceived barriers or benefits.

Herpes simplex   CH

acute Pain may be related to presence of localized inflammation and open lesions, possibly evidenced by verbal reports, distraction behaviors, and restlessness.

risk for [secondary] Infection: risk factors may include broken or traumatized tissue, altered immune response, and untreated infection or treatment failure.

risk for ineffective Sexual Dysfunction: risk factors may include lack of knowledge, values conflict, or fear of transmitting the disease.

Herpes zoster (shingles)   CH

acute Pain may be related to inflammation, local lesions along sensory nerve(s), possibly evidenced by verbal reports, guarding or distraction behaviors, narrowed focus, and changes in vital signs.

deficient Knowledge [Learning Need] regarding pathophysiology, therapeutic needs, and potential complications may be related to lack of information, misinterpretation, possibly evidenced by statements of concern, questions, and misconceptions.

High altitude pulmonary edema (HAPE)   MS

Also refer to Mountain sickness, acute

impaired Gas Exchange may be related to ventilation perfusion imbalance, alveolar-capillary membrane changes, altered oxygen supply, possibly evidenced by dyspnea, confusion, cyanosis, tachycardia, abnormal arterial blood gases.

excess Fluid Volume may be related to compromised regulatory mechanism, possibly evidenced by shortness of breath, anxiety, edema, abnormal breath sounds, pulmonary congestion.

High altitude sickness   MS

Refer to Mountain sickness, acute; High altitude pulmonary edema

High-risk pregnancy   OB

Refer to Pregnancy, high-risk

Hip replacement   MS

Refer to Total joint replacement

HIV infection   CH

Also refer to AIDS

risk-prone health Behavior may be related to life-threatening, stigmatizing condition or disease; assault to self-esteem; altered locus of control; inadequate support systems; incomplete grieving; medication side effects (fatigue, depression), possibly evidenced by verbalization of nonacceptance or denial of diagnosis, failure to take action that prevents health problems.

deficient Knowledge [Learning Need] regarding disease, prognosis, and treatment needs may be related to lack of exposure or recall, information misinterpretation, unfamiliarity with information resources, or cognitive limitation, possibly evidenced by statement of misconception, request for information, inappropriate or exaggerated behaviors (hostile, agitated, hysterical, apathetic), inaccurate follow-through of instructions, development of preventable complications.

risk for ineffective self Health Management: risk factors may include complexity of healthcare system and access to care, economic difficulties; complexity of therapeutic regimen—confusing or difficult dosing schedule, duration of regimen; mistrust of regimen and/or healthcare personnel—client and provider interactions; health beliefs or cultural influences, perceived seriousness, susceptibility, or benefits of therapy; decisional conflicts, powerlessness.

risk for complicated Grieving: risk factors may include preloss psychological symptoms, predisposition for anxiety and feelings of inadequacy, frequency of major life events.

Hodgkin's disease   CH/MS

Also refer to Cancer; Chemotherapy

Anxiety [specify level]/Fear may be related to threat of self-concept and threat of death, possibly evidenced by apprehension, insomnia, focus on self, and increased tension.

deficient Knowledge [Learning Need] regarding diagnosis, pathophysiology, treatment, and prognosis may be related to lack of information, misinterpretation, possibly evidenced by statements of concern, questions, and misconceptions.

acute Pain/impaired Comfort may be related to manifestations of inflammatory response (fever, chills, night sweats) and pruritus, possibly evidenced by verbal reports, distraction behaviors, and focus on self.

risk for ineffective Breathing Pattern/Airway Clearance: risk factors may include tracheobronchial obstruction (enlarged mediastinal nodes or airway edema).

Hospice care   CH

acute/chronic Pain may be related to biological, physical, psychological agent; chronic physical disability, possibly evidenced by verbal or coded report, preoccupation with pain, changes in appetite, sleep pattern, altered ability to continue desired activities, guarded or protective behavior, restlessness, irritability, narrowed focus—altered time perception, impaired thought processes.

Activity Intolerance/Fatigue may be related to generalized weakness, bedrest or immobility, pain, progressive disease state or debilitating condition, depressive state, imbalance between oxygen supply and demand, possibly evidenced by inability to maintain usual routine, verbalized lack of desire or interest in activity, decreased performance, lethargy.

Grieving/death Anxiety may be related to anticipated loss of physiological well-being, change in body function, perceived threat of death, or dying process, possibly evidenced by changes in communication pattern, denial of potential loss, choked feelings, anger, fear of loss of physical or mental abilities, negative death images or unpleasant thoughts about any event related to death or dying, anticipated pain related to dying; powerlessness over issues related to dying, worrying about impact of one's own death on SO(s), being the cause of other's grief and suffering, concerns of overworking the caregiver as terminal illness incapacitates.

compromised/disabled family Coping/Caregiver Role Strain may be related to prolonged disease or disability progression, temporary family disorganization and role changes, unrealistic expectations, inadequate or incorrect information or understanding by primary person possibly evidenced by client expressing despair about family reactions or lack of involvement, history of poor relationship between caregiver and care receiver; altered caregiver health status; SO attempting assistive or supportive behaviors with less than satisfactory results; apprehension about future regarding caregiver's ability to provide care; SO describing preoccupation about personal reactions; displaying intolerance, abandonment, rejection; family behaviors that are detrimental to well-being.

risk for Spiritual Distress: risk factors may include physical or psychological stress, energy-consuming anxiety, situational losses, blocks to self-love, low self-esteem, inability to forgive.

risk for moral Distress: risk factors may include conflict among decision makers, cultural conflicts, end-of-life decisions, loss of autonomy, physical distance of decision makers.

Huntington's disease   CH

Hopelessness may be related to chronic progressive debilitating condition, possibly evidenced by despondent verbalizations, withdrawal from environs, angry outbursts.

impaired Walking may be related to movement disorder (altered gait, ataxia, dystonia), possibly evidenced by inability to walk required distances, navigate curbs or uneven surfaces, climb stairs.

disturbed Thought Processes may be related to degenerative physiological changes, possibly evidenced by inaccurate interpretation of environment, cognitive dissonance, inappropriate social behavior.

imbalanced Nutrition: less than body requirements may be related to inability to ingest food (difficulty swallowing, cognitive decline), possibly evidenced by aversion to eating, inadequate food intake, weight loss, decreased subcutaneous fat or muscle mass.

total Self-Care Deficit may be related to neuromuscular impairment, cognitive decline, possibly evidenced by inability to perform desired activities of daily living.

risk for Caregiver Role Strain: risk factors may include progressive deterioration (physical and mental) of care receiver, duration of caregiving required, complexity or amount of caregiving tasks, caregiver's competing role commitments, family isolation, lack of respite or recreation for caregiver, bizarre behavior of care receiver.

Hydrocephalus   PED/MS

ineffective cerebral tissue Perfusion may be related to decreased arterial or venous blood flow (compression of brain tissue), possibly evidenced by changes in mentation, restlessness, irritability, reports of headache, pupillary changes, and changes in vital signs.

disturbed visual Sensory Perception may be related to pressure on sensory or motor nerves, possibly evidenced by reports of double vision, development of strabismus, nystagmus, pupillary changes, and optic atrophy.

risk for impaired physical Mobility: risk factors may include neuromuscular impairment, decreased muscle strength, and impaired coordination.

risk for decreased Intracranial Adaptive Capacity: risk factors may include brain injury, changes in perfusion pressure and intracranial pressure.

CH

risk for Infection: risk factors may include invasive procedure, presence of shunt.

deficient Knowledge [Learning Need] regarding condition, prognosis, long-term therapy needs, and medical follow-up may be related to lack of information, misperceptions, possibly evidenced by questions, statement of concern, request for information, and inaccurate follow-through of instructions, development of preventable complications.

Hydrophobia   CH/MS
Refer to Rabies

Hyperactivity disorder   PED/PSY
defensive Coping may be related to mild neurological deficits, dysfunctional family system, abuse or neglect, possibly evidenced by denial of obvious problems, projection of blame or responsibility, grandiosity, difficulty in reality testing perceptions.

impaired Social Interaction may be related to retarded ego development, negative role models, neurological impairment, possibly evidenced by discomfort in social situations, interrupts or intrudes on others, difficulty waiting turn in games or group activities, difficulty maintaining attention to task.

disabled family Coping may be related to excessive guilt, anger, or blaming among family members, parental inconsistencies, disagreements regarding discipline or limit-setting approaches, exhaustion of parental expectations, possibly evidenced by unrealistic parental expectations, rejection or overprotection of child, exaggerated expression of feelings, despair regarding child's behavior.

Hyperbilirubinemia   PED
neonatal Jaundice may be related to prematurity, hemolytic disease, asphyxia, acidosis, hyponatremia, hypoglycemia, difficulty transitioning to extra-uterine life, feeding pattern not well established, abnormal weight loss, possibly evidenced by abnormal blood profile (elevated blood urea nitrogen), yellow-orange skin and sclera.

risk for Injury [effects of treatment]: risk factors may include physical properties of phototherapy and effects on body regulatory mechanisms, invasive procedure (exchange transfusion), abnormal blood profile, chemical imbalances.

deficient Knowledge [Learning Need] regarding condition prognosis, treatment, and safety needs may be related to lack of exposure or recall and information misinterpretation, possibly evidenced by questions, statement of concern, and inaccurate follow-through of instructions, development of preventable complications.

Hyperemesis gravidarum   OB
deficient Fluid Volume [isotonic] may be related to excessive gastric losses and reduced intake, possibly evidenced by dry mucous membranes, decreased and concentrated urine, decreased pulse volume and pressure, thirst, and hemoconcentration.

risk for Electrolyte Imbalance: risk factors may include vomiting, dehydration.

imbalanced Nutrition: less than body requirements may be related to inability to ingest, digest, or absorb nutrients (prolonged vomiting), possibly evidenced by reported inadequate food intake, lack of interest in food or aversion to eating, and weight loss.

risk for ineffective Coping: risk factors may include situational or maturational crisis (pregnancy, change in health status, projected role changes, concern about outcome).

Hyperparathyroidism, primary   MS
risk for deficient Fluid Volume: risk factors may include excessive losses through normal routes (vomiting, diarrhea, gastric bleed).

risk for Electrolyte Imbalance: risk factors may include impaired regulatory mechanism, vomiting.

impaired Urinary Elimination may be related to anatomical obstruction (renal calculi), possibly evidenced by decreased renal function.

risk for Trauma: risk factors may include decreased calcium levels, bone fragility.

Hypertension   **CH**

deficient Knowledge [Learning Need] regarding condition, therapeutic regimen, and potential complications may be related to lack of information or recall, misinterpretation, cognitive limitations, or denial of diagnosis, possibly evidenced by statements of concern, questions, and misconceptions, inaccurate follow-through of instructions, and lack of blood pressure control.

risk-prone health Behavior may be related to condition requiring change in lifestyle, altered locus of control, and absence of feelings or denial of illness, possibly evidenced by verbalization of nonacceptance of health status change and lack of movement toward independence.

risk for Activity Intolerance: risk factors may include generalized weakness, imbalance between oxygen supply and demand.

risk for Sexual Dysfunction: risk factors may include side effects of medication.

                                                                    MS

risk for decreased Cardiac Output: risk factors may include increased afterload (vasoconstriction), fluid shifts, hypovolemia, myocardial ischemia, ventricular hypertrophy and rigidity.

acute Pain may be related to increased cerebrovascular pressure, possibly evidenced by verbal reports (throbbing pain located in suboccipital region, present on awakening and disappearing spontaneously after being up and about), reluctance to move head, avoidance of bright lights and noise, increased muscle tension.

Hypertension, intrapartum   **OB**

risk for imbalanced Fluid Volume: risk factors may include compromised regulatory mechanism, fluid shifts, excessive fluid intake, effects of drug therapy (oxytocin infusion).

risk for impaired fetal Gas Exchange: risk factors may include altered blood flow, vasospasms, prolonged uterine contractions.

impaired Urinary Elimination may be related to fluid shifts, hormonal changes, effects of medication, possibly evidenced by changes in amount and frequency of voiding, bladder distention, changes in urine specific gravity, presence of albumin.

risk for maternal Injury: risk factors may include tonic-clonic convulsions, altered clotting factors (release of thromboplastin from placenta).

acute Pain may be related to intensification of uterine activity, myometrial hypoxia, anxiety, possibly evidenced by verbalizations, altered muscle tone, distraction behaviors, autonomic responses, facial mask.

Hypertension, prenatal   **OB**

Refer to Pregnancy-induced hypertension

Hypertension, pulmonary   **CH/MS**

Refer to Pulmonary hypertension

Hyperthyroidism   **CH**

Also refer to Thyrotoxicosis

Fatigue may be related to hypermetabolic imbalance with increased energy requirements, irritability of central nervous system, and altered body chemistry, possibly evidenced by verbalization of overwhelming lack of energy to maintain usual routine, decreased performance, emotional lability and irritability, and impaired ability to concentrate.

Anxiety [specify level] may be related to increased stimulation of the central nervous system (hypermetabolic state, pseudocatecholamine effect of thyroid hormones), possibly evidenced by increased feelings of apprehension, overexcitement, or distress; irritability; emotional lability; shakiness; restless movements; tremors.

---

risk for imbalanced Nutrition: less than body requirements: risk factors may include inability to ingest adequate nutrients for hypermetabolic rate, constant activity level, impaired absorption of nutrients (vomiting, diarrhea), hyperglycemia, relative insulin insufficiency.

risk for impaired Tissue Integrity: risk factors may include periorbital edema, altered protective mechanisms of eye—reduced ability to blink.

Hypervolemia   CH/MS
excess Fluid Volume may be related to excess fluid and sodium intake, compromised regulatory mechanisms (renal failure, increased antidiuretic hormone), decreased plasma proteins, rapid or excessive administration of isotonic parenteral fluids, possibly evidenced by edema, abnormal breath sounds, S_3 heart sound, shortness of breath, positive hepatojugular reflex—elevated central venous pressure, change in mental status.

Hypochondriasis   PSY
Refer to Somatoform disorders

Hypoglycemia   CH
disturbed Thought Processes may be related to inadequate glucose for cellular brain function and effects of endogenous hormone activity, possibly evidenced by irritability, changes in mentation, memory loss, altered attention span, and emotional lability.

risk for unstable blood Glucose Level: risk factors may include dietary intake, lack of adherence to diabetes management, inadequate blood glucose monitoring, medication management.

deficient Knowledge [Learning Need] regarding pathophysiology of condition, therapy, and self-care needs may be related to lack of information or recall, misinterpretations, possibly evidenced by development of hypoglycemia and statements of questions, misconceptions.

Hypoparathyroidism (acute)   MS
risk for Electrolyte Imbalance: risk factors may include impaired regulatory mechanism.

risk for Injury: risk factors may include neuromuscular excitability—tetany and formation of renal stones.

acute Pain may be related to recurrent muscle spasms and alteration in reflexes, possibly evidenced by verbal reports, distraction behaviors, and narrowed focus.

risk for ineffective Airway Clearance: risk factors may include spasm of the laryngeal muscles.

Anxiety [specify level] may be related to threat to, or change in, health status, physiological responses.

Hypophysectomy   MS
Also refer to Surgery, general; Cancer
Fear/Anxiety may be related to situational crisis (nature of diagnosis and procedure), change in health status, perceived threat of death, separation from support system, possibly evidenced by expressed concerns, apprehension, being scared, increased tension, extraneous movement, difficulty concentrating.

risk for deficient Fluid Volume: risk factors may include failure of regulatory mechanism (decreased antidiuretic hormone).

risk for Infection: risk factors may include traumatized tissue, invasive procedure, cerebrospinal fluid leak.

Sexual Dysfunction may be related to altered body function (loss of anterior pituitary), possibly evidenced by sterility, decreased libido, impotence (male), infertility, atrophy of vaginal mucosa (female).

Hypothermia (systemic)   CH
Also refer to Frostbite

Hypothermia may be related to exposure to cold environment, inadequate clothing, age extremes (very young or elderly), damage to hypothalamus, consumption of alcohol or medications causing vasodilation, possibly evidenced by reduction in body temperature below normal range, shivering, cool skin, pallor.

deficient Knowledge [Learning Need] regarding risk factors, treatment needs, and prognosis may be related to lack of information or recall, misinterpretation, possibly evidenced by statement of concerns, misconceptions, occurrence of problem, and development of complications.

Hypothyroidism   CH
Also refer to Myxedema

Fatigue may be related to decreased metabolic energy production, possibly evidenced by verbalization of unremitting or overwhelming lack of energy, inability to maintain usual routines, impaired ability to concentrate, decreased libido, irritability, listlessness, decreased performance, increase in physical complaints.

Constipation may be related to decreased peristalsis, lack of physical activity, possibly evidenced by frequency less than usual pattern, decreased bowel sounds, hard dry stools, and development of fecal impaction.

impaired physical Mobility may be related to weakness, fatigue, muscle aches, altered reflexes, and mucin deposits in joints and interstitial spaces, possibly evidenced by decreased muscle strength or control and impaired coordination.

disturbed Sensory Perception (specify) may be related to mucin deposits and nerve compression, possibly evidenced by paresthesias of hands and feet or decreased hearing.

Hypovolemia   CH/MS
deficient Fluid Volume may be related to active fluid loss (hemorrhage, vomiting, gastric intubation, diarrhea, burns, wounds, fistulas), regulatory failure (adrenal disease, recovery phase of acute renal fialure, diabetic ketoacidosis, hyperosmolar nonketotic coma, diabetes insipidus, sepsis), possibly evidenced by thirst, weight loss, poor skin turgor, dry mucous membranes, tachycardia, tachypnea, fatigue, decreased central venous pressure.

Hysterectomy   GYN/MS
Also refer to Surgery, general

acute Pain may be related to tissue trauma, abdominal incision, edema, hematoma formation, possibly evidenced by verbal reports, guarding or distraction behaviors, and changes in vital signs.

risk for perioperative-position Injury: risk factors may include immobilization, lithotomy position.

impaired Urinary Elimination/risk for [acute] Urinary Retention: risk factors may include mechanical trauma, surgical manipulation, presence of localized edema or hematoma, or nerve trauma with temporary bladder atony.

risk for Sexual Dysfunction: risk factors may include concerns regarding altered body function and structure, perceived changes in femininity, changes in hormone levels, loss of libido, and changes in sexual response pattern.

Ileal conduit   MS/CH
Refer to Urinary diversion

Ileocolitis   MS/CH
Refer to Crohn's disease

Ileostomy   MS/CH
Refer to Colostomy

Ileus   MS
acute Pain may be related to distention, edema and ischemia of intestinal tissue, possibly evidenced by verbal reports, guarding/distraction behaviors, narrowed focus, and changes in vital signs.

Diarrhea/Constipation may be related to presence of obstruction, changes in peristalsis, possibly evidenced by changes in frequency and consistency or absence of stool, alterations in bowel sounds, presence of pain, and cramping.

risk for deficient Fluid Volume: risk factors may include increased intestinal losses (vomiting, diarrhea) and decreased intake.

Immersion foot   MS
impaired Skin/Tissue Integrity may be related to exposure to cold and wet environment (above freezing), altered circulation, presence of infection, possibly evidenced by tissue maceration, pain, soggy edema.

disturbed peripheral Sensory Perception may be related to altered sensory reception, possibly evidenced by paresthesia, numbness.

risk for ineffective self Health Maintenance: risk factors may include lack of material resources, poor coping skills, inadequate knowledge of safety needs.

Impetigo   PED/CH
impaired Skin Integrity may be related to presence of infectious process and pruritus, possibly evidenced by open, crusted lesions.

acute Pain may be related to inflammation and pruritus, possibly evidenced by verbal reports, distraction behaviors, and self-focusing.

risk for [secondary] Infection: risk factors may include broken skin, traumatized tissue, altered immune response, and virulence or contagious nature of causative organism.

risk for Infection [transmission]: risk factors may include virulent nature of causative organism, insufficient knowledge to prevent infection of others.

Impotence   CH
Refer to Erectile dysfunction

Infant (at 4 weeks)   PED
readiness for enhanced Knowledge regarding infant care, developmental expectations, safety and well-being may be related to changing needs of infant, possibly evidenced by questions, expressed concerns or desire to learn more, behaviors congruent with expressed knowledge.

risk for imbalanced Nutrition: (specify): risk factors may include failure to ingest, digest, or absorb adequate calories—insufficient intake, malabsorption, congenital problem, neglect or emotional abuse, or failure to thrive; obesity in one or both parents, rapid transition across growth percentiles.

risk for acute Pain: risk factors may include accumulation of gas in confined space with cramping of intestinal musculature.

risk for Infection: risk factors may include immature immunological response, increased environmental exposure.

risk for sudden infant Death Syndrome: risk factors may include sleeping position, secondhand smoke exposure, type of bedding used.

risk for disorganized Infant Behavior: risk factors may include immature development of sensory organs, inappropriate or inadequate environmental stimuli, effects of prenatal or intrapartal complications, drugs.

Infant of addicted mother   OB/PED

risk for Injury [central nervous system damage]: risk factors may include prematurity, hypoxia, effects of medications, substance use, or withdrawal; possible exposure to infectious agents (prenatal, intrapartal).

ineffective Airway Clearance/impaired Gas Exchange may be related to excess mucus production, depression of cough reflex and respiratory center, intrauterine asphyxia, possibly evidenced by tachypnea, tachycardia, cyanosis, nasal flaring, grunting respirations, hypoxia, acidosis.

risk for Infection: risk factors may include presence of maternal infections (Guillain-Barré syndrome, sexually transmitted diseases).

risk for imbalanced Nutrition: less than body requirements: risk factors may include inability to ingest, digest, or absorb adequate nutrients to meet metabolic needs (e.g., poor or uncoordinated sucking and swallowing, frequent gastrointestinal irritation with vomiting, diarrhea, repeated regurgitation, frequent hyperactivity).

risk for impaired Skin Integrity: risk factors may include mechanical factors (continual rubbing of face or knees against bedding, scratching face with hands), presence of excretions.

impaired Parenting may be related to lack of available or ineffective role model, unmet emotional maturation needs of parent, lack of support between or from SO, interruption in bonding process, lack of appropriate response of infant, possibly evidenced by reports of role inadequacy or inability to care for infant, inattention to infant needs, inappropriate caretaking behaviors, lack of parental attachment behaviors.

disabled family Coping may be related to SO with chronically unexpressed feelings of guilt, anxiety, hostility, despair; dissonant discrepancy of coping styles; high-risk family situations, possibly evidenced by intolerance, rejection, abandonment or desertion, neglectful relationships between family members, neglectful care of infant, distortion of reality of parent's health problem or substance use.

Infant of HIV-positive mother   OB/PED
Also refer to AIDS

risk for Infection: risk factors may include immature immune system, inadequate acquired immunity, suppressed inflammatory response, invasive procedures, malnutrition.

risk for imbalanced Nutrition: risk for less than body requirements: risk factors may include inability to ingest, digest, or absorb nutrients (e.g., impaired suck or swallow, gastrointestinal infection, malabsorption, diarrhea).

risk for delayed Development: risk factors may include separation from SO, inadequate caretaking, inconsistent responsiveness, multiple caretakers, environmental and stimulation deficiencies, effects of chronic condition or disabilities.

deficient Knowledge [Learning Need] regarding condition, prognosis, and treatment needs may be related to lack of exposure, misinterpretation, unfamiliarity with resources, lack of recall or interest in learning, possibly evidenced by questions, statements of misconceptions, inaccurate follow-through of instructions, development of preventable complications.

Infection, ear   PED
Refer to Otitis media

Infection, prenatal   OB
Also refer to AIDS

risk for disturbed Maternal/Fetal Dyad: risk factors may include presence of infection, anemia, inadequate acquired immunity, environmental exposure, rupture of amniotic membranes, treatment-related side effects.

deficient Knowledge [Learning Need] regarding treatment, prevention, and prognosis of condition may be related to lack of exposure to information or unfamiliarity with resources, misinterpretation, possibly evidenced by verbalization of problem, inaccurate follow-through of instructions, development of preventable complications, continuation of infectious process.

impaired Comfort may be related to body response to infective agent, properties of infection (e.g., skin or tissue irritation, development of lesions), possibly evidenced by verbal reports, illness-related symptoms, restlessness, withdrawal from social contacts.

Infection, puerperal   OB/CH

risk for Infection [spread/sepsis]: risk factors may include presence of infection, broken skin, traumatized tissues, high vascularity of involved area, invasive procedures/increased environmental exposure, anemia, chronic disease.

acute Pain may be related to body response to infective agent and toxins, possibly evidenced by verbalizations, restlessness, guarding behavior, self-focusing, and changes in vital signs.

imbalanced Nutrition: less than body requirements may be related to insufficient intake to meet metabolic demands (anorexia, nausea, vomiting, medical restrictions), possibly evidenced by aversion to eating, decreased or lack of oral intake, unanticipated weight loss.

risk for impaired Attachment: risk factors may include interruption in bonding process, separation, physical barriers, maternal fatigue or apathy.

Infection, wound   MS/CH

risk for Infection [sepsis]: risk factors may include presence of infection, broken skin, or traumatized tissues, stasis of body fluids, invasive procedures, increased environmental exposure, chronic disease (e.g., diabetes, anemia, malnutrition), altered immune response, and untoward effect of medications (e.g., opportunistic or secondary infection).

impaired Skin/Tissue Integrity may be related to altered circulation, presence of infection, wound drainage, nutritional deficit, possibly evidenced by delayed healing, damaged tissues, invasion of body structures.

risk for delayed Surgical Recovery: risk factors may include presence of infection, activity restrictions or limitations, nutritional deficiency.

Infertility   CH

situational low Self-Esteem may be related to functional impairment (inability to conceive), unrealistic self-expectations, sense of failure, possibly evidenced by self-negating verbalizations, expressions of helplessness, perceived inability to deal with situation.

chronic Sorrow may be related to perceived physical disability (inability to conceive), possibly evidenced by expressions of anger, disappointment, emptiness, self-blame, helplessness, sadness, feelings interfering with client's ability to achieve maximum well-being.

risk for Spiritual Distress: risk factors may include energy-consuming anxiety, low self-esteem, deteriorating relationship with SO, viewing situation as deserved or punishment for past behaviors.

Inflammatory bowel disease   CH

Refer to Colitis, ulcerative; Crohn's disease

Influenza   CH

acute Pain/impaired Comfort may be related to inflammation and effects of circulating toxins, possibly evidenced by verbal reports, distraction behaviors, and narrowed focus.

risk for deficient Fluid Volume: risk factors may include excessive gastric losses, hypermetabolic state, and altered intake.

Hyperthermia may be related to effects of circulating toxins and dehydration, possibly evidenced by increased body temperature; warm, flushed skin; and tachycardia.

risk for ineffective Breathing Pattern: risk factors may include response to infectious process, decreased energy, fatigue.

Inhalant intoxication/abuse   CH/PSY
Refer to Stimulant abuse

Insomnia, acute   CH
Insomnia may be related to daytime activity pattern, social or work schedule inconsistent with chronotype, travel across time zones, fatigue, life change, physical conditions (dyspnea, gastroesophageal reflux, night sweats), possibly evidenced by verbal reports of difficulties, not feeling well-rested, less than age-normed total sleep time, changes in behavior and performance, physical signs (dark circles under eyes, frequent yawning).

Insomnia, chronic   CH
Sleep Deprivation may be related to sustained environmental stimulation, sustained circadian asynchrony, prolonged use of pharmacological or dietary antisoporifics, prolonged pain, sleep apnea, dementia, narcolepsy, possibly evidenced by daytime drowsiness, decreased ability to perform, lethargy, slowed reaction, apathy.

Insulin resistance syndrome   CH
Refer to Metabolic syndrome

Insulin shock   MS/CH
Refer to Hypoglycemia

Intermaxillary fixation   MS/CH
Also refer to Surgery, general

risk for ineffective Airway Clearance: risk factors may include soft tissue trauma, retained secretions.

risk for Aspiration: risk factors may include facial trauma or surgery, wired jaws, difficulty swallowing.

impaired Tissue Integrity may be related to tissue trauma or damage, intraoperative manipulation, mechanical fixation device, altered circulation, nutritional deficit, possibly evidenced by edema, hematoma, ecchymosis, erythema, inflammation, delayed healing.

impaired verbal Communication may be related to wiring of jaws, edema of mouth and surrounding structures, pain, possibly evidenced by inability or reluctance to talk.

risk for imbalanced Nutrition: less than body requirements: risk factors may include facial and tissue edema, inability to chew, difficulty swallowing, decreased appetite, increased metabolic needs.

Intervertebral disc excision   MS
Refer to Laminectomy, cervical or lumbar

Intestinal obstruction   MS
Refer to Ileus

Intestinal surgery (without diversion)   MS
Also refer to Surgery, general

risk for deficient Fluid Volume: risk factors may include excessive losses through normal routes (vomiting, diarrhea), excessive losses through abnormal routes (indwelling drains, nasogastric/intestinal suctioning, hemorrhage), insufficient replacement, fever.

risk for Infection: risk factors may include chronic disease, malnutrition, opening of abdominal cavity and bowel, stasis of body fluids, altered peristalsis.

Constipation/Diarrhea may be related to effects of anesthesia, surgical manipulation, decreased dietary intake or bulk, physical inactivity, irritation, malabsorption, pain, effects of medication, possibly evidenced by change in bowel habits, change in stool characteristics, hyper-/hypoactive bowel sounds, abdominal pain.

Intracranial infections   MS
Refer to Abscess, brain [acute]; Encephalitis; Meningitis

Irritable bowel syndrome   CH
acute Pain may be related to abnormally strong intestinal contractions, increased sensitivity of intestine to distention, hypersensitivity to hormones gastrin and cholecystokinin, skin or tissue irritation, perirectal excoriation, possibly evidenced by verbal reports, guarding behavior, expressive behavior (restlessness, moaning, irritability).

Constipation may be related to motor abnormalities of longitudinal muscles, changes in frequency and amplitude of contractions, dietary restrictions, stress, possibly evidenced by change in bowel pattern—decreased frequency, sensation of incomplete evacuation, abdominal pain and distention.

Diarrhea may be related to motor abnormalities of longitudinal muscles, changes in frequency and amplitude of contractions, stress, possibly evidenced by precipitous passing of liquid stool on rising or immediately after eating, rectal urgency, incontinence, bloating.

Kanner's syndrome   PED/PSY
Refer to Autistic disorder

Kaposi's sarcoma, AIDS-related   CH/MS
Also refer to Chemotherapy

disturbed Body Image may be related to widely disseminated lesions of varied color in skin and mucous membranes, possibly evidenced by verbalizations, fear of rejection or reaction of others, negative feelings about body, hiding body parts, change in social involvement.

risk for deficient Fluid Volume: risk factors may include extensive bleeding of visceral lesions.

Kawasaki disease   PED
Hyperthermia may be related to increased metabolic rate and dehydration, possibly evidenced by increased body temperature greater than normal range, flushed skin, increased respiratory rate, and tachycardia.

acute Pain may be related to inflammation and edema or swelling of tissues, possibly evidenced by verbal reports, restlessness, guarding behaviors, and narrowed focus.

impaired Skin Integrity may be related to inflammatory process, altered circulation, and edema formation, possibly evidenced by disruption of skin surface, including macular rash and desquamation.

impaired Oral Mucous Membrane may be related to inflammatory process, dehydration, and mouth breathing, possibly evidenced by pain, hyperemia, and fissures of lips.

risk for decreased Cardiac Output: risk factors may include structural changes and inflammation of coronary arteries, and alterations in rate and rhythm or conduction.

Ketoacidosis   CH
Refer to Diabetic ketoacidosis

Kidney disease, polycystic ..... CH

risk for [urinary tract] Infection: risk factors may include inadequate primary defenses (traumatized tissue, stasis of body fluids), inadequate secondary defenses (suppressed inflammatory response), chronic disease.

acute/chronic Pain may be related to injuring agents—presence of cysts in kidneys or other organs, possibly evidenced by verbal report of back or lower side pain, headaches beyond tolerance, guarded or protective behavior, narrowed focus, sleep disturbance, distraction behaviors.

risk for excess Fluid Volume: risk factors may include compromised regulatory mechanism—kidney failure, possibly evidenced by oliguria, edema, abnormal breath sounds, jugular vein distention, hypertension.

Kidney failure, acute ..... MS
Refer to Renal failure, acute

Kidney failure, chronic ..... CH/MS
Refer to Renal failure, chronic

Kidney stone(s) ..... CH
Refer to Calculi, urinary

Knee replacement ..... MS
Refer to Total joint replacement

Kwashiorkor ..... PED

imbalanced Nutrition: less than body requirements may be related to financial or resource limitations, possibly evidenced by inadequate food intake less than recommended daily allowances, lack of food, weight loss, poor muscle tone, decreased subcutaneous fat or muscle mass, abnormal laboratory studies.

risk for Infection: risk factors may include malnutrition.

risk for disproportionate Growth: risk factors may include malnutrition, caregiver maladaptive feeding behaviors, deprivation, poverty, impaired insulin response, infection.

Labor, breech presentation ..... OB

Anxiety [specify level] may be related to situational crisis, threat to self/fetus, interpersonal transmission, possibly evidenced by increased tension, apprehension, fearfulness, restlessness, sympathetic stimulation.

risk for fetal Injury: risk factors may include entrapment of head, stretching of brachial plexus or spinal cord (nerve damage), hypoxia (brain damage).

Labor, dysfunctional ..... OB
Refer to Dystocia

Labor, induced/augmented ..... OB

deficient Knowledge [Learning Need] regarding procedure, treatment needs, and possible outcomes may be related to lack of exposure or recall, information misinterpretation, and unfamiliarity with information resources, possibly evidenced by questions, statement of concern, misconception, and exaggerated behaviors.

risk for maternal Injury: risk factors may include adverse effects or response to therapeutic interventions.

risk for impaired fetal Gas Exchange: risk factors may include altered placental perfusion, cord prolapse.

---

acute Pain may be related to altered characteristics of chemically stimulated contractions, psychological concerns, possibly evidenced by verbal reports, increased muscle tone, distraction or guarding behaviors, and narrowed focus.

Labor, precipitous   OB

Anxiety [specify level] may be related to situational crisis, threat to self/fetus, interpersonal transmission, possibly evidenced by increased tension; scared, fearful, restless, jittery; sympathetic stimulation.

    risk for impaired Skin/Tissue Integrity: risk factors may include rapid progress of labor, lack of necessary equipment.

    acute Pain may be related to occurrence of rapid, strong muscle contractions; psychological issues, possibly evidenced by verbalizations of inability to use learned pain-management techniques, sympathetic stimulation, distraction behaviors (e.g., moaning, restlessness).

Labor, preterm   OB/CH

Activity Intolerance may be related to muscle and cellular hypersensitivity, possibly evidenced by continued uterine contractions or irritability.

    risk for Poisoning: risk factors may include dose-related toxic or side effects of tocolytics.

    risk for fetal Injury: risk factors may include delivery of premature/immature infant.

    Anxiety [specify level] may be related to situational crisis, perceived or actual threats to self/fetus, and inadequate time to prepare for labor, possibly evidenced by increased tension, restlessness, expressions of concern, and autonomic responses (changes in vital signs).

    deficient Knowledge [Learning Need] regarding preterm labor treatment needs and prognosis may be related to lack of information and misinterpretation, possibly evidenced by questions, statements of concern, misconceptions, inaccurate follow-through of instruction, and development of preventable complications.

Labor, stage I (active phase)   OB

acute Pain/impaired Comfort may be related to contraction-related hypoxia, dilation of tissues, and pressure on adjacent structures combined with stimulation of both parasympathetic and sympathetic nerve endings, possibly evidenced by verbal reports, guarding or distraction behaviors (restlessness), muscle tension, and narrowed focus.

    impaired Urinary Elimination may be related to altered intake, dehydration, fluid shifts, hormonal changes, hemorrhage, severe intrapartal hypertension, mechanical compression of bladder, and effects of regional anesthesia, possibly evidenced by changes in amount and frequency of voiding, urinary retention, slowed progression of labor, and reduced sensation.

    risk for ineffective [individual/couple] Coping: risk factors may include situational crises, personal vulnerability, use of ineffective coping mechanisms, inadequate support systems, and pain.

Labor, stage I (latent phase)   OB

deficient Knowledge [Learning Need] regarding progression of labor and available options may be related to lack of exposure or recall, information misinterpretation, possibly evidenced by questions, statements of misconceptions, inaccurate follow-through of instructions.

    risk for mild Anxiety: risk factors may include situational crisis, unmet needs, stress.

    risk for ineffective Coping: risk factors may include personal vulnerability, inadequate support systems or coping methods.

Labor, stage I (transition phase)   OB

acute Pain may be related to mechanical pressure of presenting part, tissue dilation or stretching and hypoxia, stimulation of parasympathetic and sympathetic nerves, emotional and muscular tension.

Fatigue may be related to discomfort, pain, overwhelming psychological emotional demands, increased energy requirements, decreased caloric intake, possibly evidenced by verbalizations, impaired ability to concentrate, emotional lability or irritability, lethargy, altered coping ability.

risk for ineffective [individual/couple] Coping: risk factors may include sense of "work overload," personal vulnerability, inadequate or exhausted support system.

risk for imbalanced Fluid Volume: risk factors may include reduced intake, excess fluid loss, hemorrhage, excess fluid retention, rapid fluid administration.

risk for decreased Cardiac Output: risk factors may include decreased venous return, hypovolemia, changes in systemic vascular resistance.

Labor, stage II (expulsion)   OB

acute Pain may be related to strong uterine contractions, tissue stretching and dilation, and compression of nerves by presenting part of the fetus, and bladder distention, possibly evidenced by verbalizations, facial grimacing, guarding or distraction behaviors (restlessness), narrowed focus, and autonomic responses (diaphoresis).

Cardiac Output [fluctuation] may be related to changes in systemic vascular resistance, fluctuations in venous return (repeated or prolonged Valsalva's maneuvers, effects of anesthesia and medications, dorsal recumbent position occluding the inferior vena cava and partially obstructing the aorta), possibly evidenced by decreased venous return, changes in vital signs (blood pressure, pulse), urinary output, fetal bradycardia.

risk for impaired fetal Gas Exchange: risk factors may include mechanical compression of head or cord, maternal position or prolonged labor affecting placental perfusion, and effects of maternal anesthesia, hyperventilation.

risk for impaired Skin/Tissue Integrity: risk factors may include untoward stretching, lacerations of delicate tissues (precipitous labor, hypertonic contractile pattern, adolescence, large fetus) and application of forceps.

risk for Fatigue: risk factors may include pregnancy, stress, anxiety, sleep deprivation, increased physical exertion, anemia, environmental humidity, temperature, and lights.

Labor, stage III (placental expulsion)   OB

acute Pain may be related to tissue trauma, psychological response following delivery, possibly evidenced by verbalizations, changes in muscle tone, restlessness.

risk for deficient Fluid Volume/Bleeding: risk factors may include lack or restriction of oral intake, vomiting, diaphoresis, increased insensible water loss, uterine atony, lacerations of the birth canal, retained placental fragments.

risk for maternal Injury: risk factors may include positioning during delivery and transfers, difficulty with placental separation, abnormal blood profile.

risk for impaired Attachment: risk factors may include physical barriers, separation, anxiety associated with the parent role.

Labor, stage IV (first 4 hr following delivery of placenta)   OB

Fatigue may be related to increased physical exertion, sleep deprivation, stress, environmental stimuli, hormonal changes, possibly evidenced by verbalization of overwhelming lack of energy, compromised concentration, listlessness.

acute Pain may be related to effects of hormones and medications, mechanical trauma, tissue edema, physical and psychological exhaustion, anxiety, possibly evidenced by reports of cramping (afterpains), muscle tremors, guarding or distraction behaviors, facial mask.

risk for Bleeding: risk factors may include myometrial fatigue/failure of homeostatic mechanisms (e.g., continued uteroplacental circulation, incomplete vasoconstriction, effects of pregnancy-induced hypertension).

risk for impaired Attachment: risk factors may include maternal fatigue, physical barriers, separation, lack of privacy, anxiety associated with the parent role.

Laceration   CH
impaired Skin/Tissue Integrity may be related to trauma, possibly evidenced by disruption of skin layers, invasion of body structures.

risk for Infection: risk factors may include trauma, tissue destruction, increased environmental exposure.

Laminectomy, cervical   MS
Also refer to Laminectomy, lumbar

risk for perioperative-positioning Injury: risk factors may include immobilization, muscle weakness, obesity, advanced age.

risk for ineffective Airway Clearance: risk factors may include retained secretions, pain, muscular weakness.

risk for impaired Swallowing: risk factors may include operative edema, pain, neuromuscular impairment.

Laminectomy, lumbar   MS
Also refer to Surgery, general

risk for ineffective tissue Perfusion (specify) risk factors may include diminished or interrupted blood flow—pressure dressing, edema of operative site, hematoma formation; hypovolemia.

risk for [spinal] Trauma: risk factors may include temporary weakness of spinal column, balancing difficulties, changes in muscle tone and coordination.

acute Pain may be related to traumatized tissues—surgical manipulation, harvesting bone graft; localized inflammation, and edema, possibly evidenced by altered muscle tone, verbal reports, distraction or guarding behaviors, autonomic changes—changes in vital signs, diaphoresis, pallor.

impaired physical Mobility may be related to imposed therapeutic restrictions, neuromuscular impairment, and pain, possibly evidenced by limited range of motion, decreased muscle strength and control, impaired coordination, and reluctance to attempt movement.

risk for [acute] Urinary Retention: risk factors may include pain and swelling in operative area and reduced mobility, restrictions of position.

Laryngectomy   MS
Also refer to Cancer; Chemotherapy

ineffective Airway Clearance may be related to partial or total removal of the glottis—impairing ability to breath, cough, or swallow; temporary or permanent change to neck breathing (dependent on patent stoma), edema formation—surgical manipulation, lymphatic accumulation; and copious, thick secretions, possibly evidenced by dyspnea; changes in rate and depth of respiration; use of accessory respiratory muscles; weak, ineffective cough; abnormal breath sounds; and cyanosis.

impaired Skin/Tissue Integrity may be related to surgical removal of tissues and grafting, effects of radiation or chemotherapeutic agents, altered circulation or reduced blood supply, compromised nutritional status, edema formation, and pooling or continuous drainage of secretions, possibly evidenced by disruption and destruction of skin and tissue layers.

impaired Oral Mucous Membrane may be related to dehydration or absence of oral intake, decreased saliva production, poor or inadequate oral hygiene, pathological condition (oral cancer), mechanical trauma (oral surgery), decreased saliva production, difficulty swallowing and pooling of secretions or drooling, and nutritional deficits, possibly evidenced by xerostomia (dry mouth), oral discomfort, thick, mucoid saliva; decreased saliva production, dry and crusted or coated tongue, inflamed lips, absent teeth and gums, poor dental health and halitosis.

CH

impaired verbal Communication may be related to anatomic deficit (removal of vocal cords), physical barrier (tracheostomy tube), and required voice rest, possibly evidenced by inability to speak, change in vocal characteristics, and impaired articulation.

risk for Aspiration: risk factors may include impaired swallowing, facial and neck surgery, presence of tracheostomy, feeding tube.

Laryngitis   CH/PED
Refer to Croup

Latex allergy   CH
latex Allergy Response may be related to no immune mechanism response, possibly evidenced by contact dermatitis—erythema, blisters; delayed hypersensitivity—eczema, irritation; hypersensitivity—generalized edema, wheezing, bronchospasm, hypotension, cardiac arrest.

Anxiety [specify level]/Fear may be related to threat of death, possibly evidenced by expressed concerns, hypervigilance, restlessness, focus on self.

risk for risk-prone health Behavior: risk factors may include health status requiring change in occupation.

Laxative abuse   CH
perceived Constipation may be related to health beliefs, faulty appraisal, impaired cognition/ thought processes, possibly evidenced by expectation of daily bowel movement, expected passage of stool at same time every day.

Lead poisoning, acute   PED/CH
Also refer to Lead poisoning, chronic

Contamination may be related to flaking or peeling paint (young children), improperly lead-glazed ceramic pottery, unprotected contact with lead (e.g., battery manufacture or recycling, bronzing, soldering or welding), imported herbal products or medicinals, possibly evidenced by abdominal cramping, headache, irritability, decreased attentiveness, constipation, tremors.

risk for Trauma: risk factors may include loss of coordination, altered level of consciousness, clonic or tonic muscle activity, neurological damage.

risk for deficient Fluid Volume: risk factors may include excessive vomiting, diarrhea, or decreased intake.

deficient Knowledge [Learning Need] regarding sources of lead and prevention of poisoning may be related to lack of information, misinterpretation, possibly evidenced by statements of concern, questions, and misconceptions.

Lead poisoning, chronic   CH
Also refer to Lead Poisoning, acute

Contamination may be related to flaking or peeling paint (young children), improperly lead-glazed ceramic pottery, unprotected contact with lead (e.g., battery manufacture or recycling, bronzing, soldering or welding), imported herbal products or medicinals, possibly evidenced by chronic abdominal cramping, headache, personality changes, cognitive deficits, seizures, neuropathy.

imbalanced Nutrition: less than body requirements may be related to decreased intake (chemically induced changes in the gastrointestinal tract), possibly evidenced by anorexia, abdominal discomfort, reported metallic taste, and weight loss.

disturbed Thought Processes may be related to deposition of lead in central nervous system and brain tissue, possibly evidenced by personality changes, learning disabilities, and impaired ability to conceptualize and reason.

chronic Pain may be related to deposition of lead in soft tissues and bone, possibly evidenced by verbal reports, distraction behaviors, and focus on self.

Legionnaires' disease   CH/MS
Hyperthermia may be related to illness and inflammatory process, possibly evidenced by increased body temperature; flushed, warm skin; chills.

acute Pain/impaired Comfort may be related to infectious agent and inflammatory response, effects of circulating toxins, possibly evidenced by reports of headache, myalgia, high fever, diaphoresis.

ineffective Airway Clearance may be related to tracheal bronchial inflammation, edema formation, increased sputum production, pleuritic pain, decreased energy, fatigue, possibly evidenced by changes in rate and depth of respirations, abnormal breath sounds, use of accessory muscles, dyspnea, cyanosis, ineffective cough—with or without sputum production.

impaired Gas Exchange may be related to inflammatory process, collection of secretions affecting oxygen exchange across alveolar membrane, and hypoventilation, possibly evidenced by restlessness, changes in mentation, dyspnea, tachycardia, pallor, cyanosis, and arterial blood gas or oximetry evidence of hypoxia.

Diarrhea may be related to infectious process, possibly evidenced by liquid stools, abdominal cramping.

risk for Infection [spread]: risk factors may include decreased ciliary action, stasis of secretions, presence of existing infection, improper disposal of contaminated materials.

Leprosy   CH
Refer to Hansen's disease

Leukemia, acute   MS
Also refer to Chemotherapy

risk for Infection: risk factors may include inadequate secondary defenses (alterations in mature white blood cells, increased number of immature lymphocytes, immunosuppression and bone marrow suppression), invasive procedures, and malnutrition.

Anxiety [specify level]/Fear may be related to change in health status, threat of death, and situational crisis, possibly evidenced by sympathetic stimulation, apprehension, feelings of helplessness, focus on self, and insomnia.

Activity Intolerance [specify level] may be related to reduced energy stores, increased metabolic rate, imbalance between oxygen supply and demand—anemia, hypoxia; therapeutic restrictions (isolation, bedrest), effect of drug therapy, possibly evidenced by generalized weakness, reports of fatigue and exertional dyspnea, abnormal heart rate or blood pressure response.

acute Pain may be related to physical agents—infiltration of tissues, organs, central nervous system, or expanding bone marrow; chemical agents (antileukemic treatments), psychological manifestations—anxiety, fear, possibly evidenced by verbal reports of abdominal discomfort, arthralgia, bone pain, headache; distraction behaviors, narrowed focus, and autonomic responses—changes in vital signs.

risk for deficient Fluid Volume/Bleeding: risk factors may include excessive losses (vomiting, hemorrhage, diarrhea, coagulopathy), decreased intake (nausea, anorexia), increased fluid need (hypermetabolic state/fever), predisposition for kidney stone formation and tumor lysis syndrome.

Leukemia, chronic   **CH**

ineffective Protection may be related to abnormal blood profiles, drug therapy (cytotoxic agents, steroids), radiation treatments, possibly evidenced by deficient immunity, impaired healing, altered clotting, weakness.

   Fatigue may be related to disease state, anemia, possibly evidenced by verbalizations, inability to maintain usual routines, listlessness.

   imbalanced Nutrition: less than body requirements may be related to inability to ingest nutrients, possibly evidenced by lack of interest in food, anorexia, weight loss, abdominal fullness, pain.

Lice, head   **PED/CH**
Refer to Pediculosis capitis

Lice, pubic   **CH**
Refer to Pediculosis capitis

Lightning injury   **MS**
Also refer to Electrical injury

   risk for disturbed visual/auditory Sensory Perception: risk factors may include altered sensory reception (corneal laceration, retinal damage, development of cataracts, rupture of tympanic membrane).

   acute Confusion may be related to central nervous system involvement, possibly evidenced by change in level of consciousness.

   impaired Memory may be related to acute hypoxia, decreased cardiac output, electrolyte imbalance, neurological disturbance, possibly evidenced by inability to recall recent events, amnesia.

Liver failure   **MS/CH**
Refer to Cirrhosis; Hepatitis, acute viral

Liver transplantation   **MS/CH**
Refer to Transplantation, recipient

Lockjaw   **MS**
Refer to Tetanus

Long-term care   **CH**
(Also refer to condition requiring/contributing to need for facility placement.)

   Anxiety [specify level]/Fear may be related to change in health status, role functioning, interaction patterns, socioeconomic status, environment; unmet needs; recent life changes; and loss of friends/SO(s), possibly evidenced by apprehension, restlessness, insomnia, repetitive questioning, pacing, purposeless activity, expressed concern regarding changes in life events, and focus on self.

   Grieving may be related to perceived, actual or potential loss of physiopsychosocial well-being, personal possessions, and SO(s), as well as cultural beliefs about aging and debilitation, possibly evidenced by denial of feelings, depression, sorrow, guilt; alterations in activity level, sleep patterns, eating habits, and libido.

   risk for Poisoning [drug toxicity]: risk factors may include effects of aging (reduced metabolism, impaired circulation, precarious physiological balance, presence of multiple diseases and organ involvement) and use of multiple prescribed and over-the-counter drugs.

impaired Memory/disturbed Thought Processes may be related to physiological changes of aging (loss of cells and brain atrophy, decreased blood supply); altered sensory input, pain, effects of medications, and psychological conflicts (disrupted life pattern), possibly evidenced by slower reaction times, memory loss, altered attention span, disorientation, inability to follow, altered sleep patterns, and personality changes.

Insomnia may be related to internal factors (illness, psychological stress, inactivity) and external factors (environmental changes, facility routines), possibly evidenced by reports of difficulty in falling asleep, not feeling rested, interrupted sleep, awakening earlier than desired, change in behavior or performance, increasing irritability, and listlessness.

risk for Sexual Dysfunction: risk factors may include biopsychosocial alteration of sexuality; interference in psychological or physical well-being, self-image, and lack of privacy/SO.

risk for Relocation Stress Syndrome: risk factors may include temporary or permanent move that may be voluntary or involuntary, lack of predeparture counseling, multiple losses, feeling of powerlessness, lack of or inappropriate use of support system, decreased psychosocial or physical health status.

risk for impaired Religiosity: risk factors may include life transition, ineffective support or coping, lack of social interaction, depression.

LSD (lysergic acid diethylamide) intoxication   MS/PSY
Also refer to Hallucinogen abuse

risk for Trauma: risk factors may include perceptual distortion, impaired judgment, dangerous decision making, changes in mood.

Anxiety [panic attack] may be related to drug side effects, possibly evidenced by severe apprehension, fear of unspecific consequences, central nervous system excitation, central autonomic hyperactivity.

Lung cancer   MS/CH
Refer to Bronchogenic carcinoma

Lung transplantation   MS/CH
Also refer to Transplantation, recipient

risk for impaired Gas Exchange: risk factors may include ventilation-perfusion mismatch, poor healing, stenosis of bronchial or tracheal anastomosis.

risk for Infection: risk factors may include medically induced immunosuppression, suppressed inflammatory response, antibiotic therapy, invasive procedures, effects of chronic or debilitating disease.

Lupus erythematosus, systemic (SLE)   CH
Fatigue may be related to inadequate energy production, increased energy requirements (chronic inflammation), overwhelming psychological or emotional demands, states of discomfort, and altered body chemistry (including effects of drug therapy), possibly evidenced by reports of unremitting and overwhelming lack of energy, inability to maintain usual routines, decreased performance, lethargy, and decreased libido.

acute Pain may be related to widespread inflammatory process affecting connective tissues, blood vessels, serosal surfaces and mucous membranes, possibly evidenced by verbal reports, guarding or distraction behaviors, self-focusing, and changes in vital signs.

impaired Skin/Tissue Integrity may be related to chronic inflammation, edema formation, and altered circulation, possibly evidenced by presence of skin rash or lesions, ulcerations of mucous membranes and photosensitivity.

disturbed Body Image may be related to presence of chronic condition with rash, lesions, ulcers, purpura, mottled erythema of hands, alopecia, loss of strength, and altered body function, possibly evidenced by hiding body parts, negative feelings about body, feelings of helplessness, and change in social involvement.

Lyme disease   CH/MS
acute/chronic Pain may be related to systemic effects of toxins, presence of rash, urticaria, and joint swelling and inflammation, possibly evidenced by verbal reports, guarding behaviors, autonomic responses, and narrowed focus.

Fatigue may be related to increased energy requirements, altered body chemistry, and states of discomfort evidenced by reports of overwhelming lack of energy, inability to maintain usual routines, decreased performance, lethargy, and malaise.

risk for decreased Cardiac Output: risk factors may include alteration in cardiac rate, rhythm, or conduction.

Lymphedema   CH
disturbed Body Image may be related to physical changes (chronic swelling of lower extremity), possibly evidenced by verbalizations, fear of reaction of others, negative feelings about body, hiding body part, change in social involvement.

impaired Walking may be related to chronic or progressive swelling of lower extremity, possibly evidenced by difficulty walking required distances, climbing stairs, navigating uneven surfaces and declines.

risk for impaired Skin Integrity: risk factors may include altered circulation, significant edema, changes in sensation.

Macular degeneration   CH
disturbed visual Sensory Perception may be related to altered sensory reception, possibly evidenced by reported or measured change in sensory acuity, change in usual response to stimuli.

Anxiety [specify level]/Fear may be related to situational crisis, threat to or change in health status and role function, possibly evidenced by expressed concerns, apprehension, feelings of inadequacy, diminished productivity, impaired attention.

risk for impaired Home Maintenance: risk factors may include impaired cognitive functioning, inadequate support systems.

risk for impaired Social Interaction: risk factors may include limited physical mobility, environmental barriers.

Malaria   MS/CH
Hyperthermia may be related to inflammatory process, possibly evidenced by increased body temperature (106°F [41.1°C]); flushed, warm skin; tachycardia; headache; altered consciousness.

acute Pain/impaired Comfort may be related to infectious agent, inflammatory response, possibly evidenced by reports of headache, backache, myalgia, malaise, high fever, shaking chills, abdominal discomfort.

risk for deficient Fluid Volume: risk factors may include decreased intake (nausea, abdominal pain, prostration), excessive losses (vomiting, diarrhea), hypermetabolic state.

Fatigue may be related to disease state, anemia, lack of restful sleep, possibly evidenced by verbalization of unremitting or overwhelming lack of energy, inability to restore energy even after sleep, lethargy.

Mallory-Weiss syndrome   MS
Also refer to Achalasia

risk for deficient Fluid Volume [isotonic]: risk factors may include excessive vascular losses, presence of vomiting, and reduced intake.

---

deficient Knowledge [Learning Need] regarding causes, treatment, and prevention of condition may be related to lack of information, misinterpretation, possibly evidenced by statements of concern, questions, and recurrence of problem.

Malnutrition   CH
Also refer to Anorexia nervosa

adult Failure to Thrive may be related to depression, apathy, aging process, fatigue, degenerative condition, possibly evidenced by expressed lack of appetite, difficulty performing self-care tasks, altered mood state, inadequate intake, weight loss, physical decline.

ineffective Protection may be related to inadequate nutrition, anemia, extremes of age, possibly evidenced by fatigue, weakness, deficient immunity, impaired healing, pressure sores.

Marburg disease   MS
Refer to Ebola

Mastectomy   MS
impaired Skin/Tissue Integrity may be related to surgical removal of skin and tissue, altered circulation, presence of edema, drainage, changes in skin elasticity and sensation, and tissue destruction (radiation), possibly evidenced by disruption of skin surface and destruction of skin layers and subcutaneous tissues.

impaired physical Mobility may be related to neuromuscular impairment, pain, and edema formation, possibly evidenced by reluctance to attempt movement, limited range of motion, and decreased muscle mass and strength.

bathing/dressing Self-Care Deficit may be related to temporary decreased range of motion of one or both arms, possibly evidenced by statements of inability to perform or complete self-care tasks.

disturbed Body Image/situational low Self-Esteem may be related to loss of body part denoting femininity, fear of rejection or reaction of others, behaviors inconsistent with self-value system possibly evidenced by not looking at or touching area, self-negating verbalizations, preoccupation with loss, and change in social involvement or relationship.

risk for complicated Grieving: risk factors may include preloss psychological symptoms, predisposition for anxiety and feelings of inadequacy, frequency of major life events.

Mastitis   OB/GYN
acute Pain may be related to erythema and edema of breast tissues, possibly evidenced by verbal reports, guarding or distraction behaviors, self-focusing, and changes in vital signs.

risk for Infection [spread/abscess formation]: risk factors may include traumatized tissues, stasis of fluids, and insufficient knowledge to prevent complications.

deficient Knowledge [Learning Need] regarding pathophysiology, treatment, and prevention may be related to lack of information, misinterpretation, possibly evidenced by statements of concern, questions, and misconceptions.

risk for ineffective Breastfeeding: risk factors may include inability to feed on affected side, interruption in breastfeeding.

Mastoidectomy   PED/MS
risk for Infection [spread]: risk factors may include preexisting infection, surgical trauma, and stasis of body fluids in close proximity to brain.

acute Pain may be related to inflammation, tissue trauma, and edema formation, possibly evidenced by verbal reports, distraction behaviors, restlessness, self-focusing, and changes in vital signs.

disturbed auditory Sensory Perception may be related to presence of surgical packing, edema, and surgical disturbance of middle ear structures, possibly evidenced by reported or tested hearing loss in affected ear.

Measles   CH/PED

acute Pain/impaired Comfort may be related to inflammation of mucous membranes, conjunctiva, and presence of extensive skin rash with pruritus, possibly evidenced by verbal reports, distraction behaviors, self-focusing, and changes in vital signs.

Hyperthermia may be related to presence of viral toxins and inflammatory response, possibly evidenced by increased body temperature; flushed, warm skin; and tachycardia.

risk for [secondary] Infection: risk factors may include altered immune response and traumatized dermal tissues.

deficient Knowledge [Learning Need] regarding condition, transmission, and possible complications may be related to lack of information, misinterpretation, possibly evidenced by statements of concern, questions, misconceptions, and development of preventable complications.

Measles, German   PED/CH
Refer to Rubella

Melanoma, malignant   MS/CH
Refer to Cancer; Chemotherapy

Ménière's disease   CH
Also refer to Vertigo

disturbed auditory Sensory Perception may be related to altered state of sensory organ or sensory reception, possibly evidenced by change in sensory acuity, tinnitus, vertigo.

Nausea may be related to inner ear disturbance, possibly evidenced by verbal reports, vomiting.

risk for total Self-Care Deficit: risk factors may include perceptual impairment, recurrent nausea, general weakness.

Meningitis, acute meningococcal   MS

risk for Infection [spread]: risk factors may include hematogenous dissemination of pathogen, stasis of body fluids, suppressed inflammatory response (medication-induced), and exposure of others to pathogens.

risk for ineffective cerebral tissue Perfusion: risk factors may include cerebral edema altering or interrupting cerebral arterial or venous blood flow, hypovolemia, exchange problems at cellular level (acidosis).

Hyperthermia may be related to infectious process (increased metabolic rate) and dehydration, possibly evidenced by increased body temperature; warm, flushed skin; and tachycardia.

acute Pain may be related to inflammation and irritation of the meninges with spasm of extensor muscles (neck, shoulders, and back), possibly evidenced by verbal reports, guarding or distraction behaviors, narrowed focus, photophobia, and changes in vital signs.

risk for Trauma/Suffocation: risk factors may include alterations in level of consciousness, possible development of clonic-tonic muscle activity (seizures), generalized weakness, prostration, ataxia, vertigo.

Meniscectomy   MS/CH

impaired Walking may be related to pain, joint instability, and imposed medical restrictions of movement, possibly evidenced by impaired ability to move about environment as needed or desired.

deficient Knowledge [Learning Need] regarding postoperative expectations, prevention of complications, and self-care needs may be related to lack of information, possibly evidenced by statements of concern, questions, and misconceptions.

Menopause   GYN

ineffective Thermoregulation may be related to fluctuation of hormonal levels, possibly evidenced by skin flushed/warm to touch, diaphoresis, night sweats, cold hands and feet.

Fatigue may be related to change in body chemistry, lack of sleep, depression, possibly evidenced by reports of lack of energy, tired, inability to maintain usual routines, decreased performance.

risk for Sexual Dysfunction: risk factors may include perceived altered body function, changes in physical response, myths or inaccurate information, impaired relationship with SO.

risk for stress urinary Incontinence: risk factors may include degenerative changes in pelvic muscles and structural support.

readiness for enhanced self Health Management: may be related to management of life-cycle changes, possibly evidenced by expressed desire for increased control of health practice, describes reduction of symptoms.

Mental delay (formerly retardation)   CH

Also refer to Down syndrome

impaired verbal Communication may be related to developmental delay or impairment of cognitive and motor abilities, possibly evidenced by impaired articulation, difficulty with phonation, and inability to modulate speech or find appropriate words (dependent on degree of retardation).

risk for Self-Care Deficit [specify]: risk factors may include impaired cognitive ability and motor skills.

risk for imbalanced Nutrition: more than body requirements: risk factors may include decreased metabolic rate coupled with impaired cognitive development, dysfunctional eating patterns, and sedentary activity level.

risk for sedentary Lifestyle: risk factors may include lack of interest or motivation, resources; lack of training or knowledge of specific exercise needs, safety concerns, fear of injury.

impaired Social Interaction may be related to impaired thought processes, communication barriers, and knowledge or skill deficit about ways to enhance mutuality, possibly evidenced by dysfunctional interactions with peers, family, and/or SO(s), and verbalized or observed discomfort in social situation.

compromised family Coping may be related to chronic nature of condition and degree of disability that exhausts supportive capacity of SO(s), other situational or developmental crises or situations SO(s) may be facing, unrealistic expectations of SO(s), possibly evidenced by preoccupation of SO with personal reaction, SO(s) withdraw(s) or enter(s) into limited interaction with individual, protective behavior disproportionate (too much or too little) to client's abilities or need for autonomy.

impaired Home Maintenance may be related to impaired cognitive functioning, insufficient finances/family organization or planning, lack of knowledge, and inadequate support systems, possibly evidenced by requests for assistance, expression of difficulty in maintaining home, disorderly surroundings, and overtaxed family members.

risk for Sexual Dysfunction: risk factors may include biopsychosocial alteration of sexuality, ineffectual or absent role models, misinformation, lack of knowledge, lack of SO(s), and lack of appropriate behavior control.

Mesothelioma   CH/MS

Also refer to Asbestosis; Cancer

acute Pain may be related to tissue destruction, possibly evidenced by reports of chest pain (initially nonpleuritic), irritability, self-focusing, autonomic responses.

Activity Intolerance may be related to imbalance between oxygen supply and demand, possibly evidenced by dyspnea, fatigue.

Metabolic syndrome   CH

risk for unstable blood Glucose Level: risk factors may include dietary intake, weight gain, physical activity level.

sedentary Lifestyle may be related to deficient knowledge of health benefits of physical exercise, lack of interest, motivation or resources, possibly evidenced by verbalized preference for activities low in physical activity, choosing a daily routine lacking physical exercise.

risk for ineffective tissue Perfusion (specify): risk factors may include arterial plaque formation (elevated triglycerides, low levels of high-density lipoprotein), prothrombotic state, proinflammatory state.

Migraine   CH/MS
Refer to Headache

Miscarriage   OB
Refer to Abortion, spontaneous termination

Mitral insufficiency   MS/CH
Refer to Valvular heart disease

Mitral stenosis   MS/CH

Activity Intolerance may be related to imbalance between oxygen supply and demand, possibly evidenced by reports of fatigue, weakness, exertional dyspnea, and tachycardia.

impaired Gas Exchange may be related to altered blood flow, possibly evidenced by restlessness, hypoxia, and cyanosis (orthopnea, paroxysmal nocturnal dyspnea).

decreased Cardiac Output may be related to impeded blood flow as evidenced by jugular vein distention, peripheral or dependent edema, orthopnea, paroxysmal nocturnal dyspnea.

deficient Knowledge [Learning Need] regarding pathophysiology, therapeutic needs, and potential complications may be related to lack of information or recall, misinterpretation, possibly evidenced by statements of concern, questions, inaccurate follow-through of instructions, and development of preventable complications.

Mitral valve prolapse (MVP)   CH
Refer to Valvular heart disease

Mononucleosis, infectious   CH

Fatigue may be related to decreased energy production, states of discomfort, and increased energy requirements (inflammatory process), possibly evidenced by reports of overwhelming lack of energy, inability to maintain usual routines, lethargy, and malaise.

acute Pain/impaired Comfort may be related to inflammation of lymphoid and organ tissues, irritation of oropharyngeal mucous membranes, and effects of circulating toxins, possibly evidenced by verbal reports, distraction behaviors, and self-focusing.

Hyperthermia may be related to inflammatory process, possibly evidenced by increased body temperature; warm, flushed skin; and tachycardia.

deficient Knowledge [Learning Need] regarding disease transmission, self-care needs, medical therapy, and potential complications may be related to lack of information, misinterpretation, possibly evidenced by statements of concern, misconceptions, and inaccurate follow-through of instructions.

NEC PED

Refer to Necrotizing enterocolitis

Necrotizing cellulitis/fasciitis MS

Also refer to Cellulitis; Sepsis

Hyperthermia may be related to inflammatory process, response to circulating toxins, possibly evidenced by body temperature above normal range; flushed, warm skin; tachycardia; altered mental status.

impaired Tissue Integrity may be related to inflammation and edema (infection), ischemia, possibly evidenced by damaged or destroyed tissue, dermal gangrene.

Necrotizing enterocolitis PED

Also refer to Sepsis

imbalanced Nutrition: less than body requirements may be related to inability to digest or absorb nutrients (ischemia of bowel), possibly evidenced by abdominal pain and distention, gastric residuals after feedings, failure to gain weight.

risk for deficient Fluid Volume: risk factors may include vomiting, third-space fluid losses (bowel inflammation, peritonitis), lack of oral intake.

Neglect/abuse CH/PSY

Refer to Abuse, Battered child syndrome

Nephrectomy MS

acute Pain may be related to surgical tissue trauma with mechanical closure (suture), possibly evidenced by verbal reports, guarding or distraction behaviors, self-focusing, and changes in vital signs.

risk for deficient Fluid Volume: risk factors may include excessive vascular losses and restricted intake.

ineffective Breathing Pattern may be related to incisional pain with decreased lung expansion, possibly evidenced by tachypnea, fremitus, changes in respiratory depth and chest expansion, and changes in arterial blood gases.

Constipation may be related to reduced dietary intake, decreased mobility, gastrointestinal obstruction (paralytic ileus), and incisional pain with defecation, possibly evidenced by decreased bowel sounds; reduced frequency/amount of stool; and hard, formed stool.

Nephrolithiasis MS/CH

Refer to Calculi, urinary

Nephrotic syndrome MS/CH

Also refer to Renal failure, acute/chronic

excess Fluid Volume may be related to compromised regulatory mechanism with changes in hydrostatic or oncotic vascular pressure and increased activation of the renin-angiotensin-aldosterone system, possibly evidenced by edema, anasarca, effusions, ascites, weight gain, intake greater than output, and blood pressure changes.

imbalanced Nutrition: less than body requirements may be related to excessive protein losses and inability to ingest adequate nutrients (anorexia), possibly evidenced by weight loss, muscle wasting (may be difficult to assess due to edema), lack of interest in food, and observed inadequate intake.

risk for Infection: risk factors may include chronic disease and steroidal suppression of inflammatory responses.

---

risk for impaired Skin Integrity: risk factors may include presence of edema and activity restrictions.

Neuralgia, trigeminal   CH
acute Pain may be related to neuromuscular impairment with sudden violent muscle spasm, possibly evidenced by verbal reports, guarding or distraction behaviors, self-focusing, and changes in vital signs.

deficient Knowledge [Learning Need] regarding control of recurrent episodes, medical therapies, and self-care needs may be related to lack of information or recall and misinterpretation, possibly evidenced by statements of concern, questions, and exacerbation of condition.

Neural tube defect   PED
Refer to Spina bifida

Neuritis   CH
acute/chronic Pain may be related to nerve damage usually associated with a degenerative process, possibly evidenced by verbal reports, guarding or distraction behaviors, self-focusing, and changes in vital signs.

deficient Knowledge [Learning Need] regarding underlying causative factors, treatment, and prevention may be related to lack of information, misinterpretation, possibly evidenced by statements of concern, questions, and misconceptions.

Newborn, growth deviations   PED
Also refer to Newborn, premature

disproportionate Growth may be related to maternal nutrition, substance use or abuse, multiple gestation, prematurity, maternal conditions (e.g., pregnancy-induced hypertension, diabetes), possibly evidenced by birth weight at or below 10th percentile or at or above 90th percentile (considering gestational age, ethnicity, etc.).

imbalanced Nutrition: less than body requirements may be related to decreased nutritional stores, hyperplasia of pancreatic beta cells, and increased insulin production, possibly evidenced by weight deviation from expected, decreased muscle mass/fat stores, electrolyte imbalance.

risk for ineffective tissue Perfusion (specify): risk factors may include interruption of arterial or venous blood flow (hyperviscosity associated with polycythemia).

risk for Injury: risk factors may include altered growth, delayed central nervous system or neurological development, abnormal blood profile.

risk for disorganized Infant Behavior: risk factors may include functional limitations related to growth deviations (restricting neonate's opportunity to seek out, recognize, and interpret stimuli), electrolyte imbalance, psychological stress, low energy reserves, poor organizational ability, limited ability to control environment.

Newborn, normal   PED
risk for impaired Gas Exchange: risk factors may include prenatal or intrapartal stressors, excess production of mucus, or cold stress.

risk for Hypothermia: risk factors may include large body surface in relation to mass, limited amounts of insulating subcutaneous fat, nonrenewable sources of brown fat and few white fat stores, thin epidermis with close proximity of blood vessels to the skin, inability to shiver, and movement from a warm uterine environment to a much cooler environment.

risk for impaired Attachment: risk factors may include developmental transition or gain of a family member, anxiety associated with the parent role, lack of privacy (healthcare interventions, intrusive family/visitors).

risk for imbalanced Nutrition: less than body requirements: risk factors may include rapid metabolic rate, high-caloric requirement, increased insensible water losses through pulmonary and cutaneous routes, fatigue, and a potential for inadequate or depleted glucose stores.

risk for Infection: risk factors may include inadequate secondary defenses (inadequate acquired immunity, e.g., deficiency of neutrophils and specific immunoglobulins), and inadequate primary defenses (e.g., environmental exposure, broken skin, traumatized tissues, decreased ciliary action).

Newborn at 1 week   PED
Also refer to Newborn, normal

risk for Injury: risk factors may include physical (hyperbilirubinemia), environmental (inadequate safety precautions), chemical (drugs in breastmilk), psychological (inappropriate parental stimulation or interaction).

risk for Constipation/Diarrhea: risk factors may include type and amount of oral intake, medications or dietary intake of lactating mother, presence of allergies, infection.

risk for impaired Skin Integrity: risk factors may include excretions (ammonia formation from urea), chemical irritation from laundry detergent or diapering material, mechanical factors (e.g., long fingernails).

Newborn, postmature   PED
risk for impaired Gas Exchange: risk factors may include ventilation perfusion imbalances (meconium aspiration, pneumonitis).

Hypothermia may be related to decreased subcutaneous fat stores, poor metabolic reserves, exposure to cool environment, decreased ability to shiver, possibly evidenced by reduction in body temperature, cool skin, pallor.

risk for imbalanced Nutrition: less than body requirements: risk factors may include placental insufficiency, decreased subcutaneous fat stores, decreased glycogen stores at birth (neonatal hypoglycemia).

risk for impaired Skin Integrity: risk factors may include dry, peeling skin; long fingernails, absence of vernix caseous.

Newborn, premature   PED
impaired Gas Exchange may be related to alveolar-capillary membrane changes (inadequate surfactant levels), altered blood flow (immaturity of pulmonary arteriole musculature), altered oxygen supply (immaturity of central nervous and neuromuscular systems, tracheobronchial obstruction), altered oxygen-carrying capacity of blood (anemia), and cold stress, possibly evidenced by respiratory difficulties, inadequate oxygenation of tissues, and acidemia.

ineffective Breathing Pattern may be related to immaturity of the respiratory center, poor positioning, drug-related depression and metabolic imbalances, decreased energy, fatigue, possibly evidenced by dyspnea, tachypnea, periods of apnea, nasal flaring, use of accessory muscles, cyanosis, abnormal arterial blood gases, and tachycardia.

risk for ineffective Thermoregulation: risk factors may include immature central nervous system development (temperature regulation center), decreased ratio of body mass to surface area, decreased subcutaneous fat, limited brown fat stores, inability to shiver or sweat, poor metabolic reserves, muted response to hypothermia, and frequent medical/nursing manipulations and interventions.

risk for deficient Fluid Volume: risk factors may include extremes of age and weight, excessive fluid losses (thin skin, lack of insulating fat, increased environmental temperature, immature kidney/failure to concentrate urine).

risk for ineffective Infant Feeding Pattern: risk factors may include decreased energy, fatigue; poor positioning; drug-related depression; inability to coordinate sucking, swallowing, and breathing.

risk for disorganized Infant Behavior: risk factors may include prematurity (immaturity of central nervous system, hypoxia), lack of containment or boundaries, pain, overstimulation, separation from parents.

risk for Injury [central nervous system damage]: risk factors may include tissue hypoxia, altered clotting factors, metabolic imbalances (hypoglycemia, electrolyte shifts, elevated bilirubin).

Newborn, small for gestational age   PED
Refer to Newborn, growth deviations

Newborn, special needs   PED
(Also refer to specific condition.)

family Grieving may be related to perceived loss of the perfect child, alterations of future expectations, possibly evidenced by expression of distress at loss, sorrow, guilt, anger, choked feelings; interference with life activities, crying.

deficient parental Knowledge [Learning Need] regarding condition and infant care may be related to lack of or unfamiliarity with information resources, misinterpretation, possibly evidenced by questions, concerns, misconceptions, hesitancy or inadequate performance of activities.

risk for impaired Attachment: risk factors may include delay or interruption in bonding process (separation, physical barriers), perceived threat to infant's survival, stressors (financial, family needs), lack of appropriate response of newborn, lack of support between or from SOs.

risk for ineffective family Coping: risk factors may include situational crises, temporary preoccupation of SO trying to manage emotional conflicts and personal suffering, being unable to perceive or act effectively in regards to infant's needs, temporary family disorganization.

risk for parental Social Isolation: risk factors may include perceived situational crisis, assuming sole or full-time responsibility for infant's care, lack of or inappropriate use of resources.

Nicotine abuse   CH
risk-prone health Behavior may be related to lack of motivation to change behavior, low state of optimism, absence of social/SO support for change, failure to intend to change behavior, possibly evidenced by denial of health problem, failure to take action, failure to achieve optimal sense of control.

risk for Injury: risk factors may include smoking habits (e.g., in bed, while driving, near combustible chemicals or oxygen), children playing with cigarettes or matches.

risk for impaired Gas Exchange: risk factors may include progressive airflow obstruction, decreased oxygen supply (carbon monoxide).

risk for ineffective peripheral tissue Perfusion: risk factors may include reduction of arterial or venous blood flow.

Nicotine withdrawal   CH
readiness for enhanced self Health Management (smoking cessation) may be related to concern about health status, acceptance of deleterious effects of smoking, possibly evidenced by expressed concerns or desire to seek higher level of wellness.

risk for imbalanced Nutrition: more than body requirements: risk factors may include return of appetite, normalization of basal metabolic rate, eating in response to internal cues (substitution of food for activity of smoking).

risk for ineffective self Health Management: risk factors may include economic difficulties, lack of support from SO/friends, continued environmental exposure to secondhand smoke or smoking activity.

Nonketotic hyperglycemic-hyperosmolar coma   MS

deficient Fluid Volume may be related to excessive renal losses, inadequate oral intake, extremes of age, presence of infection, possibly evidenced by sudden weight loss, dry skin and mucous membranes, poor skin turgor, hypotension, increased pulse, fever, change in mental status (confusion to coma).

decreased Cardiac Output may be related to decreased preload (hypovolemia), altered heart rhythm (hyper-/hypokalemia), possibly evidenced by decreased hemodynamic pressures (e.g., central venous pressure), electrocardiogram changes, dysrhythmias.

imbalanced Nutrition: less than body requirements may be related to inadequate utilization of nutrients (insulin deficiency), decreased oral intake, hypermetabolic state, possibly evidenced by recent weight loss, imbalance between glucose and insulin levels.

risk for Trauma: risk factors may include weakness, cognitive limitations, altered consciousness, loss of large- or small-muscle coordination (risk for seizure activity).

Obesity   CH

imbalanced Nutrition: more than body requirements may be related to excessive intake in relation to metabolic needs, possibly evidenced by weight 20% greater than ideal for height and frame, sedentary activity level, reported or observed dysfunctional eating patterns, and excess body fat by triceps skinfold or other measurements.

sedentary Lifestyle may be related to lack of interest or motivation, resources; lack of training or knowledge of specific exercise needs, safety concerns or fear of injury, possibly evidenced by demonstration of physical deconditioning, choice of a daily routine lacking physical exercise.

Activity Intolerance may be related to imbalance between oxygen supply and demand, and sedentary lifestyle, possibly evidenced by fatigue or weakness, exertional discomfort, and abnormal heart rate and blood pressure response.

risk for Sleep Deprivation: risk factors may include sleep apnea.

PSY

disturbed Body Image/chronic low Self-Esteem may be related to view of self in contrast to societal values, family or subcultural encouragement of overeating; control, sex, and love issues, perceived failure at ability to control weight, possibly evidenced by negative feelings about body, fear of rejection or reaction of others, feeling of hopelessness or powerlessness, and lack of follow-through with treatment plan.

impaired Social Interaction may be related to verbalized or observed discomfort in social situations, self-concept disturbance, absence of or ineffective supportive SO(s), limited mobility, possibly evidenced by reluctance to participate in social gatherings, verbalized or observed discomfort in social situations, dysfunctional interactions with others, feelings of rejection.

Obesity-hypoventilation syndrome   CH

Refer to Pickwickian syndrome

Obsessive-compulsive disorder   PSY

[severe] Anxiety may be related to earlier life conflicts, possibly evidenced by repetitive actions, recurring thoughts, decreased social and role functioning.

risk for impaired Skin/Tissue Integrity: risk factors may include repetitive behaviors related to cleansing (e.g., hand hygiene, brushing teeth, showering).

risk for ineffective Role Performance: risk factors may include psychological stress, health-illness problems.

Opioid abuse CH/PSY
Refer to Depressant abuse; Heroin abuse/withdrawal

Oppositional defiant disorder PED/PSY
ineffective Coping may be related to situational or maturational crisis, mild neurological deficits, retarded ego development, dysfunctional family system, negative role models, possibly evidenced by inability to meet age-appropriate role expectations, hostility toward others, defiant response to requests or rules, inability to delay gratification.

impaired Social Interaction may be related to retarded ego development, dysfunctional family, negative role models, neurological impairment, possibly evidenced by discomfort in social situations, difficulty playing or interacting with others, aggressive behavior, refusal to comply with requests of others.

chronic low Self-Esteem may be related to retarded ego development, lack of positive or repeated negative feedback, mild neurological deficits, negative role models, possibly evidenced by lack of eye contact, lack of self-confidence, physical risk-taking, distraction of others to cover up own failures, projection of blame.

compromised/disabled family Coping may be related to anger, excessive guilt, blaming among family members regarding child's behavior, parental inconsistencies or disagreements regarding discipline and limit-setting, exhaustion of parental resources, possibly evidenced by unrealistic parental expectations, rejection or overprotection of child, exaggerated expressions of anger, disappointment, despair.

Organic brain syndrome CH
Refer to Alzheimer's disease

Osgood-Schlatter disease PED
acute Pain may be related to inflammation and swelling in region of patellar tendon, possibly evidenced by verbal reports, protective behavior, change in muscle tone.

impaired Walking may be related to inflammatory process (knee), possibly evidenced by impaired ability to walk desired distances, climb or descend stairs.

risk for ineffective self Health Management: risk factors may include age (adolescent), perceived seriousness or benefit, competitive nature, peer pressure.

Osteitis deformans CH
Refer to Paget's disease, bone

Osteoarthritis (degenerative joint disease) CH
Refer to Arthritis, rheumatoid
(Although this is a degenerative process versus the inflammatory process of rheumatoid arthritis, nursing concerns are the same.)

Osteomalacia CH
Refer to Rickets

Osteomyelitis MS/CH
acute Pain may be related to inflammation and tissue necrosis, possibly evidenced by verbal reports, guarding or distraction behaviors, self-focus, and autonomic responses (changes in vital signs).

Hyperthermia may be related to increased metabolic rate and infectious process, possibly evidenced by increased body temperature and warm, flushed skin.

ineffective bone tissue Perfusion may be related to inflammatory reaction with thrombosis of vessels, destruction of tissue, edema, and abscess formation, possibly evidenced by bone necrosis, continuation of infectious process, and delayed healing.

risk for impaired Walking: risk factors may include inflammation and tissue necrosis, pain, joint instability.

deficient Knowledge [Learning Need] regarding pathophysiology of condition, long-term therapy needs, activity restriction, and prevention of complications may be related to lack of information, misinterpretation, possibly evidenced by statements of concern, questions, and misconceptions, and inaccurate follow-through of instructions.

Osteoporosis   CH

risk for Trauma: risk factors may include loss of bone density and integrity increasing risk of fracture with minimal or no stress.

acute/chronic Pain may be related to vertebral compression on spinal nerve, muscles, or ligaments; spontaneous fractures, possibly evidenced by verbal reports, guarding or distraction behaviors, self-focus, and changes in sleep pattern.

impaired physical Mobility may be related to pain and musculoskeletal impairment, possibly evidenced by limited range of motion, reluctance to attempt movement, expressed fear of reinjury, and imposed restrictions or limitations.

Otitis media   PED

acute Pain may be related to inflammation, edema, pressure, possibly evidenced by verbal or coded report, guarded behavior, restlessness, crying.

disturbed auditory Sensory Perception may be related to decreased sensory reception, possibly evidenced by reported change in sensory acuity, auditory distortions, change in usual response to stimuli.

risk for delayed Development: risk factors may include auditory impairment, frequent ear infections.

Ovarian cancer   MS

Also refer to Cancer

disturbed Body Image may be related to surgical change in reproductive organs, surgical menopause, loss of hair and weight, possibly evidenced by negative feelings about body/sense of mutilation, preoccupation with change, feelings of helplessness, hopelessness, and change in social involvement.

Sexual Dysfunction may be related to change in sexual organs, postoperative menopause, vulnerability, possibly evidenced by verbalizations of problem, inability in achieving desired satisfaction, alterations in relationship with SO.

Paget's disease, bone   CH

acute Pain may be related to compression/entrapment of nerves, joint degeneration, possibly evidenced by reports of headache, back or joint pain.

Fatigue may be related to disease state and hypermetabolic condition, possibly evidenced by overwhelming lack of energy, inability to maintain usual routines, tired.

disturbed Body Image may be related to physical deformities (enlarged skull, bowing of long bones), possibly evidenced by verbalization of feelings reflecting altered view of body, negative feelings about body, fear of rejection or reaction of others, change in social involvement.

disturbed auditory Sensory Perception may be related to altered sensory reception or transmission (nerve compression), possibly evidenced by decreased auditory acuity.

risk for impaired Walking: risk factors may include bowing of long bones, hobbling gait, joint stiffness and pain, paresis or paralysis.

risk for Injury/Falls: risk factors may include bone deformity or fragility, joint stiffness and pain, altered gait.

risk for decreased Cardiac Output: risk factors may include excessive circulatory demands (metabolically active and highly vascular nature of lesions).

Palliative care   CH
Refer to Hospice care

Palsy, cerebral   PED/CH
impaired physical Mobility may be related to muscular weakness or hypertonicity, increased deep tendon reflexes, tendency to contractures, and underdevelopment of affected limbs, possibly evidenced by decreased muscle strength, control, mass, limited range of motion, and impaired coordination.

compromised family Coping may be related to permanent nature of condition, situational crisis, emotional conflicts, temporary family disorganization, and incomplete information or understanding of client's needs, possibly evidenced by verbalized anxiety or guilt regarding client's disability, inadequate understanding and knowledge base, and displaying protective behaviors disproportionate (too little or too much) to client's abilities or need for autonomy.

delayed Growth and Development may be related to effects of physical disability, possibly evidenced by altered physical growth, delay or difficulty in performing skills (motor, social, expressive), and altered ability to perform self-care or self-control activities appropriate to age.

Pancreas transplantation   MS/CH
Refer to Transplantation, recipient

Pancreatic cancer   MS
Also refer to Cancer

acute Pain/impaired Comfort may be related to pressure on surrounding organs and nerves, possibly evidenced by verbal reports, guarding or distraction behaviors, focus on self, and autonomic responses (changes in vital signs).

imbalanced Nutrition: less than body requirements may be related to inability to ingest or digest food, absorb nutrients, increased metabolic needs, possibly evidenced by inadequate food intake, anorexia, abdominal pain after eating, weight loss, cachexia.

risk for Infection: risk factors may include stasis of body fluids (biliary obstruction), malnutrition.

risk for impaired Tissue Integrity: risk factors may include poor skin turgor, skeletal prominence, presence of edema, ascites, bile salt accumulation in the tissues.

Pancreatitis   MS
acute Pain may be related to obstruction of pancreatic and biliary ducts, chemical contamination of peritoneal surfaces by pancreatic exudate, autodigestion of pancreas, extension of inflammation to the retroperitoneal nerve plexus, possibly evidenced by verbal reports, guarding or distraction behaviors, self-focusing, grimacing, changes in vital signs, and alteration in muscle tone.

risk for deficient Fluid Volume/Bleeding: risk factors may include excessive gastric losses (vomiting, nasogastric suctioning), increase in size of vascular bed (vasodilation, effects of kinins), third-space fluid transudation, ascites formation, alteration of clotting process, hemorrhage.

risk for unstable blood Glucose Level: risk factors may include decreased insulin production, increased glucagon release, physical health status, stress.

---

imbalanced Nutrition: less than body requirements may be related to vomiting, decreased oral intake, prescribed dietary restrictions, altered ability to digest nutrients—loss of digestive enzymes, possibly evidenced by reported inadequate food intake, aversion to eating, reported altered taste sensation, weight loss, and reduced muscle mass.

risk for Infection: risk factors may include inadequate primary defenses (stasis of body fluids, altered peristalsis, change in pH secretions), immunosuppression, nutritional deficiencies, tissue destruction, and chronic disease.

Panic disorder   PSY

Fear may be related to unfounded morbid dread of a seemingly harmless object or situation, possibly evidenced by physiological symptoms, mental or cognitive behaviors indicative of panic, withdrawal from or total avoidance of situations that place client in contact with feared object.

[severe to panic] Anxiety may be related to unidentified stressors, contact with feared object or situation, limitations placed on ritualistic behavior, possibly evidenced by attacks of immobilizing apprehension, physical, mental, or cognitive behaviors indicative of panic; expressed feelings of terror or inability to cope.

Paralysis, infantile   PED
Refer to Poliomyelitis

Paranoid personality disorder   PSY

risk for other-/self-directed Violence: risk factors may include perceived threats of danger, paranoid delusions, and increased feelings of anxiety.

[severe] Anxiety may be related to inability to trust (has not mastered tasks of trust vs. mistrust), possibly evidenced by rigid delusional system (serves to provide relief from stress that justifies the delusion), frightened of other people and own hostility.

Powerlessness may be related to feelings of inadequacy, lifestyle of helplessness, maladaptive interpersonal interactions (e.g., misuse of power, force; abusive relationships), sense of severely impaired self-concept, and belief that individual has no control over situation(s), possibly evidenced by paranoid delusions, use of aggressive behavior to compensate, and expressions of recognition of damage paranoia has caused self and others.

disturbed Thought Processes may be related to psychological conflicts, increased anxiety, and fear, possibly evidenced by difficulties in the process and character of thought, interference with the ability to think clearly and logically, delusions, fragmentation, and autistic thinking.

compromised family Coping may be related to temporary or sustained family disorganization/role changes, prolonged progression of condition that exhausts the supportive capacity of SO(s), possibly evidenced by family system not meeting physical, emotional, or spiritual needs of its members; inability to express or to accept wide range of feelings; inappropriate boundary maintenance; SO(s) describe(s) preoccupation with personal reactions.

Paranoid schizophrenia   PSY
Refer to Schizophrenia

Paraphilias   PSY

ineffective Sexuality Pattern may be related to conflict with sexual orientation or variant preferences, possibly evidenced by alterations in achieving sexual satisfaction, difficulty achieving desired satisfaction in socially acceptable ways.

chronic low Self-Esteem may be related to psychosocial factors (e.g., achievement of sexual satisfaction in deviant ways), substance use, possibly evidenced by expressions of shame or guilt, self-destructive behaviors, feelings of powerlessness, helplessness.

interrupted Family Processes may be related to situational crisis (e.g., revelation of sexual deviance or dysfunction), possibly evidenced by expressions of confusion about or difficulty dealing with situation, inappropriate boundary maintenance, family system does not meet emotional or security needs, failure to deal with traumatic experience constructively.

Paraplegia   MS/CH

Also refer to Quadriplegia

impaired Transfer Ability may be related to loss of muscle function and control, injury to upper extremity joints (overuse).

disturbed kinesthetic/tactile Sensory Perception may be related to neurological deficit with loss of sensory reception and transmission, psychological stress, possibly evidenced by reported or measured change in sensory acuity, change in usual response to stimuli, anxiety, disorientation, bizarre thinking, exaggerated emotional responses.

reflex urinary Incontinence/impaired Urinary Elimination may be related to disruption of bladder innervation, bladder atony, fecal impaction, possibly evidenced by lack of awareness of bladder distention, retention, incontinence or overflow, urinary tract infections—kidney stone formation, renal dysfunction.

situational low Self-Esteem may be related to situational crisis, loss of body functions, change in physical abilities, perceived loss of self or identity, possibly evidenced by negative feelings about body or self, feelings of helplessness or powerlessness, delay in taking responsibility for self-care or participation in therapy, and change in social involvement.

Sexual Dysfunction may be related to loss of sensation, altered function, and vulnerability, possibly evidenced by seeking of confirmation of desirability, verbalization of concern, alteration in relationship with SO, and change in interest in self/others.

Parathyroidectomy   MS

acute Pain may be related to presence of surgical incision and effects of calcium imbalance (bone pain, tetany), possibly evidenced by verbal reports, guarding or distraction behaviors, self-focus, and changes in vital signs.

risk for excess Fluid Volume: risk factors may include preoperative renal involvement, stress-induced release of antidiuretic hormone, and changing calcium or other electrolyte levels.

risk for ineffective Airway Clearance: risk factors may include edema formation and laryngeal nerve damage.

deficient Knowledge [Learning Need] regarding postoperative care, complications, and long-term needs may be related to lack of information or recall, misinterpretation, possibly evidenced by statements of concern, questions, and misconceptions.

Parent-child relational problem   PED/PSY

impaired Parenting may be related to lack of or ineffective role model, lack of support between or from SO, interruption in bonding process, unrealistic expectations for self/child/partner, presence of stressors, lack of appropriate response of child to parent, possibly evidenced by frequent verbalization of disappointment in child, inability to care for or discipline child, lack of parental attachment behaviors, child abuse or abandonment.

chronic low Self-Esteem/Ineffective Role Performance may be related to view self as "poor" or ineffective parent, belief that seeking help is an admission of defeat or failure, psychiatric or physical illness of the child, possibly evidenced by change in usual patterns or responsibility, expressions of lack of information, lack of follow-through of therapy, nonparticipation in therapy.

interrupted Family Process may be related to situational crisis of child/adolescent, maturational crisis (e.g., adolescence, midlife), possibly evidenced by expressions of confusion and difficulty coping with situation; family system not meeting physical, emotional, or security needs of members; difficulty accepting help; parents not respecting each other's parenting practices.

compromised/disabled family Coping may be related to individual preoccupation with own emotional conflicts and personal suffering or anxiety about the crisis, temporary family disorganization, exhausted supportive capacity of members, highly ambivalent family relationships, possibly evidenced by detrimental decisions or actions, neglected relationships, intolerance, agitation, depression, hostility, aggression.

readiness for enhanced family Coping may be related to surfacing of self-actualization goals, possibly evidenced by expressing interest in making contact with another person experiencing a similar situation, moving in direction of health-promoting or enriching lifestyle, auditing or negotiating therapy program.

Parenteral feeding   MS/CH

imbalanced Nutrition: less than body requirements may be related to conditions that interfere with nutrient intake or increase nutrient need or metabolic demand—cancer and associated treatments, anorexia, surgical procedures, dysphagia, or decreased level of consciousness, possibly evidenced by body weight 10% or more under ideal, decreased subcutaneous fat or muscle mass, poor muscle tone.

risk for Infection: risk factors may include invasive procedure and surgical placement of feeding tube, malnutrition, chronic disease.

risk for Injury [multifactor]: risk factors may include catheter-related complications (air emboli, septic thrombophlebitis).

risk for imbalanced Fluid Volume: risk factors may include active loss or failure of regulatory mechanisms (specific to underlying disease process or trauma), complications of therapy—high glucose solutions or hyperglycemia (hyperosmolar nonketotic coma and severe dehydration), inability to obtain or ingest fluids.

Fatigue may be related to decreased metabolic energy production, increased energy requirements (hypermetabolic state, healing process), altered body chemistry (medications, chemotherapy), possibly evidenced by overwhelming lack of energy, inability to maintain usual routines or accomplish routine tasks, lethargy, impaired ability to concentrate.

Parkinson's disease   CH

impaired Walking may be related to neuromuscular impairment (muscle weakness, tremors, bradykinesia) and musculoskeletal impairment (joint rigidity), possibly evidenced by inability to move about the environment as desired, increased occurrence of falls.

impaired Swallowing may be related to neuromuscular impairment, muscle weakness, possibly evidenced by reported or observed difficulty in swallowing, drooling, evidence of aspiration (choking, coughing).

impaired verbal Communication may be related to muscle weakness and incoordination, possibly evidenced by impaired articulation, difficulty with phonation, and changes in rhythm and intonation.

risk for Stress Overload: risk factors may include inadequate resources, chronic illness, physical demands.

Caregiver Role Strain may be related to illness, severity of care receiver, psychological/cognitive problems in care receiver, caregiver is spouse, duration of caregiving required, lack of respite or recreation for caregiver, possibly evidenced by feeling stressed, depressed, worried; lack of resources or support, family conflict.

Passive-aggressive personality disorder   PSY

[moderate to severe] Anxiety may be related to unconscious conflict, unmet needs, threat to self-concept, difficulty in asserting self directly, feelings of resentment toward authority figures,

possibly evidenced by difficulty resolving feelings or trusting others, passive resistance to demands made by others, extraneous movements, irritability, argumentativeness.

ineffective Coping may be related to inadequate level of confidence in ability to cope or perception of control, uncertainty, high degree of threat, inadequate social support created by characteristics of relationships, disturbance in pattern of tension release, possibly evidenced by verbalizations or inability to cope or ask for help, lack of goal-directed behavior or resolution of problem, lack of assertive behavior, use of forms of coping that impede adaptive behavior, decreased use of social supports, risk-taking.

chronic low Self-Esteem may be related to retarded ego development, unmet dependency needs, early rejection by SO, lack of positive feedback, possibly evidenced by lack of self-confidence, feelings of inadequacy, fear of asserting self, dependency on others, directing frustrations toward others by using covert aggressive tactics, not accepting responsibility for what happens as a result of maladaptive behaviors, failing to work through negative feelings.

Powerlessness may be related to interpersonal interaction, lifestyle of helplessness, dependency feelings, difficulty connecting own passive-resistent behaviors with hostility or resentment, possibly evidenced by experiencing conscious hostility toward authority figures, releasing anger or hostility through others, getting back at others through aggravation.

PCP (phencyclidine) intoxication   MS/PSY
Also refer to Hallucinogen abuse

risk for self-/other-directed Violence: risk factors may include drug abuse, psychotic symptomology, impulsivity.

risk for Trauma/Suffocation/Poisoning: risk factors may include clouded sensorium, increased muscle strength, myoclonic jerks or convulsions, ataxia, decreased pain perception, coma.

risk for ineffective cerebral tissue Perfusion: risk factors may include alterations in blood flow (hypertensive crisis).

Pediculosis capitis   PED/CH
impaired Skin Integrity related to presence of nits, intense itching and scratching; possibly evidenced by redness, excoriation, disruption of skin surface.

risk for Infection [spread]: risk factors may include insufficient knowledge to avoid exposure or transmission of parasite.

impaired Home Maintenance may be related to lack of knowledge of vermin control or transmission, lack of care assistance or resources, possibly evidenced by poor hygiene practices, accumulation of dirt, unwashed clothing or linen or personal care item; presence of vermin.

Pediculosis pubis   CH
Refer to Pediculosis capitis

Pelvic inflammatory disease   OB/GYN/CH
risk for Infection [spread]: risk factors may include presence of infectious process in highly vascular pelvic structures, delay in seeking treatment.

acute Pain may be related to inflammation, edema, and congestion of reproductive and pelvic tissues, possibly evidenced by verbal reports, guarding or distraction behaviors, self-focus, and changes in vital signs.

Hyperthermia may be related to inflammatory process and hypermetabolic state, possibly evidenced by increased body temperature; warm, flushed skin; and tachycardia.

risk for situational low Self-Esteem: risk factors may include perceived stigma of physical condition (infection of reproductive system).

deficient Knowledge [Learning Need] regarding cause/complications of condition, therapy needs, and transmission of disease to others may be related to lack of information, misinterpretation, possibly evidenced by statements of concern, questions, misconceptions, and development of preventable complications.

Periarteritis nodosa   MS/CH
Refer to Polyarteritis [nodosa]

Pericarditis   MS
acute Pain may be related to tissue inflammation and presence of effusion, possibly evidenced by verbal reports of pain affected by movement or position, guarding or distraction behaviors, self-focus, and changes in vital signs.

Activity Intolerance may be related to imbalance between oxygen supply and demand (restriction of cardiac filling and ventricular contraction, reduced cardiac output), possibly evidenced by reports of weakness, fatigue, exertional dyspnea, abnormal heart rate or blood pressure response, and signs of heart failure.

risk for decreased Cardiac Output: risk factors may include accumulation of fluid (effusion), restricted cardiac filling and contractility.

Anxiety [specify level] may be related to change in health status and perceived threat of death, possibly evidenced by increased tension, apprehension, restlessness, and expressed concerns.

Perinatal loss/death of child   OB/CH
Grieving may be related to death of fetus/infant (wanted or unwanted), inability to meet personal expectations, possibly evidenced by verbal expressions of distress, anger, loss, crying, alteration in eating habits or sleep pattern.

situational low Self-Esteem may be related to perceived "failure" at a life event, possibly evidenced by negative self-appraisal in response to life event in a person with a previous positive self-evaluation, verbalization of negative feelings about the self (helplessness, uselessness), difficulty making decisions.

risk for ineffective Role Performance: risk factors may include stress, family conflict, inadequate support system.

risk for interrupted Family Processes: risk factors may include situational crisis, developmental transition [loss of child], family roles shift.

risk for Spiritual Distress: risk factors may include loss of loved one, blame for loss directed at self/God, alienation from SO/support systems, challenged belief and value system (birth is supposed to be the beginning of life, not of death) and intense suffering.

Peripheral arterial occlusive disease   CH
Refer to Arterial occlusive disease

Peripheral vascular disease (atherosclerosis)   CH
ineffective peripheral tissue Perfusion may be related to reduction or interruption of arterial or venous blood flow, possibly evidenced by changes in skin temperature and color, lack of hair growth, blood pressure and pulse changes in extremity, presence of bruits, and reports of claudication.

Activity Intolerance may be related to imbalance between oxygen supply and demand, possibly evidenced by reports of muscle fatigue, weakness and exertional discomfort (claudication).

risk for impaired Skin/Tissue Integrity: risk factors may include altered circulation with decreased sensation and impaired healing.

Peritonitis   MS

risk for Infection [spread/septicemia]: risk factors may include inadequate primary defenses (broken skin, traumatized tissue, altered peristalsis), inadequate secondary defenses (immunosuppression), and invasive procedures.

deficient Fluid Volume [mixed] may be related to fluid shifts from extracellular, intravascular, and interstitial compartments into intestines or peritoneal space, excessive gastric losses (vomiting, diarrhea, nasogastric suction), fever, hypermetabolic state, and restricted intake, possibly evidenced by dry mucous membranes, poor skin turgor, delayed capillary refill, weak peripheral pulses, diminished urinary output, dark, concentrated urine; hypotension, and tachycardia.

acute Pain may be related to chemical irritation of parietal peritoneum, trauma to tissues, abdominal distention— accumulation of fluid in abdominal or peritoneal cavity, possibly evidenced by verbal reports, muscle guarding or rebound tenderness, distraction behaviors, facial mask of pain, self-focus, and changes in vital signs.

risk for imbalanced Nutrition: less than body requirements: risk factors may include nausea, vomiting, intestinal dysfunction, metabolic abnormalities, increased metabolic needs.

Persian Gulf syndrome   CH/MS
Refer to Gulf War syndrome

Personality disorders   PSY
Refer to Antisocial; Borderline; Obsessive-compulsive; Passive-aggressive; or Paranoid personality disorders

Pertussis   PED

ineffective Airway Clearance may be related to retained secretions, excessive thick tenacious mucus, infection, possibly evidenced by dyspnea, adventitious breath sounds, hacking/paroxysmal cough.

deficient Fluid Volume may be related to decreased intake, anorexia, vomiting, increased insensible losses (fever, diaphoresis), possibly evidenced by decreased urine output and increased specific gravity, decreased blood pressure, increased pulse rate, decreased skin and tongue turgor, dry skin and mucous membranes.

risk for Infection [transmission/secondary]: risk factors may include contagious nature of disease, stasis of body fluids, malnutrition, insufficient knowledge to avoid exposure to pathogens.

risk for imbalanced Nutrition: less than body requirements: risk factors may include inability to ingest food or absorb nutrients (anorexia, vomiting), increased metabolic demands.

risk for impaired Gas Exchange: risk factors may include compromised airways (tenacious mucus, inflammation), paroxysms of coughing, ventilation perfusion imbalance (atelectasis).

Pervasive developmental disorders   PED/PSY
Refer to Autistic disorder; Rett's syndrome; Asperger's disorder

Pheochromocytoma   MS
Anxiety [specify level] may be related to excessive physiological (hormonal) stimulation of the sympathetic nervous system, situational crises, threat to or change in health status, possibly evidenced by apprehension, shakiness, restlessness, focus on self, fearfulness, diaphoresis, and sense of impending doom.

deficient Fluid Volume [mixed] may be related to excessive gastric losses (vomiting, diarrhea), hypermetabolic state, diaphoresis, and hyperosmolar diuresis, possibly evidenced by hemoconcentration, dry mucous membranes, poor skin turgor, thirst, and weight loss.

---

decreased Cardiac Output/ineffective tissue Perfusion (specify) may be related to altered preload—decreased blood volume, altered systemic vascular resistance, and increased sympathetic activity (excessive secretion of catecholamines), possibly evidenced by cool, clammy skin, change in blood pressure (hypertension, postural hypotension), visual disturbances, severe headache, and angina.

deficient Knowledge [Learning Need] regarding pathophysiology of condition, outcome, and preoperative and postoperative care needs may be related to lack of information or recall, possibly evidenced by statements of concern, questions, and misconceptions.

Phlebitis   CH
Refer to Thrombophlebitis

Phobia   PSY
Also refer to Anxiety disorder, generalized

Fear may be related to learned irrational response to natural or innate origins (phobic stimulus), unfounded morbid dread of a seemingly harmless object or situation, possibly evidenced by sympathetic stimulation and reactions ranging from apprehension to panic, withdrawal from or total avoidance of situations that place individual in contact with feared object.

impaired Social Interaction may be related to intense fear of encountering feared object, activity or situation; and anticipated loss of control, possibly evidenced by reported change of style or pattern of interaction, discomfort in social situations, and avoidance of phobic stimulus.

Physical abuse   CH/PSY
Refer to Abuse, physical; Battered child syndrome

Pickwickian syndrome   CH
ineffective Breathing Pattern may be related to obesity, hypoventilation, possibly evidenced by decreased pulmonary function, hypercapnia, hypoxia, reduced effect of carbon dioxide in stimulating respirations.

PID   GYN/OB/CH
Refer to Pelvic inflammatory disease

Pinkeye   CH
Refer to Conjunctivitis, bacterial

Placenta previa   OB
risk for Bleeding/Shock: risk factors may include pregnancy-related complication; hypovolemia, hypotension.

impaired fetal Gas Exchange may be related to altered blood flow, altered oxygen-carrying capacity of blood (maternal anemia), and decreased surface area of gas exchange at site of placental attachment, possibly evidenced by changes in fetal heart rate and activity, and release of meconium.

Fear may be related to threat of death (perceived or actual) to self or fetus, possibly evidenced by verbalization of specific concerns, increased tension, sympathetic stimulation.

risk for deficient Diversional Activity: risk factors may include imposed activity restrictions, bedrest.

Plague, bubonic   MS
Hyperthermia may be related to illness, dehydration, possibly evidenced by increased body temperature, tachycardia, chills, confusion.

---

acute Pain may be related to inflammatory process, enlarged lymph nodes, possibly evidenced by verbal or coded reports, expressive behavior, autonomic responses.

risk for deficient Fluid Volume: risk factors may include fever, decreased oral intake.

risk for impaired Skin Integrity: risk factors may include infectious process.

Plague, pneumonic   MS

risk for Infection [spread]: risk factors may include contagious nature of disease, close contact with others

Hyperthermia may be related to illness, dehydration, possibly evidenced by increased body temperature, tachycardia, chills, severe headache, confusion.

impaired Gas Exchange may be related to alveolar-capillary membrane changes, possibly evidenced by tachypnea, dyspnea, stridor, hemoptysis, cyanosis.

deficient Fluid Volume may be related to fever, hypermetabolic state, decreased intake, bleeding diathesis (disseminated intravascular coagulation), possibly evidenced by weakness, decreased venous filling, decreased blood pressure, decreased skin turgor, dry mucous membranes, change in mental state.

Plantar fasciitis   CH

acute/chronic Pain may be related to inflammation, possibly evidenced by report of stabbing, burning pain, guarding or protective behavior, change in posture and gait, altered ability to continue previous activities.

impaired Walking may be related musculoskeletal impairment, impaired balance, pain, possibly evidenced by impaired ability to walk required distances or climb stairs.

Pleural effusion   CH/MS

Also refer to Hemothorax

acute Pain may be related to inflammation/irritation of the parietal pleura, possibly evidenced by verbal reports, guarding or distraction behaviors, self-focus, and changes in vital signs.

ineffective Breathing Pattern may be related to pain on inspiration, possibly evidenced by decreased respiratory depth, tachypnea, and dyspnea.

risk for impaired Gas Exchange: risk factors may include ventilation perfusion imbalance.

Pleurisy   CH

acute Pain may be related to inflammation and irritation of the parietal pleura, possibly evidenced by verbal reports, guarding or distraction behaviors, self-focus, and changes in vital signs.

ineffective Breathing Pattern may be related to pain on inspiration, possibly evidenced by decreased respiratory depth, tachypnea, and dyspnea.

risk for Infection [pneumonia]: risk factors may include stasis of pulmonary secretions, decreased lung expansion, and ineffective cough.

PMDD   GYN/PSY

Refer to Premenstrual dysphoric disorder

PMS   GYN/PSY

Refer to Premenstrual dysphoric disorder

Pneumoconiosis (black lung)   CH

Refer to Pulmonary fibrosis

Pneumonia   CH/MS

Refer to Bronchitis; Bronchopneumonia

Pneumonia, ventilator associated   **CH**
Refer to Bronchopneumonia

Pneumothorax   **MS**
Also refer to Hemothorax

ineffective Breathing Pattern may be related to decreased lung expansion (air accumulation), musculoskeletal impairment, pain, inflammatory process, possibly evidenced by dyspnea, tachypnea, altered chest excursion, respiratory depth changes, use of accessory muscles, nasal flaring, cough, cyanosis, and abnormal arterial blood gases.

risk for decreased Cardiac Output: risk factors may include compression or displacement of cardiac structures.

acute Pain may be related to irritation of nerve endings within pleural space by foreign object (chest tube), possibly evidenced by verbal reports, guarding or distraction behaviors, self-focus, and changes in vital signs.

Poliomyelitis   **CH**
Also refer to Postpolio syndrome

ineffective Breathing Pattern may be related to neuromuscular dysfunction and intercostal muscle impairment, hypoventilation syndrome, possibly evidenced by dyspnea, decreased depth of breathing, altered chest excursion, respiratory failure.

impaired physical Mobility related to neuromuscular dysfunction and musculoskeletal impairment, decreased muscle strength, control or mass; contracture, decreased endurance, pain, prescribed movement restriction or bracing, possibly evidenced by limited ability to move, uncoordinated or jerky movements, gait changes, exaggerated lateral postural sway, postural instability.

Self-Care Deficit [specify] may be related to neuromuscular impairment, weakness, pain, fatigue, possibly evidenced by reported or observed inability to perform specified activities.

risk for Infection [transmission]: risk factors may include inadequate acquired immunity, malnutrition, or insufficient knowledge to avoid exposure to or transmission of pathogen.

Polyarteritis nodosa   **MS/CH**
ineffective tissue Perfusion (specify) may be related to reduction or interruption of blood flow, possibly evidenced by organ tissue infarctions, changes in organ function, and development of organic psychosis.

Hyperthermia may be related to widespread inflammatory process, possibly evidenced by increased body temperature and warm, flushed skin.

acute Pain may be related to inflammation, tissue ischemia, and necrosis of affected area, possibly evidenced by verbal reports, guarding or distraction behaviors, self-focus, and changes in vital signs.

Grieving may be related to perceived loss of self, possibly evidenced by expressions of sorrow and anger, altered sleep or eating patterns, changes in activity level, and libido.

Polycythemia vera   **CH**
Activity Intolerance may be related to imbalance between oxygen supply and demand, possibly evidenced by reports of fatigue, weakness.

ineffective tissue Perfusion (specify) may be related to reduction or interruption of arterial or venous blood flow (insufficiency, thrombosis, or hemorrhage), possibly evidenced by pain in affected area, impaired mental ability, visual disturbances, and color changes of skin and mucous membranes.

Polyradiculitis, acute inflammatory   **MS**
Refer to Guillain-Barré syndrome

Postconcussion syndrome   CH

acute/chronic Pain may be related to neuronal damage, possibly evidenced by reports of headache.

disturbed Thought Processes may be related to head injury, possibly evidenced by memory deficit, cognitive dissonance, distractibility.

Anxiety [specify level] may be related to situational crisis, change in health status, ongoing nature of disability, stress, unmet needs, possibly evidenced by expressed concerns, apprehension, uncertainty, feelings of inadequacy, focus on self, difficulty concentrating.

Postmaturity syndrome   PED
Refer to Newborn, postmature

Postmyocardial syndrome   CH
Refer to Dressler's syndrome

Postoperative recovery period   MS

ineffective Breathing Pattern may be related to neuromuscular and perceptual or cognitive impairment, decreased lung expansion and energy, and tracheobronchial obstruction, possibly evidenced by changes in respiratory rate and depth, reduced vital capacity, apnea, cyanosis, and noisy respirations.

risk for imbalanced Body Temperature: risk factors may include exposure to cool environment, effect of medications and anesthetic agents, extremes of age or weight, and dehydration.

disturbed Sensory Perception (specify)/disturbed Thought Processes may be related to chemical alteration (use of pharmaceutical agents, hypoxia), therapeutically restricted environment, excessive sensory stimuli and physiological stress, possibly evidenced by changes in usual response to stimuli; motor incoordination; impaired ability to concentrate, reason, and make decisions; and disorientation to person, place, and time.

risk for deficit Fluid Volume: risk factors may include restriction of oral intake, loss of fluid through abnormal routes (indwelling tubes, drains) and normal routes (vomiting, loss of vascular integrity, changes in clotting ability), extremes of age and weight.

acute Pain may be related to disruption of skin, tissue, and muscle integrity; musculoskeletal or bone trauma; and presence of tubes and drains, possibly evidenced by verbal reports, alteration in muscle tone, facial mask of pain, distraction or guarding behaviors, narrowed focus, and autonomic responses.

impaired Skin/Tissue Integrity may be related to mechanical interruption of skin or tissues, altered circulation, effects of medication, accumulation of drainage, and altered metabolic state, possibly evidenced by disruption of skin and tissues.

risk for Infection: risk factors may include broken skin, traumatized tissues, stasis of body fluids, presence of pathogens or contaminants, environmental exposure, and invasive procedures.

Postpartum blues   OB/PSY
Refer to Depression, postpartum

Postpartum period, 4 to 48 hours   OB/CH

acute Pain/impaired Comfort may be related to tissue trauma, edema, muscle contractions, bladder fullness, and physical or psychological exhaustion, possibly evidenced by reports of cramping (afterpains), self-focusing, alteration in muscle tone, distraction behaviors, and changes in vital signs.

Breastfeeding (specify) may be related to level of knowledge, previous experiences, infant gestational age, level of support, physical structure or characteristics of the maternal breasts,

---

possibly evidenced by maternal verbalization regarding level of satisfaction, observations of breastfeeding process, infant response and weight gain.

risk for impaired Attachment: risk factors may include lack of support between or from SO(s), ineffective or no role model, anxiety associated with the parental role, unrealistic expectations, unmet social or emotional maturation needs of client/partner, presence of stressors (e.g., financial, housing, employment).

risk for deficient Fluid Volume/Bleeding: risk factors may include excessive blood loss during delivery, reduced intake or inadequate replacement, nausea, vomiting, increased urine output, and insensible losses.

impaired Urinary Elimination may be related to hormonal effects (fluid shifts, continued elevation in renal plasma flow), mechanical trauma, tissue edema, and effects of medication or anesthesia, possibly evidenced by frequency, dysuria, urgency, incontinence, or retention.

Constipation may be related to decreased muscle tone associated with diastasis recti, prenatal effects of progesterone, dehydration, excess analgesia or anesthesia, pain (hemorrhoids, episiotomy, or perineal tenderness), prelabor diarrhea and lack of intake, possibly evidenced by frequency less than usual pattern, hard-formed stool, straining at stool, decreased bowel sounds, and abdominal distention.

Insomnia may be related to pain, discomfort, intense exhilaration or excitement, anxiety, exhausting process of labor and delivery, and needs or demands of family members, possibly evidenced by verbal reports of difficulty in falling asleep or staying asleep, not feeling well-rested, interrupted sleep, lack of energy.

Postpartum period, 4 to 6 weeks   OB/CH

readiness for enhanced family Coping may be related to sufficiently meeting individual needs and adaptive tasks, enabling goals of self-actualization to surface, possibly evidenced by family member(s) moving in direction of health-promoting and enriching lifestyle.

disturbed Body Image may be related to unrealistic expectations of postpartum recovery, permanency of some changes, possibly evidenced by verbalization of negative feelings about body, feelings of helplessness, preoccupation with change, focus on past appearance, fear of rejection or reaction of others.

risk for Sexual Dysfunction: risk factors may include health-related transition, changes in body function (including lactation), lack of privacy, fear of pregnancy.

readiness for enhanced Parenting may be related to sufficiently mastering skills or adapting to new responsibilities, possibly evidenced by expressed willingness to enhance parenting, physical and emotional needs of infant/children are met, bonding evident.

Postpartum period, postdischarge to 4 weeks   OB/CH

risk for Fatigue: risk factors may include physical and emotional demands of infant and other family members, psychological stressors, continued discomfort.

Breastfeeding (specify) may be related to level of knowledge and support, previous experiences, infant gestational age, physical structure or characteristics of maternal breast, demands of home life and employment, possibly evidenced by maternal verbalizations regarding level of satisfaction, observations of feeding process, infant response and weight gain.

risk for imbalanced Nutrition: less than body requirements: risk factors may include intake insufficient to meet metabolic demands or correct existing deficiencies (e.g., lactation, anemia, excessive blood loss, infection, excessive tissue trauma, desire to regain prenatal weight).

risk for Infection: risk factors may include tissue trauma, broken skin, decreased Hb, invasive procedures, increased environmental exposure, malnutrition.

risk for ineffective Coping/compromised family Coping: risk factors may include situational or developmental changes, temporary family disorganization or role changes, little support provided by partner/family members.

risk for impaired Parenting: risk factors may include situational crisis—addition and demands of new family member, changes in responsibilities of family members; sleep disruption, lack of support from SO/family members, young parental age, life stressors—financial, employment, home environment, lack of resources.

Postpolio syndrome   CH
Anxiety [specify]/Fear may be related to change in health status, progressive and debilitating disease, change in role function and economic status, possibly evidenced by expressed concerns, uncertainty, awareness of physiological symptoms, worrisome, sleep disturbance, forgetfulness.

Fatigue may be related to disease state, stress, anxiety, sleep deprivation, depression, possibly evidenced by overwhelming lack of energy, inability to maintain usual routines or level of physical activity, difficulty concentrating.

chronic Pain may be related to chronic physical disability, joint degeneration, possibly evidenced by reports of deep aching pain, altered ability to continue previous activities, change in sleep patterns, reduced interaction with others.

impaired Walking/physical Mobility may be related to neuromuscular impairment, decreased muscle strength and atrophy, decreased endurance, pain, inability to stand erect (flat back syndrome), possibly evidenced by gait disturbances, joint or postural instability, decreased ability to perform gross motor skills.

Sleep Deprivation may be related to sleep apnea (central and obstructive), chronic pain, possibly evidenced by daytime drowsiness, decreased ability to function, inability to concentrate.

impaired Swallowing may be related to neuromuscular impairment, pharyngeal muscle weakness, possibly evidenced by coughing, choking, recurrent pulmonary infections.

ineffective Airway Clearance may be related to neuromuscular dysfunction (muscle weakness and atrophy), retained secretions, possibly evidenced by diminished or adventitious breath sounds (chronic microatelectasis), poor cough (decreased pulmonary compliance, increased chest wall tightness).

Posttraumatic stress disorder   PSY
Post-Trauma Syndrome related to having experienced a traumatic life event, possibly evidenced by reexperiencing the event, somatic reactions, psychological or emotional numbness, altered lifestyle, impaired sleep, self-destructive behaviors, difficulty with interpersonal relationships, development of phobia, poor impulse control or irritability, and explosiveness.

risk for other-directed Violence: risk factors may include startled reaction, an intrusive memory causing a sudden acting out of a feeling as if the event were occurring; use of alcohol or other drugs to ward off painful effects and produce psychic numbing, breaking through the rage that has been walled off, response to intense anxiety or panic state, and loss of control.

ineffective Coping may be related to personal vulnerability, inadequate support systems, unrealistic perceptions, unmet expectations, overwhelming threat to self, and multiple stressors repeated over a period of time, possibly evidenced by verbalization of inability to cope or difficulty asking for help, muscular tension, headaches, chronic worry, and emotional tension.

complicated Grieving may be related to actual or perceived object loss (loss of self as seen before the traumatic incident occurred as well as other losses incurred in or after the incident), loss of physiopsychosocial well-being, thwarted grieving response to a loss, and lack of resolution of previous grieving responses, possibly evidenced by verbal expression of distress at loss, anger, sadness, labile affect; alterations in eating habits, sleep or dream patterns, libido; reliving of past experiences, expression of guilt, and alterations in concentration.

interrupted Family Processes may be related to situational crisis, failure to master developmental transitions, possibly evidenced by expressions of confusion about what to do and by family having difficulty coping, family system not meeting physical, emotional, or spiritual needs of its members; not adapting to change or dealing with traumatic experience constructively, and ineffective family decision-making process.

Preeclampsia   OB
Refer to Pregnancy-induced hypertension; Abruptio placentae

Pregnancy, 1st trimester   OB/CH
risk for imbalanced Nutrition: less than body requirements: risk factors may include changes in appetite, insufficient intake (nausea, vomiting, inadequate financial resources and nutritional knowledge), meeting increased metabolic demands (increased thyroid activity associated with the growth of fetal and maternal tissues).

impaired Comfort may be related to hormonal influences, physical changes, possibly evidenced by verbal reports (nausea, breast changes, leg cramps, hemorrhoids, nasal stuffiness), alteration in muscle tone, inability to relax.

risk for disturbed Maternal/Fetal Dyad: risk factors may include environmental or hereditary factors and problems of maternal well-being that directly affect the developing fetus (e.g., malnutrition, substance use).

[maximally compensated] Cardiac Output may be related to increased fluid volume, maximal cardiac effort and hormonal effects of progesterone and relaxin (places the client at risk for hypertension and/or circulatory failure), and changes in peripheral resistance (afterload), possibly evidenced by variations in blood pressure and pulse, syncopal episodes, presence of pathological edema.

readiness for enhanced family Coping may be related to situational or maturational crisis with anticipated changes in family structure or roles, needs sufficiently met and adaptive tasks effectively addressed to enable goals of self-actualization to surface, as evidenced by movement toward health-promoting and enriching lifestyle, choosing experiences that optimize pregnancy experience and wellness.

risk for Constipation: risk factors may include changes in dietary or fluid intake, smooth muscle relaxation, decreased peristalsis, and effects of medications (e.g., iron).

Fatigue/Insomnia may be related to increased carbohydrate metabolism, altered body chemistry, increased energy requirements to perform activities of daily living, discomfort, anxiety, inactivity, possibly evidenced by reports of overwhelming lack of energy, inability to maintain usual routines, difficulty falling asleep, dissatisfaction with sleep, decreased quality of life.

risk for ineffective Role Performance: risk factors may include maturational crisis, developmental level, history of maladaptive coping, absence of support systems.

deficient Knowledge [Learning Need] regarding normal physiological/psychological changes and self-care needs may be related to lack of information or recall and misinterpretation of normal physiological or psychological changes and their impact on the client/family, possibly evidenced by questions, statements of concern, misconceptions, inaccurate follow-through of instructions, and development of preventable complications.

Pregnancy, 2nd trimester   OB/CH
Also refer to Pregnancy, 1st trimester

risk for disturbed Body Image: risk factors may include perception of biophysical changes, response of others.

ineffective Breathing Pattern may be related to impingement of the diaphragm by enlarging uterus, possibly evidenced by reports of shortness of breath, dyspnea, and changes in respiratory depth.

risk for [decompensated] Cardiac Output: risk factors may include increased circulatory demand, changes in preload (decreased venous return) and afterload (increased peripheral vascular resistance), and ventricular hypertrophy.

risk for excess Fluid Volume: risk factors may include changes in regulatory mechanisms, sodium and water retention.

Sexual Dysfunction may be related to conflict regarding changes in sexual desire and expectations, fear of physical injury to woman/fetus, possibly evidenced by reported difficulties, limitations or changes in sexual behaviors or activities.

Pregnancy, 3rd trimester   OB/CH
Also refer to Pregnancy, 1st and 2nd trimesters

deficient Knowledge [Learning Need] regarding preparation for labor/delivery and infant care may be related to lack of exposure or experience, misinterpretations of information, possibly evidenced by request for information, statement of concerns, misconceptions.

impaired Urinary Elimination may be related to uterine enlargement, increased abdominal pressure, fluctuation of renal blood flow, and glomerular filtration rate, possibly evidenced by urinary frequency, urgency, dependent edema.

risk for ineffective Coping/compromised family Coping: risk factors may include situational or maturational crisis, personal vulnerability, unrealistic perceptions, absent or insufficient support systems.

risk for disturbed Maternal/Fetal Dyad: risk factors may include presence of hypertension, infection, substance use or abuse, altered immune system, abnormal blood profile, tissue hypoxia, premature rupture of membranes.

Pregnancy, adolescent   OB/CH
Also refer to Pregnancy, 1st, 2nd, and 3rd trimesters

interrupted Family Processes may be related to situational or developmental transition (economic, change in roles, gain of a family member), possibly evidenced by family expressing confusion about what to do, unable to meet physical, emotional, or spiritual needs of the members; family inability to adapt to change or to deal with traumatic experience constructively; does not demonstrate respect for individuality and autonomy of its members, ineffective family decision-making process, and inappropriate boundary maintenance.

Social Isolation may be related to alterations in physical appearance, perceived unacceptable social behavior, restricted social sphere, stage of adolescence, and interference with accomplishing developmental tasks, possibly evidenced by expressions of feelings of aloneness, rejection, or difference from others; uncommunicative; withdrawn; no eye contact; seeking to be alone; unacceptable behavior; and absence of supportive SO(s).

situational/chronic low Self-Esteem may be related to situational or maturational crisis, biophysical changes, and fear of failure at life events, absence of support systems, possibly evidenced by self-negating verbalizations, expressions of shame or guilt, fear of rejection or reaction of other, hypersensitivity to criticism, and lack of follow-through or nonparticipation in prenatal care.

deficient Knowledge [Learning Need] regarding pregnancy, developmental/individual needs, and future expectations may be related to lack of exposure, information misinterpretation, unfamiliarity with information resources, lack of interest in learning, possibly evidenced by questions, statement of concern, misconception, sense of vulnerability, denial of reality, inaccurate follow-through of instruction, and development of preventable complications.

risk for impaired Parenting may be related to chronological age and developmental stage, unmet social, emotional, or maturational needs of parenting figures; unrealistic expectation of

---

self/infant/partner, ineffective role model or social support, lack of role identity, and presence of stressors (e.g., financial, social).

Pregnancy, high-risk   OB/CH
Also refer to Pregnancy, 1st, 2nd, and 3rd trimesters

Anxiety [specify level] may be related to situational crisis, threat of maternal/fetal death (perceived or actual), interpersonal transmission or contagion, possibly evidenced by increased tension, apprehension, feelings of inadequacy, somatic complaints, difficulty sleeping.

deficient Knowledge [Learning Need] regarding high-risk situation and preterm labor may be related to lack of exposure to or misinterpretation of information, unfamiliarity with individual risks and own role in risk prevention and management, possibly evidenced by request for information, statement of concerns, misconceptions, inaccurate follow-through of instructions.

risk for disturbed Maternal/Fetal Dyad: risk factors may include maternal health problems, substance use or abuse, exposure to teratogens or infectious agents.

risk of maternal Injury: risk factors may include preexisting medical conditions, complications of pregnancy.

risk for Activity Intolerance: risk factors may include presence of circulatory or respiratory problems, uterine irritability.

risk for interrupted Family Processes: risk factors may include situational crisis, change in health status of family member, family role shift, economic stressors.

risk for ineffective self Health Management: risk factors may include client value system, health beliefs, cultural influences, issues of control, presence of anxiety, complexity of therapeutic regimen, economic difficulties, perceived susceptibility.

Pregnancy-induced hypertension   OB/CH
Also refer to Eclampsia

deficient Fluid Volume [isotonic] may be related to a plasma protein loss, decreasing plasma colloid osmotic pressure allowing fluid shifts out of vascular compartment, possibly evidenced by edema formation, sudden weight gain, hemoconcentration, nausea, vomiting, epigastric pain, headaches, visual changes, decreased urine output.

decreased Cardiac Output may be related to hypovolemia, decreased venous return, increased systemic vascular resistance, possibly evidenced by variations in blood pressure and hemodynamic readings, edema, shortness of breath, change in mental status.

risk for disturbed Maternal/Fetal Dyad: risk factors may include compromised oxygen transport—vasospasm of spiral arteries and relative hypovolemia.

deficient Knowledge [Learning Need] regarding pathophysiology of condition, therapy, self-care, nutritional needs, and potential complications may be related to lack of information or recall, misinterpretation, possibly evidenced by statements of concern, questions, misconceptions, inaccurate follow-through of instructions, development of preventable complications.

Pregnancy, postmaturity   OB
Anxiety [specify level] may be related to situational crisis, threat to maternal/fetal health status (perceived or actual), interpersonal transmission or contagion, possibly evidenced by increased tension, apprehension, irritability, feelings of inadequacy, somatic complaints.

ineffective [uteroplacental] tissue Perfusion may be related to placental involution, multiple infarcts, and villous degeneration, possibly evidenced by decrease in fetal motion, meconium staining of amniotic fluid, intrauterine growth restriction, late decelerations on fetal monitor.

risk for maternal Injury: risk factors may include dysfunctional or prolonged labor.

risk for impaired fetal Gas Exchange: risk factors may include altered placental perfusion, cord compression (oligohydramnios).

risk for fetal Injury: risk factors may include prolonged labor (tissue hypoxia, acidosis), meconium aspiration.

Premature ejaculation   CH

Sexual Dysfunction may be related to altered body function, partner-related issues, possibly evidenced by reports of disruption of sexual response pattern, inability to achieve desired satisfaction.

situational low Self-Esteem may be related to functional impairment, perceived failure to perform satisfactorily, rejection of other(s), possibly evidenced by self-negating verbalizations, expressions of helplessness, powerlessness.

Premature infant   OB/PED

Refer to Newborn, premature

Premenstrual dysphoric disorder   GYN/PSY

chronic Pain may be related to cyclic changes in female hormones affecting other systems (e.g., vascular congestion, spasms), vitamin deficiency, fluid retention, possibly evidenced by increased tension, apprehension, jitteriness, verbal reports, distraction behaviors, somatic complaints, self-focusing, physical and social withdrawal.

[moderate to panic] Anxiety may be related to cyclic changes in female hormones affecting other systems, possibly evidenced by feelings of inability to cope or loss of control, depersonalization, increased tension, apprehension, jitteriness, somatic complaints, and impaired functioning.

ineffective Coping may be related to personal vulnerability, threat to self-concept, multiple stressors (premenstrual symptoms) repeated over period of time, poor nutrition, possibly evidenced by verbalization of difficulty coping or problem-solving, inability to meet role expectation or seek help, emotional and muscular tension, chronic fatigue, insomnia, lack of appetite or overeating, high illness rate, decreased societal participation.

excess Fluid Volume may be related to abnormal alterations of hormonal levels, possibly evidenced by edema formation, weight gain, and periodic changes in emotional status/irritability.

deficient Knowledge [Learning Need] regarding pathophysiology of condition and self-care and treatment needs may be related to lack of information, misinterpretation, possibly evidenced by statements of concern, questions, misconceptions, and continuation of condition, exacerbating symptoms.

Premenstrual tension syndrome   GYN/PSY

Refer to Premenstrual dysphoric disorder

Prenatal substance abuse   OB

Refer to Substance dependence/abuse, prenatal

Pressure ulcer or sore   CH

Also refer to Ulcer, decubitus

ineffective peripheral tissue Perfusion may be related to reduced or interrupted blood flow, possibly evidenced by presence of inflamed, necrotic lesion.

deficient Knowledge [Learning Need] regarding cause, prevention of condition, and potential complications may be related to lack of information or misinterpretation, possibly evidenced by statements of concern, questions, misconceptions, and inaccurate follow-through of instructions.

Preterm labor   OB/CH

Refer to Labor, preterm

Prostate cancer   MS

Also refer to Cancer; Prostatectomy

[acute/chronic] Urinary Retention may be related to blockage of urethra, possibly evidenced by sensation of bladder fullness, dysuria, small and frequent voiding, residual urine, bladder distention.

acute Pain may be related to destruction of tissues, pressure on surrounding structures, bladder distention, possibly evidenced by verbal reports, restlessness, irritability, autonomic responses.

Prostatectomy   MS

Also refer to Surgery, general

impaired Urinary Elimination may be related to mechanical obstruction (blood clots, edema, trauma, surgical procedure, pressure or irritation of catheter and balloon) and loss of bladder tone, possibly evidenced by dysuria, frequency, dribbling, incontinence, retention, bladder fullness, suprapubic discomfort.

risk for Bleeding/deficient Fluid Volume: risk factors may include trauma to highly vascular area with excessive vascular losses, restricted intake, postobstructive diuresis.

acute Pain may be related to irritation of bladder mucosa and tissue trauma/edema, possibly evidenced by verbal reports (bladder spasms), distraction behaviors, self-focus, and autonomic responses (changes in vital signs).

disturbed Body Image may be related to perceived threat of altered body and sexual function, possibly evidenced by preoccupation with change or loss, negative feelings about body, and statements of concern regarding functioning.

                                                                CH

risk for Sexual Dysfunction: risk factors may include situational crisis (incontinence, leakage of urine after catheter removal, involvement of genital area) and threat to self-concept, change in health status.

Prostatitis, acute   CH

Also refer to Cystitis

acute Pain/impaired Comfort may be related to inflammatory response, possibly evidenced by reports of low back and pelvic pain, arthralgia, myalgia.

impaired Urinary Elimination may be related to localized swelling, urinary tract infection, possibly evidenced by dysuria or burning on urination, frequency, urgency, nocturia, obstructed voiding.

Hyperthermia may be related to illness, possibly evidenced by high fever; chills; flushed, warm skin.

risk for ineffective self Health Management: risk factors may include length of therapy, perceived seriousness or benefits.

Prostatitis, chronic   CH

Also refer to Cystitis

impaired Comfort/acute Pain may be related to inflammatory response, possibly evidenced by reports of back, pelvic, or scrotal discomfort; low-grade fever.

impaired Urinary Elimination may be related to localized swelling, urinary tract infection, possibly evidenced by dysuria, frequency, urgency.

Pruritus   CH

acute Pain may be related to cutaneous hyperesthesia and inflammation, possibly evidenced by verbal reports, distraction behaviors, and self-focus.

risk for impaired Skin Integrity: risk factors may include mechanical trauma (scratching) and development of vesicles or bullae that may rupture.

Psoriasis   CH

impaired Skin Integrity may be related to increased epidermal cell proliferation and absence of normal protective skin layers, possibly evidenced by scaling papules and plaques.

disturbed Body Image may be related to cosmetically unsightly skin lesions, possibly evidenced by hiding affected body part, negative feelings about body, feelings of helplessness, and change in social involvement.

Psychological abuse   CH/PSY
Refer to Abuse, psychological

PTSD   PSY
Refer to Posttraumatic stress disorder

Pulmonary edema   MS

impaired Gas Exchange may be related to alveolar-capillary membrane changes (fluid collection or shifts into interstitial space or alveoli), possibly evidenced by dyspnea, restlessness, irritability, abnormal rate and depth of respirations, lethargy, confusion.

[moderate to severe] Anxiety may be related to change in health status, threat of death, interpersonal transmission, possibly evidenced by expressed concerns, distressed, apprehension, extraneous movement.

risk for impaired spontaneous Ventilation: risk factors may include respiratory muscle fatigue, problems with secretion management.

Pulmonary edema, high altitude   MS
Refer to High altitude pulmonary edema

Pulmonary embolus   MS

Ineffective Breathing Pattern may be related to tracheobronchial obstruction (inflammation, copious secretions or active bleeding), decreased lung expansion, inflammatory process, possibly evidenced by changes in depth or rate of respiration, dyspnea, use of accessory muscles, altered chest excursion, abnormal breath sounds (crackles, wheezes), and cough (with or without sputum production).

impaired Gas Exchange may be related to altered blood flow to alveoli or to major portions of the lung, alveolar-capillary membrane changes (atelectasis, airway or alveolar collapse, pulmonary edema and effusion, excessive secretions, active bleeding), possibly evidenced by profound dyspnea, restlessness, apprehension, somnolence, cyanosis, and changes in arterial blood gas or pulse oximetry (hypoxemia and hypercapnia).

ineffective [pulmonary] tissue Perfusion may be related to interruption of blood flow (arterial or venous), exchange problems at alveolar level or at tissue level (acidotic shifting of the oxyhemoglobin curve), possibly evidenced by radiology and laboratory evidence of ventilation-perfusion mismatch, dyspnea, and central cyanosis.

Fear/Anxiety [specify level] may be related to severe dyspnea, inability to breathe normally, perceived threat of death, threat to or change in health status, physiological response to hypoxemia, acidosis, and concern regarding unknown outcome of situation, possibly evidenced by restlessness, irritability, withdrawal or attack behavior, sympathetic stimulation (cardiovascular excitation, pupil dilation, sweating, vomiting, diarrhea), crying, voice quivering, and impending sense of doom.

Pulmonary fibrosis   CH

impaired Gas Exchange may be related to alveolar-capillary membrane changes (inflammation, development of scar tissue), ventilation-perfusion imbalance (retained secretions), possibly evidenced by dyspnea, adventitious breath sounds, nonproductive cough, cyanosis.

Anxiety [specify]/Fear may be related to situational crisis, change in health status, threat of death, interpersonal transmission, possibly evidenced by expressed concerns, apprehension, uncertainty, ruminations, increased tension.

Activity Intolerance may be related to imbalance between oxygen supply and demand, generalized weakness, possibly evidenced by exertional dyspnea, abnormal heart rate and blood pressure response to activity, cyanosis.

risk for Infection: risk factors may include stasis of secretions, chronic disease, drug therapies (corticosteroids, cytotoxins).

Pulmonary hypertension   CH/MS

impaired Gas Exchange may be related to changes in alveolar membrane, increased pulmonary vascular resistance, possibly evidenced by dyspnea, irritability, decreased mental acuity, somnolence, abnormal arterial blood gases.

decreased Cardiac Output may be related to increased pulmonary vascular resistance, decreased blood return to left side of heart, possibly evidenced by increased heart rate, dyspnea, fatigue.

Activity Intolerance may be related to imbalance between oxygen supply and demand, possibly evidenced by reports of weakness, fatigue, abnormal vital signs with activity.

[mild to moderate] Anxiety may be related to change in health status, stress, threat to self-concept, possibly evidenced by expressed concerns, uncertainty, anxiety, awareness of physiological symptoms, diminished productivity and ability to problem-solve.

Pulmonic insufficiency   MS/CH
Refer to Valvular heart disease

Pulmonic stenosis   MS/CH
Refer to Valvular heart disease

Purpura, idiopathic thrombocytopenic   CH

ineffective Protection may be related to abnormal blood profile, drug therapy (corticosteroids or immunosuppressive agents), possibly evidenced by altered clotting, fatigue, deficient immunity.

Activity Intolerance may be related to decreased oxygen-carrying capacity, imbalance between oxygen supply and demand, possibly evidenced by reports of fatigue, weakness.

deficient Knowledge [Learning Need] regarding therapy choices, outcomes, and self-care needs may be related to lack of information, misinterpretation, possibly evidenced by statements of concern, questions, and misconceptions.

Pyelonephritis   MS

acute Pain may be related to acute inflammation of renal tissues, possibly evidenced by verbal reports, guarding or distraction behaviors, self-focus, and changes in vital signs.

Hyperthermia may be related to inflammatory process and increased metabolic rate, possibly evidenced by increase in body temperature; warm, flushed skin; tachycardia; and chills.

impaired Urinary Elimination may be related to inflammation and irritation of bladder mucosa, possibly evidenced by dysuria, urgency, and frequency.

deficient Knowledge [Learning Need] regarding therapy needs and prevention may be related to lack of information, misinterpretation, possibly evidenced by statements of concern, questions, misconceptions, and recurrence of condition.

Pyloric stenosis   PED

deficient Fluid Volume may be related to excessive projectile vomiting, possibly evidenced by decreased, concentrated urine; poor skin turgor, dry skin and mucous membranes, lethargy.

imbalanced Nutrition: less than body requirements may be related to inability to digest or absorb nutrients, possibly evidenced by weight loss, poor muscle tone, pale conjunctiva and mucous membranes.

Quadriplegia   MS/CH

Also refer to Paraplegia

ineffective Breathing Pattern may be related to impairment of innervation of diaphragm—lesions at or above C5, complete or mixed loss of intercostal muscle function, reflex abdominal spasms, gastric distention, possibly evidenced by decreased respiratory depth, dyspnea, cyanosis, and abnormal arterial blood gases.

risk for Trauma [additional spinal injury]: risk factors may include temporary weakness, instability of spinal column.

Grieving may be related to perceived loss of self, anticipated alterations in lifestyle and expectations, and limitation of future options and choices, possibly evidenced by expressions of distress, anger, sorrow; choked feelings; and changes in eating habits, sleep, communication patterns.

total Self-Care Deficit related to neuromuscular impairment, evidenced by inability to perform self-care tasks.

Bowel Incontinence/Constipation may be related to disruption of nerve innervation, perceptual impairment, changes in dietary and fluid intake, change in activity level, possibly evidenced by inability to evacuate bowel voluntarily; increased abdominal pressure and distention; dry, hard formed stool; change in bowel sounds.

impaired bed/wheelchair Mobility may be related to loss of muscle function and control.

risk for Autonomic Dysreflexia: risk factors may include altered nerve function (spinal cord injury at T6 or above); bladder, bowel, or skin stimulation (tactile, pain, thermal).

impaired Home Maintenance may be related to permanent effects of injury, inadequate or absent support systems and finances, and lack of familiarity with resources, possibly evidenced by expressions of difficulties, requests for information and assistance, outstanding debts or financial crisis, and lack of necessary aids and equipment.

Rabies   CH/MS

Hyperthermia may be related to infection, possibly evidenced by fever, malaise.

risk for ineffective Airway Clearance: risk factors may include excessive salivation, muscle spasms (laryngeal, pharyngeal).

deficient Fluid Volume related to inability to drink (severe painful pharyngeal muscle spasms), excessive salivation, possibly evidenced by extreme thirst, decreased skin turgor, decreased output/concentrated urine.

risk for trauma: risk factors may include progressive restlessness, uncontrollable excitement, inability to utilize physical restraints for safety.

Radiation syndrome/poisoning   MS

(Dependent on dose and duration of exposure)

[severe] Anxiety/Fear may be related to situational crisis, threat of death, interpersonal transmission and contagion, unmet needs, possibly evidenced by expressed concerns, fearfulness, hopelessness, restlessness, agitation, anguish, increased tension, awareness of physiological symptoms.

deficient Fluid Volume may be related to intractable nausea, vomiting, diarrhea (gastrointestinal tissue necrosis and atrophy), interference with adequate intake (stomatitis, anorexia),

---

hemorrhagic losses (thrombocytopenia), possibly evidenced by dry skin and mucous membranes, poor skin turgor, decreased venous filling, reduced pulse volume and pressure, hypotension, weakness, change in mentation.

acute Confusion may be related to central nervous system inflammation, decreased circulation/hypotension, effects of circulating toxins, possibly evidenced by fluctuations in cognition or level of consciousness, agitation.

ineffective Protection may be related to effects of radiation, abnormal blood profile (leukopenia, thrombocytopenia, anemia), inadequate nutrition, possibly evidenced by neurosensory alterations, anorexia, deficient immunity, impaired healing, altered clotting, disorientation.

risk for Infection: risk factors may include inadequate primary defenses (traumatized or necrotic tissues, stasis of body fluids, altered peristalsis), inadequate secondary defenses (anemia, leukopenia).

Sexual Dysfunction may be related to altered body function, possibly evidenced by amenorrhea, decreased libido, infertility.

risk for disturbed visual Sensory Perception: risk factors may include altered sensory reception (development of cataracts).

Radiation therapy   CH
Also refer to Brachytherapy; Cancer; Radiotherapy

Nausea may be related to therapeutic procedure, irritation to gastrointestinal system, possibly evidenced by verbal reports, vomiting, gastric stasis.

imbalanced Nutrition: less than body requirements may be related to inability to ingest adequate nutrients (nausea, stomatitis, and fatigue), hypermetabolic state, possibly evidenced by weight loss, aversion to eating, reported altered taste sensation, sore, inflamed buccal cavity, diarrhea.

impaired Oral Mucous Membrane may be related to side effects of radiation, dehydration, and malnutrition, possibly evidenced by ulcerations, leukoplakia, decreased salivation, and reports of pain.

ineffective Protection may be related to inadequate nutrition, radiation, abnormal blood profile, disease state (cancer), possibly evidenced by impaired healing, deficient immunity, anorexia, fatigue.

Radical neck surgery   MS
Refer to Laryngectomy

Rape   CH
deficient Knowledge [Learning Need] regarding required medical/legal procedures, prophylactic treatment for individual concerns (sexually transmitted diseases, pregnancy), and community resources and supports may be related to lack of information, possibly evidenced by statements of concern, questions, misconceptions, and exacerbation of symptoms.

Rape-Trauma Syndrome (acute phase) related to actual or attempted sexual penetration without consent, possibly evidenced by wide range of emotional reactions, including anxiety, fear, anger, embarrassment, and multisystem physical complaints.

risk for impaired Tissue Integrity: risk factors may include forceful sexual penetration and trauma to fragile tissues.

                                                             PSY
ineffective Coping may be related to personal vulnerability, unmet expectations, unrealistic perceptions, inadequate support systems or coping methods, multiple stressors repeated over time, overwhelming threat to self, possibly evidenced by verbalizations of inability to cope or difficulty asking for help, muscular tension/headaches, emotional tension, chronic worry.

Sexual Dysfunction may be related to biopsychosocial alteration of sexuality (stress of posttrauma response), vulnerability, loss of sexual desire, impaired relationship with SO, possibly evidenced by alteration in achieving sexual satisfaction, change in interest in self/others, preoccupation with self.

Raynaud's disease   CH
acute/chronic Pain may be related to vasospasm and altered perfusion of affected tissues, and ischemia or destruction of tissues, possibly evidenced by verbal reports, guarding of affected parts, self-focusing, and restlessness.

ineffective peripheral tissue Perfusion may be related to periodic reduction of arterial blood flow to affected areas, possibly evidenced by pallor, cyanosis, coolness, numbness, paresthesia, slow healing of lesions.

deficient Knowledge [Learning Need] regarding pathophysiology of condition, potential for complications, treatment, and self-care needs may be related to lack of information, misinterpretation, possibly evidenced by statements of concern, questions, and misconceptions; development of preventable complications.

Raynaud's phenomenon   CH
Refer to Raynaud's disease

Reactive attachment disorder   PED/PSY
Refer to Anxiety disorders—PED

Reflex sympathetic dystrophy   CH
Refer to Complex regional pain syndrome

acute/chronic Pain may be related to continued nerve stimulation, possibly evidenced by verbal reports, distraction or guarding behaviors, narrowed focus, changes in sleep patterns, and altered ability to continue previous activities.

ineffective peripheral tissue Perfusion may be related to reduction of arterial blood flow (arteriole vasoconstriction), possibly evidenced by reports of pain, decreased skin temperature and pallor, diminished arterial pulsations, and tissue swelling.

disturbed tactile Sensory Perception may be related to altered sensory reception (neurological deficit, pain), possibly evidenced by change in usual response to stimuli, abnormal sensitivity of touch, physiological anxiety, and irritability

risk for ineffective Role Performance: risk factors may include situational crisis, chronic disability, debilitating pain.

risk for compromised family Coping: risk factors may include temporary family disorganization and role changes and prolonged disability that exhausts the supportive capacity of SO(s).

Regional enteritis   CH
Refer to Crohn's disease

Renal disease, end-stage   CH/MS
Also refer to Renal failure, chronic

death Anxiety may be related to progressive debilitating disease, unmet needs, inadequate support system, personal vulnerability, past negative experiences, possibly evidenced by fear of the process of dying or loss of abilities, concerns of unfinished business, powerlessness, loss of control, denial of impending death.

Renal failure, acute   MS
excess Fluid Volume may be related to compromised regulatory mechanisms (decreased kidney function), possibly evidenced by weight gain, edema, anasarca, intake greater than output, venous

congestion, changes in blood pressure and central venous pressure, altered electrolyte levels, decreased hemoglobin and hematocrit, pulmonary congestion on x-ray.

risk for imbalanced Nutrition: less than body requirements: risk factors may include inability to ingest or digest adequate nutrients—anorexia, nausea, vomiting, ulcerations of oral mucosa, and increased metabolic needs; protein catabolism, therapeutic dietary restrictions.

risk for Infection: risk factors may include depression of immunological defenses, invasive procedures or devices, and changes in dietary intake, malnutrition.

risk for disturbed Thought Processes: risk factors may include accumulation of toxic waste products and altered cerebral perfusion.

Renal failure, chronic   CH/MS
Also refer to Dialysis, general

risk for decreased Cardiac Output: risk factors may include fluid imbalances affecting circulating volume, myocardial workload, and systemic vascular resistance; alterations in rate, rhythm, and cardiac conduction (electrolyte imbalances, hypoxia); accumulation of toxins (urea); soft-calcification.

risk for Bleeding: risk factors may include abnormal blood profile—suppressed erythropoietin production and secretion, decreased red blood cell production and survival, altered clotting factors; increased capillary fragility.

disturbed Thought Processes may be related to physiological changes—accumulation of toxins (e.g., urea, ammonia), metabolic acidosis, hypoxia, electrolyte imbalances, calcifications in brain, possibly evidenced by disorientation, memory deficit, altered attention span, decreased ability to grasp idea, impaired ability to make decisions or problem-solve, changes in sensorium, irritability, psychosis.

risk for impaired Skin Integrity: risk factors may include altered metabolic state, circulation (anemia with tissue ischemia), and sensation (peripheral neuropathy), decreased skin turgor, reduced activity, immobility, accumulation of toxins in the skin.

risk for impaired Oral Mucous Membrane: risk factors may include decreased or lack of salivation, fluid restrictions, chemical irritation (conversion of urea in saliva to ammonia).

Renal transplantation   MS
Also refer to Transplantation, recipient

risk for excess Fluid Volume: risk factors may include compromised regulatory mechanism (implantation of new kidney requiring adjustment period for optimal functioning).

disturbed Body Image may be related to failure and subsequent replacement of body part and medication-induced changes in appearance, possibly evidenced by preoccupation with loss or change, negative feelings about body, and focus on past strength and function.

Fear may be related to potential for transplant rejection or failure and threat of death, possibly evidenced by increased tension, apprehension, concentration on source, and verbalizations of concern.

risk for Infection: risk factors may include broken skin or traumatized tissue, stasis of body fluids, immunosuppression, invasive procedures, nutritional deficits, and chronic disease.

                                                      CH
risk for ineffective Coping/compromised family Coping: risk factors may include situational crises, family disorganization and role changes, prolonged disease exhausting supportive capacity of SO/family, therapeutic restrictions/long-term therapy needs.

Repetitive motion injury   CH
Refer to Carpal tunnel syndrome

Respiratory distress syndrome, acute   MS

ineffective Airway Clearance may be related to loss of ciliary action, increased amount and viscosity of secretions, and increased airway resistance, possibly evidenced by presence of dyspnea, changes in depth and rate of respiration, use of accessory muscles for breathing, wheezes, crackles, cough with or without sputum production.

impaired Gas Exchange may be related to changes in pulmonary capillary permeability with edema formation, alveolar hypoventilation and collapse, with intrapulmonary shunting, possibly evidenced by tachypnea, use of accessory muscles, cyanosis, hypoxia per arterial blood gases or oximetry, anxiety and changes in mentation.

risk for deficient Fluid Volume: risk factors may include active loss from diuretic use and restricted intake.

risk for decreased Cardiac Output: risk factors may include alteration in preload (hypovolemia, vascular pooling, diuretic therapy, and increased intrathoracic pressure, use of ventilator, and positive end-expiratory pressure [PEEP]).

Anxiety [specify level]/Fear may be related to physiological factors (effects of hypoxemia), situational crisis, change in health status/threat of death, possibly evidenced by increased tension, apprehension, restlessness, focus on self, and sympathetic stimulation.

risk for [pulmonary] Injury: risk factors may include increased airway pressure associated with mechanical ventilation (PEEP).

Respiratory distress syndrome (premature infant) PED

Also refer to Newborn, premature

impaired Gas Exchange may be related to alveolar-capillary membrane changes (inadequate surfactant levels), altered oxygen supply (tracheobronchial obstruction, atelectasis), altered blood flow (immaturity of pulmonary arteriole musculature), altered oxygen-carrying capacity of blood (anemia), and cold stress, possibly evidenced by tachypnea, use of accessory muscles and retractions, expiratory grunting, pallor or cyanosis, abnormal arterial blood gases, and tachycardia.

impaired Spontaneous Ventilation may be related to respiratory muscle fatigue and metabolic factors, possibly evidenced by dyspnea, increased metabolic rate, restlessness, use of accessory muscles, and abnormal arterial blood gases.

risk for Infection: risk factors may include inadequate primary defenses (decreased ciliary action, stasis of body fluids, traumatized tissues), inadequate secondary defenses (deficiency of neutrophils and specific immunoglobulins), invasive procedures, and malnutrition (absence of nutrient stores, increased metabolic demands).

risk for ineffective gastrointestinal Perfusion: risk factors may include persistent fetal circulation and exchange problems.

risk for impaired Attachment: risk factors may include premature/ill infant who is unable to effectively initiate parental contact (altered behavioral organization), separation, physical barriers, anxiety associated with the parental role and demands of infant.

Respiratory syncytial virus   PED

impaired Gas Exchange may be related to inflammation of airways, ventilation perfusion imbalance (areas of consolidation), apnea, possibly evidenced by dyspnea, abnormal arterial blood gases/hypoxia.

ineffective Airway Clearance may be related to infection, retained secretions, exudate in alveoli, inflammation of airways, possibly evidenced by dyspnea, adventitious breath sounds, cough.

risk for deficient Fluid Volume: risk factors may include increased insensible losses (fever, diaphoresis), decreased oral intake.

Restless leg syndrome   CH

Refer to Myoclonus, nocturnal

Retinal detachment   CH

disturbed visual Sensory Perception related to decreased sensory reception, possibly evidenced by visual distortions, decreased visual field, and changes in visual acuity.

[mild to moderate] Anxiety may be related to situational crisis, change in health status and role function, possibly evidenced by expressed concerns, apprehension, uncertainty, focus on self.

deficient Knowledge [Learning Need] regarding therapy, prognosis, and self-care needs may be related to lack of information, misconceptions, possibly evidenced by statements of concern and questions.

risk for impaired Home Maintenance: risk factors may include visual limitations, activity restrictions.

Rett's syndrome   PED/PSY

Also refer to Autistic disorder

delayed Growth and Development may be related to effects of physical and mental disability, possibly evidenced by altered physical growth; delay or inability in performing skills and self-care or self-control activities appropriate for age.

impaired Walking/physical Mobility may be related to neuromuscular impairment, joint stiffness, contractures, disuse, possibly evidenced by limited range of motion, inability to perform gross motor skills, walk, or reposition self.

risk for Trauma: risk factors may include cognitive deficits, lack of muscle tone and coordination, seizure activity.

imbalanced Nutrition: less than body requirements may be related to poor muscle tone, dependence on others and inability to meet own needs, possibly evidenced by weak and ineffective sucking or swallowing and observed lack of adequate intake with weight loss or failure to gain.

risk for complicated Grieving: risk factors may include loss of "the perfect child," chronic condition requiring long-term care, and unresolved feelings.

Reye's syndrome   PED

deficient Fluid Volume [isotonic] may be related to failure of regulatory mechanism (diabetes insipidus), excessive gastric losses (pernicious vomiting), and altered intake, possibly evidenced by increased and dilute urine output, sudden weight loss, decreased venous filling, dry mucous membranes, decreased skin turgor, hypotension, and tachycardia.

ineffective cerebral tissue Perfusion may be related to diminished arterial or venous blood flow and hypovolemia, possibly evidenced by memory loss, altered consciousness, and restlessness, agitation.

risk for Trauma: risk factors may include generalized weakness, reduced coordination, and cognitive deficits.

ineffective Breathing Pattern may be related to decreased energy and fatigue, cognitive impairment, tracheobronchial obstruction, and inflammatory process (aspiration pneumonia), possibly evidenced by tachypnea, abnormal arterial blood gases, cough, and use of accessory muscles.

Rheumatic fever   PED

acute Pain may be related to migratory inflammation of joints, possibly evidenced by verbal reports, guarding or distraction behaviors, self-focus, and changes in vital signs.

Hyperthermia may be related to inflammatory process, hypermetabolic state, possibly evidenced by increased body temperature; warm, flushed skin; and tachycardia.

Activity Intolerance may be related to generalized weakness, joint pain, and medical restrictions or bedrest, possibly evidenced by reports of fatigue, exertional discomfort, and abnormal heart rate in response to activity.

risk for decreased Cardiac Output: risk factors may include cardiac inflammation, enlargement, and altered contractility.

Rheumatic heart disease   PED/MS
Also refer to Valvular heart disease

Activity Intolerance may be related to imbalance between oxygen supply and demand, generalized weakness, and prolonged bedrest or sedentary lifestyle, possibly evidenced by reported or observed weakness, fatigue, changes in vital signs, presence of dysrhythmias, dyspnea, pallor.

risk-prone health Behavior may be related to health status requiring change in lifestyle or restriction of desired activities, unrealistic expectations, negative attitudes, possibly evidenced by denial of situation, demonstration of nonacceptance of health status, failure to achieve optimal sense of control.

risk for ineffective self Health Management: risk factors may include complexity and duration of therapeutic regimen, imposed restrictions or limitations, economic difficulties, family patterns of healthcare, perceived seriousness or benefits.

risk for impaired Gas Exchange: risk factors may include alveolar-capillary membrane changes (fluid collection or shifts into interstitial space or alveoli).

Rhinitis, allergic   CH
Refer to Hay fever

Rickets   PED
delayed Growth and Development may be related to dietary deficiencies/indiscretions, malabsorption syndrome, and lack of exposure to sunlight, possibly evidenced by altered physical growth and delay or difficulty in performing motor skills typical for age.

deficient Knowledge [Learning Need] regarding cause, pathophysiology, therapy needs and prevention may be related to lack of information, possibly evidenced by statements of concern, questions, misconceptions, and inaccurate follow-through of instructions.

Ringworm, tinea   CH
Also refer to Athlete's foot

impaired Skin Integrity may be related to fungal infection of the dermis, possibly evidenced by disruption of skin surfaces and presence of lesions.

deficient Knowledge [Learning Need] regarding infectious nature, therapy, and self care needs may be related to lack of information, misinformation, possibly evidenced by statements of concern, questions, and recurrence and spread.

Rocky Mountain spotted fever   CH/MS
Refer to Typhus

RSD   CH
Refer to Reflex sympathetic dystrophy

RSV   PED
Refer to Respiratory syncytial virus

Rubella   PED/CH

acute Pain/impaired Comfort may be related to inflammatory effects of viral infection and presence of desquamating rash, possibly evidenced by verbal reports, distraction behaviors, restlessness.

deficient Knowledge [Learning Need] regarding contagious nature, possible complications, and self-care needs may be related to lack of information, misinterpretations, possibly evidenced by statements of concern, questions, and inaccurate follow-through of instructions.

Rubeola   PED/CH
Refer to Measles

Ruptured intervertebral disc   CH/MS
Refer to Herniated nucleus pulposus

Sarcoidosis   CH
Also refer to Pulmonary fibrosis

Fatigue may be related to disease state, anemia, possibly evidenced by lack of energy, lethargy, decreased performance, inability to maintain usual routines.

risk for disturbed visual Sensory Perception: risk factors may include altered sensory reception—inflammation of the eye, increased intraocular pressure.

risk for Injury: risk factors may include autoimmune dysfunction, abnormal blood profile—thrombocytopenia, leukopenia, anemia; sensory dysfunction.

SARS (sudden acute respiratory syndrome)   MS

Hyperthermia may be related to inflammatory process, possibly evidenced by high fever, chills, rigors, headache.

acute Pain/impaired Comfort may be related to inflammation and circulating toxins, possibly evidenced by reports of myalgia, headache, malaise.

impaired Gas Exchange may be related to ventilation perfusion imbalance (interstitial infiltrates, areas of consolidation), possibly evidenced by dyspnea, changes in mentation or level of consciousness, restlessness, hypoxemia.

risk for impaired spontaneous Ventilation: risk factors may include hypermetabolic state, infection, depletion of energy stores, respiratory muscle fatigue.

death Anxiety may be related to uncertainty of prognosis, possibly evidenced by report of apprehension; increased pulse and respiratory rate, muscle tension, pupil dilation.

risk for ineffective Protection: risk factors may include inadequate nutrition, abnormal blood profile (leukopenia, thrombocytopenia).

Scabies   CH

impaired Skin Integrity may be related to presence of invasive parasite and development of pruritus, possibly evidenced by disruption of skin surface and inflammation.

deficient Knowledge [Learning Need] regarding communicable nature, possible complications, therapy, and self-care needs may be related to lack of information, misinterpretation, possibly evidenced by questions and statements of concern about spread to others.

Scarlet fever   PED

Hyperthermia may be related to effects of circulating toxins, possibly evidenced by increased body temperature; warm, flushed skin; and tachycardia.

acute Pain/impaired Comfort may be related to inflammation of mucous membranes and effects of circulating toxins (malaise, fever), possibly evidenced by verbal reports, distraction behaviors, guarding (decreased swallowing), and self-focus.

risk for deficient Fluid Volume: risk factors may include hypermetabolic state (hyperthermia) and reduced intake.

Schizoaffective disorder   PSY

risk for other-/self-directed Violence: risk factors may include depressed mood, feelings of worthlessness, hopelessness, unsatisfactory parent-child relationship, feelings of abandonment by SOs, anger turned inward or directed at the environment, punitive superego, irrational feelings of guilt, numerous failures, misinterpretation of reality.

Social Isolation may be related to developmental regression, depressed mood, feelings of worthlessness, egocentric behaviors (offending others and discouraging relationships), delusional thinking, fear of failure, unresolved grief, possibly evidenced by sad, dull affect; absence of support systems; uncommunicative, withdrawn, or catatonic behavior; absence of eye contact; preoccupation with own thoughts; repetitive or meaningless actions.

imbalanced Nutrition: less than body requirements may be related to energy expenditure in excess of intake, refusal or inability to take time to eat, lack of attention to or recognition of hunger cues, possibly evidenced by lack of interest in food, weight loss, pale conjunctiva and mucous membranes, poor muscle tone and skin turgor, amenorrhea, abnormal laboratory studies.

Schizophrenia (schizophrenic disorders)   PSY

disturbed Thought Processes may be related to disintegration of thinking processes, impaired judgment, presence of psychological conflicts, disintegrated ego boundaries, sleep disturbance, ambivalence and concomitant dependence, possibly evidenced by impaired ability to reason or problem-solve, inappropriate affect, presence of delusional system, command hallucinations, obsessions, ideas of reference, cognitive dissonance.

Social Isolation may be related to alterations in mental status, mistrust of others, delusional thinking, unacceptable social behaviors, inadequate personal resources, and inability to engage in satisfying personal relationships, possibly evidenced by difficulty in establishing relationships with others, dull affect, uncommunicative or withdrawn behavior, seeking to be alone, inadequate or absent significant purpose in life, and expression of feelings of rejection.

risk for self-/other-directed Violence: risk factors may include disturbances of thinking and feeling (depression, paranoia, suicidal ideation), lack of development of trust and appropriate interpersonal relationships, catatonic or manic excitement, toxic reactions to drugs (alcohol).

ineffective Coping may be related to personal vulnerability, inadequate support system(s), unrealistic perceptions, inadequate coping methods, and disintegration of thought processes, possibly evidenced by impaired judgment, cognition, and perception; diminished problem-solving or decision-making capacities, poor self-concept, chronic anxiety, depression, inability to perform role expectations, and alteration in social participation.

CH

interrupted Family Processes/disabled family Coping may be related to ambivalent family system or relationships, change of roles, and difficulty of family member in coping effectively with client's maladaptive behaviors, possibly evidenced by deterioration in family functioning, ineffective family decision-making process, difficulty relating to each other, client's expressions of despair at family's lack of reaction or involvement, neglectful relationships with client, extreme distortion regarding client's health problem, including denial about its existence and severity, or prolonged overconcern.

ineffective Health Maintenance/impaired Home Maintenance may be related to impaired cognitive and emotional functioning, altered ability to make deliberate and thoughtful judgments, altered communication, and lack of or inappropriate use of material resources, possibly evidenced by inability to take responsibility for meeting basic health practices in any or all functional areas

---

and demonstrated lack of adaptive behaviors to internal or external environmental changes, disorderly surroundings, accumulation of dirt, unwashed clothes, repeated hygienic disorders.

Self-Care Deficit [specify] may be related to perceptual and cognitive impairment, immobility (withdrawal, isolation, or decreased psychomotor activity), and side effects of psychotropic medications, possibly evidenced by inability or difficulty in areas of feeding self, keeping body clean, dressing appropriately, toileting self, or changes in bowel and bladder elimination.

Sciatica   CH

acute/chronic Pain may be related to peripheral nerve root compression, possibly evidenced by verbal reports, guarding or distraction behaviors, and self-focus.

impaired physical Mobility may be related to neurological pain and muscular involvement, possibly evidenced by reluctance to attempt movement and decreased muscle strength and mass.

Scleroderma   CH

Also refer to Lupus erythematosus, systemic (SLE)

impaired physical Mobility may be related to musculoskeletal impairment and associated pain, possibly evidenced by decreased strength, decreased range of motion, and reluctance to attempt movement.

ineffective tissue Perfusion (specify) may be related to reduced arterial blood flow (arteriolar vasoconstriction), possibly evidenced by changes in skin temperature and color, ulcer formation, and changes in organ function (cardiopulmonary, gastrointestinal, renal).

imbalanced Nutrition: less than body requirements may be related to inability to ingest, digest, or absorb adequate nutrients (sclerosis of the tissues rendering mouth immobile, decreased peristalsis of esophagus and small intestines, atrophy of smooth muscle of colon), possibly evidenced by weight loss, decreased intake, and reported or observed difficulty swallowing.

risk-prone health Behavior may be related to disability requiring change in lifestyle, inadequate support systems, assault to self-concept, and altered locus of control, possibly evidenced by verbalization of nonacceptance of health status change and lack of movement toward independence or future-oriented thinking.

disturbed Body Image may be related to skin changes with induration, atrophy, and fibrosis, loss of hair, and skin and muscle contractures, possibly evidenced by verbalization of negative feelings about body; focus on past strength, function, or appearance; fear of rejection or reaction by others; hiding body part; and change in social involvement.

Scoliosis   PED

disturbed Body Image may be related to altered body structure, use of therapeutic device(s), and activity restrictions, possibly evidenced by negative feelings about body, change in social involvement, and preoccupation with situation or refusal to acknowledge problem.

deficient Knowledge [Learning Need] regarding pathophysiology of condition, therapy needs, and possible outcomes may be related to lack of information, misinterpretation, possibly evidenced by statements of concern, questions, misconceptions, and inaccurate follow-through of instructions.

risk-prone health Behavior may be related to lack of comprehension of long-term consequences of behavior, possibly evidenced by minimizing health status change, failure to take action, and evidence of failure to improve.

Seasonal affective disorder   PSY

Refer to Affective disorder, seasonal

Sedative intoxication/abuse   CH/PSY

Refer to Depressant abuse

Seizure disorder   **CH**

deficient Knowledge [Learning Need] regarding condition and medication control may be related to lack of information, misinterpretations, scarce financial resources, possibly evidenced by questions, statements of concern, misconceptions, incorrect use of anticonvulsant medication, recurrent episodes or uncontrolled seizures.

chronic low Self-Esteem/disturbed Personal Identity may be related to stigma associated with condition, perception of being out of control or helpless, possibly evidenced by verbalization about changed lifestyle, fear of rejection, negative feelings about "brain" or self, change in usual pattern of responsibility, denial of problem resulting in lack of follow-through or nonparticipation in therapy.

impaired Social Interaction may be related to unpredictable nature of condition and self-concept disturbance, possibly evidenced by decreased self-assurance, verbalization of concern, discomfort in social situations, inability to receive or communicate a satisfying sense of belonging and caring, and withdrawal from social contacts and activities.

risk for Trauma/Suffocation: risk factors may include weakness, balancing difficulties, cognitive limitations, altered consciousness, loss of large- or small-muscle coordination (during seizure).

Separation anxiety disorder   **PED/PSY**
Refer to Anxiety disorders—PED

Sepsis   **MS**
Also refer to Sepsis, puerperal

risk for deficient Fluid Volume: risk factors may include marked increase in vascular compartment—massive vasodilation, vascular shifts to interstitial space, and reduced intake.

risk for decreased Cardiac Output: risk factors may include decreased preload (venous return and circulating volume), altered afterload (increased systemic vascular resistance), negative inotropic effects of hypoxia, complement activation, and lysosomal hydrolase.

risk for Shock: risk factors may include infection/sepsis, hypovolemia—fluid shifts or third spacing; hypotension, hypoxemia.

Sepsis, puerperal   **OB**

risk for Infection [spread]: risk factors may include presence of infection, broken skin, or traumatized tissues, rupture of amniotic membranes, high vascularity of involved area, stasis of body fluids, invasive procedures, or increased environmental exposure, chronic disease (e.g., diabetes mellitus, anemia, malnutrition), altered immune response, and untoward effect of medications (e.g., opportunistic or secondary infection).

Hyperthermia may be related to inflammatory process, hypermetabolic state, dehydration, effect of circulating endotoxins on the hypothalamus, possibly evidenced by increase in body temperature, warm, flushed skin; increased respiratory rate and tachycardia.

risk for impaired Attachment: risk factors may include interruption in bonding process, physical illness, perceived threat to own survival.

risk for ineffective peripheral tissue Perfusion: risk factors may include interruption or reduction of blood flow—presence of infectious thrombi.

risk for Shock: risk factors may include infection, hypovolemia, hypotension, hypoxemia.

Septicemia   **MS**
Refer to Sepsis

Serum sickness   **CH**
acute Pain may be related to inflammation of the joints and skin eruptions, possibly evidenced by verbal reports, guarding or distraction behaviors, and self-focus.

deficient Knowledge [Learning Need] regarding nature of condition, treatment needs, potential complications, and prevention of recurrence may be related to lack of information, misinterpretation, possibly evidenced by statements of concern, questions, misconceptions, and inaccurate follow-through of instructions.

Severe acute respiratory syndrome   MS
Refer to SARS

Sexual desire disorder   PSY
Sexual Dysfunction may be related to boredom or conflict in relationship, depression, hormonal imbalance, harmful relationships, traumatic events in childhood, possibly evidenced by loss of sexual desire, disruption of sexual response pattern, alteration in relationship with SO.

Anxiety [specify] may be related to situational crisis, stress, unconscious conflict about essential values, unmet needs, possibly evidenced by expressed concerns, distress, feelings of inadequacy, fear of unspecific consequences.

situational low Self-Esteem may be related to perceived functional impairment, emotional insecurity, rejection by SO, possibly evidenced by expressions of helplessness, self-negating verbalizations, change in involvement with partner.

Sexual dysfunctions   PSY
Refer to Dyspareunia; Erectile dysfunction; Sexual desire disorder; Vaginismus

Sexually transmitted disease   GYN/CH
risk for Infection [transmission]: risk factors may include contagious nature of infecting agent and insufficient knowledge to avoid exposure to or transmission of pathogens.

impaired Skin/Tissue Integrity may be related to invasion of and irritation by pathogenic organism(s), possibly evidenced by disruptions of skin and tissue, and inflammation of mucous membranes.

deficient Knowledge [Learning Need] regarding condition, prognosis, potential complications, therapy needs, and transmission may be related to lack of information, misinterpretation, lack of interest in learning, possibly evidenced by statements of concern, questions, misconceptions, inaccurate follow-through of instructions, and development of preventable complications.

Shingles   CH
Refer to Herpes zoster

Shock   MS
Also refer to Shock, cardiogenic; Shock, hypovolemic/hemorrhagic; Sepsis

ineffective tissue Perfusion (specify) may be related to changes in circulating volume or vascular tone, possibly evidenced by changes in skin color and temperature and pulse pressure, reduced blood pressure, changes in mentation, and decreased urinary output.

Anxiety [specify level] may be related to change in health status and threat of death, possibly evidenced by increased tension, apprehension, sympathetic stimulation, restlessness, and expressions of concern.

Shock, cardiogenic   MS
Also refer to Shock

decreased Cardiac Output may be related to structural damage, decreased myocardial contractility, and presence of dysrhythmias, possibly evidenced by electrocardiogram changes, variations in hemodynamic readings, jugular vein distention, cold and clammy skin, diminished peripheral pulses, and decreased urinary output.

risk for impaired Gas Exchange: risk factors may include ventilation perfusion imbalance, alveolar-capillary membrane changes.

Shock, hypovolemic/hemorrhagic   MS
Also refer to Shock

deficient Fluid Volume [isotonic] may be related to excessive vascular loss, inadequate intake or replacement, possibly evidenced by hypotension, tachycardia, decreased pulse volume and pressure, change in mentation, and decreased, concentrated urine.

Shock, septic   MS
Refer to Sepsis

Sicca syndrome   CH
Refer to Sjögren syndrome

Sick building syndrome   CH
Contamination may be related to presence of atmospheric or environmental contaminants in building (e.g., volatile organic compounds, carbon monoxide, asbestos, dust, fungi, molds, pollens, tobacco smoke), flooring surface (carpeted surfaces hold contaminant residue more than hard floor surfaces), poorly ventilated areas, lack of effective protection, possibly evidenced by headaches; eye, nose, or throat irritation; dry cough; dry or itchy skin; dizziness; nausea; difficulty in concentrating; fatigue.

Fatigue may be related to occupation or employment in a specific building or zone within a building as evidenced by reports of being tired, lethargic; decreased performance

Sick sinus syndrome   MS
Also refer to Dysrhythmia, cardiac

decreased Cardiac Output may be related to alterations in rate, rhythm, and electrical conduction, possibly evidenced by electrocardiogram indication of dysrhythmias, reports of palpitations, weakness, changes in mentation or consciousness, and syncope.

risk for Trauma: risk factors may include changes in cerebral perfusion with altered consciousness, loss of balance.

SIDS   PED
Refer to Sudden infant death syndrome

Sinusitis, chronic   CH
acute/chronic Pain may be related to inflammatory process, possibly evidenced by reports of headache and facial pain, irritability, change in sleep, fatigue.

risk for Infection [spread]: risk factors may include chronic irritation and inflamed tissues, stasis of body fluids, improper handling of infectious material.

Sjögren syndrome   CH
impaired Oral Mucous Membrane related to decreased salivation, possibly evidenced by xerostomia (dry mouth), oral pain or discomfort, self-report of bad or diminished taste, difficulty eating and swallowing.

risk for impaired Tissue Integrity (cornea, mucous membranes): risk factors may include impaired production of tears, mucus.

risk for Infection: risk factors may include decreased secretions, tissue dryness and damage.

risk for disturbed visual Sensory Perception: risk factors may include altered sensory reception (light sensitivity, blurred vision, corneal ulcers).

Skin cancer   **CH**

impaired Skin Integrity may be related to invasive growth, surgical excision may be evidenced by disruption of skin surface, destruction of dermis.

    risk for acute Pain: risk factors may include ulceration of skin, surgical incision.

    risk for disturbed Body Image: risk factors may include skin lesion, surgical intervention.

    deficient Knowledge [Learning Need] regarding condition, prognosis, treatment, and prevention may be related to lack of information, misinterpretation, possibly evidenced by statements of concern, questions, misconceptions, inaccurate follow-through of instructions, development of preventable complications, or recurrence.

SLE   **CH**

Refer to Lupus erythematosus, systemic

Sleep apnea   **CH**

Sleep Deprivation may be related to sleep apnea (recurrent apneic episodes followed by gasping arousal), possibly evidenced by daytime drowsiness, tiredness, decreased ability to perform, slowed mentation.

    impaired Gas Exchange may be related to altered oxygen supply (recurrent apneic episodes lasting 10 seconds to 2 minutes), possibly evidenced by morning headache, decreased mental acuity, abnormal arterial blood gases (hypoxemia, hypercapnia), dysrhythmias (e.g., extreme bradycardia, ventricular tachycardia).

    risk for ineffective self Health Management: risk factors may include duration of therapy, associated discomfort, perceived seriousness or benefit.

Smallpox   **MS**

risk of Infection [spread]: risk factors may include contagious nature of organism, inadequate acquired immunity, presence of chronic disease, immunosuppression.

    deficient Fluid Volume may be related to hypermetabolic state, decreased intake (pharyngeal lesions, nausea), increased losses (vomiting), fluid shifts from vascular bed, possibly evidenced by reports of thirst; decreased blood pressure, venous filling, and urinary output; dry mucous membranes; decreased skin turgor; change in mental state; elevated hematocrit.

    impaired Tissue Integrity may be related to immunological deficit, possibly evidenced by disruption of skin surface, cornea, mucous membranes.

    Anxiety [specify level]/Fear may be related to threat of death, interpersonal transmission or contagion, separation from support system, possibly evidenced by expressed concerns, apprehension, restlessness, focus on self.

                                                           CH

interrupted Family Processes may be related to temporary family disorganization, situational crisis, change in health status of family member, possibly evidenced by changes in satisfaction with family, stress-reduction behaviors, mutual support, expression of isolation from community resources.

    ineffective community Coping may be related to man-made disaster (bioterrorism), inadequate resources for problem-solving, possibly evidenced by deficits of community participation, high illness rate, excessive community conflicts, expressed vulnerability or powerlessness.

Snake bite, venomous   **MS**

[severe] Anxiety/Fear may be related to situational crisis, threat of death, interpersonal transmission, possibly evidenced by expressed concerns, apprehension, irritability, jitteriness, increased tension, tremors.

acute Pain/impaired Comfort may be related to effects of toxins (edema formation, erythema, enlargement of lymph nodes, nausea, fever, diaphoresis, muscle fasciculations), possibly evidenced by reports of pain and paresthesias, guarded behavior, restlessness, autonomic responses.

impaired Skin Integrity may be related to trauma, inflammation, altered circulation, possibly evidenced by disruption and destruction of skin layers (skin tense, discolored, necrosis around bite).

risk for deficient Fluid Volume: risk factors may include excessive losses (vomiting, edema formation, hemorrhage from mucous membranes).

Snow blindness   CH

disturbed visual Sensory Perception may be related to altered status of sense organ (irritation of the conjunctiva, hyperemia), possibly evidenced by intolerance to light (photophobia) and decreased or loss of visual acuity.

acute Pain may be related to irritation and vascular congestion of the conjunctiva, possibly evidenced by verbal reports, guarding or distraction behaviors, and self-focus.

Anxiety [specify level] may be related to situational crisis and threat to or change in health status, possibly evidenced by increased tension, apprehension, uncertainty, worry, restlessness, and focus on self.

Somatoform disorders   PSY

ineffective Coping may be related to severe level of anxiety that is repressed, personal vulnerability, unmet dependency needs, fixation in earlier level of development, retarded ego development, and inadequate coping skills, possibly evidenced by verbalized inability to cope or problem-solve, high illness rate, multiple somatic complaints of several years' duration, decreased functioning in social and occupational settings, narcissistic tendencies with total focus on self and physical symptoms, demanding behaviors, history of "doctor shopping," and refusal to attend therapeutic activities.

chronic Pain may be related to severe level of repressed anxiety, low self-concept, unmet dependency needs, history of self or loved one having experienced a serious illness, possibly evidenced by verbal reports of severe, prolonged pain; guarded movement or protective behaviors, facial mask of pain, fear of reinjury, altered ability to continue previous activities, social withdrawal, demands for therapy and medication.

disturbed Sensory Perception (specify) may be related to psychological stress (narrowed perceptual fields, expression of stress as physical problems or deficits), poor quality of sleep, presence of chronic pain, possibly evidenced by reported change in voluntary motor or sensory function (paralysis, anosmia, aphonia, deafness, blindness, loss of touch or pain sensation), la belle indifférence (lack of concern over functional loss).

impaired Social Interaction may be related to inability to engage in satisfying personal relationships, preoccupation with self and physical symptoms, altered state of wellness, chronic pain, and rejection by others, possibly evidenced by preoccupation with own thoughts, sad, dull affect; absence of supportive SO(s), uncommunicative or withdrawn behavior, lack of eye contact, and seeking to be alone.

Spina bifida   PED

Also refer to Paraplegia; Newborn, special needs

Bowel Incontinence/Constipation may be related to disruption of nerve innervation, perceptual impairment, reduced activity level, possibly evidenced by inability to evacuate bowel voluntarily, increased abdominal pressure or distention, dry and hard formed stool, change in bowel sounds.

risk for impaired Walking/physical Mobility: risk factors may include neuromuscular impairment, developmental delay, musculoskeletal impairments—clubfoot, hip dislocation, joint deformities, kyphosis.

risk for decreased Intracranial Adaptive Capacity: risk factors may include structural changes (aqueductal stricture, malformation of brain stem).

risk for Infection: risk factors may include increased environmental exposure, invasive procedures, traumatized tissues (cerebrospinal fluid leak).

Spinal cord injury (SCI)   MS/CH
Refer to Paraplegia; Quadriplegia

Splenectomy   MS/CH
Refer to Surgery, general

risk for Infection: risk factors may include inadequate secondary defenses (decreased antibody synthesis, reduced immunoglobulin M), insufficient knowledge or motivation to avoid exposure to pathogens.

risk for ineffective self Health Management: risk factors may include length of therapy, economic difficulties, perceived benefits.

Spongiform encephalopathy   CH
Refer to Creutzfeldt-Jakob disease

Sprain of ankle or foot   CH
acute Pain may be related to trauma to and swelling in joint, possibly evidenced by verbal reports, guarding or distraction behaviors, self-focusing, and changes in vital signs.

impaired Walking may be related to musculoskeletal injury, pain, and therapeutic restrictions, possibly evidenced by reluctance to attempt movement, inability to move about environment easily.

Sprue, nontropical   CH
Refer to Celiac disease

Stapedectomy   MS
risk for Trauma: risk factors may include increased middle-ear pressure with displacement of prosthesis and balancing difficulties, dizziness.

risk for Infection: risk factors may include surgically traumatized tissue, invasive procedures, and environmental exposure to upper respiratory infections.

acute Pain may be related to surgical trauma, edema formation, and presence of packing, possibly evidenced by verbal reports, guarding or distraction behaviors, and self-focus.

Stasis dermatitis   CH
Also refer to Venous insufficiency

impaired Skin Integrity may be related to altered circulation, presence of edema, extremely fragile epidermis, pigmentation, possibly evidenced by erythema, scaling, brown discoloration, disruption of skin surface.

risk for Infection: risk factors may include circulatory stasis, edema formation (small-vessel vasoconstrictive reflexes) in lower extremities, persistent inflammation, tissue destruction.

STD   CH
Refer to Sexually transmitted disease

Stillbirth   OB
Refer to Perinatal loss/death of child

Stimulant abuse   **CH**

Also refer to Cocaine hydrochloride poisoning, acute, Substance dependence/abuse rehabilitation

imbalanced Nutrition: less than body requirements may be related to anorexia, insufficient or inappropriate use of financial resources, possibly evidenced by reported inadequate intake, weight loss or less than normal weight gain, lack of interest in food, poor muscle tone, signs and laboratory evidence of vitamin deficiencies.

risk for Infection: risk factors may include injection techniques, impurities of drugs, localized trauma and nasal septum damage, malnutrition, altered immune state.

Insomnia may be related to central nervous system sensory alterations, psychological stress, possibly evidenced by constant alertness, racing thoughts preventing rest, denial of need to sleep, reported inability to stay awake, initial insomnia then hypersomnia.

PSY

Fear/Anxiety [specify] may be related to paranoid delusions associated with stimulant use, possibly evidenced by feelings or beliefs that others are conspiring against or are about to attack or kill client.

ineffective Coping may be related to personal vulnerability, negative role-modeling, inadequate support systems, ineffective or inadequate coping skills with substitution of drug, possibly evidenced by use of harmful substance despite evidence of undesirable consequences.

disturbed Sensory Perception (specify) may be related to exogenous chemical, altered sensory reception, transmission, or integration (hallucination), altered status of sense organs, possibly evidenced by responding to internal stimuli from hallucinatory experiences, bizarre thinking, anxiety, panic changes in sensory acuity (sense of smell, taste).

Stomatitis   **CH**

impaired Oral Mucous Membrane may be related to infection, vitamin deficiency, excessive alcohol or tobacco use, ill-fitting dentures, jagged teeth, orthodontic appliances, mouth breathing, nursing bottles with hard or too long nipples, possibly evidenced by oral pain, lesions, ulcers, white patches or plaques, sensitive tongue.

risk for deficient Fluid Volume: risk factors may include oral pain, difficulty swallowing.

Strep throat   **CH**

Hyperthermia may be related to illness and effects of toxins, inability to ingest sufficient fluids, possibly evidenced by body temperature above normal range, flushed dry skin, decreased urine output.

acute Pain may be related to injuring biological agent, possibly evidenced by report of throat, head, and abdominal pain, change in ability to eat, crying.

risk for Infection [transmission]: risk factors may include insufficient knowledge to avoid exposure to or transmission of pathogen.

Stress disorder, acute   **PSY**

Refer to Posttraumatic stress disorder

Substance dependence/abuse, prenatal   **OB**

imbalanced Nutrition: less than body requirements may be related to insufficient dietary intake to meet metabolic needs, inadequate or improper use of financial resources, possibly low-weight gain, decreased subcutaneous fat and muscle mass, reported altered taste sensation, lack of interest in food, protein or vitamin deficiencies.

risk for disturbed Maternal/Fetal Dyad: risk factors may include alcohol or drug use, treatment related side effects.

ineffective Denial/Coping may be related to personal vulnerability, difficulty handling new situations, use of drugs for coping, inadequate support systems, possibly evidenced by denial, lack of acceptance of consequences of drug use, manipulation to avoid responsibility for self, impaired adaptive behaviors.

Powerlessness may be related to substance addiction, episodic compulsive indulgence, failed attempts at recovery, lifestyle of helplessness, possibly evidenced by statements of inability to stop behavior, continuous thinking about drug, alterations in personal, occupational, and social life.

chronic low Self-Esteem may be related to social stigma attached to substance abuse, social expectation that one controls own behavior, continual negative evaluation of self, personal vulnerabilities, possibly evidenced by not taking responsibility for self, lack of follow-through, self-destructive behavior, denial that substance use is a problem.

compromised/disabled Family Coping may be related to codependency issues, situational crisis of pregnancy and drug abuse, family disorganization, exhausted supportive capacity of family members, possibly evidenced by denial or belief that all problems are due to substance use, financial difficulties, severely dysfunctional family, codependent behaviors.

Substance dependence/abuse rehabilitation   PSY/CH
(Following acute detoxification)

ineffective Denial may be related to threat of unpleasant reality, lack of emotional support from others, overwhelming stress, possibly evidenced by lack of acceptance that drug use is causing the present situation, delay in seeking or refusal of healthcare attention to the detriment of health, use of manipulation to avoid responsibility for self, projection of blame or responsibility for problems.

Powerlessness may be related to substance addiction with/without periods of abstinence, episodic compulsive indulgence, attempts at recovery, and lifestyle of helplessness, possibly evidenced by ineffective recovery attempts, statements of inability to stop behavior, requests for help, constantly thinking about drug or obtaining drug, alteration in personal, occupational, or social life.

imbalanced Nutrition: less than body requirements may be related to insufficient dietary intake to meet metabolic needs for psychological, physiological, or economical reasons, possibly evidenced by weight less than normal for height and body build, decreased subcutaneous fat and muscle mass, reported altered taste sensation, lack of interest in food, poor muscle tone, sore and inflamed buccal cavity, laboratory evidence of protein or vitamin deficiencies.

Sexual Dysfunction may be related to altered body function (neurological damage and debilitating effects of drug use), changes in appearance, possibly evidenced by progressive interference with sexual functioning; a significant degree of testicular atrophy, gynecomastia, impotence and decreased sperm counts in men; and loss of body hair, thin soft skin, spider angiomas, and amenorrhea and increase in miscarriages in women.

dysfunctional Family Processes may be related to abuse, history of alcoholism or drug use, inadequate coping skills, lack of problem-solving skills, genetic predisposition or biochemical influences, possibly evidenced by feelings of anger, frustration, responsibility for alcoholic's behavior, suppressed rage, shame, embarrassment, repressed emotions, guilt, vulnerability, disturbed family dynamics, deterioration in family relationships, family denial or rationalization, closed communication systems, triangulating family relationships, manipulation, blaming, enabling to maintain substance use, inability to accept or receive help.

OB

risk for fetal Injury: risk factors may include drug or alcohol use, exposure to teratogens.

deficient Knowledge [Learning Need] regarding condition, effects on pregnancy, prognosis, and treatment needs may be related to lack or misinterpretation of information, lack of recall, cognitive limitations, interference with learning, possibly evidenced by statements of concern, questions, misconceptions, inaccurate follow-through of instructions, development of preventable complications, continued use in spite of complications.

Sudden infant death syndrome   PED

complicated Grieving may be related to unexpected loss of child, lack of anticipatory grieving, possibly evidenced by expressions of distress, guilt, anger; idealization of child, reliving past with little reduction of intensity of grief, labile affect, crying, prolonged interference with life functioning, withdrawal.

risk for impaired Parenting: risk factors may include recent crisis, change in family unit, maladaptive coping strategies, sleep disruption, depression.

risk for interrupted Family Processes: risk factors may include situational crisis, loss of a family member.

risk for chronic Sorrow: risk factors may include death of a loved one, anniversary dates (birth, death, etc.), trigger events (e.g., infants on TV, at play).

Suicide attempt   MS
Also refer to specific means, e.g., Drug overdose, acute; Wound, gunshot

                                                                 PSY

Hopelessness may be related to long-term stress, abandonment (actual or perceived), deteriorating physical or mental condition, challenged value or belief system, possibly evidenced by verbal cues, passivity, lack of involvement or withdrawal, angry outbursts.

risk for Suicide: risk factors may include prior or current attempt, marked changes in behavior, attitude, or performance, impulsiveness, sudden euphoric recovery from major depression, living alone, loss of independence, economic instability, substance abuse, has a plan and available means.

chronic/situational low Self-Esteem may be related to losses, functional impairment, developmental changes, failures or rejection, possibly evidenced by evaluating self as unable to deal with events, expressions of helplessness, uselessness, shame, or guilt; self-negating verbalizations.

compromised family Coping may be related to temporary family disorganization, role changes, prolonged disease or disability, situational or developmental crises, possibly evidenced by client expressing concern about SO's response to problems, SO confirms ineffective supportive behaviors, SO withdraws from client at the time of need.

Sunstroke   MS
Refer to Heatstroke

Surgery, general   MS
Also refer to Postoperative recovery period

deficient Knowledge [Learning Need] regarding surgical procedure and expectation, postoperative routines, therapy, and self-care needs may be related to lack of information, misinterpretation, possibly evidenced by statements of concern, questions, and misconceptions.

Anxiety [specify level]/Fear may be related to situational crisis, unfamiliarity with environment, change in health status or threat of death and separation from usual support systems, possibly evidenced by increased tension, apprehension, decreased self-assurance, fear of unspecific consequences, focus on self, sympathetic stimulation, and restlessness.

risk for perioperative-positioning Injury: risk factors may include disorientation, immobilization, muscle weakness, obesity, edema.

risk for Injury: risk factors may include wrong client, procedure, site, implants, equipment or materials; interactive conditions between individual and environment; external environment—physical design, structure of environment, exposure to equipment, instrumentation, positioning, use of pharmaceutical agents; internal environment—tissue hypoxia, abnormal blood profile or altered clotting factors, broken skin.

risk for imbalanced Fluid Volume: risk factors may include preoperative fluid deprivation, blood loss, and excessive gastrointestinal losses—vomiting or gastric suction; inappropriate or rapid replacement.

Syndrome X   CH
Refer to Metabolic syndrome

Synovitis (knee)   CH
acute Pain may be related to inflammation of synovial membrane of the joint with effusion, possibly evidenced by verbal reports, guarding or distraction behaviors, self-focus, and changes in vital signs.

impaired Walking may be related to pain and decreased strength of joint, possibly evidenced by reluctance to attempt movement, inability to move about environment as desired.

Syphilis, congenital   PED
Also refer to Sexually transmitted disease

acute Pain may be related to inflammatory process, edema formation, and development of skin lesions, possibly evidenced by irritability or crying that may be increased with movement of extremities and autonomic responses (changes in vital signs).

impaired Skin/Tissue Integrity may be related to exposure to pathogens during vaginal delivery, possibly evidenced by disruption of skin surfaces and rhinitis.

delayed Growth and Development may be related to effect of infectious process, possibly evidenced by altered physical growth and delay or difficulty performing skills typical of age group.

deficient Knowledge [Learning Need] regarding pathophysiology of condition, transmissibility, therapy needs, expected outcomes, and potential complications may be related to caretaker/parental lack of information, misinterpretation, possibly evidenced by statements of concern, questions, and misconceptions.

Syringomyelia   MS
disturbed Sensory Perception (specify) may be related to altered sensory perception (neurological lesion), possibly evidenced by change in usual response to stimuli and motor incoordination.

Anxiety [specify level]/Fear may be related to change in health status, threat of change in role functioning and socioeconomic status, and threat to self-concept, possibly evidenced by increased tension, apprehension, uncertainty, focus on self, and expressed concerns.

impaired physical Mobility may be related to neuromuscular and sensory impairment, possibly evidenced by decreased muscle strength, control, and mass; and impaired coordination.

Self-Care Deficit [specify] may be related to neuromuscular and sensory impairments, possibly evidenced by statement of inability to perform care tasks.

Tarsal tunnel syndrome   CH
acute/chronic Pain may be related to pressure on posterior tibial nerve at ankle, possibly evidenced by verbal reports, reluctance to use affected extremity, guarding behaviors, expressed fear of reinjury, altered ability to continue previous activities.

impaired Walking may be related to neuromuscular impairment and increased pain with walking, possibly evidenced by inability to walk desired distances, climb stairs, navigate curbs or uneven surfaces.

Tay-Sachs disease   PED

delayed Growth and Development may be related to effects of physical condition, possibly evidenced by altered physical growth, loss of or failure to acquire skills typical of age, flat affect, and decreased responses.

disturbed visual Sensory Perception may be related to neurological deterioration of optic nerve, possibly evidenced by loss of visual acuity.

CH

family Grieving may be related to expected eventual loss of infant/child, possibly evidenced by expressions of distress, denial, guilt, anger, and sorrow; choked feelings; changes in sleep or eating habits; and altered libido.

family Powerlessness may be related to absence of therapeutic interventions for progressive and fatal disease, possibly evidenced by verbal expressions of having no control over situation or outcome, and depression over physical and mental deterioration.

risk for Spiritual Distress: risk factors may include challenged belief and value system by presence of fatal condition with racial or religious connotations and intense suffering.

compromised family Coping may be related to situational crisis; temporary preoccupation with managing emotional conflicts and personal suffering; family disorganization; and prolonged, progressive disease, possibly evidenced by preoccupations with personal reactions, expressed concern about reactions of other family members, inadequate support of one another, and altered communication patterns.

TBI   MS/CH
Refer to Traumatic brain injury

Temporal arteritis   CH
acute Pain may be related to arterial inflammation, possibly evidenced by reports of severe headache, scalp tenderness, pain with chewing, myalgia.

risk for disturbed visual Sensory Perception: risk factors may include altered reception (arterial inflammation, ischemic optic neuropathy).

risk for ineffective self Health Management: risk factors may include medication side effects, economic difficulties, perceived seriousness or benefits.

Temporomandibular joint syndrome   CH
chronic Pain may be related to pressure on nerves, possibly evidenced by reports of pain in temporomandibular joint area worsened with chewing, muscle tension headache.

risk for imbalanced Nutrition: less than body requirements: risk factors may include inability to ingest food (pain worsened by chewing, limited movement of joint).

risk for disturbed auditory Sensory Perception: risk factors may include altered sensory reception (tinnitus, occasional deafness).

Tendonitis   CH
acute/chronic Pain may be related to inflammation, swelling of tendon, possibly evidenced by verbal reports, guarding or protective behavior, fear of reinjury, altered ability to continue previous activities.

impaired physical Mobility may be related to pain, joint stiffness, musculoskeletal impairment, prescribed movement restrictions, possibly evidenced by limited range of motion, limited ability to perform fine or gross motor skills.

risk for ineffective Role Performance: risk factors may include health alterations, fatigue, pain.

Health Conditions and Client Concerns With Associated Nursing Diagnoses   **1087**

Testicular cancer   MS

Also refer to Cancer

disturbed Body Image may be related to surgical change in reproductive organs, loss of hair and weight, possibly evidenced by negative feelings about body and sense of mutilation, preoccupation with change, feelings of helplessness or hopelessness, and change in social environment.

Sexual Dysfunction may be related to change in sexual organs, postoperative impotence, vulnerability, possibly evidenced by verbalizations of problem, inability in achieving desired satisfaction, alterations in relationships.

Tetraplegia   MS/CH

Refer to Quadriplegia

Thoracotomy   MS

Refer to Surgery, general; Hemothorax

Thrombophlebitis   CH/MS/OB

ineffective peripheral tissue Perfusion may be related to interruption of venous blood flow, venous stasis, possibly evidenced by changes in skin color and temperature over affected area, development of edema, pain, diminished peripheral pulses, slow capillary refill.

acute Pain/impaired Comfort may be related to vascular inflammation and irritation, and edema formation (accumulation of lactic acid), possibly evidenced by verbal reports, guarding or distraction behaviors, restlessness, and self-focus.

Anxiety [specify level] may be related to change in health status, perceived or actual threat to self, situational crisis, interpersonal transmission, possibly evidenced by increased tension, apprehension, restlessness, sympathetic stimulation.

risk for impaired physical Mobility: risk factors may include pain and discomfort and restrictive therapies and safety precautions.

deficient Knowledge [Learning Need] regarding pathophysiology of condition, therapy, self-care needs, and risk of embolization may be related to lack of information or misinterpretation, possibly evidenced by statements of concern, questions, inaccurate follow-through of instructions, and development of preventable complications.

Thrombosis, venous   MS

Refer to Thrombophlebitis

Thrush   CH

impaired Oral Mucous Membrane may be related to presence of infection as evidenced by white patches or plaques, oral discomfort, mucosal irritation, bleeding.

risk for imbalanced Nutrition: less than body requirements: risk factors may include inability to ingest adequate amount of nutrients (oral pain).

Thyroidectomy   MS

Also refer to Hyperthyroidism; Hypoparathyroidism, Hypothyroidism

risk for ineffective Airway Clearance: risk factors may include tracheal obstruction—edema, hematoma formation, laryngeal spasms.

impaired verbal Communication may be related to tissue edema, pain or discomfort, and vocal cord injury or laryngeal nerve damage, possibly evidenced by impaired articulation, does not or cannot speak, and use of nonverbal cues or gestures.

risk for Injury [tetany]: risk factors may include chemical imbalance—hypocalcemia, increased release of thyroid hormones; excessive central nervous system stimulation.

risk for head/neck Trauma: risk factors may include loss of muscle control and support, and position of suture line.

acute Pain may be related to presence of surgical incision, manipulation of tissues and muscles, postoperative edema, possibly evidenced by verbal reports, guarding or distraction behaviors, narrowed focus, and autonomic responses—changes in vital signs.

Thyrotoxicosis   MS
Also refer to Hyperthyroidism

risk for decreased Cardiac Output: risk factors may include uncontrolled hypermetabolic state increasing cardiac workload; changes in venous return and systemic vascular resistance; and alterations in rate, rhythm, and electrical conduction.

Anxiety [specific level] may be related to physiological factors and central nervous system stimulation (hypermetabolic state and pseudocatecholamine effect of thyroid hormones), possibly evidenced by increased feelings of apprehension, shakiness, loss of control, panic, changes in cognition, distortion of environmental stimuli, extraneous movements, restlessness, and tremors.

risk for disturbed Thought Processes: risk factors may include physiological changes—increased central nervous system stimulation, accelerated mental activity; and altered sleep patterns.

deficient Knowledge [Learning Needs] regarding condition, treatment needs, and potential for complications or crisis situation may be related to lack of information or recall, misinterpretation, possibly evidenced by statements of concern, questions, misconceptions, and inaccurate follow-through of instructions.

TIA   CH
Refer to Transient ischemic attack

Tic douloureux   CH
Refer to Neuralgia, trigeminal

TMJ syndrome   CH
Refer to Temporomandibular joint syndrome

Tonsillectomy   PED/MS
Refer to Adenoidectomy

Tonsillitis   PED
acute Pain may be related to inflammation of tonsils and effects of circulating toxins, possibly evidenced by verbal reports, guarding or distraction behaviors, reluctance/refusal to swallow, self-focus, and changes in vital signs.

Hyperthermia may be related to presence of inflammatory process, hypermetabolic state and dehydration, possibly evidenced by increased body temperature; warm, flushed skin; and tachycardia.

deficient Knowledge [Learning Need] regarding cause/transmission, treatment needs, and potential complications may be related to lack of information, misinterpretation, possibly evidenced by statements of concern, questions, inaccurate follow-through of instructions, and recurrence of condition.

Total joint replacement   MS
risk for Infection: risk factors may include inadequate primary defenses (broken skin, exposure of joint), inadequate secondary defenses or immunosuppression (long-term corticosteroid use),

invasive procedures and surgical manipulation, implantation of foreign body, and decreased mobility.

impaired physical Mobility may be related to pain and discomfort, musculoskeletal impairment, and surgery and restrictive therapies, possibly evidenced by reluctance to attempt movement, difficulty with purposefully moving within the physical environment, reports of pain or discomfort on movement, limited range of motion, and decreased muscle strength and control.

risk for ineffective peripheral tissue Perfusion: risk factors may include reduced arterial or venous blood flow, direct trauma to blood vessels, tissue edema, improper location or dislocation of prosthesis, and hypovolemia.

acute Pain may be related to physical agents (traumatized tissues, surgical intervention, degeneration of joints, muscle spasms) and psychological factors (anxiety, advanced age), possibly evidenced by verbal reports, guarding or distraction behaviors, self-focus, and changes in vital signs.

risk for Constipation: risk factors may include insufficient physical activity, decreased mobility, weakness, insufficient fiber or fluid intake, dehydration, poor eating habits, decreased gastrointestinal motility, effects of medications—anesthesia, opiate analgesics; environmental changes, inadequate toileting.

Tourette's syndrome   CH

chronic low Self-Esteem may be related to inherited disorder, continual negative evaluation of self and capabilities, personal vulnerability, possibly evidenced by self-negating verbalizations, expressed shame, exaggerated negative feedback about self, hesitancy to try new situations.

Social Isolation may be related to unaccepted social behaviors, inability to engage in satisfying personal relationships, rejection or ridicule by others.

risk for Injury: risk factors may include adverse side effects of medications, negative response of uneducated individuals.

Toxemia of pregnancy   OB

Refer to Pregnancy-induced hypertension

Toxic enterocolitis   PED/MS

Also refer to Colostomy

deficient Fluid Volume may be related to fulminating losses into the bowel, diarrhea, lack of intake evidenced by decreased concentrated urine, dry mucous membranes, poor skin turgor, decreased venous filling, change in mentation.

risk for decreased Cardiac Output: risk factors may include decreased venous return, altered heart rate and rhythm.

Toxic megacolon   MS

Refer to Toxic enterocolitis

Toxic shock syndrome   MS

Also refer to Sepsis

Hyperthermia may be related to inflammatory process, hypermetabolic state and dehydration, possibly evidenced by increased body temperature; warm, flushed skin; and tachycardia.

deficient Fluid Volume [isotonic] may be related to increased gastric losses (diarrhea, vomiting), fever, hypermetabolic state, and decreased intake, possibly evidenced by dry mucous membranes, increased pulse, hypotension, delayed venous filling, decreased concentrated urine, and hemoconcentration.

acute Pain may be related to inflammatory process, effects of circulating toxins, and skin disruptions, possibly evidenced by verbal reports, guarding or distraction behaviors, self-focus, and changes in vital signs.

impaired Skin/Tissue Integrity may be related to effects of circulating toxins and dehydration, possibly evidenced by development of desquamating rash, hyperemia, and inflammation of mucous membranes.

Traction   MS
Also refer to Casts; Fractures

acute Pain may be related to direct trauma to tissue and bone, muscle spasms, movement of bone fragments, edema, injury to soft tissue, traction or immobility device, anxiety, possibly evidenced by verbal reports, guarding or distraction behaviors, self-focus, alteration in muscle tone, and changes in vital signs.

impaired physical Mobility may be related to neuromuscular and skeletal impairment, pain, psychological immobility, and therapeutic restrictions of movement, possibly evidenced by limited range of motion, inability to move purposefully in environment, reluctance to attempt movement, and decreased muscle strength and control.

risk for Infection: risk factors may include invasive procedures (including insertion of foreign body through skin and bone), presence of traumatized tissue, and reduced activity with stasis of body fluids.

deficient Diversional Activity may be related to length of hospitalization or therapeutic intervention and environmental lack of usual activity, possibly evidenced by statements of boredom, restlessness, and irritability.

Transfusion reaction, blood   MS
Also refer to Anaphylaxis

risk for imbalanced Body Temperature: risk factors may include infusion of cold blood products, systemic response to toxins.

Anxiety [specify level] may be related to change in health status and threat of death, exposure to toxins, possibly evidenced by increased tension, apprehension, sympathetic stimulation, restlessness, and expressions of concern.

risk for impaired Skin Integrity: risk factors may include immunological response.

Transient ischemic attack   CH
ineffective cerebral tissue Perfusion may be related to interruption of blood flow (e.g., vasospasm), possibly evidenced by altered mental status, behavioral changes, language deficit, change in motor and sensory response.

Anxiety [specify level]/Fear may be related to change in health status, threat to self-concept, situational crisis, interpersonal contagion, possibly evidenced by expressed concerns, apprehension, restlessness, irritability.

risk for ineffective Denial: risk factors may include change in health status requiring change in lifestyle, fear of consequences, lack of motivation.

Transplant, living donor   MS
Also refer to Surgery, general; Nephrectomy

decisional Conflict may be related to multiple or divergent sources of information, family system (demands, expectations, or responsibilities to others), risk to self, possibly evidenced by verbalized uncertainty about choices, questioning personal values or beliefs, delayed decision making, increased tension.

[moderate to severe] Anxiety/Fear may be related to situational crisis, unconscious conflict about essential beliefs or values, familial association, threat to health status or death, possibly evidenced by expressed concerns, apprehension, uncertainty, increased tension, fear of failing family member (e.g., organ rejection), sympathetic stimulation.

Health Conditions and Client Concerns With Associated Nursing Diagnoses   **1091**

Transplantation, recipient   MS

Also refer to Surgery, general; Cardiac surgery

Anxiety [specify level]/Fear may be related to unconscious conflict about essential values/ beliefs, situational crisis, interpersonal contagion, threat to self-concept, threat of organ rejection or death, side effects of medication, possibly evidenced by increased tension, apprehension, uncertainty, expressed concerns, somatic complaints, sympathetic stimulation, insomnia.

risk for Infection: risk factors may include medically induced immunosuppression, suppressed inflammatory response, antibiotic therapy, invasive procedures, broken skin and traumatized tissue, effects of chronic and debilitating disease.

(Refer to specific conditions relative to compromise or failure of individual transplanted organ, e.g., Renal failure, acute; Heart failure, chronic; Pancreatitis.)

CH

ineffective Coping/compromised family Coping may be related to situational crisis, high degree of threat, uncertainty, family disorganization or role changes, prolonged disease exhausting supportive capacity of family/SO, possibly evidenced by verbalizations, sleep disturbance, fatigue, poor concentration, protective behaviors disproportionate to client's needs, SO describes preoccupation with personal reaction.

risk for ineffective Protection: risk factors may include drug therapies, compromised immune system, effects of debilitating disease.

readiness for enhanced self Health Management may be related to desire to live life more fully, engage in healthy lifestyle, possibly evidenced by expressed desire to manage treatment and prevention of sequelae, reduction of risk factors, no unexpected sequelae.

risk for ineffective self Health Management: risk factors may include complexity of therapeutic regimen and healthcare system, economic difficulties, family patterns of healthcare.

Transurethral resection of prostate   MS

Refer to Prostatectomy

Traumatic brain injury (TBI)   MS

ineffective cerebral tissue Perfusion may be related to interruption of blood flow—hemorrhage, hematoma, cerebral edema (localized or generalized response to injury, metabolic alterations, drug or alcohol overdose), decreased systemic blood pressure—hypovolemia, cardiac dysrhythmias; hypoxia, possibly evidenced by altered level of consciousness, memory loss, changes in motor or sensory responses, restlessness, changes in vital signs.

risk for decreased Intracranial Adaptive Capacity: risk factors may include brain injuries, systemic hypotension with intracranial hypertension.

risk for ineffective Breathing Pattern: risk factors may include neuromuscular dysfunction—injury to respiratory center of brain; perception or cognitive impairment, tracheobronchial obstruction.

disturbed Sensory Perception (specify) may be related to altered sensory reception, transmission or integration (neurological trauma or deficit), possibly evidenced by disorientation to time, place, person; motor incoordination; altered communication patterns; restlessness or irritability; change in behavior pattern.

risk for Infection: risk factors may include traumatized tissues, broken skin, invasive procedures, decreased ciliary action, stasis of body fluids, nutritional deficits, suppressed inflammatory response—steroid use; altered integrity of closed system—cerebrospinal fluid leak.

risk for imbalanced Nutrition: less than body requirements: risk factors may include altered ability to ingest nutrients—decreased level of consciousness; weakness of muscles for chewing or swallowing, hypermetabolic state.

impaired physical Mobility may be related to perceptual or cognitive impairment, decreased strength or endurance, restrictive therapies, safety precautions, possibly evidenced by inability to purposefully move within physical environment—including bed mobility, transfer, ambulation, impaired coordination, limited range of motion, decreased muscle strength and control.

disturbed Thought Processes may be related to physiological changes, psychological conflicts, possibly evidenced by memory deficits, distractibility, altered attention span or concentration, disorientation to time, place, person, circumstances, or events; impaired ability to make decisions, problem-solve, reason or conceptualize; personality changes.

interrupted Family Processes may be related to situational transition and crisis, uncertainty about ultimate outcome and expectations, possibly evidenced by difficulty adapting to change, family not meeting needs of all members, difficulty accepting/receiving help, inability to express or to accept feelings of members.

Self-Care Deficit (specify) may be related to neuromuscular or musculoskeletal impairment, weakness, pain, perceptual or cognitive impairment, possibly evidenced by inability to perform desired or appropriate activities of daily living.

Trench foot   MS
Refer to Immersion foot

Trichinosis   CH
acute Pain may be related to parasitic invasion of muscle tissues, edema of upper eyelids, small localized hemorrhages, and development of urticaria, possibly evidenced by verbal reports, guarding/distraction behaviors (restlessness), and changes in vital signs.

deficient Fluid Volume [isotonic] may be related to hypermetabolic state (fever, diaphoresis); excessive gastric losses (vomiting, diarrhea); and decreased intake and difficulty swallowing, possibly evidenced by dry mucous membranes, decreased skin turgor, hypotension, decreased venous filling, decreased concentrated urine, and hemoconcentration.

ineffective Breathing Pattern may be related to myositis of the diaphragm and intercostal muscles, possibly evidenced by resulting changes in respiratory depth, tachypnea, dyspnea, and abnormal arterial blood gases.

deficient Knowledge [Learning Need] regarding cause, prevention of condition, therapy needs, and possible complications may be related to lack of information, misinterpretation, possibly evidenced by statements of concern, questions, and misconceptions.

Tricuspid insufficiency   CH
Refer to Valvular heart disease

Tricuspid stenosis   CH
Refer to Valvular heart disease

Tubal pregnancy   OB
Refer to Ectopic pregnancy

Tuberculosis (pulmonary)   CH
risk for Infection [spread/reactivation]: risk factors may include inadequate primary defenses (decreased ciliary action, stasis of secretions, tissue destruction and extension of infection), lowered resistance or suppressed inflammatory response, malnutrition, environmental exposure, insufficient knowledge to avoid exposure to pathogens, or inadequate therapeutic intervention.

ineffective Airway Clearance may be related to thick, viscous, or bloody secretions; fatigue with poor cough effort; and tracheal or pharyngeal edema, possibly evidenced by abnormal respiratory rate, rhythm, and depth; adventitious breath sounds—rhonchi, wheezes; stridor and dyspnea.

  risk for impaired Gas Exchange: risk factors may include decrease in effective lung surface; atelectasis; destruction of alveolar-capillary membrane; bronchial edema; thick, viscous secretions.

  Activity Intolerance may be related to imbalance between oxygen supply and demand, possibly evidenced by reports of fatigue, weakness, and exertional dyspnea.

  imbalanced Nutrition: less than body requirements may be related to inability to ingest adequate nutrients (anorexia, effects of drug therapy, fatigue, insufficient financial resources), possibly evidenced by weight loss, reported lack of interest in food or altered taste sensation, and poor muscle tone.

  risk for ineffective self Health Management: risk factors may include complexity of therapeutic regimen, economic difficulties, family patterns of healthcare, perceived seriousness or benefits (especially during remission), side effects of therapy.

TURP   MS
Refer to Prostatectomy

Twin-twin transfusion syndrome   OB
decreased Cardiac Output may be related to altered preload (hypovolemia, anemia) to donor fetus, possibly evidenced by oliguria, oligohydramnios.

  excess Fluid Volume may be related to excess fluid intake (shunting of circulation) to recipient fetus, possibly evidenced by polyuria, polyhydramnios.

  risk for disproportionate Growth: risk factors may include multiple gestation with imbalanced circulation and nutrition to both fetus.

Tympanoplasty   MS
Refer to Stapedectomy

Typhoid fever   MS
Also refer to Sepsis

  risk for Infection [spread]: risk factors may include presence of bacteria in excretions, inadequate knowledge to avoid exposure to pathogen (food or water, fecally contaminated objects).

  risk for deficient Fluid Volume [isotonic]: risk factors may include gastric irritation, ulcers.

  imbalanced Nutrition: less than body requirements: risk factors may include inability to ingest, digest, or absorb nutrients; hypermetabolic state, possibly evidenced by anorexia, abdominal pain, weight loss.

Typhus   CH/MS
Hyperthermia may be related to generalized inflammatory process (vasculitis), possibly evidenced by increased body temperature, warm flushed skin, and tachycardia.

  acute Pain may be related to generalized vasculitis and edema formation, possibly evidenced by verbal reports, guarding or distraction behaviors, self-focus, and autonomic responses (changes in vital signs).

  ineffective tissue Perfusion (specify) may be related to reduction or interruption of blood flow—generalized vasculitis or thrombi formation, possibly evidenced by reports of headache, abdominal pain, changes in mentation, and areas of peripheral ulceration or necrosis.

Ulcer, decubitus   CH/MS
impaired Skin/Tissue Integrity may be related to altered circulation, nutritional deficit, fluid imbalance, impaired physical mobility, irritation of body excretions or secretions, and sensory impairments, evidenced by tissue damage or destruction.

acute Pain may be related to destruction of protective skin layers and exposure of nerves, possibly evidenced by verbal reports, distraction behaviors, and self-focus.

risk for Infection: risk factors may include broken or traumatized tissue, increased environmental exposure, and nutritional deficits.

Ulcer, peptic (acute)   MS/CH

risk for Shock: risk factors may include hypovolemia, hypotension

Fear/Anxiety [specify level] may be related to change in health status and threat of death, possibly evidenced by increased tension, restlessness, irritability, fearfulness, trembling, tachycardia, diaphoresis, lack of eye contact, focus on self, verbalization of concerns, withdrawal, and panic or attack behavior.

acute Pain may be related to caustic irritation and destruction of gastric tissues, reflex muscle spasms in stomach wall, possibly evidenced by verbal reports, distraction behaviors, self-focus, and changes in vital signs.

deficient Knowledge [Learning Need] regarding condition, therapy, self-care needs, and potential complications may be related to lack of information or recall, misinterpretation, possibly evidenced by statements of concern, questions, misconceptions; inaccurate follow-through of instructions; and development of preventable complications or recurrence of condition.

Ulcer, pressure   CH/MS

Refer to Ulcer, decubitus

Ulcer, venous stasis   CH

Also refer to Venous insufficiency

impaired Skin/Tissue Integrity may be related to altered venous circulation, edema formation, inflammation, decreased sensation, possibly evidenced by destruction of skin layers, invasion of body structures.

decreased peripheral tissue Perfusion may be related to interruption of venous flow—small-vessel vasoconstrictive reflex, possibly evidenced by skin discoloration, edema formation, altered sensation, delayed healing.

Ulnar neuropathy   CH

Refer to Cubital tunnel syndrome

Unconsciousness   MS

Refer to Coma

Upper GI bleeding   MS

Refer to Gastritis, acute or chronic; Ulcer, peptic

Urinary diversion   MS/CH

risk for impaired Skin Integrity: risk factors may include absence of sphincter at stoma, character and flow of urine from stoma, reaction to product or chemicals, and improperly fitting appliance or removal of adhesive.

disturbed Body Image related factors may include biophysical factors—presence of stoma, loss of control of urine flow; and psychosocial factors—altered body structure, disease process and associated treatment regimen, such as cancer, possibly evidenced by verbalization of change in body image, fear of rejection or reaction of others, negative feelings about body, not touching or looking at stoma, refusal to participate in care.

acute Pain may be related to physical factors—disruption of skin and tissues, presence of incisions and drains; biological factors—activity of disease process, such as cancer, trauma;

and psychological factors—fear, anxiety, possibly evidenced by verbal reports, self-focusing, guarding or distraction behaviors, restlessness, and autonomic responses—changes in vital signs.

impaired Urinary Elimination may be related to surgical diversion, tissue trauma, and postoperative edema, possibly evidenced by loss of continence, changes in amount and character of urine, and urinary retention.

Urinary tract infection   **CH**
Refer to Cystitis

Urolithiasis   **MS/CH**
Refer to Calculi, urinary

Uterine bleeding, dysfunctional   **GYN/MS**
Anxiety [specify level] may be related to perceived change in health status and unknown etiology, possibly evidenced by apprehension, uncertainty, fear of unspecified consequences, expressed concerns, and focus on self.

Activity Intolerance may be related to imbalance between oxygen supply and demand, decreased oxygen-carrying capacity of blood (anemia), possibly evidenced by reports of fatigue, weakness.

Uterine myomas   **GYN**
Also refer to Anemia

acute Pain/impaired Comfort may be related to growth, size, and degeneration or twisting of tumors, possibly evidenced by reports of pressure, cramping, guarding behavior, irritability.

impaired Urinary Elimination may be related to uterine pressure on bladder, possibly evidenced by frequency, urgency.

risk for deficient Fluid Volume: risk factors may include excessive or chronic blood loss.

Uterus, rupture of, in pregnancy   **OB**
risk for Shock: risk factors may include hypovolemia, hypotension.

acute Pain may be related to tissue trauma and irritation of accumulating blood, possibly evidenced by verbal reports, guarding or distraction behaviors, self-focus, and autonomic responses—changes in vital signs.

Anxiety [specify level] may be related to threat of death of self/fetus, interpersonal contagion, physiological response—release of catecholamines, possibly evidenced by fearful or scared affect, sympathetic stimulation, stated fear of unspecified consequences, and expressed concerns.

UTI   **CH**
Refer to Cystitis

Vaginal hysterectomy   **MS**
Refer to Hysterectomy

Vaginismus   **GYN/PSY**
acute Pain may be related to muscle spasm and hyperesthesia of the nerve supply to vaginal mucous membrane, possibly evidenced by verbal reports, distraction behaviors, and self-focus.

Sexual Dysfunction may be related to physical or psychological alteration in function (severe spasms of vaginal muscles), possibly evidenced by verbalization of problem, inability to achieve desired satisfaction, and alteration in relationship with SO.

Vaginitis   GYN/CH

impaired Tissue Integrity may be related to irritation or inflammation and mechanical trauma (scratching) of sensitive tissues, possibly evidenced by damaged or destroyed tissue, presence of lesions.

acute Pain may be related to localized inflammation and tissue trauma, possibly evidenced by verbal reports, distraction behaviors, and self-focus.

deficient Knowledge [Learning Need] regarding hygienic needs, therapy, and sexual behaviors or transmission of organisms may be related to lack of information, misinterpretation, possibly evidenced by statements of concern, questions, and misconceptions.

Vaginosis, bacterial   GYN

risk for impaired Tissue Integrity: risk factors may include vulvar or vaginal irritation, itching.

risk for [secondary] Infection: risk factors may include prescribed antibiotic therapy, insufficient knowledge to avoid exposure to pathogens.

Valvular heart disease   MS

decreased Cardiac Output may be related to alteration in preload, increased arterial pressure and venous congestion, increased afterload, changes in electrical conduction, possibly evidenced by variations in hemodynamic parameters, dysrhythmias and electrocardiogram changes, dyspnea, adventitious breath sounds, cyanosis or pallor, jugular vein distention, fatigue.

Activity Intolerance may be related to imbalance between oxygen supply and demand (decreased or fixed cardiac output), possibly evidenced by reports of fatigue, weakness, abnormal heart rate and blood pressure in response to activity, exertional discomfort or dyspnea.

Anxiety may be related to threat to or change in health status (chronicity of disease), physiological effects, situational crisis (changes in lifestyle, hospitalization), possibly evidenced by expressed concerns, increased tension, apprehension, uncertainty, sympathetic stimulation, insomnia.

risk for excess Fluid Volume: risk factors may include increased sodium and water retention, changes in glomerular filtration.

risk for ineffective tissue Perfusion (specify): risk factors may include interruption of arterial-venous flow (systemic emboli), venous thrombosis (venous stasis, decreased activity).

VAP   MS/CH

Refer to Ventilator assist/dependence; Bronchopneumonia

Varices, esophageal   MS

Also refer to Ulcer, peptic [acute]

risk for Bleeding/deficient Fluid Volume [isotonic]: risk factors may include presence of varices, reduced intake, and gastric losses—vomiting; vascular loss.

Anxiety [specify level]/Fear may be related to change in health status and threat of death, possibly evidenced by increased tension, apprehension, sympathetic stimulation, restlessness, focus on self, and expressed concerns.

Varicose veins   CH

chronic Pain may be related to venous insufficiency and stasis, possibly evidenced by verbal reports.

disturbed Body Image may be related to change in structure (presence of enlarged, discolored tortuous superficial leg veins), possibly evidenced by hiding affected parts and negative feelings about body.

---

risk for impaired Skin/Tissue Integrity: risk factors may include altered circulation, venous stasis and edema formation.

Varicose veins ligation/stripping   MS

risk for ineffective peripheral tissue Perfusion: risk factors may include localized edema, vascular irritation, inadequate venous return, dressings.

impaired Skin Integrity may be related to surgical procedure, pressure dressings, tissue edema, vascular engorgement, possibly evidenced by incisions, development of complications (e.g., ulcerations).

Varicose veins sclerotherapy   MS

risk for impaired Skin Integrity: risk factors may include pressure wraps, extravasation of sclerosing agent.

risk for ineffective self Health Management: risk factors may include perceived seriousness or benefit, required lifestyle and activity changes, postprocedure dressings.

Variola   MS
Refer to Smallpox

Vasculitis   CH
Refer to Polyarteritis nodosa; Temporal arteritis

Vasectomy   CH/MS

acute Pain/impaired Comfort may be related to manipulation of delicate tissues, edema/hematoma formation, possibly evidenced by verbal reports, guarding behavior, irritability.

deficient Knowledge [Learning Need] regarding self-care and future expectations (issues of reproduction, safety/sexually transmitted diseases) may be related to information misinterpretation, lack of recall, possibly evidenced by verbalizations, misconceptions, inaccurate follow-through of instructions.

Venereal disease   CH
Refer to Sexually transmitted disease

Venous insufficiency   CH
Also refer to Stasis dermatitis; Ulcer, venous stasis

chronic Pain/impaired Comfort may be related to altered venous circulation, edema formation, possibly evidenced by reports of aching, fullness, tiredness of lower extremities with activity.

risk for risk-prone health Behavior: risk factors may include health status requiring change in lifestyle, lack of motivation to change behaviors.

risk for ineffective self Health Management: risk factors may include economic difficulties, perceived seriousness or benefit, social support deficit.

Ventilator assist/dependence   MS/CH

ineffective Breathing Pattern/impaired spontaneous Ventilation may be related to neuromuscular dysfunction, respiratory muscle fatigue, spinal cord injury, hypoventilation syndrome, possibly evidenced by dyspnea, increased work of breathing/use of accessory muscles, reduced vital capacity and total lung volume, changes in respiratory rate, decreased PO_2/SaO_2, increased PCO_2.

ineffective Airway Clearance may be related to artificial airway in trachea, inability to or ineffective cough, possibly evidenced by changes in rate and depth of respirations, abnormal breath sounds, anxiety, restlessness, cyanosis.

impaired verbal Communication may be related to physical barrier (artificial airway), neuromuscular weakness or paralysis, possibly evidenced by inability to speak.

Fear/Anxiety [specify] may be related to situational crisis, threat to self-concept, threat of death or dependency on machine, change in health status, socioeconomic status, or role functioning; interpersonal transmission, possibly evidenced by increased muscle or facial tension, hypervigilance, restlessness, fearfulness, apprehension, expressed concerns, insomnia, negative self-talk.

risk for impaired Oral Mucous Membrane: risk factors may include inability to swallow oral fluids, decreased salivation, ineffective oral hygiene, presence of endotracheal tube in mouth.

risk for imbalanced Nutrition: less than body requirements: risk factors may include inability to ingest nutrients, increased metabolic demands.

risk for dysfunctional Ventilatory Weaning Response: risk factors may include limited or insufficient energy stores, sleep disturbance, pain or discomfort, perceived inability to wean, decreased motivation, inadequate support or adverse environment, history of ventilator dependence greater than 1 week or unsuccessful weaning attempts.

Ventricular fibrillation   MS
Also refer to Dysrhythmias

decreased Cardiac Output may be related to altered electrical conduction and reduced myocardial contractility, possibly evidenced by absence of measurable cardiac output, loss of consciousness, no palpable pulses.

Ventricular tachycardia   MS
Also refer to Dysrhythmias

risk for decreased Cardiac Output: risk factors may include altered electrical conduction and reduced myocardial contractility.

Vertigo   CH
disturbed kinesthetic Sensory Perception may be related to altered status of sensory organ (middle or inner ear), altered sensory integration, possibly evidenced by visual distortions, altered sense of balance, falls.

risk for Falls: risk factors may include presence of postural hypotension, acute illness, medications, substance abuse.

West Nile Fever   CH/MS
Hyperthermia may be related to infectious process, possibly evidenced by elevated body temperature, skin flushed and warm to touch, tachycardia, increased respiratory rate.

acute Pain may be related to infectious process, circulating toxins, possibly evidenced by reports of headache, myalgia, eye pain, abdominal discomfort.

risk for deficient Fluid Volume: risk factors may include hypermetabolic state, decreased intake, anorexia, nausea, losses from normal routes (vomiting, diarrhea).

risk for impaired Skin Integrity: risk factors may include hyperthermia, decreased fluid intake, alterations in skin turgor, bedrest, circulating toxins.

Whooping cough   PED
Refer to Pertussis

Wilms' tumor   PED
Also refer to Cancer; Chemotherapy

Anxiety [specify level]/Fear may be related to change in environment and interaction patterns with family members and threat of death with family transmission and contagion concerns, possibly evidenced by fearful/scared affect, distress, crying, insomnia, and sympathetic stimulation.

risk for Injury: risk factors may include nature of tumor (vascular, mushy with very thin covering) with increased danger of metastasis when manipulated.

interrupted Family Processes may be related to situational crisis of life-threatening illness, possibly evidenced by a family system that has difficulty meeting physical, emotional, and spiritual needs of its members, and inability to deal with traumatic experience effectively.

deficient Diversional Activity may be related to environmental lack of age-appropriate activity (including activity restrictions) and length of hospitalization or treatment, possibly evidenced by restlessness, crying, lethargy, and acting-out behavior.

Withdrawal, drugs/alcohol   CH/MS
Refer to Alcohol intoxication, acute; Drug overdose, acute; Drug withdrawal

Wound, gunshot   MS
(Depends on site and speed/character of bullet.)

risk for Bleeding/deficient Fluid Volume: risk factors may include trauma, vascular losses, restricted oral intake.

acute Pain may be related to destruction of tissue (including organ and musculoskeletal), surgical repair, and therapeutic interventions, possibly evidenced by verbal reports, guarding or distraction behaviors, self-focus, and changes in vital signs.

impaired Tissue Integrity may be related to mechanical factors—yaw of projectile and muzzle blast, possibly evidenced by damaged or destroyed tissue.

risk for Infection: risk factors may include tissue destruction and increased environmental exposure, invasive procedures, and decreased hemoglobin.

CH

risk for Post-Trauma Syndrome: risk factors may include nature of incident (catastrophic accident, assault, suicide attempt) and possibly injury or death of other(s) involved.

Zollinger-Ellison syndrome   MS/CH
Also refer to Ulcer, peptic

Diarrhea may be related to intestinal irritation—hypersecretion of gastric acid, possibly evidenced by at least three loose liquid stools per day, abdominal pain, change in bowel sounds.

risk for impaired Skin/Tissue Integrity: risk factors include frequent bowel movements, hyperacidity of liquid stools, esophageal regurgitation.

acute/chronic Pain may be related to acidic irritation of esophageal mucosa (GERD), muscle spasm, possibly evidenced by reports of heartburn, distraction behaviors.

risk for ineffective self Health Management: risk factors may include length of therapy, economic difficulties, perceived susceptibility.

Definitions of Taxonomy II Axes

AXIS 1 DIAGNOSTIC CONCEPT: The principal element or the fundamental and essential part, the root, of the diagnostic statement.

AXIS 2 SUBJECT OF THE DIAGNOSIS: The person(s) for whom a nursing diagnosis is determined. Values are:

Individual: A single human being distinct from others, a person.

Family: Two or more people having continuous or sustained relationships, perceiving reciprocal obligations, sensing common meaning, and sharing certain obligations toward others; related by blood and/or choice.

Group: A number of people with shared characteristics.

Community: A group of people living in the same locale under the same governance, such as neighborhoods, cities, census tracts. When the unit of care is not explicitly stated, it becomes the individual by default.

AXIS 3 JUDGMENT: A descriptor or modifier that limits or specifies the meaning of the diagnostic concept. Values are:

Complicated: Intricately involved, complex

Compromised: Damaged, made vulnerable-

Decreased: Lessened (in size, amount, or degree)

Defensive: Used or intended to defend or protect

Deficient: Insufficient, inadequate

Delayed: Late, slow, or postponed

Disabled: Limited, handicapped

Disorganized: Not properly arranged or controlled

Disproportionate: Too large or too small in comparison with norm

Disturbed: Agitated, interrupted, interfered with

Dysfunctional: Not operating normally

Effective: Producing the intended or desired effect

Enhanced: Improved in quality, value, or extent

Excessive: Greater than necessary or desirable

Imbalanced: Out of proportion or balance

Impaired: Damaged, weakened

Ineffective: Not producing the intended or desired effect

Interrupted: Having its continuity broken

Low: Below the norm

Organized: Properly arranged or controlled

Perceived: Observed through the senses

Readiness for: In a suitable state for an activity or situation

Situational: Related to a particular circumstance

AXIS 4 LOCATION: Consists of parts/regions of the body and/or their related functions—all tissues, organs, anatomical sites or structures. Values are:

Auditory	*Olfactory*
Bladder	*Oral*
Bowel	*Peripheral neurovascular*
Cardiac	*Peripheral vascular*
Cardiopulmonary	*Renal*
Cerebral	*Skin*
Gastrointestinal	*Tactile*
Gustatory	*Tissue*
Intracranial	*Vascular*
Kinesthetic	*Visual*
Mucous membranes	*Urinary*

AXIS 5 AGE: The age of the person who is the subject of the diagnosis. Values are:

Fetus	*School-age child*
Neonate	*Adolescent*
Infant	*Adult*
Toddler	*Older adult*
Preschool child	

AXIS 6 TIME: The duration of the diagnostic concept. Values are:

Acute: Lasting less than 6 months

Chronic: Lasting more than 6 months

Intermittent: Stopping or starting again at intervals, periodic, cyclic

Continuous: Uninterrupted, going on without stop

AXIS 7 STATUS OF THE DIAGNOSIS: The actuality or potentiality of the problem or the categorization of the diagnosis as a wellness/health promotion diagnosis. Values are:

Actual: Existing in fact or reality, existing at the present time

Health Promotion: Behavior motivated by the desire to increase well-being and actualize human health potential (Pender, Murdaugh, & Parsons, 2006)

Risk: Vulnerability, especially as a result of exposure to factors that increase the chance of injury or loss

Wellness: The quality or state of being healthy

Permission from NANDA International. (2009). *NANDA-I Nursing Diagnoses: Definitions & Classification 2009–2011*. Philadelphia: NANDA-I.

Doenges & Moorhouse's Diagnostic Division Index

Nursing Diagnoses Index

Index